P9-DKE-359

Surgical Technology for the Surgical Technologist

A Positive Care Approach

FOURTH EDITION

Association of Surgical Technologists, Inc.

EXECUTIVE EDITOR
KEVIN B. FREY, CST, MA
Director, Continuing Education Department, Association of Surgical Technologists, Inc.

SENIOR EDITOR
TRACEY ROSS, CST, ED.D
Patient & Employee Safety & Quality Officer, Perioperative Services, Lancaster General Hospital

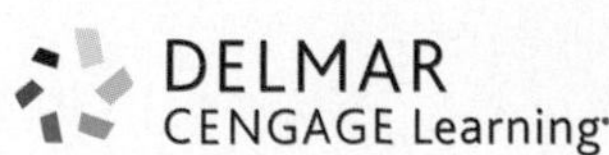

DELMAR
CENGAGE Learning

Australia • Brazil • Japan • Korea • Mexico • Singapore • Spain • United Kingdom • United States

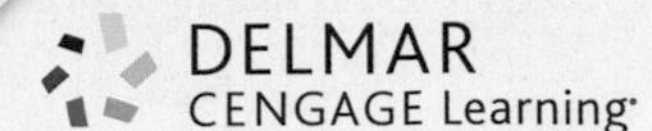

Surgical Technology for the Surgical Technologist: A Positive Care Approach, 4th Edition

Association of Surgical Technologists, Inc

Vice President, Careers & Computing: Dave Garza

Publisher: Stephen Helba

Senior Acquisitions Editor: Tari Broderick

Director, Development—Careers & Computing: Marah Bellegarde

Senior Product Manager: Juliet Steiner

Editorial Assistant: Nicole Manikas

Brand Manager: Wendy Mapstone

Market Development Manager: Jonathan Sheehan

Senior Production Director: Wendy A. Troeger

Production Manager: Andrew Crouth

Senior Content Project Manager: Kenneth McGrath

Senior Art Director: Jack Pendleton

Media Editor: William Overocker

For product information and technology assistance, contact us at
Cengage Learning Customer & Sales Support, 1-800-354-9706
For permission to use material from this text or product,
submit all requests online at **www.cengage.com/permissions.**
Further permissions questions can be e-mailed to
permissionrequest@cengage.com

Example: Microsoft® is a registered trademark of the Microsoft Corporation.

Library of Congress Control Number: 2012947504

ISBN-13: 978-1-1110-3756-7
ISBN-10: 1-1110-3756-6

Delmar
5 Maxwell Drive
Clifton Park, NY 12065-2919
USA

Cengage Learning is a leading provider of customized learning solutions with office locations around the globe, including Singapore, the United Kingdom, Australia, Mexico, Brazil, and Japan. Locate your local office at: **international.cengage.com/region**

Cengage Learning products are represented in Canada by Nelson Education, Ltd.

To learn more about Delmar, visit **www.cengage.com/delmar**

Purchase any of our products at your local college store or at our preferred online store **www.cengagebrain.com**

Printed in the United States of America
1 2 3 4 5 6 7 16 15 14 13 12

Brief Table of Contents

CONTENTS

SECTION 2
PRINCIPLES AND PRACTICE OF SURGICAL TECHNOLOGY

CHAPTER 7 Preventing Perioperative Disease Transmission 127

CHAPTER 8 Hemostasis, Emergency Situations, and All-Hazards Preparation 177

CHAPTER 9 Surgical Pharmacology and Anesthesia 198

CHAPTER 10
Instrumentation, Equipment, and Supplies 264

CHAPTER 11
Wound Healing, Sutures, Needles, and Stapling Devices 289

CHAPTER 12 Surgical Case Management 321

CHAPTER 15 Obstetric and Gynecologic Surgery 511

CHAPTER 16 Ophthalmic Surgery 595

CHAPTER 17 Otorhinolaryngologic Surgery 630

CHAPTER 18 Oral and Maxillofacial Surgery 700

CHAPTER 19 Plastic and Reconstructive Surgery 725

CHAPTER 20 Genitourinary Surgery 805

CHAPTER 24
Neurosurgery 1136

List of Tables

List of Techniques

PREFACE

INTRODUCTION

Surgical Technology for the Surgical Technologist represents a significant change in the field of surgical technology education. Surgical technology faculty and students have long depended on textbooks prepared by and for the nursing student or nursing graduate to serve as the foundation text for surgical technology education. These textbooks, although excellent texts for their primary audience, contained a significant amount of information not related to the role of the surgical technologist. More significantly, these texts lacked the subtle observations and nuances that come from years of experience in the role of surgical technologist. *Surgical Technology for the Surgical Technologist is* written by surgical technologists and surgical technology educators with many years of experience and commitment to the field of surgical technology.

Surgical Technology for the Surgical Technologist approaches the surgical technology student and instructor in an innovative manner. First and foremost, the textbook focuses on the knowledge and cognitive skills required of the surgical technologist. Many specific practices and techniques are described, but all are placed in the context of the *A POSitive CARE Approach.* This approach provides a consistent and reliable way for students to learn and instructors to teach the knowledge and skills required of the surgical technologist.

The *A POSitive CARE Approach* focuses on the cognitive process used by the surgical technologist who is serving in the traditional role called "first scrub." The *A POSitive CARE Approach* for the surgical technologist finds its foundations in the following assumptions:

- The surgical technologist serves the patient's interest primarily by providing assistance to the surgeon.
- The surgical technologist's primary task during an operative procedure is to *anticipate* the intraoperative needs of the surgeon and surgical patient.
- To accomplish the primary task efficiently and effectively, the surgical technologist must learn to "think like the surgeon" intraoperatively.
- To accomplish the primary task efficiently and effectively, the surgical technologist must be well grounded in the basic sciences, especially anatomy, microbiology, and pathophysiology.
- The surgical technologist contributes to global patient care by serving as a team member who monitors the surgical environment along with the other team members.

The intraoperative team commonly makes these same assumptions and uses them to judge the competency of surgical technologists. Educators struggle to get students to anticipate the surgeon's next move or the effects of a given surgical action. Surgical technology graduates suddenly feel at home in the operating room when they begin to plan many steps ahead during an operative procedure. More important, the surgical technologist can be observed time and again to follow a specific sequence of cognitive steps. The cognitive steps require an adequate preparatory education. The surgical technologist must be well grounded in anatomy, pathophysiology, and microbiology. These studies are the foundation of all practices in the operating room. This information is the springboard to the cognitive activity of the surgical technologist.

The basic steps of the cognitive process are easy to define. The surgical technologist:

- has a mental image of normal anatomy
- makes a mental comparison of the normal anatomy with the actual anatomy of a specific patient
- knows the operative procedure used to correct the pathological condition
- makes adjustments in instrumentation, supplies, and equipment according to variations in the pathology and the surgeon's needs
- anticipates and prepares to meet the needs of the surgeon and surgical patient prior to the need being verbalized

The cognitive sequence described is an anticipatory model. Its basis is the scientific method, and it differs only by type and depth of information from other models. The more information the surgical technologist has, the better she or he will be able to anticipate needs in the surgical setting and to contribute to better patient care.

THE SURGICAL TECHNOLOGIST

Surgical Technology for the Surgical Technologist is written by surgical technologists and for surgical technologists. More specifically, it is written with the surgical technology student and instructor in mind, and it is focused on the surgical technologist in the first scrub role. Some of the underlying beliefs about the role of surgical technologists are:

- Surgical technologists are allied health professionals.
- Surgical technologists primarily render care to the patient by providing assistance to the surgeon.
- Surgical technologists primarily work in the role traditionally referred to as "first scrub."
- Surgical technologists work within a synergistic team to provide care to the patient.
- Surgical technologists' knowledge, skills, and tasks sometimes overlap with the scope of practice of other health care providers in the operating room.
- Surgical technologists best serve the patient when they have as much knowledge as possible to serve as an "extra pair of professional eyes and ears" in the operating room environment.

SURGICAL TECHNOLOGY EDUCATION

Surgical technology programs vary in format, length of time, and type of educational institution. Surgical technology programs are found in community colleges, vocational-technical schools, hospitals, universities, and the military. The programs vary in length from 11 to 24 months. The programs award certificates, diplomas, and associate-level degrees. In spite of the differences, there is a *Core Curriculum for Surgical Technology,* common accreditation standards, and considerable curriculum stabilization in terms of what topics are covered. Educationally, *Surgical Technology for the Surgical Technologist* is written with the following presumptions in mind:

- The necessary scope, sequence, and balance for surgical technology education are best delivered via an associate degree curriculum.
- The necessary scope, sequence, and balance for surgical technology education should be a *minimum* of 12 months for proper execution.
- Surgical technology students are best served when they have a solid background in the basic sciences.
- Students are best served when introductory anatomy and physiology with a focus on systemic anatomy and microbiology courses, with attendant lab sections, are taken as full-credit college-level courses, preferably as prerequisites.
  - Surgical anatomy should be taught within the context of surgical procedures without regard for the number of systemic anatomy courses that are taken.
  - Due to the variance in surgical technology programs, some basic microbiology should be included in the chapter on preventing disease transmission. (The authors do not suggest that it is inclusive.)
- A separate introductory pharmacology course is preferred. Due to the variance in surgical technology programs, some basic pharmacology should be included in the chapter on pharmacology and anesthesia. (The authors do not suggest that it is inclusive.)
- Surgical technology students (and their future patients) are worthy of the best educational program that can be provided.

Establishing a Cognitive Model

The question to ask is namely, what is the cognitive process used by the surgical technologist to perform the first scrub role during the surgical procedure? Physicians, for example, are educated according to what is commonly called the *medical model.* In other words, physicians are educated to think about health and health care in a certain way. Thinking this way does not guarantee a proper solution to a medical problem or exclude an error in judgment. Thinking this way does provide for a consistent method for approaching every medical question. Likewise, nursing has established a model for approaching the planning of nursing care. This model is commonly referred to as the *nursing process*. These models serve the instructor because they allow for educational material to be organized in a reasonable and consistent manner. The models serve the student because they provide a way of thinking that can be used in every situation. The models serve the patient not by guaranteeing right solutions but by reducing errors in thought processes. This book establishes and uses a cognitive model for the surgical technologist performing the scrub role to describe how a surgical technologist approaches the kinds of problems faced daily in the operating room. The cognitive model is based on the fact that the primary task of the surgical technologist in the first scrub role is to anticipate a series of events and needs given specific kinds of information.

Surgical Procedures

Every textbook is limited in terms of space. However, a goal of the fourth edition is to present every procedure that is listed in the sixth edition *Core Curriculum for Surgical Technology*, and this edition achieves that goal. Over 100 new procedures are offered in a comprehensive new format utilizing the cognitive model for surgical technology.

THE *A POSITIVE CARE* APPROACH

This book will use a memory tool to reinforce the principles of the cognitive model. The memory tool is **"A POSitive CARE Approach."** The A POSitive CARE Approach is provided in two phases. The **A POS** phase comes directly from the cognitive model—Anatomy, Pathology, Operative Procedure, and Specific Variations. This phase directly relates to operative procedures. However, even technical information and skills serve a higher purpose. Logically, the psychological and philosophical desire to care for others precedes the development of knowledge and skills.The **CARE** phase is from the moral obligation to the surgical patient. This phase reinforces in the student's mind that caring attitudes and behaviors are a prerequisite to being a professional health care provider.

Using the *CARE* Acronym

The first 12 chapters are related to the CARE acronym. CARE is intended to remind the surgical technologist that all of his or her activities affect the care given to the patient. Caring behavior is primarily exhibited by consistent and professional concern for the technical tasks for which the surgical technologist is responsible. An improperly monitored surgical environment that leads to a contaminated surgical field resulting in a wound infection is inherently uncaring. The very nature of surgical intervention requires a heightened awareness of the effects of given behaviors.

C Care directed toward the patient and/or team
A Aseptic principles and technique
R Role of the surgical technologist
E Environmental awareness and concern

In the nonprocedural chapters, objectives will be oriented to the CARE acronym. For instance, the physical environment might have objectives such as these:

CARE

1. Discuss the relationship between the physical environment, safety procedures, and patient care outcomes.
2. Explain the relationship between asepsis and operating room design.
3. Discuss the relationship between proper operating room attire and asepsis.
4. Discuss the role of the surgical technologist in the maintenance of the operative environment.
5. Describe the physical layout of the operating room.
6. Describe the piped-in systems and the electrical outlets in an operating room.
7. State the proper ranges for temperature and humidity.
8. Explain the air ventilation system in the operating room, including laminar flow.
9. Discuss principles of environmental safety procedures.

Both the instructor and the student should be aware that the highly variable topics of these chapters do not allow for a simple one-to-one correlation of the CARE memory tool, but that it is a conceptual tool intended to help organize the information.

Using the *A POS* Acronym

The last 12 chapters relate to the A POS acronym and focus on operative procedures by surgical specialty. This systematic approach to intraoperative problem solving focuses on the ability of the surgical technologist to anticipate the surgeon's and patient's needs. **A POS** is defined as follows:

A Anatomy
P Pathology
O Operative procedure
S Specific variations

Each category has specific components. For instance, the surgical technologist is concerned with the following:

- Anatomy
  - Incision options
  - General systemic anatomy
  - Positioning
- Pathology
  - Diagnostic procedures
  - General pathology
  - Intended surgical outcomes
  - Potential morbidity
- Operative procedure
  - Patient safety
  - Procedural steps
  - Nonsterile equipment needed
  - Sterile instrumentation, supplies, and equipment
  - Suture and needles
  - Dressings
  - Immediate postoperative considerations
  - Troubleshooting of equipment problems
- Specific variations
  - Common patient variations (such as age, size, gender, and other conditions)
  - Common equipment and instrumentation variations
  - Most common emergency conditions

Both the instructor and student will have the best results if they reinforce this format every time a procedure is addressed. The Study Guide and the Instructor's Manual will assist you in this effort.

GUIDELINES FOR THE STUDENT: LEARNING SURGICAL PROCEDURES

Surgical procedures are important to the surgical technologist for several reasons:

- Surgical procedures are the medical intervention taken to restore health to the surgical patient.
- Surgical procedures are the event around which most of the knowledge and skills of a surgical technologist are focused.
- Surgical procedures provide the best educational experience for learning "to think like a surgeon."
- Learning to think like a surgeon is the best way to organize the knowledge and skills required.

So how do you learn to think like a surgeon and apply it to the role of the surgical technologist? You learn it by repeated practice. As you will learn in this textbook, the process of becoming a health care professional, at every level, involves intellectual and physical development. The process includes developing specific knowledge, attitudes, perspectives, and physical skills. The following pattern is one that summarizes a specific approach to learning surgical procedures and serves as a mental checklist prior to each surgical procedure:

- Patient identification (name of patient, age, sex, allergies, prostheses)
- Surgeon and other team members
- Preoperative diagnosis
- Preoperative tests or diagnostic studies (results; available in operating room, such as X-rays)
- Preoperative routines
- Anesthesia and anticipated challenges
- Surgical patient positioning and devices needed
- Surgical procedure to be performed, including anticipation of anatomical variations, incision, drains, closure, dressings
- Postoperative diagnosis
- Initial status of patient following completion of the surgical procedure

It is helpful for the surgical technology student to consistently follow this pattern of organization with variations that reflect the needs of the first scrub role until it becomes second nature. (See the student handbook for sample forms.) The student should notice that this process provides a consistent format for remembering information. It also allows the student to compare anesthesia, positioning, anatomy, procedure, and postoperative results learned in the classroom with what is seen in the operating room (OR). The student will discover that he or she remembers more information as experience is gained. As cases accumulate, the student will be able to identify variables such as different surgeons, anatomical situations, pathological conditions, and environmental conditions that resulted in variances.This helps the student to account for the variables and make better predictions about the patient's and surgeon's needs on the next similar case.

CORE CURRICULUM COMPLIANCE

The *Standards and Guidelines for an Accredited Educational Program in Surgical Technology* state that a program that is accredited by the Commission on Accreditation of Allied Health Education Programs (CAAHEP) must demonstrate by comparison that the curriculum offered meets or exceeds the content demands of the latest edition of the *Core Curriculum for Surgical Technology,* published by the Association of Surgical Technologists (AST) This textbook offers the essential elements of the core curriculum (with the exception of the in-depth basic sciences that we believe require full-length courses for proper introduction to the core surgical technology courses, as described previously).

ORGANIZATION OF THE TEXTBOOK

This textbook comprises 24 chapters divided into three major content areas:

- Introduction to Surgical Technology
- Principles and Practice of Surgical Technology
- Surgical Procedures

Each chapter opens and closes with a case study to help apply material to real-life situations, and a key terms listing with glossary is provided to help improve vocabulary.

NEW TO THE FOURTH EDITION

The changes to the fourth edition were based on extensive market feedback from surgical technology educators across the country. The publisher and authors have made every effort possible to consider and implement suggestions from current users of the textbook, and to improve the overall package.

In the fourth edition, new topics have been added, and others have been expanded and updated, including:

- All-hazards preparation
- New content in Chapter 7: Preventing Perioperative Disease and Transmission
- Updated surgical equipment information
- Updated laser information
- Updated pharmacology information
- Updated computer and robotic information
- Cardiopulmonary resuscitation (CPR) information updated based on American Heart Association (AHA) course material

The theme for revising the textbook was "combine and streamline." The following improvements were made to the overall textbook content in the fourth edition to reflect the theme:

- Over 100 new surgical procedures added
- A new format is introduced for the surgical procedures chapters; the anatomy, pathology, and diagnostic tests are presented at the beginning of each procedure in order to prevent the student from having to go back to the beginning of the chapter for information. For each surgical specialty chapter, the routine instruments, equipment, and supplies are provided in the beginning material in order to avoid repeating this information in each surgical procedure. New additional lists of instrument sets have been added to the chapters. The procedural considerations are now listed directly under the steps of the surgical procedure. Lastly, wound classification has been added to the postoperative considerations.
- Three new comprehensively illustrated procedures have been added: coronary artery bypass graft surgery, extracapsular cataract extraction, and thyroidectomy
- Chapter 7 renamed to reflect a focus on preventing surgical site infection, and reformatted to improve the order of learning by the student
- Comprehensive all-hazards preparation section added to Chapter 8
- Chapter 2 has a new title to better reflect the content, "Legal Concepts, Risk Management, and Ethical Issues"
- Combined information on electrosurgery and lasers previously found throughout the text into Chapter 6
- Condensed pharmacology information previously found throughout other chapters into a comprehensive new Chapter 9

TEACHING AND LEARNING PACKAGE

The publisher has provided a complete learning package to accompany the fourth edition of *Surgical Technology for the Surgical Technologist: A Positive Care Approach.* Each supplement is authored by qualified educators currently teaching in surgical technology programs around the country.

Student Resources

The following resources were developed to aid students in the learning and practice of information essential to becoming a surgical technologist.

Study Guide and Lab Manual to Accompany Surgical Technology for the Surgical Technologist

ISBN-13: 978-1-1110-3758-1

With extensive revisions to reflect the changes in the core text, the addition of numerous new questions, and new question types including Group Assignments and Analyze the Situation activities, the Study Guide is a robust resource for practicing surgical technology skills and concepts. A lab manual portion inspires creative learning, skill assessments track mastery of procedural skills, case studies develop critical thinking, and review questions build knowledge and confidence.

CourseMate to Accompany Surgical Technology for the Surgical Technologist ISBN-13: IAC 978-1-1115-4407-2 ISBN-13: PAC 978-1-1115-4406-5

Cengage Learning's CourseMate brings course concepts to life with interactive learning, study, and exam preparation tools that support the printed textbook. Watch reader comprehension soar as your class works with the printed textbook and the textbook-specific website. CourseMate goes beyond the book to deliver what you need! The *Coursemate for Surgical Technology for the Surgical Technologist,* Fourth Edition includes:

- Interactive e-book with highlighting and note taking abilities
- Quizzes for each chapter providing additional opportunities to test student comprehension of content.
- Glossary games such as crossword puzzles and flash cards to challenge comprehension of important terminology and increase comfort with new vocabulary.
- Engaging support materials such as Chapter Objectives, FAQs, Class Notes, and Learning Links giving you additional opportunities for learning and study.
- Dynamic Video Case Studies help improve critical thinking.
- Additional Surgical Instrumentation image bank to help you master this important component of the curriculum.
- Engagement Tracker allows instructors to see how much time students spend in different components of the CourseMate, which can be used to help remediate students who are struggling.

Instructor Resources

The following comprehensive tools are available to instructors to enhance the planning and implementation of their instructional program.

Instructor Resources to Accompany Surgical Technology for the Surgical Technologist CD-ROM, ISBN-13: 978-1-1110-3761-1

Spend less time planning and more time teaching with Delmar Cengage Learning's *Instructor Resources to Accompany Surgical Technology for the Surgical Technologist,* Fourth Edition. This electronic resource provides a number of tools to aid with course management, testing, and evaluation.

- The *Instructor's Manual to Accompany Surgical Technology for the Surgical Technologist,* fourth edition, contains a number of aids designed to simplify course management tasks and evaluation of learner progress. The manual includes a correlation chart that maps text content to the requirements of the *Core Curriculum for Surgical Technology,* sixth edition. Also provided is a list of Skill Assessments that appear in the Study Guide. Answer keys are given for the Case Studies and Questions for Further Study that appear in the textbook, and answer keys for all Study Guide exercises are also provided. Numerous new Chapter Pop Quizzes have also been provided, along with answer keys, which can be printed and passed out to students for quick assessments. Additional new instructor support materials include Sample Syllabus and Lesson Plans, Teaching Notes for instructors personal development, and Handouts for students.
- PowerPoint® presentations for each chapter containing key concepts and images from the textbook.
- Computerized Testbank in ExamviewPro® test-generating software with over 1700 questions organized by chapter allows instructors to create quizzes and tests as well as monitor learner progress.

Instructor Companion Website to Accompany Surgical Technology for the Surgical Technologist ISBN-13: 9781285187099

The password-protected Instructor Resources Companion Website includes everything found on the Instructor Resource CD in an easy-to-access online format. The Instructor Companion Website can be accessed by going to www.cengage.com/login to create a unique user log-in. Once your instructor account is activated you'll have the Instructor's Manual, PowerPoints, Test Bank Questions and more right at your fingertips.

BIBLIOGRAPHY

Neurological Foundations to Cognition

Brodal, P. (2010) . *The central nervous system: Structure and function* (4th ed.). New York: Oxford University Press.

Calvin, W. H. (2001). *The cerebral symphony: Seashore reflections on the structure of consciousness.* Bloomington, IN: iUniverse.

Churchland, P. S. (2002). *Brainwise: Studies in neurophilosophy.* Cambridge, MA: MIT Press.

Edelman, G. M. (1990). *Neural Darwinism: Theory of neuronal group selection.* Oxford, England: Oxford Paperbacks.

Joseph, R. (2011). *Frontal lobes.* Lanham, MD: University Press.

Mason, P. (2011). *Medical neurobiology.* New York: Oxford University Press—USA.

Shepherd, G. M. (2003). *The synaptic organization of the brain* (5th ed.). New York: Oxford University Press—USA.

Cognition

Glass, A. L. (2007). *Cognition* (3rd ed.). New York: Random House.

Gregory, R. L. (Ed.). (2004). *The Oxford companion to the mind* (2nd ed.). New York: Oxford University Press—USA.

Contributors

Connie Bell, CST, FAST

Chapter 1: Orientation to Surgical Technology
Chapter 4: Special Populations

Bill Hammer, CST, MEd

Chapter 2: Legal Concepts, Risk Management, and Ethical Issues

Rebecca Hall, CST, CSA, FAST, MS

Chapter 3: The Surgical Patient

Tammy Mangold, CST, CSFA, FAST, MEd

Chapter 3: The Surgical Patient
Chapter 10: Instrumentation, Equipment, and Supplies

Tracey Ross, CST, Ed.D.

Chapter 5: Physical Environment and Safety Standards
Chapter 11: Wound Healing, Sutures, Needles, and Stapling Devices
Chapter 14: General Surgery
Chapter 15: Obstetric and Gynecologic Surgery
Chapter 19: Plastic and Reconstructive Surgery
Chapter 20: Genitourinary Surgery
Chapter 22: Cardiothoracic Surgery
Chapter 23: Peripheral Vascular Surgery

Kevin Frey, CST, MA

Chapter 6: Biomedical Science
Chapter 13: Diagnostic Procedures
Chapter 15: Obstetric and Gynecologic Surgery
Chapter 17: Otorhinolaryngologic Surgery
Chapter 21: Orthopedic Surgery

Margaret Rodriguez, CST, CSFA, FAST, BS

Chapter 7: Preventing Perioperative Disease Transmission

Joseph Long, CST, Ed.D

Chapter 8: Hemostasis, Emergency Situations, and All-Hazards Preparation
Chapter 12: Surgical Case Management

Ann McGuiness, CST, FAST, RN, CNOR, MSEd

Chapter 9: Surgical Pharmacology and Anesthesia

Kathy Duffy, CST, CSFA, CSA

Chapter 16: Ophthalmic Surgery
Chapter 18: Oral and Maxillofacial Surgery

Holly Falcon, CST, FAST, BS

Chapter 24: Neurosurgery

Reviewers of Proof Chapters

Connie Bell, CST, FAST
Chapters1 & 4

Mary McNaron, CST, RN, CNOR, MSN, MSHRM
Chapters 2, 15, 22, 23

Rebecca Hall, CST, CSA, FAST, MS
Chapters 3, 6, 11, 18, 20, 21

Angie Burton, CST
Chapters 5, 10, 13, 16, 17

Margaret Rodriguez, CST, CSFA, FAST, BS
Chapters 6, 7, 10, 11, 14, 15

Gemma Fournier, CST, FAST, RN, MSN
Chapters 8 & 10

Ann McGuiness, CST, FAST, RN, CNOR, MSEd
Chapter 9

Tracey Ross, CST, Ed.D.
Chapters 12, 14, 19, 24

Reviewers

Debra Bradley, CST
Surgical Technology Program Director
Spartanburg Community College
Spartanburg, SC

Kathy Gelety, RN, CNOR, CST
Program Director
Indian River State College
Fort Pierce, FL

Janayah Hudson, RN, MPH, CST, CNOR
Program Coordinator
Aiken Technical College
Graniteville, SC

Amy Kennedy, RN, MSN, CNOR
Program Director, Surgical Technology
Harrisburg Area Community College
Harrisburg, PA

Richard A. Lopez, BSN, RN
Director, Surgical Technology
Northern Michigan University
Marquette, MI

Wendy McClellan, CST
Program Director
Central Florida Community College
Ocala, FL

Joyce Moyer, CRCST, CST, RN
Department Head, Surgical Technology
Greenville Technical College
Greenville, SC

Carolyn Steinhorst, RN, CST
Program Director/Instructor, Surgical Technology
Madison Area Technical College
Madison, WI

Rob Surles
Faculty and Clinical Coordinator
Cape Fear Community College
Wilmington, NC

Linda VanDyke, CST, CFA
Program Coordinator, Surgical Technology
Hillyard Technical Center
St. Joseph, MO

Technical Reviewers

Raquel L. Altmann, RN, BSN, CNOR
Surgical Technologist, Central Service Program Director
Mid-State Technical College
Marshfield, WI

Joseph Charleman, CST, CRCST, LPN, MS
Chair, Surgical Technology and Sterile Processing Programs
Dover Business College
Clifton, NJ

Jeff Feix, CST, CSFA, LVN, FAST
Surgical Technology Program Coordinator, Instructor
Vernon College
Wichita Falls, TX

Janice Lovekamp, CST, CSFA
Program Director, Surgical Technology
Lincoln Land Community College
Springfield, IL

Tedd Lupella, CST
Surgical Technology Instructor
Gateway Technical College
Burlington, WI

Beth Mayfield
Surgical Technology Program Director
Monongalia County Technical Education Center
Morgantown, WV

Deborah Pearson, CST, SA, CRCST, BCT
Surgical Technology Program Director, Instructor
Erwin Voc-Tech
Tampa, FL

Katherine J. Wolfer, RN, MEd, MSN, CNOR
Surgical Technology Instructor
Cincinnati State Technical and Community College
Cincinnati, OH

HOW TO USE THIS BOOK

***Surgical Technology for the Surgical Technologist: A Positive Care Approach,* fourth edition**, presents the core physical and biological concepts and technical surgical information needed for the surgical technologist to perform efficiently and effectively in the surgical environment. A problem-solving methodology is used consistently throughout the text. The purpose of the methodology is to develop the surgical technologist's ability to anticipate the surgeon's and patient's needs and to plan ahead during the operative procedure to achieve the best possible outcome. The features shown on these pages are integrated throughout the text and all contribute to the development of the surgical technologist.

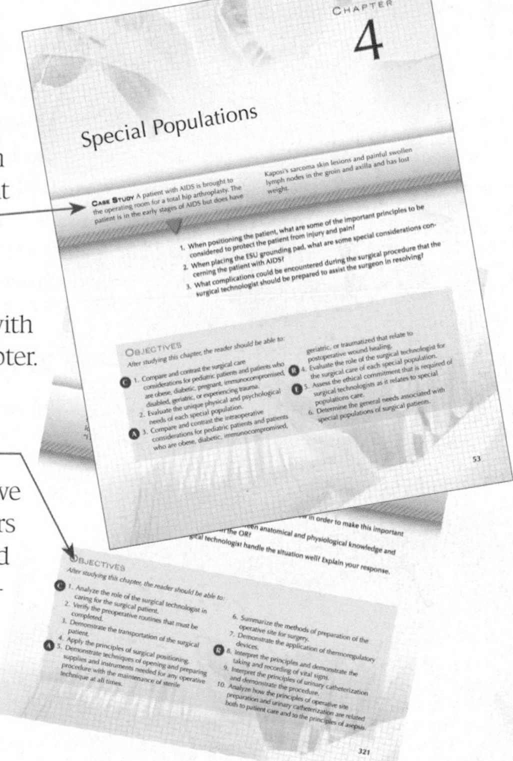

1. Case Study

Two case studies are presented in each chapter. They describe clinical situations with related questions that require the learner to apply information presented in the chapter. Their intent is to help the learner develop critical thinking skills.

2. Objectives

The text uses a systematic approach to problem solving using the **CARE** and **A POS**itive acronyms. The objectives are identified by the components of these acronyms. Chapters 1–12 apply the **CARE** components. These chapters introduce surgical technology and its principles and practices. They emphasize that the care of the patient in the operating room is the surgical technologist's highest priority. The **CARE** components provide a framework for placing the specific technical information presented in these chapters. **CARE** represents:

- **C** Care (directed toward the patient and/or surgical team)
- **A** Aseptic Principles (guiding the practice of sterile technique)
- **R** Role (of the surgical technologist during the preoperative, intraoperative, and postoperative phases)
- **E** Environmental Awareness (and concern)

Chapters 13–24 on operative procedures by surgical specialty apply the **A POS**itive components, as follows:

- **A** Anatomy
- **P** Pathology
- **O** Operative Procedure
- **S** Specific Variations

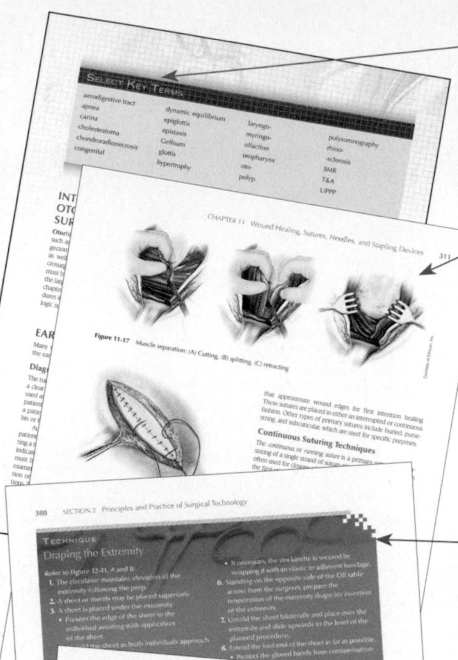

3. Select Key Terms

Each chapter contains a list of terms to be learned. Each term is emphasized in the chapter in boldface type. Definitions of these terms appear in the glossary for ready reference.

4. Art

Full-color illustrations are used throughout the text. Illustrations and photos used in the **CARE** chapters show steps used in specific skills and identify general equipment and supplies common to many operative procedures.

Illustrations in the **A POS** chapters (operative procedures) show the anatomy of the surgical field for specific operative procedures. The correct placement of instruments during the procedure is also illustrated. Equipment and supplies specific to a surgical specialty or procedure are also shown.

5. Techniques

Techniques represent skills required in most operative procedures, such as the surgical scrub, donning and removing surgical attire and personal protective equipment, and setting up the OR. Each technique lists the necessary steps in sequence.

6. Procedures

The procedure format is based on the concept that allows one procedure to highlight several important steps that appear in related procedures. Many procedures are also included in step-by-step outline and paragraph formats in order to reflect the content in the *Core Curriculum for Surgical Technology* published by AST. Procedures are presented in detail with information organized by Equipment, Instruments, Supplies, Operative Preparation, Practical Considerations, Operative Procedure with Technical Considerations, and Postoperative Considerations.

7. Pearl of Wisdom

Following each procedure, these tips are based on the authors' years of experience as surgical technologists. They offer practical suggestions and cautions to be observed during the procedure.

8. Questions for Further Study

These questions at the end of each chapter encourage you to seek and apply additional related information.

Section 1

Introduction to Surgical Technology

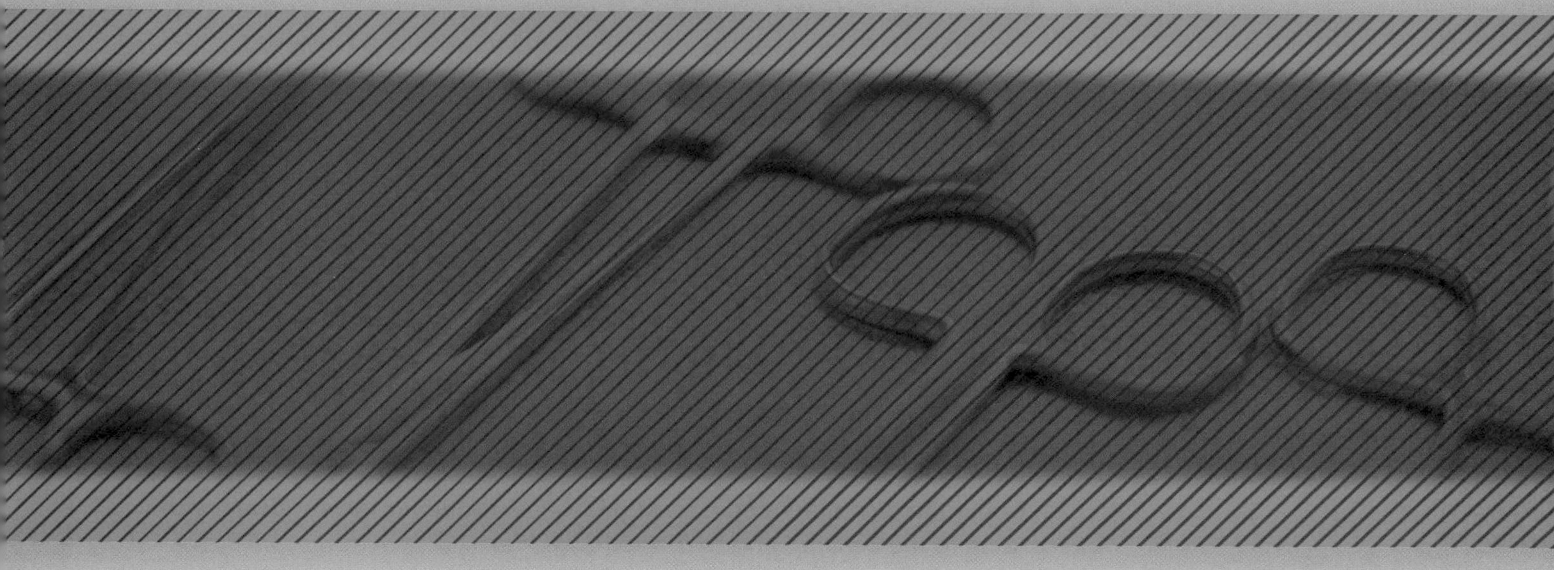

CHAPTER

1

Orientation to Surgical Technology

CASE STUDY Gloria is a 43-year-old woman. She is scheduled for diagnostic laparoscopy for chronic pelvic pain. She has been resting for 30 minutes in the preoperative holding area where a registered nurse has performed a nursing evaluation; has checked her paperwork, history and physical, allergies, special needs, and informed consent; and has provided emotional support. The anesthesia provider has reviewed the steps that will be taken and started an IV line. A registered nurse and an OR nursing assistant maneuver a stretcher with Gloria on it into OR 5. Gloria notices an individual who is wearing a surgical gown, gloves, cap, mask, and protective eyewear. This strangely clad person is moving surgical instruments into place on a large, flat table. The individual steps back from the table, turns slightly toward Gloria, and says, "Hello, I'm Sarah. I'm a surgical technologist and I'll be assisting Dr. J. today."

1. The registered nurse is functioning in a classic OR nursing role. This role is referred to by what common term?
2. The surgical technologist who is gowned, gloved, and working at the back table is functioning in the classic role of the surgical technologist. This role is commonly referred to by what term?
3. Determine the recommended educational background for the surgical technologist according to the *Recommended Standards of Practice*.
4. Name the entity responsible for verifying that the school attended by the surgical technologist meets national standards.
5. Name the organization or governing body responsible for the examination taken by the surgical technologist to verify that she has an adequate entry level of knowledge to perform in the role of a certified surgical technologist.

OBJECTIVES

After studying this chapter, the reader should be able to:

C 1. Demonstrate the principles of communication in the surgical setting.
A 2. Trace the historical development of surgical technology.
3. Recognize members of the surgical team and their roles.
R 4. Describe the surgical technology professional organizations: AST; ARC/STSA; NBSTSA.
5. Compare and contrast the various roles of the surgical technologist.
6. Interpret the components of a job description for the surgical technologist.
7. Analyze the components of effective teamwork and communication.
8. Discuss the meaning of "surgical conscience" and its application to surgical technology.
E 9. Summarize the different types of health care facilities.
10. Analyze a typical hospital organizational structure.
11. Classify hospital departments and their relationship to surgical services.

SELECT KEY TERMS

acronym	competency	HMO	preceptor
ambulatory surgical center	*Core Curriculum for Surgical Technology*	intraoperative	preoperative
ARC/STSA	DO	The Joint Commission	professional
AST	elective	NBSTSA	proprietary
circulator	emergent	optional	urgent
		postoperative	Vesalius

HISTORY OF SURGERY

The history of surgery in the Western world is closely tied to the broader history of medicine, science, and intellectual development. The earliest records indicate some amazing insights into the nature of certain illnesses and some unbelievably inaccurate observations and theories. The Classical Period revolutionized thinking in the Western world. Hippocrates, Aristotle, and Galen were insightful and influential; however, their scientific thought was subservient to their philosophical and theological biases. The so-called Dark Ages comprised a long period of arrested development in many areas of thought. The human mind is never content to ignore what it does not know, and the Renaissance issued in a new era of thought and development. **Vesalius**, almost single-handedly, overthrew 1500 years of established anatomical teaching. Others rose to the task and the development of science began. In many instances, the observations remained inaccurate because modern scientific tools were not available, but the attitude with which the observations were made was remarkably different. Slowly but surely, physicians began to understand and control the mechanisms of pain, hemorrhage, and infection. Except in the crudest of forms, surgery is not possible without the control of pain, hemorrhage, and infection. Parallel and correlated discoveries in microbiology, anatomy, and physiology were necessary to reach the period of modern surgery. In fact, surgery as we know it today is a 20th-century phenomenon. Given the rapid development of technology, surgical intervention will be radically changed in the next quarter century. The quest for better and safer patient care will ensure that change is a constant in surgical practice. A select review of the history of surgery is presented in Table 1-1.

TABLE 1-1 Select History of Surgery Time Line (Dates Are Approximations)

4000 B.C.	Cuneiform script	First anatomical descriptions of human organs tablets from Nineveh
2500 B.C.	Imhotep	Revered Egyptian physician (declared divine); wrote an early "book" on surgery
2000 B.C.	Code of Hammurabi	Medical practices of the day described; some reflect real insight into disease; most are religious in nature
1500 B.C.	*Vedas* (Hindu)	Correlates "sweet smell" of urine with a specific disease
1000 B.C.	Homer	Early Greek history/myth provides a view of military medicine of the day
500 B.C.	Aristotle	Established an early "scientific" mindset; founder of comparative anatomy
25000 B.C.	Celsus	Described the signs of inflammation
A.D. 500	Galen	First great anatomist; controlled thought, unchallenged, for 1500 years; biology made to serve theology
1500	Pare	Greatest surgeon of the 16th century; began to ligate arteries after amputation; stopped cauterizing wounds with hot irons and oil
1500	Vesalius	Father of modern anatomy; challenged Galen openly and correctly; performed dissections on human cadavers himself; used illustrators to create permanent records; changed the whole approach to anatomical studies
1800	Jenner	Inventor of the vaccination for smallpox
1850	Pasteur	Father of microbiology, virology, and immunology
	Lister	Developed technique of antiseptic surgery
	Billroth	Responsible for advances in surgical procedures; best known for gastrectomy procedures
	Halsted	Developed meticulous closure of wounds
	Biejerinick	Developed the concept of a virus
	Roentgen	Developed the X-ray machine
1900	Cushing	Father of neurosurgery; reduced mortality rate for meningiomas from 96% to 5%
1950	Cooley	Perfected the heart-lung machine; performed first U.S. heart transplant and first total artificial heart implant
	DeBakey	Developed the first ventricular assist pump
1980s		Technological revolution begins; endoscopic surgery becomes routine
1990s		Computer age changes surgery; stereotactic approach to neurosurgery; virtual reality offers promise for education and clinical practice
2000s		Minimally invasive surgical (MIS) techniques, including lasers and robotic-assisted surgery, continue to evolve with the advances in biotechnology

SURGERY TODAY

A key factor associated with advancements in the practice of surgery has been the number of surgical services, specialties, and subspecialties that have become established. The surgical procedures available to the patient are classified into broad categories that cross specialty areas:

- **Emergent**: Surgical pathology threatening life or limb within a relatively short time period (e.g., ruptured aneurysm of the abdominal aorta)
- **Urgent**: Surgical pathology requiring treatment within a relatively short period of time (e.g., unruptured ectopic pregnancy with stable vital signs)
- **Elective**: Surgical intervention that does not have to be performed immediately or within a short period of time (If the surgical intervention can be scheduled at a future date, it is elective; e.g., a torn meniscus in the knee.)
- **Optional**: Surgical intervention that does not have to be performed in order to preserve life or function (e.g., rhytidectomy)

Surgical Specialties

Medicine today is a field of specialization and subspecialization. The same is true for modern surgery. The field called "general" surgery is actually a specialty (see Chapter 14). It is general only in the sense that it is not exclusively focused on one body system. General surgeons typically perform surgery on the digestive system, including the hepatobiliary system, thyroid and parathyroid glands, general skin lesions, and breast lesions (may vary by region). Some general surgeons may subspecialize, only performing surgery on the hepatobiliary system or gastrointestinal system. Other specialties include obstetric and gynecologic surgery (see Chapter 15), ophthalmic surgery (see Chapter 16), otorhinolaryngology (see Chapter 17), oral and maxillofacial surgery (see Chapter 18), reconstructive surgery (see Chapter 19), genitourinary surgery (see Chapter 20), orthopedics (see Chapter 21), cardiothoracic surgery (see Chapter 22), peripheral vascular surgery (see Chapter 23), and neurosurgery (see Chapter 24). Each specialty has subspecialties (e.g., pediatric cardiovascular, hand and wrist (orthopedics), and neuro-oncology (neurosurgery). No body system is immune to surgical intervention, and each represents a specialization in modern surgery. Each specialty must account for specific variations in the population, such as age in pediatric and geriatric patients. Trauma presents unique variations to normal procedures and specific patient care demands. Finally, the procurement of donated organs and their transplantation into other humans affects many specialties, thereby producing variations in patient care.

HISTORY OF SURGICAL TECHNOLOGY

The history of surgical technology is difficult to trace with certainty. Surgeons have had nonphysician and non-nursing assistants since the beginning of surgical history. The military, in particular, used nonphysician and non-nursing assistants in various roles, partly because women were excluded from the battlefield. The more modern version of surgical technology, that is, an allied health professional serving predominantly in the scrub role, began to develop in Britain and the United States following World War II. The history of surgical technology is presented in a table format. Key events in surgical technology history have been selected to demonstrate general themes, key issues of the day, and general development (Table 1-2).

FIELD OF SURGICAL TECHNOLOGY

Surgical technology is part of the allied health field in the United States. **The Joint Commission** defines *surgical technologist* (ST) in its *Lexikon: Dictionary of Health Care Terms, Organizations, and* ***Acronyms*** *for the Era of Reform* as follows:

> An allied health **professional** who works closely with surgeons, anesthesiologists, registered nurses and other surgical personnel delivering patient care and assuming appropriate responsibilities before, during, and after surgery.

This textbook accepts the definitions of *profession* and *professional* as defined by The Joint Commission as the most precise descriptors for the field of surgical technology and the role of the ST. Additionally, each of the terms specifies the relationship between the professional and the physician and contributes to our understanding of surgical technology.

Working Conditions

The surgical environment is brightly lit, relatively quiet, and temperature controlled. Most of the duties of the ST require standing for extended periods of time and the ability to lift and move heavy objects. Attention must be focused. The ST can be exposed to communicable diseases, unpleasant sights, odors, and hazardous materials. Most surgical procedures are carried out during the day, and a 40-hour workweek is common. The ST may be required to work the evening or night shift, weekends, and holidays and to periodically take "call" (be available to work on short notice in case of an emergency surgical procedure [e.g., cesarean section]).

Personal Characteristics

As part of the surgical team, the ST must be able to work quickly and accurately, with a commitment to detail. A number of activities must be integrated according to priority when under pressure in stressful and emergency situations. Therefore, a stable temperament and a strong sense of responsibility are qualities essential to the ST. Considerable patience and concern for order are required. Manual dexterity, good vision and hearing, and physical stamina are vital. Sensitivity to the needs of the patient as well as other members of the surgical team must be demonstrated. Individuals who practice this profession have a strong desire to help others and make a valuable contribution to society. Honesty and moral integrity are essential in upholding standards for providing safe surgical patient care.

Problem-solving Skills

A key characteristic that the ST should exhibit and constantly improve upon is problem-solving skills, which are applied during all phases of surgical patient care. This is especially important in regard to avoiding medical errors in the care of the patient. The problems encountered by the ST can, obviously, range from simple to complex and from technically oriented to patient care–related concepts, both direct and indirect. Some individuals view a problem as an opportunity that presents the possibility of making a positive change in

Table 1-2 Select History of Surgical Technology Time Line

Date	*Place or Actor*	*Event or Information*
Late 19th century	London Hospital	Mr. Rampley employed in the operating room (OR) as "surgery beadle" (theater technician)
1948	Britain	Formation of the Operating Theater Technicians
Early 1950s	United States	Early development parallels Britain: • Many OR technicians educated in the military • Civilian education predominantly on the job and widely varying in expectations
1954	American Hospital Association	Publication of first book focused on OR technicians: *Surgical Technical Aide—Instructor's Manual* (Ginsberg)
1959	Association of Operating Room Nurses (AORN) Board of Directors	Forms survey group to study the needs of OR technicians
Dec. 1967	AORN Manual Committee	A new publication: *Teaching the Operating Room Technician*
Feb. 1969	AORN House of Delegates	A critical proposal: "The Association of Operating Room Nurses, Inc. (AORN) shall structure an associated organization for Operating Room Technicians, under the auspices of AORN. This organization will be known as the Association of Operating Room Technicians (AORT) and the two associations shall relate to each other through an Advisory Board at both the Local and National levels"
July 19–20, 1969	New York Conference	Formal Organization: Association of Operating Room Technicians (AORT)
Dec. 1970	AORT Board of Directors and Advisory Committee	• Certification selected over licensure • First examination given
1972	American Medical Association House of Delegates	Fundamentals of an education program for the OR technician adopted
1972	AORT	First edition of *O.R. Tech* magazine
1973	AORT and AORN	National Advisory Board dissolved "as AORT was able to assume the responsibilities of managing its own association."
1974	The Liaison Council on Certification for Surgical Technology (LCC-ST)	LCC becomes arm of AST responsible for certification
1974	Accreditation Review Committee on Education in Surgical Technology (ARC-ST)	ARC on Education for the ORT appointed (Commission on Accreditation of Allied Health Education Programs [CAAHEP] system)
1978	AORT National Conference	AORT changes name to Association of Surgical Technologists (AST); *O.R. Tech* magazine changes to the journal *The Surgical Technologist*
1981	AST	***Core Curriculum for Surgical Technology*** (1st ed.) published
1985	AST	Code of Ethics published
Nov. 1986	*The Surgical Technologist*	Claire Olsen introduces associate degree discussion
May 1988	AST House of Delegates	First edition AST Standards of Practice adopted
Nov. 1990	AST	Job description for Surgical First Assistant published; revised in 2008
Mar. 1992	AST	Surgical assisting core curriculum published; revised in 2006
2006	LCC-ST	LCC-ST changes name to National Board of Surgical Technology and Surgical Assisting (NBSTSA)
2006–Present	AST	Comprehensive "Recommended Standards of Practice for Surgical Technology & Surgical Assisting" published
2009	ARC/STSA	ARC-ST changes name to Accreditation Review Council on Education in Surgical Technology and Surgical Assisting

the care of the patient. Good problem-solving skills include the following:

- Ability to prioritize and choose those problems that can be solved within the time allowed
- If time is short and the optimal solution cannot be implemented, ability to consider alternative solutions that still solve the problem with positive results
- Ability to evaluate one's own abilities to possibly solve the problem on an individual basis or determine if others need to be involved
- Ability to work with others as a team to consider alternate solutions to problems and choose the best solution or solutions
- Ability to assess the results of the solution; identify, with team members, improved solutions to implement in case the problem is reencountered in the future; and accept in a positive manner feedback from other individuals, possibly including the patient

Surgical Team Members

An ST works as a member of the surgical team to ensure that the operative procedure is conducted under optimal conditions (Figure 1-1). Surgical team members are responsible for the three phases of surgical patient care. The team functions in one of two capacities—nonsterile and sterile. All surgical team members must adhere to the principles of asepsis and the practice of sterile technique (refer to Chapter 7). While the ST in the first scrub role is the focus of this textbook, an overview of the roles and responsibilities of each surgical team member is provided.

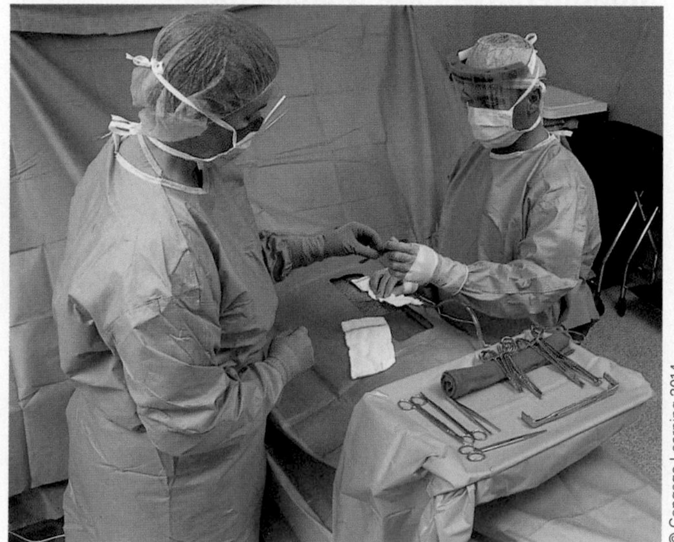

Figure 1-1 Surgical technologist passing a scalpel to the surgeon

THE THREE PHASES OF SURGICAL CASE MANAGEMENT

The three phases of surgical case management are the **preoperative**, **intraoperative**, and **postoperative** phases.

1. **Preoperative:** The preoperative case management phase occurs prior to initiation (creation of the incision or insertion of an endoscope) of the surgical procedure.
2. **Intraoperative:** The intraoperative case management phase occurs while the surgical procedure is being performed.
3. **Postoperative:** The postoperative case management phase begins when the surgical procedure is terminated (application of the sterile dressing or extraction of the endoscope).

NONSTERILE SURGICAL TEAM MEMBERS

The nonsterile team members are the **circulator** and the anesthesia provider. Additionally, other personnel, such as the radiology technologist or pathologist, may also be present in the operating room (OR).

The circulator is a registered nurse (RN), licensed practical or vocational nurse (LPN or LVN), or ST. Some of the duties of the circulator include:

- Assisting with preparing the OR
- Ensuring needed diagnostic and laboratory reports are available
- Conducting the preoperative patient interview
- Confirming surgical consents
- Transporting the patient to the OR
- Verifying correct patient
- Assisting with transferring the patient to the operating table
- Assisting in positioning the patient
- Assisting the anesthesia provider
- Assisting with initiating the surgical "time out"
- Assisting with verifying correct surgical site
- Prepping the patient
- Assisting with draping the patient
- Connecting various cords and tubings
- Performing surgical counts with the first scrub ST
- Providing additional items to the sterile field during the surgical procedure
- Maintaining the patient's operative record
- Caring for specimens

- Securing dressings
- Assisting with transferring the patient from the operating table
- Completing surgical record
- Assisting with transporting the patient to the postanesthesia care unit (PACU)
- Assisting with preparing the OR for the next patient

The anesthesia provider may be either a physician (medical doctor [MD] or doctor of osteopathy [**DO**]) or a certified registered nurse anesthetist (CRNA). Some of the duties of the anesthesia provider include:

- Assessing the patient preoperatively
- Determining the type of anesthetic to be administered
- Discussing the risks and benefits of the planned anesthetic with the patient and obtaining informed consent
- Offering alternative anesthetic options to the patient, if necessary
- Managing all phases of anesthesia (refer to Chapter 9)
- Monitoring the patient's vital signs during the surgical procedure
- Providing any supportive measures (e.g., fluid and airway management)

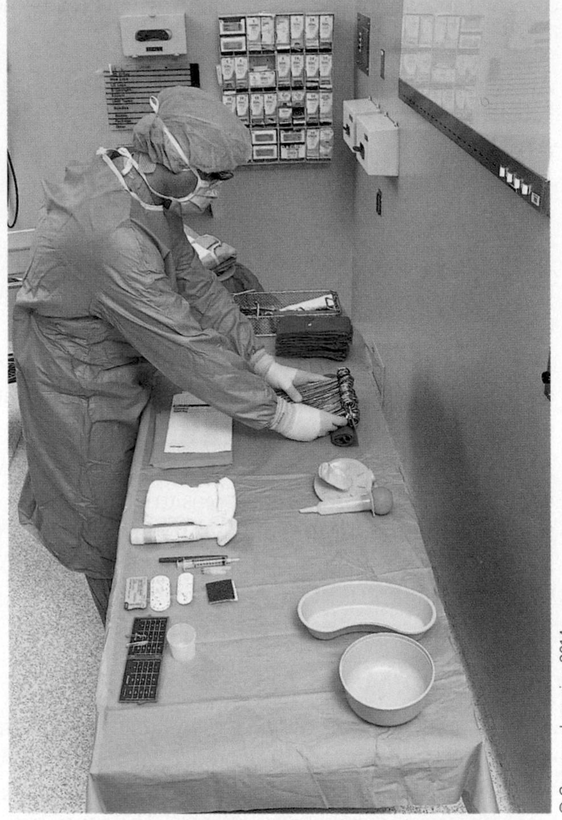

Figure 1-2 Surgical technologist organizing the back table

STERILE SURGICAL TEAM MEMBERS

The first scrub ST, the surgeon, and the surgical first assistant are the sterile team members. Traditionally, the ST functions in the sterile capacity, referred to as the first scrub surgical technologist, during the surgical procedure but also performs many nonsterile duties (known as assisting circulating duties) throughout the course of the workday. Some of the duties of the first scrub ST include the following descriptions.

Preoperative Case Management

- Donning OR attire and personal protective equipment (PPE)
- Assisting with surgical site verification
- Assisting with correct patient verification (i.e., "time out")
- Assisting with preparing the OR
- Gathering necessary equipment and supplies
- Opening sterile supplies, instruments, and equipment
- Creating and maintaining the sterile field
- Performing surgical scrub and donning sterile gown and gloves
- Organizing the sterile field for use (Figure 1-2)
- Performing initial sponge, sharps, and instrument count
- Assisting team members during entry of the sterile field
- Assisting with placing sterile drapes to expose the operative site
- Securing tubing, cords, and other sterile accessories

Intraoperative Case Management

- Maintaining the sterile field, including establishing neutral zone
- Passing instrumentation, equipment, and supplies to the surgeon and surgical assistant as needed
- Assessing and anticipating the needs of the patient and surgeon to provide the necessary items in order of need
- Preparing irrigation fluids
- Preparing and handling medications
- Counting necessary items
- Caring for the specimen
- Initiating final count of necessary items
- Clearing residual blood and skin prep solutions from patient's skin
- Preparing and applying sterile surgical dressing as directed by the surgeon

Postoperative Case Management

- Maintaining the sterile field until the patient is transported from the OR
- Separating instruments and disassembling the sterile field
- Removing used instruments, equipment, and supplies from the OR
- Caring for and maintaining instruments (instrument cycle), equipment, and supplies following use
- Placing sharps in secured and contained sharps container
- Placing contaminated items in biohazards bags
- Preparing and transporting used instruments and equipment to the decontamination area
- Assisting with room turnover, cleaning, and preparing the OR for the next patient (OR cycle)

The surgeon may be an MD, DO, doctor of podiatric medicine (DPM), or doctor of dental science (DDS). Some of the duties of the surgeon include the following:

- Determining the necessity of surgical intervention and the type of procedure to be performed
- Discussing the risks and benefits of the planned procedure with the patient and obtaining consent for the procedure
- Offering alternative treatment options to the patient, if available
- Identifying the correct surgical site
- Performing the surgical procedure
- Providing follow-up patient care

The surgical assistant may be a physician (MD or DO) or a nonphysician (physician assistant [PA], Certified Registered Nurse First Assistant [CRNFA], or a Certified Surgical First Assistant [CSFA]). Some of the duties of the surgical assistant include the following:

- Assisting in positioning the patient
- Assisting with draping the patient (Figure 1-3)
- Providing visualization of the surgical site through retraction of tissue, suctioning, and sponging
- Assisting in identifying anatomical structures and landmarks
- Assisting with achieving temporary or permanent hemostasis
- Participating in volume replacement or autotransfusion techniques
- Closing body planes
- Selecting and applying wound dressings
- Assisting in transferring patient to the stretcher

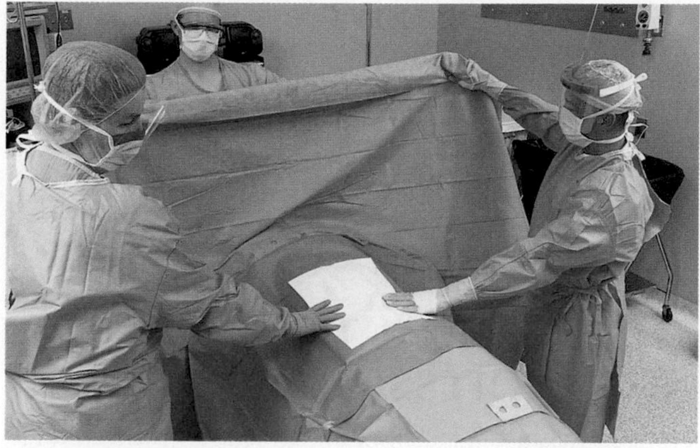

Figure 1-3 Surgical assistant helping to drape the patient

Surgical Technology Education and Certification

Educational programs for STs are accredited by the Commission on Accreditation of Allied Health Education Programs (CAAHEP) (Table 1-3). The Accreditation Review Council on Education in Surgical Technology and Surgical Assisting (**ARC/STSA**) directly oversees academic accreditation for the field of surgical technology. The National Board of Surgical Technology and Surgical Assisting (**NBSTSA**) is responsible for the credentials (Certified Surgical Technologist [CST] and CSFA) and the national certification examination for both credentials.

Eligibility to take the certification examination is restricted to graduates of CAAHEP and Accrediting Bureau of Health Education Schools (ABHES) accredited programs (and currently

TABLE 1-3 Agencies Related to Surgical Technology Education

Association of Surgical Technologists (AST) (303-694-9130; www.ast.org)
• Provides general services and educational products Accreditation Review Council on Education in Surgical Technology and Surgical Assisting (ARC/STSA) (303-694-9262; www.arcstsa.org)
• Part of the CAAHEP system of program accreditation Commission on Accreditation of Allied Health Education Programs (CAAHEP) (727-210-2350; www.caahep.org)
National Board of Surgical Technology and Surgical Assisting (NBSTSA) (800-707-0057; www.nbstsa.org)
• Responsible for all aspects of individual certification, including *recertification*

or previously CSTs). Since certification is voluntary at this time, although it may be required as a condition of employment by an employer or state legislation, an ST professional chooses to take the national examination. Additional information about the three organizations, AST, ARC/STSA, and NBSTSA, is provided in Table 1-3.

THE SURGICAL TECHNOLOGIST AS A PROFESSIONAL

Professionalism is a lifelong commitment for the ST. Professionalism, as applied to the ST, denotes maintaining competence in a specialized body of knowledge and skills. It means that the ST has specific duties and responsibilities for the provision of quality surgical patient care. Also included are the relevant attitudes, values, and behaviors of the professional ST.

STs must strive to learn, understand, and exhibit the characteristics that foster surgical technology as a profession and not merely an occupation. STs must continually seek opportunities for personal and professional growth.

This section looks at some of the expectations the ST will encounter in his or her career. Some of the expectations are professional, while others are predominantly personal.

Professionalism

Professionalism begins with **competency** and commitment in the workplace. Both employers and patients deserve a dependable health care professional. Some important professional traits include:

- Conscientiousness
- Professional honesty
- Consistent attendance
- Punctuality
- Understanding of employer policies/procedures and standards
- Skills competency
- Ability to obey rules
- Spirit of cooperation
- Being a team member
- Commitment to continuing education
- Ability to problem solve and prioritize
- Willingness to serve on committees
- Willingness to learn and cope with change
- Demonstration of flexibility and organizational skills
- Ability to communicate effectively
- Willingness to learn from constructive criticism and suggestions
- Respect for patient decisions
- Being nonjudgmental
- Maintenance of patient confidentiality

Being a health care professional entails more than competency in the workplace. Professionals are obligated to support and develop their profession.

PROFESSIONAL ORGANIZATION

The **AST** is the national nonprofit professional organization for STs. For four decades, the primary purpose of AST has been to ensure that STs have the knowledge and skills required to administer patient care of the highest quality.

The AST's mission statement summarizes this obligation well: "Enhancing the profession to ensure quality patient care." Obviously the role of a professional organization is to enhance the profession it represents; however, there is a qualifier when it is a health care profession. The actions must be intended to provide better patient care. Being an active health care professional means many things for the ST. The ST receives the benefits of the activities of the professional organization. Membership in the AST and participation in the activities of the professional association offer support. Continuing education is important to the ST for two reasons: (1) continuing education is necessary for continued personal development and improved patient safety and (2) continuing certification requires demonstration of continuing education. Finally, professionals must always behave in a mature, honest, and ethical manner.

The AST logo features the roles that the ST performs within the OR (Figure 1-4). The circles that are filled represent common roles. The filled circle with the arc extending from it represents the assistant circulator (the term "circulator" arises from the fact that this individual can move about the OR). The large rectangle represents the operating table and the three empty circles represent the patient, the surgeon, and the anesthesia provider. The filled circle to the left of the dark rectangle

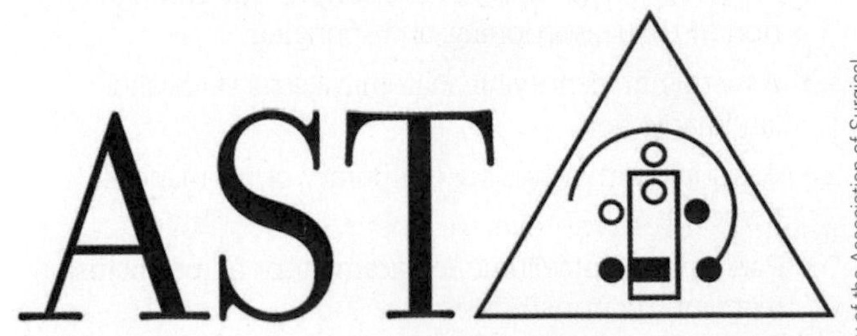

Figure 1-4 Association of Surgical Technologists logo

represents the first scrub ST. The dark rectangle represents the Mayo stand. The filled circle opposite the empty circle is the surgical first assistant.

The Surgical Technologist's Lifestyle

As an ST, life will change in ways that the student probably never considered.

In the ethical and legal section of Chapter 2, the student will learn more about the concepts of duty and obligation. For the purposes of this chapter, it is enough to understand that health care professionals have duties and obligations that differ from those of the general population. There is a moral and legal duty and obligation to the patient. This means that each individual's actions are counted or evaluated against a standard of practice. Accountability, for the ST, extends beyond the OR into one's personal life.

Some simple illustrations demonstrate how the ST's professional obligations affect his or her personal life. Consider the following:

- The ST may be leaving his or her family at inconvenient times because of "on call" responsibilities.
- The ST has a greater obligation to protect himself or herself from communicable disease than the general population.
- The ST will know details of other people's lives that cannot be shared with family and friends.
- The ST may find that most of the exciting "world of the OR" cannot be shared because others do not want to know about it.

The ST cannot act in such a way that increases the chance of injury to a patient and cannot afford to be mentally or physically impaired in any way. The ST must think about this and make adjustments to account for this obligation to be prepared to provide the best patient care possible.

The ST has access to confidential information about patients and their families. The ST must not share this information with family, friends, or news media. Additionally, many individuals, including family members, do not want to know or hear about what you do in the OR. It may be too upsetting, especially if a family member or close friend recently underwent surgery, or it may be "gross," even though you find working in surgery challenging and fascinating.

Roles and Competencies

AST developed a list of roles to serve as guidelines for the ST and for employers looking for appropriate criteria to develop a clinical ladder. Note that a *role* is defined as a set of responsibilities or expected results associated with a job; a job usually includes several roles (see Table 1-4). Additionally, entry into the profession anticipates (1) graduation from an accredited program in surgical technology and (2) successful completion of the certification examination in order to meet the competencies or abilities needed to perform the roles of the surgical technology job (see Table 1-5).

Job Descriptions for the Surgical Technologist

Role descriptions are broad in scope. Job descriptions, however, are produced and approved by the facility for which one works. Depending on the type of job, they may be written broadly but are usually quite specific. The ST should be familiar with the job description in the facility of employment.

STs have traditionally been assigned to the nursing department when employed by a facility such as a hospital or ambulatory surgical center. With the increased use of private STs and the "traveling" ST, the employer may be a physician, a physician's group, or an agency. In some locales, an ST who is employed outside the facility is required to seek permission to work at that facility through the medical credentials committee. Regardless of the employment situation, the job description may establish the criteria by which the ST will be judged in a case concerning alleged negligence or malpractice. STs should keep a copy of the job description in their own files and update it as necessary. Should the ST find any of the components of a standard job description to be missing from the institution's job description, it should be reported to the supervisor and included in the formal job description.

The ST should identify the following components of the job description:

- Job title (e.g., surgical technologist level I)
- Requirements (e.g., graduation from an accredited program and national certification)
- Nature of position (e.g., the surgical technologist is a member of the intraoperative surgical team)
- Duties (e.g., the surgical technologist, level I, shall perform in the scrub role and shall be responsible for . . .)
- Accountability (e.g., the ST shall be directly accountable to the director of surgical services)
- Immediate supervisor (e.g., the immediate supervisor for all surgical services personnel is the OR charge nurse)

Career Development and Opportunities

Most STs are employed in hospital surgery departments, labor and delivery departments, and ambulatory surgical centers to perform the scrub role. The roles of circulator and surgical assistant provide additional career opportunities for the ST. With additional education, training, or experience, the ST can assume a challenging career by specializing, management opportunities, or advancement in other related fields of expertise. The education completed by an ST provides a solid background

Table 1-4 Role Definitions of the CST

Role	*Description*	*Examples of Duties*
Certified Surgical Technologist First Scrub	Sterile surgical team member who prepares the surgical environment, maintains and monitors the sterile field, and passes instrumentation, supplies, and equipment to the surgeon and other team members	• Anticipates needs of the surgeon and patient • Organizes the sterile field • Applies sterile surgical drapes • Passes sterile instruments, equipment, and supplies to surgeon and other sterile team members • Prepares, labels, and handles medications at the sterile field • Performs sponge, sharps, and instrument counts • Handles surgical specimens • Applies sterile dressings to surgical wounds
Certified Surgical Technologist Second Scrub	Sterile surgical team member who assists the surgeon by providing visualization of the surgical wound and assists with hemostasis and wound closure	• Provides visualization of the surgical site through retraction of tissue or manipulation of endoscope • Suctions blood and body fluids from wound • Sponges the surgical site • Assists with opening and closing the surgical incision
Certified Surgical Technologist Assistant Circulator	Nonsterile surgical team members who are responsible for providing an optimal surgical environment for the patient	• Prepares the OR • Transports the patient to the OR • Positions the patient • Performs the surgical skin prep • Dispenses additional items to the sterile field • Maintains the patient's operative record • Assists the anesthesia provider

Surgical Assistant	Sterile surgical team member, CST, or CSFA who has obtained additional knowledge and experience and obtained an appropriate surgical assistant credential	• As defined by the American College of Surgeons (ACS), the surgical assistant provides aid in exposure, hemostasis, and other technical functions that will help the surgeon carry out a safe operation with optimal results for the patient.
		• Additional functions include, but are not limited to,
		  • Positioning the patient
		  • Suturing and closure of body planes and skin
		  • Application of dressings

for career development. Employment options available to the experienced ST include:

- Specialization in a surgical specialty such as orthopedics, cardiovascular surgery, or trauma
- Employment in material management or sterile processing areas (Figure 1-5)
- Surgical technology educator and/or program director (Figure 1-6)
- Surgical first assistant
- Medical services and equipment salesperson
- Organ and tissue procurement technician
- Private employment by a surgeon
- Research and product development assistant
- Veterinary assistant
- Endoscopy technician
- Labor and delivery technician
- Office manager
- Surgery scheduler
- Anesthesia technologist
- Employment as a traveling ST to fill temporary staffing needs for health care facilities
- Volunteer opportunities (e.g., Peace Corps)

Table 1-5 Surgical Technologist: Nature of the Position

The surgical technologist must be able to:

- Stand, bend, stoop, and/or sit for long periods of time in one location with minimal/no breaks
- Lift a minimum of 20 pounds
- Refrain from nourishment or rest room breaks for periods up to 8 hours
- Demonstrate sufficient visual and tactile ability to load a fine (10–0) suture onto needles and needle holders with/without corrective lenses and while wearing safety glasses
- Demonstrate sufficient peripheral vision to anticipate and function while in the sterile surgical environment
- Hear and understand muffled communication without visualization of the communicator's mouth/lips and within 20 feet
- Hear activation/warning signals on equipment
- Detect odors sufficient to maintain environmental safety and patient needs
- Manipulate instruments, supplies, and equipment with speed, dexterity, and good eye–hand coordination
- Ambulate/move around without assistive devices
- Assist with and/or lift, move, position, and manipulate, with or without assistive devices, the patient who is unconscious
- Communicate and understand fluent English both verbally and in writing
- Be free of reportable communicable diseases and chemical abuse
- Demonstrate immunity to rubella, rubeola, tuberculosis, and hepatitis B, or be vaccinated against these diseases, or be willing to sign a waiver of release of liability with regard to these diseases
- Possess short- and long-term memory sufficient to perform tasks such as, but not limited to, mentally tracking surgical supplies and performing anticipation skills intraoperatively
- Make appropriate judgments and decisions
- Demonstrate the use of positive coping skills under stress
- Demonstrate calm and effective responses, especially in emergency situations
- Exhibit positive interpersonal skills in patient, staff, and faculty interactions

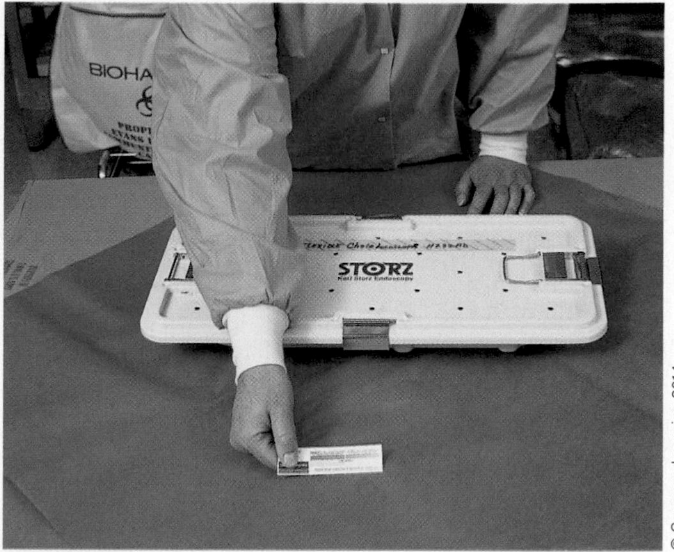

Figure 1-5 Surgical technologist preparing supplies for sterilization in the sterile processing department

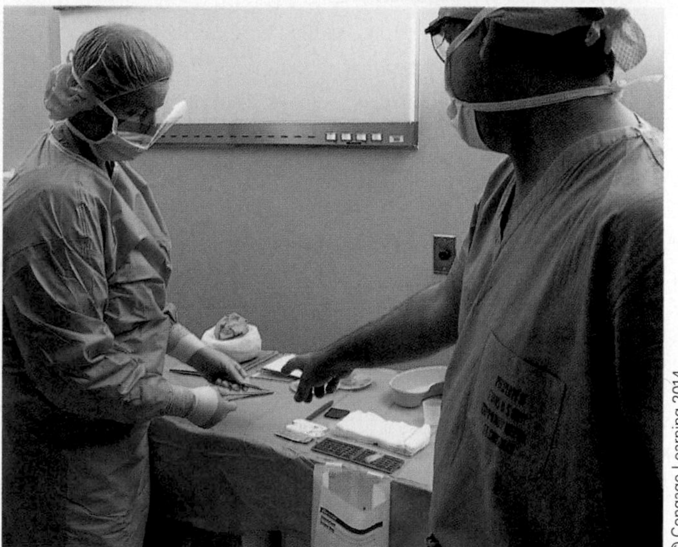

Figure 1-6 Surgical technology educator demonstrating the technique for placing a scalpel blade on a scalpel handle

- Military service
- Technical writing, illustration, and photography
- Employment as a private consultant

CLINICAL LADDER PROGRAM

Clinical ladder programs (see Table 1-6) allow an ST to move upward to positions of increased responsibility within an organization. They offer employers a long-term strategy for

Table 1-6 AST Recommended Clinical Ladder for the Surgical Technologist

Level I: Entry-Level Practitioner

The Level I practitioner is a recent graduate of an accredited surgical technology program who has been employed as a surgical technologist for 1 year or less.

1. Has graduated from an accredited surgical technology program
2. Independently scrubs basic surgical procedures
3. Demonstrates ability to problem solve in relation to the procedure being performed
4. Applies base knowledge of anatomy and physiology, medical terminology, microbiology, and pharmacology for optimal surgical patient care
5. Applies basic knowledge of computers, robotics, and lasers
6. Demonstrates knowledge and practice of patient care concepts
7. Applies the principles of asepsis during surgical procedures
8. Participates in orientation program to attain competency in complex cases and achieve Level II: Proficient Practitioner
9. Becomes certified within 1 year of graduation
10. Maintains certification by participating in continuing education activities

Level II: Proficient Practitioner

The Level II practitioner is a Certified Surgical Technologist who has been employed as a surgical technologist for 1 year or more and who takes on greater responsibility in providing patient care than a Level I practitioner. Level II practitioners demonstrate higher-level critical thinking and problem-solving skills than do Level I practitioners.

1. Meets the criteria stated in Level I
2. Demonstrates advanced knowledge and proficient practice in the first scrub role in a majority of surgical procedures
3. Applies knowledge of advanced surgical techniques
4. Applies knowledge related to emergency situations and surgical procedures
5. Demonstrates critical thinking skills in relation to anticipating the perioperative needs of the patient and surgeon
6. Exhibits a higher level of collaboration with peers in making decisions related to surgical patient care
7. Assists in performing circulating skills and tasks
8. Participates in program to achieve Level III: Expert Practitioner

Level III: Expert Practitioner

The Level III practitioner is an advanced practitioner who thinks on a more global level and is more involved in endeavors related to, but outside of, the surgery department.

1. Meets the criteria stated in Level II
2. Demonstrates superior knowledge of the various surgical equipment and advanced surgical instrumentation
3. Demonstrates superior knowledge and expert practice in the first scrub role in advanced surgical procedures
4. Performs the preceptor role for surgical technology students
5. Demonstrates leadership abilities
6. Serves as a mentor and role model
7. Member of at least one department or hospital committee
8. Involved with community health promotional efforts and other related community services
9. Demonstrates knowledge of department fiscal requirements
10. Participates in decision-making activities related to evaluating and acquiring surgical equipment, instruments, and supplies
11. Collaborates with other health care professionals in the development of surgical budgetary requirements
12. Demonstrates skills in organizing and coordinating the effective use of personnel and materials
13. Develops, organizes, and delivers continuing education topics and/or courses

Courtesy of the Association of Surgical Technologists

employee retention and maintaining good department morale. They also serve as motivation for STs to continually improve their knowledge, skills, and competencies.

The goals of the clinical ladder program are to:

- Enhance quality surgical patient care
- Encourage employer recognition and reward advanced competency
- Promote accountability and responsibility of the ST toward the patient as well as broaden the role
- Provide new staff the means for advancement to encourage the professional growth of the ST
- Increase the visibility of the role of the ST in the hospital and other facilities

EMPLOYABILITY SKILLS

To make the transition from student to employee, basic employability skills are needed to obtain and maintain a job:

- Work ethic: professional and personal honesty
- Communication skills: verbal and nonverbal
- Dedication: empathy, devotion, and vocation
- Adaptability: ability to change to accept positive outcomes
- Conflict resolution: making a difference between positive and negative results
- Personal appearance and hygiene: important grooming habits for health care professionals
- Accountability: responsibility for your own actions
- Commitment to continuing education: enhancing your knowledge and personal growth

Resume Preparation

A resume is an overview or a summary about your past experiences and implies what you can achieve in the future.

Required Elements

A typical resume should include the following:

- Career objective
- Qualifications
- Work experience
- Education
- Skills and accomplishments

When conducting a job search, there are several letter styles recommended for use:

- Cover letter: introduces your resume
- Professional reference: letter of recommendation from someone of importance familiar with your skills, capabilities, experience, etc.
- Thank-you letter: thanks the interviewer and expresses appreciation for the chance to meet and discuss the job opening
- Acceptance letter: thanks the interviewer for the opportunity to work with his or her business and accepts the position and terms offered
- Letter of refusal: thanks the interviewer for the opportunity to interview but indicates not accepting the position

A business's application must be prepared and completed prior to the interview. All application forms must be completed honestly and legibly. Any untruthful information may be terms for immediate dismissal.

Interview Preparation

The more prepared you are for the interview, the easier it is to communicate effectively with the interviewer and present your message in a clear and concise manner.

The following list summarizes the "to do" list before an interview:

- Learn about the organization.
- Review qualifications for the specific job.
- Prepare answers about yourself (education, experience, availability).
- Review and know your own resume.
- Practice mock interviews.
- Arrive before the scheduled time for the interview.
- Dress for success.

Resignation

Just as you take time to prepare for an interview, careful consideration must be given when resigning from a job. Resignation notice may be written or verbal. Even though most employments are "at will," 2 weeks, notice is desirable. The most important job-search rule to remember when resigning from any job is not to leave on bad terms with the employer. Some companies may require an exit interview with a representative of the company's human resources (HR) department and the departing employee. The HR representative might ask the employee questions, complete a questionnaire, or both.

COMMUNICATION SKILLS AND TEAMWORK

Technical skills are critical to surgical patient care. However, they are only part of the skills required of an efficient and effective ST. Appropriate body language and verbal and nonverbal communication skills are very important. The modern surgical environment is clinically and technologically complicated and surgery is inherently dangerous. Even though the surgeon bears primary responsibility for the patient, the surgeon can neither see nor do everything required for safe patient care alone. Many important facts must be shared with various surgical team members. Some examples of necessary communication are shown in Table 1-7.

Communication

Effective communication contributes to positive teamwork and patient safety. Principles of effective communication include:

- Always speak respectfully and professionally.
- Keep communication focused on the patient and the procedure.
- Express needs clearly. (Example: "May I have another package of lap sponges, please?")
- Always repeat complicated orders, names of medications or solutions, and count information. (Example: "The syringe contains 1% lidocaine with epinephrine.")
- If unsure, ask. (Example: "Are you ready to switch from irrigation solution to contrast medium?")
- If concerned about an action that another individual is about to take, state the concern in the form of a question. (Example: "Should we switch from the monopolar to the bipolar electrosurgical unit at this point?")
- Always tell the truth. The patient's well-being may depend on it. (Example: "I did not verify what medication is in that syringe during the relief report. It must be discarded.")

All members of the surgical team know their individual roles and typically do not have to be told what to do or when to do it by another team member. Every team member has the best interest of the patient in mind and all must work together to ensure patient safety. Everyone must be observant of the events occurring around them and use effective verbal and nonverbal skills to communicate with one another.

But just as important is ensuring effective, open, and honest communication between patients and the health care staff. In particular, the ST often only has brief contact with the surgical patient, such as when transporting the patient on the stretcher from the hospital ward to the surgery department. The ST must quickly establish a professional relationship with the patient, based upon open and effective communication, which in turn establishes the level of trust the patient will have in the ST. The following discussion provides some basic background information pertaining to communication, including body language signals.

There are three basic types of relationships that the ST will effect:

- Social: Relationship established with peers and friends
- Professional: Relationship with co-workers, surgeon, and other health care providers
- Therapeutic: Relationship with the patient and the patient's family

For these relationships to work, effective communication is a key component, including recognizing the needs of the patient and meeting those needs.

There are five broad goals of communication:

- Provide information to an individual or a group of people
- Obtain information from an individual or a group of people
- Express one's feelings
- Solve problems
- Persuade an individual or a group of people to change a behavior or opinion about a specific subject

However, in relation to the surgical patient, the goals of effective communication are more specific, including:

- Maintaining teamwork among health care providers to ensure that the care provided to the patient is constant and consistent (e.g., during a shift change STs going off-shift must communicate information concerning any patients to the STs coming on-shift).
- Creating an environment where patients are comfortable in communicating their feelings, emotions, physical needs, and fears to the surgical team.
- Communicating with the patient in a positive and open manner, because effective communication can influence the patient's behavior in the OR, the patient's level of anxiety, and the patient's cooperativeness with the surgery team.

Table 1-7 Examples of Communication of Important Information

Information Needed by	*Information Needed from First Scrub Surgical Technologist*
Anesthesia provider: checking blood loss	"500 mL of irrigation has been used."
Anesthesia provider: beginning of craniotomy	"We have 25 mL of 1% lidocaine with epinephrine in the scalp."
Surgeon: as cholangiocath is passed	"Cholangiocath has been irrigated with normal saline. Syringe contains normal saline."
Surgeon: as peritoneum is being closed	"First closing count is correct."
Circulator: change in expected procedure	"We are going to need the GI suture after all. 3-0 chromic and 3-0 silk please."

To achieve these goals, communication is used either in oral or written form, or as nonverbal communication such as body language, crying, shivering, or nodding the head in a sign of agreement or disagreement.

The four components of communication are sender (encoder), message, receiver (decoder), and feedback (Figure1-7). The following is a brief description of each of the components:

- Sender
  - The sender has an idea or message that needs to be shared with an individual or a group of people.
  - The sender "encodes" the idea or message by choosing the method in which to send the message. The message can be sent verbally or nonverbally.
- Receiver
  - The receiver gets the message.
  - The receiver "decodes" the message using his or her knowledge, background, and environment.
  - The receiver also has the responsibility of using active listening skills when receiving the message from the sender.
- Feedback
  - Probably the most important part of the communication process occurs when the sender receives feedback from the receiver that the message was understood. For example, the receiver may say, "What I understood was said . . ."
  - This can also be awkward because asking for feedback, either verbally or nonverbally, can make the communication process uncomfortable for both parties.
  - However, using open-ended questions beginning with the words *who, what, how,* etc., as opposed to closed-ended questions such as *Do you understand?* works best. Additionally, creating a culture or environment of feedback eases the process.

Effective verbal communication with the patient must be combined with effective listening skills. Often, surgical patients need someone who will listen to them, which helps patients to alleviate some of their anxiety. Effective listening skills include the following:

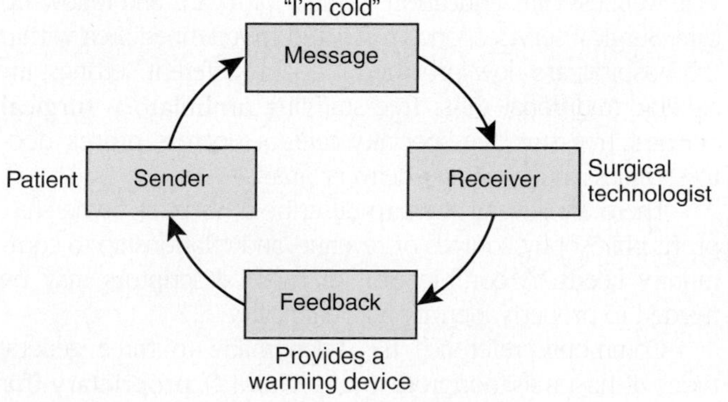

Figure 1-7 Components of communication

- Eye contact: Focus on what the speaker is saying. Eye contact cannot always be maintained, for example, when transporting the patient on the stretcher down the hall, but when possible it lets the patient know you are attentive.
- Receptive: Be open-minded and objective about what the patient is saying; he or she may be providing some important information related to his or her medical condition, status, or ethical beliefs.
- Sensitive: Think about your response; respond in a positive, sincere manner that does not belittle or "cut down" the patient.

Body language is a type of nonverbal communication that is important for the ST to recognize when used by the patient. Body language can provide clues to the patient's feelings and attitudes, as well as reinforce what he or she is saying. Additionally, one's own body language can be recognized by the patient and interpreted as either positive or negative. Positive body language signals include:

- Eye contact
- Smiling
- Arms unfolded
- Leaning slightly toward patient
- Head nodding in agreement
- Therapeutic touch

Negative body language can include:

- Tightly folded arms
- Distancing oneself from the patient
- Frowning or eye rolling
- Lips pressed tightly together
- Tapping foot, indicating impatience with the situation

The qualities of communication include:

- Respect for yourself and others
- Active listening
- Sensitivity and assertiveness
- Clarity in delivering information
- Clear feedback

Teamwork

Effective use of communication skills is essential to teamwork. In order to achieve team building, group interaction, and positive teamwork, the following principles are needed:

- Positive team interaction
- Discussion of conflict, project, etc.
- Yielding toward others' points of view
- Acceptance of change during the process

- Politeness and respect
- Collaboration toward a common goal
- Willingness to reach a compromise

A model for conflict resolution developed by Bruce Tuckman in 1965 is commonly followed and contains four stages:

- Forming: Individuals form a team
- Storming: Ideas, perspectives, option, plans begin to be discussed
- Performing: Individuals start working as a team with little supervision
- Adjourning: Completion of the task and break-up of the team

Conflict management and problem behavior in the OR involves:

- Verbal abuse
- Lateral violence and bullying collectively referred to as "workplace violence"
- Complaints, rumors, and gossip
- Feedback and criticism
- Sexual harassment and hostile environment

Conflict resolution may result in one of the following:

- Win-Win: It is the desired outcome with a solution acceptable to all involved.
- Win-Lose: Only one party involved in the conflict is satisfied.
- Lose-Lose: All parties end up worse off.

Refer to the AST position statement on teamwork that further reinforces the above-mentioned principles of communication and teamwork in the care of the surgical patient.

AST Position Statement on Teamwork

Teamwork is an essential part of the surgical environment. The Association of Surgical Technologists (AST) recognizes the importance of a collaborative teamwork environment. The primary focus of all surgical team members is to provide a seamless, safe, and efficient surgical experience with a positive patient outcome.

The surgical arena is a highly technical and fast-paced environment. In many cases, this technological environment has decreased the amount of time that the patient spends within the OR. This time reduction has resulted in the need for increased proficiency, team collaboration, and the use of interpersonal skills to provide safe, quality outcomes for the surgical patient.

Team-building skills aid in the ability of a group to work together effectively. Team players need to learn and refine their skills in communication, conflict negotiation and resolution, and consensual decision making. AST promotes the development of these skills within the surgical environment, as this is imperative to achieving exceptional team and patient outcomes.

SURGICAL CONSCIENCE

An ST committed to professional honesty, patient confidentiality, nondiscriminatory treatment, cost consciousness, and sterile technique will provide the greatest level of safety to the patient that can be expected. For the ST, surgical conscience is rooted in the following principles:

1. An ST must be willing to accept responsibility for his or her own actions and be willing to be held liable for his or her actions and to provide the information needed for an accurate evaluation of those actions.
2. The ST must be committed to maintaining the confidentiality of patient information. Patients should never have to question that their care will be in the hands of individuals of good faith who handle information properly.
3. A surgical conscience dictates nondiscriminatory treatment of all patients. Personal values, feelings, and principles take a secondary position to the patient's need for the highest quality of treatment.
4. Modern medicine is very expensive and both the patient and hospitals should be committed to cost control. Cost containment is the responsibility of everyone involved: the health care facility, health care providers, and the patient.
5. A surgical conscience is rooted in the fundamental understanding of the principles of asepsis and a commitment to practice sterile technique. Of all the tasks and roles that an ST fulfills during his or her career, the most important is that of strictly practicing sterile technique in the OR.

HEALTH CARE FACILITIES ORGANIZATION AND MANAGEMENT

Traditionally, surgical care was provided in a hospital, that is, a facility that provided many medical services. However, health care has changed dramatically; even hospitals that still provide the traditional style of services look outside their walls to provide wellness care, education, home health care, and follow-up care. Surgical services, once restricted to a defined area within the hospital, are now provided in many different settings, including traditional ORs, free-standing **ambulatory surgical centers**, free-standing specialty centers, doctors' offices, doctors' clinics, and labor and delivery units.

There are several ways to describe a hospital: ownership, profit philosophy, sources of revenue, and relationship to community needs. A combination of these descriptors may be needed to properly identify a given facility.

Commonly, reference has been made to three general types of hospitals: nonprofit (not-for-profit), **proprietary** (for profit), and tax supported.

A hospital is an organization with a governing body, medical staff, professional staff, and in-patient facilities. Hospitals provide medical, nursing, and related services on a permanent, around-the-clock basis. States may have varying legal definitions of a hospital to distinguish them from other health care organizations for licensing purposes.

Not-for-profit hospitals are general, acute-care hospitals defined as nontaxable by the federal government. A private corporation owns these facilities. Profits are turned back into the maintenance and improvement of the hospital, including its physical facility and services. A community, church, or other organization that views its primary purpose as community service may own these facilities. Tax revenues may support some of them. In that case, the hospital is both tax supported and not-for-profit. A federal, state, county, or city hospital is an example.

Proprietary or investor-owned hospitals are owned and operated by an individual or corporation. The primary intent of these facilities is to provide good patient care. However, they differ from the nonprofit hospitals in that profits are returned to the investors. The profits are also taxable.

As mentioned, any tax-levying government body might provide support for a hospital. These are less common in the current environment as governments at all levels are attempting to divest themselves of hospital ownership. Community agencies and organizations provide financial support through dispersal of private funds or grants.

In many hospitals, surgery may be performed in more than one setting. It is not uncommon for a hospital to have a traditional OR to serve in-patient needs; a free-standing surgical ambulatory center for outpatient surgery; separate ORs for cesarean sections, dilation and curettage, and tubal ligation within the labor and delivery unit; and possibly a separate area for pediatric surgery. Even then, surgical services are not limited to hospitals. Several other types of facilities provide surgical services.

The ambulatory surgical center is physically or geographically separate from a hospital. It provides surgical services to patients who do not require hospitalization.

A preferred provider organization (PPO) is a collection of private-practice donors, labs, patient care facilities, and hospitals that contract with insurance companies and receive an agreed set rate for their services. The patient has more control over his or her own medical needs and does not need a referral as long as the doctor he or she is seeing is a member of the PPO. A health maintenance organization (**HMO**) is a collection of hospitals, health professionals, and doctors who work for a set fee. The HMO may require the patients to use a primary care physician for all referrals.

Both organizations act as insurer and provider of medical services. A group of physicians, defined by contractual arrangement, provides services to a population of clients who are enrolled in the program. A clinic is a facility or part of a facility designed for diagnosis and treatment of outpatients. Some clinics may perform a limited range of procedures. Like the clinic, certain procedures may be performed in the physician's office. Typically, a room is set aside within the office space for a limited range of procedures.

HOSPITAL ORGANIZATION

Although surgical services are provided outside the traditional hospital setting, most hospitals continue to have some features that resemble the traditional hospital organizational structure. With that in mind, we now look briefly at the way in which hospitals typically organize themselves.

Hospital philosophy and policies are typically established by a board of directors or a board of trustees. Given the type of hospital, boards of directors are elected or appointed. The board will hire a chief executive officer (CEO), whose job it is to put the philosophy and policies into practice (Figure 1-8).

Hospitals typically have several layers of administration. At the top administrative level, several vice presidents oversee broad areas. For example, each of the following areas might have a vice president assigned to it: administration, medical affairs, patient services, legal services, finances, and building and environment. Depending on the size of the hospital, these areas may be subdivided.

Typically, under medical affairs there will be a second division—medical services and nursing services. The physicians are organized under medical services. The chief physician in the hospital is called the chief of staff. Medical services are also subdivided. Often there is a chief of medicine and a chief of surgery. These divisions are organized by specialty. In the case of surgery, one may find the surgical staff committee composed of one representative from each surgical specialty at the hospital. The representative of the specialty is called, for example, the chief of orthopedics. Usually, all other nursing and allied health services are organized under nursing services.

One of the functions of the medical staff committee is to verify the credentials of the physicians and specified health care personnel. The ST who holds the CSFA credential may be required to submit an application for privileges to this committee.

Most hospitals place STs under nursing services. The director of nursing (DON) oversees nursing services. Nursing services is typically large and divided into subunits. Surgical services is one of those units, commonly referred to as the surgery *department*. The director of surgical services represents the surgical nurses and allied health personnel at the nursing services meetings.

The surgical services department may also be divided into units. A head nurse oversees the day-to-day activity in the unit. Surgical specialty areas may have a coordinator. Sterile processing may be a separate unit with its own coordinator. These coordinators communicate needs, concerns, and decisions in their assigned areas.

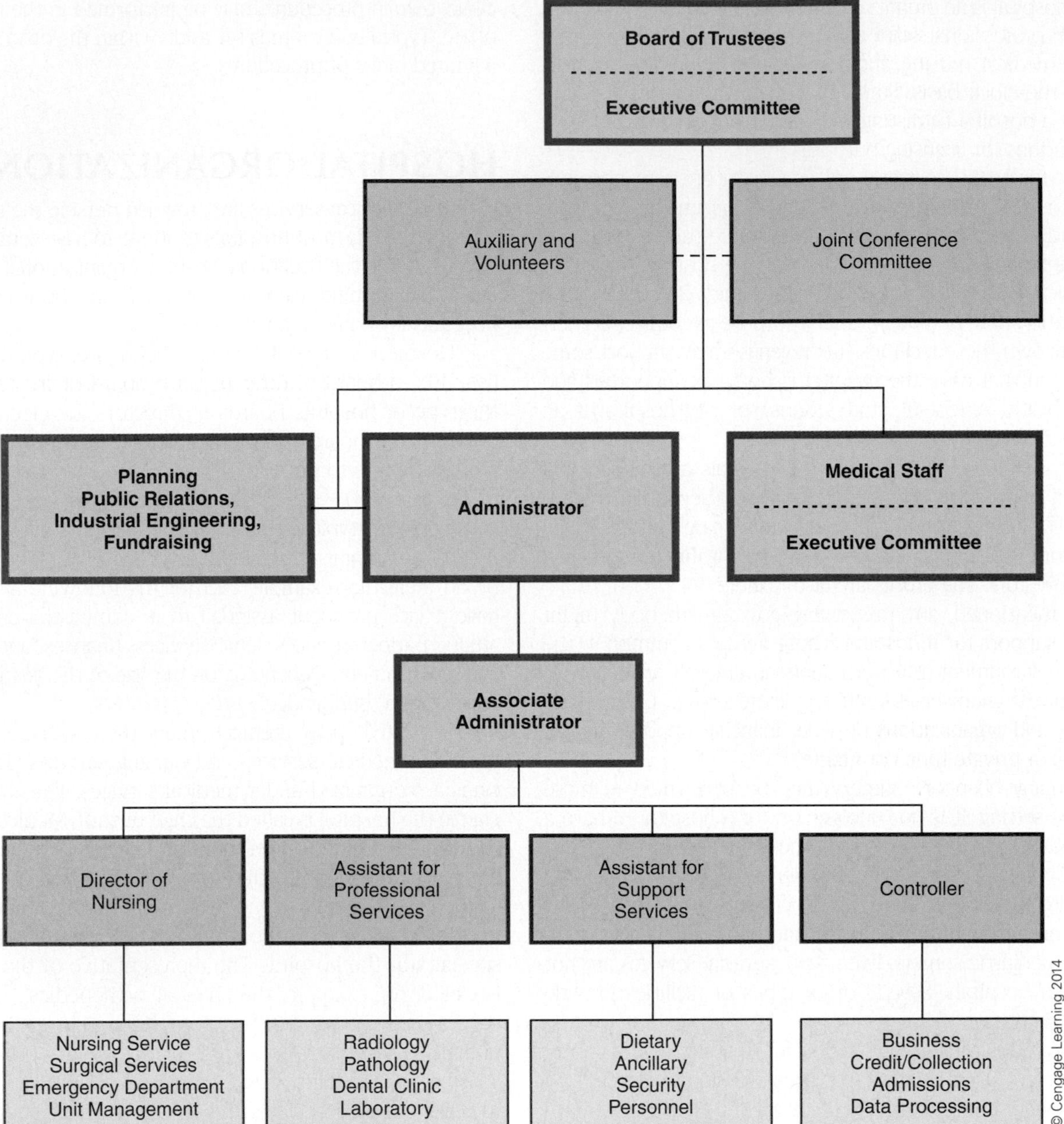

Figure 1-8 Sample hospital organization chart

In its day-to-day activities, surgeons, nursing personnel, anesthesia personnel, allied health personnel, and ancillary personnel staff the surgical services department.

Surgeons are medical doctors, doctors of osteopathy (DOs), or doctors of podiatric medicine (DPMs) who completed a designated course of education and training and have surgical privileges. The surgeons have 4 years of premedical college, 4 years of medical school, and 4 to 8 years of residency training in a surgical specialty. Surgeons with whom the ST works are or will become board certified in their specialty.

The nursing staff an ST may work with may be LPNs, LVNs, or RNs who completed an associate degree in nursing (ADN) or bachelor of science in nursing (BSN). Some of the nurses may hold a voluntary credential, CNOR (Certified Nurse Operating Room), awarded by the Association of periOperative Nurses (AORN) to RNs who pass the certification examination. Today, one may see the credential Certified Registered Nurse First Assistant (CRNFA). This credential is awarded to the registered nurse who has passed the certification examination.

The anesthesia staff may include anesthesiologists (MDs/DOs), certified registered nurse anesthetists (CRNAs), an anesthesiologist's assistant (AAs), and anesthesia technicians. The anesthesiologist is a physician who has been through a residency program in anesthesia. Like the surgeon, the anesthesiologist will be board certified. The CRNA is a registered nurse with several years of experience in critical care nursing and specialty training in anesthesia. The anesthesiologist's assistant is an allied health professional who works under the direction of an anesthesiologist. The tasks performed vary but may include collecting preoperative data, assisting with the insertion of intravenous (IV) and arterial catheters, assisting with airway management, and other tasks for which the AA is approved. The anesthesia technician is also an allied health professional who supports the anesthesiologist and CRNA by caring for equipment and supplies. The anesthesia technician may be trained to assist in certain specified procedures performed by the anesthesiologist or CRNA.

Physician assistants (PAs) may also work in the OR. These are allied health personnel who have bachelor's or master's degrees. PA programs are usually 20 to 24 months long and often are affiliated with a medical school. The PA is a physician extender. One may see the PA in the role of surgical first assistant and/or communicating with the physician about other patients under the physician's care.

There may be representatives of several different allied health professions in the OR. It is not uncommon to see the following allied health support personnel in the OR: diagnostic imaging technician, perfusionist, cell saver technician, bioelectrical technician, medical laboratory technician, EEG technician, medical service representative, radiology technician, and orthopedic and ophthalmic technician.

Hospital Departments and Interdepartmental Communication

The surgical services department and the OR team do not work in a vacuum. Many related departments and personnel are involved in patient care and safety in a modern hospital. Hospital departments can be categorized as having direct or indirect patient care responsibilities. The following departments have direct patient care responsibilities:

- Patient care units (e.g., medical-surgical units, critical care units)
- Diagnostic imaging (e.g., radiology, computerized axial tomography, magnetic resonance imaging, and sonography)
- Medical laboratory (includes clinical laboratories, pathology, and blood bank)
- Pharmacy
- Physical and occupational therapy

Departments that contribute to patient care through secondary means include:

- Hospital administration
- Hospital maintenance and security services
- Housekeeping and environmental services
- Dietitian and food services
- Purchasing, central supply, and materials management
- Medical records and admissions

Tables 1-8 and 1-9 describe the departments in the hospital and their services to the patient.

The department of surgical services has daily contact with most departments of the hospital. Some interactions may exist based on the type of service supplied by the department or its relationship to the patients in surgery. Typical interactions are defined in Table 1-10.

Each department must communicate with the other departments. Patient safety and hospital efficiency and effectiveness are related to the consistency and clarity with which these communications are carried out. Hospital departments communicate through several means: medical records, requisitions for services, computer records and requisitions, verbal communication (telephone and individual to individual), and

Table 1-8 Direct Patient Care Departments

Department	*Hospital Administrator*	*Direct Oversight*	*Contribution*
Patient care units/intensive and critical care units	Director of nursing	Charge nurse	Direct nursing care
Diagnostic imaging	Contracted physician, contracted company	Radiologist	Diagnostic support for all departments
Medical laboratory, blood bank, and pathology	Contracted physician, contracted company	Pathologist	Diagnostic support for all departments
Pharmacy	Hospital administrator	Pharmacist	Drug intervention advice and control for all departments
Physical/occupational therapy	Varies	Therapist	Rehabilitation services

TABLE 1-9 **Indirect Patient Care Departments**

Department	Hospital Administrator	Direct Oversight	Contribution
Administration	Chief executive officer	Vice president of area	Fiscal and policy oversight
Maintenance and security	Vice president of physical environment	Shift supervisor	Care and maintenance of the building and grounds
Environmental services	Vice president of physical environment	Shift supervisor	Daily upkeep of rooms and furniture, including patient rooms
Dietitian and food services	Vice president of food services	Chef/dietitian/supervisor	Food preparation for patients, family, and staff
Purchasing/central services and materials management	Vice president of finances	Purchasing agent	Control, purchase, storage, and dispersal of equipment and supplies
Medical records and admissions	Varies	Supervisor	Maintenance of all legal records of patient care

interhospital department meetings. Specifically, STs should know the forms that are used daily in surgical services and their role and responsibility in relation to each.

Financial Considerations and Reimbursement

Surgical intervention can be very costly. However, in some special instances surgical intervention is provided free of charge or as a charitable mission. For instance, some surgeons may donate a portion of their time to treating children whose families lack the financial resources to gain treatment. Additionally, as part of maintaining proprietary status, organizations may waive some portion of costs as charitable donations, including the cost of surgical care. In general, surgical care is based upon a fee-for-service system. However, based on the recent passage of *The Patient Protection and Affordable Care Act (2010)*, the delivery of health care is undergoing major changes to attempt to ensure health care coverage and access for all individuals.

Insurance designates a contractual relationship that exists when one party or entity agrees to pay another for a specified loss or condition. Typically, with health insurance, the individual and the insurance provider enter into a contract, where the individual pays a fee to the insurer on an ongoing basis and the insurer agrees to cover health care expenses, which are outlined in the insurance policy or contract. Historically, the most common type of health insurance is private insurance, where a private citizen and private insurance agency enter into a contractual agreement for health care coverage. This type of insurance may also evolve from a contractual agreement between a business and an insurer for the benefit of the employee, where the employer pays for all or a portion of the insurance premium.

Private insurance is still used today as a means for reimbursing hospitals, physicians, and other health care professionals for their services. However, most health care coverage today is provided through HMOs and PPOs. Although many types of these programs exist, their primary purpose is to control costs through contractual agreements with health care providers (hospitals and physicians), limiting the payment to an agreed amount or capitated payment. Additional health care coverage may be provided in the form of government-sponsored programs, such as Medicare and Medicaid. Table 1-11 describes the various types of health care reimbursement programs in today's society.

Health care reimbursement has been influenced by the implementation of Medicare diagnosis-related groups (DRGs), which were implemented in 1983. Within this system, providers are reimbursed through a prospective payment system. Providers are reimbursed based upon the average charges for treating conditions within certain DRGs, or upon the DRG defined upon hospital discharge. For instance, if the average cost for treating a patient with acute cholelithiasis is $5000, then the hospital is reimbursed at that rate no matter how long the patient is admitted.

Government financial assistance (DRGs, PPOs, and HMOs) changed health care significantly. Historically, the cost of health care has been escalating and Americans still continue to demand high quality and advanced technology. Additionally, the number of uninsured Americans continues to increase. In response, the U.S. government passed *The Patient Protection and Affordable Care Act* in 2010 with the goal of all individuals having access to affordable health care coverage and needed treatments. The ST and every member of the surgical team must develop both cost awareness and quality conscience in order to ensure cost-effective care with positive surgical outcomes for the patient.

TABLE 1-10 Special Relationships

Department	*Surgical Services Interactions or Relationship*
Patient care units	Patient preparation Informed consent Transportation of patient to and from unit to OR Coordination of information for family Postoperative recovery and care (Several units may be specialty units, such as orthopedics)
Diagnostic imaging	Preoperative diagnostic studies Communication of studies and diagnostic findings to OR Intraoperative studies Stereotactic assistance Postoperative studies
Medical/clinical laboratory Blood bank Pathology department	Preoperative diagnostic studies Communication of studies and diagnostic findings to OR Intraoperative studies (e.g., blood gases, electrolytes) Blood replacement Pathological studies (e.g., frozen section) Postoperative studies
Pharmacy	Control and dispensing of medications Response to special needs Response to emergency needs
Physical/occupational therapy/home health and hospice services	Rehabilitation (may begin in the postanesthesia care unit)
Maintenance and biomed	Control of physical environment Repair of broken equipment Safety checks
Environmental services Purchasing/central services	General housekeeping tasks Purchasing and dispensing of surgical services equipment and supply needs Typically has a central sterile supply unit Oversees sterilization needs May perform basic case cart preparation Restocking of basic supplies for OR
Medical records	Transcription of history and physical Maintains and verifies all patient records Requires proper signatures May provide past medical information when needed
Risk management	Establishment of policies for patient and employee safety Identification of patient hazards and developing solutions
Infection control	Tracking postoperative infection rates Identifying causes of postoperative infections Instituting preventive measures
Administration	Budget Human resources Policies and procedures

TABLE 1-11 Types of Health Care Reimbursement

Insurance Provider	*Description*	*Key Reimbursement Points*
Private insurance	Type of insurance agreement where a private citizen and private insurance agency enter into a contract for health care coverage	Patient or their employers pay an ongoing *premium* contribution to the insurer, who agrees to cover health care expenses as outlined in the insurance policy agreement.
HMOs and PPOs	Provide insurance coverage and a designated range of medical services at a *capitated* rate of payment	Within this system, a set of contracted physicians provides services for the insurance plan enrollees. The physician fees are predetermined and established in the contract (or capitated). The individual's primary care physician serves to refer the patient to other medical specialty physicians, such as a cardiologist, for treatment. Within this system, access to some services and providers may be restricted.
Medicare	Program administered by the federal government through the Centers for Medicare and Medicaid Services (CMS)	Provides reimbursement to both hospital and physicians for the following categories: • Qualifying individual >65 years of age • People eligible for Social Security disability payments for at least 2 years • Renal failure patients and most transplantation patients *Medicare Part A:* Hospital insurance *Medicare Part B:* Supplemental insurance that covers physician costs and other services *Medicare Part D:* Prescription drug coverage *Medicare Advantage* and *Medigap:* Additional supplemental coverage choices
Medicaid	Government assistance program that is funded jointly by the state and federal governments	Reimburses hospitals and physicians for services rendered to low-income persons.

PROFESSIONAL MANAGEMENT

To gain a better understanding of health care in the United States, it helps the student to have a beginning knowledge of various national health organizations as well as those organizations directly related to surgical technology.

Professional Organizations

- Accreditation Review Council on Education in Surgical Technology and Surgical Assisting (ARC/STSA): This organization reviews surgical technology education programs to determine adherence to the CAAHEP standards in education as well as the AST ***Core Curriculum in Surgical Technology***.
- Association of Surgical Technologists (AST): The national nonprofit organization for STs dedicated to the improvement of surgical patient care by promoting standards in surgical technology education and practice.
- Commission on Accreditation of Allied Health Education Programs (CAAHEP): This organization reviews and accredits surgical technology programs upon recommendation of the ARC/STSA.

Credentialing Organizations

- National Board for Surgical Technology and Surgical Assisting (NBSTSA): Organization solely responsible for the development of the national surgical technology and surgical first assisting national certification examinations, including establishing policies for eligibility to take the exam and awarding and renewal of the credential.

Related Professional Organizations

- American College of Surgeons (ACS): professional organization dedicated to the improvement of surgical care by elevating standards of surgical education and practice.
- American Medical Association (AMA): professional physician organization that focuses its efforts on professional and public health issues.
- American National Standards Institute (ANSI): national organization that establishes recognized standards that directly impact businesses and professions in nearly every sector, including health care.
- Association for Professionals of Infection Control and Epidemiology (APIC): international organization that promotes wellness and worldwide infection prevention.
- Association for the Advancement of Medical Instrumentation (AAMI): professional organization that represents an international alliance of members to increase the understanding and use of medical instrumentation through effective standards.
- Association of peri-Operative Registered Nurses (AORN): professional organization of OR nurses dedicated to the improvement of patient care by elevating educational standards and practice for surgical nurses
- Centers for Disease Control and Prevention (CDC): U.S. government organization under the federal Department of Health and Human Services dedicated to protecting the health of individuals through research and control of disease.
- Council on Surgical and Perioperative Safety (CSPS): consists of seven health organizations, including AST, that promote excellence in surgical patient safety.
- Emergency Services Advanced Registry for Volunteer Health Professionals (ESAR-VHP): federal program to establish and implement guidelines and standards for the registration, credentialing, and deployment of medical professionals in the event of a large-scale national emergency.
- Environmental Protection Agency (EPA): agency of the federal government of the United States charged with protecting human health and the environment, by writing and enforcing regulations based on laws passed by Congress.
- Food and Drug Administration (FDA): agency of the U.S. Department of Health and Human Services responsible for promoting public health through the regulation of food safety, tobacco products, medications, blood transfusions, medical devices, and cosmetics.
- International Association of Healthcare Central Service Materiel Management (IAHCSMM): professional association that represents central sterile supply technicians and advances quality in central sterile supply.
- The Joint Commission: an independent, nonprofit national organization that develops standards for health care organizations and accredits over 17,000 health care organizations in the United States.
- Medical Reserve Corps (MRC): national network dedicated to improving the health and safety of communities across the country by organizing and utilizing public health, medical, and other volunteers.
- National Disaster Life Support Education Consortium (NDLSEC): organization dedicated to achieving and promoting excellence in education, training, and research related to disaster medicine and public health preparedness for all health professionals.
- National Fire Protection Association (NFPA): organization dedicated to establishing fire safety standards for all public sectors, including health care.
- National Institute of Occupational Safety and Health (NIOSH): U.S. federal agency responsible for conducting research and making recommendations for the prevention of work-related injury and illness; is within the U.S. Department of Health and Human Services.
- Occupational Safety and Health Administration (OSHA): agency of the U.S. Department of Labor; dedicated to preventing work-related injuries, illnesses, and occupational fatalities by issuing and enforcing standards for workplace safety and health.
- World Health Organization (WHO): a division of the United Nations that promotes health activities worldwide.

Case Study Ian is a surgical technologist at a busy metropolitan hospital. He has several years of experience and often serves as a **preceptor** (a surgical technologist employed by the hospital or surgery center that trains the students during their clinical rotation) for surgical technology students from the local community college.

A new student is observing Ian. On this day, he is assisting the registered nurse in a room dedicated to orthopedic surgery. They have just completed positioning the patient, and the registered nurse asks Ian if he will "prep" the patient's leg while she performs the final checks of the video monitors.

1. **What role is being performed by Ian? Are there any restrictions to the role?**
2. **Describe the various roles of the OR team members and state how they interrelate.**

Questions for Further Study

1. What is the difference between a job description and a role description?
2. How does health care financing affect the services that health care professionals provide?
3. List several reasons why a surgical technologist might need to communicate with the diagnostic imaging department, medical laboratory department, or a medical-surgical floor nurse.
4. Describe a "typical" workday for the surgical technologist.
5. Define the term *competency* as it relates to the role of the surgical technologist.
6. In addition to the traditional role of the surgical technologist in the surgical setting, list at least two other related employment options.

BIBLIOGRAPHY

Association of Surgical Technologists (2006). *Core curriculum for surgical assisting* (2nd ed.). Littleton, CO: Association of Surgical Technologists.

Association of Surgical Technologists (2011). *Core curriculum for surgical technology* (6th ed.). Littleton, CO: Association of Surgical Technologists.

Association of Surgical Technologists (2011). *Surgical technologist certifying exam study guide* (3rd ed.). Littleton, CO: Association of Surgical Technologists.

Bilchik, G. (1998, May 20). When the saints go marching out: Is American health care losing its religion? *Hospitals and Health Networks*, 37–42.

Cragg, G. R. (1990). *The church and the age of reason 1648–1789.* New York: Penguin Books.

Eiseley, L. (1961). *Darwin's century.* New York: Anchor Books.

Ginsberg, F. (1983, January/February). *Surgical technical aide—instructor's manual reference journal.*

Greene, J. (1998, April 20). Blue skies or black eyes? Hedis puts non-for-profit plans on top. *Hospitals and Health Networks*, 27–30.

Haugh, R. (1998, June 5). Who's afraid of capitation now? *Hospitals and Health Networks*, 30–37.

Mayr, E. (1985). *The growth of biological thought.* Cambridge, MA: Belknap.

McKeon, R. (Ed.). (2001). *Basic works of Aristotle.* New York: Modern Library.

Nuland, S. B. (1995). *Doctors: The biography of medicine.* New York: Vintage Books.

O'Leary, M. R. (1998). *Lexikon: Dictionary of health care terms, organizations and acronyms for the era of reform* (2nd ed.). Oakbrook Terrace, IL: Joint Commission on Accreditation of Healthcare Organizations.

Serb, C. (1998, July 20). Is remaking the hospital making money? *Hospitals and Health Networks*, 32–33.

Tuckman, B. W. (1965). Developmental sequence in small groups. *Psychological Bulletin, 63*(6), 384–399.

CHAPTER

2

Legal Concepts, Risk Management, and Ethical Issues

CASE STUDY Bret, a surgical technologist, has been asked by the surgeon to inject contrast medium into the cystic duct during an open cholecystectomy.

1. What scope of practice issues can you identify?
2. Is this act any different from injecting a medication into an IV line? If so, how?
3. What do you think Bret should do in this situation?
4. How do you think the surgeon may respond if Bret refuses?
5. How can Bret know if he should perform this act?

OBJECTIVES

After studying this chapter, the reader should be able to:

C 1. Analyze the concepts of law.
2. Interpret the legal responsibilities of the surgical technologist and other surgical team members.
3. Compare and contrast criminal and civil liabilities and the consequences for these acts.
4. Analyze the American Hospital Association's Patient Care Partnership.
5. Describe the need for professional liability insurance policies.

A 6. Analyze the key elements related to developing a surgical conscience.

R 7. Assess the resources that aid the surgical technologist in interpreting and following professional standards of conduct.
8. Develop an increased sensitivity to the influence of ethics in professional practice.
9. Analyze the role of morality during ethical decision making.
10. Cite examples of ethical situations and problems in the health professions.
11. Analyze scope of practice issues as they relate to surgical technology.

12. Interpret prevention, correction, and documentation techniques that may positively affect risk management issues.
13. Analyze the recommended practices and legal elements of proper documentation.
14. (E) Apply principles of problem solving in ethical decision making.
15. Assess errors that may occur in the operating room and devise a plan for investigation, correction, and notification.

Select Key Terms

abandonment	credentialing	malpractice	Safe Medical Device Act
accreditation	ethics	moral principles	scope of practice
advance directive	incident report	negligence	surgical conscience
Affidavit	informed consent	Patient Care Partnership	tort law
Code of Ethics	liability	risk management	

LEGAL ISSUES

In the health care environment, there is considerable agreement over basic values and their applications for patient care. The laws, standards, and guidelines developed for health care practice reflect these basic values. As one becomes more specific (e.g., a given law or a given case) disagreement may grow, but the general intent of health care legislation has been accepted for many years, and is reflected in the American Hospital Association (AHA)'s Patient Care Partnership, which is discussed later in the chapter. These rights reflect a generally accepted view of the patient as an autonomous individual who is in need of a service that he or she cannot provide for himself or herself.

This chapter explores legal aspects of health care and the ethical and moral behavior necessary for proper patient care. **Risk management** and scope of practice concepts are also explored. To understand some of the concepts related to legal aspects in medicine, the surgical technologist should be familiar with basic legal terminology and procedures.

Definitions of General Legal Terms

Accountability—Obligation to disclose details for evaluation; commonly used to mean "to be held responsible for"

Affidavit—Voluntary statement of facts sworn to be true before an authority

Allegation—Statement one expects to prove true

Bona fide—In good faith or innocently

Case law—All legal decisions reported on a given legal subject

Complaint—First pleading filed by plaintiff's attorney in a negligence action

Defendant—In criminal cases, the person accused of the crime; in civil matters, the person or organization being sued

Deposition—Method of pretrial discovery in which questions are answered under oath

Federal law—Jurisdiction is given to federal courts in cases involving the interpretation and application of the U.S. Constitution, acts of Congress, and treaties

Guardian—Court-appointed protector for an individual incapable of making his or her own decisions

Iatrogenic injury—Injury resulting from the activity of health care professionals

Indictment—Formal written accusation from a grand jury

Jury—Group of citizens who decide the outcome of a criminal or civil trial

Larceny—Taking another's property without consent

Law, common—Principles that have evolved and continue to evolve on the basis of court decisions

Law, statutory—Any law prescribed by the action of a legislature

Liability—Obligation to do or not do something

Liability, corporate—Obligation to do or not do something that is the responsibility of the corporate body

Liability, personal—Obligation by the individual to do or not do something

Malpractice—Professional misconduct that results in harm to another; negligence of a professional; the following definitions interrelate with malpractice:

Negligence—Omission (not doing) or commission (doing) of an act that a reasonable and prudent individual would not do under the same conditions; may be associated with the phrase "departure from the standard of care"

Negligence, criminal—Reckless disregard for the safety of another; willful indifference

Perjury—Intentionally providing false testimony under oath

Plaintiff—Person who initiates a lawsuit

Precedent—Legal principle, created by a court decision, that provides an example or authority for judges deciding similar issues later

Standard of care—Description of conduct that is expected of an individual or professional in a given circumstance

State law—State statutes, regulations, principles, and rules having the force of law

Subpoena—Court order to appear and testify or produce required documents

Tort—Civil wrong; may be intentional or unintentional

Trial—When parties to a dispute present evidence in a court of law in order to achieve a resolution or, in a criminal act, to determine a person's innocence or guilt

Definitions of Legal Doctrines and Traditional Principles

Aeger primo—"The Patient First" (motto of the AST)

Doctrine of corporate negligence—Health institution may be found negligent for failing to ensure that an acceptable level of patient care was provided. This means that potential employees and medical staff should be carefully screened and that competent staff should be maintained and monitored for proper performance.

Doctrine of borrowed servant—One who is controlling or directing the employee has greater responsibility than the one who is paying the employee. Courts frequently found that the surgeon was liable for any negligent act committed in his or her presence in the operating room under the *captain of the ship* doctrine. However, some rulings have found that the surgeon, under the *borrowed servant* rule, is not always responsible if a surgical technologist or registered nurse on the surgical team fails to carry out a routine procedure that he or she was properly educated to perform.

Doctrine of foreseeability—Foreseeability is the ability to see or know in advance; the ability to reasonably anticipate that harm or injury may result because of certain acts or omissions. The courts expect you to anticipate risks to patients. In other words, health care providers can be held liable for failure to recognize and/or failure to act on a critical event that was foreseeable.

Doctrine of personal liability—Each person is responsible for his or her own conduct, even though others may be liable as well. For example, an authority figure such as a physician assures the medical professional that he or she will take responsibility for an action; however, the health professional is still responsible.

Doctrine of the reasonably prudent person—Persons should perform an action as would any reasonable person of ordinary prudence. In law, the reasonable person is not a typical person but a collection of the community's judgment as to how the typical community member should behave in situations that might pose a threat of harm to the public. A standard of conduct is not established simply because the majority of people in the community behave in a certain way.

Primum non nocere—"Above all, do no harm."

Res ipsa loquitur—"The thing speaks for itself;" harm obviously came from a given act or thing of which the defendant had sole control.

Respondeat superior—"Let the master answer"; employer is responsible for the actions of his or her employees.

Torts

Tort law describes any civil wrong independent of a contract. Tort law provides a remedy in the form of an action for damages. Most actions against operating room personnel are civil actions rather than criminal and may be either intentional or unintentional.

INTENTIONAL TORTS

Intentional acts are willful and violate the civil rights of a patient. These types of torts include:

Assault—Act that causes another person to fear that he or she will be touched in an offensive, insulting, or physically injurious manner without consent or authority to do so.

Battery—Actual act of harmful or unwarranted contact with a person, including contact without proper consent.

Defamation—Slander (oral statement) or libel (written statement) that damages a person's reputation or good name.

False imprisonment—Illegal detention of a person without consent (e.g., use of restraints), or forcing a person to stay in an area by not allowing him or her to leave.

Intentional infliction of emotional distress—Disparaging remarks made about a patient that result in emotional distress.

Invasion of privacy—Disclosure of private information concerning a patient or photographing a patient without consent.

An intentional tort requires proof of the willful action of the following three elements:

1. The defendant's action was intended to interfere with the plaintiff or plaintiff's property.
2. The consequences of the act were also intended.
3. The act was a substantial factor in bringing about the consequences.

UNINTENTIONAL TORTS

Despite the surgical team's best efforts, individuals make mistakes. Unintentional torts are the most common types of patient care errors committed by operating room personnel and include negligence and malpractice. To establish negligence, a plaintiff must prove that the defendant had a duty to the plaintiff, the defendant breached that duty by failing to conform to the required standard of conduct, the defendant's negligent conduct was the cause of the harm to the plaintiff, and the plaintiff was, in fact, harmed or damaged.

If an individual engages in an activity requiring special skills, education, or experience, such as working in an operating room, the standard by which his or her conduct is measured is the conduct of a reasonably skilled, competent, and experienced person who is a qualified member of the group authorized to engage in that activity.

The following list identifies some of the errors and incidents that occur in the operating room:

- *Patient misidentification*—Check and cross-check procedures should be in place to prevent patient misidentification. All patients who enter the operating room should have an identification (ID) band firmly attached to their wrist. Transportation personnel should always check the ID band before the patient leaves the unit. The preoperative holding area nurse should check the ID band and compare it to the chart when the patient arrives (the patient should be asked to repeat his or her name to verify identification with the wristband). The circulator and anesthesia provider are the next to verify patient identity in the same manner before taking the patient to the operating room and the surgeon should do the same as he or she enters the room. Each cross-check ensures that the patient undergoing the surgical procedure is the correct patient.
- *Performing an incorrect procedure (often related to limbs)*—Surgical team must take great precautions to prevent the removal of the wrong body part or to prevent performing any surgical procedure on the wrong site or side. Identification of the correct limb and/or surgical site should be verbally confirmed by the patient. Information in the patient's chart should be checked by the circulator, anesthesia provider, surgical technologist, and surgeon to verify the correct area or side. Diagnostic tests (especially radiography, computed tomography [CT], or magnetic resonance imaging [MRI]) should be checked by the surgeon and surgical assistant and the proper area or side confirmed before the incision is made. Finally, a "time-out" period involving all members of the surgical team should take place immediately before starting the procedure, so that a final verification of the correct patient, procedure, and, when applicable, implant placement is completed. No procedure should start until any and all questions or concerns held by any member of the surgical team can be resolved (JCAHO, 2003). All surgical team members in the operating room must agree with the correct patient, correct site and side, and procedure.
- *Foreign bodies left in patients secondary to incorrect sponge, sharps, and instrument counts*—The circulator and surgical technologist must count all items that the hospital policy specifies for counting before the procedure begins, at the time that wound closure begins, and during skin closure.
- *Patient burns*—Burn wounds occur when there is contact between tissue and energy sources, such as heat, electrical current, radiation, or chemicals. Burns in the operating room can occur from the following situations:
  - Hot instruments from a steam autoclave (The surgical technologist is responsible for cooling the instrument with cool sterile water before use.)
  - Improper placement of the dispersive electrode for the electrosurgical unit (Placement is typically the responsibility of the circulator.)
  - Malfunctioning of the electrosurgical unit (The unit should be tested for proper functioning before the procedure begins.)
  - Other electrical device malfunctions (Electrical equipment must be properly grounded to reduce the risk of burns and should be tested frequently.)
  - Improper use of lasers (Special endotracheal tubes are required to prevent laryngeal injury. Wet towels are to be placed around an operative area to prevent burns from an improperly discharged laser beam.)
  - Pooled flammable prep solutions
  - Flammable anesthesia gases
  - Irrigation fluid that is too hot
- *Falls or positioning errors resulting in patient injury*—Unattended patients can fall from a stretcher that has its side rails down, and patients can also fall when being transferred to the operating table from the transportation stretcher if safe procedures for transfer are not followed. A safety strap should be applied as soon as the patient is moved to the operating table to prevent a fall. Nerve, skin, joint, and vascular injuries can occur due to incorrect positioning or padding after the patient is anesthetized. Adequate support is necessary and pressure points should be properly padded. The anesthetized patient cannot report to the team that a position is causing

pain, so constant vigilance and an understanding of proper positioning techniques and adequate support are imperative.

- *Improper handling, identification, or loss of specimens*—Negligence occurs if a specimen is lost, improperly prepared or "fixed" for analysis, or inaccurately labeled. Loss of a specimen would prevent diagnosis and may require another surgical procedure, as could improper specimen preparation for lab analysis.
- *Incorrect drugs or incorrect administration*—To reduce the risk of incorrect administration or use of an incorrect drug, the circulator and surgical technologist in the first scrub role must follow hospital policy for transfer of drugs to the sterile field (refer to "Transfer of a Medication to the Sterile Field" in Chapter 9). All medications and solutions on the sterile setup should be labeled. If the surgical technologist has more than one drug on the back table, the drugs should be separated and labeled. The members of the surgical team share equal responsibility for transfer of a drug to the sterile field.
- *Harm secondary to use of defective equipment/ instrument*—Malfunctioning equipment and instrumentation can cause injury to a surgical patient. The manufacturer's recommendations for service and operation should always be followed. Instrumentation and power equipment (e.g., saws, drills, reamers) are maintained by the surgical staff and sterile processing department staff. Electrical equipment must be tested and maintained on a regular schedule. Liability for malfunctioning equipment and instrumentation may lie with the institution if it can be proven that the equipment was not properly maintained and tested (refer to the later section in this chapter on the Safe Medical Device Act of 1990).
- *Loss of or damage to patient's property*—Surgical personnel can be held liable for the loss of a patient's personal property. A patient occasionally arrives at the surgical services department with personal property or prostheses, such as dentures, hearing aids, or glasses. Each item must be removed by the circulator or holding area nurse and placed in a protective container that is clearly marked as property of the patient. The container should be placed with the patient's chart and sent along with the chart and patient to the postanesthesia care unit after completion of the procedure. The holding area nurse may want to send the property back to the patient's room before the patient is anesthetized and should follow proper hospital procedures for return of the item to the unit.
- *Harm secondary to a major break in sterile technique*—Improper practice of sterile technique can lead to a postoperative infection that can cause debilitation and even death. The surgical technologist, through the application of a strong **surgical conscience**, should apply all principles of asepsis and must report any breaks that may occur to reduce the risk of postoperative infections.
- *Exceeding authority or accepted functions; violation of hospital policy*—The surgical technologist should be aware of state medical practice acts and laws and hospital policies. The surgeon should delegate tasks to be performed by the surgical technologist in the first scrub role that are not prohibited by hospital policy or state law.
- *Abandonment of a patient*—If a member of the surgical team leaves a patient who is dependent on his or her presence as a caregiver, then the caregiver can be held liable for **abandonment**. The danger that harm could befall a patient who is not closely monitored is great because patients are often under the effects of medication and dependent on the caregiver for their safety. A confused patient could fall from an operating table or transportation stretcher or could suffer a seizure or cardiac arrest.

Prevention is truly the best medicine, and a vigilant surgical conscience should prevent every one of the incidents listed here. It is the moral and legal responsibility of everyone on the surgical team to render the best and safest care possible to the patient.

Consent for Surgery: A Basic Right

The Joint Commission (TJC)'s definition of a *patient* is as follows: "A person who receives health services from a health care provider and who gives *consent* for the provider to provide those services." Inherent in the definition of *patient* is the concept of personal decision. The right to make personal decisions extends from the concept of autonomy, and autonomy is central to the understanding of the patient in the AHA's Patient Care Partnership. Autonomy is the state of having control over one's life.

Consent is a term that refers to permission being given for an action. Proper consent requires that the party granting permission has the capability and authority to do so. Consent presumes that at least two individuals are involved. One is the proposed recipient of an action; the other will perform the action. Under the circumstances with which we are concerned, the recipient is typically the patient. This may vary according to certain legal situations. In the case of a minor, for instance, the authorized party may be the parent. The individual performing the action is the health care provider. Consent, then, is a voluntary and informed act in which one party gives permission to another party to "touch." Given the nature of surgical intervention, surgical procedures are not performed without the written and **informed consent** of the patient except in a narrow range of legally defined situations. To perform surgery without consent can be the commission of battery.

Consent may be given in either of two formats: express and implied. *Express consent* is a direct verbal or written statement granting permission for treatment. *Implied consent* is consent in which circumstances exist that would lead a reasonable health care provider to believe that the person, or patient, had given consent although no direct or verbally expressed words of consent had been given. In health care, express consent in written form is the desired form of consent.

INFORMED CONSENT

The requirement to obtain written, informed consent for all invasive procedures is an example of an action taken by the health care industry to protect both the patient and the health care provider. TJC defines *informed consent* as "agreement or permission accompanied by full notice about what is being consented to." Expanding the definition to its use in tort law, TJC says that informed consent refers to "the requirement that a patient be apprised of the nature and risks of a medical procedure before the physician or other health professional can validly claim exemption from liability for battery or from responsibility for medical complications and other undesirable outcomes."

Written, informed consent protects the patient in that it guarantees that the patient is aware of his or her condition, the proposed intervention, the risks, and variables that may occur. Patients may be psychologically or educationally ill prepared to understand this information. Language and cultural differences may affect the understanding. Nevertheless, the best option exists when the health care providers follow the guidelines precisely. They can then verify an honest, good-faith effort to inform the patient, answer questions, and allow a free decision.

Two categories of consent are used in the hospital setting: general and special. On admission to the hospital, every patient signs a general consent for treatment (Figure 2-1). In this case, the patient consents to all routine services, general diagnostic procedures, medical treatment, and other normal and routine "touching" that may be expected to result from any hospitalization. The general consent is for treatment defined in its broadest form. General consent cannot be substituted for special consent. To do so is to sidestep the patient's right to make informed decisions. Special consent must be given for any procedure that entails a higher-than-normal risk—surgical procedures, fertility and sterilization procedures, anesthesia, transfusions, chemotherapy, and participation in experimental programs. Additionally, patients must give special consent when receiving an implant such as a heart valve, plate and screws for fracture repair, or coronary artery stent.

The final responsibility for securing written, informed surgical consent belongs to the surgeon. The surgeon will discuss the condition, proposed treatment, risks, and alternatives with the patient and possibly family. Once agreement is reached, this communication is relayed to the hospital staff and the proper documents are prepared. The documents are then signed by the patient, witnessed by the hospital staff, and made part of the patient's record.

The physician's responsibility for securing an informed consent requires that the following conditions be met:

- Information must be given in understandable language.
- There can be no coercion or intimidation of the patient.
- The proposed surgical procedure or treatment must be explained.
- Potential complications must be explained.
- Potential risks and benefits must be explained.
- Alternative therapies and their risks and benefits must be explained.

Because surgical patients vary in age, condition, psychological makeup, language usage, and cultural background, the amount and type of information supplied may vary from patient to patient.

A critical feature of informed consent is the language used. Even highly educated patients may have little experience with medical terminology. *Cholecystitis* may be meaningless to the patient, whereas *inflamed gallbladder* is understood clearly. All health care providers should accustom themselves to responding to patients with clear and understandable language.

More subtle, but equally important, is the tone of the presentation. Patients should not be made to feel as if they have no choice. This may become a critical factor if the patient is elderly, for instance, or if there is some disagreement within the family about a prospective treatment plan. The physician must carefully present the plan he or she thinks best but must not present it in such a way as to make the patient feel as if there are no other options.

The specific provisions for written consent are dictated by medical practice acts and state law, which vary slightly from state to state, but in general a properly written informed consent should contain the following information:

- Patient's legal name
- Surgeon's name
- Procedure to be performed, including side if applicable
- Risks of anesthesia and procedure, including complications
- Patient's legal signature
- Signature of witness(es)
- Date and time of signatures

The patient must meet the following conditions:

- Of legal age or a legally emancipated minor
- Mentally alert
- Legally competent
- Not under the influence of alcohol or drugs

The surgical consent must be signed prior to entry into surgery or the treatment area. Special circumstances such as illiteracy, sensory impairment, language barrier, and emergency considerations will be cause to vary from the normal consent procedure. For example, illiterate individuals may sign the form with an "X," with another authorized individual signing the consent form as witness that the patient did mark the consent form. When a patient speaks a foreign language an interpreter must be present. In some instances, the patient may be physically unable or legally incompetent to give

SAMPLE

Standard Consent to Surgery or Special Procedure

Patient Name ______________________________

Attending Physician ______________________________

Surgeon or Supervising Physician ______________________________

1. (*Name of facility*) maintains personnel and facilities to assist your/the patient's physicians and surgeons in their performance of various surgical or other special diagnostic or therapeutic procedures. These operations and procedures may involve risks of unsuccessful results, complications, injury, or death, from known and/or unforeseen causes, and no warranty or guarantee is made as to results or cure.

   You have the right to be informed of such risks as well as the nature of the operation or procedure; the expected benefits of such; and any available alternatives and their risks and benefits. Except in case of emergency, operations or procedures are not performed until you have had the opportunity to receive this information and have given your consent. You have the right to consent or refuse any proposed operation or procedure any time prior to its performance.
2. Your/the patient's physician/surgeon has recommended the operation or procedure set forth below. Upon your authorization and consent, the operation or procedure set forth below, together with any different or further procedures which in the opinion of the supervising physician/surgeon may be indicated due to an emergency, will be performed on you/the patient. The operation or procedure will be performed by the supervising physician or surgeon named above (or in the event of an emergency causing his/her inability to complete the procedure, a qualified substitute supervising physician or surgeon), together with associates and assistants, including anesthesiologists, pathologists and radiologists from the medical staff of (*name of facility*) to whom the supervising physician or surgeon may assign designated responsibilities. The persons in attendance for the purpose of performing specialized medical services such as anesthesia, radiology, or pathology are not agents, servants, or employees of the facility and your/the patient's supervising physician or surgeon, but are independent contractors, and therefore your agents, servants, or employees.
3. The pathologist is hereby authorized to use his/her discretion in disposing any member, organ, or other tissue removed from your/the patient's person during the operation or procedure set forth below.
4. Your signature below constitutes your acknowledgment that: you have read and agree to the foregoing; that the operation or procedure set forth belowhas been adequately explained to you by the above-named physician/surgeon and by your/the patient's anesthesiologist and that you have received all of the information that you desire concerning such operation or procedure; and that you authorize and consent to the performance of the operation or procedure.

Procedure: ______________________________

____

____

Signature (Patient/Parent/Conservator/Guardian) Relationship (if other than patient)

____

Date Time Witness

I have been informed of the risks/benefits and alternatives of blood product infusions. I consent to the use of blood product infusions.

____

Signature (Patient/Parent/Conservator/Guardian) Relationship (if other than patient)

____

Date Time Witness

(Name of Facility
Address of Facility)

(Patient Identification–Stamp)

Figure 2-1 Sample of a standard consent to surgery or special procedures form

permission. In this situation, under nonemergency conditions, another authorized individual must provide the consent. The same guidelines for an informed consent apply to this authorized person.

Informed consent may be given by any of the following:

- A competent adult speaking for himself or herself
- Parent or legal guardian of a minor
- Guardian in the case of physical inability or legal incompetence
- Temporary guardian
- Hospital administrator
- The courts

When normal procedure cannot be followed, state law will determine who may be the witness or consenting party. Emergency circumstances may alter the consent process. State law dictates the methods for securing consent under these conditions, some of which include:

- Telephone
- Electronic
- Agreement of two consulting physicians (not to include the operating surgeon)
- Administrative consent

In each case, state law and facility policy will dictate how many people are needed for securing the consent, who may be a witness, and how the consent will be documented.

Implied consent is never the preferred option in a health care environment, but the law allows for implied consent in emergency situations when no other authorized person may be contacted. Implied consent may apply when conditions are discovered during a surgical procedure. For example, if the procedure performed extends beyond what is in the informed consent, the surgeon may be liable for assault and battery unless it can be proved that good judgment was used when unexpected conditions were encountered. This is covered by the extension doctrine, which implies that the patient has given implicit consent for correction or treatment of pathologic conditions that were not expected or anticipated by the surgeon.

Patients have the right to change their mind and withdraw consent. Withdrawal of consent or any refusal of consent for a procedure should be noted in the patient's medical record. If possible, a form releasing the hospital and the health care team from responsibility for the decision should be signed and placed in the patient's medical record.

Documentation

In the health care field, the term *documentation* is used broadly to refer to the placing of information into a patient's medical record (chart). The medical record is the combined account of the interaction between the patient and the health care providers during a given incidence of illness or treatment. The medical record will typically include:

- Identification of the patient
- Identification of the physician(s), nurse(s), and other health care providers involved in the patient's care (e.g., the operating room record will name each member of the surgical team)
- Patient's medical history and physical examination
- Diagnosis
- Treatment plan, details, and results
- Medication record
- Physical findings during the hospital stay
- Discharge condition
- Possible follow-up treatment plan

Anything of clinical significance should be recorded in the chart so that anyone who is involved with patient care can provide for continuity. Events should only be recorded after the fact. For legal purposes, the chart can be used to discover the source of a negligent act.

In the case of the surgical patient, special documentation is required that is focused on the surgical intervention and recovery usually referred to as the intraoperative record. Prior to surgery, every patient must have a history and physical record in his or her medical record and an informed consent for the surgery. All of the patient's personal physical data, the surgical procedure, anesthetic procedure, and postanesthesia care are placed in the patient's medical record. There are different styles of operative patient records, but the record always includes information about the surgical team; patient's condition before, during, and after surgery; patient position; patient skin prep; insertion of urinary catheter (if performed); time out before the surgical skin incision; time of initiation and termination of the procedure; documentation of counts; and information concerning drains and dressings. Some facilities may use separate count sheets for monitoring sponges, sharps, and instruments. If so, these sheets may become part of the record. Since most procedures produce a tissue specimen of some sort and require pathological study, pathology and laboratory forms will be used for interdepartmental communication and will become part of the medical record. The anesthesia team will maintain an anesthesia record.

Other records are part of the patient's medical record and may require reporting to government agencies. The hospital provides a legal record of all births and deaths that take place there. Patient charges are made part of the record, and patients and insurance providers receive detailed reports of charges. Department order forms are used to secure items for patient care and to verify the accuracy of the charges.

Even though this is not a part of the medical record, the surgeon's preference cards contribute to what is included in the medical record. A preference card is maintained in a central file or in a computer in the operating room; it is a list of the supplies and equipment a surgeon requires for the various procedures he or she performs as well as variances to the procedure that are unique to the surgeon's preference.

As mentioned earlier, proper medical record keeping protects the patient and the hospital and its employees. Proper documentation and record keeping are used for legal, accounting, and quality assurance purposes. For legal purposes, several rules for proper documentation exist. All reports, notations, and summaries are to be written using standard terminology and approved abbreviations (see Box 2-1). Spelling is to be correct and hand writing legible. Information presented in medical documents should be factual in nature and not subjective.

Box 2-1 THE JOINT COMMISSION "DO NOT USE" ABBREVIATION LIST

In 2004, The Joint Commission created the "do not use" list:

Do Not Use	Use Instead
U (unit)	Write "unit"
IU (international unit)	Write "international unit"
Q.D., QD, q.d., qd (daily)	Write "daily"
Q.O.D., QOD, q.o.d., qod (every other day)	Write "every other day"
Trailing zero (X.0 mg)	Write X mg
Lack of a leading zero (.X mg)	Write 0.X mg
MS	Write "morphine sulfate"
MSO_4 and $MgSO_4$	Write "magnesium sulfate"

Abbreviations for **possible** future inclusion on "Do Not Use" List

Do Not Use	Use Instead
> (greater than)	Write "greater than"
< (less than)	Write "less than"
Abbreviations for drug names	Write drug names in full
Apothecary units	Use metric units
@	Write "at"
cc	Write "mL", "ml" or "milliliters"
µg	Write "mcg" or "micrograms"

Errors, obviously, can occur in documentation. These can be corrected following a proper legal procedure. Errors are to be marked through with a single line, never erased. The correct information is placed immediately above the error. The correction is verified with the initials of the reporter. The individual who made the initial error must make the correction. All reports, notations, and summaries include the legal signature of the reporter.

Sentinel Event/Incident Reports

Most hospitals have a mechanism for reporting incidents related to any adverse patient occurrence. **Incident reports** or sentinel events reports constitute much of the information used by the hospital in risk management. Risk management is the effort by the hospital to collect and use data to decrease the chance of harm to patients and staff or damage to property.

Falls, medication errors, intraoperative burns, and loss of specimens are examples of events that would require reporting. If the behavior of any member of the surgical team is such that a lawsuit could result (e.g., sexual harassment, aggressive behavior toward other team members), then a report would be required before the offender is confronted.

These reports are forwarded to the risk management department, where representatives from various departments attempt to identify the factors that caused the incident and what can be done to prevent it from happening again.

Advance Directives

In health care, an **advance directive** is a written instruction dealing with the right of an incapacitated patient to self-determination. This directive carries the weight of state law and expresses a patient's wishes about the kinds and amount of medical treatment provided in the event that the patient can no longer make those types of decisions. Two examples of advanced directives are a living will and a durable power of attorney.

AHA Patient Care Partnership

In 1972 the AHA adopted the 12 rights known as the Patient's Bill of Rights that emphasized collaboration between patients, physicians, and hospitals is essential to optimal patient care. However, the AHA has now replaced the Patient's Bill of Rights with the **Patient Care Partnership**, which contains plainer language that informs the patient about what he or she should expect during a hospital stay with regard to his or her rights and responsibilities. The AHA is also emphasizing through this revision that the patient needs to be involved in his or her health care and ask questions of health care providers at any time, because unasked or unanswered questions can add to the stress of a stay in the hospital. The following is a list of the partnership's six expectations, rights, and responsibilities (AHA, 2003):

- High-quality hospital care
- A clean and safe environment
- Involvement in the patient's care
- Protection of patient privacy
- Help when leaving the hospital by preparing the patient and family
- Help with bill and insurance claims

The Patient Care Partnership is reinforced in *The Patient Self-Determination Act of 1990.* This act says that each patient has a right under state law to make decisions concerning his or her care, including the right to refuse treatment.

RISK MANAGEMENT AND LIABILITY

Risk management is an integrated system developed by hospitals for the prevention and control of areas of potential liability. Identification and reporting of unsafe conditions and hazards is the most critical aspect of every risk management process, because all subsequent phases of risk management depend on it. After the risk is identified, it should be assessed for severity and frequency.

Risk management objectives for a hospital are to:

- Minimize risks to patients, visitors, and hospital employees.
- Avoid or control financial loss to the hospital.
- Identify actual or potential causes of patient and employee accidents through risk detection, evaluation, and prevention.
- Implement programs, policies, and procedures to eliminate or reduce occurrences.
- Collect and use data to decrease harm to patients and staff or damage to property.

Two issues that have an impact on the hospital's risk management policies and plans are reduced staffing and employee rights. Many health care professions, including physicians, are experiencing dramatic shortages that place added stresses on the health care system, delivery of quality health care to an expanding population that is also getting older, and health care personnel. Health care providers are being asked to do more with fewer resources as well as keep costs down for the patient and deal with increased patient loads due to workforce shortages, which can lead to patient safety issues. However, health care employees have rights that the employer must recognize and support as well as rights related to risk management and safety issues, such as number of hours a health care provider should work, for example, covering two work shifts (e.g., 7:00 A.M.–3:00 P.M. and 3:00–11:00 P.M.).

Medical Errors

In-patient error reduction in medicine began to gain attention in the second half of the 1990s with the release of the Institute of Medicine's (IOM's) *To Err Is Human: Building a Better Health System.* The IOM claimed that more people die each year from medical errors than from car accidents, AIDS, and breast cancer combined (making medical errors the country's eighth leading cause of death).

Technology has become the best weapon for the reduction of medical errors. Some of these technologies include bar-coded medications and identification strips, handheld wireless devices, and computer drug-order-entry systems. A study at two Veterans Administration (VA) hospitals in Kansas found that these devices reduced medication error rates by 70% over a 5-year period.

In the operating room, the surgical technologist can help prevent medical errors by closely following written policies and procedures and by following standard precautions related to the use of personal protective equipment. The surgical technologist should be aware of the location and proper use of all emergency equipment. Prevention practices include routine preventive maintenance for all surgical equipment (faulty or malfunctioning equipment or devices should be removed from service) and professional development/continuing education programs for employees. Most employers require employees to complete an annual in-service in which updates on safety practices and patient care are provided as well as review updates in policies and procedures as part of the hospital's risk management program.

An emphasis has also been placed on the reduction of medical errors by many organizations such as AST, The Joint Commission, and the Council on Surgical and Perioperative Safety (CSPS), a joint effort of ACS, AST, ASA, AANA, ASPAN, and AORN. These organizations have published many statements concerning the use of abbreviations in the health care setting, time out in the OR, retained foreign objects, labeling of all medications and medication containers, and use of the neutral zone (See table 2-1 and Box 2-2). One example includes the 2006 *National Patient Safety Goals* published by The Joint Commission. One provision of the goals is the requirements as related to the labeling of medications. The Joint Commission has stated that all medications and medication containers should be labeled, including syringes, medicine cups and basins, and solutions that are on and off the sterile field in the perioperative setting. AST has backed The Joint Commission requirements by establishing the *AST Guideline for Safe Medication Practices in the Perioperative Area.*

Another statement that AST has established that is important to the practice of surgical technology is the AST Guideline Statement for the Implementation of the Neutral Zone in the Perioperative Environment (Box 2-2).

TABLE 2-1 **Strategies for Exposure Prevention (from Lancaster General Hospital, 2004)**

Strategy	*Implementation*
1. The neutral zone is dedicated for sharps only. All other instruments are passed hand-to-hand. Only one sharp in the neutral zone at a time.	Identify the neutral zone in consultation between the first scrub surgical technologist and the surgeon.
2. Do not hold the neutral zone device.	Place the neutral zone device in the designated, area keeping the fingers out of the way.
3. Orient the sharp in the neutral zone to facilitate the surgeon being able to pick it up with her or his dominant hand without having to turn or reposition body.	Alert the surgeon that the sharp item has been placed in the neutral zone and is ready to be picked up.
4. Avoid need to reposition the needle holder in the surgeon's right or left hand.	Ensure that suture needles are correctly positioned and clamped.
5. Move neutral zone as needed to accommodate the surgeon.	Open and positive verbal communication is maintained between the first scrub surgical technologist and surgeon.
6. Avoid contact with the suture needle when surgeon has finished using it.	Keep sharp end of suture needles grasped between the needle holder when finished with use.
7. Use no-touch technique when placing drains.	Use a grasping instrument to position drains.
8. When finished using a sharp the surgeon continues to use the neutral zone.	Surgeon returns the sharp to the neutral zone and avoids passing it back directly to the first scrub surgical technologist.

BOX 2-2 **AST GUIDELINE STATEMENT FOR THE IMPLEMENTATION OF THE NEUTRAL ZONE IN THE PERIOPERATIVE ENVIRONMENT**

Introduction

The perioperative environment poses several challenges for reducing the risks of sharps-exposure injuries. According to Davis (2001), one-fourth of suture needle injuries and more than half of scalpel injuries occur during passing between surgical team members. The perioperative environment is a high-risk environment and surgical team members routinely face the risk of contamination of blood-borne pathogens from sharps and percutaneous injuries. The establishment of the neutral zone is an evidenced-based practice implemented to reduce sharps and percutaneous injuries in the perioperative environment. The neutral zone, also referred to as the "no pass" or "no touch" technique, is used for the placement of sharps during the surgical procedure to prevent person-to-person transfer of sharps.

AST Guideline Statement

A neutral zone should be established for the placement of sharps during a surgical procedure to ensure that no person-to-person passing of sharps occurs. The creation of a neutral zone will assist in the reduction of percutaneous injuries and blood exposures commonly caused by the hand-to-hand transfer of sharps during surgical procedures. The establishment of a neutral zone is only effective when a team approach is used and positive communication occurs among the perioperative team members (Price, 2004).

Exceptions to the Use of the Neutral Zone

There are situations in which use of the neutral zone is negated and hand-to-hand transfer of

continues

Box 2-2 (continued)

sharps remains an appropriate action. Examples include:

1. Surgeon's discretion when he or she cannot avert his or her eyes from the surgical field to the neutral zone.
2. Surgeon cannot reach the neutral zone due to patient positioning.
3. Microscope or loops are being used by the surgeon.

Examples of Neutral Zone Devices

Any device used as the neutral zone should be large enough to adequately contain the sharps used, should not be easily tipped over, and preferably should be mobile. Examples include the following:

- Instrument/magnetic mat
- Emesis basin or transfer basin
- Designated area for neutral zone on designated portion of the sterile field, Mayo stand, or back table

Additional Sharps Safety Techniques

- Never recap hypodermic needles. When recapping is unavoidable, a one-handed technique or safety device should be used.
- Sharps on the Mayo stand or back table should be placed in a central location.
- Utilize a small sharps container to store needles and to promote a safe and accurate count of sharps such as needles and knife blades.
- Load needles just prior to use to avoid open needles on the Mayo stand or back table.
- Avoid using hands or fingers to retract or for any skills for which an instrument could be used.
- Provide verbal notification when passing a sharp.
- When possible, keep hands away from the surgical field when sharps are in use.
- When pulling a drain trocar through an exit wound, replace the guard onto the sharp tip using a grasping instrument rather than fingers.

The Safe Medical Device Act

The **Safe Medical Device Act** became effective November 28, 1990. The act expanded the U.S. Food and Drug Administration's (FDA) authority to regulate medical devices. The reason for the act was concerns by the U.S. Congress about the FDA's ability to quickly learn and act on information when a medical device caused an adverse patient event and ensure that hazardous devices are removed from hospitals and other health care facilities in a timely manner.

A medical device includes, but is not limited to, electronic equipment such as ventilators and monitors, implants, syringes, needles, catheters, and disposables. A key provision of the act is called device tracking. Hospitals are required to participate in tracking medical devices whose failure could result in a serious adverse patient outcome. The law also requires hospitals and distributors and manufacturers of devices to cooperate in implementing methods of device tracking. For example, hospitals are required to provide device manufacturers with information about patients with permanently implanted devices and life-sustaining and life-supporting devices. The act requires that medical device users report to the manufacturer and the FDA incidents that reasonably suggest the probability that a medical device has caused or contributed to the death, serious injury, illness, or other adverse experience of a patient.

Managing Patient and Employee Injuries

As previously mentioned, sentinel events include patient and employee injuries. Managing injuries involves two key components: injury is immediately reported and the individual is rendered medical treatment if necessary. Obviously, the longer the delay in reporting an injury, the longer treatment is delayed; recall of the incident decreases as well. Documentation of the details of the incident contributes to the ability of the employer to analyze the situation and implement controls in order to avoid a repeat of the situation. Additionally, the report serves as legal documentation in instances of patient injury or if the employee files for worker's compensation.

Malpractice Insurance

Hospital employees who commit negligent acts are typically covered by insurance polices provided by the facility, as long as the negligent act was committed within the scope of the institution's policies and procedures. If the surgical technologist is sued as an individual, however, personal malpractice insurance (professional liability) will be required to cover any discrepancy between the hospital's and the individual's policies. All practicing surgical technologists and surgical assistants should carry professional liability insurance because the odds that they will be sued for malpractice are greater than in the past.

When a negligence suit is filed, all those who may have had a part in the injury or death will be named in the suit. If there is a settlement against a specific health care provider and there is no malpractice insurance to cover the settlement, the judge may attach a lien on property owned by the defendant, or the money may be obtained from future earnings.

Health Insurance Portability and Accountability Act (HIPAA)

The Health Insurance Portability and Accountability Act (HIPAA) is the first federal act to establish privacy standards to protect patients' medical records and other health-related information. It took effect on April 14, 2003. The standards were developed by the Department of Health and Human Services (HHS). The standards provide the ability for patients to easily access their medical records and have more control over how their personal health information is disclosed. HIPAA standards represent a major step forward in providing additional privacy protections and control to the health consumers across the United States.

The privacy regulations ensure a national floor of privacy protections for patients by limiting the ways that health plans, pharmacies, hospitals, and other covered entities can use patients' personal medical information. The regulations protect medical records and other individually identifiable health information, whether it is on paper, in computers, or communicated orally. The privacy rule requires health plans, pharmacies, physicians, and other covered entities to establish policies and procedures to protect the confidentiality of protected health information about patients. The main objectives of HIPAA include:

1. Ensure health insurance portability even in the face of preexisting medical conditions.
2. Guarantee the privacy of health information of all patients.
3. Decrease the incidences of fraud and abuse in the health care community.

Key provisions of the standards include:

1. *Access to medical records:* Patients should be able to see and obtain copies of their medical records and request corrections if they identify errors and mistakes.
2. *Notice of privacy practices:* Covered health plans, physicians, and other health care providers must provide a notice to their patients of how they may use personal medical information and their rights under the new privacy regulation.
3. *Limits on use of personal medical information:* The privacy rule sets limits on how health plans and covered providers may use individually identifiable health information.
4. *Prohibition on marketing:* The privacy rule sets new regulations and limits on the use of patient information for marketing purposes.
5. *Confidential communications:* Under the privacy rule, patients can request that their physicians, health plans, and other covered entities take steps to ensure their communications with the patient are confidential.
6. *Complaints:* Consumers may file a formal complaint regarding the privacy practices of a covered health plan or provider.

Overall, the aim of HIPAA is to provide improved patient service, protect the privacy of patients, and reduce fraud and abuse. Even though implementing the rules results in expenditures and training of health care personnel, the importance of *Aeger primo*—"The Patient First"—remains first and foremost when complying with HIPAA standards.

ETHICAL AND MORAL ISSUES

Surgical technologists are constantly challenged by important decisions that require an understanding of the concepts of right or wrong for matters involving the operative patient. Knowing that each decision we make may have a huge impact on our patients, safety and well-being should give us pause with our decision making. In philosophy, **ethics** defines what is good for the individual and for society and establishes the nature of duties that people owe themselves and one another. Ethics is the *system* of moral principles and rules that become standards for professional conduct, and should not be confused with morality. Morality dictates *codes of conduct*, which are put forward by a society and used as a guide to behavior by the members of that society.

Moral Principles

Basic **moral principles** are the guides for ethical decision making, the principles that we try to instill in our children (such as benevolence, trustworthiness, and honesty). These principles include the concern that we have for the well-being of others and respect for their autonomy. The principles also include those that deal with basic justice and the prevention of harm, as well as the refusal to take unfair advantage.

Individuals acting in a professional capacity take on an additional burden of ethical responsibility. The codes of ethics of professional associations (described in detail later in this chapter) provide rules of conduct and standards of behavior that include principles such as impartiality, objectivity, duty of care, confidentiality, and full disclosure. Surgical technologists should be trustworthy and honest. These are the basic tenets of a sound surgical conscience found at the professional level of ethical behavior.

Elements of Ethical Decision Making

Ethics has deep roots in our legal system; in fact, legal doctrines are often used to interpret ethical concepts. However, ethics can be difficult to define. In simplest terms, it has been identified as the moral obligations that one person owes another

(Garner, 1999). TJC defines *ethics* as "the branch of philosophy that deals with systematic approaches to moral issues, such as the distinction between right and wrong and the moral consequences of human actions. Ethics involves a system of behaviors, expectations, and morals composing *standards of conduct* for a population or a profession."

At its beginning, the principles of problem solving in ethical decision making begin with five basic questions:

1. What makes a "right act" right?
2. To whom is moral duty owed?
3. What "kinds" of acts are right?
4. What is the relationship between specific situations and ethical principles or guidelines?
5. What action is to be taken in the situation at hand?

Ethics begins with a decision about *right* and *wrong* leading the individual to consider several factors in making an ethical decision, including:

- Personal values
- Accountability for one's actions
- Responsibility for one's actions
- Religious beliefs
- Cultural beliefs
- Corporate integrity
- Method(s) of problem solving

How, then, can one summarize what a health care professional should do in the complicated world of medical ethics? The following practical guidelines will help when faced with ethical dilemmas: Spend some time thinking about the five major questions listed previously so that you can identify your own value system. Pay attention to illustrative arguments in society and read broadly about them, and mentally play out scenarios in which various decisions are made. Ask what the outcomes might be for the patient, family, physician, surgical technologist, nurse, and so forth.

Be aware that other well-intentioned individuals will have different viewpoints. The surgical technologist will be exposed to many issues that may create personal or vocational discomfort. These are just some of the issues that arise today:

- Animal experimentation
- Assisted suicide
- Care of individuals with human immunodeficiency virus (HIV) infection and acquired immunodeficiency syndrome (AIDS) or other communicable diseases
- Elective abortion
- Elective sterilization
- Gender reassignment
- Genetic engineering
- Good Samaritan law
- Human experimentation
- Newborn with a severe disability
- Organ donation/transplantation
- Quality versus quantity of life
- Refusal of treatment (especially for a child)
- Reproductive procedures
  - In vitro fertilization
  - Artificial insemination
- Stem cell research
- Substance abuse
  - Self
  - Knowledge of impaired health care provider
- Termination of care and right to die
- Workplace violence

A wealth of information is available on these subjects. The health care professional should be well informed about these topics and others that may require ethical decision making.

Professional Codes of Conduct

Most professions have adopted highly detailed codes of conduct along with methods for enforcement of breaches of those codes. In some cases, these codes are spoken of as *professional ethics* or, in the case of law, *legal ethics*. The American Medical Association has the Principles of Medical Ethics. Nurses often refer to the International Code of Nursing Ethics, a code established by their own professional association.

Many professional codes have been incorporated into law, and all codes can have some effect on judgments about professional conduct for litigation. Failure to comply with a code of professional conduct often results in expulsion from the profession.

In 1985 the AST established a **Code of Ethics** that provides guidelines for the surgical technologist (Table 2-2).

SCOPE OF PRACTICE

Scope of practice is a legal term that identifies the knowledge and skills required for the profession in order to provide effective and reliable services. Scope of practice refers to our core accountabilities. For the health care provider, this refers to those services for which the provider is accountable, based on education, experience, national credentialing, and state licensure. For those in health care support roles, these accountabilities may be based on formal education or job-related training.

Professional scopes of practice and standards of conduct derive from a number of different sources, including:

- Federal law
- Federal agencies
- State law and regulations

Table 2-2 AST Code of Ethics for Surgical Technologists

1. To maintain the highest standards of professional conduct and patient care
2. To hold in confidence, with respect to the patient's beliefs, all personal matters
3. To respect and protect the patient's legal and moral rights to quality patient care
4. To not knowingly cause injury or any injustice to those entrusted to our care
5. To work with fellow technologists and other professional health groups to promote harmony and unity for better patient care
6. To always follow the principles of asepsis
7. To maintain a high degree of efficiency through continuing education
8. To maintain and practice surgical technology willingly, with pride and dignity
9. To report any unethical conduct or practice to the proper authority
10. To adhere to the Code of Ethics at all times with all members of the health care team

- Legal precedent
- Hospital policy
- Professional organizations

The surgical technologist functions in an environment in which each of the listed entities affects the understood standard of care. AST has both Recommended Standards of Practice and a Code of Ethics, which are statements of basic principles. In general, codified scopes of practice are broad and define many of the tasks the professional may perform, but they also allow the professional to use some personal and professional judgment and allow for delegation to other professions.

The surgical technologist in the first scrub role performs surgical tasks intraoperatively under the supervision and broad delegatory authority of the surgeon, for which specific provisions vary from state to state. The basis for this is usually found in state medical practice acts or as rendered through the state attorneys' general offices. The underlying principle is that the physicians/surgeons may delegate tasks to nonphysicians when the tasks are performed under the direct supervision and in the physical presence of the physician and the physician and/or employer has made a reasonable determination that the person to whom those tasks are to be delegated has the appropriate skills and knowledge to safely perform those tasks. This principle supports the discretion of the surgeon and the facility in determining the first scrub and surgical assistant roles, what tasks will be performed, and to what extent, throughout the conduct of the surgeon's case. The surgeon has the ability to observe the surgical technologist's competency and performance and to ensure that the surgical technologist is performing tasks and procedures in the manner preferred for proper intraoperative patient care.

1. Finally, the best assurance of safe and professional behavior is a well-developed surgical conscience. The surgical technologist using surgical conscience (along with a thorough knowledge of state law and hospital policy) may ask the following questions: Is the skill not allowed to be performed by the surgical technologist by hospital policy or state law?
2. Does performing the skill meet the "reasonable and prudent" standard? Is performing the skill within an acceptable standard of care provided by a reasonable and prudent person who has similar education, training, and experience?
3. Are there professional association standards of practice, guideline statements, or position statements that support the performance of the skill with additional education and experience?
4. Are you prepared to accept responsibility and accountability for performing the skill competently and safely?

In the absence of specific statutory or regulatory prohibition, it is within the scope of practice for surgical technologists to perform generally accepted intraoperative activities for which they have been prepared through basic education, appropriate continuing education, and experience *and* for which they have demonstrated competence to perform safely and effectively.

Credentialing

One of the ways in which the public is protected from unqualified health care professionals is through the process of **credentialing**. Credentialing does not verify competency because competency is an ongoing evaluation. Credentialing does establish a minimum knowledge base for a given health care profession. Many types of credentials are used in the health care community. Some types of credentialing that apply to an individual are (in order of least to most restrictive):

- *Registration:* Formal process by which qualified individuals are listed in a registry
- *Certification:* Recognition by an appropriate body that an individual has met a predetermined standard
- *Licensure:* Legal right granted by a government agency in compliance with a statute that authorizes and oversees the activities of a profession

Upon graduation from an accredited surgical technology program, surgical technologists may sit for the national certification examination administered by the National Board of

Surgical Technology and Surgical Assisting (NBSTSA). Although *certification* is a term that is sometimes used to refer to facilities and educational programs, surgical technology programs that are verified by CAAHEP and ABHES as meeting minimum educational standards are said to be *accredited*.

Accreditation and Core Curriculum

As discussed in detail in Chapter 1, most surgical technology programs are accredited through CAAHEP or ABHES. **Accreditation** contributes to the protection of the public by assessing educational programs for their quality and effectiveness in educating and training students. Accreditation is an important indicator for employers who are evaluating the credentials of a potential employee.

The accreditation standards for surgical technology require that programs base their program curriculum on the *Core Curriculum for Surgical Technology*. The core curriculum attempts to set a standard in curriculum quality and standardize the education of the surgical technology student.

Case Study A 5-year-old child presents to the hospital emergency department after a motor vehicle accident. She is hypotensive and in shock. The physician suspects that her spleen is ruptured. He recommends to the parents that she undergo an emergency exploratory laparotomy for possible splenorrhaphy or splenectomy, and he writes orders to type and cross-match blood for possible replacement. The parents refuse all treatment on religious grounds.

1. What legal and ethical issues can you identify?
2. Could the parents be charged if the child were to die?
3. How could the physician resolve this situation?

Questions for Further Study

1. Under what principle are most health care providers usually sued? Identify the two terms most often associated with this principle.
2. Explain the fundamental change the Patient Care Partnership introduced as related to the patient.
3. A surgical technologist believes that genetic engineering is wrong and bad for society. What belief does the surgical technologist hold: formalism or utilitarianism? Explain why.
4. Classroom Discussion: Is it within the scope of practice of the surgical technologist to administer medications to the surgical patient under the supervision of the surgeon? Use the four questions stated on p. 41 as a guide. Items to consider include irrigating a cavity with antibiotic solution, applying hemostatic chemical agents to tissue, and parenteral injection.

BIBLIOGRAPHY

Adler, M. J. (1997). *Ten philosophical mistakes*. New York: Touchstone.

American Hospital Association. (2003). The Patient Care Partnership. Retrieved October 20, 2006, from http://www.aha.org/aha/content/2003/pdf/pcp_english_030730.pdf

Aquinas, T. (1987). *On politics and ethics* (P. E. Sigmund, Ed.). New York: Norton.

Aristotle. (1974). In R. McKeun (Ed.), *Introduction to Aristotle* (2nd ed.). Chicago: University of Chicago Press.

Association of Surgical Technologists. AST Code of Ethics. Available at http://www.ast.org

Association of Surgical Technologists. (2011). *Core curriculum for surgical technology* (6th ed.). Littleton, CO: Association of Surgical Technologists.

Atkinson, L. J., & Fortunato, N. (2007). *Berry and Kohn's operating room technique* (11th ed.). St. Louis, MO: Mosby.

Berger, F. R. (1989). Classical utilitarianism. In W. C. Starr & R. C. Taylor (Eds.), *Moral philosophy: Historical and contemporary essays*. Milwaukee, WI: Marquette University Press.

Colero, L. *A framework for universal principles of ethics.* Crossroads Programs Inc. Retrieved April 1999, from http://www.ethics.ubc.ca/papers/invited/colero.html

DeLaune, S. C., & Ladner, P. K. (2010). *Fundamentals of nursing: Standards and practice* (4th ed.). Clifton Park, NY: Delmar Cengage Learning.

Department of Health and Human Services. (2003, April 14). *Health Insurance Portability and Accountability Act.* Washington, DC: HHS.

Frankena, W. K. (1988). *Ethics* (2nd ed.). Upper Saddle River, NJ: Pearson Education.

Garner, B. (Ed.). (1999). *Black's Law dictionary: Deluxe seventh edition.* St. Paul, MN: West Publishing Company.

Irving, D. (2001). *The bioethics mess.* Washington, DC: The Morley Institute. Available from http://www.lifeissues.net/writers/irv/irv_37bioethicsmess.html

The Joint Commission. (2008). *Comprehensive accreditation manual for hospitals: The official handbook.* Oakbrook Terrace, IL: The Joint Commission.

Joint Commission on Accreditation of Healthcare Organizations. (2003). *Universal protocol for preventing wrong site, wrong procedure, wrong person surgery.* Retrieved December 5, 2005, from http://www.jcaho.org/accredited+organizations/patient+safety/universal+protocol/wss_universal+protocol.htm

Kant, I. (1989). *Foundations of the metaphysics of morals: Text and critical essays* (R. P. Wolff, Ed.). Upper Saddle River, NJ: Prentice Hall.

Lancaster General Hospital, Department of Nursing Services. (2004). Policies and procedures for exposure prevention. Unpublished manuscript.

McNamara, C. Employee staffing: Specifying jobs, roles, and competencies. Available from http://managementhelp.org/staffing/specify/specify.htm

Mill, J. S. (1987). *Utilitarianism.* New York: Prometheus.

O'Leary, M. (1998). *Lexikon: Dictionary of health care terms, organizations, and acronyms for the era of reform* (2nd ed). Oakbrook Terrace, IL: The Joint Commission.

Outka, G. (1977). *Agape: An ethical analysis.* New Haven: Yale University Press.

Pieper, J. (1965). *The four cardinal virtues.* Notre Dame, IN: Notre Dame Press.

Pozgar, G. D. (2006). *Legal aspects of health care administration* (10th ed.). Sudbury, MA: Jones & Bartlett Learning.

Ramsey, P. (1970). *Fabricated man: The ethics of genetic control.* New Haven, CT: Yale University Press.

Ramsey, P., Farley, M., Jonsen, A. R., Wood, M. R., & May, W. F. (2002). *The patient as person: Explorations in medical ethics.* New Haven, CT: Yale University Press.

Tokarski, C. (2000). Medical error-prevention strategies face barriers to acceptance. *Medscape Money & Medicine,* Medscape, Inc. Retrieved March 3, 2001, from http://www.ahcpr.gov/news/medscap2.htm

Veateh, R. M. (1977). *Case studies in medical ethics.* Cambridge, MA: Harvard University Press.

White, L., Duncan, G., & Baumle, W. (2011). *Foundations of Nursing* (3rd ed.). Clifton Park, NY: Delmar Cengage Learning.

White, N., Denise, T. C., & Peterfreund, S. P. (2007). *Great traditions in ethics* (12th ed.). Belmont, CA: Wadsworth.

CHAPTER

3

The Surgical Patient

CASE STUDY Following an automobile accident, Juan, a 37-year-old man, was in the operating room with a fractured left femur, left tibia, and fibula. He also had a severe compound fracture of the right tibia and fibula with a near amputation. While the anesthesia personnel were starting intravenous lines, two surgeons and the circulator were standing near the patient's right leg. The surgeons were laying out their operative approach to the circulator and the surgical technologist in the first scrub role. Juan asked three consecutive times, "What is wrong with my left leg?" The first two times the anesthesia provider said, "Your left leg will be fine." Upon the third asking, the surgical technologist said, "Juan, your left leg is severely injured, but it is not as severely injured as your right leg. We will operate on both legs tonight." Juan noticeably relaxed and said, "Thank you."

1. What do you think Juan was concerned about when he asked, "What's wrong with my left leg?"
2. At age 37, what is Juan's developmental stage?
3. After surgery, Juan's first nonphysical concerns will probably focus on what area of his life?
4. Identify Juan's patient care needs. Which need will the surgical team address first during surgery?
5. What spiritual issue may be raised by this incident for Juan?

OBJECTIVES

After studying this chapter, the reader should be able to:

(C) 1. Assess the patient's response to illness and hospitalization.
(A) 2. Demonstrate awareness that all surgical patients have the right to the highest standards and practices in asepsis.
(R) 3. Distinguish and assess the physical, spiritual, and psychological needs of a patient.
(E) 4. Distinguish and assess cultural and religious influences on the surgical patient.
5. Compare and contrast the patient's responses to the process of death.
6. Discuss the procedure for a patient death in the operating room.

SELECT KEY TERMS

Maslow's hierarchy of needs
patient
physical need
psychological need
social need
spiritual need

THE SURGICAL TECHNOLOGIST AND THE SURGICAL PATIENT

In Chapter 1, the surgical technologist was described using the common definition of a professional, that is, an individual who has specialized education and training in a given field and who meets certain competency-based and ethical criteria. The primary role of the surgical technologist in rendering care to the surgical **patient** is assisting the surgeon during the surgical procedure—the establishment and protection of a sterile field, the care and handling of surgical instrumentation, and assistance with technical tasks throughout the surgical procedure. When surgical technologists refer to the tasks they perform as preoperative, intraoperative, or postoperative, they typically mean tasks performed within the operating room The surgical technologist commonly has only a short period of contact with the conscious surgical patient. Even with this limited amount of time spent with the conscious patient, every surgical team member can relate stories in which the short but intense interactions were important to patient care and safety.

The information provided in this chapter is designed to help the entry-level surgical technologist understand from the patient's perspective what it means and how it feels to face the prospect of surgery.

PHYSICAL, PSYCHOLOGICAL, SOCIAL, AND SPIRITUAL NEEDS OF THE SURGICAL PATIENT

For the surgical patient, surgical intervention is a physical, psychological, social, and spiritual event. Imagine for a moment the questions that pass through the mind of a young woman who is about to undergo a hysterectomy: What changes will my body go through? Who will I be as a wife and mother? Why did God let this happen to me? These are profound questions: one physical (Will my body be the same?), one psychological (Who am I?), one social (Who am I in my social role of wife and mother?), and one spiritual (What does this say about my belief system?).

The following definitions will be used when referring to the components that make up the needs of an individual:

- **Physical need:** Any need or activity related to genetics, physiology, or anatomy
- **Psychological need:** Any need or activity related to the identification and understanding of oneself
- **Social need:** Any need or activity related to one's identification or interaction with another individual or group
- **Spiritual need:** Any need or activity related to the identification and understanding of one's place in an organized universe (expressions may involve theology, philosophy, mythology, and intuition)

None of these human features exists alone. They function together in a dynamic state. **Maslow's hierarchy of needs** establishes a means of prioritizing needs effective for basic understanding of individuals and for quick recognition of patient concerns.

UNDERSTANDING THE SURGICAL PATIENT AS A HUMAN BEING

Surgical patients are, first and foremost, people. They have a whole life outside the role of patient. That life is at risk with every surgical intervention. The person who is brought into your operating room is not "the hysterectomy in room 5" but rather Jane Doe, single mother of three, bank executive, aspiring vocalist, Episcopalian, African-American, Democrat, practical jokester, and a lot more. Health care is no place for someone who cannot or chooses not to care for the total individual, despite his or her own personal beliefs. One must never "lose sight" of the total person. To do so is to violate the ethical and moral obligations that every health care professional has to every patient.

Causes of Surgical Intervention

Every surgical patient is a unique individual; however, all surgical patients have something in common. Given all options, they would elect not to be having surgery. Even when a surgical procedure is selected for cosmetic reasons, it is selected because the patient is dissatisfied with his or her body as it is. Most are having surgery because genetic factors, trauma or disease have presented them with a condition that can only be or best be corrected with surgical intervention. Surgery is often the last resort after other treatment options have been exhausted.

Common factors that result in surgical intervention are:

Factor	Example
Genetic malformation	Cheiloschisis (cleft lip)
Trauma	Anterior cruciate ligament tear
Nonmalignant neoplasm	Uterine fibroid
Malignant neoplasm	Colon cancer
Disease	Cholecystitis (gallbladder infection)
Condition	Kidney stone
Psychological state	Rhytidectomy (facelift)

The surgical patient, then, is an individual who became a patient because of an illness, disease, or condition. The patient became a surgical patient because surgical intervention offers the hope of a cure or correction.

Patient Responses to Illness and Hospitalization

As previously mentioned, every surgical patient is a unique individual. In order to meet the needs unique to each patient, the surgical technologist should be aware of and sensitive to the patient's feelings about the illness and upcoming surgery. Human behavior in reaction to health, illness, and hospitalization varies with the age of the patient, but two broad factors that apply to the majority of patients are adaptation and stress. These two factors can then be further broken down into coping mechanisms.

Sister Callista Roy is best known for the development of what is referred to as the Roy Adaptation Model. Roy's model views the patient as a biopsychosocial individual that is constantly interacting with the environment with the ability to adapt by using coping skills in dealing with internal and external stressors. Roy then interprets the environment as "all conditions, circumstances, and influences that surround and affect the development and behaviour of the person" (Roy & Andrews, 2005). She also states that health involves becoming an integrated and whole person (Roy & Anderson, 2005). Placed in context with the surgical patient, this can refer to the mind and body being in sync in order to successfully adapt to the situation and promote recovery. The adaptive process involves both physiological and psychological changes that indicate the person's attempt to adapt to and counter the stressors of illness or trauma. Adaptation occurs in a rapid or slow fashion based on the nature and type of illness or trauma, family support, patient's culture, level of the patient's social development, level of the patient's intelligence, patient's personality, and learned responses.

Dr. Hans Selye, a recognized expert in the study of stress, defines *stress* as a "nonspecific response of the body to a demand" (2006). Stress can take the form of a physical, chemical, or emotional phenomenon that causes tension. Further, stress can be divided into two types: distress and eustress. Distress is the most commonly referred to type of stress—the type that has negative implications. Eustress, whose prefix "eu" means "well" or "good," is the term for the positive, desirable form of stress. Both types of stress can be equally taxing on the body and mind, but the outcome is different. Examples of eustress that illustrate its positive nature include coming in first during a race, receiving a promotion, getting married, and having a baby. Distress, which is what will be discussed for the remainder of this section and referred to herein as "stress," is the result of a perceived or real threat to the person and is characterized by particular physiological and psychosocial behaviors. Individuals vary in their reaction and tolerance to stress, and one's reaction also depends on the intensity, type, and duration of the stressor. For example, a small cut may produce a high level of intensity, but the duration may be short, whereas a long and deep surgical incision can produce a much higher level of intensity with a longer duration.

As mentioned, stress is physiological and psychological. The patient feels vulnerable and threatened by his or her illness, trauma, possible loss of a body part, temporary or permanent loss of a body function, or potential death. The patient can manifest stress in several manners, including loss of appetite and weight; changes in body functions, including digestion, fluid, and electrolyte balance; changes in mental status; increase in blood pressure and heart rate; and changes in metabolism. For example, the patient's secretion of adrenocortical hormones may increase, which can contribute to a delay in wound healing and decreases the body's resistance to infection. The surgical technologist must be aware of these stressors and how they affect the patient physically and mentally. Factors to be aware of include the following:

- Type, nature, and severity of the illness, trauma, or disease
- Patient's previous experiences with illness, trauma, or disease, including previous experience with surgery
- Age of patient. Pediatric patients feel much more threatened, especially when taken from their parents to be transported to the operating room. Adolescents are much more conscious about their bodies and privacy, whereas older adults are worried about multiple concerns, such as death, infirmity, family, paying the bills, and job security.
- Environmental differences. The hospital and surgical environment is definitely not the same as home, and the patient has to quickly adapt to a different schedule, such as waking up by 7:30 a.m. for breakfast, being constantly woken at night postoperatively to take vital signs, etc.

- Family role. An individual who is the primary "money maker" may now be in a highly dependent role, relying on health care providers; postoperatively he or she may have to rely on other family members for care and assistance.
- Economic factors: How will the bills be paid; how can we take our planned vacation; who is going to pay for the groceries; will I still have a job after a lengthy postoperative recovery? These are the patient's concerns.
- Religious beliefs: Religion can affect attitudes and views of illness, life, and death, and how illness or trauma should be approached. Religious beliefs may determine the treatment options available to the patient. For example, Jehovah's Witnesses do not believe in or permit the transfusion of whole blood or blood components.

When faced with these types of stressors, the patient may exhibit one or more coping mechanisms. The mechanisms, whether positive or negative, represent the individual working at accepting and coping with the situation, eventually being able to make decisions related to his or her care, and looking forward to a resolution and/or recovery. Common types of coping mechanisms include the following:

- *Denial:* Patient does not want to accept the truth of what is occurring.
- *Rationalization:* Patient attempts to rationalize illness or disease. For example, a diabetic patient who is facing amputation of his or her foot due to a gangrenous ulcer may say "diabetes runs on my father's side of the family."
- *Regression:* Patient regresses to an earlier stage of life, such as adolescence, and exhibits behaviors unique to that stage, such as assuming a fetal position, excessive crying, and pouting. This can also be associated with dependency on others.
- *Repression:* Patient represses thoughts and feelings about illness or disease and does not want to hold any discussions concerning what is happening. This can also be associated with escaping or avoiding the situation.

Death and Dying

Death is one part of the natural progression of life. As health deteriorates and treatments fail, a slow but steady shift takes place near the end of life and the focus of care changes from cure, to palliative treatment, to comfort care.

There are three accepted definitions of death:

1. **Cardiac death:** The irreversible loss of cardiac and respiratory function. This is the permanent absence of heartbeat and respiration.
2. **Higher-brain death:** This is the irreversible loss of higher-brain function. The lower brain stem continues to provide respiration, blood pressure, and a heartbeat without the assistance of a respirator.
3. **Whole-brain death:** The irreversible loss of all functions of the entire brain. Whole-brain death is the current law as to what defines death in most jurisdictions of the world and reflects the standard set by the Harvard School of Medicine. It includes a flat EEG, unresponsiveness, lack of pupil reflexes, and low body temperature.
   - Spiritual or religious practices and rituals play important roles in end-of-life care. It is important that the health care provider be sensitive to any religious or cultural practices that honor the patient in death. For example, the Roman Catholic ritual known as Anointing of the Sick may be performed on a seriously ill person. Last rites may be given to Catholic or Protestant patients before death. Muslim tradition might request that immediately after death, the patient's body be turned east to face Mecca, their holiest city. If the patient is Jewish, the dying patient (*goses*) should not be left alone. The nurse cannot touch the body until the rabbi offers final rites. After death, a son or relative will close the eyes and mouth of the deceased and wash and dress the body. Buddhists believe in reincarnation and that the last thoughts of a person before death determine the rebirth condition. Hindus feel that cremation is the best way for the soul to begin its journey.

People cope with grief in distinct stages. These stages were introduced by Elizabeth Kübler-Ross and have become to be known as the *Five Stages of Grief.* These stages apply to any form of personal loss, such as the death of a loved one. These stages may not occur in order and not everyone will go through all the stages.

1. **Denial:** This is the initial stage. Patients may be saying something such as "It can't be happening to me." Denial is usually a temporary defense and a means of coping for the patient.
2. **Anger:** When the first stage cannot be continued, it is replaced by feelings of anger, rage, envy, and resentment. The patient is asking, "Why me?"
3. **Bargaining:** If a patient has been unable to face the reality and has gone through the stage of being angry, he or she may move to the stage of bargaining to postpone the inevitable. The patient may say, "Just let me live to see my son graduate."
4. **Depression:** When a terminally ill person can no longer deny the illness as it progresses, his or her anger is replaced with a sense of great loss. The patient may be thinking, "Please don't take me away from my family."
5. **Acceptance:** When a patient has had enough time to work through the first four stages, he or she will reach a stage of being neither depressed nor angry. The statement of resolution may be, "I know I will be in a better place."

Any unexpected death is tragic, but when the death is due to non-natural causes, the burden on the family is much greater. Families are wise to seek out support groups to assist in handling the grief process. The following are the general categories of causes of death:

- **Accidental:** These deaths can be caused by nature (floods, lightening, earthquake) or humans (motor vehicle, gunshot). The family is left to deal with the emotional trauma. These cases may engender wrongful death suits. The surgical technologist should be aware of the protocol of preserving evidence. Photographs of hospital scenes or physical injuries to the individual may need to be obtained.
- **Terminal:** A patient who is *terminal* is suffering from a disease that is progressive and incurable. Death will be the final outcome. Palliative treatment is often prescribed for these patients to improve their quality of life during the course of the illness. These patients often feel they have imposed an economic burden on their family members. Examples of terminal illnesses include metastatic cancer and liver cirrhosis.
- **Prolonged (chronic):** A condition that is long-lasting (more than 4–6 weeks and in many cases lifelong), and needs to be managed on a long-term basis. Two examples of chronic illnesses are asthma and high blood pressure. These types of illnesses are often managed through lifelong medical treatment.
- **Sudden:** Any death that occurs without warning, such as a cardiac arrest or SIDS (sudden infant death syndrome).

Each of us has different values and morals guided by our culture, religion, and family values. When faced with a terminal condition, these values become prevalent. The extent to which we are willing to endure treatment becomes a personal matter. Extending life because we have the technology to do so may not fit into our value system if the quality of our life is more important. Palliative procedures are intended to provide the patient with symptom relief, the avoidance of symptoms, or relief from conditions secondary to the progressive local disease. Palliative care is not just for those at the end of life; it can improve quality of life for those with a terminal illness. An example of a palliative treatment may be placement of a stent in the common bile duct to restore bile flow in a patient with liver cancer.

Therapeutic procedures are used to treat or manage a disease. These procedures fall into several categories. These include elective and nonelective surgeries. Elective surgeries include placement of a cardiac stent, pacemaker insertion, and Novasure or a D&C for dysmenorrhea; an example of nonelective surgery would be a live organ donor transplant.

Life support refers to a set of therapies that preserve a patient's life when body systems are not functioning sufficiently to sustain life. Life-support therapies may utilize some combination of several techniques including feeding tubes, intravenous drips, total parenteral nutrition, mechanical respiration, heart/lung bypass, defibrillation, urinary catheterization, and dialysis. Life-support therapies can be further broken down into "ordinary" or "extraordinary" means of care. Ordinary means are often used to illustrate care given to prolong life that the physician is morally obligated to provide. They do not impose any additional burden to the patient. Extraordinary measures include those therapies that may pose an undue burden on the patient and may be costly. A treatment can be extraordinary because it is simply futile. For example, those who are dying of one illness have no obligation to accept treatment for a second life-threatening condition that is at a less advanced stage. A treatment will be extraordinary not because that treatment will be altogether futile, but because its burdens will be disproportionate to the benefits it will bring, and the physician would not be morally obligated to provide it.

The term *euthanasia* comes from the Greek for "good death," and Americans have recast its meaning as "easy death" or "painless inducement of quick death." The two categories of easy death are:

1. *Passive euthanasia,* which is when the physician does nothing to preserve life.
2. *Active euthanasia,* which requires actions that speed the process of dying, such as the administration of morphine. Active euthanasia is further divided into *voluntary euthanasia,* where the patient initiates facilitation of his or her death, and *involuntary euthanasia,* where the patient's autonomous rights are violated.

The AHA Patient Care Partnership allows patients the right to refuse treatment. The Patient Self-Determination Act, passed in 1990, requires medical facilities to inform patients of their right to choose the type and extent of their medical care and to provide patients with information concerning living wills and powers of attorney. Health care providers must make a conscious effort to refrain from imposing their value system on a patient. If a competent patient's request seems irrational, but his or her reasons for it are rational, we must honor the patient's request, even if that request results in death.

Advance directives is a general term that refers to one of two legal documents used to speak for patients in the event that they cannot make decisions for themselves. A *living will* allows patients to state in writing exactly what medical interventions they are willing to endure to sustain life. A power of attorney is a legal way to appoint a health care proxy who will make medical decisions for the patient in the event that he or she cannot do so. A Do Not Resuscitate/Do Not Intubate (DNR/DNI) order, which is written by a physician, states that resuscitation should not be attempted if a patient suffers a cardiac or respiratory arrest. The DNR/DNI must be initiated by the patient. The DNR/DNI is recognized in the medical setting but a patient should re-emphasize if the DNR/DNI is to be honored during surgical procedures. Many hospitals rescind the DNR/DNI during surgery, so this should be discussed with the surgeon, anesthesia provider, and other surgical team members.

Death of a patient in the operating room can be sudden, such as cardiac arrest during a scheduled procedure, or may be anticipated by the patient, family, and surgical team: for example, a patient brought into the operating room with an abdominal aortic aneurysm that has a good chance of rupturing. However, when a patient death occurs in the operating room the hospital policy and procedure must be followed by the surgical team and consistently applied. Procedures will vary according to health care facility; however, the following are broad guidelines (the order can vary according to the situation):

- Notify the surgery department supervisor of the patient death and the implementation of postmortem patient care.
- Family and significant others, who may be at the hospital, are immediately notified by the surgeon.
- The religious leader of the patient's faith may be notified by hospital personnel unless the family has already done so.
- In instances of homicide or other types of situations that would involve law enforcement, the surgical team will need to carefully follow procedures for the preservation of evidence, including turning over the body to the coroner for autopsy.
- The surgery team may be responsible for preliminary preparation of the body for the family to view.
- The surgery team may be responsible for postmortem care of the body for transportation.

Surgical team members, obviously, can be psychologically affected by a death in the operating room, in particular multiple deaths that occur during an all-hazards situation. It is important for the team members to understand that talking to others, such as peers, counselors, and/or religious leaders, is okay and that one may need to share one's feelings and fears as related to the traumatic situation that occurred. Some health care facilities may have support groups for staff members or can refer the surgical technologist to an outside support group. It has been recognized that having counselors immediately available during an all-hazards situation is important in order to provide services to those affected as well as health care providers. However, students who do ask, "how do you handle the death of a patient in the operating room?" should understand a key factor:

- As mentioned earlier, it is okay for the surgical team members to realize that particular feelings could be associated with losing a patient in the operating room and to have empathy for the family and friends. However, the surgical technologist will have to realize that he or she cannot become overwhelmed by the loss of a patient that he or she probably did not know. The surgical technologist, in particular during all-hazards situations, must move on to patients who are alive and have a chance at living. If the surgical technologist becomes consumed by a patient's death, he or she could become a non-effective member of the surgical team.

When a patient dies, the donation of organs is a choice that he or she may have made at some point in life. Organ transplantation began in the early 1950s. Under Title XI of the Omnibus Budget Reconciliation Act of 1986, hospitals are required to establish organ procurement protocols or lose Medicare and Medicaid funding. Until recently, a patient had to be declared dead according to the whole-brain death criterion. Currently, however, in reaction to the shortage of available organs for transplant and the fact that more people are completing an advance directive to make it known that they do not wish to be maintained on mechanical ventilator if they become gravely ill, the decision to discontinue mechanical support will allow a patient to donate organs by means of Donation After Cardiac Death (DCD). A patient is considered a candidate for DCD only if it is predicted that the heart will cease functioning within 90 minutes of removal from mechanical support. There are several steps to organ donation after cardiac death. Once a patient is declared dead, the family is consulted about organ donation. The participants in the discussion may include the attending physician, nurse, clergy, and social worker. The next of kin must consent to the donation by signing the consent for donation documentation. The facility's Gift of Life Coordinator determines the patient's suitability for organ donation and organizes the process. The Gift of Life Coordinator and medical team coordinate the donation process, including a respiratory drive assessment, organ function assessment, and review of medical/social history; schedule the operating room time and arrange for the surgical team to arrive; as well as decide when ventilator support will be removed. For patients who were not placed on or were removed from life support, various tissues can be recovered, including:

- Corneas
- Skin
- Bone

Prioritizing Needs: Maslow's Hierarchy

Maslow (1968, 1971) constructed a model of human development. The developmental stages for human progression are expressed in terms of a hierarchy. The simple but powerful point of the hierarchical structure is that all the requisite needs of each prior level must be met in order to achieve the next level (Figure 3-1):

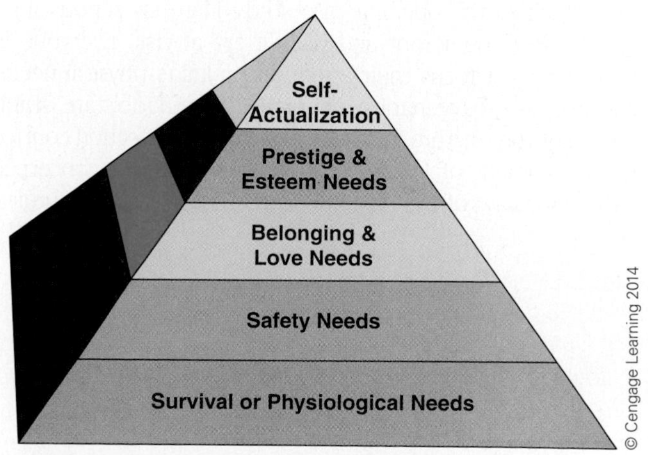

Figure 3-1 Maslow's hierarchy of needs

- *Physiological needs:* The most basic needs are biological needs, such as the need for water, oxygen, food, and temperature regulation.
- *Safety needs:* These needs refer to the perception on the part of the individual that his or her environment is safe.
- *Love and belonging needs:* These are basic social needs—to be known and cared for as an individual and to care for another.
- *Esteem needs:* This level of need refers to a positive evaluation of oneself and others, a need to be respected and to respect others.
- *Self-actualization:* This is the need to fulfill what one believes is one's purpose.

If physiological needs are not being met, the individual must spend energy meeting the basic needs of food, water, and temperature regulation. Without these needs being met, the individual dies. Likewise, it is easy to see that an individual who is consumed with safety needs will not have the time and energy required to develop the emotional and intellectual pursuits necessary for higher-level development. The individual who believes the environment is inherently dangerous cannot trust. Without trust, one cannot experience or give love and affection. If physiological and safety needs are met but love and affection are not found within the social group, the individual will not be able to generate positive self-regard. It is only when physical, safety, affective, and self-esteem needs are effectively met that individuals can turn their thoughts and energy to becoming all that they are capable of being.

This hierarchy is especially important in the field of health care. The nature of surgery requires that the surgical team concentrate on physiological needs first, followed by environmental, then affective, then self-esteem, and then self-actualization needs.

A SAMPLE APPLICATION OF MASLOW'S HIERARCHY

Think back to the opening case study. Juan has serious injuries. Both his right foot and his life are at risk. Everyone in the room must focus their attention on Juan's physical needs: blood volume, oxygenation, pain relief, anesthetic state, stabilization of the fracture, revascularization, and infection control. At the moment of Juan's question, everyone was concerned with taking care of the physical needs. In this case the surgical technologist in the first scrub role, who had completed the case setup and was protecting the sterile field and listening to the surgeon state his plan for the procedure, had the time to allow Juan's question to sink in and to reflect on what he was asking. It dawned on him that Juan was afraid that his left leg, a leg that was hurting and obviously damaged, was amputated. Why? No one was paying any attention to that leg. The surgical technologist could respond to Juan's question at a higher level than the physical—at the level of his fear.

Cultural and Religious Influences

Every culture expresses different value orientations. The surgical technologist should be aware of these fundamental values and beliefs. Maslow's hierarchy establishes guidelines for responding to patients' needs. Cultural values will specify the way the patient thinks and feels about these issues.

Religious values are always expressed within a culture, but they reach across cultures, too. Religious values can easily conflict with modern medicine. These create both ethical and legal problems for patients and health care providers. The patient population in the United States is both multicultural and multireligious. The surgical technologist should have a basic understanding of various faith statements and their relationship to surgical care (Table 3-1).

SAMPLE APPLICATION: USING RELIGIOUS AND CULTURAL INFORMATION IN THE OPERATING ROOM

Think about Juan again. His concerns about life and death, family responsibility, amputation, and so forth will be expressed in a specific language and context. His cultural and religious beliefs will determine these. For instance, Juan may believe that his existence is the result of a universal action organized by a central mind and power. What he calls this universal action will depend on his cultural background, the religious story he believes, and his personal life experiences. Whether he understands the accident as ordained, punishment, or something else will arise from this foundation. Guilt will be determined by his beliefs. Postoperatively, his family and friends, clergy and counselors, physicians, and other health care providers will hear all his needs and concerns and his solutions expressed in this form.

TABLE 3-1 Religion and Religious Values

Item	*Roman Catholic*	*Protestant*	*Jehovah's Witness*
Leaders	Bishop, priest	Bishop, priest, minister, pastor	Elders
Holy text	*Bible*	Bible	*New World Bible*
Weekly holy day	Sunday	Sunday	None
Dietary restrictions	Fish on Fridays, fasting during Lent	Generally none; some variance	No blood-containing food
View of medical treatment	Encouraged	Generally encouraged; sect variance	Encouraged; no blood transfusion
Birth control	Not allowed	Allowed	Allowed
Infertility treatment	Allowed with some rules	Allowed	Allowed
Abortion	Not allowed	Some circumstances	Not allowed
Removal of life support	Specific conditions	Specific conditions	Specific conditions
Organ donation	Permitted	Permitted	Allowed
Item	*Mormon*	*American Indian*	*Islam*
Leaders	Bishop	Medicine man/elder	Imam
Holy text	Bible, *Book of Mormon*, other writings	Oral tradition	*koran, shari'a Hadith*
Weekly holy day	Sunday	None	Friday
Dietary restrictions	Drugs, alcohol, tea, coffee, tobacco	Varies	Pork, alcohol, other rules
View of medical treatment	Encouraged	Varies	Encouraged (privacy very important)
Birth control	Allowed	Discouraged	Allowed
Infertility treatment	Allowed	Allowed	Allowed with some rules
Abortion	Specific conditions	Not allowed	Some circumstances
Removal of life support	Personal choice	Not necessary	Specific conditions
Organ donation	Allowed	Discouraged	Permitted

CASE STUDY Chandra is a 13-year-old who was involved in an automobile accident. She has a severe facial laceration but was not rendered unconscious and has no negative neurological signs. She is coming to the operating room where a plastic surgeon will repair her facial laceration.

1. What psychological concerns might Chandra have? Which concerns may take priority?
2. How can the surgical team help ease Chandra's experience?

Questions for Further Study

1. Are there any differences in the Roman Catholic and American Indian views of transplant surgery?
2. During a surgical procedure in which general anesthesia is being administered, which level of Maslow's hierarchy is the surgical team meeting, and why?
3. As surgical technologists, we are taught to treat every operative patient the same, without regard to background, past history, culture, or reason for surgery. Does this hold in every situation? (a) Compare and contrast the type of conversation that the surgical technologist might have when transporting a female patient who will be undergoing a mastectomy, and the conversation with a female patient who will be undergoing a rhinoplasty for cosmetic reasons. (b) Would a prisoner who has killed a police officer and is brought to the operating room to repair a gunshot wound be treated any differently than a 12-year-old girl who is to have a tonsillectomy?
4. Alternative therapy treatments have been on the rise for the last few years. Should a physician consider consulting with (and possibly employing the therapies advocated by) a healing priest from a patient's nontraditional religion? What factors would prevent a physician from doing so, even at the patient's request? Could the physician's refusal affect the outcome of the treatment he or she prescribes?

BIBLIOGRAPHY

Association of Surgical Technologists. (2006). *Core curriculum for surgical assisting* (2nd ed.). Littleton, CO: Association of Surgical Technologists.

Association of Surgical Technologists. (2010). *Core curriculum for surgical technology* (6th ed.). Littleton, CO: Association of Surgical Technologists.

Brehm, S. S., & Kassin, S. M. (2004). *Social psychology* (6th ed.). Boston: Houghton Mifflin.

Edge, R. S., & Groves, J. R. (2005). *A guide for clinical practice* (3rd ed.). Clifton Park, NY: Delmar Cengage Learning.

Estes, M. E. Z. (2010). *Health assessment and physical examination* (4th ed.). Clifton Park, NY: Delmar Cengage Learning.

Flavell, J. H. (2001). *Cognitive development* (4th ed.). Englewood Cliffs, NJ: Prentice Hall.

Ford, R. D. (Ed.). (1990). *Diagnostic tests handbook.* Springhouse, PA: Springhouse.

Fowler, J. (1995). *Stages of faith: The psychology of human development and the quest for meaning.* New York: Harper One.

Gilligan, C. (1993). *In a different voice: Psychological theory and women's development.* Cambridge: Harvard University Press.

Goulet, L. R., & Baltes, P. B. (Eds.). (1970). *Life-span developmental psychology: Research and theory.* New York: Academic.

Guyton, A. C. (2005). *Textbook of medical physiology* (11th ed.). Philadelphia: Saunders.

Hartshorne, H., & May, M. (1928–1930). *Studies in the nature of character. Vol.1: Studies in deceit, Vol. 2: Studies in self-control, Vol. 3: Studies in the organization of character.* New York: Macmillan.

Health Encyclopedia—Disease and Conditions. (n.d.). Stress. Retrieved November 1, 2006, from www.healthscout.com/ency/68/103/main.html

Kagan, J. (1994). *The nature of the child* (10th ed.). New York: Basic Books.

Kane, R. L., Ouslander, J. G., & Abrass, I. B. (2008). *Essentials of clinical geriatrics* (6th ed.). New York: McGraw-Hill.

Kübler-Ross, E. (1970). *On death and dying.* New York: Simon and Schuster.

Livingston, E. A. (2006). *The concise Oxford dictionary of the Christian church* (2nd ed.). London: Oxford University Press.

Maslow, A. H. (1992). *Toward a psychology of being* (3rd ed.). Hoboken, NJ: Wiley.

Maslow, A. H. (1993). *The farther reaches of human nature.* New York: Penguin Books.

Mazanec, P., & Tyler, M. K. (2003). Cultural considerations in end of life care: How ethnicity, age, and spirituality affect decisions when death is imminent. *American Journal of Nursing, 102*(3), 50–58.

McCance, K. L., & Huether, S. E. (2005). *Pathophysiology: The biologic basis for disease in adults and children* (5th ed.). St. Louis: CV Mosby.

McGaa, E. (1990). *Mother Earth spirituality.* San Francisco: Harper.

McLuhan, T. C. (1971). *Touch the Earth: A self-portrait of Indian existence.* New York: Simon and Schuster.

Phillips, N. F. (2007). *Berry & Kohn's operating room technique* (11th ed.). St. Louis: Mosby.

Pitorak, E. F. (2003). Care at the time of death. *American Journal of Nursing, 103*(7), 42–52.

Roy, C., & Andrews, H. A. (2008). *The Roy Adaptation Model* (3rd ed.). Upper Saddle River, NJ: Prentice Hall.

Scott, A. S., & Fong, E. (2008). *Body structures and functions* (11th ed.). Clifton Park, NY: Delmar Cengage Learning.

U.S. Department of State Foreign Affairs Manual, Vol. 7. (2007, November). Deaths of non-natural causes—homicide, suicide, accidental death. Retrieved March 13, 2007, from http://foia.state.gov/masterdocs/07fam/07fam0230.pdf

CHAPTER

4

Special Populations

CASE STUDY A patient with AIDS is brought to the operating room for a total hip arthroplasty. The patient is in the early stages of AIDS but does have Kaposi's sarcoma skin lesions and painful swollen lymph nodes in the groin and axilla and has lost weight.

1. When positioning the patient, what are some of the important principles to be considered to protect the patient from injury and pain?
2. When placing the ESU grounding pad, what are some special considerations concerning the patient with AIDS?
3. What complications could be encountered during the surgical procedure that the surgical technologist should be prepared to assist the surgeon in resolving?

OBJECTIVES

After studying this chapter, the reader should be able to:

C 1. Compare and contrast the surgical care considerations for pediatric patients and patients who are obese, diabetic, pregnant, immunocompromised, disabled, geriatric, or experiencing trauma.

2. Evaluate the unique physical and psychological needs of each special population.

A 3. Compare and contrast the intraoperative considerations for pediatric patients and patients who are obese, diabetic, immunocompromised, geriatric, or traumatized that relate to postoperative wound healing.

R 4. Evaluate the role of the surgical technologist for the surgical care of each special population.

E 5. Assess the ethical commitment that is required of surgical technologists as it relates to special populations care.

6. Determine the general needs associated with special populations of surgical patients.

Select Key Terms

arterial blood gases (ABGs)
autoimmune diseases
central venous catheter
diabetes mellitus
enterocolitis
golden hour
human immunodeficiency virus (HIV)
hypothermia
immunocompetence
intra-arterial measurement
Kaposi's sarcoma
kernicterus
kinematics
penetrating trauma
pneumothorax
Revised Trauma Score
septic shock
splenectomy
splenomegaly
torticollis
urine output
venous compression device

INTRODUCTION

Surgical patients with special needs present various challenges in which the specifics of care must be adjusted to meet the particular needs of the patient. The surgical technologist must be aware of the needs of special populations and proper responses to these. Special populations present with unique physical and psychological needs. For example, infants and older adults have increased difficulty in adjusting to the stresses of traumatic injuries, loss of body temperature, and loss of intravascular fluids. Above all else, the surgical technologist must be ethically committed to providing the same quality standard of care and empathy for all surgical patients.

Although many surgical patients have special needs, space limits the mention of all of them. The special needs groups to be discussed in this chapter include pediatric, obese, diabetic, pregnant, immunocompromised, disabled, and geriatric patients. Trauma patients are included as well due to the unique circumstances that accompany traumatic injury.

PEDIATRIC PATIENTS

A patient is considered a pediatric patient if he or she is between birth and the age of 18 years. The common terms applied to the pediatric population that are related to their chronological age are as follows:

Neonate: The first 28 days of life outside the uterus

Infant: 1–18 months

Toddler: 18–30 months

Preschooler: 30 months to 5 years

School age: 6–12 years

Adolescent: 13-18 years

Pediatric patients require surgery for the same reasons as anyone else—congenital anomalies, disease, and trauma. The commonly used cliché "Children are not little adults" does indeed apply. The medical and surgical care of pediatric patients is a specialty focused on the unique problems and challenges presented by this special needs group.

The surgical technologist must be familiar with the specific conditions and needs of the pediatric patient. Anatomical and physiological differences are of primary importance to the surgical team (Table 4-1). Vital signs are listed in Tables 4-2 and 4-3.

Psychological factors must be accounted for in pediatric patients. An important factor is the ability to use language to understand their situation, the environment, and procedure. The neonate and infant are startled easily, so a quiet environment is essential. The preschool and school-aged child may use language to the same general ends as adults—to inform, persuade, distract, or manipulate—but they will not use language the same way. Their descriptions of pain, for instance, are likely to be imprecise in terms of both symptoms and location. Learning to "hear" the child takes considerable experience. Members of the surgical team must also be aware of their personal and communal psychological response to the pediatric patient. Almost every individual feels protective of a child. The surgical team will and should feel protective of all patients. Despite that emotional response, the surgical team cannot explain to neonates, infants, and toddlers the nature of the condition, the procedure, or the complications. The surgical team can only explain some small portion of these to the preschool and school-aged child. These issues are, however, appropriately conveyed to the parents of the child.

In pediatric surgery, the surgical team is forced to focus on the physiological needs of the patient in a more dramatic way than it is with any other age group. In most cases, it is the role of the surgical team to efficiently and effectively achieve a state of anesthesia, complete the surgical procedure, and return the child to his or her family as quickly as possible.

An overwhelming feeling that most pediatric patients feel is that of anxiety due to separation from the parent(s). A feeling of permanent abandonment can occur. The challenge for the surgical technologist who greets and cares for the child is to form, in a very short period, a bond of trust to allay some of the child's fears. The following are suggestions to help reduce the anxiety level of the child:

- Let the child bring a favorite toy or stuffed animal into surgery.
- During the preoperative visit, introduce the child to all of the individuals who will be involved in his or her surgical care.

TABLE 4-1 Pediatric Anatomical and Physiological Considerations

Issue	*Child*
Temperature regulation	Child less than 6 months of age cannot shiver and therefore at risk for hypothermia, bradycardia, and acidosis.
Pulse and respiration	Rates decline with age, reaching adult norms at adolescence
Blood pressure	Child of 1 year and older: systolic pressure in mm Hg = 80 + (2 × age) and diastolic = ⅔ systolic
Head	Suture ridges palpable until 6 months of age
	Posterior fontanel closes by 3 months
	Anterior fontanel closes by 19 months
Eyes	Visual acuity 2/200 at birth
	No tears produced until 2–3 months of age
Ears	Shorter external auditory canal is positioned upward
	Eustachian tube more horizontal, wider, and shorter, leading to more infections
Sinuses	Only ethmoid and maxillary sinuses present at birth
	Frontal sinuses develop at 7 years
	Sphenoid sinuses develop after puberty
Mouth	Systematic development of teeth
	Salivation starts at 3 months
Breasts	Breast tissue develops between 9 and 13 years
	Mature adult tissue achieved between 13 and 16 years
Thorax and lungs	Chest is circular and does not reach adult ratios until age 6
	Chest wall is thin in infants
	Ribs are horizontally displaced in infants
	Trachea is short in the newborn and only reaches adult length near end of adolescence
	Infant to 3–4 months dependent on breathing through their noses
	Infants and toddlers prefer abdominal breathing
Abdomen	Liver proportionately larger in abdominal cavity in the infant
Bone growth	Epiphyses not closed until age 20
Neurological	Neurological system not fully developed
Genitalia (male)	Testes descend by 1 year of age

TABLE 4-2 Normal Heart Rate Ranges for Children

Age	*Heart Rate Range*	*Average Heart Rate*
Infants to 2 years	80–130	110
2–6 years	70–120	100
6–10 years	70–110	90
10–16 years	60–100	85

TABLE 4-3 Normal Respiratory Rate Ranges for Children

Age	*Respiratory Rate per Minute*
1 year	10–40
3 years	20–30
6 years	16–22
10 years	16–20
17 years	12–20

- Take the child into the front part of the surgery department to see how it looks.
- Let the parent(s) walk alongside while transporting the patient to the surgery department. They can accompany the child into the preoperative area.
- Allow the parents to come into the pediatric acute care unit (PACU) after the child arrives and the first set of vital signs has been recorded.

Another primary fear of the pediatric patient is fear of anesthesia. Children do not understand the meaning of unconsciousness and may fear that they are going to sleep and will never wake up. Again, the preoperative visit is helpful; it allows the anesthesia provider to show the child the equipment, and even let the child hold a mask on his or her face to know ahead of time what will be occurring. Just as with the adult surgical patient, the child should be dealt with in a truthful manner, and questions concerning needles used for injection and postoperative pain should be truthfully answered. Children are generally very quick to recognize deception, and the caregiver can quickly lose the trust of the child by trying to deceive.

Since the development of rapid induction, the child no longer has to be subjected to long induction times. Patients who are 2 years of age and younger are usually held by the anesthesia provider during induction. The circulator should stand nearby to assist the anesthesia provider by holding the mask on the face of the child or by holding the child's hands or arms, and by making sure that the room is kept very quiet during the induction.

Monitoring the Pediatric Patient

The pediatric patient must be closely monitored during the surgical procedure. Distinct differences exist for physiological measurement between the pediatric and adult patient. The critical parameters to monitor for the pediatric patient include temperature, **urine output**, cardiac function, and oxygenation.

Temperature

In comparison with adults, pediatric patients, in particular neonates, lack the ability to shiver and have little subcutaneous fat and therefore poor thermal insulation. They also have less lean body mass, which is required for retaining and generating heat. Newborns lose heat through radiation, convection, conduction, and evaporation. Incubators aid in minimizing heat loss by radiation and convection by decreasing the airflow across the skin of the newborn.

Temperature is monitored by measuring the rectal, esophageal, tympanic, axillary, and skin temperature. In the operating room (OR), skin temperature is the primary means of monitoring the temperature. Maintaining proper body temperature is critical in the OR, so the temperature of the room is increased prior to the patient entering. An overhead radiant heater is often used for patients 2 years and younger. However, the most effective means for maintaining body temperature is to keep the infant's extremities wrapped and covered. Warm air- or water-filled blankets may be used during the surgical procedure.

Urine Output

For fluid management, urine output measurement is highly useful for all patient age groups. Neonates and infants are not usually catheterized due to the high risk of trauma to the small urethra; a collection bag is just as useful in obtaining an accurate measurement. An appropriate urine output is 1 to 2 mL/kg/hr.

Cardiac Function

The use of the sphygmomanometer and stethoscope has disadvantages with pediatric patients due to the reliance on cuff size, which varies considerably among children. For very ill infants and children who require constant electrocardiographic (ECG) monitoring, **intra-arterial measurement** is recommended. In infants and children, a cutdown approach to the radial artery is most commonly used. In neonates, the umbilical artery is most commonly used due to easy accessibility.

When no cardiac abnormalities are present, a **central venous catheter** is inserted percutaneously into the subclavian or internal jugular vein in older children. In neonates and infants, a cutdown approach to the external jugular vein is preferred. Due to higher incidences of contamination when procedures are performed in the groin region, the saphenous vein is the route least used.

Oxygenation

The standard for monitoring oxygenation for all age groups of surgical patients is measuring the **arterial blood gases (ABGs)**. However, with the introduction of pulse oximetry, the monitoring of oxygenation has been made considerably easier. Its advantages include immediate blood oxygen saturation information and low cost. The elimination of the necessity for an indwelling probe also decreases the possibility of infection. In surgery, it can be difficult to obtain a blood specimen from the small artery of a neonate or infant; consequently, pulse oximetry has reduced the waiting time for collecting monitoring data.

Shock

The two common types of shock seen in all age groups are septic and hypovolemic shock. In infants and children, **septic shock** is most commonly seen. It is highly important for the surgical technologist to be aware that the neonate and infant respond to shock differently from the older child and adult. For the neonate affected by hypovolemic shock, bradycardia is a physiological response, whereas tachycardia is the typical adult response. Neonates' blood pressure is normally low, so shock does not significantly decrease the blood pressure. However, hypovolemia does result in decreased venous return that lowers cardiac output and leads to poor tissue perfusion with eventual lactic acidosis.

In infants, dehydration is the most common cause of hypovolemic shock; therefore, the main treatment of hypovolemic shock is quick fluid and blood replacement. As a rule of thumb, more water is lost than electrolytes. Emergency treatment is the infusion of a hypotonic solution of sodium chloride.

Septic shock is usually caused by gram-negative bacteria. Peritonitis due to intestinal perforation is a common cause of shock in neonates and infants. Other causes of septic shock include urinary tract infection (UTI), upper respiratory infection (URI), and a contaminated intravascular catheter.

Septic shock also presents with reduced circulating blood volume; therefore initial treatment is the infusion of colloid solutions. Clinical research supports the infusion of colloid solutions as preferable to crystalloid solutions for treating septic shock in all age groups. In addition, the infection is treated with broad-spectrum antibiotics. If the infusion of fluids has achieved its purposes of elevating the central venous pressure (CVP), but hypotension is still present, dopamine is the agent of choice to increase cardiac output.

Fluids and Electrolytes

The management of fluids and electrolytes in neonates and infants requires an understanding of the changes in body fluids that occur before and after birth. The normal physiological processes presented in Table 4-4 are interrupted in premature neonates who must eliminate excess postnatal total body water in a very short period of time after birth. This has a significant effect on the premature neonate who must undergo surgery. An increased extracellular fluid (ECF) volume in a "preemie" is a stimulus for the release of prostaglandin E_2, which will maintain the patency of a ductus arteriosus.

Newborns and infants do not tolerate dehydration well. In addition, their immature kidneys cannot excrete water as effectively as mature kidneys, making fluid management difficult in a surgical setting.

A major concern in the OR is insensible water loss (usually transepithelial). Reasons for insensible water loss include water loss through the skin and lungs caused by overhead radiant heaters and phototherapy. The insensible water loss from the skin in the OR is decreased by covering the extremities; water loss from the lungs is decreased by the humidification of the inspired gases.

Infection

Immediately after birth, bacterial colonization of the newborn's skin and gastrointestinal tract begins. By the 10th day after birth, newborns have the same common aerobic and anaerobic bacteria as that found in the gastrointestinal (GI) tract of adults. However, the normal microbial barriers, the skin and GI tract, are still underdeveloped in the newborn, as are the host defense mechanisms; therefore the newborn is at risk for developing infections.

The initial sign of postoperative infection is fever. The most common sites of postoperative infection are the lungs, surgical wound, urinary tract, and vascular access sites. Treatment for infected surgical wounds includes incision, debridement, and placement of antibiotic-impregnated packing. Frequent dressing changes are required until the wound has healed. Vascular access site infections and urinary catheter infections are treated by removing the catheter and administering antibiotics.

Generally, the indications, uses, and choices of antibiotics are the same for neonates, infants, and children as they are for adults. For clean-contaminated elective surgical procedures, such as a colon operation, the antibiotics of choice are penicillin in combination with aminoglycoside or third-generation cephalosporin. The first dose of antibiotics is given just before the skin incision is made, and doses are continued postoperatively for 24–48 hours. The side effects are similar to those seen in adults, except for three important differences:

1. Sulfonamides (such as Bactrim or Septra) are associated with an increased incidence of **kernicterus** in neonates. Kernicterus is an excess of bilirubin in the blood. Sulfonamides should *not* be administered to newborns.
2. Chloramphenicol (Chloromycetin) is the synthetic form of an antibiotic originally isolated from *Streptomyces venezuelae* and is associated with the cause of "gray syndrome" in which the infant's skin turns gray from

TABLE 4-4 Changes in Body Fluids Before and After Birth

Trimester or Age	*Percent of Total Body Water*	*Percent of Extracellular Fluid Volume*
First trimester	95% of body weight	
32 weeks' gestation	80%	60%
Term	78%	45%
First postnatal week	75%	
Next 1–2 years	60%	20%

drug toxicity. Chloramphenicol should *not* be administered to newborns.

3. Tetracycline causes staining and hypoplasia of the enamel of the developing teeth; therefore, it should *not* be administered to children.

Practically every antibiotic has been associated with the development of pseudomembranous **enterocolitis**, most likely from the overgrowth of *Clostridium difficile* due to antibiotic suppression of the growth of normal bacteria in the colon. One treatment consists of discontinuing the antibiotic that contributed to the cause of the enterocolitis (infection of the small and large bowel), and oral administration of vancomycin.

Metabolic and Nutritional Responses

The caloric requirements of infants are much higher than those of children and adults. Surgery increases the caloric requirements (a 20% to 30% increase with a major operation). Since the work of feeding (sucking and swallowing) accounts for a large portion of the infant's caloric use in the first few months of life, gastrostomy tube feedings are often used postoperatively for procedures of the GI tract.

Trauma

Accidents are the number one cause of death in children aged 1–15. In 2007, 2,800 children aged 1–14 died from an unintentional injury (Centers for Disease Control and Prevention, National Center for Injury Prevention and Control, 2009). Obviously, the emphasis should be on prevention, such as the design of better restraint devices in automobiles and the wearing of helmets when riding a bike.

The causes of trauma in children are most often the result of blunt trauma. Head trauma is much more common in children than adults and accounts for the majority of morbidity and mortality in pediatrics. Motor vehicle accidents are the major cause of trauma in children. Other causes seen more often in children than adults include falls, bicycle accidents, drowning, burns, and poisonings. Childbirth trauma and child abuse are also unique trauma circumstances.

Key Differences in Treatment

Children's emotional reactions to trauma differ from those of an adult. They experience communication barriers in indicating the origin of pain. They may give misleading information, such as exhibiting signs that their abdominal region hurts when there is no abdominal injury. Children also often display signs of developmental regression, especially if the parents are not present.

A second key difference is the metabolic and nutritional differences of children as compared to adults:

- Postoperative metabolic management of the pediatric patient is important, especially if the patient is being treated for trauma.
- What seems to be an insignificant loss of blood can result in marked hemodynamic changes in the child.
- Water and heat loss can occur quickly in children, who lack insulating subcutaneous fat.
- **Hypothermia** intensifies the effects of acidosis, an abnormal increase in hydrogen ion concentration in the body that is a result of the accumulation of acid in the body, reflected by a pH that is below normal.
- Vomiting due to gastric dilatation is common in children who experience trauma and/or surgical procedures; consequently, aspiration is of concern.
- Increased nutritional requirements that were previously discussed must not be forgotten.

GENERAL PRINCIPLES OF PEDIATRIC EMERGENCY TREATMENT

As with all trauma patients, the first priority is to make sure that the patient has an open airway and that it is maintained. The airway should be cleared of any obstacles, such as blood or broken teeth. If the patient is having breathing difficulties, the best treatment is to intubate the child immediately by placing an uncuffed endotracheal tube. If a neck injury is suspected, the cervical spine must be stabilized with a collar or sand bags.

If breathing continues to be difficult, **pneumothorax** (accumulation of air in the pleural cavity) can be a possibility. It is difficult to diagnose pneumothorax in children, but a chest radiograph will aid in diagnosis. A pediatric chest tube is placed to treat the pneumothorax. Hyperventilation is a common response by children to injury, resulting in gastric dilatation. This is easily resolved by inserting a nasogastric tube.

An intravenous (IV) catheter should be placed next. If it is difficult to place a needle in a peripheral vein, it is recommended that a cutdown be performed to the greater saphenous vein at the ankle. Fluids can then start to be infused to treat the pediatric patient for shock. The insertion of a central venous or arterial line may be considered.

Bleeding must also be controlled to prevent severe hypovolemia. Pressure placed on lacerations as soon as possible is important in the management of blood and body fluid loss.

Trauma During Birth

A small percentage of births result in a traumatic injury to the neonate. The use of prenatal ultrasonography has greatly reduced the incidence of birth trauma. The injuries typically seen are bone fractures; injuries to the liver, spleen, and adrenal glands; and nerve injuries.

The most common bone fracture is of the clavicle, usually as a result of shoulder dystocia. *Dystocia* is the term used for difficult labor or delivery of a baby. Shoulder dystocia occurs when the baby's head is delivered, but the shoulders cannot be delivered because they are too wide and are stuck behind the mother's pubic bone or the opening to the birth canal. Upper brachial plexus palsy can occur secondary to shoulder dystocia or breech presentation. Peripheral facial nerve paralysis occasionally occurs due to direct pressure on the infant's face by the mother's pelvis or from the use of forceps. Complete recovery from the nerve paralysis most often occurs by 1 year of age.

Injuries to the liver, spleen, or adrenal glands are caused by direct pressure on the infant's abdomen from the mother's birth canal. However, this rarely requires surgical intervention. Birth trauma can injure the sternocleidomastoid muscle, which leads to the formation of a hematoma and **torticollis** (a contracted state of the muscle). Surgery is necessary if the injury is not recognized in time to correct the condition.

Child Abuse

Child abuse is a tragic event that often presents with multiple traumatic injuries, some of which may have already healed, especially in the case of fractures. The abuse takes the form of physical and/or mental injury, sexual abuse, nutritional neglect, verbal abuse, and delayed treatment of disease and injuries. Surgery is often required to treat soft tissue injuries, fractures, burns, and head trauma. Visceral injuries include internal liver and splenic lacerations, internal pancreatic damage, and duodenal hematomas.

PATIENTS WITH OBESITY

Morbid obesity refers to patients whose body weight is 100 pounds greater than ideal body weight and have an increased susceptibility to morbidity and mortality caused by the physical difficulties of carrying extra weight. The number of complications and morbidity varies according to the severity of the obese condition. Physiological and disease conditions as related to obesity include:

- Myocardial hypertrophy (enlargement of the heart) due to the increased demands placed on the heart, leading to congestive heart failure
- Coronary artery disease (CAD)
- Hypertension (high blood pressure) and vascular changes in the kidneys, affecting elimination of protein wastes and the maintenance of normal fluid and electrolyte balance
- Varicose veins and edema in lower extremities due to poor venous return (venous pooling can lead to thromboembolism and thrombophlebitis)
- Pulmonary function complications, including decreased tidal volume leading to hypoxemia, shortness of breath, sleep apnea, and decrease in lung expansion, making the patient susceptible to postoperative pulmonary infection and embolism
- Liver and gallbladder disease
- Osteoarthritis
- **Diabetes mellitus**
- Pituitary abnormalities
- Arteriosclerosis
- Dysfunctional uterine bleeding

The following section provides an overall review of considerations for the surgical technologist who works with patients who are obese. The following section focuses on specific issues to consider when performing bariatric surgery and the safety precautions needed to prevent injury to the patient and surgical team.

Review of Surgical Considerations

Lifting and transporting the patient who is obese present the first set of challenges. In many instances, the patient will require mechanical lifters from the hospital bed to the stretcher, or the patient may be transported to the OR on the bed because the stretcher may not be large enough. An adequate number of individuals should be available for transport to avoid injury to hospital personnel.

When transferring the patient to the operating table, a mechanical lifting device may be required if the patient cannot move on his or her own. Obese patients tend to be self-conscious; therefore, respect for the patient should be shown and exposure kept to a minimum when transporting and transferring. Once the patient is on the operating bed, a pillow should be placed under the patient's knees and the safety belt should be placed about 2 inches above the knees.

A venous cutdown may be required to insert an intravenous (IV) line if peripheral veins are not visible. Intubation may be difficult due to limited mobility of the cervical spine. Due to decreased pulmonary functions, lower concentrations of anesthetic gases reach the lungs, therefore increasing the induction time. Higher concentrations of anesthetic agents are required due to their uptake by large amounts of adipose tissue; therefore, postoperative anesthesia recovery time is increased because adipose tissue retains fat-soluble anesthetic agents. In addition, poor blood supply to adipose tissue contributes to the slow elimination of these agents.

Care must be taken when positioning the obese patient on the operating room table. Extra personnel should be present to help prevent injury to personnel and to prevent the patient from falling. In many instances, two operating tables are situated next to each other to accommodate the larger patient. Tissue must be protected from injury because folds of tissue can be caught in the crevices of the operating table. Skin wrinkles should be smoothed out when positioning to avoid cutting off the blood supply to the tissue, possibly causing skin ulcers and tissue necrosis. Areas of concern should be padded to prevent bruising and pressure injuries.

The proper principles of grounding pad placement must be followed. Avoid skin wrinkles when placing or the pad will not be in full contact with the patient. One surgical technologist may have to use both hands to slightly "stretch" the skin to remove wrinkles and provide a smooth surface, while the other applies the pad to the patient. To avoid tissue burns, the pad should not be surrounded by overlapping skin folds.

For many procedures, long and deep instruments will be required, such as long needle holders, large retractors, large blades for self-retaining retractors, and long hemostats. Ties may have to be cut longer than usual for use by the surgeon in the deep wound, and longer carriers may be required for ties. The surgical technologist should be prepared for a lengthier procedure than normal.

As previously mentioned, healing is delayed due to the poor blood supply to the adipose tissue. Obese patients are prone to an increased incidence of postoperative wound infections. They are also more disposed to wound disruptions, such as wound dehiscence or evisceration. The surgical technologist should be prepared for various closure preferences of surgeons, such as the use of Montgomery straps or retention suture devices such as retention suture bridges and looped sutures.

Specific Considerations of Bariatric Surgery

Many patients with obesity who come to surgery have preoperative morbidity, primarily respiratory insufficiency and insulin-dependent diabetes. Surgery itself increases the risks of the patient who is obese, including postoperative wound infection, dehiscence, pulmonary embolism, anesthetic complications, acute respiratory failure, thrombophlebitis, ventricular failure, postoperative asphyxia in patients with obstructive sleep apnea syndrome, and anastomotic leaks.

Obese patients are high-risk patients for coronary artery disease because of hypertension and diabetes. Cardiac dysfunction is also associated with respiratory insufficiency. Perioperative ECGs are very important throughout the process of caring for these patients.

Obese patients present numerous difficulties for the anesthesia provider. The patient is at significant risk for anesthesia complications, in particular during induction. This risk is increased for patients with respiratory insufficiency. Obese patients tend to have short, large necks with limited mobility, making intubation and ventilation more of a challenge. The anesthesia provider may need assistance when intubating the patient; the assistant should elevate the jaw and hyperextend the neck while the anesthesia provider performs the intubation. Placing the patient in the reverse Trendelenburg position expands total lung volume and aids in ventilation. However, this leg-down position predisposes the patient to venous stasis and thrombophlebitis. Therefore, when setting up the room prior to the procedure, the surgical technologist should make sure that a **venous compression device** is in the room and that the patient is fitted with intermittent venous compression boots.

As previously mentioned, obese patients are at risk for deep venous thrombosis (DVT). This risk increases with a prolonged surgical procedure or postoperative period in which the patient is immobile and when the patient is in the supine position during surgery. Prophylactic anticoagulant therapy, such as heparin, is typically administered subcutaneously 30 minutes before the procedure and at intervals for at least 2 days postoperatively. As mentioned, the reverse Trendelenburg position significantly improves pulmonary function, but intermittent venous compression boots must be used to reduce the incidence of DVT. The patient should also attempt to walk as soon as possible postoperatively to aid the prevention of thrombosis.

Postoperatively, the obese patient should be kept in the reverse Trendelenburg position. When respiratory insufficiency is not present, most patients can be extubated in the OR or PACU and returned to their hospital rooms.

Complications After Gastric Surgery

The three most common complications after gastric bypass or gastroplasty surgery are abdominal catastrophes, internal hernia, and acute gastric distention. It can be difficult to diagnose an abdominal catastrophe in obese patients. The symptoms and the complaints of the patient are of great importance, and signs of infection may not be present. Often acute respiratory failure indicates peritonitis. If visceral perforation is suspected, an exploratory laparotomy will be performed.

Gastric bypass patients are at risk for internal hernia with a closed-loop obstruction leading to bowel strangulation. Left untreated, necrosis can result. The primary symptom is periumbilical pain, and, again, exploratory laparotomy will be performed for repair.

Postoperatively, gastric bypass patients can develop severe gaseous distention in the distal bypassed stomach. This can lead to gastric perforation or can damage the gastrojejunostomy. Symptoms include hiccups, bloated feeling, severe left shoulder pain, and shock. Diagnosis is made by taking an upright abdominal radiograph that will show the dilated stomach. An emergency laparotomy with insertion of a gastrostomy tube is performed along with examination of the jejunostomy.

Gallstones

During abdominal procedures on obese patients, gallstones are often found (in addition to the original pathology) and the gallbladder is removed. Therefore, when performing an abdominal procedure on these patients, the surgical technologist should have the instrumentation and other supplies available for a cholecystectomy with possible cholangiography.

Degenerative Osteoarthritis

Degenerative osteoarthritis of the back, hips, and knees is common in individuals who are obese. Weight reduction may help reduce the pain and increase the mobility of the patient, but often the damage is extensive, requiring a total joint arthroplasty. However, in very large patients (250 pounds or more), loosening of the prosthesis is common. Often, the surgeon requires the patient to lose a sufficient amount of weight before the arthroplasty is performed.

PATIENTS WITH DIABETES

Diabetes mellitus is a disorder of the endocrine system. It affects the production of insulin in the pancreas and glucose tolerance in the body. Insulin is the hormone that aids in breaking down sugars and carbohydrates. The origin of the disorder is most often genetic. There are two types of diabetes mellitus:

1. *Type 1—insulin-dependent diabetes mellitus (IDDM):* The pancreas produces little or no insulin, and the individual must have daily, regular doses of insulin.
2. *Type 2—non-insulin-dependent diabetes mellitus (NIDDM):* The pancreas produces different amounts of insulin. The individual is not required to take insulin and blood glucose levels are usually controlled by diet.

When performing surgery on patients who are diabetic, the following conditions must be prevented:

- Ketonuria
- Hyperglycemia
- Ketoacidosis
- Acetonuria
- Hypoglycemia and hypoglycemic shock

Preoperative preparation of the patient includes:

- Fasting
- Urinalysis to determine presence of sugar and acetone
- Complete blood count (CBC)
- Blood urea nitrogen (BUN)
- Postprandial blood sugar level
- Serum electrolyte level
- Chest radiograph
- ECG

Complications Associated with Diabetes

Surgery affects the normal caloric intake of the patient and daily dosage of insulin. Anesthesia also affects the normal metabolic processes of the patient with diabetes. Blood glucose can increase while the serum insulin levels decrease. NIDDM patients usually go through surgery without any difficulties. Perioperative metabolic control of the IDDM patient presents the surgery team with unique challenges and difficulties, especially when the operation is lengthy and involves a large amount of tissue trauma. The diabetic patient is at a higher risk for the following:

- *Infection* (Ulcers that develop on the extremities, particularly the foot, heal slowly or not at all and are prone to infection. Many elderly patients with diabetes must undergo extremity amputation to control an infection of the extremity that is not responding to antibiotics or other surgical interventions.)
- *Dehydration*
- *Poor circulation combined with vascular disease*
- *Hypertension and myocardial infarction*
- *Delayed wound healing and infection*
- *Nephropathy*
- *Control of postoperative blood glucose level*
- *Neuropathic musculoskeletal disease resulting in severe bone destruction*
- *Neurogenic bladder resulting in frequent (UTIs)*
- *Retinopathy resulting in blindness*
- *Coronary artery disease*
- *Thrombophlebitis and peripheral edema*
- *Tachycardia*
- *Peripheral edema*

Care of the Patient with Diabetes in Surgery

Diabetic patients require specific preoperative, intraoperative, and postoperative procedures to ensure their safety:

Preoperative

- A blood sample for the fasting serum glucose test is taken to provide data for postoperative care of the patient.
- The normal dosage of preoperative medication is decreased since narcotics can induce vomiting, which predisposes the patient to fluid and electrolyte imbalance, causing a hypoglycemic reaction.
- The preoperative insulin dose is reduced to prevent intraoperative hypoglycemia or insulin shock.
- When positioning the patient, bony prominences and other areas of concern must be adequately padded to prevent pressure sores and ulcers, particularly if the operation will be lengthy.
- Procedures on diabetic patients should be the first cases of the day so these patients can get back on their regular dietary schedule as soon as possible.

Intraoperative

- IV access is accomplished by the anesthesia provider to monitor insulin and glucose levels. Electrolytes can be added to the IV fluids to maintain balance. Insulin can be added to the IV fluids or given as a subcutaneous injection.
- Monitoring, especially during long procedures, is important to avoid a metabolic crisis. Monitoring is necessary to determine the patient's needs for insulin, glucose, or both. A glucometer is used to measure the blood glucose level. Urine specimens are monitored for the presence of ketones.
- Antiembolic stockings are worn by the patient during surgery to prevent thromboembolism.
- Adherence to strict sterile techniques is of paramount importance when operating on the diabetic patient.

Postoperative

An increased rate of infection is one of the most common postoperative complications of diabetes, primarily due to diminished levels of blood flow to the affected area. Postoperative stress hormone levels predispose the patient to hyperglycemia, as do changes in activity level and some medications or their interactions with other drugs administered postoperatively. In addition, glucose-lowering agents used to control hyperglycemia preoperatively should influence decisions regarding perioperative glucose management.

Postoperatively, the patient should be:

- Provided with proper nutrients (either intravenously or orally) for healing and glucose control
- Administered the proper type and dose of antihyperglycemic medications
- Fitted with intermittent/sequential venous compression boots to prevent thromboembolism or DVT

PREGNANT PATIENTS

There are approximately 4.31 million live births per year in the United States. Approximately 1% to 2% of pregnancies require surgery for reasons other than cesarean section or spontaneous abortion. When planning surgery on the pregnant patient, two patients must be taken into consideration: the mother and the fetus. Immediate operative intervention is done for emergencies, such as ectopic pregnancy, appendicitis, trauma injury, or incompetent cervix. Urgent surgical procedures are delayed until after the second or third trimester, or until the mother delivers. Elective procedures are definitely delayed until after delivery and the mother has had some time to recover from the ordeal of pregnancy and delivery.

Surgical procedures performed in the first trimester should be postponed if possible, due to the increased chances of spontaneous abortion. Abdominal procedures are best performed in the second trimester. In the second trimester, the fetus is stable and the tissue of major organs is well differentiated. In addition, since the uterus has not greatly enlarged, the abdominal organs have not been displaced from their normal position to any great degree, making it easier to expose the wound, retract, and manipulate the organs. For procedures performed in the third trimester, there is a 40% risk of premature labor, and further difficulties are encountered due to the displacement of organs by the enlarged uterus.

Considerations When Caring for Pregnant Patients

Due to the size of the late-term uterus, the abdominal organs are displaced from their normal anatomical location; additionally, anatomical landmarks are difficult to locate. This can make trauma and disease diagnoses difficult. When surgery is being contemplated, the anatomical changes must be considered. For example, a pregnant patient with appendicitis may initially be thought to have cholecystitis since the appendix is displaced to the lower region of the upper right quadrant (appendicitis and acute cholecystitis are the two most common nonobstetric emergencies in the pregnant patient). Results of laboratory tests are skewed by the hormonal and physiological changes of pregnancy, and the results vary according to the gestational stage.

Physiological assessment is difficult since pregnancy alters vital signs. The pulse rate increases to compensate for the increase in circulatory volume. The arterial blood pressure is lower as compared to prepregnancy levels. The diagnosis of hypovolemic shock is especially challenging. The pregnant patient may not immediately display the classic physiological signs of shock (such as cool and clammy skin) because of decreased peripheral vascular resistance. Circulating blood volume may decrease as much as 30% before the patient has signs of hypovolemic shock (such as decreased blood pressure and increased pulse rate). By that time, blood is being shunted away from the placental circulation and the fetus becomes hypoxic. The intraoperative and postoperative use of the electronic fetal heart monitor (EFM) is vital for prevention of hypovolemic shock.

Postoperatively, the patient must be observed for vaginal bleeding, ruptured membranes, or uterine irritability. These symptoms can indicate preterm labor. Bladder distention can also cause uterine irritability and preterm labor; therefore, the indwelling catheter should be left in place for monitoring fluid status. The EFM should continue to be used as well.

Anesthesia

The three important items to remember are the increase in preterm labor, fetal death, and low birth weight when general anesthesia must be used. With this in mind, the following are considerations for the safe delivery of anesthesia to the pregnant patient.

Anesthetic agents cross the placental barrier and enter the fetal circulation. The fetal liver is not developed; therefore, it slowly metabolizes narcotics and tranquilizers. Preferably, only short-acting drugs should be used. Drugs that have an adverse effect on the fetus in the first trimester include sedatives, tranquilizers, halogenated agents, and nitrous oxide (also a consideration for the pregnant team member who breathes in these scattered fumes). Fetal respiratory depression is a common occurrence with the use of any of these drugs. Other adverse effects of drugs on the fetus include bradycardia (bupivacaine) and central nervous system depression (lidocaine).

The most important consideration in the delivering of anesthetic agents is to prevent preterm labor. Halogenated agents decrease the uterine tone and aid in preventing uterine contractions. On the other hand, vasopressors and neostigmine (reversed muscle relaxation) can stimulate preterm labor.

Intraoperative Considerations for the Surgical Technologist

The surgical technologist must be prepared to assist the surgeon in intraoperative monitoring activities and be prepared for any untoward events. The following are important considerations for the surgical technologist to remember:

- Without compromising patient care or violating the principles of asepsis, the surgical technologist should move as quickly as possible when assisting the surgeon to keep general anesthesia time to a minimum.
- The surgical technologist should aid the surgeon by palpating the uterus during the surgical procedure to detect contractions.
- The circulating surgical technologist should be available to assist the anesthesia provider by providing cricoid pressure during induction.
- When positioning the patient in the supine position, a small rolled sheet or pad should be placed under the right hip to slightly laterally shift the uterus to the left (Figure 4-1). Additionally, the operating room table may be tilted 30 degrees to the left and placed in slight Trendelenburg position to aid with venous return. This takes the weight of the uterus off the vena cava and abdominal aorta to aid in maintaining a normotensive level.
- If irrigation is used during the procedure, the assistant circulating surgical technologist should accurately document the amount used so that the anesthesia provider can estimate blood loss.
- Before the patient enters the OR, the assistant circulating surgical technologist should raise the temperature of the room to prevent maternal hypothermia. Plenty of warm blankets should be available to cover the patient.
- The surgical technologist should have the instrumentation, supplies, and equipment immediately available in the event that an emergency cesarean section must be performed.
- The surgical technologist should be aware that the transducer of the Doppler ultrasound scanner for fetal heart rate monitoring has been placed on the maternal abdominal wall away from the operative site.
- A sterile Doppler device may be necessary.

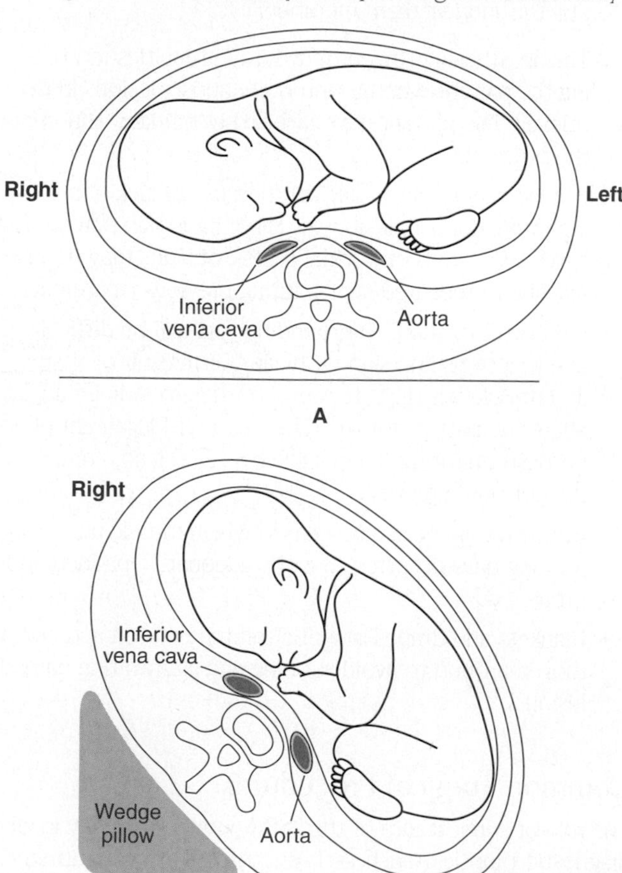

Figure 4-1 Relief of pressure: (A) pressure on aorta and vena cava caused by gravid uterus; (B) pressure is relieved by placing a wedge under right hip

IMMUNOCOMPROMISED PATIENTS

Immunocompetence is the degree of function for an immune system that is designed to keep a patient from infection by pathogens. The immunocompromised status of a patient can be influenced by many factors. Typically, the old or very young have immune systems that are compromised to a certain degree. Certain diseases, especially chronic ones that target the immune system, can decrease the body's ability to fight off infection by pathogens. The immune system can be intentionally suppressed by specific drugs to combat an overactive immune system that is attacking the body's own tissues instead of the foreign invaders for which it was intended. These **autoimmune diseases** include multiple sclerosis, lupus erythematosus, and rheumatoid arthritis. Immunosuppressant drugs are also administered to recipients of organ transplants to prevent the recipient's immune system from rejecting the newly transplanted organ. Patients who are receiving antineoplastic agents to combat cancer are also immunosuppressed.

It is extremely important for the surgical technologist to remember the immunocompromised patient's decreased ability to fight infection. Therefore, strict adherence to sterile technique is imperative. Additionally, the surgical technologist should be cognizant of the following physical manifestations of the patient in order to provide the needed physical and emotional support to the patient and family members:

- skin rashes
- skin lesions

- poor nutritional status
- painful joints
- possible cardiovascular complications
- generalized malaise

Acquired Immunodeficiency Syndrome

Patients with AIDS have tested positive for the **human immunodeficiency virus (HIV)** and are symptomatic, usually of an opportunistic disease that the compromised immune system has allowed to take hold. In fact, AIDS patients are often inflicted with several opportunistic infections, many of which were not commonly seen until AIDS arrived, including **Kaposi's sarcoma**, severe psoriasis rash of the body, *Pneumocystis carinii* pneumonia (PCP), and other fungal and parasitic infections. HIV is grouped in the family of retroviruses and may remain inactive and undetected for a long period of time before causing disease. Once active, the virus disrupts the normal functions of the T-lymphocytes of the body, thus impairing the patient's immune system. However, during the time of inactivity in which there are no outward signs of infection, the individual can transmit the virus through blood or body fluids.

At one point in time, HIV/AIDS was considered an exclusive disease of homosexual male behavior, intravenous drug users, or recipients of transfused blood containing HIV. We now know that anyone is susceptible to transmission, especially during unprotected sex or through the sharing of contaminated needles. In addition, infected pregnant females can transmit the virus to the unborn fetus.

Complications

As previously mentioned, surgical patients with AIDS may present with multiple opportunistic infections by parasites, fungi, viruses, or bacteria; overall, the general poor health demands special care of the patient. The patient often experiences pain from various complications and should be carefully handled and made as comfortable as possible.

A common complication is the presence of multiple external and internal lesions due to Kaposi's sarcoma. The external Kaposi's sarcoma lesions are often painful, open infectious wounds, so care must be taken not to aggravate these lesions when transporting patients and positioning them in surgery. Internal Kaposi's sarcoma can cause the following complications, providing additional challenges to the surgery team:

- If located in the esophagus, the lesions can make it difficult for the patient to swallow or can prevent swallowing altogether.
- Intestinal lesions can cause bowel obstruction and prevent the normal absorption of nutrients. Chronic nausea, vomiting, anorexia, and diarrhea are common symptoms of the AIDS patient, contributing to overall tissue and muscle wasting of the body.

Considerations for the Surgical Team Members

Surgical technologists must keep in mind the poor physical condition of the AIDS patient. Most systems of the body will be involved either directly or indirectly in the disease process, requiring a comprehensive plan of care that addresses all concerns. All members of the surgical team must show compassion, empathy, and professionalism without allowing personal feelings about the stigma attached to AIDS to impact the care that they are providing. As with all surgical patients, the need for confidentiality of patient information is critical.

As discussed, the patient may present with extreme muscle and tissue wasting; additional personnel should be available to lift and move from the hospital bed to the stretcher and from the stretcher to the operating table. The patient may not be able to move due to weakness, painful joints, and skin lesions. The use of extra personnel will ensure a smooth transfer, causing as little pain as possible for the patient.

Many routine procedures are going to be difficult to perform. The following are examples of the difficulties encountered by the surgical team members:

- The anesthesia provider may have difficulties intubating the patient who has internal Kaposi's lesions in the trachea. The patient may have to be "masked" throughout the procedure.
- IV placement will be difficult because of lack of a suitable vein. Kaposi's lesions or candidiasis skin patches may cover large areas of normal access, or veins may be "used up" due to repeated sticks during previous treatments.
- Placement of the ESU grounding pad will be difficult due to lesions and skin wrinkling (as a result of tissue and muscle wasting). Removal of the grounding pad can injure the patient for the same reasons. Placement of adhesive monitoring devices (such as ECG leads) may also disrupt skin integrity.
- Bony prominences and areas in which muscle and tissue wasting have occurred must be adequately padded and protected.
- Blankets and drapes must be carefully placed and not moved around to avoid rubbing and aggravating painful lesions.

Common Surgical Procedures

The role of surgical care of the AIDS patient primarily involves diagnostic biopsies (such as bronchoscopy) and treatment of complications of malignancies and infections. Cryptosporidiosis and cytomegalovirus infections frequently occur in the biliary tree, causing acute cholecystitis and cholangitis, requiring emergency repair (a choledochoenteric bypass may also be performed). *Candida* infection and Kaposi's sarcoma have also been documented as causing cholangitis, requiring bypass surgery.

Acute perforations of the GI tract from cytomegalovirus infection, cryptosporidiosis, and candidiasis have been documented, requiring bowel resection, bypass, or colostomy. GI obstruction due to Kaposi's sarcoma lesions also requires bowel surgery. A study of AIDS patients requiring an abdominal operation described four clinical syndromes that require surgical intervention:

1. Peritonitis secondary to cytomegalovirus infection
2. Non-Hodgkin's lymphoma of the GI tract resulting in obstruction and/or bleeding
3. Kaposi's sarcoma lesions of the GI tract
4. Mycobacterial infection of the retroperitoneum or spleen

Thrombocytopenia is another complication of AIDS patients. **Splenectomy** (removal of the spleen) obtains very good results in these patients and for those experiencing **splenomegaly** (enlargement of the spleen). Debilitating fevers are associated with splenomegaly, and the patient experiences positive palliative effects after splenectomy.

A frequent procedure performed by the general surgeon is placement of an indwelling catheter. The primary care physician will request the surgery in order to have long-term access for the treatment of fungal infections and for nutritional support of AIDS patients with debilitating diarrhea.

PHYSICALLY CHALLENGED OR SENSORY IMPAIRED PATIENTS

Often, surgical technologists encounter patients who have various sensory, physical, or mental challenges that can cause increased levels of anxiety for the patient preoperatively and postoperatively. Patients may be physically, developmentally, or mentally impaired and surgical technologists should be aware of the psychosocial and physical needs of these patients.

Patients with hearing impairments may be totally deaf or impaired to varying degrees. Patients who are partially deaf are typically required to remove their hearing aid devices prior to surgery, so they may not be able to understand spoken commands. In this case, or if the patient is totally deaf, the surgical team may be required to communicate via hand signals or sign language (an interpreter may be necessary). Occasionally, written commands may be necessary. Nonverbal communication is very important, and a gentle touch goes a long way in the transmission of a comforting emotion. It is often helpful for a surgical team member to make a preoperative visit to the unit while the patient still has a hearing aid in place, or while family members are available to translate for the totally deaf, and give details of what will transpire in the OR. This will relieve some anxiety on the part of the patient.

Patients with visual impairments may be blind or have a visual impairment that can be corrected with eyeglasses. Eyeglasses are typically not allowed to accompany the patient to the OR, but should be available for the patient upon awakening from the anesthesia. Contact lenses are removed in the unit because they can cause corneal damage if the surgical team forgets to remove them before anesthesia is administered. Patients with visual impairments can usually hear verbal commands, but may require assistance (and possibly extra personnel) in carrying out those commands. An explanation of their surroundings, including a description of who is in the room, will ease anxiety about unfamiliar areas.

Physical challenges, such as the absence of an extremity or severe arthritis, contractures, deformities, paralysis, tremors, and stiffness, may require the surgical team to take extra precautions when moving the patient from the stretcher to the operating table, and when positioning the patient after the administration of anesthesia. Extra personnel and positioning/padding devices that protect the patient may be necessary. The surgical team should be aware of any chronic disease that could affect respiration or circulation and thus require extra precautions during positioning to protect those systems and the tissues that they serve.

A paralyzed patient will require extra personnel for transport from the stretcher to the operating table, and should be carefully positioned due to chronic wasting of muscles that can lead to skin injury or compression of nerves or vessels. Special care must be taken to ensure patient safety during the transfer and to prevent falls and injury.

Surgical technologists may come in contact with patients who have a cognitive impairment. "Cognitive impairment" is the term used to describe a condition that limits an individual's ability to learn and to reason. Individuals who are developmentally delayed may have cognitive disabilities, but this group also includes many people who have normal intelligence. These individuals exhibit a delay in their physical or cognitive development.

Members of the surgical team may struggle to communicate with patients who have impaired cognitive function. These patients may show a reduced capacity to learn, remember, think, or solve problems. It may be challenging to provide explanations about the surgical procedure and the surgical environment. The patient with a cognitive impairment may become anxious or fearful of all aspects of the surgical experience. It may become difficult to obtain cooperation from the patient before, during, and after the surgical procedure. The surgical team should make every attempt to communicate with the patient at the patient's level of understanding. The surgical team must communicate with the parent or legal guardian in these instances, especially when referencing the surgical consent and any additional information related to the surgical intervention. Caring for patients with cognitive impairment requires a team approach to meeting their individual needs throughout their treatments and procedures. Box 4-1 provides a specific example of caring for a mentally challenged patient.

CARING FOR THE PATIENT WITH DOWN'S SYNDROME IN SURGERY

Down's syndrome (DS) is associated with some impairment of cognitive abilities and growth. Individuals with DS tend to have a lower-than-average cognitive ability ranging from mild to moderate disabilities. A small number may have severe mental disabilities, and for the most part DS patients adapt very well to life in general, including learning independent living skills (including a few DS individuals who have been given major awards as actors and actresses). However, there are health concerns that the DS patient can face, including congenital heart defects, gastroesophageal reflux disease (GERD), recurrent ear infections, obstructive sleep apnea, and thyroid dysfunctions. The surgical technologist must remember that DS patients undergoing surgery at an early age may be very frightened, and time should be taken with the patient to establish a rapport as well as comfort when transporting to the OR. The language skills of the DS patient may be lacking; there could be a noticeable difference between understanding what is being said and expressing speech because DS patients often have a speech delay. Therefore, patience is of utmost importance as well as slow, deliberate movements so as not to startle the patient. The parent(s) or legal guardian should be present while transporting to the surgery department, and allowed in preoperative holding and brought into PACU as soon as feasible. In the OR, again, patience is key; gaining the trust of the DS patient can go a long way in securing cooperation. The OR should be kept quiet; the surgical technologist in the first scrub role may need to stop setting up the back table and Mayo stand until the patient is under anesthesia to avoid noise. Talking slowly with the DS patient and holding his or her hand builds trust; DS patients tend to be "clingy" and to an appropriate degree returning the affection can go a long way toward securing the trust and cooperation of the DS patient. Physically, DS patients tend to have microgenia, muscle hypotonia, a flat nasal bridge, macroglossia, a short neck, and excessive joint laxity. Obviously, these physical traits must be taken into consideration by the anesthesia provider and PACU personnel; additionally, the surgical team must be well aware of the muscle hypotonia and joint laxity when positioning the patient.

ISOLATION PATIENTS

Obviously, surgical technologists come into contact with patients on a daily basis. Therefore, it is important for the surgical technologist to be aware of the risk of transmission of microorganisms among patients, from patients to hospital staff, and among hospital staff. The Occupational Safety and Health Administration (OSHA) along with the Centers for Disease Control and Prevention (CDC) and its division, the National Institute for Occupational Safety and Health (NIOSH), have established policies and regulations such as the OSHA Bloodborne Pathogens Final Rule and the CDC Standard Precautions that hospital departments must implement. These policies are discussed in detail in Chapters 5 and 7. The following section addresses on a general basis the isolation precautions the surgical team members should follow; these precautions are based on CDC guidelines.

The primary routes of transmission of microorganisms include:

- Contact: direct or indirect
- Droplet
- Airborne
- Common vehicle (food, water, medications, medical devices, and equipment)
- Vector-borne (mosquitoes, flies, rats)

Isolation precautions are intended to prevent the transmission of pathogenic microorganisms in the hospital through the routes listed above. Patients who are identified as being infected with a serious and epidemiologically important microorganism, such as *Mycobacterium tuberculosis,* which causes tuberculosis, must be isolated to prevent transmission to other patients and hospital staff. However, the surgical technologist must be aware of the challenges the patient faces when in isolation and be empathetic to these factors, including limited contact with family and friends, which can be psychologically harmful, especially for the pediatric patient. Additionally, due to the precautions that health care providers must take, such as wearing respirators, gowns, etc., the patient can perceive his or her care as being cold and impersonal, and may feel disconnected from others. If the isolation patient requires surgery, the surgical team should put forth extra effort to communicate and reassure the patient to show that a caring environment is still critical to a positive surgical outcome for the patient.

The basic fundamentals of care of the isolated patient in the surgical environment include:

- Frequent handwashing
- Wearing gloves (sterile surgical team members wear sterile gloves; nonsterile team members wear nonsterile exam gloves)
- Wearing gowns (sterile surgical team members wear sterile gowns; nonsterile team members wear some type of nonsterile gown. Nonsterile gowns are worn by health care providers who work in the preoperative holding area and PACU.)
- Wearing eye protection or face shields
- Wearing masks (HEPA)

The wearing of protective attire is mandated by the OSHA bloodborne pathogens final rule. However, the CDC also requires the wearing of a NIOSH-certified respirator through its tuberculosis standards. The minimum allowable respiratory protection device is a filtering (nonpowered, air-purifying, half-facepiece) respirator, such as the N95 disposable respirator model. Of extreme importance is the fit testing of the respirator. The facial size and characteristics of the health care worker must be taken into consideration to achieve the proper fit of the respirator or its effectiveness will be negated. Additionally, it must be ensured that the health care worker knows how to properly don the respirator.

Two last items of general concern that relate to the surgical team are transport of the isolation patient and handling of surgical instruments, equipment, supplies, and linen. When the patient is to be transported from the isolation room to the surgery department, the following are recommended precautions:

- Health care workers and patient are wearing appropriate barriers including masks, gowns, respirator (if necessary), and gloves, and if patient has had a previous invasive procedure, the wound site has the proper impervious dressing applied.
- All surgery personnel, including preoperative holding, anesthesia, and PACU personnel, are notified that the isolation patient will be arriving into the department and told to take the necessary precautions to reduce the risk of transmission of infectious microorganisms.
- Patients are provided preoperative teaching of the ways they can assist in preventing the transmission of their infectious microorganism(s) during transport to the surgery department.

In most instances, the surgical instruments, equipment, supplies, and linen do not require any additional special handling other than what is routinely done. The dirty surgical instruments should be transported to the decontamination room in an enclosed container and disinfected and sterilized according to hospital policy. Sharps, including needles, scalpels, trocars, and electrosurgical tips, should be disposed of in a puncture-resistant container. Patient care equipment should be wiped down and cleaned with the proper type of broad-spectrum disinfectant according to hospital policy; particular attention should be focused on equipment that comes into contact with the patient, such as tourniquets. Linen should be placed in a leak-proof bag and all attempts should be made to prevent contaminating the outside of the bag when placing the linen inside; otherwise, double bag the linen. Contaminated single-use and disposable patient care equipment and supplies should be handled and transported in a manner to reduce the risk of transmission of microorganisms and decrease the chances of environmental contamination in the hospital. Environmental services personnel should be notified as soon as possible to remove the trash and linen from the surgery department.

GERIATRIC PATIENTS

Geriatric patients are those in a specific age group (usually over the age of 65 years), although the label is meaningless as the only indicator for surgical risk because many patients over the age of 65 are healthier than some young adults. However, for the typical older patient, some form of chronic debilitation or decreased physiologic status (especially cardiovascular and respiratory) is present that requires special consideration and precautions by the surgical team (Table 4-5). Preoperative assessment and planning that take this status into consideration are imperative for proper surgical outcomes, as is evidenced by the fact that emergency procedures on geriatric patients are associated with much higher mortality rates than elective ones, primarily because proper planning was not possible (Figure 4-2). The geriatric population represents a challenge to the entire surgical team, in particular since approximately 80% of geriatric patients present with one or more comorbid conditions when entering the surgical environment.

Geriatric patients may come to the OR with visual and hearing impairments that require the considerations

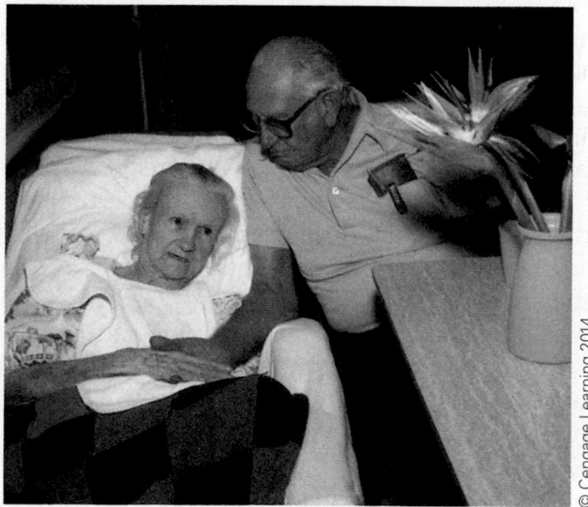

Figure 4-2 Geriatric patient

Table 4-5 Physiological Changes in the Elderly Patient

System	*Normal Physiological Changes*
Integumentary	Loss of skin elasticity
	Loss of subcutaneous fat
	Skin more prone to damage from pressure and shear forces
	Skin lesions, tags, and warts
Musculoskeletal	Loss of bone mass
	Skeletal instability
	Curvature of the spine
	Arthritis and osteoporosis
	Decreased range of motion and balance
Cardiovascular	Decreased coronary artery blood flow
	Increased blood pressure
	Decreased ability to tolerate insult
Respiratory	Decreased lung elasticity
	Increased rigidity in the chest wall
	Reduced tidal exchange
Digestive	Decreased salivary and digestive gland secretion
	Decreased peristalsis and gastric motility
	Decreased body water and plasma volume
Genitourinary	Decreased nephron function
	Decreased tone in ureters, bladder, and urethra
	Decreased bladder capacity
Nervous	Decreased cerebral blood flow with accompanying psychological changes
	Decreased position sense in extremities
	Increased tolerance to pain
	Numerous sensory changes related to both central nervous system and sensory organ change

discussed in the previous section. To facilitate psychologic security, items such as dentures, hearing aids, and eyeglasses should be returned to the geriatric patient as soon as possible. In addition, elderly patients are often arthritic and suffer from restricted movements of extremities and fragile skin that require special consideration when lifting, transporting, and positioning. Cardiovascular and respiratory impairments must be considered during anesthesia and surgical positioning. Elderly patients can easily become hypothermic in an OR, so warm blankets are imperative. A forced-air warming blanket may be applied to the patient during anesthesia. Geriatric patients may have slow circulation and hypotension, which may place them at an increased risk of emboli and thrombus formation. The application of antiembolic stockings or sequential compression devices helps to decrease this risk.

Watters and McClaran list the following eight critical factors for obtaining the best outcomes from surgical treatment on geriatric patients:

1. Careful preoperative preparation of the patient and optimization of medical and physiological status
2. Appropriate anesthesia and physiological monitoring
3. Recognition of alterations in clinical pharmacology
4. Minimization of the postoperative stresses of hypothermia, hypoxemia, and pain
5. Prevention of alterations in blood pressure and heart rate
6. Avoidance of perturbations of fluid, electrolyte, and acid–base status
7. Careful surgical technique
8. Optimization of functional level

Convalescence issues for the elderly are influenced by the possible lack of immediate family to provide postoperative care, which can increase the length of hospital stays. Nursing home or home health care may need to be arranged by hospital personnel.

SUBSTANCE ABUSE PATIENTS

Substance abuse patients (e.g., alcoholism, illegal drugs, prescription drugs) challenge the skills of all health care workers due to the range of difficult situations that must be managed, such as behavioral problems and the co-morbid disorders associated with the substance abuse. The two primary difficulties encountered by the surgical team are the behavior of the patient that contributes to the level of communication that can be established. Often the substance abuse patient is brought to the OR as a trauma victim, which adds to the intensity of the situation. The behavior of the patient can range from violent to somewhat calm to catatonic based on the patient's drug of choice and how much has been ingested. Violent patients are going to be very difficult to communicate with in the OR, and it is difficult to gain any level of cooperation, whereas the "calm" patient (one who may have taken depressants such as a tranquilizer or barbiturate) may be more willing to cooperate.

A significant factor to be remembered by the surgical team is the co-morbid psychiatric disorders that often drove the patient to abuse alcohol and/or medications in the first place. Studies suggest that 30% to 80% of substance abusers suffer from coexisting psychiatric illness (Scimeca, Savage, Portenoy, & Lowinson, 2000). A high prevalence of anxiety disorder, panic disorder, depression, and bipolar syndrome is seen in substance abuse patients (Scimeca et al.). Add to this the pain the patient is experiencing from trauma or need for urgent surgery (e.g., gallstones, hernia, etc.).

The surgical team would benefit from the presence of a counselor or social worker to provide assistance to the team and patient. If the patient is in treatment and the procedure is urgent or elective, it is recommended the patient's counselor be included in the preoperative conversations with the patient as well as accompany the patient to the preoperative holding and PACU on the day of surgery. The day of surgery it also helps if the counselor and/or family members communicate the "mood" of the patient to the surgery team prior to transport to the OR so the team knows what to expect and how to properly react.

TRAUMA PATIENTS

In 2008, over 29 million people in the United States were affected by nonfatal trauma, and in 2007 182,479 trauma deaths occurred (CDC, 2009). Treating the trauma patient is a challenge due to the multiple injuries that can be sustained by the individual. A single bullet or a car accident can injure several body structures, requiring the efforts of several surgeons and more than one surgical team. The surgical technologist must be prepared to assist on any type of surgical procedure when treating a trauma patient.

THE "GOLDEN HOUR" AND TRAUMA SYSTEM

Military physicians became aware, when treating those injured during war (e.g., World Wars I and II, the Korean and Vietnam conflicts), that the shorter the response time, the greater is the chance for survival of the trauma patient. Recent studies have also shown that the sooner CPR is begun for a heart attack victim, the greater is the chance that the heart rhythm will return to normal with less damage to the heart muscle. This concept, when applied to the civilian population, is classically referred to as the **golden hour**, meaning that reaching the trauma victim and providing treatment within the first hour following injury is critical in determining the patient's outcome. The time immediately after an injury has been sustained is the best time for rapid and aggressive interventions to effectively reduce morbidity and mortality.

The emergency medical services (EMS) system has also greatly facilitated the treatment of trauma patients by providing a system for rapid transportation to a facility designated as being able to provide optimal treatment. Facilities that are designated as trauma centers have met certain criteria indicating that they can meet the specialized treatment needs of the various types of trauma injuries. In the United States, trauma centers are ranked by the American College of Surgeons (ACS) as Level I, Level II, and Level III. Some states have independent rankings separate from the ACS. Trauma centers are commonly designated as one of four trauma levels:

- *Level I trauma center:* Can meet all needs required for treating trauma patients, including qualified personnel and equipment on a 24-hour basis, offering a comprehensive service and the highest level of surgical care.
- *Level II trauma center:* Can treat seriously injured or ill patients, but does not have all of the resources that a Level I facility would have. Level II trauma centers work in collaboration with Level I centers.
- *Level III trauma center:* Most often a community or rural hospital in an area that does not have a Level I or II facility. These centers offer limited care and have resources for immediate care until the trauma patient is stabilized and then transported to a Level I or II hospital.
- *Level IV trauma center:* Available in some states, the center can provide advanced trauma life support to stabilize the patient before the patient is transported to a Level I or II hospital. It provides initial evaluation, stabilization, diagnostic capabilities, and transfer to a higher level of care.

KINEMATICS

Compared to elective surgical procedures, little information is usually available to the health care team about the trauma patient and preparation time can be short. What does provide valuable information is the **kinematics** or *mechanism of injury (MOI)*. MOI is the action and effect of a particular type of force on the human body. By knowing the types of injuries caused by certain types of forces, the health care team can be better prepared to treat the trauma patient. For example, a bullet wound will produce a different action and effect on the body than a knife wound.

Three factors are important when considering the resulting injury the patient will sustain due to these various forces:

1. Velocity of the injuring force
2. Flexibility of the tissue
3. Shape of the injuring force

For example, bones have little flexibility, resulting in fractures and shattering, whereas a soft tissue injury due to blunt trauma often results in organ damage and bruising.

Blunt Trauma

Blunt trauma results from forces such as deceleration, acceleration, compression, and shearing. Breaks in the integrity of the skin are often not present, making diagnosis difficult. Examples in which blunt trauma is sustained include motor vehicle accidents (MVAs), falls, assaults (hit with a fist or blunt object), and sports injuries. MVAs account for a large percentage of blunt trauma injuries. The spleen is the number one organ injured in an MVA. Three types of collisions can occur during an MVA:

1. Car collides with another object.
2. Person inside car collides with objects such as steering wheel or dashboard.
3. Internal body structure collides with a rigid bony surface. For example, a motorcyclist is thrown from the motorcycle and hits a tree. The brain is accelerating forward and when the person hits the tree, the brain tissue rapidly decelerates by colliding with the frontal portion of the cranium, causing severe blunt trauma.

Common injuries sustained in MVAs include the following:

- Not wearing a seat belt
  - Head and neck injuries
  - Facial injuries
  - Fractures of the sternum, clavicle, patella, and femur
  - Liver or spleen lacerations
  - Bruising of the heart muscle
- Wearing a seat belt that is a combination of lap and shoulder belts, and airbag inflation
  - Liver and spleen lacerations
  - Pelvic fractures
  - Neck injuries, including cervical bone fractures
  - Bruising of the heart muscle
  - Rupture of the diaphragm
  - Facial fractures
  - Humeral, radial, and ulnar fractures (airbag related)

Penetrating Trauma

Penetrating trauma results when a foreign object passes through tissue. The most common foreign objects are bullets and knives. The extent of the injury depends on the:

- Type of foreign object
- Size of foreign object, such as the caliber of the bullet, or a pocket knife versus a Bowie knife
- Distance the victim was from the foreign object
- Body structures that were penetrated
- Amount of energy (velocity) of the penetrating foreign object

Bullet injuries are classified as being low velocity (bullet travels 1,000 feet per second or slower) or high velocity (3,000 feet per second; commonly seen with military weapons). Factors that affect the extent of the injury include:

- High-velocity bullets, obviously, will cause more damage to tissue.
- The closer the victim is to the bullet as it leaves the weapon, the more damage that will result due to the increased speed of the bullet.
- Different bullets result in different types and severities of injury. For example, a hollow-point bullet mushrooms on impact, causing more tissue damage than other types of bullets.

If the bullet travels completely through the body (referred to as a *through and through*), the entrance wound tends to be smaller than the exit wound. For example, the bullets fired from an M-16 gun have a tumbling motion that produces a small entrance wound, but the exit wound is usually very large.

Stab wounds are low-velocity wounds. The width and length of the penetrating object influence the extent of the traumatic injury. The penetrating object must not be removed at the scene or in the emergency department; removal is done in the OR. The retained object provides a tamponade effect for bleeding. In addition, if removed at the scene, the course of entry cannot be exactly followed upon removal and additional damage to body organs and tissue can occur.

TRAUMA SCORING

Injuries are scored using the **Revised Trauma Score** (RTS) to assess the severity of the trauma. Assigning an RTS assists in the triage process and provides a standardized method of communicating between facilities if, for instance, the patient has to be transported. The RTS involves the Glasgow Coma Scale as well as other physiological factors.

CONSIDERATIONS FOR THE SURGICAL TECHNOLOGIST

Severely injured patients most likely will require multiple procedures, performed simultaneously or in succession. For example, a patient who has sustained severe fractures of the right leg and head trauma may have a neurosurgeon performing a craniotomy at the same time as an orthopedic surgeon is repairing the fractures. This presents a challenge to the surgical technologist as far as preparation. The surgeon(s) will communicate to the surgical technologist the order of procedures, which is based on treating those injuries that are life threatening or possibly permanently debilitating before other, lesser injuries. The typical order of priority is head, chest, abdomen, and extremities.

Preservation of Evidence

If the patient is a victim of a violent crime, many items will need to be preserved for the law enforcement officials as evidence against the perpetrator of the crime. All physical evidence must be carefully handled and facility policy must be followed for purposes of documentation. Evidence includes the patient's clothes, bullets and bullet fragments, knife fragments, trace evidence (hair), and biologic evidence (blood and body fluids).

As previously mentioned, the policies and procedures of the surgery department and law enforcement agency must be followed. The following are some general recommendations:

- Remove clothing by cutting along the seams and around bullet or stab wound holes. The shape of the hole can provide evidence as to the type of weapon that was used. The clothes should be placed in a paper bag or wrapped in a clean sheet and given to the law enforcement officials.
- Hair, tissue, and gunpowder residue may be found on the hands of the victim. If the hand(s) does not require surgery, a bag should be placed around the hand(s) and taped in place.
- Bullets must be carefully handled since the lead can be easily scratched. They should not be handled with metal forceps or clamps so as not to alter the ballistic markings. After removal, the surgical technologist should place the bullet(s) on a clean gauze sponge and pass it from the sterile field to the circulator for placement in a dry plastic specimen container.
- A chain of custody of evidence must be documented in writing. This accounts for the identification of all individuals on the surgical team who handled the evidence and the order of handling. The anatomical site from which the evidence is retrieved must be documented and the time. The documentation will serve as legal documents.

Hypothermia

Often trauma patients have been exposed to the environment for a prolonged period and become hypothermic at the scene. Hypothermia is typically defined as a core body temperature that is below 35°C. Upon arrival in surgery, the patient should be kept as warm as possible by using warm blankets and by increasing the temperature in the OR. The surgical team should only use warm irrigating solutions, both externally when performing the skin prep and internally when the surgeon is irrigating the surgical wound.

Infection

The wounds of trauma patients are frequently contaminated with debris, dirt, grass, and, if penetrating trauma, the foreign object that was used to cause the injury. If the stomach, gallbladder, or intestines are perforated, they will spill their contents into the abdominal cavity, putting the patient at a high risk for peritonitis.

If time permits, the surgical team may be able to perform a skin prep to decontaminate the skin using sterile scrub brushes or pulse-lavage. However, care must be taken to avoid further damage to the traumatic wound. When presented with life-threatening circumstances, the only thing there may be time for is to quickly pour or spray some antiseptic solution over a large area.

PREPARATION OF THE CASE

The majority of Level I trauma centers will have two or more ORs designated for trauma surgery. The facility will also have preassembled emergency instrument sets such as craniotomy, abdominal, and chest sets. The trauma ORs are stocked with necessary supplies and equipment such as sponges, catheters, sutures, a crash cart, and monitoring devices.

Many facilities have a fluoroscopic operating table to facilitate taking radiographs during surgery. The table also aids in positioning the patient. Positioning is always a concern in surgery, but for trauma patients it is of utmost concern, particularly if they have been involved in a situation such as an MVA in which the spine may have been injured. Before the patient is removed from the backboard to the operating table, the surgical team must confirm that the surgeon has communicated that the spine is either injury free or is injured, requiring extra positioning precautions. However, any time the patient's position is changed, the anesthesia provider will direct the team effort. The anesthesia provider is also responsible for moving the head and neck of the patient and keeping the cervical spine stable and in-line during positioning. If multiple procedures are to be performed, the patient position may be changed, again requiring the guidance of the anesthesia provider.

When performing multiple procedures, the surgical technologist will be required to organize several setups. If possible, the surgical technologist should have more than one Mayo stand and back table on which to set up the different procedures, time allowing. In addition to proper instrumentation and equipment, the surgical technologist must have an adequate supply of sponges, suture, and ties opened onto the back table, especially when the patient has sustained abdominal trauma. In such a case, more than the usual number of hemostatic clamps will most likely be needed. Hemostatic agents such as gelatin sponges and topical thrombin should be available if the need arises. In life-threatening situations in which there is not much time for preparation, the surgical technologist may not be able to perform the initial sponge, instrument, and sharp counts. The circulator should document this on the patient's OR record and postoperative radiographs may have to be taken to confirm that nothing was inadvertently retained within the patient.

Post-Traumatic Stress Disorder Patient

Post-traumatic stress disorder (PTSD) is the result of prolonged exposure to traumatic situations or a series of traumatic situations that is characterized by the patient suffering from long-lasting emotional, psychological, and social problems. It has most often been associated with military personnel who, during times of war, are constantly exposed to prolonged high-stress situations as well as the tragedies of war. PTSD had been called by different names over time. During the Civil War, it was referred to as "soldier's heart"; World War I called it "combat fatigue"; and World War II referred to as "gross stress reaction." Vietnam veterans who have PTSD symptoms were at the time of the war said to have "post-Vietnam syndrome." However, since 1980 it has been recognized as a formal diagnosis and officially called PTSD. But military personnel are not the only group that can suffer from PTSD; rape victims can suffer from PTSD, as well as adolescents who live in lower economic conditions and are exposed to the violence of gangs.

Obviously, the prospect of surgery can be very frightening to the PTSD patient who may associate the act of surgery, such as cutting and dissecting, with the violence he or she previously faced. There are many aspects of PTSD that cannot be addressed in this section of the textbook due to the complexity of the disorder, but the following are important points for the surgical team when providing care to the PTSD patient:

- The level of PTSD varies from patient to patient; the symptoms are the same, including "flashbacks" (reexperiencing traumatic events), inability to interact socially and avoidance of people, sleep disorders, etc. However, the level of the symptoms can vary. The surgery team should meet with the patient's counselor(s) to determine at what level the patient is suffering from PTSD, when the patient was diagnosed, and the treatment progress.
- The surgery team should take the initiative to learn as much as possible about PTSD.
- The surgery team should be aware that the patient can be irritable, angry, and aggressive; have poor concentration; and not relate well to people. The patient may even be severely disassociated and often nonresponsive. It may be difficult to gain any level of trust with the patient. It is recommended that a counselor experienced in treating PTSD patients accompany the patient to preoperative holding and be available to go into PACU.
- The surgery team, in particular, the anesthesia provider, should be informed of the medications that the patient is taking to treat the PTSD, as well as a history of substance abuse, which is prevalent among PTSD patients.
- PTSD patients have an increased tendency and reaction to being startled due to chronic hyperarousal. The preoperative holding room should be kept as quiet as possible; the patient may need to be isolated. The first scrub surgical technologist should stop setting up the back table and Mayo stand once the patient is brought into the OR to prevent making any noises that may disturb the patient; once the patient is under anesthesia the surgical technologist can resume activities.
- Some PTSD patients may be hypervigilant to perceived threats. Preoperative personnel should be careful in displaying any sharps the patient may see, such as when placing an IV line, and the surgery team should be aware of the same. Sharps must be kept out of reach of the PTSD patient.
- The surgery team should approach the patient slowly so as to convey a nonthreatening environment. The anesthesia provider could have difficulties masking the patient who may feel confined or claustrophobic.
- Many PTSD patients have a constant sense of doom, despair, helplessness, and hopelessness, leading to suicidal thoughts and an overall belief that one will not live much longer so life does not matter. The surgical team needs to be cognizant of the mental condition of the patient who, while being transported to the surgery department, may frequently comment "I know I'm doing to die today."
- Last, don't fight the patient; if the patient is having a "bad" day, it may be best for the surgical team and counselor to consult one another to determine if the surgery should or should not be performed, if it is a nonemergency procedure.

Case Study A female in the third trimester of pregnancy is brought to the operating room for an emergency appendectomy. It will be necessary for the patient to receive general anesthesia in order to perform the procedure.

1. Anatomically, what changes have taken place in the patient that must be taken under consideration for the surgical procedure?
2. Why might the results of laboratory tests be abnormal when the patient actually has normal values?
3. During the appendectomy, the surgical technologist should be ready to quickly set up and assist the surgeon with what additional emergency procedure?
4. Postoperatively, what symptoms should be closely watched for in the patient that could indicate preterm labor?

Questions for Further Study

1. Name some methods that can be used to reduce a pediatric patient's level of anxiety.
2. A neonate who is very ill requires surgery. What artery will most likely be used to insert an intra-arterial monitor?
3. In the immediate postoperative period, in what position should the bariatric patient be placed to aid pulmonary function?
4. A bariatric patient has recently undergone a gastric bypass procedure and complains of periumbilical pain. What complication is the patient possibly experiencing and what type of surgical procedure will be performed to repair it?
5. What device is frequently used during a surgical procedure and postoperatively to prevent thrombophlebitis in the patient who is diabetic?
6. What physiological occurrence is difficult to recognize in the pregnant patient and may result in the fetus becoming hypoxic? What device should be used intraoperatively and postoperatively to avoid the complication?

BIBLIOGRAPHY

Association of Surgical Technologists (2011). *Core curriculum for surgical technology* (6th ed.). Littleton, CO: Author.

Barone, J. E., Gingold, B. S., Arvantis, M. L., et al. (1986). Abdominal pain in patients with acquired immunodeficiency syndrome. *Annals of Surgery, 204,* 619.

Barron, W. M. (1984). The pregnant surgical patient: Medical evaluation and management. *Annals of Internal Medicine, 101,* 683.

Bell, E. F., Weinstein, M. R., & Oh, W. (1980). Heat balance in premature infants: Comparative effects of convectively heated incubator and radiant warmer with and without plastic heat shield. *Journal of Pediatrics, 96,* 460.

Centers for Disease Control and Prevention, National Center for Injury Prevention and Control. (2009). *Injury prevention & control: Data and statistics.* Retrieved from http://www.cdc.gov/injury/wisqars/dataandstats.html

Champion, H. R., Sacco, W. J., Copes, W. S., et al. (1989). A revision of the Trauma Score. *Journal of Trauma, 29*(5), 623–629.

Drain, C. B. (2008). *Perianesthesia nursing: A critical care approach* (5th ed.). St. Louis: Elsevier Saunders.

Friis-Hansen, B., Holiday, M., Stapleton, T., et al. (1951). Total body water in children. *Pediatrics, 7,* 321.

Frisenda, R., Roty, A. R., Jr., Kilway, J. B., et al. (1979). Acute appendicitis during pregnancy. *American Surgery, 45,* 503.

Garner, J. S. (1996). *Guideline for isolation precautions in hospitals.* Retrieved November 13, 2006, from http://www.cdc.gov/ncidod/dhqp/g1_isolation_ptII.html

Jensen, P. A., Lambert, L. A., Iademarco, M. F., & Ridzon, R. (2005, December 30). *Guidelines for preventing the transmission of Mycobacterium tuberculosis in health-care settings, 2005.* Retrieved November 14, 2006, from http://www.cdc.gov/mmwr/preview/mmwrhtml/rr5417a1.htm

Kanne, A. F. (2006). Trauma surgery. In M. Meeker & J. Rothrock (Eds.), *Alexander's care of the patient in surgery* (13th ed., pp. 1301–1330). St. Louis, MO: Mosby.

Phillips, N. (2007). *Berry & Kohn's operating room technique* (11th ed.). St. Louis, MO: Mosby.

Potter, P. A., & Perry, A. G. (2008). *Fundamentals of nursing: Concepts, process, and practice* (7th ed.). St. Louis, MO: Mosby.

Robinson, G., Wilson, S. E., & Williams, R. A. (1987). Surgery in patients with acquired immunodeficiency syndrome. *Archives of Surgery, 22,* 170.

Rutledge, R., & Fakhry, S. M. (1993). Injury severity scoring in trauma patients. In K. Maull (Ed.), *Advances in trauma and critical care* (Vol. 8, pp. 117–143). St. Louis, MO: Mosby-Year Book.

Sanerkin, N. G., & Edwards, P. (1966). Birth injury to the sternomastoid muscle. *Journal of Bone Joint Surgery, 48B,* 441.

Scimeca, M. M., Savage, S. R., Portenoy, R., & Lowinson, J. (2000). Treatment of pain in methadone-maintained patients. *The Mount Sinai Journal of Medicine, 67*(5 & 6), 412–422.

Trunkey, D. (1983). Trauma. *Scientific American, 249,* 28–35.

United States Department of Health and Human Services, Centers for Disease Control and Prevention. (2005, Sept. 8). *Births: Final data for 2003.* Retrieved November 7, 2006, from http://www.wonder.cdc.gov/wonder/sci_data/natl/.../type_txt/Natal03/Births03.pdf

Wilson, S. E., Robinson, G., Williams, R. A., et al. (1989). Acquired immune deficiency syndrome (AIDS): Indications for abdominal surgery, pathology, and outcome. *Annals of Surgery, 210,* 428–434.

CHAPTER

5

Physical Environment and Safety Standards

CASE STUDY Larry is a certified surgical technologist who works in the general surgery unit of a local OR. One night he was serving as the first scrub on a trauma case in which the patient had suffered several gunshot wounds to the abdomen. The patient was known to be an IV drug user. The case went well and the patient was stabilized. The count began as the peritoneum was being closed. As the case was nearing its end, a surgeon tossed a loaded needle holder onto the Mayo stand, without warning. The needle holder landed near Larry's hand, and as he turned, the needle punctured his single glove and skin.

Larry immediately reported the needle-stick injury and the circulator helped him remove the glove to assess the wound. Another team member scrubbed in and replaced Larry at the Mayo stand. Larry washed the wound with soap and water. Since it was late at night and the occupational health office was not open, he reported to the emergency department for treatment. All appropriate reports were filed.

1. What should be done with the needle and the needle holder that have become contaminated by piercing Larry's glove and skin?
2. Should Larry have waited until the end of the case to "break scrub" and wash his hand?
3. What could Larry have done to afford himself extra protection from this needle-stick injury?

OBJECTIVES

After studying this chapter, the reader should be able to:

(C) 1. Recognize the hazards to the patient in the operative environment.
2. Distinguish among the support services that work with the operating room (OR) team in the care of the patient.

(A) 3. Review the type of air-handling system required in the OR and the temperature and humidity required to maintain a sterile field.
4. Indicate cleaning procedures, traffic patterns, and routines required in the operative environment.

R 5. Analyze the role of the surgical technologist in the protection of self, patients, and others from hazards in the operative environment.

E 6. Recognize the design types of the OR.

7. Classify hospital departments that relate to surgical services.
8. Recognize the working environment of the OR.
9. Determine the physical components of the OR.

Select Key Terms

airborne bacteria
back table
Breakpoints
Decontamination Room
electrosurgical unit
high-efficiency particulate air (HEPA) filter
ionizing radiation
laminar air flow
linen hamper
Mayo stands
Occupational Safety and Health Administration (OSHA)
pathology department
perfusionist
personal protective equipment (PPE)
plume
polymethyl methacrylate (PMMA)
postanesthesia care unit (PACU)
prophylaxis
restricted areas
ring stands
Standard Precautions
suction outlet
surgical site infection (SSI)

PHYSICAL DESIGN OF THE SURGERY DEPARTMENT

When a hospital is designed, the location of the surgery department is usually such that it is easily accessible to and from the various surgical patient support departments, such as the intensive care unit (ICU), the emergency department (ED), labor and delivery, and central sterile supply. Obviously, the size of the hospital will determine location and it may not be feasible to locate every department close to the surgery department. However, a key factor is locating the surgery department in an area where traffic is limited and the general public does not have access.

Several basic design types are used in surgical services departments, depending on the age of the facility and the physical design of the areas outside the department. All surgery departments are designed with the idea of controlling traffic patterns and quickly providing each operating room (OR) with the necessary supplies during and after each case, while keeping clean and contaminated traffic patterns separate. Among these designs are:

- Race track plan
- Hotel plan
- Specialty grouping plan

The "race track" plan, recently favored by many facilities, involves a series of ORs around a clean central core (Figure 5-1). In this design, the front entrance to each OR is from the outer corridor, and supplies are retrieved through a rear entrance to the room leading to the central-core storage and work areas. The soiled entrance areas are situated outside this central-core area to allow for separation of the two areas and related traffic. Scrub sinks are also situated in the outer corridor with easy access through the main entrances to the OR.

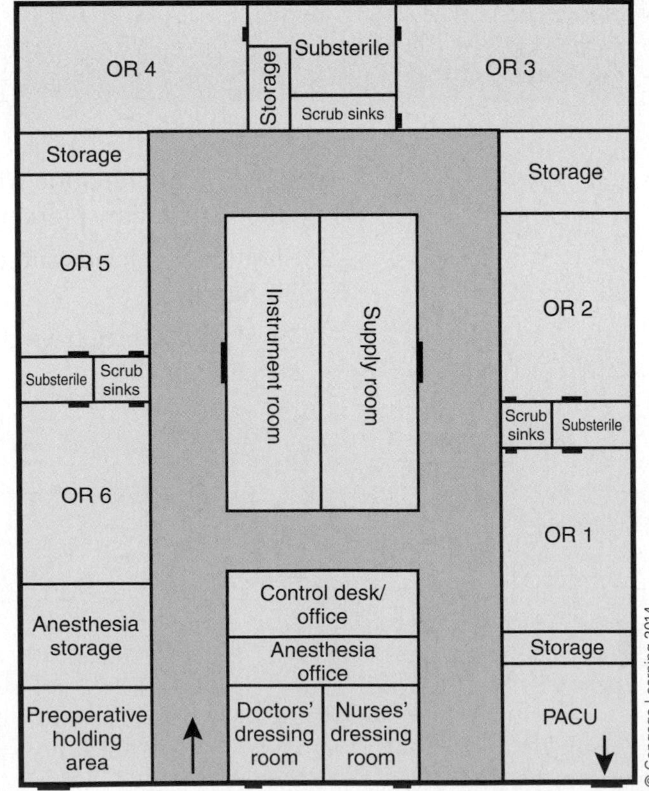

Figure 5-1 Standard surgery department plan

The "hotel plan" is a variation of this, in which the ORs are situated along a central corridor, with separate clean core and soiled work areas. The primary difference in this plan is that all traffic enters and exits the surgery department through a single entrance or a primary entrance and holding area entrance situated along the same corridor.

The "specialty grouping" plan is simply a variation on the hotel or race track plan, in which ORs are grouped by specialty (e.g., neurosurgery, general surgery), each with its own closely associated clean storage areas and, in some cases, each with its own soiled instrument work area.

Each department, regardless of design type, is equipped with a supply room in a restricted area. This room contains sterile supplies either for the entire department or for an entire specialty area if multiple storage rooms are used. Supplies stored within this area include towels, linens, sponges, gloves, and supplies used on a daily basis in every case. These areas also contain special prefabricated sterile case packs and instrument sets. Proper storage techniques should be followed in these storage areas, such as not placing sterile packs too close to ceilings or floors (see Chapter 7). As in the OR, temperature should be controlled between 68° and 73°F. Humidity should be maintained between 20% and 60% to help protect the sterility of packaged items (ANSI/ASHEA/ASHRAE, 2010). Separate storage rooms are used for large equipment such as special OR tables and attachments and endoscopic carts.

The design of any surgery department revolves around environmental control, traffic control, and the desire to prevent **surgical site infection (SSI)**. Such factors as the separation of clean and soiled work areas and areas of the department specified as restricted and unrestricted assist in the promotion of this idea. Efficiency is increased with strategic placement of computers, preparation areas, and staff areas.

AREAS OF THE OPERATING ROOM

Regardless of the design chosen by the facility, certain principles apply universally. Traffic control follows predetermined traffic patterns that all persons entering the department are expected to follow. The department is divided into unrestricted, semirestricted, and **restricted areas**, with particular attire required for each.

The unrestricted area is usually located near the entrance and is isolated from the main hospital corridor by doors. This area often contains dressing rooms for physicians and surgery staff, an anesthesia office, a main office, and a main desk. In this area, street clothes are allowed.

Operating room attire is required in the semirestricted and restricted areas (see Chapter 7). Surgical scrub suits as well as hats are required. Because there are often no doors to separate these areas, many hospitals designate the semirestricted area from the unrestricted area with the use of signage and/or a red line painted on the floor. Anyone passing this line is expected to be in proper OR attire and to observe the rules of the semirestricted area.

The restricted area includes the ORs as well as the sterile storage areas. In addition to proper OR attire, masks are required in this area. Some hospital policies require masks to be worn in the OR only when a sterile procedure is in progress, meaning sterile supplies are being opened and/or have been opened or the patient is in the room.

Instrument Room

A separate room for storage of nonsterile equipment and instrumentation is necessary. Single instruments are stored in this room and can be pulled for use as needed. In some hospitals, the area where instruments are reassembled into sets after decontamination and prior to sterilization may also be referred to as the *instrument room*.

Utility and Decontamination Room

The department is also equipped with a separate utility and **decontamination room** with sinks for gross decontamination of instrumentation. This room often contains an ultrasonic washer for cavitation of instruments prior to sending them to central sterile for processing. In some cases this area is divided by a wall into a cleaning area and a separate preparation area. In this setup, a washer-sterilizer is used to clean the instruments and they are removed to the other side of the wall in the preparation area. The preparation area may be used to reassemble and wrap instrument sets, basin sets, and trays prior to sending them to central sterile for final processing.

PHYSICAL COMPONENTS OF THE OPERATIVE SUITE

The individual rooms where surgical procedures are performed are referred to as ORs or sometimes suites. (We will restrict the use of *suite* to refer to the physical location of the entire surgical department. *OR* will refer to a single room.) The standard size of an OR has traditionally been at least 400–600 ft^2, but as technology progresses and new equipment has been put into use, there has been a need in some specialties to increase the size of the room (Figure 5-2). For example, an OR that is specifically designed for trauma patients may be at least 800 ft^2. Advanced imaging technology and the added need for equipment generally require additional space.

Equipment

Each OR is equipped with certain standard equipment plus any additional equipment and supplies that are necessary for the specialty use of the room.

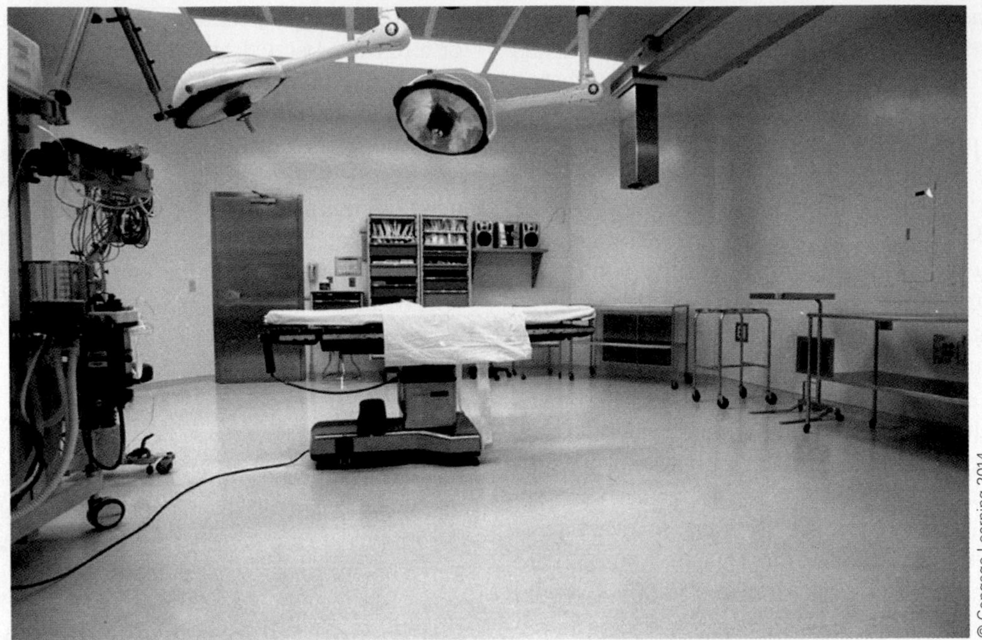

Figure 5-2 Operating room

Electrical Outlets

The majority of ORs contain both 110-volt and 220-volt outlets. Electrical outlets are mounted well above the floor and must be on a monitored electrical system. All outlets must have ground-fault interrupters and be explosion proof. Emergency outlets are designated in red and are connected to the hospital's backup generator system in case of power outage. These outlets should be used for such equipment as anesthesia equipment and other equipment vital to the procedure and to the safety of the patient.

Suction Outlets

Each OR must have at least two **suction outlets**. In some cases more suction outlets are present or required. At least one outlet is used by the surgical team for suctioning in the sterile field and one is used by anesthesia.

Gas Outlets

In addition to suction outlets, each OR is provided with several gas outlets, including outlets for compressed/medical air, oxygen, and nitrous oxide. These outlets are placed on walls or ceilings within the OR. Emergency manual shut-off valves must be located in the outside corridor. The outlets are designated by color: compressed air—yellow; oxygen—green; and nitrous oxide—blue.

Lights

Each OR is equipped with regular overhead lighting as well as surgical lights. Surgical lights should be designed to provide a range of intensity and focus with a minimum of heat and should be freely moveable. Track lights are no longer recommended because of the danger of fallout contamination. Surgical lights should be freely adjustable in both the horizontal and vertical planes and should provide a light color approximating normal sunlight. The focus point of the surgical lights should not leave a dark center spot on the surgical field. The lights must be easily accessible for cleaning and accumulated dust on the suspension system must be easily removed. Surgical lights should be equipped with handles that adjust intensity or focus of the lights and that also may be used when covered with sterile handle covers to reposition the lights intraoperatively.

Viewing Box for Diagnostic Images

A viewing box for diagnostic images is positioned at eye level so it can be seen by the surgeon without leaving the operating table. Radiographs, isotope, and computed tomography (CT) and magnetic resonance imaging (MRI) scans are routinely displayed on the view boxes.

Operating Table

The operating table is narrow, padded, and flexible. The traditional operating table was operated manually, but the modern operating table is maneuvered by an electrical control system by either the circulator or anesthesia provider. The table has ***breakpoints***, or bendable points, at the knee, waist, and head. In addition, the operating table has removable sections at the head point and at the footboard for use in procedures where the legs are placed in stirrups. The height of the table may be adjusted preoperatively and intraoperatively to aid the surgeon in visualization of the surgical site. The table should be constructed in such a manner that all surfaces are easily cleaned between cases. Small parts must be removable for terminal cleaning.

The operating table has a wide base to prevent tipping under uneven weight distribution. Rails are situated along the sides for attachment of arm boards and other accessories such as a Mayfield headrest used for craniotomy procedures (Figure 5-3). The table is always well padded prior to patient positioning, and additional padding is added when necessary.

Special operating tables are used for specific procedures. The Wilson frame operating table is used for procedures in which the patient is placed in the prone position, such as for an anterior-posterior spinal fusion. Special fracture tables are used in some orthopedic procedures. The urology or cystoscopy table is used for genitourinary surgical procedures, such as endoscopic prostate surgery. The table top is usually radiolucent, to facilitate taking radiographs. A fluid drain pan with a mesh bottom can be attached to the end of the table.

Other Items

Many procedures are time critical. Each OR should have a wall-mounted clock with an easily readable face and a sweep second hand for the timing of certain procedures and for the timing of cardiac or respiratory arrests. Many are equipped with an additional start/stop timer.

An intercom system allows for communication by the surgical team with areas outside the OR and within the surgical department without going out of the room. This can also be used for discussions with the pathology department or for calling for diagnostic imaging. Some rooms are equipped with foot-activated intercom switches so that a scrubbed member of the surgical team may operate the device.

Increasingly, ORs are equipped with one or more computer terminals to be used by the circulator and/or the anesthesia provider. The circulator may use this terminal in some cases to complete all patient chart data entry, to view previous or current laboratory work values, and to order supplies for the room, radiographs, or further tests for the patient. Further, the computer may provide access to reference information such as surgeon's preference cards, the daily schedule, and common laboratory values. The computer may also be used to record operating times and room turnover times and to assist with patient tracking. The patient's family or friends may be able to track the patient's progress via a computer screen in the waiting area. The patient's identity is protected by assigning each patient a specific identification number. As technology evolves, systems within the hospital are increasingly integrated into computer networks, decreasing the paper load and increasing the speed with which vital patient information may be shared within the facility.

Many ORs are now equipped with permanently installed closed-circuit television capability. This may be used to assist members of the team in viewing endoscopic procedures and in some cases is connected to the pathology department so that the surgeon may have a discussion with the pathologist without leaving the OR. Additionally, closed-circuit television allows the surgical procedure to be viewed from a remote location and is used in many academic centers.

Increasingly, ORs include surgical equipment "booms." Surgical equipment booms are ceiling-mounted, articulating arms that contain a variety of surgical equipment, such as electrical, gas, and communication devices. Surgical booms take the place of mobile carts and offer an opportunity to reduce clutter and to better position the surgical devices and their connections as the surgical procedure requires (Figure 5-4).

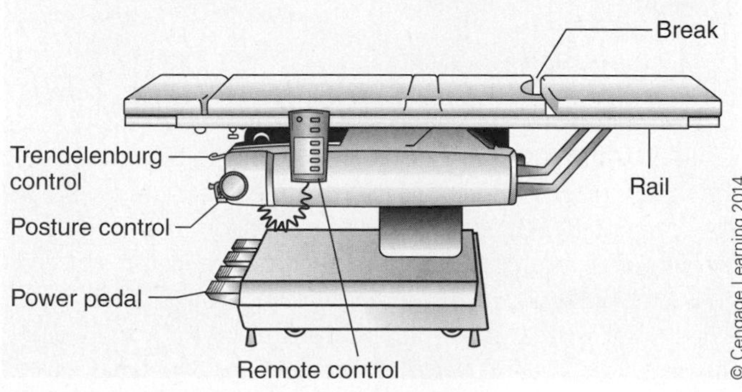

Figure 5-3 Operating table

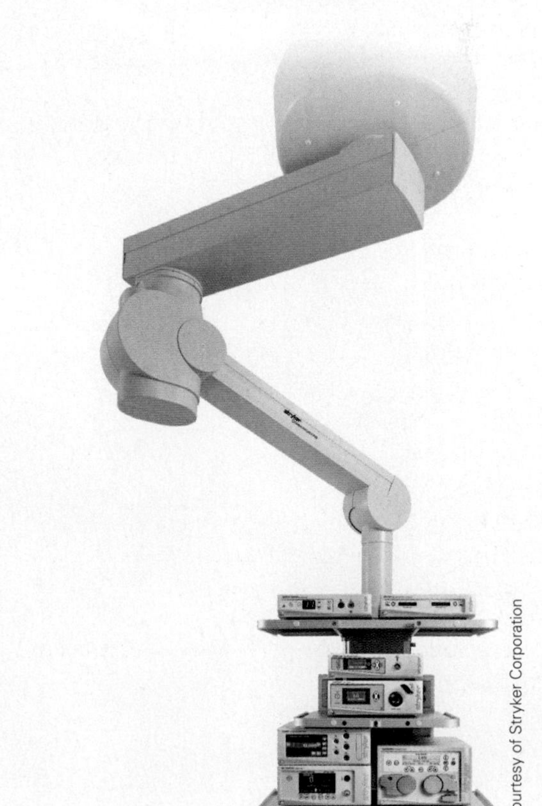

Figure 5-4 Surgical equipment boom

Standard Operating Room Furniture

Each OR should be equipped with a standard set of furniture and equipment, including the operating table, a **back table**, one or more **Mayo stands, ring stands,** and a kick bucket. Each room will also be equipped with accessories particular to the specialty or the procedure to be performed in that room, such as positioning devices for orthopedic procedures.

A Mayo stand is the stand that is moved up to the operative field and extends across the patient's body. The surgical technologist works from this stand to supply immediately necessary instrumentation to the surgeon. Prior to the procedure, a separate small table or Mayo stand is used to set up gowns and gloves for the surgical technologist (Figure 5-5).

The back table is a large table on which the back table pack is placed and opened to create a sterile field. Sterile supplies, equipment, and instruments are placed on this table, and it is the responsibility of the surgical technologist to arrange the items on the back table while setting up for the surgical procedure. The surgical technologist obtains the surgical instruments that will be used most often from the back table and places them on the Mayo stand. Supplies such as suture and sponges are obtained from the back table and it serves as a large area where the circulating person can open additional sterile supplies that are needed during the procedure (Figure 5-6).

Ring stands are four-wheeled stands with one or two metal rings at the top (Figure 5-7). They are used to hold sterile basins and are covered with a sterile drape prior to the procedure.

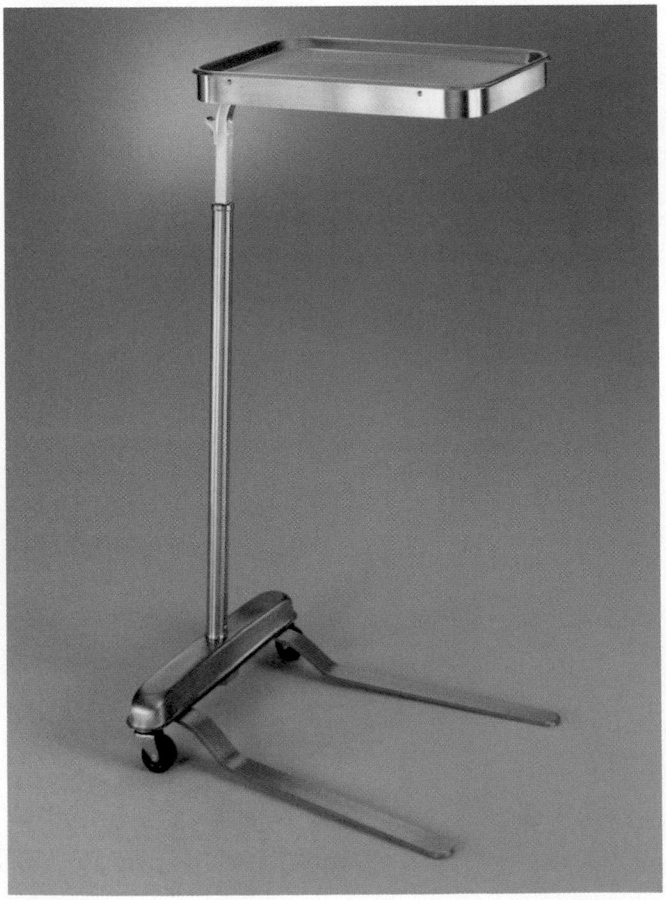

Courtesy of Blickman Health Industries

Figure 5-5 Mayo stand

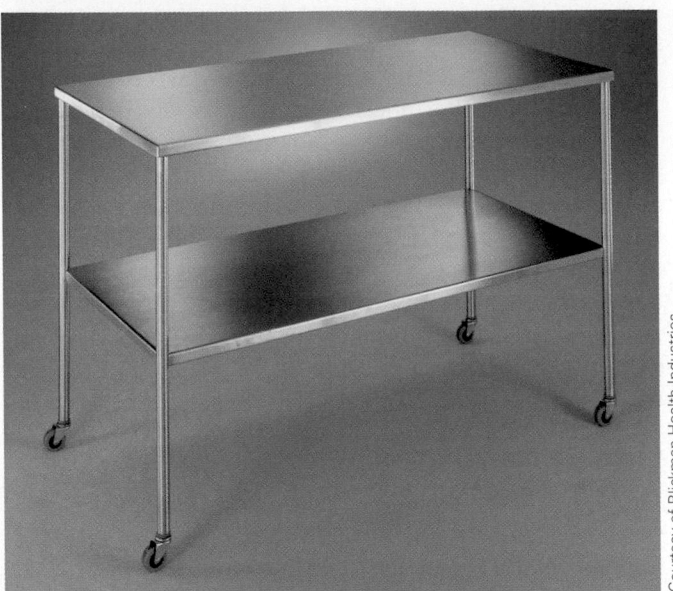

Courtesy of Blickman Health Industries

Figure 5-6 Back table

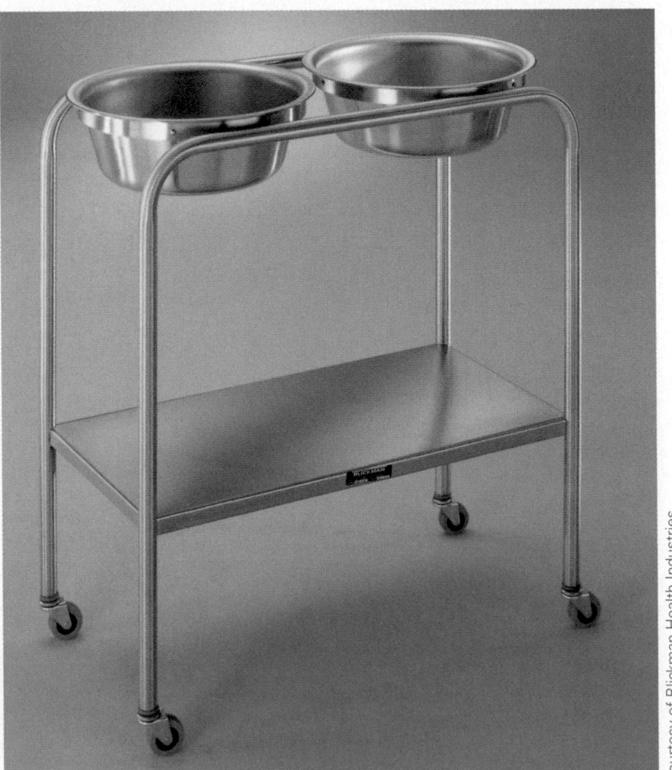

Courtesy of Blickman Health Industries

Figure 5-7 Double ring stand

These basins hold the various fluids to be used during the procedure, including saline and/or sterile water for rinsing instruments and for irrigation. In some cases, such as cardiac cases, these basins may be used to hold a sterile ice/slush solution for hypothermia in the absence of a *slush machine*.

Kick buckets are also four-wheeled stands, but they are very low to the floor and can be maneuvered with the foot (kicked) (Figure 5-8). These are buckets lined with biohazard trash bags. The sterile team member tosses soiled counted sponges into these buckets. The kick bucket is not for paper waste but for counted sponges only.

A **linen hamper** and trash containers are typically four-wheeled stands but are large enough that soiled linens and trash from the sterile field may be placed into them by the surgical technologist. They too may be lined with biohazardous designator bags.

Suction sets are low-wheel-based stands on which the suction canisters rest. Sterile suction tubing from the field may be attached to the canister by the circulator (Figure 5-9). The canisters are connected to the suction outlet by another plastic tube. They may be lined with plastic liners and have measurements marked on the side to help estimate fluid use and/or

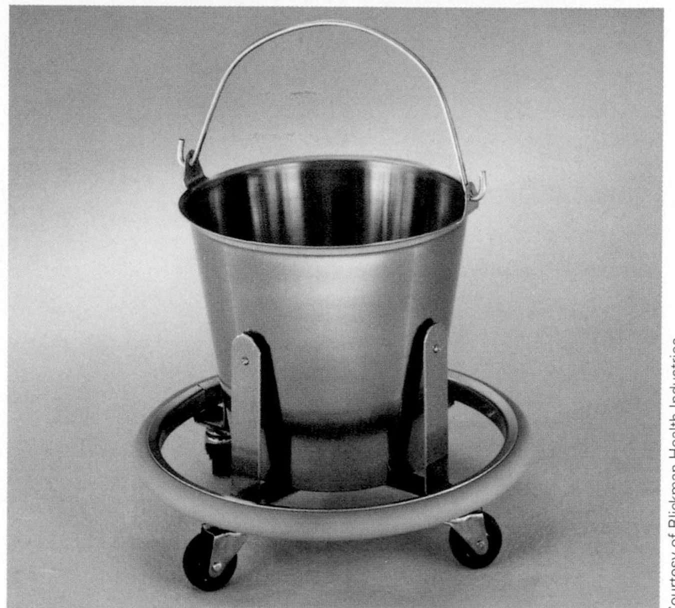

Courtesy of Blickman Health Industries

Figure 5-8 Kick bucket

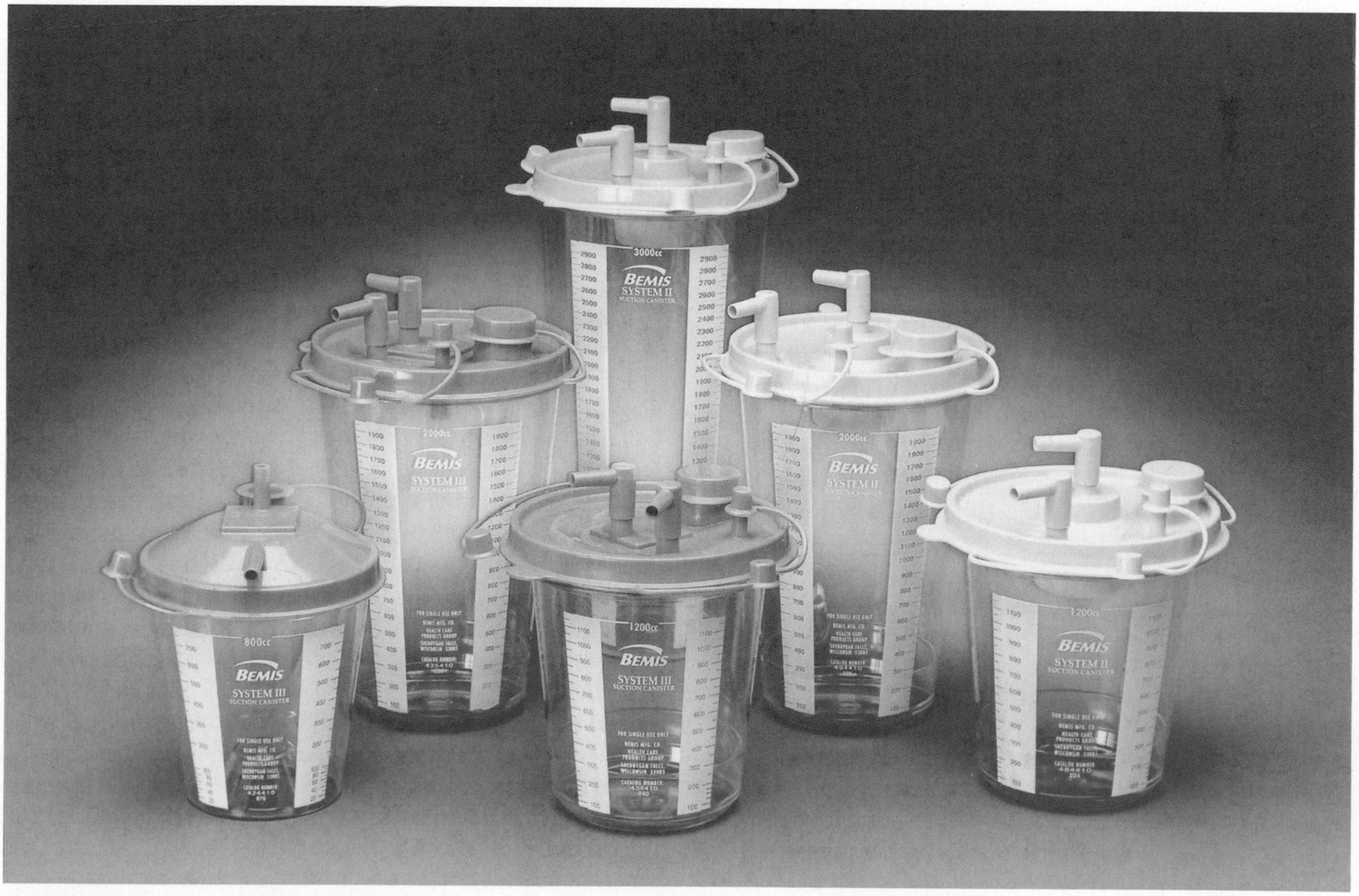

Courtesy of Bemis Manufacturing Co.

Figure 5-9 Suction system

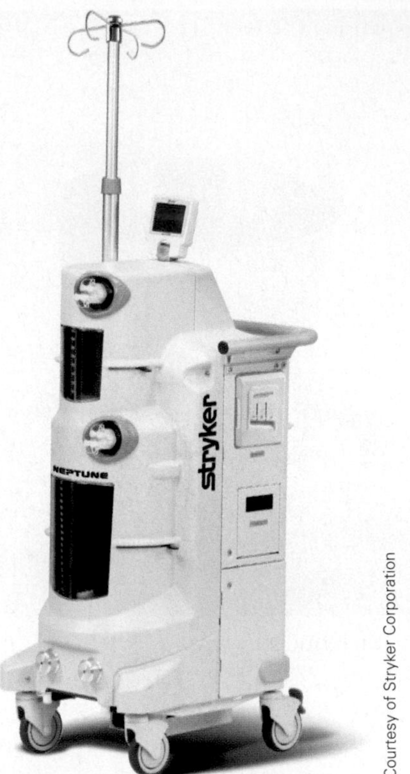

Courtesy of Stryker Corporation

Figure 5-10 Stryker Neptune 2 waste management system

blood loss. Some ORs use a waste management system that is a totally closed unit, meaning it collects fluid with minimal operator assistance. These systems may provide suction as well as smoke evacuation for the surgical field (Figure 5-10).

In addition to this equipment, each OR is equipped with an *anesthesia cart* and supplies. This will include patient monitoring equipment to keep the surgical team aware of the patient's physiological status and it is primarily used by the anesthesia provider. A writing surface is provided on the wall within easy view of the sterile members of the surgical team. This surface is used to provide the team with vital information about the patient, such as age, weight, name, etc., as well as to provide a surface on which to write and maintain sponge, sharps, and instrument counts.

Surfaces in the Operating Room

The walls of the OR should have the following characteristics:

- Nonglare
- Fireproof
- Nonporous
- Waterproof
- Nonreflective
- Pleasant in color
- Easy to clean with antimicrobial solution

Floors should also be nonporous and waterproof, which makes them easier to clean by wet vacuuming. Tile floors are undesirable (though often seen in older ORs) because the grout tends to harbor bacteria and is difficult to clean. Many new ORs are using cushioned flooring systems to decrease personnel fatigue. If cushioned rubber standing mats are used around the table, they should be of the solid and smooth type with no grooves to allow for easy and thorough cleaning.

Cabinets and Doors

Cabinets and doors within the OR should be recessed into the wall when possible to avoid dust accumulation on their top surfaces. Storage cabinets should be provided with doors to lower dust accumulation on supplies and for ease of terminal cleaning of the room. Doors on cabinets should be of the surface-mounted sliding type when possible, because swinging doors move air within the room and disturb microorganisms that have settled on floors and surfaces within the room into the operative field. Cabinets and doors, like walls and floor, should be nonporous and waterproof for easy cleaning.

Doors

Access doors to the OR should be kept closed during all procedures to protect the room from outside contamination. When possible, surface-mounted sliding doors that can swing open in an emergency situation should be used. Sliding doors lower the incidence of swinging-door air disturbance in the room, which can redistribute contaminant microbes onto the operative field. Traffic into and out of the OR should be limited during any procedure for this purpose, and particularly during open-joint orthopedic procedures; many ORs place signage to this effect on the doors.

Ventilation System

The ventilation system in the OR should provide a supply of clean air; remove airborne contamination that is produced within the room; remove waste anesthetic gases, toxic fumes, and vapors; and provide a comfortable working environment for surgical personnel.

Studies in the 1940s showed that when air for the ORs was brought in through intakes in the corridors and other areas of the hospital, bacteria could be introduced into the OR. These findings led to the practice of creating a *positive-pressure* air supply for each OR. The air-handling system should provide for positive **laminar airflow**, a unidirectional positive-pressure flow of air that captures microbes to be filtered. This means that the air pressure in the OR is kept by ventilation at a higher level than that of the surrounding corridors. When a door is opened out to the corridor, air from the room rushes outward into the corridor rather than from the corridor into the room. This process helps keep **airborne bacteria** from entering the room. To keep air movement into the OR at a minimum, no windows that may be opened are allowed in the OR.

Air Changes in OR

A minimum of 15 air exchanges per hour are required for the OR, with a recommended range of 20 to 25 air exchanges per hour. Studies have shown that 20 to 25 air exchanges per hour helps keep the amount of airborne contamination in the OR to a minimum. The Centers for Disease Control and Prevention (CDC) guidelines recommend that the air is filtered. **High-efficiency particulate air (HEPA) filters** are usually the filter of choice. These filters are capable of removing bacteria as small as 0.5–5 μm. The CDC guidelines also recommend that at least 20% of the air change per hour be from fresh outside air.

Temperature and Humidity

The temperature in the OR is kept between 68° and 73°F. The recommended range for relative humidity is 20% to 60% (ANSI/ASHEA/ASHRAE, 2010). These levels provide comfort for the patient and surgical team, and also contribute to preventing infection control. Care should be taken to prevent patient hypothermia; studies have shown decreased incidences of SSI and shorter recovery times in patients who were kept at a normal body temperature intraoperatively.

SUBSTERILE AREA

Each OR or group of ORs is provided with a scrub sink area and a *substerile room*. This substerile area is a workroom for that particular OR or group of adjacent rooms and contains a sink and a steam sterilizer. The substerile room may also contain a blanket and solution warmer. It may be used in emergent situations to clean and immediate-use steam sterilize instruments that were contaminated (e.g., dropped on the floor) for return to the sterile field. This room is situated so that the circulator or surgical technologist is able to remove instruments directly from the sterilizer and will not have to transport these instruments through the "nonsterile" corridors. This room not only provides for easy immediate-use steam sterilization but also provides a small storage area that allows the circulator to remain in or close to the OR at all times. Doors to this room should remain closed during the operation to prevent cross-contamination from adjacent rooms. Positive air pressure is defeated in this case because adjacent rooms also are under this same system.

DIRECT SUPPORT SERVICES

As mentioned in Chapter 1, many departments of the hospital interact with surgical services. Some are directly related to surgical services and some are related indirectly. Some departments may have a physical presence in the surgery department, for instance, diagnostic imaging. Others may communicate by other means from a distant location.

Preoperative or "Same-Day" Check-in Unit

Many hospitals have established a preoperative "same-day" check-in unit, when separate same-day surgery facilities are not used. This is the area the patient is directed and admitted to on arrival at the hospital. The patient is provided with a private dressing room to change clothes. Lockers are provided for the patient to safeguard personal items, although any jewelry or money should either be left with a family member or turned over to hospital security for safekeeping. In this area, a designated family waiting area is provided. After admission and any necessary preoperative laboratory work, the patient is taken to the preoperative holding area.

Preoperative Holding Area

The *preoperative holding* area is a designated room where patients wait within the surgery department before entering the OR. Depending on design, this may be a large area where all patients are held until transport to the specific OR or a small room just outside each OR. Regardless of the location, this room or area should be shielded from noise and views into the OR. Patients should not be held in the main corridor, because this is typically noisy and quite frightening to the surgical patient. In this area, intravenous (IV) lines and invasive monitoring devices may be inserted. The anesthesia provider often uses this room for a preoperative interview and assessment of patient status, and regional blocks such as epidural anesthesia may be administered while the OR is being cleaned or "turned over" from the previous case. For pediatric cases, this room is often equipped with a rocking chair, and a parent is allowed to sit and wait in the room with the child to assist in the alleviation of both parent and child anxiety.

Postanesthesia Care Unit

Postoperatively, the patient is usually transported to the **postanesthesia care unit (PACU)**, where he or she is "recovered" just after surgery, until transport to a nursing unit (or discharge, in the case of same-day surgery patients) is possible. For cases in which the patient has not yet been extubated, this is performed in the PACU when the patient has regained consciousness and can breathe unassisted.

The PACU is a large room that may be located adjacent to the surgery department or in the unrestricted area of the department. The room is divided into a series of individual cubicles, usually separated by curtains but in some facilities separated by walls. It is preferable that the number of cubicles should at least equal the number of ORs in the department. However, the number of cubicles needed is also based on the surgical caseload, OR turnover times, and length of procedures. For example, at a teaching hospital the procedures may take longer than normal. Some facilities may have isolation rooms in the PACU for patients with an epidemiologically important disease or infection. If the PACU does not have an isolation room, the patient should be placed in a designated area of the PACU away from other patients with curtains drawn completely around the stretcher. Isolation precautions and hospital policy should be followed when providing care to the patient and handling bedding and equipment; see Chapter 4 for detailed information concerning care of isolation patients.

Each PACU cubicle has the following equipment for patient care:

- Pulse oximeter
- Blood pressure cuff
- Wall suction and tubing
- Wall oxygen and tubing
- Electrocardiographic (ECG) monitor

Supplies and equipment that are kept in the PACU include:

- Warmer for blankets and IV solutions
- IV administration sets
- Various types of wound dressing supplies
- Medications, including narcotics
- Various types of urinary catheters
- Emesis basins
- Bedpans
- Airway management supplies
- Crash cart with defibrillator and medications; depending on the number of cubicles there may need to be more than one crash cart located in the PACU
- Malignant hyperthermia (MH) emergency cart
- Tracheotomy trays

Laboratory Department

The laboratory department provides the surgical team with perioperative laboratory values used when monitoring the patient. Certain laboratory procedures may be performed within the surgery department, such as blood gas monitoring, which is often performed by **perfusionists** during cardiovascular procedures. Other laboratory work is sent out of the OR to the laboratory, where it is assigned a value of time importance (stat, critical, and noncritical) and values are returned to the OR. This may be accomplished via telephone, via intercom, and, increasingly, via computer. When the laboratory and OR are linked by computer network, values may be posted online as they become available and may also be compared with previous values to help in identifying a trend.

Radiology Department

The radiology department provides the OR with radiologic patient studies, including plain x-ray films, CT scans, and MRI, and intraoperative techniques such as fluoroscopy, which provides real-time radiographic monitoring for orthopedic and other cases. Larger hospitals often provide the surgery department with a dedicated radiology technician staff for ease and speed, and the department is usually equipped with mobile radiographic equipment and a C-arm (fluoroscope). The radiology department is usually contacted via a telephone or intercom system and radiographs are returned to the room as soon as they have been developed. The radiology department may be called on to take x-ray films to assist when a sponge, instrument, or sharps count has been found to be incorrect.

The surgical technologist must always oversee any activity around the patient while radiological studies are being performed. Radiology personnel may have little awareness of aseptic principles and techniques, and it is therefore the duty of the surgical technologist to supervise personnel movement around the sterile field. It is also important for surgical technologists in cases utilizing x-ray or fluoroscopy to wear protective lead shields such as leaded aprons and/or thyroid shields to prevent exposure to **ionizing radiation**.

Pathology Department

Specimens are sent to the **pathology department** for testing, processing, and diagnosis. This department is not located within the surgery department, but communication systems such as closed-circuit television, computer networking, and direct intercoms link them closely to communicate quickly and directly. Pathology results, like laboratory results, are easily accessible by computer. Care should be taken by the surgical technologist when sending specimens to pathology that they are placed in the proper type of containers and fluids. The surgical technologist should always double check with the surgeon and circulator to ensure proper labeling and handling of the specimen. Permanent specimens are usually sent to the pathology laboratory in formalin solutions and frozen sections are sent dry. For a better understanding of the handling of specimens, refer to Chapter 13.

Environmental Services

Environmental services is the ancillary department charged with cleaning the surgery department. In some cases, this includes cleaning the OR for turnover between cases, but increasingly, the surgical team is being used for this purpose for speed and efficiency. In many cases, the environmental services department is charged primarily with terminal cleaning of the ORs at night. This department is also in charge of the removal of soiled linens and regular as well as biohazard-classified trash. These workers should be well versed in **Standard Precautions**, because they could potentially come in contact with blood and other body fluids. They should also be trained in decontamination and terminal cleaning of ORs and equipment.

Central Sterile Supply and Processing

The central sterile supply and processing department (CSPD) is usually located outside of the surgical department. Many hospitals place this department a floor above or below the surgery department and use a dumbwaiter system to transport sterile and dirty supplies (in separate dumbwaiters) between departments. In some cases, hospitals will use a specified elevator to transport contaminated surgical instruments and equipment via a case cart system. While primary decontamination of instruments (removal of gross blood and debris) is usually the responsibility of the surgical team, final wrapping of instrument sets and sterilization usually take place in this department.

In addition to sterilization, the CSPD is used for storing and distributing supplies and equipment and often for processing supplies as they arrive from the manufacturers. Supplies are maintained in the surgery department storage areas at a particular level and the materials management staff orders supplies from central sterile to maintain these levels. Increasingly, computers are being used between the two departments for use in patient charging and inventory control. Other hospitals have implemented a computerized storage cabinet system that automatically tracks supplies as they are used and reports stock levels within the surgery department to ancillary departments such as materials management and CSPD. Some hospitals use a "case cart" system, in which a cart of dirty supplies and instruments is sent to the decontamination room and then on to sterile supply and exchanged for a cart containing the same supplies that have been processed to replace the dirty ones.

The design of the CSPD must be such that traffic flow patterns will allow for a separation of clean or sterile instruments and supplies from dirty or contaminated instruments and supplies to be reprocessed.

HAZARDS AND REGULATORY AGENCIES

The surgical department is an environment containing hazards to the patient and surgical team. Of utmost concern is the safety of patients, but equally important is the safety of the surgical team. For a safe environment to exist:

1. Equipment must be properly handled and operated.
2. The surgical team must have knowledge of the possible hazards that exist in the OR and the methods of ensuring a safe surgical environment.

Potential safety hazards in the surgery department can be placed in one of the following categories:

Physical hazards—Noise, ionizing radiation, electricity, injury to the body, fire, explosion, and injuries from sharps

Biological hazards—Laser and electrosurgical **plume,** pathogens found in body fluids, latex sensitivity

Chemical hazards—Disinfecting agents, waste anesthetic gases, and vapors and fumes from chemical agents

Surgery department policies and procedures for reducing the risks of the above three hazards are based on standards and guidelines established by numerous local, state, and federal agencies. The following is a short description of six key agencies:

National Fire Protection Agency (NFPA)—Organization whose mission is to reduce the frequency of fires through the establishment of fire prevention standards, research, and public fire safety education.

Occupational Safety and Health Administration (OSHA)—Federal organization that is dedicated to protecting the health of workers by establishing standards that address issues related to safety in the workplace. The standards are legally enforceable in order to protect workers, and many of the standards are based on the findings of other agencies, such as NFPA, ANSI, and NIOSH. Areas of OSHA regulation include noise levels, exposure to ionizing radiation, laser safety standards as established by ANSI, and fire safety standards for health care facilities as established by NFPA.

National Institute for Occupational Safety and Health (NIOSH)—Organization whose responsibilities are similar to OSHA but tends to be more research oriented in establishing permissible exposure limits (*PELs*) for chemical vapors and gases. NIOSH is an arm of the CDC that is under the U.S. Department of Health and Human Services.

American National Standards Institute (ANSI)—Organization of industry experts who promote and facilitate voluntary consensus standards in technical fields. An example is the laser safety standard that is intended for use by all health care facilities that use lasers in the treatment of patients.

American Society for Testing and Materials (ASTM)—Similar to ANSI, it is also an organization of industry experts who develop and provide voluntary consensus standards for medical equipment by testing the equipment.

Association for the Advancement of Medical Instrumentation (AAMI)—Organization that establishes standards that reach across the spectrum of the health care field, including sterilization, electrical safety, levels of device safety, and use of medical devices.

SAFETY CONSIDERATIONS

The modern OR is a complex and technologically sophisticated environment. Each of the systems involved in creating a modern surgical environment also creates safety considerations.

Surgical Lights

The beam from surgical lights should be nonglare to prevent eye fatigue (Figure 5-11). Most manufacturers of surgical lights have placed emphasis on trying to produce lights that emit a blue-white beam that still adequately illuminates the surgical site yet produces little glare and approximates the color

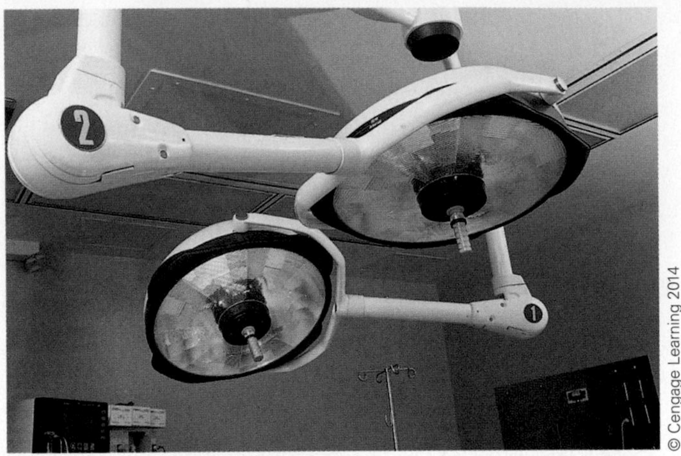

Figure 5-11 Surgical lights

intensities of normal sunlight. Some surgical instruments are manufactured with a satin or ebony finish to decrease surgical light reflection and glare off the instrument. Drapes and towels are designed in nonreflective colors such as blue or green in order to reduce glare.

Noise in the Operating Room

Noise can be irritating to patients and the surgical team. Noise from a combination of sources can lead to interference with communication or prevent the ability to hear monitor alarms. Sources of noise include music, suction, power instruments, clattering of surgical instruments, and conversation. The circulator must make sure the door to the OR is closed to eliminate external noise. Conversation should be kept to a minimum and, if necessary, carried on in a low to normal tone of voice. Music can be relaxing to the patient and may serve as a stimulant for the surgical team. For patients undergoing local anesthesia, it can be of particular benefit. However, much like conversation, it should be played in a low tone and the type of music should be appropriate for the environment and not be distracting to the surgical team.

Ergonomics and Safety Considerations

Proper posture and body mechanics can help protect the body, especially the lumbar region of the back. Back injury and/or pain is usually the result of a number of factors that may include:

1. Lifting with the back bowed out
2. Bending and reaching with the back bowed out
3. Jerking or twisting at the hips
4. Obesity
5. Loss of strength and flexibility
6. Poor nutrition

The nature of the surgical technologist's job places abnormal strains on the body, in particular the lower back, knees, and feet. Proper body mechanics helps prevent injury and discomfort. The following are guidelines to aid in preventing pain and injury due to poor body mechanics:

1. Stand with legs approximately shoulder width apart. This allows the ligaments of the hips and knees to naturally support the body and the wider stance is less fatiguing for the surgical technologist.
2. Avoid weight bearing on one foot for a prolonged period of time. The wide stance will prevent this from happening. If weight bearing on one foot is necessary, shift the weight as often as possible.
3. The surgical technologist should stand next to the OR table in an erect manner with arms relaxed from the shoulder down. The use of a standing stool(s) may be necessary.
4. For surgical procedures that require sitting, the surgical technologist should sit in an erect fashion with the spinal column straight. Do not lean forward from the shoulders, but from the hips.
5. Push, do not pull, heavy equipment such as microscopes, OR tables, gurneys, and laser equipment.

Most of the lifting done by the surgical technologist is relatively light. However, instrument sets can be quite heavy. The Association for the Advancement of Medical Instrumentation (AAMI) recommends a 25-pound weight limit on instrument trays and sets (ANSI/AAMI, 2006). One of the more difficult tasks for the team is moving an anesthetized or incapacitated patient. Teamwork and proper body mechanics are important of the patient and the surgical team members. Proper lifting technique is summarized next:

1. Squat to lift and lower. Do not bend at the waist.
2. Lift with the legs and abdominal muscles, not the lower back.
3. Keep the weight as close to the body as possible.
4. Bow your back in and raise up with the head first; heels flat; lift with a smooth, even motion.
5. If a turn must be made while holding the weight, turn the whole body, not at the waist.
6. Keep the lower back bowed in when lowering the object.
7. Keep the feet shoulder width apart.

Fire Hazards and Safety

An estimated 550 to 650 surgical fires occur in the United States each year, including an estimated 10 to 20 cases per year where patients are seriously burned or disfigured (ECRI Institute, 2009). The danger of fire in the surgery department has been reduced with the introduction of halogenated anesthetic agents and the elimination of flammable cyclopropane. However, nitrous oxide, which itself is nonflammable, supports combustion in the presence of oxygen. Combined with a source of ignition, the potential for explosion and fire in the OR is an issue of significant importance.

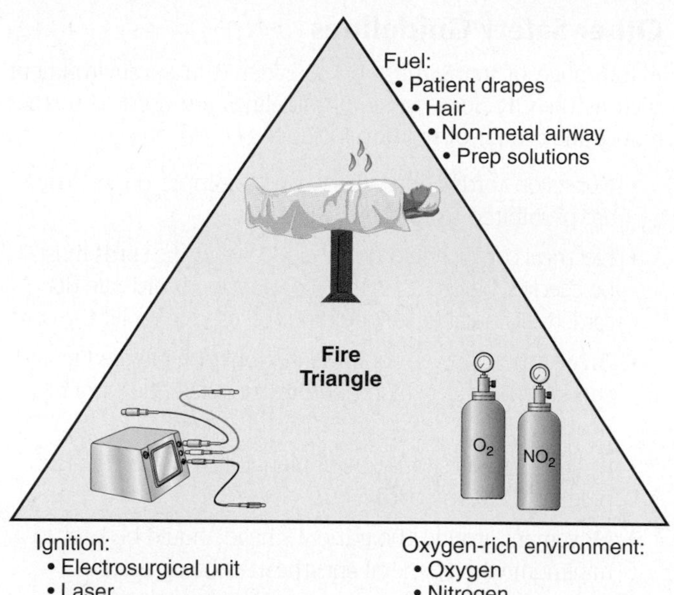

Figure 5-12 Three components of fire: fuel, source of ignition, and oxygen

A combination of three components referred to as the fire triangle can result in a fire and/or explosion (Figure 5-12):

1. Source of ignition, for example, electrosurgery, electrocautery, lasers, fiber-optic light sources, defibrillators, sparks from dental or orthopedic burs, or sparks from metal hitting metal (e.g., two metal retractors coming into contact)
2. Oxygen-rich environment
3. Fuel—flammable chemical gas, vapor, or liquid such as ethyl alcohol and skin prep solutions containing isopropyl alcohol; surgical drapes; disposable surgical supplies

Standards established by the NFPA and AAMI aid in the prevention of fires in the OR. One of the NFPA standards of particular importance to health institutions is the *Standard for Health Care Facilities*.

Sources of Ignition

The nature of modern surgery creates many potential sources of ignition. Specific procedures and guidelines are in place for many of these.

Lasers

Laser is an acronym for "light amplification by the stimulated emission of radiation." This refers to (1) the process in which light energy is produced and (2) the device that generates the laser energy or beam. However, as with most technology, the laser light presents hazards that must be understood in order to protect the patient, not the least of which is the potential to cause a fire.

Fire prevention is critical during laser surgery. The surgical team must be aware of the precautions to follow to prevent a fire.

Sterile water must be available for the surgical team to use in the event of a small fire. The sterile water is also used to keep the sponges and towels wet during the procedure to prevent them from igniting.

Portable fire extinguishers must be immediately available. The *halon fire extinguisher* is recommended for laser fires due to its low toxicity and because residue is not produced.

The laser beam can ignite surgical drapes, but laser-retardant drapes are available commercially. To decrease the chance of fire, wet towels can be placed on the drapes around the surgical site.

The anesthesia provider must use a nonexplosive anesthetic agent. During oral or laryngeal surgery, the anesthesia provider must use a flame-resistant type of endotracheal (ET) tube, which is commercially available. The ET tube balloon must be inflated with sterile water instead of air and wet sponges placed around the tube and cuff.

Special caution should be used when laser surgery is performed in the head and neck area. Nitrous oxide and oxygen can build up beneath the surgical drapes, presenting an environment conducive to fire or explosion. Flammable alcohol-based preparation solutions should not be used. Excess solution may pool under the patient, causing vapors to be trapped beneath the surgical drapes. The volatility of these vapors increases the risk of surgical drape fires. The patient's hair should be covered with wet sponges or towels to prevent ignition if close to the laser site. The patient should be given preoperative instructions not to use hair spray that can easily ignite.

During laser procedures in the anorectal area, the rectum must be packed with a sterile-water-soaked sponge to prevent a methane gas explosion or fire.

Finally, it is important to remember that a fire can be started by a reflected beam as readily as by a direct-beam impact. Nonreflective instrumentation must be used in the vicinity of the laser site.

For additional safety, signs warning that a laser is in use are posted on all entrances to the OR to limit traffic in and out of the room (Figure 5-13). The surgical team should wear the appropriate eye protection and high-filtration masks when the laser is in use. The eye is highly susceptible to damage by lasers. The eyes are affected differently according to the laser's wavelength; for example, the CO_2 laser is absorbed by and can cause corneal burns and the Nd:YAG laser is absorbed by and damages the retina, causing blindness. The eye protection should be of the correct optical density. Optical density is the ability of the protective lens of the eyewear to absorb a specific wavelength. Each type of laser has a unique wavelength; therefore the optical density will vary. The color of the lenses does not provide the eye protection; the color simply provides an indication of the optical density of the lenses. The surgical team members should follow the recommendations of the laser manufacturer as to the selection of the correct-density

DANGER
Laser in use
Safety eyewear required
Class IV laser
© Cengage Learning 2014

Figure 5-13 Warning sign that laser is in use and safety eyewear must be worn before entering the operating room

eyewear to use according to the type of laser. Other eye safety factors to follow include the following:

- The eyewear must completely shield the eyes, including top, bottom, and sides. The surgical team member should be fitted for the eyewear to ensure a snug and secure, but not uncomfortable, fit.
- Goggles are to be worn over prescription glasses unless prescription lenses of the correct density are available.
- Surgical team members who wear contact lenses must also wear protective eyewear.
- If the lenses of the eyewear have one or more scratches, they should not be worn because the protection of the lenses is now compromised.
- Patients' eyes must be protected with the same type of eyewear that is worn by the surgical team members.

Electrosurgical Unit

The **electrosurgical unit** generates considerable heat. If inadvertently activated, the electrosurgical pencil may burn or smolder the surgical drapes. When not in use, the handpiece should be placed in a holder attached to the drapes or positioned so that the handpiece will not be inadvertently activated.

Fiberoptic Beam

The fiberoptic beam at the end of endoscopes must not be focused on the drapes. The heat from the beam can burn or smolder the drapes.

Static Electricity

Static electricity can ignite a flame under the right conditions. The humidity of the OR should be no higher than 60%. Humidity lower than 20% may be conducive to spark transmission.

Other Safety Guidelines

A full range of items must be considered in an environment such as the OR. Some general guidelines are used to further reduce the chance of ignition include:

- Extension cords and power strips (multiple-outlet strip) are prohibited from use in the OR.
- Electrical cords should be rubber coated. The cords must be checked before use. Frayed or damaged cords are discarded; electrical tape should not be used to repair the cord.
- All electrical power equipment should be plugged in and checked prior to use and before anesthetic delivery has begun.
- Electrical cords should be unplugged by pulling on the plug only, not the cord.
- Movement around the patient's head should be kept to a minimum when general anesthesia is being used.
- Only cotton blankets should be used to cover the patient. Wool or blankets manufactured from other material tend to produce static electricity.
- The patient's hair should be covered to prevent static discharge.
- Never attach the active electrode cord to the drapes with a metal device.

Fire Safety Guidelines

The surgical technologist should be familiar with the health institution's fire policy and procedure. The Surgical Technologist should know the procedure for reporting a fire, where the fire alarms and fire extinguishers are located, and routes of evacuation. Surgical technologists should know how to operate a fire extinguisher and know the three classes of extinguishers:

1. *Class A*: Pressurized water; suitable for fires involving solid materials, e.g., wood, paper, or textiles
2. *Class B*: Carbon dioxide or dry chemical for fires involving flammable liquids, oils, and gas
3. *Class C*: Halon for electrical or laser fires

The PASS mnemonic is used when operating a fire extinguisher:

P—Pull the pin at the top of the fire extinguisher

A—Aim the nozzle toward the base of the fire

S—Squeeze the handle to discharge the extinguisher while standing approximately 8 feet away from the fire

S—Sweep the nozzle in a back-and-forth motion at the base of the fire until the fire is extinguished

The three main concerns if a fire should occur in the OR are to (1) protect the patient, (2) contain the fire if possible, and (3) move the anesthesia equipment as far away as possible from the fire source. The patient should be moved from the room as quickly as possible. Surgery personnel must be available to assist the anesthesia provider in moving the patient. Activate the fire alarm system and use the proper fire extinguisher to extinguish the fire if possible. Some health care facilities identify specific employees who have received additional education to respond to fires and to take responsibility for the operation of the fire extinguisher.

Education of the surgical team is imperative to fire preparedness and fire safety. Health care facilities should have designated fire evacuation strategies and plans for patient care in these situations. Routine fire drills help to prepare the entire surgical team for their role in a surgical fire and help to identify fire evacuation routes, gas shutoff valves, and fire alarm pull boxes. Many health care facilities use the acronym "RACE" to prepare employees in the event of a fire:

R—Remove/rescue anyone from fire or smoke danger to a safe area

A—Alert/sound the alarm

C—Contain the fire

E—Extinguish/evacuate

ELECTRICAL HAZARDS

The use of electrical equipment in the surgical environment has increased with the advent of minimally invasive surgical techniques and the use of lasers, robots, and electrosurgical equipment. Surgical technologists must be trained in the use of the equipment, safety measures, and equipment troubleshooting methods.

The manufacturer's instructions should always be followed when operating electrical equipment. AAMI and The Joint Commission have developed safety standards for electrical equipment used in the OR. These instructions and standards are helpful in training surgical technologists to avoid human error or equipment malfunctions that may cause injury to the patient and staff.

Electrical Current

To prevent harm to the surgical patient, *grounding* of the electrical equipment is critical. Grounding prevents the passage of the electrical current through the patient by directing the current to the ground, therefore bypassing the patient. A common example of a grounding system is the three-prong plug. Electricity is supplied through the two upper prongs and the third prong is the grounding prong. This allows the current to have a return path to the ground. Manufacturers' instructions emphasize that this third prong should not be removed in order to make it fit a nongrounded outlet. If this is done, ground protection will not be provided.

Preventing Electrical Burns

An electrosurgical unit (ESU), also called the cautery or Bovie machine, produces an electrical current that is converted into thermal heat for cutting or coagulating tissue. To complete the monopolar circuit, the active electrode (formerly called Bovie pencil or electrosurgical pencil) is connected to the ESU; the electrical current travels through the active electrode and patient to the patient return electrode (formerly called grounding pad) and the current returns to the ESU.

It is important that the patient return electrode be in place prior to the beginning of the procedure. It should be affixed firmly to the patient. If the patient return electrode is not firmly affixed, the patient could suffer first-, second-, or third-degree electrical burns in the area of the pad or on other areas of the body that come into contact with metal parts of the operating table or equipment, or at the site of rings, such as wedding bands and ECG electrodes. Care is taken in positioning the patient so that the body does not come into contact with the operating table or other metal or conductive surfaces.

Static Electricity

Static electricity can be a source of ignition leading to explosion, especially in the presence of oxygen and anesthetic gases. There are two processes by which static charge buildup can occur. The first is by friction between two surfaces; the second is by proximity to an electrostatic field. Friction is the concern of the OR and is described as follows (Simco, 1998):

> When substances become charged, electrons migrate from the surface of one material to the surface of the other. Upon separation of the two surfaces, one surface loses electrons and becomes positively charged. The other surface gains electrons and becomes negatively charged. As the friction increases, the amount of static buildup increases. Separating the two surfaces causes a spark(s) from the production of heat. Sparks can ignite flammable gases or substances.

Sterile surgical drapes are made of static-resistant material; however, care must be taken to avoid static buildup, especially if the surgery site is in the head and neck region where waste anesthetic gases can accumulate. The surfaces of draping materials should not be rubbed together.

IONIZING RADIATION

Ionizing radiation can have therapeutic as well as harmful effects. When used in therapeutic doses, it can be used in the treatment of cancer, causing the death of cancer cells. Surgical technologists must be aware of the harmful effects of ionizing radiation, specifically x-rays.

Surgical technologists and patients are exposed to radiation during surgical procedures that require the use of the C-arm (fluoroscopy) and/or intraoperative x-rays. Ionizing radiation can cause changes in the cell membrane, enzymes, protein, and genetic material. These changes can lead to the development of bone, thyroid, and gonad cancer and cataracts and cause spontaneous abortion. Safety measures should be taken to protect the surgical patient as much as possible from the x-rays. The surgical technologist should use protective radiation protective gloves, aprons, thyroid shields, and glasses to minimize exposure to radiation.

Protection of the Surgical Patient

The following guidelines aid in reducing the patient's exposure to x-rays and fluoroscopy:

- When possible, shield the patient's body with a lead apron. The lead shield should always be used for pregnant patients to protect the fetus. Low levels of ionizing radiation can also be harmful to the fetus.
- When fluoroscopy is not being used, it should be turned off. When fluoroscopy is turned on, the patient is continuously being exposed to the radiation.
- Cover the patient's thyroid and/or reproductive areas with lead shields made specifically for those areas.

Protection of the Surgical Technologist

The three most important factors to remember concerning the safety of the surgical technologist and ionizing radiation are time, shielding, and distance. Surgical technologists who constantly work in surgical specialties in which x-rays and the use of fluoroscopy are routine, such as orthopedics, need to be aware of the safety precautions. Surgical team members should follow the radiation monitoring and safety policies and procedures that are established by their health care facility; the policies and procedures will be based on ANSI, CDC, NIOSH, and OSHA regulations and guidelines as well as The Joint Commission standards. The following guidelines aid in reducing the surgical technologist's exposure to x-rays and fluoroscopy:

- Time
  - When not in use, make sure the fluoroscope is turned off.
  - Avoid overexposure to ionizing radiation. The shorter the time of exposure, the less amount of radiation absorbed. When possible, a mechanical device that is designed to hold x-ray cassettes in position should be utilized to prevent exposure of the surgical team members' hands.
  - Surgical technologists exposed to ionizing radiation on a frequent basis or during a long surgical procedure should wear an x-ray–monitoring device. The most popular type is the film badge. The badge measures the accumulated exposure to ionizing radiation. Where the monitor is worn determines the area of the body being monitored. Individual data are collected weekly or monthly.
- Shielding
  - Pregnant surgical technologists should avoid exposure. Staff assignments should be made accordingly to allow the surgical technologist and fetus to be protected. If exposure must occur, the surgical technologist should either leave the room or wear a lead shield that adequately covers the body and fetus. To prevent exposure to the same radiation dose as other surgical personnel, the voluntary declaration of pregnancy must be in writing. Upon notification, the health care facility and Radiation Safety Officer (RSO) must take measures to ensure the occupational exposure does not exceed 0.5 rem during the entire pregnancy. The pregnant surgical technologist may be required to wear an additional x-ray–monitoring device (film badge) to track fetal exposure; the device should be worn under the apron at the waist.
  - All members of the sterile surgical team should wear lead aprons, especially if fluoroscopy will be used throughout the surgical procedure. The lead apron is worn under the sterile gown and must be donned prior to scrubbing.
  - Sterile and nonsterile lead gloves are available to protect the long bones of the hand. The gloves should be worn if it is necessary to hold an x-ray cassette for a single x-ray exposure or during the surgical procedure if an extremity must be held or manipulated during the use of fluoroscopy.
  - Lead thyroid shields should be worn during fluoroscopy.
  - Lead aprons should be laid flat or preferably hung on the apron rack when not in use. Allowing the apron to fold or bend can cause cracks in the lead, rendering the lead apron inefficient.
- Distance
  - If possible, whether sterile or nonsterile, leave the room during exposure of x-rays.
  - Surgical technologists who are a part of the sterile team and cannot leave the room should stand as far away as possible (6 ft or more) from the patient, avoiding the direct beam of ionizing radiation. Stand behind the x-ray machine if possible, behind a portable lead screen, or behind someone wearing a lead shield.

BIOLOGICAL HAZARDS AND SAFETY CONSIDERATIONS

Surgical technologists should be aware of the biohazards that exist in the surgical environment and their ability to cause infectious diseases. Hospital policy and procedures and federal regulations must be followed to protect patients, the public, and health care providers. OSHA and the CDC have established policies to govern the disposal of infectious wastes and prevention of bloodborne diseases.

Standard Precautions

Standard Precautions were defined by the CDC in 1996 apply to blood and *all* body fluids, secretions, and excretions (except sweat). Whether or not they contain visible blood, all body fluids should be treated as if they were potentially infectious, and the skin and mucous membranes of health care workers are to be protected from these fluids to reduce the risk of transmission of microorganisms. Gloves should be worn at all times when working with all body fluids. A description of potential pathogen hazards in the OR is in Chapter 7, including hepatitis virus B, C, and D; HIV; tuberculosis; and other infectious diseases. Anyone in the operative environment is at risk.

Because workers in the operative environment, and especially those in the sterile field, often handle sharp instruments contaminated with blood, the likelihood of accidents is increased.

Causes of Injury Leading to Exposure in the Operative Environment

The majority of sharps injuries in the hospital occur in the OR, and most of these are from scalpel and suture needle injury. Davis indicates other commonly used devices that have caused percutaneous injuries include all sharp and moderately sharp instruments used in operative procedures (Davis, 2001). Injuries occur in common situations such as the following:

- Suturing
- Manual tissue retraction
- Dropping needle on worker's foot
- Placing a sharp in the disposal container
- Reaching for device that is sliding off drapes
- Poorly designed or overfilled sharps container
- Positioning and passing a needle in a needle holder
- Leaving needle on field, which contacts worker's hand

In summary, any handling of a sharp or semisharp instrument or item is potentially dangerous. Proper technique and vigilance are required at all times. The strategies of Standard Precautions, including the proper use of **personal protective equipment (PPE),** will help to minimize risk.

Strategies for Exposure Prevention

PPE must be provided by every facility for all workers, and OR personnel should assume a share of the responsibility for their own protection. Individual concerns and needs as to adequate protection and fit of items provided should be addressed.

In response to the increasing numbers of exposures experienced by health care workers, an increasing number of safety devices have been and are being developed, including blunt suture needles, a suturing device to avoid manual handling of needles, double-gloving, and "no-touch" techniques during wound closure. In addition, safety syringes, IV catheters, lancets, and needleless IV connection systems have been developed. A general safety checklist is presented in Table 5-1.

TABLE 5-1 General Safety Checklist

Absolute Prerequisites
Complete hepatitis B vaccination series.
Use Standard Precautions with all patients.
Use personal protective equipment.
Wear fluid-resistant headwear when appropriate.
Use adequate eye and face protection.
Use appropriate neck protection. Consider recently shaved skin to be nonintact.
Wear fluid-resistant or fluid-impervious gowns as appropriate to expected exposure risk.
Choose gloves appropriately.
Wear appropriate footwear or shoe covers.
Remove gloves carefully to avoid splatter.
Wash hands with antiseptic soap after removing gloves.
Remove eye protection last.
Remove contaminated PPE before leaving the room.
Carefully remove and discard mask following each procedure.
Safety Techniques
Wear gloves when handling surgical specimens.
Wear eye protection if surgical specimen container is opened or splashing is anticipated.
Apply dressings and handle drains or packs with clean gloves.
Avoid touching any surface with contaminated gloves.
Avoid touching existing contaminated surfaces.

Numerous strategies and procedures are used by every hospital to assist the employee with safety issues. These strategies and procedures must be taught and reevaluated on an ongoing basis. Some of these strategies include:

- Have extra PPE readily available should replacement be needed.
- Position sharps disposal containers at point of use.
- Use engineering controls (sharps safety devices) to reduce the risk of percutaneous injury.
- Have a plan for sharps management.
- Continuously evaluate sharps safety devices (safety scalpels, blunt suture needles, other safety needles, and sharps containers).
- Discourage unauthorized entry into the OR.

- Secure a signed preoperative consent for HIV testing, in case of exposure.
- Store a tube of blood preoperatively for all surgical patients to be held in the laboratory for possible HIV testing should an exposure occur.

Neutral Zone

In addition to the previously noted safety practices and devices, a "neutral zone" strategy should be deployed in each procedure. Because many puncture injuries occur during hand-to-hand transfer, we recommend the use of a neutral zone in which sharps may be safely placed by one person and retrieved by another. This may be any of a number of devices, such as magnetic mats, trays, an instrument stand, or a designated area on the sterile field. Small basins are not recommended because items are deep within the basin and hard to pick up and the basin may tip over.

The neutral zone is selected and agreed on prior to the beginning of the procedure by the surgeon and the surgical technologist. This zone is a "sharps-only" zone, and all other instruments are passed directly hand to hand. It is suggested that the surgical technologist announce the sharp by name when placing it in the neutral zone so that the surgeon is aware that a sharp object occupies that space. The sharp object is placed in the neutral zone in a position such that the surgeon may pick up the instrument with the dominant hand and use it without repositioning it, much as with hand-to-hand instrument transfer. The surgeon returns the instrument in like fashion to the neutral zone, rather than passing it back directly. Above all, a team approach should be taken with the neutral zone and communication is key.

Other Sharps Safety Techniques

Hypodermic needles should never be recapped. In the rare occasion where recapping is unavoidable, a safety device or one-handed technique should be used.

Sharps on the Mayo stand should be kept in a central location and always in the same place. A small magnetic sterile sharps container should be used to store used needles for safety and for counting, and loaded needles should be placed at a position as far as possible from the hands of the surgical technologist. Load needles just prior to use to avoid open needles on the Mayo stand.

Hazardous Waste Disposal

Two basic microbiological concepts govern the transmission of disease:

1. A sufficient number of microorganisms must be present in order to cause infection.
2. The microorganisms must have a path for entry into the host.

Health care providers are at risk of contracting infectious disease presented by infectious wastes and from exposure to blood and body fluids from patients. Local, state, and federal government regulations address the issues of how infectious waste material is to be disposed of by health institutions. Infectious waste includes but is not limited to blood and body fluids and disposable surgical supplies contaminated by blood, such as gloves, gowns, sponges, drapes, and sharps. These blood-contaminated items must be disposed of separately from routine surgery department waste material. Sharps must be placed in containers that are resistant to puncture and can be tightly sealed. Blood-contaminated disposable items may be placed in bags, and it may be necessary to double-bag the contaminated items. The bags should also be of a color, usually red, that distinguishes the waste material as separate from routine waste (Figure 5-14).

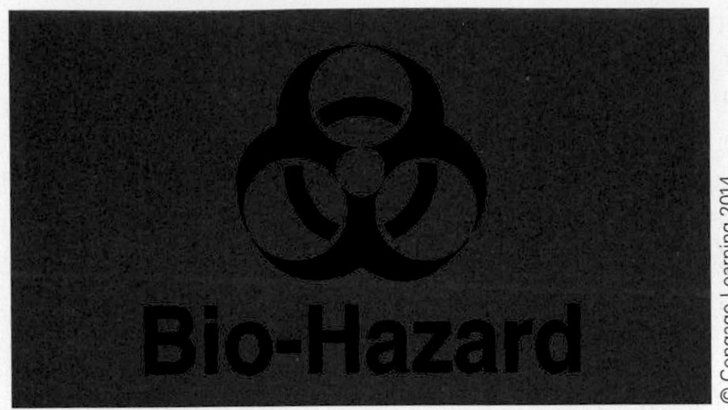

Figure 5-14 Universal biohazard symbol to indicate infectious waste material

Standard Precautions state that all surgical patients are considered a source of infection. Therefore, surgical technologists must follow the biohazard exposure control plan that the surgery department has established as mandated by OSHA outlined earlier in this chapter. By enforcing the policies, such as hand washing after removing surgical gloves, surgical technologists' exposure risk should be reduced.

MANAGEMENT OF EXPOSURE

Despite the best efforts of everyone in the operative environment, accidents do happen. Health care professionals should know how to respond to exposure incidents immediately. Appropriate postexposure measures, including HIV postexposure **prophylaxis** (PEP), are important for the prevention of occupationally acquired HIV and other diseases. The CDC has published updated guidelines and recommendations for the care of occupationally exposed health care workers. These were published in May 1998, and further updates will follow as more information becomes available. Each institution should have a PEP protocol and a list of names of individuals who are experts in infection control readily available for consultation. Some individual on this list should be available 24 hours per day and some PEP treatments should be started within hours of an injury.

When an exposure occurs, surgical personnel should immediately assess the severity of the exposure. If a needle stick or sharps injury has occurred to a person in the sterile field, the glove should be removed to assess the injury. The exposure site should be treated immediately (see later section). As soon as the wound is treated, the exposure should be reported and assessment of the risk of infection should be made by the appropriate clinical personnel, usually the occupational health department of the hospital and the OR supervisor. When indicated, PEP should be initiated within 2 hours of exposure. In high-risk and HIV-risk situations, appropriate counseling as to the risk factors should be provided.

Treatment

If the skin is broken, the wound should be washed with soap and water or a suitable scrub solution. If the exposure is to the oral or nasal mucosa, the area should be flushed with water. Eye exposures are treated by flushing with water or saline.

Risk Assessment

Hospitals should have a well-established system of risk assessment based on CDC recommendations. After exposure, the patient and the exposed health care worker are evaluated to determine the need for HIV PEP. Newer rapid HIV tests are helpful, as the health care worker may need to make a decision within hours as to whether to initiate HIV PEP. The exposure is evaluated based on a set of "risk factors" for potential to transmit HIV, which is determined by the body substance that was involved in the exposure and the route of the exposure (e.g., hollow needle stick, solid needle stick). The patient is evaluated for HIV infection, viral load, and risk factors for infection. When this information is not available, PEP should not be delayed while information is gathered. It is better to start PEP and stop it later than not to have started it within the time window recommended.

Prophylaxis for HIV

If prophylactic drug therapy is indicated based on the risk factors involved, the exposed surgical technologist or health care worker is informed that:

1. Knowledge is not yet complete about the effectiveness or toxicity of the drugs used for PEP. Health care workers must be informed of the possible side effects and toxicity of the drugs.
2. Only zidovudine (ZDV) has been shown to prevent HIV transmission in humans (as of this writing).
3. Although the data are inconclusive, combination drug regimens are recommended at this time because of increased potency.
4. All PEP drugs may be declined.

If PEP is to be used, it should be begun as soon as possible after the exposure. Health care workers exposed to HIV or HBV should receive follow-up counseling and postexposure testing and evaluation. Further testing should be performed at 6 weeks, 12 weeks, and 6 months postexposure.

LASER AND ELECTROSURGICAL PLUME

When a laser beam strikes tissue, the tissue is coagulated, or a powered surgical instrument such as a saw cuts bone, a plume of smoke is produced depending on the power, duration of exposure, and tissue type. Research has been conducted over the years on the plume emitted during surgical procedures. Experiments have documented the content of the plume, particulate matter size, and toxicity of such plumes when inhaled by surgical personnel.

Electrosurgical plume causes an offensive odor and may produce watery eyes and respiratory irritation in surgical personnel. The main area of concern is the viability of the cells in the plume. Many studies have been conducted to answer the question of viability of the cellular contents, especially in the area of laser plume. Studies have not been conclusive but have proved that the laser plume contains water, carbonized particles, and intact strands of DNA. In 1998, Garden and associates discovered intact DNA strands of human papillomavirus in laser plume after using a CO_2 laser at low and high settings to vaporize verrucas (benign viral warts caused by the virus) in seven patients. The study concluded that target tissue can become aerosolized and could possibly be infectious.

Recommendations for protection from plume is the wearing of specially manufactured laser masks that can filter particles as small as 0.1–0.3 μm; proper eye protection such as face shield, goggles, or eyewear that has side shields; and a smoke evacuator.

Currently, electrosurgical plume is evacuated with regular suction often held by the surgical technologist, a practice that may change as increasing attention is given to the possible hazards posed to the surgical team by electrosurgical plume. Special evacuator units are required for laser surgery and may soon be required for electrosurgical plume. Units available on the market filter laser plume from 0.1 to 0.5 μm. Usually the unit has a HEPA or ULPA (ultra-low-penetration air) filter combined with a charcoal filter. The charcoal absorbs hydrocarbons and the offensive odor produced by the plume.

When the filter needs to be changed, it should be done as soon as possible. The individual changing the filter should treat it as contaminated infectious waste, wearing gloves, protective eyewear, and a mask and using clean technique in discarding the biohazardous contaminated filter into a biohazardous waste container.

Positioning the evacuation wand or tip is the duty of the surgical technologist during a laser procedure. The tip must be held very close to the laser tissue impact site in order to efficiently remove the smoke. When the tip is held within 1 cm of the impact site, approximately 98% of the plume is removed. If the distance from the impact site is doubled to 2 cm, the efficiency rate of plume removal is reduced by half.

In summary, the optimal methods to control laser or electrosurgical plume and decrease the surgical team's hazard of inhaling the plume are to:

1. Use an evacuation unit.
2. Change the filter when required.
3. Use filters that evacuate plume particulate matter a minimum of 0.3 μm but ideally 0.1 μm.
4. Ensure the surgical technologist holds the evacuation wand or suction tip as close as possible to the tissue impact site.
5. Wear gloves, masks, and proper eye guards.

LATEX ALLERGY

Latex is made from the natural rubber harvested from trees found in warm tropical climates. It was first discovered by the British in the mid-18th century but did not come into wide use until about 50 years ago. William Halstead introduced natural rubber latex gloves into surgery in 1890. In 1979 a British medical journal reported the first case of latex allergy—a woman had reacted to the rubber in household gloves.

About 1% of the general population is reported to have allergic reactions to latex. Of that percentage, the FDA estimates that 6% to 7% of all direct patient care personnel are sensitive to latex, representing the largest occupational group of individuals who are known to be latex sensitive. Many of the items used in surgery contain latex, and surgical team members who are exposed on a daily basis can become sensitized. Some of the items containing latex include tape, shoe covers, and electrode pads.

Two types of latex allergic responses have been identified: Type I and Type IV. Type IV is the less serious, more localized reaction characterized by skin irritation and discomfort. The common benign reactions associated with Type IV are allergic contact dermatitis and irritant dermatitis. Type I is immunoglobulin E (IgE) mediated and is the most serious reaction, possibly leading to respiratory arrest. Rubber contains proteins, resins, and sugars. Clinical research has shown that water-soluble proteins in the latex itself appear to be the primary cause of allergic reactions attaching to the skin from glove powder absorption or the allergic reaction may also result from inhalation of airborne allergens bound to the glove powder. Refer to Table 5-2 for a comparison of the allergic responses.

Individuals at risk include health care providers, patients who have had multiple surgeries, and children with spina bifida. Surgical technologists should know and recognize the signs and symptoms of possible allergic reaction so immediate action can be taken by the surgical team.

Important points to remember include:

1. All high-risk patients and health care providers should be latex allergy tested.
2. A latex-safe environment should be provided for latex-allergic patients. Only nonlatex products should be used.
3. Latex-allergic patients should be scheduled in the OR as the first surgical procedure. This allows latex dust from the previous day's surgeries to be removed during end-of-day cleaning.
4. All departments involved in the care of the patient, such as the pharmacy and central sterile supply, should be notified so precautions will be taken.
5. The patient's chart should be properly marked signifying latex allergy, and a red ID bracelet should be worn.

Diagnosing latex allergy consists of detailed patient history, skin-prick tests, and the RAST (radioallergosorbent testing) immunoassay. There are drawbacks to both the RAST and the skin-prick test. The RAST blood test, while safe, can render

TABLE 5-2 Comparison of Types of Latex Allergic Responses

Irritant Contact Dermatitis	*Allergic Contact Dermatitis*	*Latex Allergy (Type I)*

• Most common reaction
• Skin reaction
  • Red
  • Raw
  • Cracking
	• Occurs after sensitization period
	• Rash appears 6–48 hours after contact with latex
	• Characterized by fluid-filled vesicles on outer skin layer
		• Reaction occurs within very short period (seconds to minutes) after latex exposure
		• Characterized by
		  • Hives
		  • Edema
		  • Hypotension
		  • Tachycardia
		  • Wheezing
		  • Respiratory distress
		  • Laryngospasms and bronchospasms
		  • Circulatory collapse

Table 5-3 Items Used in Surgery that Contain Latex

- Asepto syringe
- Bulb syringe
- Blood pressure cuffs and blood pressure tubing
- Catheters and tubing
- Disposable face masks
- Esmarch bandage
- Oral airway
- Sterile and nonsterile gloves
- Stethoscopes
- Stopcocks
- Syringes
- Tape
- Tubing
- Urinary catheters and accessory items (bags, tubing, etc.)
- Various types of tourniquets
- Wound drainage devices
- Yankauer suction tip

false negatives, and skin-prick tests can be dangerous to the latex-allergic person if the latex extract's dilution is not carefully controlled. Presently, no cure or desensitization exists for latex allergy. The latex-allergic individual may be prescribed steroids, epinephrine pens, and antihistamines by an allergist. These regimes only treat the symptoms and not the disease. The only true treatment for latex allergy is to avoid the allergen.

Refer to Table 5-3 for examples of items used in surgery that have latex. Manufacturers of disposable surgical supplies generally use a visual symbol on the product packaging to denote that the product is latex free. The types of manufacturing materials used in place of latex to produce items such as those listed in Table 5-3 include Nitrile, neoprene, vinyl, nonpowdered low-protein gloves, polyvinylchloride, and styrene ethylene butylene.

CHEMICAL HAZARDS AND SAFETY CONSIDERATIONS

Many important chemicals used in medical care, such as ethylene oxide and formaldehyde, are potentially hazardous. The chemicals are capable of causing effects ranging from mucous membrane irritation to cancer and adverse genetic damage.

Surgical technologists should be familiar with the chemicals used in the OR and general information concerning the chemicals. Information can be gained from the Material Safety Data Sheets (MSDS) that the surgery department must have available to workers.

Waste Anesthetic Gases

Waste anesthetic gases are vapors that escape from the anesthesia machine and tubing. Studies have indicated that chronic exposure to the gases could pose health hazards such as cancer, hepatic and renal complications, nerve and brain damage, and spontaneous abortion. OSHA enforces NIOSH recommendations for setting the standards determining the occupational limits of exposure for surgical team members.

In addition to good anesthetic techniques employed by anesthesia personnel, a gas-scavenging system should be used and proper maintenance of all anesthesia equipment should occur. The gas-scavenging system, which should be connected to every anesthesia machine used in the surgery department, removes waste anesthetic gases to be filtered and then dispersed to the outside atmosphere. Combined with the scavenger system, the OR ventilation system should aid in preventing the buildup of waste anesthetic gases.

Polymethyl Methacrylate

Polymethyl methacrylate (PMMA) is a chemical compound composed of a mixture of liquid and powder. The common name of PMMA used in surgery is bone cement. It is used for cementing metal prostheses in place during total joint arthroplasties. The liquid and powder components are combined by the surgical technologist at the sterile back table. The vapors released from the mixture are noxious and irritating to the eyes and mucous membranes of the respiratory tract and can damage soft contact lenses, thus damaging the eyes. PMMA has potential health effects that have not been proved. They could include mutagenic effects and carcinogenic and hepatic disorders. The liquid portion of the mixture can permeate through the sterile latex gloves, causing contact dermatitis. Self-contained vapor evacuation systems are available to contain the fumes while mixing the cement.

PMMA also poses a risk to the patient in the form of a pathology known as bone cement implantation syndrome. PMMA infiltrates the interstices of cancellous bone and binds the prosthetic device to the patient's bone. As the cement hardens within the medullary canal of the long bone, it also expands, causing an increase in the intramedullary hypertension. It is thought that this hypertension can cause the microembolization of fat, bone marrow, PMMA cement, and air into the femoral venous vessels; the microemboli are then transported to the lungs.

PMMA cement can also cause vasodilatation and a decrease in systemic vascular resistance, which is thought to be the cause of hypotension frequently associated with the use of PMMA. The syndrome is characterized by one or more of the following:

- Hypoxia (increased pulmonary shunt)
- Hypotension
- Cardiac arrhythmias
- Cardiac arrest

- Pulmonary hypertension
- Decreased cardiac output

Strategies to minimize the effects of this complication and avoid patient death include:

- Increasing the inspired oxygen concentration prior to injecting the PMMA cement
- Maintaining normovolemia in the patient by close monitoring of blood loss
- Surgically venting the distal femur to relieve intramedullary pressure
- Using uncemented prostheses

Formalin

Formalin is a commonly used preservative for tissue specimens to be sent to the pathology department. The vapors from the liquid are an irritant to the mucous membranes of the respiratory tract. It is known to be a mutagen, a carcinogen, and toxic to the liver. Both OSHA and NIOSH have established standards for the permissible exposure limits (PEL) in the surgery department. If exposure to formalin is necessary, it should only be handled in a well-ventilated area with mask and gloves worn.

Ethylene Oxide

Ethylene oxide (EtO) is a liquid chemical converted to a gas for sterilization purposes. Surgical equipment and instruments that are heat sensitive may be sterilized with the use of EtO. The hazards associated with the use of EtO are as follows:

1. Exposure to the gas can cause nausea, vomiting, and vertigo.
2. Ethylene oxide is known to be highly mutagenic and carcinogenic.
3. If EtO combines with water, the toxic byproducts ethylene glycol and ethylene chlorohydrin will form. (Ethylene glycol is easily absorbed through the skin, causing systemic difficulties.)

Glutaraldehyde

Glutaraldehyde is a liquid disinfectant and sterilizing agent. Commercially known as Cidex®, the fumes can be irritating to the eyes and mucous membranes. When not in use, glutaraldehyde must be kept in a covered container system. It must be used in a well-ventilated area, and many health facilities have installed commercial ventilation systems for the removal of the fumes.

Case Study Johanna, CST, is scheduled to be the first scrub on a procedure at 8:00 AM in which a laser will be used to obliterate abnormal tissue in the larynx. She is preparing for the case.

1. What specific safety issues should she consider in preparing for this case?
2. What procedures should be in place to ensure the patient's safety?
3. Are there any anesthetic concerns?

Questions for Further Study

1. Name four ancillary departments in the hospital that directly support the OR.
2. At what temperature and humidity levels should the OR be maintained?
3. What agency is dedicated to protecting the health and safety of the workers in the OR?
4. Should a latex-sensitive patient be scheduled in the OR as the first patient or the last patient of the day?
5. What are the three important safety factors for surgical technologists to consider when exposed to ionizing radiation?

BIBLIOGRAPHY

American National Standards Institute (ANSI). (1996). *Standard Z136.3-1996: Safe use of lasers in health care facilities.* Available from http://web.ansi.org

Ansell Health Care. (1998). *Management of the latex-sensitive patient & health care workers.* Available from http://www.ansell.com/ america/latamer/source/jan93-2.htm

ANSI/AAMI. (2006). ANSI/AAMI ST77*: 2006 Containment devices for reusable medical device sterilization.* Arlington, VA: Author.

ANSI/ASHEA/ASHRAE. (2010). *Standard 170: Ventilation of health care facilities.* Washington, DC: Author.

Association of Surgical Technologists. (2011). *Core curriculum for surgical technology* (6th ed.). Littleton, CO: Author.

Ball, K. A. (2004). *Lasers the perioperative challenge* (3rd ed.). Denver, CO: Association of Perioperative Nurses.

Davis, M. S. (2001). *Advanced precautions for today's OR.* (2nd ed.). Atlanta, GA: Sweinbinder Publications.

Dickerson, J., & Strickland, B. (2003). Low temperature sterilization. In J. D. Ninemeier (Ed.), *Central service technical manual* (pp. 165–175). Chicago, IL: International Association of Healthcare Central Service Material Management.

ECRI. (2003, January). A clinician's guide to surgical fires. *Health Devices, 32*(1), 5–24.

ECRI. (2009, October). New clinical guide to surgical fire prevention. *Health Devices, 38*(10), 5–8.

Garden, J. M., O'Bannon, K., & Shelnitz, L. (1998). Papillomavirus in the vapor of carbon dioxide laser-treated verrucae. *Journal of the American Medical Association, 8,* 1199–1202.

Harris, H. R. (1994). Anesthetic gas: Danger in the OR. *The Surgical Technologist, 26*(10), 14–15.

Kanich, D. G., & Byrd, J. (1996, July/Aug.). How to increase OR efficiency. *OR Reports, 5*(4), 3–8.

Klacik, S., & Strickland, B. (2003). Disinfection. In J. D. Ninemeier (Ed.), *Central service technical manual* (pp. 83–100). Chicago, IL: International Association of Healthcare Central Service Material Management.

Kurz, A., Sessler, D. I., & Lenhardt, R. (1996). Perioperative normothermia to reduce the incidence of surgical-wound infection and shorten hospitalization. *New England Journal of Medicine, 334,* 1209–1215.

Lenehan, G. P. (2004). Latex allergy: Separating fact from fiction. *Nursing, 34,* 12–17.

Marquette University. (1997). *Lifting and proper body mechanics.* Retrieved from http://www.mu.edu/dept/pt/lift.htm

Mercy Hospital Medical Center. (1997). *Are you allergic to latex?* Retrieved from http://www.mercydesmoines.org/health/articles/latex.htm

National Fire Protection Agency (NFPA). (2005). *Standard for health care facilities.* Available from http://www.nfpa.org/freecodes/free_access_document.asp

Occupational Safety and Health Administration (OSHA). (1992). *Bloodborne pathogens and acute care facilities.* Available from http://www.osha.gov

Occupational Safety and Health Administration (OSHA). (1998). *Hazardous medications.* Available from http://www.osha.gov

Patterson, P. (1993). OSHA steps up action on waste anesthetic gases; OR exposure to electrosurgical smoke a concern; efficiency of evacuators depends on filtration system. *OR Manager, 9*(6), 6–11.

Phillips, N. F. (2004). *Berry & Kohn's operating room technique* (10th ed.). St. Louis, MO: Mosby.

Primary electrical circuits (n.d.). Available from http://www.innerbody.com

Simco. (2006). *Understanding static electricity.* Available from http://www.simco.nl/info/about-simco/static-electricity-machinery-j/

Smith, K., Wallace, A., & Smith-Campbell, B. (2004). What you should know about latex allergy. *The Nurse Practitioner, 29*(12), 24.

Stehlin, D. (1992). *Latex allergies: When rubber rubs the wrong way.* Available from http://www.encyclopedia.com/doc/1G1-12535648.html

Strickland, B., & Klacik, S. (2003). Cleaning and decontamination. In J. D. Ninemeier (Ed.), *Central service technical manual* (pp. 67–82). Chicago, IL: International Association of Healthcare Central Service Material Management.

Taylor, L. S. (1996). *What you need to know about radiation.* Available from http://www.physics.isu.edu/radinf/1st.htm

Wenzel, R. P. (2002). *Prevention and control of nosocomial infections* (4th ed.). Baltimore, MD: Williams & Wilkins.

SECTION 2

Principles and Practice of Surgical Technology

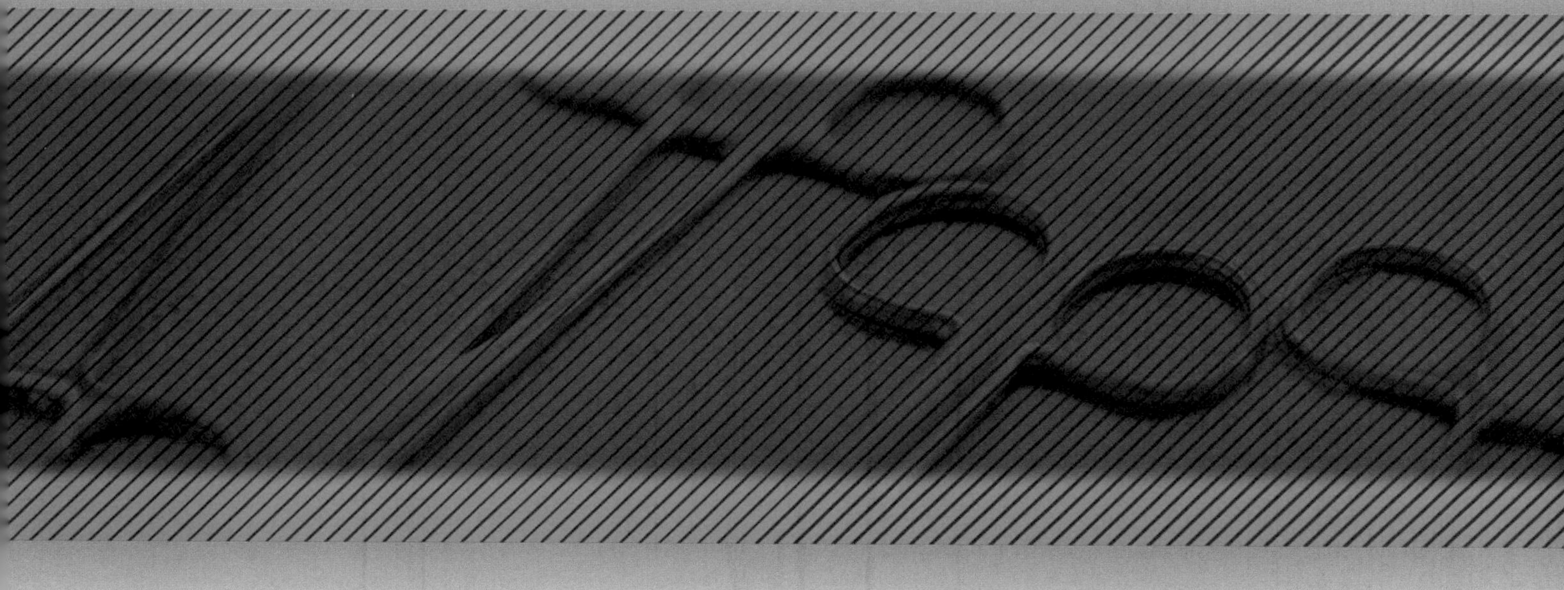

CHAPTER

6

Biomedical Science

CASE STUDY During an open colon resection, the surgeon encounters a small bleeding vessel. A Crile hemostat is applied to occlude the vessel. While the surgeon is holding the clamp, the surgical technologist applies the tip of the activated electrosurgical pencil to the hemostat to coagulate the vessel and stop the bleeding. Suddenly, the surgeon pulls her hand away, yelling aloud. Upon examination, she discovers a pinpoint third-degree burn on her right index finger.

1. Where should the tip of the electrosurgical pencil be placed in relation to the surgeon's hand to reduce the risk of injury?
2. List two possible causes for the burn suffered by the surgeon. Explain both principles.
3. What complications may result from the burn?
4. What is acting as the insulator in this situation?
5. What three factors contributed to the outcome of this situation?

OBJECTIVES

After studying this chapter, the reader should be able to:

1. Recognize basic components of a computer system.
2. Demonstrate basic word processing, Internet, and e-mail functions.
3. Apply computer knowledge to safe patient care.
4. Apply electrical safety precautions.
5. Cite the basic principles of electricity and their application in the operating room (OR).
6. Interpret the basic concepts of robotics.

7. Analyze the geometrical concepts of robotics and the mechanisms of the robotic system.

R

8. Apply the principles of robotics to safe patient care practices in the OR.

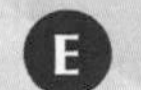

9. Demonstrate principles of sterile technique during robotic surgical procedures.

SELECT KEY TERMS

active electrode
Cartesian coordinate geometry
central processing unit (CPU)
circuit
degrees of freedom
electrons
free electrons
generator
grounding pad
insulators
load
mass
modem
monitor
mouse
neutrons
patient return electrode
plasma
power
pressure
protons
switch

INTRODUCTION

This chapter provides a broad base of knowledge for the entry-level surgical technologist in the areas of computers, electricity, and robotics. As surgical equipment becomes more sophisticated, understanding the fundamental principles of these technologies is essential.

COMPUTERS

Hardware

Hardware is the overall term used to describe the components of a computer, such as the **central processing unit (CPU), monitor, modem**, and memory storage devices (see Tables 6-1 and 6-3).

Using the Computer

The first step is to switch on the computer and the related hardware. Typically, a power button located on the front of each item must be depressed. Once the power is turned on, the CPU goes through a start-up process (sometimes referred to as "booting") and opens the desktop. For security purposes, a login screen that requests the user's name and password may be required. Passwords can be easily changed and updated. Additionally, if users need to be switched, the login screen must be used again for the new user to type in his or her name and password.

For the remainder of this section on computers, the information will be of a general nature and not specific to any one type of operating system (such as Macintosh® or Windows®) or software program (such as Microsoft Word®). Some terms may slightly differ depending on the type of computer and/or software being used, but all attempts have been made to describe terms that are used on a daily basis.

Desktop

The first thing that will pop up on the monitor screen is the desktop, the general background on which windows, dialog boxes, and icons appear. Shortcuts to programs can be placed on the desktop, the screen background (called *wallpaper*) changed, and the taskbar customized.

Software

Computer software are programs that operate the computer system and its individual hardware components, as well as the user's programs, such as word processing, e-mail, or Internet access. Software or computer programs are available on CD-ROMs to facilitate loading (installation) on the computer or may be downloaded from the Internet via the software manufacturer or consolidated software download websites (i.e., www.downloads.com).

Many varieties of software are on the market. Most computer systems are factory equipped with software programs. An example of a popular word processing program is Microsoft Word®. When buying or using a computer, it is important to use one that contains software programs that can be used interchangeably between home, school and work.

Word Processing

Word processing is a term that means creating a document. There are many functions that can be used when creating a document. The functions may be displayed in toolbars (either as words or symbols, called icons, that can be clicked) (see Table 6-4). To reemphasize, the following information is not specific to any one computer program; the terms vary according to the type of computer and software, but every attempt is made to define and describe commonly used computer terminology (see Table 6-5).

INTERNET BASICS

Just as a single computer in a hospital is one of many computers connected via cables to the same server creating a network, the Internet is a gigantic international network connected via millions of servers (including providers for thousands of individual computers). E-mail began as a form of communication

Table 6-1 Components of Tower or Desktop Case

Component	*Location*	*Function(s)*
Central processing unit (CPU)	Silicon chip located within case	• Coordinates operations of computer • Manages computer systems • Facilitates exchange of date with computer memory
Ports	Usually located in back of case, but could be located in front or top	• Serve as attachment points for computer components, e.g. keyboard, speakers, printer and USB thumb drive (Figure 6-1)
Expansion slots	Back of case	• Provide ability to upgrade computer
Network or Ethernet card	Internal or installed in expansion slot	• Provides ability to communicate over network or to Internet
Hard drive	Internal	• Stores information on long term basis; can be magnetic or solid-state
CD-ROM/DVD/ Blu-Ray drive	Generally internal with button on front of case to open and close the drawer that accepts the disk; can be external.	• Disk inserted into drive • Another convenient portable method of storage • Large storage capacity • Files and documents can be "read only" • CD-RW (read-write), DVD+R, DVD−R, DVD+RW, DVD−RW allow recording of files to disk
USB port	Opening in front and/or back of computer tower to insert USB thumb drive or additional peripherals such as mouse, printer, camera, keyboard and iPhone.	• USB is a communication technology. • Referred to as USB thumb drive or USB flash drive; it is a type of USB storage device
Modem	Internal or external device	• Facilitates sending information (e.g., Internet searches and e-mail) over telephone line

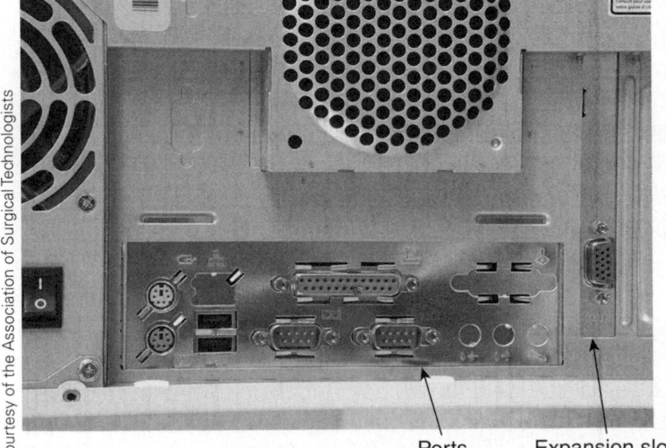

Figure 6-1 Expansion slots and ports

Table 6-2 Bytes of Memory

Name	*Size of Memory*
Byte	Equals to or holds 1 character
Kilobyte (KB)	1024 bytes
Megabyte (MB)	1024 kilobytes
Gigabyte (GB)	1024 megabytes
Terabyte (TB)	1024 gigabytes

TABLE 6-3 **External Computer Accessory Devices**

Device Name	*Functions*
Monitor	• Screen that displays output of computer • Viewable space is measured diagonally • Resolution refers to clarity of the screen image, e.g., 640 × 480, 800 × 600
Keyboard	• Similar to old typewriter keyboard; contains keys with functions to enter characters and commands into the computer • Divided into four areas: alphabet keys, function keys, number keys, and cursor control keys • On desktop devices, keyboards may have a cord that is plugged into a port on the back of the computer case or may be wireless • On laptops (also called notebooks) and netbooks, the keyboard is installed directly onto the unit
Mouse	• Used to move cursor to different areas on screen • Used to select text or commands • Laptops and netbooks have a mouse pad, touch screen, or roller ball to navigate around the screen • Has right and left buttons; pressing on button is called "clicking" • Roller in middle of mouse allows scrolling through a document • Wired and wireless available
Scanner (Figure 6-2)	• Plugs into port at back of computer case • Converts printed text or graphics into digital format (electronic reproduction) so it can be used by computer
Speakers	• Plug into back of computer case • Some monitors have built-in speakers • Require installation of sound card inside the computer case • Facilitate audio functions
Printer	• Plugs into port at back of computer • Prints paper version (called hard copy) of documents and images • Black-and-white or color printers available • Laser printer most commonly used
Surge protector	• Electrical power strip that accepts several appliances • Provides buffer against damage from high-voltage surges, protecting computer and accessories
Battery backup	• Combination battery and surge protector • If electricity is interrupted, the battery's stored energy allows continued use of computer for a short period of time

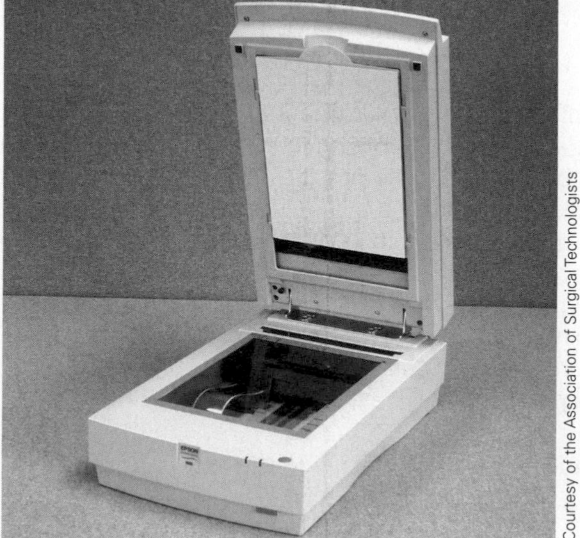

Figure 6-2 Scanner

on the Internet. Now, most e-mail exchange is done through World Wide Web (WWW)–based software.

The WWW is an easy-to-navigate, user-friendly format for browsing Internet pages. The web features computer graphics, text formatting, and even some programming functions that make a logo flash or a word spin. Each photograph or article stored on the web has a different address where the information is stored. These addresses usually start with *http://* and usually contain the letters *www.* (*Note*: Internet software programs do not require the user to type in the *http://* part of the address.) The address ending typically tells the user what type of organization owns the information. Addresses ending in *.com* are usually corporations, those ending in *.org* are nonprofit organizations, and those ending in *.gov* are government agencies. Addresses ending in *.edu* typically signify educational institutions. For example, the web address for the Association of Surgical Technologists is http://www.ast.org. E-mail addresses are similar to Internet addresses and are discussed later in this chapter.

Table 6-4 Basics of Using the Computer

Item or Activity	*Description*
Taskbar	• Shows applications or documents that are open or running • Provides ability to switch between applications or documents, and keep multiple applications or documents open on desktop
Opening a program	• Open menu that lists all installed computer programs • Using mouse, open program by clicking title
Opening a document	• Open documents menu • Click title of document to open
Changing the desktop	• Open control panel (As previously mentioned, we are using general terms. However, here is one specific example. On a Macintosh®, control panels appear as "preference panes" accessible through the systems preference utility; preference panes are small documents rather than independent applications.) • Control panel includes functions such as desktop options, time and date settings, and printers
Getting help (called application menu in Mac)	• Source of information about the computer system • Source of commands for an overall program
Shutting down the computer	• Following correct shutdown process (according to type of computer and the software being used) to prevent losing files • Close all files prior to shutting down the computer
Minimizing and maximizing	• Buttons let user minimize/reduce a window or document. The item is restored by clicking its icon at the bottom of the screen • A window/document can be made smaller on the monitor screen and restored to normal size by clicking minimize or maximize
Opening multiple windows or documents	• Opening two documents simultaneously lets user view and/or compare information as well as move information between documents (see cut/copy/paste function in Table 6-5)
Scrolling	• Term for moving up and down within a document using the mouse or up and down arrows on the keyboard
Dragging and dropping folders or files	• Term for moving folders and files on the desktop or in drives for organizational purposes • Mouse cursor placed over folder or file; while holding down the left mouse button item can be "dragged" (moved) • Mouse button is released to "drop" the folder or file in desired place

Accessing the Internet

To access the Internet, users must set up an account with an Internet service provider (ISP) directly or through their school or library. There are many Internet providers, local and national. Some national Internet providers include AOL and MSN. Each requires the user's computer to contain Internet browser software, such as Microsoft Explorer® or Mozilla Firefox®. This section describes Internet access using Microsoft Explorer®.

The home page appears on the screen whenever the user accesses the Internet. Additionally, the user can always click on the "Home" icon to return to the designated home page.

The phrase *surfing the Internet* refers to looking at many different web pages and jumping from one to another. This is similar to browsing through a magazine; therefore, software for accessing the web is often referred to as a *browser.* Surfing or browsing is made possible using *hyperlinks*—the bold or underlined words on a particular web page. Clicking on one of these words (sometimes an icon) immediately takes the user to a different page. Notice that when a **mouse** points to a link, the arrow changes to a hand with the index finger pointing to the item. Browsing is also performed by using a search engine such as Google®, which is discussed later in the chapter.

Favorites and History Features

Several methods are available to archive website addresses for easy referencing, such as the Favorites and History features.

Table 6-5 Word Processing Functions

- Menu Bar: Includes functions such as File, Edit, View, and Insert. When a name is clicked a menu appears from which various functions can be selected.
  - File: Lists functions including Open, Close, Print Preview, and Print
  - Edit: Cut/Copy/Paste functions are located in this menu
  - View: Provides options to display various other toolbars
  - Insert: Two important functions listed here are page numbering and footnotes
  - Window menu: Menu items allow user to switch between documents or split the screen to view two documents at once
  - Help menu: Allows user to ask questions pertaining to the particular program that is open; also may have Internet help access
- Creating a Document: Each time a user opens a word processing program a new document is automatically created.
- Saving a Document: It is highly important for the user to frequently save his or her work so that entered information is not lost in case of a power outage or computer malfunction. When shutting down a computer the user will be asked if he or she wants to save the current document if is has not already been saved; the user has the choice of clicking "yes" or "no."
- Printing a Document: Click File; click Print in the drop-down menu; a box with various options will appear.
- Previewing a Document: Click File; click Print Preview in drop-down menu. The Print Preview function is used to view how each page of a document will look when printed.
- Spell Checker: This function is used to search for spelling, grammatical, and sentence structure errors. A spell checker will not catch a word that is spelled correctly, but is not the correct word usage in a sentence (i.e., "patience" instead of "patients"). Always proofread the document for errors. Medical term spell-check software is available on the market to download into a computer.
- Cutting/Copying/Pasting: These functions provide the ability to move words, sentences, or whole documents to another place within a document or to another document. In addition, the user can use these functions to repeat a phrase instead of having to retype it or move it.
- Bold: This function darkens words for emphasis.
- Highlight: The electronic version of using a highlighter to emphasize words, sentences, or paragraphs.
- Italics and Underlining: These functions are also used for emphasis.
- Fonts: Fonts are styles of lettering; there are many options, such as Times New Roman, Arial, and Garamond.
- Font Size: This refers to the size of letters; one of the most common font sizes is 12 points.
- Font Color: Used to change the color of the characters or letters.
- Center/Align: Using these commands, the text or images may be aligned to the left, centered, aligned to the right, or set to fill the width of the document.
- Numbering: Numbering is used to number sequential items.
- Bullets: Bullets are used to emphasize items in a list.
- Track Changes: Feature in Word® that allows monitoring of what has been added and deleted from a document; useful when revising a document or policy.

The Favorites feature allows the user to save addresses permanently for easy access; the Favorites heading is clicked and the list comes up for viewing. The list can be arranged in a desired order by the user by dragging and dropping the address. The History feature displays sites that have been accessed within the period of time selected.

Forward and Back Buttons

To move back and forth among pages of a website, use the Back and Forward buttons in the standard toolbar. After surfing through several websites, the user can return to previously viewed pages by clicking these buttons. These buttons only access very recently viewed websites. If the user closes the Internet for any reason, these buttons lose the stored memory of recent pages. In this case, the user can access the History function to return to a particular page.

Importing Images from the Internet

Photographs and drawings can be imported into a document from the Internet. Be aware, however, that material placed on the Internet, in particular documents and photographs, is often copyrighted. Unless a website specifically states that copying is permitted, it is always advisable to contact the publisher, author, photographer, or artist for permission to use the article or image. The following are general steps for importing an image from the Internet into a document or presentation:

- Place the mouse pointer within the image and right-click.
- A menu will appear with several options, such as Save Picture As, E-mail Picture, Print Picture, and Copy.
- Click Copy.
- Open the document or presentation in which you want to import the image. Click Edit in the File menu; click Paste. The image will appear in the document.

The size and location of the graphic can be easily manipulated. Click the image and several small squares or circles will be displayed around the perimeter of the image. Place the mouse pointer over one of the circles and it will change into an arrow; move the arrow up, down, right, or left to increase the size of the image. To move the image, place the cursor over the image. The cursor will change to two crossed arrows. Depress the left button of the mouse and move the image. Release the mouse button once you have placed the image where you want it.

Internet Research

The WWW contains so much information that the user would quickly be frustrated if he or she could not search for a specific topic. Research is conducted by means of a *search engine* (the user's Internet browser always contains a Search function with instant access to one of these engines). Some of the more popular search engines are Google and Yahoo.

The biggest challenge to doing research on the web is helping the search engine understand what exactly to look for. It takes the key word(s) or phrase you type in and finds any links associated with the subject. Consequently, many links will be useless for research purposes, since it may lead to an advertisement or an unrelated article. As a rule of thumb, the first 20 to 30 articles listed pertain directly to the subject area.

When performing a search, keep the subject to one word or a short and succinct phrase. More words will result in a larger search and lead to many unrelated articles and documents being listed. Use quotation marks around the phrase to tell the search engine to search only for those exact words. For instance, a search for "laparoscopic cholecystectomy" would produce a listing of web pages that contain those exact words. Specifically, a search engine works as follows:

- Search engine website is opened
- User types in key word(s) and clicks *Search*
- Page listing websites that match the key word(s) will come up
- User can click on various websites to open

Using E-Mail

Individuals who communicate by e-mail are assigned an e-mail address similar to a home street address. The e-mail address always employs the symbol @ within the address. The first portion of the address is usually personalized by the user and the last portion indicates the Internet/e-mail provider, for example, johndoe@msn.com or janedoe@aol.com (MSN represents Microsoft Network; AOL denotes America Online).

Internet providers often include an e-mail software program. Other types of e-mail programs are also available via certain websites. These include Hotmail and Yahoo.

Several functions can be performed within an e-mail program, including saving a message and replying to, forwarding, printing, or deleting it.

- *Saving*—To save the message, use the File function as previously described for saving other types of files.
- *Replying*—To reply to the sender, simply click on Reply, type your reply, and click Send.
- *Forwarding*—To send a particular message to others, click Forward. The cursor will appear in the To line. This allows the user to input the e-mail addresse(s) of the individual(s) who should receive copies of the e-mail.
- *Carbon Copy (cc)*—The term *carbon copy* is from the days of manual typewriters. It indicates to the persons being copied that they do not need to reply, but they should read the message. The appropriate address is typed in the cc box.
- *Blind carbon copy (bcc)*—Allows the message sender to copy one or more person, but the receiver cannot see who else received the message.
- *Printing*—To print the message, use the Print icon as previously described.
- *Deleting*—To delete an e-mail click the X with the message open. The message is sent to the Delete box and the next new message is automatically opened. Alternatively, close the message by clicking the X. Click once to highlight the message, and then click the X.
- *Address Book*—Used to avoid typing the same addresses repeatedly. The address is entered into the Address Book and can then be accessed automatically for all future use.

SURGICAL APPLICATIONS

Advanced application of computer technology in the hospital setting adds a new dimension to surgical patient care.

Scheduling Surgical Patients

Scheduling of surgical patients has been streamlined because of computer technology. Communication via e-mail or fax from the physician's office instantly provides necessary patient information. The information saved in the computer is easily updated and can be printed or sent by e-mail prior to surgery in order to disseminate the information to surgical personnel and to other pertinent hospital departments. The surgery schedule can be scanned, saved, and sent as an e-mail attachment.

Surgeon's Preference Card

In the past, surgeon's preference cards were handwritten, with additional notes scribbled in the margins, and often became illegible. In addition, if the surgeon had privileges at more than one hospital, it was difficult to get copies of the cards or, if the surgeon moved, the cards would be left behind at the previous hospital. Now, the majority of surgical facilities develop and save preference cards electronically. Consequently, it is easier to update the cards and obtain an accurate copy when preparing for a surgical procedure (preoperative case management) as well as e-mail as an attachment to other health care facilities.

Patient Charts

Centers for Medicare and Medicaid Services (CMS) has mandated that health care facilities use an electronic medical record (EMR) system. Computers facilitate storing, updating, and sharing of patient information among hospital departments and the physician's office. The patient's chart is easily accessed to confirm results of diagnostic studies or other information vital to providing quality care to the surgical patient. Additionally, using these systems have proved to reduce transcription errors and to increase communication between caregivers.

Surgical Records

Many facilities install a computer in each operating room (OR) to facilitate completion of the OR record and save it to the patient's hospital record (chart). The computer can also be used to send laboratory or radiology requisitions and receive the results of the tests in the OR, and other requests and orders can be e-mailed to various related departments (e.g., sterile processing, oncology).

Computers are also helpful for interdepartmental communication. An example is receiving the results of a frozen section specimen from the pathology department. Prior to the availability of and easy access to computers, the pathology report would be called into the surgery department and the information would be written down for the surgeon to review in the OR. (Such information should not be verbalized to the surgeon in case the patient has received local anesthesia and is awake; hearing the results of a negative report could upset the patient and it is best for the surgeon to communicate such information to the patient and family postoperatively.) Now the information can be sent via computer to the surgery department or directly into the OR for the surgeon to read.

Sterile Processing

Computers have substantially reduced the paperwork of the sterile processing department. Supplies can be ordered online, inventory records maintained electronically, and records related to the sterilization of supplies and equipment saved on the computer. Additionally, just as with the surgeon's preference cards, the instrument list/count sheet for the assembly of instrument trays can be entered, saved, updated, and printed.

ELECTRICITY

Physicians have long recognized the benefits of using heat on wounds with electrocautery, which uses a heated wire in direct contact with tissue, eventually being developed to accelerate blood clotting. In the 1920s, the physicist W. T. Bovie developed the first spark-gap tube generator, which culminated in the electrosurgical generator now commonly used in surgery to coagulate or cut tissue. Although the electrosurgical unit (ESU) is completely different from the original machine developed by Bovie, many facilities still refer to the ESU as the *Bovie*.

To ensure patient safety, it is crucial to study the basic terminology and principles of electricity and examine its applications as they relate to the OR. Ultimately, the surgical technologists of the future must be comfortable with theories relating to electricity and its usage. Medicine in the 21st century will increasingly be electronic and, in many cases, robotic.

Basic Principles of Electricity

The principles that govern the behavior of tiny particles known as **electrons** are called the *electron theory*, which helps to explain electricity and serves as the basis for design of all electrical equipment.

Atoms, Electrons, and Matter

Matter is anything that has **mass** and occupies space. All matter consists of atoms and all atoms are composed of small particles: **protons**, electrons, and **neutrons**. The center of the atom is called the *nucleus* and contains protons, positively charged electric particles, and neutrons, neutral particles. Electrons are negatively charged particles that travel in concentric paths or orbits around the nucleus.

Electrons revolve around the nucleus in paths called *shells* or *orbits*. Electrons located closer to the nucleus demonstrate a stronger attraction to the nucleus, whereas electrons moving in the outer orbits are less attracted. In certain atoms, if these outer electrons are exposed to light, heat, or electric energy, they will speed up and leave the atom. These outer electrons are referred to as **free electrons**, and it this movement of free electrons that creates electric current. The term *electricity* describes the free electrons moving or flowing from the ring of one atom to another. Materials that allow the flow of free electrons are called *conductors*. Examples of conductors are silver, copper, aluminum, zinc, brass, iron, saltwater, carbon, and some acids. Copper is the most commonly used conductor because it is the most economical. Examples of devices that use copper wire as a conductor in the OR include surgical lamps, ESU, and power drills.

Insulators

Materials that inhibit the flow of electrons are called **insulators**. Insulators are simply poor conductors. Conductors, such as copper and other metals, are wrapped with an insulating material that does not conduct electricity in order to prevent leakage of electrons while the current flows to the device that will use it. Examples of insulators in the OR are the rubber and plastic covers around the cords of the ESU or x-ray machine.

Because water is a conductor of electricity, the amount of humidity in the air within an environment is important to consider. High humidity often results in static charge leakage and low humidity results in the formation of sparks; therefore, humidity in the OR should be maintained between 20% and 60%.

Electrical Charge

Electrical charges can be either negative or positive and are simply defined as too many or too few electrons on an atom, respectively. One important rule to remember is the law of electric charges: *like* charges repel each other; *unlike* charges attract each other. In other words, two negative charges (materials that have more electrons than protons) or two positive charges (substances that have more protons than electrons) will repel each other. Conversely, unlike charges are attracted to each other. Just remember: opposites attract!

Electrical Current

Electric current is movement of the electrical charge (Figure 6-3). For example, a light bulb illuminates because the electrons move through the conductor and the tungsten filament in the bulb. The filament heats up and brightens. The electrical current travels through conductors by movement of the free electrons that migrate from atom to atom inside the conductor.

Magnetism and Electricity

Electricity and magnetic fields share an important relationship. Today, generators depend on this relationship to produce most of our electricity. Other methods of producing electricity include heat, gas, and solar.

Magnetic Fields

In all atoms, electrons create a magnetic field or electric charge as they orbit the nucleus. In most substances, the effect is neutral since electrons are traveling in different directions. However, in some materials, they line up in the same direction and their magnetic fields are combined and strengthened. Naturally occurring magnetic substances include iron, nickel, and cobalt. Even the earth is one super-size magnet.

Like the earth, magnets have two ends or poles. The north pole of a magnet is located at the end that would point north if the magnet could swing freely. The opposite end is the south pole. A magnetic field is the lines of magnetic force that flow between the north and south poles on a magnet. If two like poles are placed together (north to north), the magnetic force will push the two apart. Conversely, if two unlike poles are placed near each other, the two would move quickly together.

The magnetic field also causes metallic objects, such as paperclips, to be attracted to the magnet or to follow the magnet when it is moved in a certain direction. Another familiar item is the needle in a compass that rotates to align with the magnetic north of the earth.

Two principles are briefly discussed that have important applications in the OR: (1) Magnetism can generate an electric current and (2) electricity is used to generate magnetism.

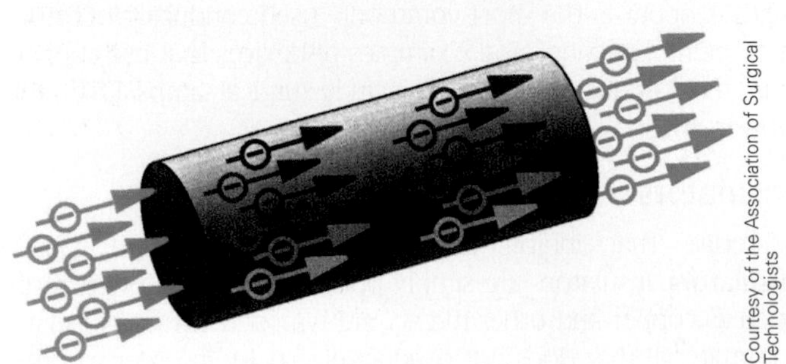

Courtesy of the Association of Surgical Technologists

Figure 6-3 Electrical current

Electromagnets

Electromagnets are metals that become magnetic when a conductor, such as copper wire, is wrapped around them. Current flowing through the wire creates a magnetic field in the metal. A magnetic field can also create electricity. Remember, electricity does not produce power; it is only the means for transporting it. The interaction between the wires and magnets is what produces the power. An example is a rotating magnet that creates an electrical current in a wire conductor. This is how a power plant works. In a coal- or oil-powered hydroelectric plant, water from a dam or waterfall is heated to form steam that is used to turn the turbines. Turbines are simply **generators**—devices that convert mechanical energy (from steam or water) to electric energy. The turbines rapidly spin magnets that create the electricity used by hospitals and clinics, businesses, and homes.

Volts

The term *volt* defines electrical potential. Voltage is the potential energy of electrons (or the electric charge) at any given time between two points. An electric system uses a battery or generator to create a force or voltage to move the electricity from one point to another. The path that electricity travels from the energy source to a device and then back to the energy source is defined as a **circuit**. A simple electrical circuit is comprised of a source of **power**, conductor, **load**, and **switch**.

Current

Current is measured in amperes (amps). *Current* is the flow of electric charge or the rate of flow of electrons. For example, a single strand of copper wire is laid on a table; one end of the wire is negative, and the other is positive. All free electrons in the wire will be attracted to the positive end and consequently flow in the same direction. Free electrons will always be attracted from a point of excess electrons to a point that lacks them.

Power, Load, and Switch

Power is defined as "the rate at which work is done." Power is measured in watts (W), and to facilitate usage, watts are converted to kilowatts (kW). One kilowatt equals 1,000 W.

In a simple electrical circuit, the device that transforms the electrical energy into a useful function, such as heat or light, is the load. The load is the device that uses the electricity to perform some type of function. The load can also change the amount of energy that is delivered from the power source. Examples of loads are surgical lamps, ESU, surgical power drills, surgical robots, and video monitors.

Surgical lamps are resistive energy loads. The conductor material, such as the filament in a light bulb, has a high resistance to the flow of electricity. Resistance refers to restricting the flow of current. The electricity has to force its way through the resistance and the energy causes the conductor to glow or heat up. When the load increases or decreases, the power source is delivering more or less power.

A switch is the device used to open or close a circuit and controls the flow of electricity. Examples in the OR include switches for the surgical lights, operating table, endoscopic camera, and computer monitor.

A flashlight is another common example of a simple electrical circuit (Figure 6-4). The source of power for the flashlight is the batteries. Wires (conductors) are connected to the battery, which is connected to a switch activated by the user. The bulb at the end of the flashlight is the load. The bulb must have voltage in order to work. The voltage is carried by the conductor, and the switch controls the flow of the current to the load. When the switch is "open," there is no flow and the flashlight is not on. When the switch is "closed," the flashlight is on.

When a surgical lamp burns out, the resistance to the current flow will increase and prevent the flow of current. When the voltage remains constant, resistance increases, and the watts decrease. When the current ceases, the bulb is not lit.

Wall Outlets

In the OR, wall outlets are usually 110 volts (V), excluding the outlet for the mobile x-ray unit, which is 220 V. Plugs used in surgery have three prongs. Components of the three-prong plug are

- First prong (positive)
- Second prong (negative)
- Third prong (ground)

If an electrical short occurs, the electrical current will flow through the grounded plug, reducing the risk of current passing through the surgical team or the patient. The third prong should never be removed (cut off) to accommodate plugging into the electrical outlet.

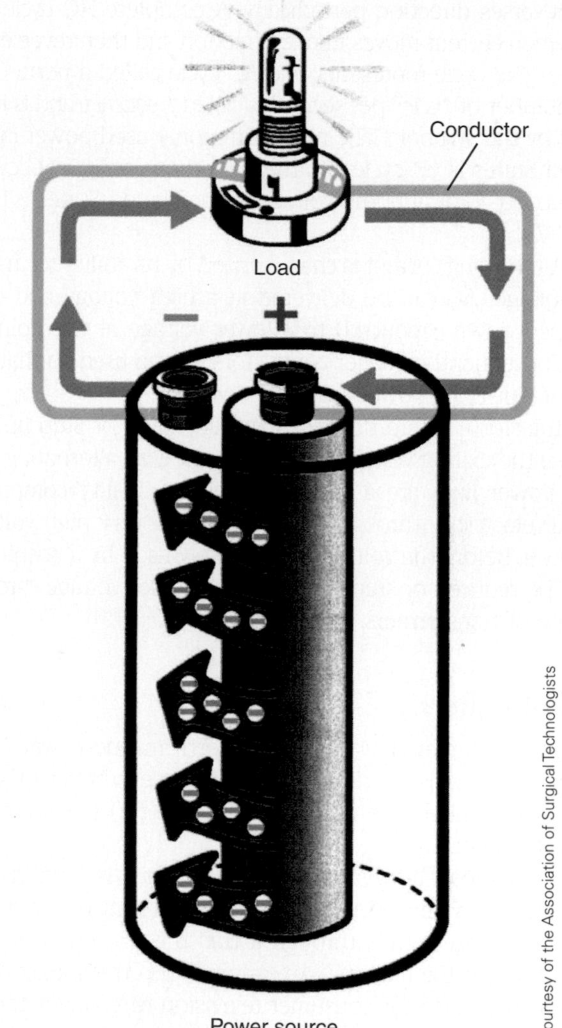

Figure 6-4 Electrical circuit

Direct Current and Alternating Current

There are two types of electrical systems: direct current (DC) and alternating current (AC). Direct current (DC) indicates electrical current that flows in one direction from the negative pole to the positive pole. Batteries are a common example of DC current. Batteries have a negative (−) terminal and a positive (+) terminal. When the switch is closed, current flows from one terminal to the other. Current ceases when the switch is open.

The four components of a DC circuit are:

- Source of electricity (e.g., battery)
- Conductor (e.g., wire from source to load)
- Control device (e.g., switch)
- Load (e.g., bulb, heater, or other load)

Alternating current (AC) describes the flow of current that reverses direction periodically. A complete AC cycle occurs when current moves in one direction and then reverses its course. The cycle represents one AC cycle called a hertz (Hz). The number of cycles per second is called *frequency* and is indicated by the symbol *f*. The most commonly used power in the United States is 60-cycle AC, meaning there are 60 AC cycles per second. Typical home voltage in the United States is 110 V or 120 V.

Alternating current is characterized by its ability to change the voltage. AC can be delivered at a high voltage and then "stepped down" (reduced) to a lower voltage at the point of use. Consequently, smaller conductors can be used so that the cost of delivering power is lower.

Transformers are devices that step down or step up (increase) the exiting voltage and only work with alternating current. Power lines are a common example. Utility companies deliver electricity through power lines at a very high voltage. However, before the voltage can be safely used by a hospital, it must be reduced or stepped down to a lower voltage through the use of transformers.

Radiofrequency

All radio and television signals are electromagnetic waves. An important concept to remember is that the number of wave cycles (remember, one cycle is called a hertz) per second is called frequency.

The radio or television transmitter output is connected to the antenna system located at a distance from the transmitter. The energy travels through a transmission line from the transmitter to the antenna. An example of a transmission line is the cables used for consumer television receiving antennas. Depending on the frequency, the waves travel through the atmosphere or space.

Isolated Circuit

One of the least understood concepts in electricity is protection against electric shock from an isolated or floating circuit. The energy source, or AC generator, is grounded. The secondary circuit contains hazardous current due to the isolated circuit. The secondary circuit is isolated from other circuits by the transformer insulation. However, if a person touches both poles of the isolated circuit in the area where insulation is absent, current will flow through the body to the ground, producing an electrical shock or burn.

Two simple methods are used to prevent shocks from isolated circuits. In the first, a person is prevented from access to all parts of the circuit by the placement of a barrier of basic insulation, usually solid insulation. The second method involves a conductive barrier of insulation between the isolated circuit and conductive barrier that prevents access to all parts of the circuit. The conductive barrier does not require grounding.

Electrosurgery

One of the occupational hazards of working in the OR is electrical burn or shock during electrosurgery. The surgeon or surgical technologist who experiences a shock or burn usually attributes it to a hole in the surgical glove. However, other causes exist for shocks and burns during electrosurgery.

As mentioned earlier, electrosurgery is the application of electrical current through tissue to coagulate or cut tissue. The electrosurgical generator (ESU) is the device that provides the power for electric current to travel to the tissue. Components of the ESU include the generator, optional foot pedal, cords, an **active electrode**, and a **patient return electrode**.

ESU Circuit

The circuit of the ESU consists of

- Generator (power source)
- Active electrode (electrosurgical pencil)
- Patient
- Patient return electrode (PRE)

Current flows from the generator through a conductor cord to the active electrode. The active electrode delivers the electric current to the surgical site through the tissue. The ESU is used to apply electrical current through the patient's tissue to cut and/or coagulate the tissue (Figure 6-5). The electric current is channeled back to the generator via the PRE **(grounding pad)**. Results at the surgical site are dependent on the size of the active electrode, amps, and duration for which the ESU is activated.

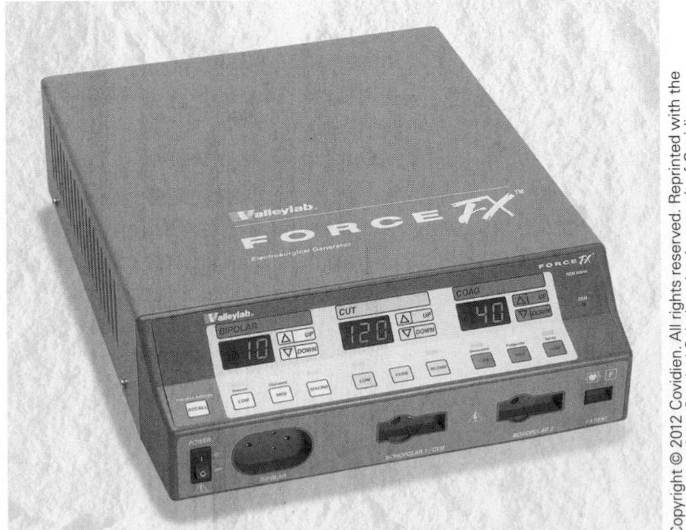

Figure 6-5 Combination bipolar and monopolar ESU

The ESU uses two modes to deliver the electrical current to the tissue: monopolar and bipolar. The *monopolar* mode is the most commonly used. Monopolar electrosurgery is more frequently used for coagulation, but may also be used to cut tissue. The generator is capable of blending the coagulation and cutting functions to achieve a combined result. Monopolar electrosurgery is used when large surgical areas are involved. The *bipolar* mode is used less frequently and is only used for the purposes of coagulation, not cutting. Bipolar electrosurgery is used for delicate surgical procedures, at sites where moisture is nearby, or to prevent damage to delicate tissue and nerves.

MONOPOLAR ELECTROSURGICAL UNITS

The monopolar mode consists of three main components: generator, active electrode, and PRE, also called the grounding pad. (For purposes of clarity and to make the information easier to remember, the term *grounding pad* will be used for the remainder of the discussion, because that is the most common term used in the OR.)

The pathway of the monopolar current is as follows (Figure 6-6):

- Current travels from the generator to the active electrode.
- The active electrode is activated by the surgeon to deliver the cutting or coagulating current to the tissue or vessel.

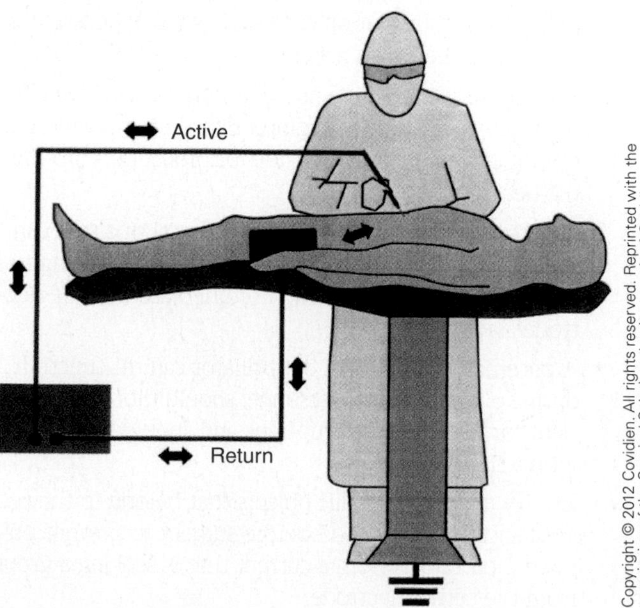

Figure 6-6 Monopolar electrosurgery

- The electrical current passes through the patient's body to the grounding pad.
- The current exits the patient's body via the grounding pad and returns to the generator.

The *generator* is the main unit that provides the source of electrical current to the active electrode and completes the pathway for the returning current from the grounding pad. The generator is activated by the surgeon with a hand control located on the active electrode or with a foot pedal. The power or electrical cord is attached to the back of the ESU. The electrical cord is plugged into a wall outlet in the OR. An electrical cord with a three-prong hospital-grade plug must be used; additionally, an extension cord must never be used with the electrical cord or any electrically driven equipment in the OR. The power cords for the monopolar (and bipolar) foot pedals are attached to the back of the generator. Also located on the back of the generator is the volume control. When the active electrode is in use, the generator emits a sound; if the active electrode is inadvertently activated, the sound alerts the surgical team to stop the activation and prevent burning the drapes and/or patient. Therefore, for safety reasons, the volume should never be completely turned off.

The control panel is located on the front of the generator; located on the front panel is the on/off switch, plug-ins for the active electrode and grounding pad, power level adjustment, and blend (cutting/coagulating) adjustment. Some generators are equipped to handle two active electrodes at the same time. This feature is useful when multiple procedures are simultaneously performed on a patient. The surgeon determines the power and blend settings and communicates the settings to the surgical team.

Some generators are capable of operating in either monopolar or bipolar mode. If this is the case, a separate area on the control panel is dedicated to the functions related to the bipolar mode, such as power level adjustment. For purposes of safety, when turned on the generator performs a self-check prior to entering the "ready" mode.

The *active electrode,* also called the *electrosurgical pencil* or Bovie pencil, is a sterile disposable item that is packaged and sterilized by the manufacturer. It includes a pencil-shaped device (active electrode) with a removable metal tip and a protective holster.

To prepare the Bovie pencil for use, the surgical technologist removes it from the sterile package and sets the entire unit (Bovie pencil with tip and holster) aside on the back table for placement on the sterile field following the application of sterile drapes on the patient. After draping is completed, the cord and holster are attached to the sterile drapes with a nonperforating towel clip. The cord from the Bovie pencil is passed, using aseptic technique, off the sterile field to the circulator for attachment to the generator. Once connected, the power settings are adjusted by the circulator according to the surgeon's orders. When the Bovie pencil is not in use, it should be placed in the holster to prevent inadvertent activation and to prevent the Bovie tip from penetrating the drapes and possibly injuring the patient.

The Bovie pencil is activated by the surgeon by pushing on one of the buttons; there is a cutting button and a coagulating button. Some of the new models of Bovie pencils have a third button that allows the surgeon to adjust the power setting up or down at the sterile field rather than having to request the circulator to adjust the setting located on the generator's front panel.

Various types of tips are available for placement on the end of the Bovie pencil. They include blade-shaped, ball-tipped, loop, and needle tips. Long extended tips are available for deep surgical wounds. Some surgical procedures may call for the use of more than one type of tip; therefore, the tips can be removed and replaced on the end of the pencil by the surgical technologist. The blade or tip of the pencil must be kept clean and free of charred tissue in order to allow the current to freely flow and work efficiently. Sterile "scratch pads" are commercially available that consist of a small square with adhesive on the bottom for attachment to the drapes and a rough, sandpaper topping that the blade or tip can be scraped upon to remove debris and tissue. The surgical technologist must make sure the scratch pad does not come loose and enter the surgical wound. Teflon-coated Bovie tips are available, which allow charred tissue to be wiped away cleanly with a sponge. The tip, no matter what kind is used, is considered a sharp and is included in the sharps count. Dispose of it in the sharps container in the OR.

The flexible, disposable grounding pad is supplied in a protective package with a conductive cord and conductive gel. It is available in adult and pediatric patient sizes. The gel supports the conductivity of the current from the patient back to the generator and allows the pad to stick uniformly to the patient without damaging the skin upon removal; therefore, it should not be rubbed off and the pad should be handled as little as possible. Note that the grounding pad is *only* used when the ESU is operated in monopolar mode. The grounding pad is removed by the circulator from its package and securely placed on the skin of the patient; the flexible conducting cord is then connected to the front panel of the generator. An improperly placed grounding pad can be the cause of severe patient burns.

General safety and patient considerations include the following:

- Even though the patient has received preoperative medications, he or she is still sensitive to what is occurring in the OR. Since ORs are kept relatively cool, the grounding pads can be cold when applied to the skin of the patient. If the patient is receiving general anesthesia, it is recommended to apply the grounding pad after he or she is anesthetized. If he or she is receiving local anesthesia, warn the patient that you are applying a cold pad to the skin.
- Apply the pad *after* the patient has been positioned to prevent wrinkling or movement of the pad.
- Apply the pad to a large, fleshy area, preferably over a muscle mass that is clean and dry. Avoid placing the pad over a bony area or prominence that could contribute to an uneven placement. If the patient is placed in supine position, avoid placing the pad on the buttocks because uneven placement could occur and the pad cannot be seen.
- Do not apply the pad over a metal prosthesis. Doing so may cause the electrical current to travel through the metal and internally and externally burn the patient.
- Handle the pad as little as possible.
- Make sure the entire pad is making full contact with the skin and there is no wrinkling or tunneling. Spaces between the pad and skin can contribute to a break in the electrical current's ability to exit the body and can cause patient burns.
- The packaging may have an expiration date because the conductive gel can become dry. Make sure to check for an expiration date or, if the gel is dry, throw away the pad and open a new package. Do not apply gel to the pad to replace dried gel.
- Place the grounding pad as close to the operative site as possible so that the electrical current traveling through the body is kept to a minimum.
- If a pad is placed but the placement is not satisfactory, remove the pad and apply a new pad; do not use the pad that was removed.
- Do not let skin prep solutions pool around or under the grounding pad. The solutions can burn the patient's skin, causing the pad to fail to adhere to the skin, and the fumes from the solution can ignite when exposed to a spark from the Bovie pencil.
- Flammable anesthetics should not be used during electrosurgery. Precautions should be taken to prevent ignition of oxygen or nitrous oxide for procedures around the head.
- Electrocardiogram electrodes have metal tips that can serve as an errant pathway for the current traveling to a ground, burning the patient. Careful placement of electrodes is necessary.
- A pacemaker or internal defibrillator can malfunction during electrosurgery. Personnel should monitor the patient for potential interruptions and should be prepared with a defibrillator.
- Jewelry or other metallic objects that belong to the patient should be removed before surgery to prevent possible patient burns from a current that is seeking a ground from the active electrode.

BIPOLAR ELECTROSURGICAL UNITS

Bipolar electrosurgery is actually bipolar electrocautery because it is only used for coagulating, not cutting. Bipolar mode uses the same three basic components as monopolar mode, except in a different configuration. The active and inactive electrodes consist of the two prongs of a forceps, eliminating the need to use a grounding pad. Typically, the forceps and cord are reusable and reprocessed by gas sterilization. The surgical technologist sets up the forceps and cord in the same method as the Bovie pencil by preparing it for use at the back table and securing it to the sterile drape at the sterile field. The end of the cord is passed off to the circulator for attachment to the generator and the circulator adjusts the power settings according to surgeon preference. The surgeon will activate the bipolar forceps with the use of a foot pedal.

The bipolar current is as follows:

- Current flows from generator to the active electrode (one of the prongs of the forceps).
- The active electrode delivers the coagulating current to the surgical site.
- Electrical current passes through the tissue between the tips of the forceps prongs.
- Current returns to the generator via the inactive electrode/prong.

ACCESSORIES TO ELECTROSURGERY

Argon gas can be used to enhance the effectiveness of the electrosurgical current. Argon gas is inert and incapable of combustion, allowing electric current to pass safely through the gas. Argon gas is delivered from a portable tank that is attached to a specialized ESU; the gas is emitted from the distal end of a specialized electrosurgical pencil. When the gas is ionized by electric current, it becomes more conductive than air and provides a more efficient pathway along which the current can travel. The energized argon gas appears as a bright beam of light. Because argon gas is heavier than air, the "beam" displaces the air, causing less tissue damage, which in turn produces less vaporized tissue plume than traditional electrosurgery. Since electrical current still passes through the patient, a grounding pad specific for the argon beam coagulator must be placed on the patient.

The harmonic scalpel uses ultrasonic energy rather than electricity to cut and coagulate tissue at the point of impact. Ultrasonic energy is precise and tissue coagulates at a lower temperature compared to traditional electrosurgery; therefore, the surrounding tissues suffer less thermal damage (charring) and less vaporized tissue plume is produced. A grounding pad is not necessary because no electricity passes through the patient.

ADVANTAGES OF ELECTROSURGERY

The advantages of electrosurgery include the following:

- Reduces blood loss and bleeding is quickly controlled
- Saves time since it is faster to use than applying suture ligatures (also called "ties")
- Cutting current burns tissue as it is divided, reducing the need to stop and control bleeding
- Cutting current seals small spaces in the tissue and lymphatic vessels that would normally ooze fluid postoperatively, reducing resorption of toxic fluids, edema, and postoperative pain

HAZARDS TO THE PATIENT AND SURGICAL TEAM

One of the dangers of electrosurgery is electrical burn. In addition to the patient, the surgical team members are also at risk. Possible causes for surgical team members sustaining burns include resonant frequency (RF) capacitive coupling and dielectric breakdown.

RF capacitive coupling occurs when an alternating current travels from the active electrode, across intact insulation, and into the skin. For example, this may happen when a surgeon clamps a hemostat onto a bleeding vessel. While holding the hemostat, the surgeon's skin and the metal hemostat act like two conductors. The surgeon or assistant applies the tip of the Bovie pencil to the hemostat and activates it to coagulate the vessel. The current travels down the hemostat to the vessel. Normally, the surgeon's glove would function as an insulator, protecting the surgeon from the current moving through the metal conductor (hemostat). However, if the glove is thin, thus providing little resistance, the current may travel through the glove (following the path of least resistance) to the surgeon's skin, causing a painful burn. In addition to the thickness of insulation, the risk of RF capacitive coupling is influenced by the size of the active electrode, the duration of activation of the electrode, and the strength of the current. To aid in preventing RF capacitive coupling, the tip of the Bovie pencil should be placed below the fingers of the surgeon or assistant who is holding the clamp or forceps.

Dielectric breakdown occurs when high voltage breaks down some insulating material, such as the sterile gloves. During electrosurgery, it may result when the material in the gloves is unable to withstand the leakage of current generated by the ESU. A high voltage can produce a hole in the glove and consequently the surgeon will sustain a burn. Again, thickness of the insulation, duration of activation of the electrode, and strength of the current influence the outcome.

Vaporized tissue plume (smoke and aerosolized tissue) is formed when tissue is thermally destroyed and vaporized through the use of the ESU, laser, or other surgical devices such as power equipment used to cut bone. Vaporized tissue plume is known to contain harmful chemical and biological byproducts, including carcinogens, blood-borne pathogens, and mutagens, and therefore is considered potentially hazardous to the surgical team members. It is recommended that a smoke evacuator system be used by the sterile surgical team members. The tip of the evacuator wand should be positioned as close as possible to the surgical site to allow maximum removal of the plume. Removal of the plume aids the surgeon in visualizing the surgical site.

SURGICAL APPLICATIONS

Electricity is used in numerous ways in the OR environment. The following examples represent just a few applications encountered while working in the OR.

X-ray Machine

The x-ray machine uses electromagnetic radiation to view internal structures. In the OR, radiographs are used to determine the presence of abnormalities and foreign bodies, to locate retained sponges or sharps, to verify the presence of fluid or air, to confirm correct location of the surgical site, to assist in bone realignment, to aid in prosthesis placement, and to identify the placement of catheters, tubes, and drains.

Endoscopes

A flexible or rigid endoscope is a viewing instrument that is used for diagnosis, biopsy, visualization, repair, retrieval of an object, and hemorrhage control in a hollow structure, such as the abdomen, thorax, heart, ureters, and ventricles of the brain. Endoscopes are attached to a camera and light cord to produce images on a video monitor, and can be used in conjunction with an ESU for coagulation and dissection or paired with a laser for better coagulation and treatment of tumors.

Robotics

Robotics seeks to extend and enhance human capabilities by using powerful computers and robots. Surgical technologists will be encountering robotic arms, the voice-activation control system, and the remote surgical manipulator. Robotics is discussed in more detail later in this chapter.

Lasers

Lasers have been used in the OR with greater frequency since the first practical model was built in 1960. Virtually all surgical specialties have incorporated the use of lasers into their surgical armamentarium as the technology has advanced. The acronym "laser" means *light amplification by the stimulated emission of radiation* and refers to the process of converting some form of energy into light energy that extends from the near-ultraviolet portion to the far-infrared portion of the electromagnetic spectrum.

Laser light is different from ordinary light. Laser light is monochromatic, which means that the photons that compose the light are all of the same color or wavelength. Its color will decide how it will react with various tissues; in other words, red laser light is absorbed by red-pigmented tissue. As the laser energy is absorbed by the tissue, heat energy is produced and the tissue is damaged. Laser light is *collimated,* which means that its waves are parallel to each other and do not spread out as they travel away from their source. This property of laser light allows for pinpoint precision for surgical applications. Laser light is also *coherent,* meaning that the light waves travel in the same direction and in phase with each other, increasing its amplitude and its power.

Another important concept to understand is *fluence.* Fluence refers to the precision of the laser beam and consists of three properties: spot size, watts, and time. Fluence = (watts × time) × spot size. The effect of the laser beam on the tissue will vary if any of the three properties are changed. For example, a laser beam contacts the tissue at 75 watts for 5 seconds. A second laser beam contacts the tissue at 5 watts for 75 seconds, thus delivering the same amount of energy as the first laser beam. However, in the second instance there will be more adjacent thermal tissue damage due to the longer length of time that the laser beam contacts and heats the tissue. Therefore, the concept of fluence emphasizes the importance of the surgeon using the highest safest wattage for the shortest time possible to keep damage to the adjacent tissue to a minimum.

Four Interactions of Laser with Tissue

When the laser beam contacts the tissue, there are four interactions that can occur: absorption, transmission, reflection, or scattering. Thermal damage to tissue due to the absorption of the laser energy depends on the fluence and wavelength of the laser beam, tissue color and consistency, and cellular water content. As the laser energy is absorbed by the tissue, heat is produced and damage to the tissue can occur. The spread of the heat energy is dependent on the tissue consistency and the quality of blood flow to the tissue, which aids in cooling the laser impact site.

When the laser energy impacts the tissue and is absorbed, the cellular water content is heated, causing the water to be converted to steam. The **pressure** within the cell increases, and eventually the cell bursts, releasing debris and smoke from the tissue, which is referred to as laser plume.

The factors that decide the penetration depth of the beam include power of the laser beam, color and consistency of the tissue, laser wavelength, and duration of beam exposure. As the laser beam penetrates the tissue, it continues to heat the deeper tissues. To prevent damage to adjacent tissues and limit the absorption of the laser energy, a backstop is used. Wet sponges, titanium, or quartz rods are used as backstops.

The absorption of the laser energy of the argon and Nd:YAG lasers depends on the chromophores hemoglobin and melanin. The wavelength of the laser beams is absorbed by the chromophores, causing heating of the surrounding tissue. CO_2 laser energy is absorbed by cellular water and is not dependent on tissue color. The majority of the energy is absorbed by and heats the cellular water.

Transmission is best described by the following two examples. The Nd:YAG energy can be transmitted through the distending media, such as glycine that has been introduced into the bladder to vaporize bladder wall tumors. The argon laser energy travels through the clear aqueous humor contained in the anterior chamber of the eye to coagulate blood vessels on the retina.

The laser beam can be reflected from the impact site. The reflection can either cause harm by hitting inadvertent tissue or be purposefully diverted, as in the case of specular reflection. Specular reflection is when the angle of the reflection is equal to the angle of the oncoming light, thus maintaining the beam. This type of reflection is used when the beam is reflected off a laser mirror to direct it toward hard-to-reach tissue. Specular reflection can be a hazard if the laser beam reflects off a surgical instrument, causing it to impact tissue elsewhere. Therefore, when a surgical laser is being used the surgical technologist must make sure that nonreflective instruments are available for the surgeon to use.

Laser Parts

The parts of a laser system include the energy pump or excitation source, laser head, *ancillary* (auxiliary) components, control panel, and delivery system. These are the parts that should undergo annual maintenance, and if the laser does not properly work, they are inspected to determine the problem.

The excitation source is responsible for delivering the energy to the laser head to produce the laser light. The source of a laser's energy can come from any energy form, including electrical or chemical energy or flash lamps. Solid lasers are excited with flash lamps and gas lasers with electricity.

The laser head contains the active medium, which is the substance that is energized and produces the laser energy. Lasers are named according to the active medium, so Nd:YAG is neodymium, yttrium–aluminum–garnet. Refer to Table 6-6 for further information concerning the types of active media.

Mirrors are positioned at both ends of the laser head. The laser energy is reflected off these mirrors. The mirror at one end of the laser head is completely reflective and the mirror at the other end is partially reflective, which allows the laser light to exit as a narrow beam that is focused by a lens or passes into the delivery system.

The ancillary components include the console, cooling system, and vacuum pump. The ancillary components can vary according to the type of laser. The console is the outer cover that houses and protects the inner components of the laser system. It may have a lock in order to prevent unauthorized access to the system. The cooling system prevents the laser head from overheating. Laser systems are either air cooled or water cooled. Air-cooled systems involve an internal fan. Water-cooled systems use either water from an external source or from a continual flow system. The vacuum pump is used in the CO_2 laser; it provides the power to draw out the CO_2 from the gas tank to be delivered to the laser head.

Table 6-6 Active Media

Media	*Characteristic*
Gas	This active medium is energized by electricity to produce the laser light. Examples include carbon dioxide, helium-neon, krypton, argon, and excimer.
Solid	An energy-producing element on a rod is energized by flash lamps to produce the laser light. Examples include ruby and Nd:YAG.
Liquid	An organic dye is energized by a laser beam to produce the laser light in various wavelengths.
Semiconductor crystals	Laser energy is delivered directly to tissue through a filter or slit-lamp microscope.

The control panel is self-explanatory; it contains the controls for operating the laser system, including wattage, duration, and mode. Some control panels have dials that are turned to adjust the parameters, and the newer laser systems have push buttons. A master key must be inserted into the control panel to make the laser operational.

The delivery system is the attachment that transports the laser energy to the tissue from the laser head. The types of delivery systems are articulated arm, fixed optical array, and fiber.

CO_2 Laser

The CO_2 laser has been one of the most frequently used lasers in surgery (see Figure 6-7). The beam is invisible and is located in the middle of the infrared region of the electromagnetic spectrum. Because the beam is invisible, a helium–neon laser beam is transmitted with the CO_2 laser beam to aid the surgeon in aiming. The helium–neon laser beam is a red color. It follows the path of the laser beam. The helium–neon beam has no effect on the tissue.

The advantage of the CO_2 laser beam is that it permits precise cutting and coagulating due to the absorption of the energy by the cellular water content. Therefore, the absorption is not dependent upon tissue color or consistency. Lighter tissue will absorb the energy just as well as dark tissue. Additionally, the CO_2 beam does not scatter. However, since the

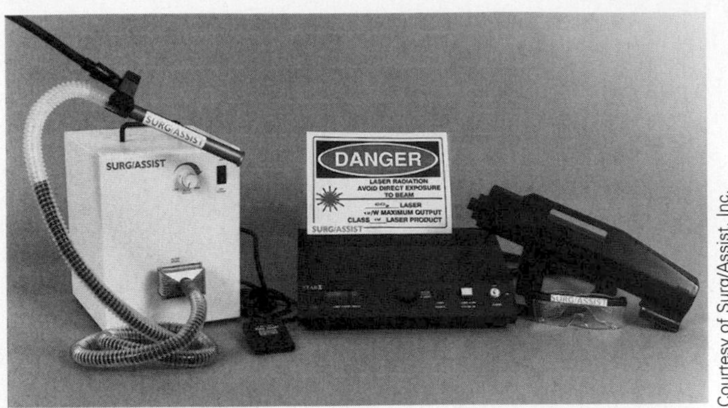

Courtesy of Surg/Assist, Inc.

Figure 6-7 Carbon dioxide laser with plume evacuator

laser beam is absorbed by water, the CO_2 laser is not effective for use if the laser light needs to be transmitted through clear fluids.

The depth of tissue penetration by the laser beam is controlled by the power density and fluence (duration of exposure). When the surgeon wants to cut, higher power with a focused beam is used with short exposure, which decreases the thermal damage to adjacent tissues. For coagulation the beam is enlarged, thus increasing the spot size and spreading the energy. During cutting or coagulation, the beam will continue to go through to the deeper tissue. Therefore, some type of backstop must be used.

The CO_2 and helium–neon beams are delivered through an articulated arm that is a hollow tube. Mirrors are positioned inside the tube at the articulations (joints) and the beams are reflected off the mirrors down the tube. When transporting the laser to the OR and setting it up, the surgical technologist must be very careful to prevent the arm from hitting the wall or anything else so as not to disrupt the alignment of the beams. If the alignment is not correct, the helium–neon aiming beam could appear at one point of the tissue, but the invisible CO_2 beam impacts the tissue at a different point. The options for the delivery of the beam include pulsed, repeat pulse, superpulse, and continuous wave (CW).

A handpiece is attached to the end of the arm, which allows the surgeon to use the laser in a freehand style. The focusing lens is inside the arm, which narrows and focuses the beam onto the target site. The lens must be carefully handled. The lens must never be sterilized by any method or soaked in any type of solution. The manufacturer's recommendations must be followed when caring for the lens.

Nd:YAG Laser

The Nd:YAG wavelength is located in the near-infrared region of the electromagnetic spectrum. The laser consists of an yttrium–aluminum–garnet solid crystal that is laced with the element neodymium. The neodymium is what produces the light energy when it is exposed to flash lamps. The laser beam is invisible, thus requiring a helium–neon laser aiming beam.

The laser–tissue interaction is such that when the laser energy strikes the tissue, there is a slow heating of the tissue at the site of impact and a slowly progressive coagulation of the deeper tissue. The Nd:YAG laser beam is absorbed by darker pigmented tissue, causing a greater coagulation reaction. A significant advantage of the Nd:YAG laser is that the beam can be transmitted through clear fluids because it is not absorbed by fluids. Therefore, the Nd:YAG is often used to vaporize bladder tumors.

The electrical requirements of the Nd:YAG laser may vary. Systems may require a 110-, 208-, or 220-volt line. Older models require an external water-cooling system to cool the laser tube. Newer models are air cooled with an internal water supply that is cooled by the fan.

The laser beam can be delivered to the tissue either by a noncontact fiber delivery system or contact fiber delivery system. The noncontact system uses a quartz fiber. The laser light travels through the fiber end aided by a lens system. As the beam exits the fiber, it impacts the tissue. The fibers must not come into contact with the tissue. If tissue is present on the fibers, due to the heat it will be baked onto the fibers and the fibers will be permanently damaged. The farther the fiber is held from the tissue, the larger the area of tissue that is impacted, but there is a decrease in power density. Handpieces have been developed that have a lens just in front of the beam as it exits, allowing the beam to be focused by adjusting the distance of the lens from the site. The fibers are either reusable or single use. The reusable fibers should always be calibrated prior to the use of the laser by following the manufacturer's instructions. Manufacturers recommend discarding a fiber that has more than 25% loss of power transmission.

Contact fiber systems are facilitated by the use of special tips that deliver the laser energy and are held directly against the tissue. The tips are screwed onto a handpiece fiber or catheter endoscopic fiber, allowing the interchangeability of tips. The tip converts the laser energy into heat at the target area. Laser tips of varying shapes are available that produce the desired shape of laser energy distribution. Tips are chosen based on whether the surgeon wants to cut, vaporize, or coagulate tissue. The tip must always be in contact with the tissue while the laser is in use or the tip will overheat and break. Additionally, the surgeon should not place lateral stress on the tip or it can break. The concept to be remembered is that the laser energy and not the movement of the laser scalpel through the tissue must be used to cut the tissue.

Fluid or air will flow through the length of the fiber and exit at the tip. This aids in cooling the tip while the laser is being used. The side holes on the tip must be kept from being clogged in order to maintain the continuous flow of fluid or air.

The surgical technologist should clean, handle, and store contact tips according to the manufacturer's recommendations. The tips can be soaked in hydrogen peroxide to loosen any tissue and debris prior to cleaning. The majority of tips can be steam sterilized. Additionally, since the tips are small, the surgical technologist should account for all tips when breaking down the sterile field and ensure no tips are lost and thrown away with the disposable surgical drapes.

Holmium:YAG Laser

A type of YAG laser is the holmium:YAG laser, which discharges a pulsed beam. The laser energy travels to the tissue through a flexible fiber. The tip of the fiber should be held less than 5 mm away from the tissue in order to have any effect. The holmium:YAG laser is popular for use among orthopedic surgeons during arthroscopic procedures because the laser beam is transmitted through clear fluids. It is also used in dentistry, for atherectomy, and for radial keratoplasty. The laser system does not require water cooling, but it does have special electrical needs, such as 208-volt service.

Krypton Laser

The krypton laser is a gas laser. An electrical current activates the krypton medium to create the laser energy. The krypton laser has special electrical requirements and requires a water-cooling system.

The wavelengths vary, including green, yellow, and red laser beam colors. The red light is the most frequently used. The krypton laser beam is absorbed less by hemoglobin than the argon laser beam; therefore, ophthalmologists are increasingly using the krypton laser to destroy tissue on the retina of the eye.

Excimer Laser

Excimer laser systems use gases and halogens as the active medium. The laser beam is ultraviolet in color and is absorbed by protein with minimal thermal spread, so the system is used to reshape the cornea for radial keratoplasty and to destroy plaque within a stenotic artery for angioplasty. The four gases used most often are argon fluoride, xenon fluoride, krypton fluoride, and xenon chloride.

The primary advantage of the excimer laser system is the excellent precision that can be achieved in cutting and coagulating tissue with no noticeable spread of thermal damage to the adjacent tissues. However, there are two concerns associated with the laser system. The first is the gases that are used in the unit, which are very toxic and fatal. The excimer laser unit is large due to the large console (protective housing) needed to contain the gases and exhaust system and protect from external electricity. The second concern relates to the possibility of harmful effect of exposure to ultraviolet (UV) radiation. Research is ongoing to determine if the UV rays have mutagenic and/or carcinogenic effects on cells.

Argon Laser

The argon laser produces a blue light or green light in the electromagnetic spectrum. Both blue and green light contribute to excellent tissue absorption of the laser energy. The primary component of the laser system is a **plasma** tube that contains the argon. An electrical current travels down the tube through the gas to excite the argon atoms to produce the laser energy. However, a disadvantage of the argon laser is that the plasma tube must be replaced on a periodic basis and the tube is very expensive. The chromophores (hemoglobin and melanin) selectively absorb the argon laser energy. The laser energy is converted to heat when absorbed and this produces the effects of coagulation or vaporization.

Since the argon laser beam is visible, an aiming beam is not necessary. The low-power argon laser systems require 208 or 220 volts and are internally air cooled by fans. The high-power argon laser systems require higher-voltage connections as well as an external water-cooling system.

The argon laser beam can travel through clear fluids and tissues. Therefore, it is useful for the treatment of diabetic retinopathy, a condition in which bleeding vessels on the retina impair vision. The posterior bleeding vessels can be coagulated since the laser beam can travel through the clear anterior chamber of the eye. Additionally, the argon laser can be used through a cystoscope to vaporize bladder tumors.

Lasers in Endoscopy

With development of the quartz fiberoptic delivery system in the 1970s, lasers could finally be attached to endoscopes for less invasive repair. The first application for endoscopic laser technology was for gastrointestinal hemorrhage control. An argon laser attached to a gastroscope was used to coagulate bleeding vessels in the stomach for a patient with advanced gastritis, eliminating the need for a major surgical procedure to open the abdomen.

Today, the laser of choice for gastrointestinal endoscopy is the Nd:YAG laser system because its beam penetrates deeply into the tissues for better coagulation and destruction of tumor masses. The argon laser, with its shallow beam, is still used to treat angiodysplasias within the thin wall of the intestine.

Laser microlaryngoscopy is routinely used for the endoscopic treatment of many benign and malignant tumors of the larynx. Because of the proximity of the laser to the endotracheal tube, precautions must be taken to prevent combustion during anesthesia administration.

Laser bronchoscopy, first described in 1974, has improved access for treatment of certain diseases of the tracheobronchial tree. The CO_2 and Nd:YAG lasers are the instruments of choice for laser bronchoscopy.

Stereotactic laser endoscopy is used for treatment of certain brain tumors to preserve adjacent neural tissue and to reduce postoperative cerebral edema and recovery time.

Arthroscopy is occasionally performed with Nd:YAG, CO_2, or Ho:YAG laser systems to vaporize protein and bond collagen and to cut or smooth cartilage or tissues within joints. Percutaneous disk procedures can also be performed with the Nd:YAG laser.

Endoscopic transurethral prostatectomy is occasionally achieved with an Nd:YAG laser system. Urethral strictures can be released with an Nd:YAG laser attached to a cystoscope. Bladder tumors can be vaporized with an Nd:YAG laser attached to a cystoscope. A fiberoptic ureteroscope introduced through the urethra and bladder can be used to direct a pulsed dye laser beam into the ureters to fragment calculi.

Hysteroscopes can be coupled with an Nd:YAG laser system to excise and vaporize uterine septa, sessile polyps, and smaller fibroids. Menorrhagia can also be treated with this combination. Laparoscopic laser applications for other gynecological conditions include endometriosis vaporization with the Nd:YAG/laparoscope combination, neosalpingostomy, uterosacral transection, ovarian cystectomy, and certain instances of ectopic pregnancy.

Laparoscopic laser applications can be used for certain general surgery procedures, such as laparoscopic cholecystectomy, which can be performed with an Nd:YAG, KTP, Ho:YAG, or argon laser system.

Colonoscopes combined with argon or Nd:YAG laser systems are used to treat polyps, arteriovenous malformations, and bleeding disorders and to perform the ablation of certain types of tumors.

SURGICAL ROBOTS

A *robot* is a sophisticated machine developed to perform specific tasks. Most robots are used in factories, but with advances in technology, robots are functioning in agriculture, construction, retailing, and other services. This section deals with surgical robots and their applications in the OR.

A machine is defined as a robot if it features some degree of mobility and, once programmed, operates automatically and performs a large variety of tasks.

Robots are classified by generations. First-generation robots are simple mechanical arms without artificial intelligence (AI). They perform precise repetitive motions at high speeds for industrial applications and require consistent oversight.

Second-generation robots incorporate a level of AI. Characteristically, these machines may include pressure or tactile sensors and some type of vision and hearing. While not requiring constant supervision, occasional monitoring is necessary.

Third-generation robots include autonomous and insect robots. An autonomous robot works independently, without supervision by human controllers or an overseeing computer. The insect robots are controlled by a larger central AI computer.

Fourth-generation robots are not yet fully developed but will be distinguished from the other generations by their ability to learn, reproduce, and evolve. Eventually, the intelligence of these robots will exceed the collective computing power of every human brain on the planet.

Surgical robots improve surgical patient care by helping to overcome limitations in human precision and reliability. Although surgical robots are increasingly complex, they still require surgeon control and input, primarily by remote control and voice activation. Experts believe that a robot can be designed that will be autonomous with the ability to operate on patients without human interaction, as well as able to diagnose a disease without human intervention, in the near future.

Robots help control the cost of health care not only by replacing expensive surgical personnel but also by enabling surgeons to perform surgical procedures from a distance. Another cost-saving benefit is the shorter period of convalescence resulting from the minimally invasive procedures performed by robots. Robots can also mitigate the hand tremors of the surgeon and surgical technologist that can result from fatigue.

Terminology

Before a discussion can take place concerning the clinical applications of robotics in surgery, basic robotic concepts must be understood. The robotic "language" presented next will be frequently used by OR personnel:

- *Articulated*—Broken into sections by joints. Many robot arms have articulated geometry and the versatility is measured in **degrees of freedom**.
- *Binaural hearing*—Ability of humans and robots to determine the direction from which sound is coming. Humans have two ears that provide this ability; robots are given two sound transducers that provide the ability.
- ***Cartesian coordinate geometry***—Derived from the Cartesian system used for graphing mathematical functions. The axes are always perpendicular to each other. Also called rectangular coordinate geometry.
- *Cylindrical coordinate geometry*—Refers to the plane that is used in combination with a plane coordinate system and elevation in conjunction with a robotic arm.
- *Degrees of freedom*—Number of ways that a robot manipulator can move. The majority of manipulators move in three dimensions but have more than three degrees of freedom.
- *Degrees of rotation*—Extent that a robot joint or a set of joints can move clockwise or counterclockwise about an axis. A reference point is established and the angles of the joint are stated in degrees.
- *Expert systems*—Method of reasoning in AI used to control smart robots. The expert system consists of facts or data supplied to the robot about the robot's environment; also called rule-based system.
- *Manipulators*—Technical term for robot arms (Figure 6-8).

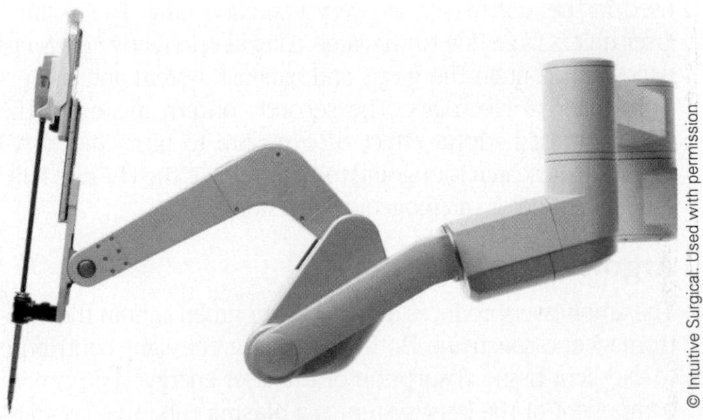

Figure 6-8 da Vinci S® instrument arm

- *Resolution*—Extent to which a machine, microscope, human, or robot can differentiate between two objects.
- *Revolute geometry*—Refers to a robotic arm that can move in three dimensions, resembling the movements of a human arm, such as rotating through a full circle (360 degrees).
- *Sensitivity*—Ability of a machine or robot to see in dim light or detect weak impulses at invisible wavelengths.
- *Telechir*—Name given to remotely controlled robots.
- *Telepresence*—Refers to the operation of a robot at a distance, meaning the operator is situated in one location, usually miles apart, and the robot is on-site with the patient.

da Vinci® Robotic System

One of the most frequently used surgical robots is the da Vinci® system by Intuitive Surgical® (Figure 6-9). The system consists of the following components: console where the surgeon sits to control the manipulators and perform the surgical procedure; patient-side cart where the patient lays during surgery; four manipulators; high-definition three-dimensional vision system (Figure 6-10). The system allows the surgeon to perform minimally invasive surgery through 1- to 2-mm incisions. An innovation by Intuitive Surgical® is the development of the EndoWrist® surgical instruments that are placed in the manipulators for the surgeon to perform the procedure. The instruments provide a full range of motion like the human

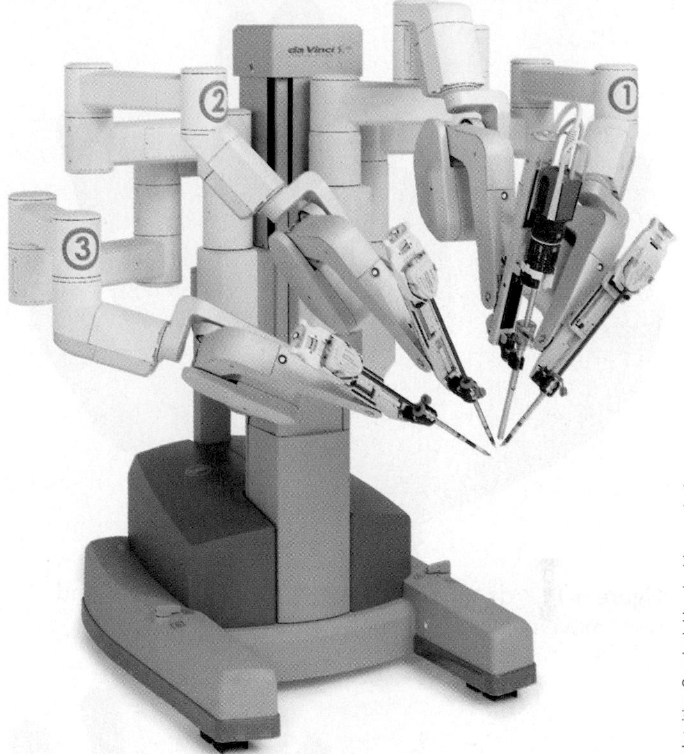

Figure 6-9 da Vinci Si HD® surgical robot

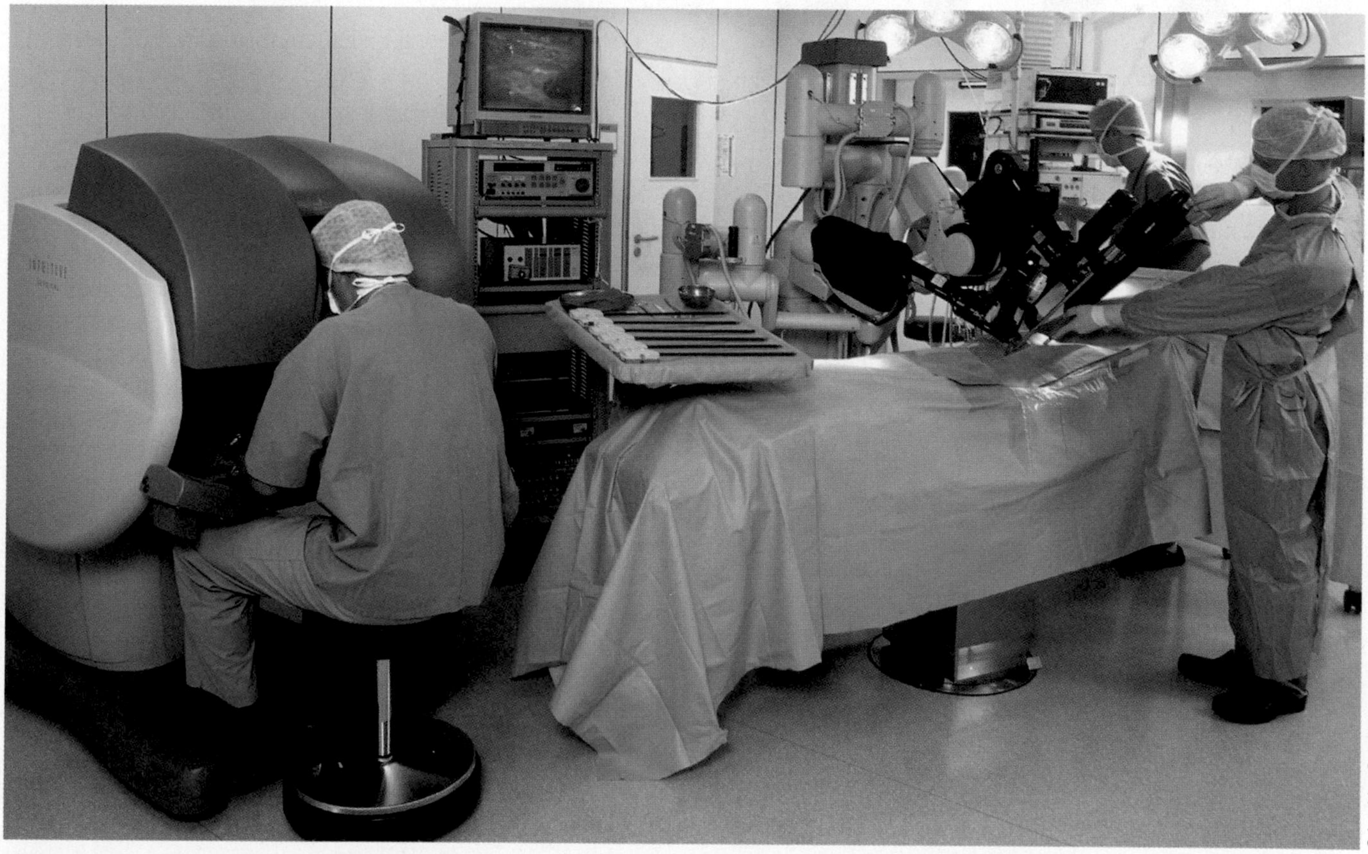

Figure 6-10 da Vinci® surgical system

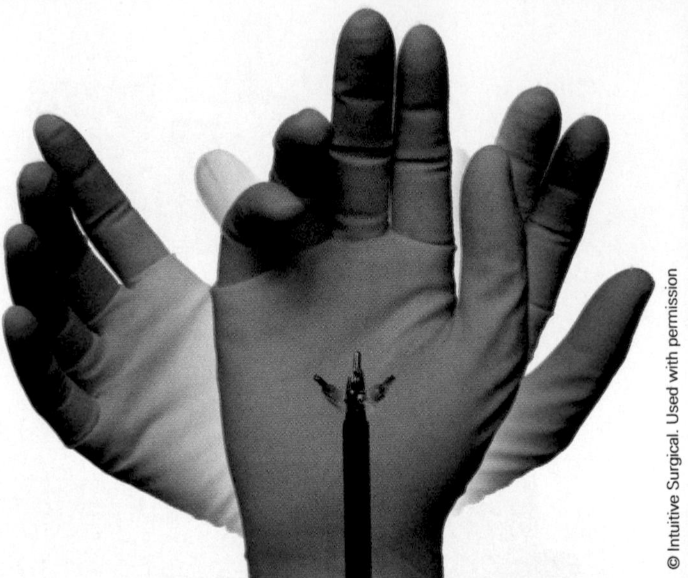

Figure 6-11 da Vinci® surgical system: EndoWrist® and wrist movements of surgeon's hand

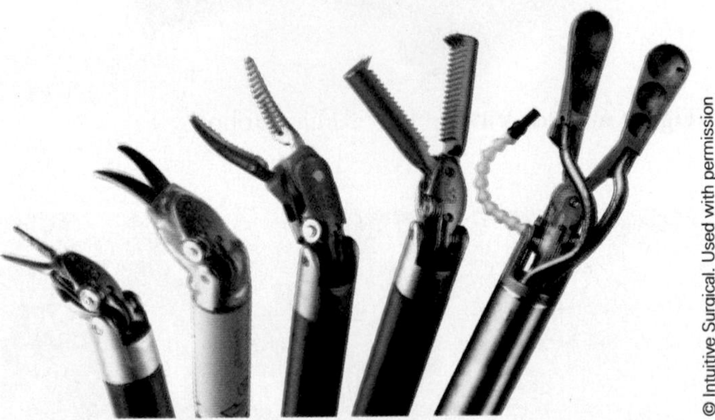

Figure 6-12 EndoWrist® instruments

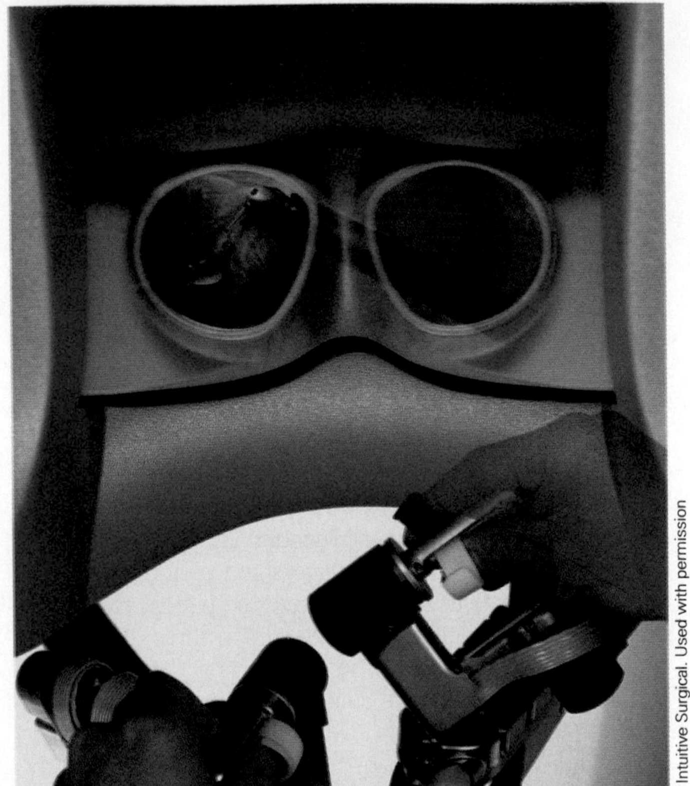

Figure 6-13 da Vinci® surgical system: In-site vision

wrist joint (Figure 6-11). The instruments have seven degrees of freedom and 90 degrees of articulation, providing surgeons with precision ability in performing surgery. Examples of EndoWrist® instruments include the following (Figure 6-12):

- Advanced energy instruments: Provide the surgeon with electrosurgery capability, including monopolar and bipolar energy as well as laser.
- Grasping instruments: Forceps and clamps of various types for use on delicate to heavy fibrous tissues.
- Needle holders: Various sizes available to hold delicate needles such as for cardiovascular surgery to large needles used for suturing the uterus. SutureCut™ needle holders are a combination needle holder and cutting blade to cut the suture after the surgeon has tied the knot.
- Retractors: Various types of retractors with or without serrations.
- Hemostatic clip appliers: Different sizes available to accommodate the various sizes of clips.
- The 5-mm EndoWrist® instruments: Design allows use of smaller incision ports such as during pediatric surgery.

The surgeon sits at the console and views the image of the inside of the patient's body (Figures 6-10 and 6-13). The controls are below the monitor for the surgeon to use; the surgeon's fingers, hands, and wrist movements translate into movement of the surgical instruments positioned in the manipulators (Figures 6-14 and 6-15). The specially designed patient side cart, as previously mentioned, allows the patient to be positioned next to the robotic system under the manipulators; the patient position is according to the procedure to be performed (Figures 6-16 through 6-19). For example, for cardiothoracic procedures, the side cart will be positioned so the manipulators are positioned over the patient's chest.

The surgical technologist who is involved with robotic surgery must have a thorough understanding of the robotic system:

- Positioning the system, including use of the patient side cart and correctly positioning the patient according the procedure to be performed (Figure 6-20)
- Connecting the electrical cords and equipment
- Testing the system

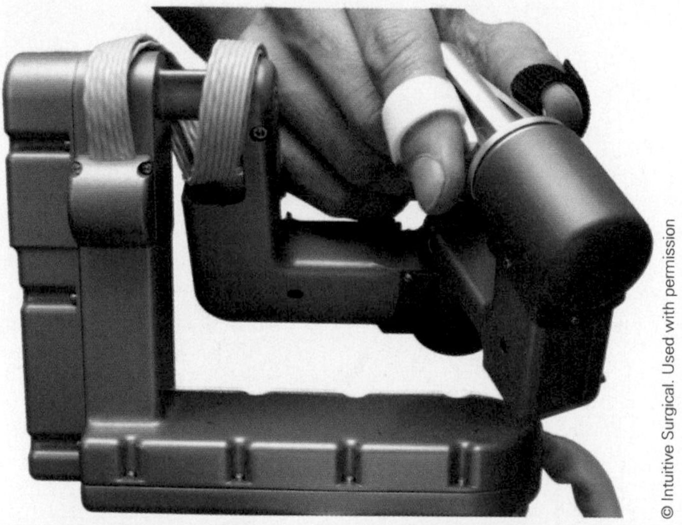

Figure 6-14 da Vinci® surgical system: Hand on control

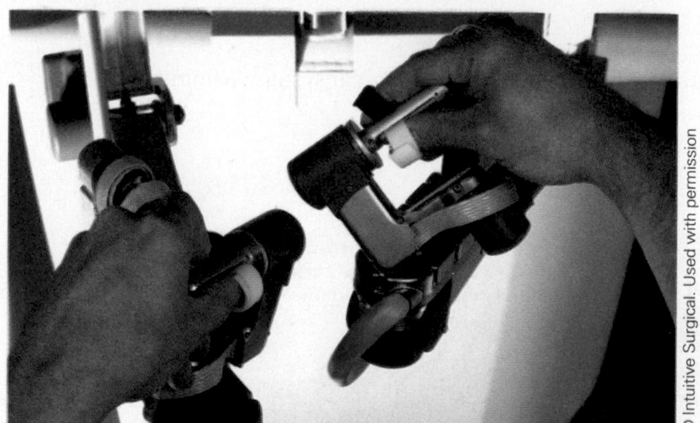

Figure 6-15 da Vinci® surgical system: Console masters

- Loading and switching out the surgical instruments on the manipulators
- Troubleshooting the robotic system and instrumentation

A viewing monitor (referred to as the "slave" monitor) positioned at the patient's side should be used by the surgical team, in particular the surgical technologist, to watch the progression of the procedure (see Figure 6-10). This allows the surgical technologist to anticipate the surgical instruments that will be needed and loading suture. It provides for troubleshooting malfunctioning equipment and instruments.

With advances in robotic technology, the surgeon may perform a surgical procedure from miles away. The surgeon can remotely control the robotic arms at a computer station in Washington, D.C., for a patient and robot located in Las Vegas. Performing a surgical procedure in real time at a distance is termed *telesurgery*. A major obstacle of telesurgery has been the time delay between the surgeon's hand movements and the robotic arms' responses.

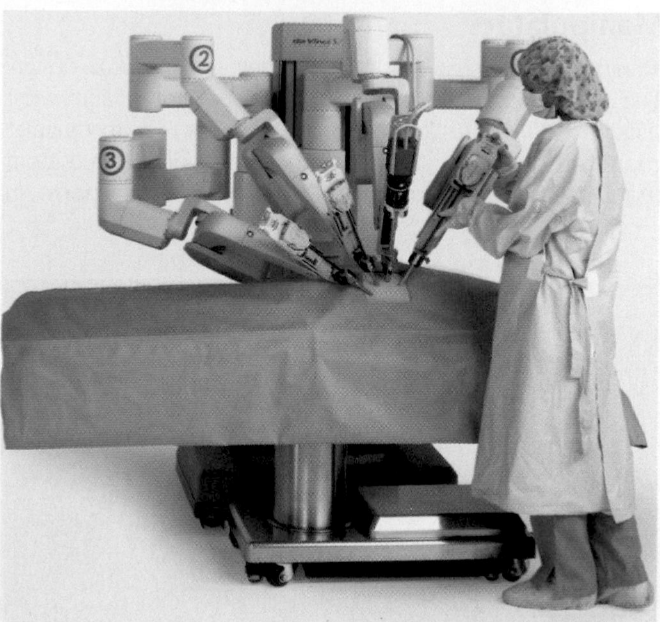

Figure 6-16 da Vinci Si HD® surgical system: Patient side cart

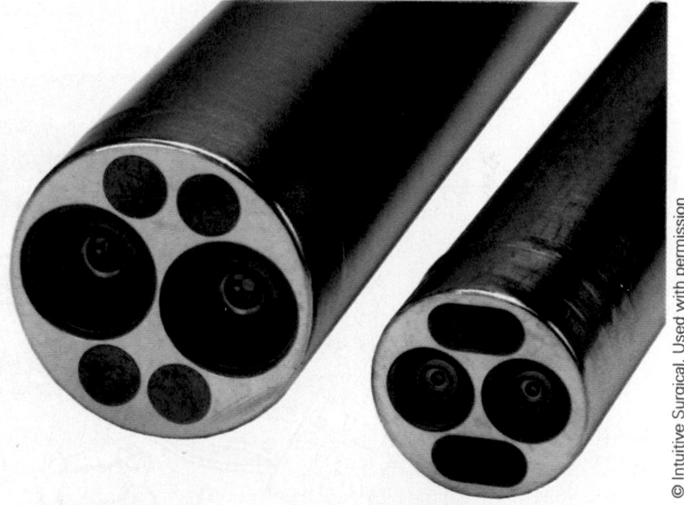

Figure 6-17 The 12-mm and 8-mm endoscopes–distal end

Advantages of Remote Manipulation

- Eliminates hand tremor for more precise surgical technique and fewer errors.
- Allows the surgeon to effectively perform complex interventions within a confined space via small access portals (1.5 mm).
- Affords better visualization of the operative site through three-dimensional imaging.
- Fosters telesurgery, which is a benefit to small rural hospitals.

Manipulators

Manipulators are categorized by their geometrical design. The joints are referred to as shoulders, elbow, and wrist (Figure 6-21). Cartesian coordinate geometry, or rectangular coordinate geometry, is a manipulator design derived from the Cartesian system for graphing mathematical functions. An

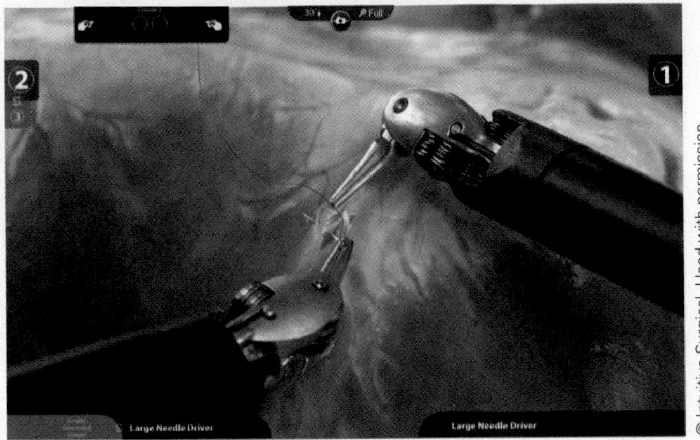

Figure 6-18 da Vinci® surgical system: Operative field view

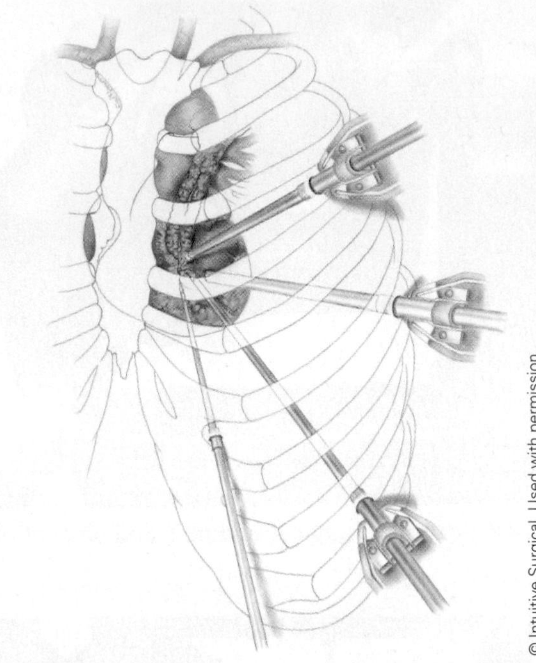

Figure 6-19 da Vinci® surgical system: Minimally invasive ports

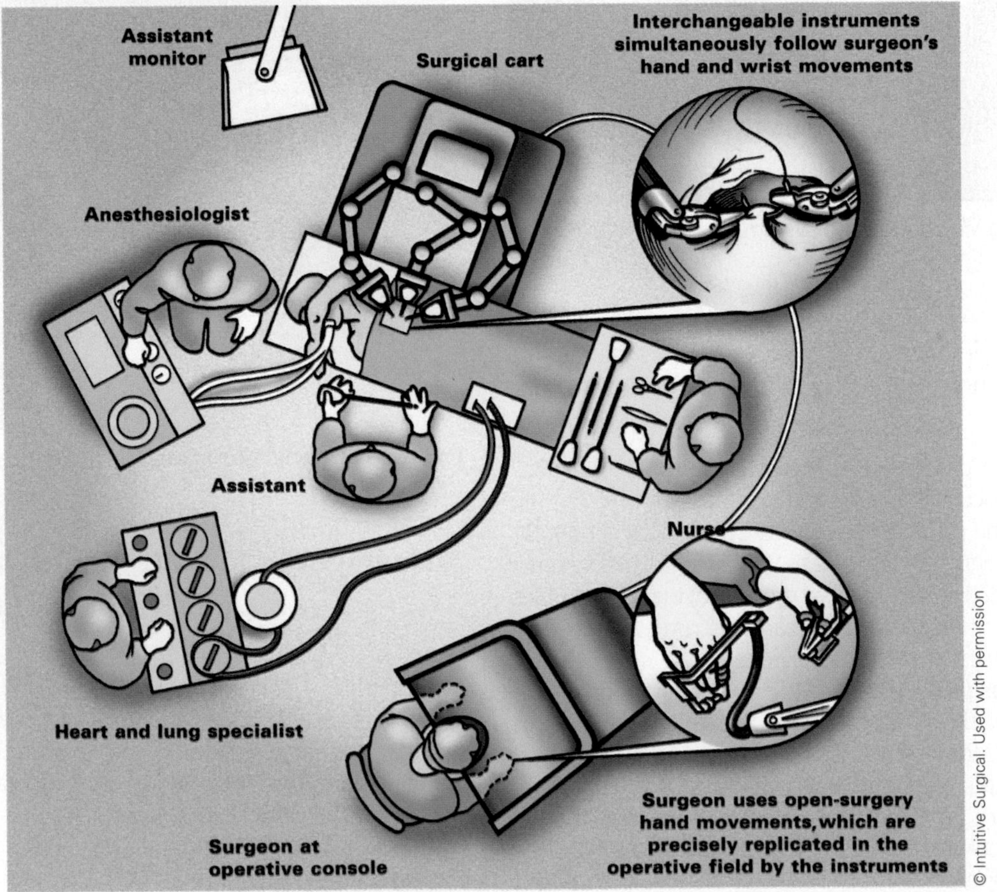

Figure 6-20 da Vinci® surgical system: Operating room set-up

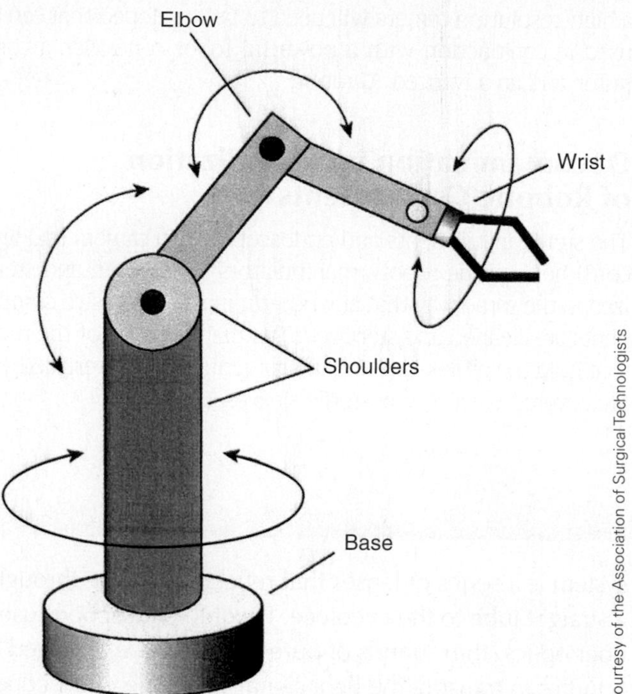

Figure 6-21 Rotation of the manipulator

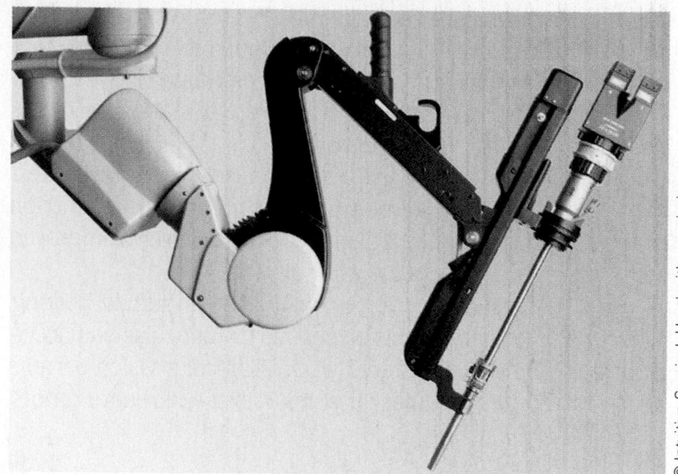

Figure 6-22 da Vinci® surgical system: Camera arm

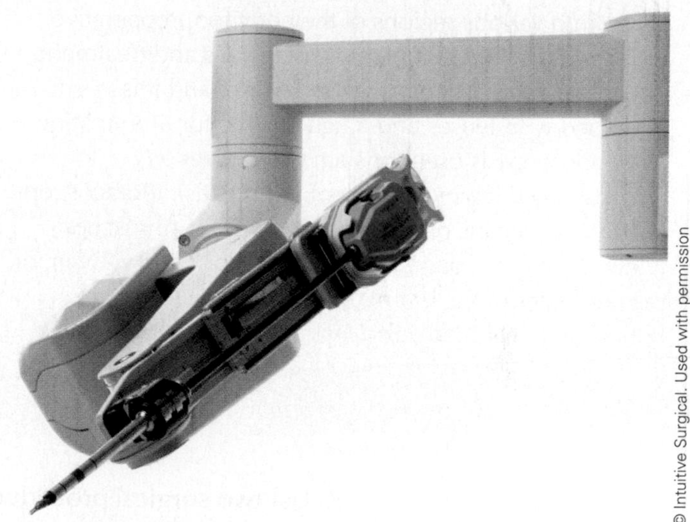

Figure 6-23 da Vinci S® instrument arm—angled

arm with Cartesian geometry moves along the *x*, *y*, and *z* axes (up-down, right-left, and front-back).

The manipulator has a definite number of degrees of freedom and rotation. Degrees of freedom refer to the number of dimensions in which a manipulator can move (most have three dimensions). An up-and-down movement is known as *pitch*, whereas right and left movements are called *yaw*. A rotating movement is a *roll*. By comparison, the human arm has seven degrees of freedom. Degrees of rotation relate to a manipulator's clockwise and counterclockwise movements around an axis.

Other manipulator geometry designs include cylindrical coordinate geometry, a manipulator design that incorporates a plane polar coordinate system with an elevation dimension added; and revolute geometry, a design that allows an arm to move in three dimensions with 360-degree rotation and 90-degree elevation from the shoulder (Figure 6-22). An elbow joint moves through 180 degrees (from a straight position to double back on itself), and a wrist joint revolves and flexes like the elbow (Figure 6-23).

Voice-Activated Control System, Hearing and Vision

Another component of the surgical robotics system is the voice-activated control system. It is a master control unit that is activated by the surgeon's hand or voice via a headset and microphone. The unit controls the manipulator and other surgical applications, such as the shaver and fluid pump in arthroscopic surgery, the light controls in the OR suite, or the printer and computer for storage of intraoperative photographic documentation. It is programmed to ignore casual conversation.

Machine hearing is analogous to human hearing. A robot can distinguish from which direction sound originates and the actual type of sound, such as a human voice. To accomplish this, robots are built with binaural hearing, the same type of hearing humans possess. To provide a robot with binaural hearing, robots, particularly voice-controlled units employed in surgery, are equipped with two sound transducers. This makes it possible for the robot to determine the source of the sound and its origin. Each human voice produces a unique waveform. A recording of the voice (waveform) can be made. The robot will be able to analyze the waveform and interpret commonly spoken commands issued by specific individuals.

Two important concepts must be understood when discussing robotic vision: sensitivity and resolution. *Sensitivity* is the ability of the robot to see in dim light. In some instances, a high level of sensitivity is necessary. For example, during endoscopic procedures, the lights in the OR, including the surgical overhead lights, are either dimmed or turned off. A robot would require a level of sensitivity designed to see in such dim lighting. *Resolution* is the ability to differentiate between two objects and resolution capabilities vary. Obviously, the better the resolution, the better the vision.

However, sensitivity and resolution have a negative effect on each other. If the resolution is improved, the vision function of the robot will decrease in dim light, and vice versa: Improved sensitivity causes a decrease in resolution.

Just as binaural hearing is analogous to human hearing, binocular machine vision is analogous to binocular human vision, also referred to as stereo vision. Binocular vision permits depth perception. In surgery, if vision is ever realized for robots, a high-resolution camera will need to be developed that can be used in conjunction with a powerful robot controller, a computer, and an advanced AI robot.

Decontamination and Sterilization of Robotic Components

The sterile instruments and endoscope (with camera and light cord) held by the robot's manipulators are cleaned and sterilized in the same way that any other minimally invasive components are cleaned and sterilized. The manipulators of the robot that hold the endoscope and instruments are not sterilized, but are covered with special sterile sleeves.

CASE STUDY Endoscopy involves the insertion of a scope into various regions of the body for preoperative, intraoperative, or postoperative diagnosis and treatment. The endoscope may be rigid or flexible, and it is equipped with lenses and a light source for illumination. The endoscope is used for such procedures as laparoscopy (viewing of abdominal organs), thoracoscopy (viewing of organs of the thoracic cavity), arthroscopy (viewing of joint spaces), and ventriculoscopy (viewing of the ventricles of the brain). Rigid endoscopes use an optical system called a *rod lens system*. The rod lens system is a series of lenses that reflect the image through a straight tube to the eyepiece. Flexible endoscopes use fiber optics, thin strands of pure glass that are arranged in bundles to transmit the light signals. Flexible endoscopes are equipped with controlling wires to allow for a wider range of motion. Fiber-optic endoscopes work through a physics principle called *total internal reflection*. The light in a fiber-optic cable travels through the endoscope core by bouncing (reflecting) from the glass cladding along its walls. The cladding does not absorb any light from the core, so the light wave can travel great distances.

1. **List two surgical procedures that would most likely require the use of a rigid endoscope.**
2. **List two surgical procedures that would most likely require the use of a flexible endoscope.**
3. **Why does the light emitted by a laser create different results than a light emitted by an endoscope?**

QUESTIONS FOR FURTHER STUDY

1. Briefly describe the function used to move up and down within a document on the computer.
2. What are some of the consequences of high humidity in the OR?
3. Why might a patient's jewelry be hazardous in the OR?
4. What is the purpose of the patient return electrode?
5. What are the four factors that determine the penetration depth of the laser beam?
6. What kind of surgical instruments must the surgical technologist make sure are used during laser surgery?

BIBLIOGRAPHY

Association of Surgical Technologists. (2011). *Core curriculum for surgical technology* (6th ed.). Littleton, CO: Author.

Baaea, I., Schultz, C., Grzybowski, L., & Gotzen, V. (1999, March). Voice-controlled robotic arm in laparoscopic surgery. *Croatian Medical Journal, 40*(3), 409–412.

Ball, K. A. (2004). *Lasers, the perioperative challenge* (3rd ed.). Denver, CO: Association of Perioperative Room Nurses.

Basic electricity. (n.d.). Retrieved August 22, 2002, from http://www.actechelp.com/Electrical/basic_electricity_lesson.htm

Computertime technologies. (n.d.). Retrieved July 29, 2002, from http://www.computertim.com/howto

Cosgrove, D. M., & Sabik, J. F. (1996). Minimally invasive approach for aortic valve operations. *Annals of Thoracic Surgery, 62,* 596–597.

Cosgrove, D. M., Sabik, J. F., & Navia, J. L. (1998). Minimally invasive valve operations. *Annals of Thoracic Surgery, 65,* 135–138.

Donnelly, S. (1998). *Solids, liquids, and gases, oh why?* Retrieved October 16, 2002, from http://www.cpo.com/Weblabs/solig.htm

Felger, J. E., Nifong, L. W., & Chitwood, W. R. (2001, March). Robotic cardiac valve surgery: Transcending the technologic crevasse! *Current Opinions in Cardiology, 16*(2), 146–151.

Feynman, R. P. (2005). *Six easy pieces.* New York: Basic Books.

Freeman, I. A. (1989). *Physics made simple.* New York: Doubleday Dell Publishing.

Geis, W. P. (1995). Efficiency & outcomes improve with AESOP. *Computer Motion Review,1*(1).

Getting results with Microsoft Office 97. (1997). Redmond, WA: Microsoft Press.

Gibilisco, S. (2006). *Teach yourself electricity and electronics* (4th ed.). New York: McGraw-Hill.

Goldwasser, S. A. (1998). *A practical guide to lasers for experiments and hobbyists.* Retrieved October 16, 2002, from http://www.eio.com/repairfaq/sam/laserfaq.htm#faqwi

Gussow, M. (2007). *Schaum's outline of basic electricity.* New York: McGraw-Hill.

Harada, K. (2002). *Basic electrical principles.* Retrieved October 7, 2002, from http://www.harada-sound.com/sound/handbook/basicelec.html

Henderson, T. (1996). *The physics classroom: Work, energy, and power.* Retrieved October 7, 2002, from http://www.glenbrook.k12.il.us/gbssci/phys/Class/energy/energtoc.html

INT Media Group, Inc. (2002). *Webopedia.* Retrieved July 29, 2002, from http://www.webopedia.com

Intuitive Surgical, Inc. (2000). *da Vinci surgical system.* Retrieved November 14, 2000, from http://www.intuitivesurgical.com/html/index.html

John Hopkins University Office of News and Information. (1998). *John Hopkins University launches research center to expand role of computers.* Retrieved September 24, 1998, from http://www.hopkinsmedicine.org

Karney, J. A. (2006). *A+ certification training kit* (3rd ed.). Redmond, WA: Microsoft Press.

Kasser, B. (1999). *Using the Internet* (4th ed.). Indianapolis, IN: Que Corporation.

Konecny, C. (1995). Laparoscopic cholecystectomy setup. *Computer Motion Preview, 1*(1).

Konecny, C. (1995). Scrub nurse (tech) considerations for laparoscopic cholecystectomy. *Computer Motion Preview, 1*(1).

Kozierok, C. M. (2002). *The PC guide.* Retrieved July 29, 2002, from http://www.PCGuide.com

Kuhn, K. F. (1996). *Basic physics: A self-teaching guide* (2nd ed.). New York: John Wiley & Sons.

Law, C., Taralekar, C., & Wang, J. (2002). *Basic electricity and magnetism.* Retrieved October 7, 2002, from http://www.library.thinkquest.org/16600/beginner/electricity.shtml

Lawson, P. (1996). Laparoscopic Nissen fundoplication. *Computer Motion Preview, 1*(2).

Lehrman, R. L., (1998). *Physics the easy way* (3rd ed.). Hauppauge, NY: Barron's Educational Series.

Marion, J. B. (1985). *General physics with bioscience essays* (2nd ed.). New York: John Wiley & Sons.

Massillon, O. H. (2006). *Understanding the relationship between surgical gloves and electrosurgery.* Red Bank, NJ: Ansell Healthcare Products, Inc.

Medical Robotics at University of California-Berkeley. (2002). *Surgical robotics.* Retrieved November 14, 2000, from http://robotics.eecs.berkeley.edu/medical

Meyer, L. A. (1995). *Basics of electricity.* Hayward, CA: LAMA Books.

MIT Medical Vision Group. (2001). *Project on image guided surgery: A collaboration between the MIT AI Lab and Brigham and Women's Surgical Planning Laboratory.* Retrieved November 14, 2000, from http://www.ai.mit.edu/projects/medical-vision

Nute, R. (2002). *Floating circuits—protection against electric shock.* Retrieved October 7, 2002, from http://www.ewh.ieee.org/soc/emcs/pstc/TechSpk/floating.html

Oman, D. M., & Oman, R. M. (1998). *Physics for the utterly confused.* New York: McGraw-Hill.

Padwick, G., et al. (1997). *Using Microsoft Outlook 97.* Indianapolis, IN: Que Corporation.

Person, R., & Rose, K. (1995). *Using Word for Windows 95.* Indianapolis, IN: Que Corporation.

Phillips, N. F. (2007). *Berry & Kohn's operating room technique* (11th ed.). St. Louis, MO: Mosby.

Rothrock, J. C. (Ed.). (2006). *Alexander's care of the patient in surgery* (13th ed.). St. Louis, MO: Mosby.

Sullivan, L. (1993, July). *Autoclaves. Safe science newsletter.* Lansing, MI: Office of Radiation, Chemical and Biological Safety, Michigan State University. Retrieved October 16,

2002, from http://www.orcbs.msu.edu/newsletters/July1993/autoclave.html

Tusczynski, J. A., & Dixon, J. M. (2001). *Biomedical applications of introductory physics.* New York: John Wiley & Sons.

Valkenburgh, V. (1995). *Basic electricity.* Clifton Park, NY: Delmar Cengage Learning.

Valley Lab. (2002). *Principles of electrosurgery.* Retrieved October 7, 2002, from http://www.valleylab.com

Woods, J., Yong, W. J., Sutton, A., & Hopkins, W. (1999). *Light and lasers: Behavior of light.* Retrieved January 12, 1999, from http://www.ece.utexas.edu/projects/ k12-fall98/14540/Group7/Behavior.html

Chapter

7

Preventing Perioperative Disease Transmission

Case Study It was a Thursday morning in operating room 10. The room, instrumentation, and patient were prepared for a left frontal craniotomy for the removal of a meningioma. The neurosurgeon had just made the skin incision when the unit charge nurse opened the OR door and said, "Stop where you are! Central Sterile Processing just called. There was a malfunction of the steam sterilizer during the night shift. The sterilizer chart does not confirm that the instruments went through a complete cycle. All the external indicators are turned and, thus far, all the internal indicators have turned."

1. What steps should be taken at this point?
2. If all the indicators are "turned," why is the unit charge nurse concerned?
3. What mistake or mistakes were made that allowed the instruments to reach the OR?

Objectives

After studying this chapter, the reader should be able to:

C 1. Discuss the relationship between the principles of asepsis and practice of sterile technique and surgical patient care.
2. Define and discuss the concept of surgical conscience.
A 3. Discuss the principles of asepsis.
4. Define the terms related to asepsis.
5. Discuss the sterile practices related to the principles of asepsis.
6. Identify the principles and procedures related to disinfection and sterilization.
R 7. Demonstrate competency related to the practice of sterile technique.
8. Demonstrate competency in the procedures related to disinfection and sterilization.
E 9. Discuss the surgical environment and the application of the principles of asepsis to the environment.

SELECT KEY TERMS

asepsis
autoclave
bioburden
biological indicator
Bowie-Dick
cavitation
chelation
chemical indicator
colonization
contaminated
endoscope
event-related sterility
immediate-use steam sterilization
immersion
integrity
Intermediate-level disinfection
Julian date
lumen
pathogen
permeability
SSIs
sterile field
sterile technique
sterilization
ultrasonic cleaner

PART I: Surgical Microbiological Principles

CASE STUDY

A patient who recently underwent abdominal surgery has developed a postoperative SSI. The surgeon orders the antibiotic gentamicin to be administered to the patient, but the infection worsens. The patient is next administered linezolid (Zyvox®), an antibiotic in the class of synthetic antibiotics called oxazolidinones, and the infection begins to resolve.

1. What microorganism is most likely the cause of the postoperative SSI?
2. What other diseases can this microorganism cause?
3. The microorganism stains purple when subjected to the Gram stain test. Is the microbe gram-positive or gram-negative?
4. The microorganism can grow aerobically on the skin's surface and anaerobically in the pores of the skin. What is the oxygen classification of this microbe?

PATHOGENS AND INFECTION

Microorganisms, minute life forms invisible to the naked eye, are a natural part of the world in which we live. They include nonpathogenic and parasitic life forms. In nature, microorganisms serve to convert complex organic compounds such as animal and plant matter into more simple forms through the process of decay. Some microorganisms take inorganic compounds and convert them to higher forms that can be used as nutrients by plants and animals. These organisms are used beneficially by humans in the production of food products such as yogurt and cheese, in nutrient compounds, and even in antibiotics. This chapter provides an overview of the microorganisms encountered in the operating room (OR).

Human–Microbe Relationships

When a person becomes sick or develops infection in a wound, he or she typically notices the interaction of the microbial world with humans but usually does not understand the types of relationships that exist between humans and microbes. This section briefly discusses these various relationships, including symbiosis, mutualism, commensalism, parasitism, and pathogenicity.

Microbes that live on the skin and inside the human body, referred to as *indigenous microflora*, include bacteria, fungi, viruses, and protozoa. Indigenous microflora are also referred to as *opportunistic pathogens*. Under normal circumstances these microflora are harmless, but given an "opportunity," such as the ability to enter the body through a surgical wound, they become pathogens. The relationship between human hosts and indigenous flora is called *symbiosis*. The term *symbiont* refers to both organisms. The relationship may be harmless, harmful, or beneficial to one or both symbionts. *Mutualism, commensalism,* and *parasitism* are the categories of symbiosis (see Box 7-1).

PATHOGENS ASSOCIATED WITH SURGICAL SITE INFECTION

The multiplication of organisms in the tissues of a host is called *infection*. Any infection that develops while a patient is in

Box 7-1 CATEGORIES OF SYMBIOSIS

Mutualism

Both organisms benefit from and depend on one another to a certain extent.

Example

- *Escherichia coli*, which colonizes within the human intestine, obtains nutrients from the food that humans eat.
- *E. coli* produces vitamin K, which is essential to the blood-clotting process in humans.

Synergism: Subcategory of mutualism

- Two organisms work together to achieve a result neither could obtain alone.
- Example: Fusobacteria and spirochetes work together to cause a disease known as trench mouth.

Commensalism

- One organism benefits but second organism neither benefits nor is harmed.

Example: Indigenous microflora on the skin of humans obtain nutrients, but do not affect the skin or human body. To a certain extent they benefit humans by occupying space and preventing other potentially harmful microbes from colonizing, a process referred to as *competitive exclusion*.

Neutralism: Subcategory of commensalism

- Two organisms occupy the same area with no effect on each other.

Antagonism: Second subcategory of commensalism

- One microorganism inhibits or interferes with the growth of another.
- Example: A microbe produces waste products that are toxic to the neighboring microbes.

Parasitism

- One organism benefits and the host is harmed.

Example: Endoparasites, such as intestinal worms, cause an infection and deplete the body of nutrition.

Microorganisms that cause an infection are called **pathogens**. Examples of pathogenic relationships include the following:

- Commensal microbes that become opportunistic by entering through a surgical skin incision.
- Nosocomial infections (infections acquired in a hospital) such as urinary tract infections.
- Airborne viruses, such as the virus that causes the common cold.

the health care facility is termed a *nosocomial* infection. More recently, government agencies involved with patient care, infection control, and public health have broadened the categorization of infection and termed them health care–associated infections (HAIs). These infections may affect not only a patient but also any individual who has contact with the health care facility, including health care workers and visitors. HAIs may become apparent during inpatient stays; however, as many as 25% of infections acquired intraoperatively do not become evident until the patient has been discharged from the hospital. The Centers for Disease Control and Prevention (CDC) compiled recent data estimating that HAIs accounted for 1.7 million infections and 99,000 associated deaths per year. Of these:

- 32% of all HAIs are urinary tract infections
- 22% are surgical site infections **(SSIs)**
- 15% are pneumonia (lung infections)
- 14% are bloodstream infections

The primary goal of the surgical technologist, as well as all surgical team members, is to be vigilant with sterile technique to prevent the transmission of microbes perioperatively, therefore preventing SSIs.

In this chapter, we describe only the most commonly occurring pathogens associated with SSIs. The types of microorganisms that may cause infection are numerous, and for a more in-depth look, the reader should refer to a standard microbiology text.

Bacteria

All living cells are classified into two groups: *prokaryotes* and *eukaryotes*. The eukaryotes' cellular structure is complex, and this classification includes protozoa; fungi; green, brown and red algae; and all plant and animal cells. The prokaryotes are less complex organisms whose organelles are not membrane bound like those of the eukaryotes. All bacteria are prokaryotes. Bacteria divide by the process of binary fission, which is a simple division that results in two identical cells.

Bacteria are classified based on specific characteristics that are observed in the laboratory. The identification of these characteristics not only aids in classifying the bacteria, but also identifies the relationship of the microbe to other microbes and humans. For example, if a patient develops an SSI and a culture and sensitivity of the infection is taken, the laboratory should be able to identify the bacterium causing the infection. The information is communicated to the physician, who is then able to order the antibiotic that is most effective in fighting the infection, based upon the characteristics of the infectious microorganism and the specific antibiotics to which the organism is sensitive. Another example would be the identification of a new type of bacteria; based on the observations of the bacterial cell, microbiologists would be able to classify the microorganism. Table 7-1 provides information on the characteristics that are examined when identifying and classifying bacteria.

Table 7-2 lists common bacterial pathogens. Table 7-3 provides an overview of pathogens most commonly associated

Table 7-1 Characteristics of Bacteria

Morphology: size, shape, and arrangements of bacteria

- Coccoid: round-shaped bacteria (*coccus*, singular form; *cocci*, plural form)
  - Diplococci: paired bacteria
  - Streptococci: chain of bacteria
  - Staphylococci: cluster of bacteria
  - Coccobacilli: a bacterial cell intermediate in morphology between a coccus and a bacillus. While still rod shaped, coccobacilli are so short and wide that they resemble cocci.
- Bacillus: rod-shaped bacteria (*bacillus*, singular form; *bacilli*, plural)
- Spirilla: spiral-shaped bacteria
- L-form: bacteria that lose normal shape due to adverse environmental conditions; once normal conditions are reestablished cells revert to normal shape

Growth: varies with type of agar medium

- Shape, size, and color of a bacterial colony will be specific to the bacterial species grown on or in a particular nutrient medium
- Rate at which bacteria multiply is a key characteristic

Motility: ability of a microbe to move by itself

- Flagella: long thin structure attached to the outside of the cell; uses whipping motion to provide motility to the cell
- Cilia: fine, short, hairlike extensions located on the surface of the cell; their coordinated, rhythmic movement allows the cell to move

Nutritional requirements: bacterial species are classified according to their nutritional needs

- Examples of nutritional needs: carbon, oxygen, sulfur, nitrogen, hydrogen, phosphorus, vitamins, iron, calcium, copper, zinc

Oxygen requirements: bacterial species classified according to oxygen and carbon dioxide needs

- Obligate aerobes: require level of oxygen found in a typical room
- Microaerophiles: require oxygen but at level lower than that found in room air (about 5% oxygen)
- Obligate anaerobes: will not grow if there is any amount of oxygen present in the environment
- Facultative anaerobes: able to survive in an environment that contains oxygen or no oxygen
- Aerotolerant anaerobes: grow best in environment without oxygen, but can survive in atmosphere that contains up to 15% oxygen
- Capnophiles: grow best in high concentrations of carbon dioxide

Pathogenicity: ability to cause disease

- Release of exotoxins or endotoxins
- Release of enzymes
- Presence of a protective capsule
- Direct damage by attaching to the host cells to invade tissues of the body

Metabolism: secretion of waste products

- Secretion of enzymes, oxygen, methane, or carbon dioxide

Proteins: some proteins are specific to a bacterial species

- Microbiologists examine amino acid sequences of these proteins to determine the relationship of species to other types of bacteria.

Genetics: DNA is unique to each bacterial species

- Determining DNA and/or RNA sequence aids the microbiologist in determining the relationship between two different species or establishing information as related to a new strain of bacteria.

Staining: used to prepare specimens for microscopic examination

- Simple stain: used to determine basic shape and structures of cell; single dye such as methylene blue is used and the cell is rinsed with water.
- Gram stain: cells are stained with crystal violet; washed with ethanol that removes purple stain from bacteria that don't retain the stain; red dye safranin is applied; specimen is rinsed with water. Gram-positive bacteria retain the crystal violet and therefore are a purple color; gram-negative bacteria do not retain the crystal violet and are red from the safranin stain. Gram-variable bacteria, such as *Mycobacterium tuberculosis*, do not consistently stain red or purple.
- Acid-fast stain: used to identify bacteria classified in the genus *Mycobacterium*. Red dye (carbolfuchsin) is retained by acid-fast bacteria.

(continues)

Table 7-1 (continued)

Spore forming (sporulation): bacterial species capable of forming spores

Clostridium is one example.

- When environmental conditions are unfavorable, including extremes in temperature, dry environment, and a total lack of a source of food, the genetic material of the cell is enclosed in a protein capsule.
- Spores can survive for a long time until favorable conditions are reestablished; the bacteria returns to its vegetative state and is able to grow and reproduce again.
- Not to be confused with reproduction, sporulation is a method of bacterial survival.
- Spores are difficult to destroy; therefore sterilization processes must also be able to kill spores.

Table 7-2 Common Bacterial Pathogens

Microorganism	Infections
Staphylococcus	
S. aureus	Toxic shock syndrome
	Osteomyelitis
	Endocarditis
	Postoperative SSI
S. epidermis	IV catheter infections
	UTIs
	Prosthetic device infections
	Subacute bacterial infections
	Endocarditis
Streptococcus	
S. pneumoniae	Bacterial pneumonia
	Bacterial meningitis
	Otitis media
	Bacteremia
S. pyogenes	Strep throat
	Tonsillitis
	Rheumatic fever
	Scarlet fever
	Necrotizing fasciitis
S. agalactiae	Neonatal septicemia
	Neonatal meningitis
S. mutans	Dental caries
Aerobic Gram-Negative Cocci, Coccobacilli	
Bordetella pertussis	Whooping cough (pertussis)
Neisseria gonorrhoeae	Pelvic inflammatory disease leading to salpingitis
N. meningitides	Bacterial meningitis
Moraxella catarrhalis	Otitis media in children

Microorganism	Infections
Aerobic Gram-Positive Bacilli, Coccobacilli, Coryneform Bacilli	
B. anthracis	Cutaneous, inhalation, and GI anthrax
Listeria monocytogenes	Meningitis
	Bacteremia
Lactobacillus species	Endocarditis
Corynebacterium diphtheriae	Respiratory and cutaneous diphtheria
Aerobic, Microaerophile Gram-Negative Bacilli, Spirochetes	
Acinetobacter	Respiratory and urinary tract infections
	Wound infections; septicemia
Bartonella species	Bartonellosis
	Endocarditis
	Bacteremia
Legionella pneumophila	Pontiac fever (influenza-like illness)
	Legionnaires' disease (severe form of pneumonia)
Pseudomonas aeruginosa	Deep-tissue health care–associated infections in patients with burns, deep puncture wounds, and open bone fractures
	External otitis
	Keratitis
	UTIs
	Endocarditis in patients with prosthetic heart valves
Helicobacter pylori	Chronic gastritis
	Stomach ulcers
	Peptic ulcers

(continues)

Table 7-2 (continued)

Microorganism	Infections
Rickettsia rickettsii	Rocky Mountain spotted fever
Campylobacter jejuni	Leading cause of diarrheal illness
Treponema pallidum	Venereal syphilis
Facultative Anaerobic Gram-Positive Cocci	
Enterococcus	Enterococcal infections of the urinary tract and bloodstream; associated with intra-abdominal abscesses and wound infections
Facultative Anaerobic Gram-Negative Bacilli	
Haemophilus influenzae	Bacterial meningitis (primary cause in infants and children)
	Respiratory tract infections
	Bacterial pneumonia (elderly)
	Otitis media
	Eye infections
	Septic arthritis
	Cellulitis
Gardnerella vaginalis	Vaginosis that can also cause fallopian tubal adhesions
	Pelvic inflammatory disease
	Postpartum endometriosis
Escherichia coli	UTIs
	Sepsis
	Neonatal meningitis
Klebsiella pneumoniae	Health care–associated UTIs
	Wound and burn infections
	Ankylosing spondylitis (sequelae of a *Klebsiella* infection)
Salmonella enterica	Salmonellosis (*Salmonella* gastroenteritis)
Salmonella typhi	Typhoid fever (*S. typhi* tends to remain in gallbladder and biliary tract and patient may undergo cholecystectomy)
Vibrio cholerae	Cholera
Proteus	UTIs
Anaerobic Gram-Positive Bacteria	
Clostridium perfringens	Gas gangrene infection
	Cellulitis
	Fasciitis
C. botulinum	Food-borne botulism
	Wound botulism
	Infant botulism
C. difficile	Antibiotic-associated GI diseases (self-limiting diarrhea to life-threatening pseudomembranous colitis)
Anaerobic Gram-Negative Bacilli, Coccibacilli	
Bacteroides fragilis	Peritonitis
Porphyromonas gingivalis	Gingivitis
	Periodontitis
Mycobacteria	
Mycobacterium leprae	Leprosy (Hansen's disease)
Mycobacterium tuberculosis	Tuberculosis
Chlamydia	
C. trachomatis	Conjunctivitis
	Ocular lymphogranuloma venereum
	Lymphogranuloma venereum
	Nongonococcal urethritis
	Postgonococcal urethritis
	Infant pneumonia
***Mycoplasma* (facultative anaerobe)**	
M. hominis	Gastrourinary tract infections

with SSIs. In addition to bacteria, fungi, such as *Candida albicans*, and viruses, such as the hepatitis virus and human immunodeficiency virus, may cause infections.

As shown in Table 7-3, the most commonly transmitted pathogen in the operating room is *Staphylococcus aureus*, a gram-positive coccus. This bacterium is common in the flora of the skin, hair, and nares of the nose; 25% of all people are colonized with this microorganism. Studies have shown that the skin of the patient can be a cause of SSI, and the skin, hair, and nares of surgical personnel can be the source of infection.

Tuberculosis

Tuberculosis (TB), caused by *Mycobacterium tuberculosis* and transmitted through airborne droplet nuclei, usually infects the lungs but may also infect the kidneys, bone, joints, or skin. Elective operations on patients with TB are postponed until drug therapy is effective. Surgical procedures performed on known TB carriers require implementing isolation precautions, including the wearing of gloves, protective eyewear, gown, and National Institute of Occupational Safety and Health (NIOSH)–approved

Table 7-3 Pathogens Commonly Associated with SSI

January 2006–October 2007 Pathogen	*Percentage of Infections*
Staphylococcus aureus	30.0
Coagulase-negative staphylococci	13.7
Enterococcus spp.	11.2
Escherichia coli	9.6
Pseudomonas aeruginosa	5.6
Enterobacter spp.	4.2
Klebsiella pneumoniae	3.0
Candida albicans	2.0
Klebsiella oxytoca	0.7
Acinetobacter baumannii	0.6
	N = 7.025

Table from the *Surgical Site Infection (SSI) Toolkit* 12/2009 http://www.cdc.gov/HAI/pdfs/toolkits/SSI_toolkit021710SIBT_revised.pdf Courtesy of the Centers for Disease Control

respirators. The patient must also be advised of precautions, including how he or she can prevent cross-contamination, and must wear a mask. Chapter 4 provides further details about the care of isolation patients.

Viruses

Unlike bacteria, which are living microorganisms, viruses are nonliving particles that are completely reliant on the host cell for survival. The largest virus measures 300 nm, approximately the size of a small bacterium, and the smallest virus is the poliovirus, measuring 30 nm. The characteristics that are unique to viruses are as follows:

- Viruses are obligate intracellular parasites.
- Viral replication is directed by the viral nucleic acid within the host cell.
- Viral cells contain either DNA or RNA and a protein coat that encases the nucleic acid.
- Viral cells depend on the protein production of the host cell; the viral cell does not contain the enzymes required for the production of energy.

The DNA or RNA is surrounded by a protein covering called the *capsid* that is composed of protein molecules called *capsomeres.* The protein coat protects the DNA or RNA and contains components that aid in the attachment of the viral cell to the host cell. The nucleic acid–capsid combination is referred to as a *nucleocapsid.* Nucleocapsids have a variety of symmetrical shapes, including icosahedrons (20 sides), helices, or even more complex shapes (see Figure 7-1).

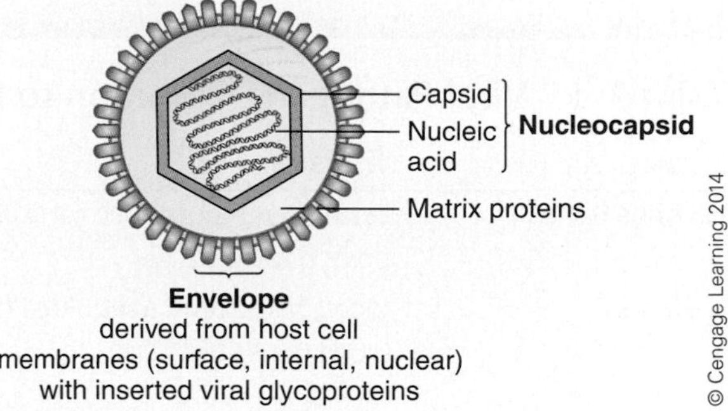

Figure 7-1 Envelope derived from host cell membranes (surface, internal, nuclear) with inserted viral glycoproteins

Viruses enter the body through the following methods:

- Inhalation of respiratory droplets
- Exchange of body fluids (for example, HIV is transmitted by blood, semen, and mother's breast milk)
- Ingestion of food or water
- Bites by arthropod vectors

The viral cell first attaches to the host cell with the aid of receptors on the capsomere. The virus then enters the cell by penetrating the cytoplasmic membrane or through receptor-mediated endocytosis. The viral nucleic acid is now freed and viral replication begins. To further illustrate the process of infection, the following example lists the steps of infection by the rhinovirus, the causative agent of the common cold.

1. An infected individual sneezes, thus releasing thousands of viral particles into the air.
2. A noninfected person inhales some of the viral particles and becomes infected with the rhinovirus.
3. The viral particles bind to the host cells lining the nasal sinuses and begin to rapidly replicate.
4. The host cells lyse and new viral particles are released to continue replicating in the sinuses and travel to the lungs.
5. The infected sinus cells are induced by the viral particles to release fluid, which enters the throat, where the viral particles invade the cells that line the throat, causing a sore throat.
6. The body's immune response begins to fight the infection by releasing pyrogens that cause the body temperature to rise; the increased temperature helps to slow the rate of viral replication.

The surgical technologist is often exposed to deadly viruses in the OR, including hepatitis B (HBV) and human immunodeficiency virus (HIV) (see Table 7-4). The surgical technologist should be aware that he or she not only can be infected by a patient, but can pass an infection on to a patient. Surgical technologists should follow hospital procedures and policies and Standard Precautions. Additionally, surgical technologists should be vaccinated against HBV and follow the proper procedure if an exposure incident occurs, such as sustaining a needle-stick injury.

TABLE 7-4 Viral Pathogens Common to the Operating Room

Virus	*Transmission*	*Description*
Hepatitis B (HBV)	Percutaneous or permucous in blood, serum, and other body fluids	Causes inflammation of the liver, jaundice, cirrhosis, and, in some cases, liver cancer
Hepatitis C	Blood-borne RNA; transmitted through blood and blood products	Asymptomatic when acute; may be carried for 25 years; causes chronic hepatitis, cirrhosis, liver cancer
Hepatitis D (Delta)	Coexists with HBV	Causes liver disease, superinfection of HBV, death
Human immunodeficiency virus (HIV)	Blood or other body fluids	Compromises immune system
Herpes simplex virus (HSV)	Contact with fluid from lesions	Causes localized blisterlike eruptions; can also cause keratoconjunctivitis, acute retinal necrosis, meningoencephalitis
Papillomavirus	Direct contact with another person	Warts
Cytomegalovirus (CMV)	Direct contact with body fluids	Infects salivary glands or viscera; opportunistic infection in patients with HIV or hepatitis
Creutzfeldt-Jakob Disease (CJD)	Exact mode of transmission unknown; thought to be by percutaneous inoculation with brain tissue or cerebral spinal fluid from infected persons; transmission has been associated with use of contaminated instruments; longer sterilization times required.	Rapidly progressive fatal central nervous disease characterized by dementia, myoclonus

Emerging Infectious Diseases

Humans are more mobile than ever before, allowing microorganisms to be easily transmitted and infect on a global basis. This is a major change from the past, when breakouts of infection tended to be localized. Additionally, there is an increase in bacterial multidrug–resistant (MDR) strains. For example, tuberculosis is receiving worldwide attention due to MDR strains of *M. tuberculosis*. Traditional first-line medications including streptomycin, rifampin, and isoniazid can be ineffective against MDR-TB. A more recent development is a virulent strain labeled extensively drug-resistant TB (XDR-TB) that has risen out of misuse or mismanagement of second-line defense drugs such as fluoroquinolone, amikacin, and kanamycin, rendering them ineffective as well.

Viruses, in particular, are able to constantly mutate and evolve in order to adapt to changing environments. This ability to mutate, along with the transmission of mutated viruses from animals, has contributed to the emergence of new viruses that infect on a global basis. Examples of viruses that at one point were typically localized, but now are considered global threats, include the hantavirus and the group of viral hemorrhagic fevers including Ebola virus, Dengue virus, and Lassa virus.

If an infected patient requires surgical care, the surgical technologist along with the other surgical team members must practice meticulous technique in the care of the patient to prevent infection of the team and cross-contamination of other patients. Hospital policy and procedures pertaining to the care of these types of patients must be followed and the surgical technologist should make sure to implement safety methods such as the use of the neutral zone.

Prions

The term *prion* is short for "proteinaceous infectious particle." Prions are entirely different from other infectious agents in that they are built of proteins and do not contain DNA or RNA. The human body produces the same protein, called PrP, that is responsible for CJD but the normal protein's structure is slightly different from that of the infectious prion. The PrP changes from a noninfectious spiral shape, called the alpha-helical form, to the infectious folded shape called the beta-sheet. When a prion contacts the normal PrP it starts a chain reaction in which the prion is replicated by folding the alpha-helical into the beta-sheet form.

Prions attack the brain, which is why the diseases they cause are called subacute spongiform encephalopathies. Within the brain the PrP converts the alpha-helical form to the beta-sheet inside the neurons. The beta-sheet prions accumulate in the lysosomes and eventually kill the neuron. The death of the neurons creates holes in the brain tissue, which aids in the release of prions to further invade and infect healthy neurons.

Although prions are an infectious agent, they are not transmitted or contagious in the same way as other microorganisms.

Human-to-human transmission is not direct, but rather occurs through the use of surgical instruments that are contaminated with the prion or tissue transplantation from an infected individual. Prion diseases are more common in animals, and include the two common forms of scrapie (a disease that infects sheep and goats) and bovine spongiform encephalopathy (commonly called mad cow disease). The disease that affects humans, as mentioned, is CJD. CJD can also be inherited as a mutant gene or as a sporadic case; this is rare, but precautions should be used in caring for patients demonstrating possible signs and symptoms of disease in whom a family history of CJD has been confirmed.

CJD develops very slowly, with an incubation time of up to 20 years. Symptoms early in the course of the disease mimic those of Alzheimer's disease and include depression and poor memory; later stages are characterized by dementia and progressive loss of physical functions. A diagnosis of CJD is obtained by observing changes in electroencephalogram results and magnetic resonance imaging (MRI) changes; definitive diagnosis is through histologic examination of affected brain and lymphoid tissue. There is no vaccine or cure for CJD.

A new variant strain of CJD called vCJD or nvCJD has a much younger median age of onset at 28 years of age, compared to 68 years for CJD. However, the duration of symptoms is longer, with 13 to 14 months for vCJD and 4 to 5 months for CJD. The other clinical characteristic that sets vCJD apart is the more apparent chemical indicators of prion accumulation in the neural and lymphoid tissues.

As previously mentioned, transmission of CJD is possible through the use of surgical instruments, in particular, instruments used during neurosurgical procedures. The tissues that have been identified as high risks for transmission include eye tissue, dura mater, brain tissue, and spinal cord. Recommendations and guidelines concerning the postoperative decontamination and sterilization of surgical instruments and equipment that are used on patients suspected of or are diagnosed as having CJD are not well established or universal. Prions are very resistant to chemical and physical sterilization methods such as steam under pressure, ethylene oxide, and dry heat. The World Health Organization's Infection Control Guidelines for Transmissible Spongiform Encephalopathies recommends the use of single-use, disposable instruments and the destruction of all reusable instruments. See Table 7-5 for a sample guideline for CJD cases.

Parasites

The study of invertebrates that cause disease is called parasitology. There are two categories of parasitic human pathogens: unicellular protozoans and multicellular protozoans. The helminth and arthropod groups belong in the metazoans category and are endoparasites. Helminths are popularly known as worms. Those that are most common in the human population are tapeworms, flukes, and roundworms. The primary route of transmission is ingestion of contaminated food or water that contains the worms or eggs, but also includes penetration through the skin, fecal-oral contamination, and arthropod bite.

The chances of a surgical technologist encountering a helminth infection have increased due to the mobility of the world population and immigration from Third World countries. Worms can damage body tissues and organs to the point that they require surgery. For example, cysticeri (*Taenia solium*)

TABLE 7-5 Sample Guidelines for Suspected or Known CJD Patients

Preoperative Preparation

- Notify all units that will be involved, including nursing, pharmacy, central sterile processing department, infection control, environmental services, laboratory, surgical services, and pathology.
- Remove all unnecessary equipment and supplies from the OR as possible. Move everything else as far from the OR table as possible.
- Cover all surfaces in the OR, including anesthetic equipment and OR table, with impervious sheets.
- Cover electrical cords with sterile plastic sleeves.

Intraoperative Case Management

- Use disposable equipment and instruments as much as possible.
- Try to avoid use of power instruments to prevent aerosolization of contaminates.
- Use neutral zone when passing sharps.
- Sterile attire should include double gloves, face shields, and knee-high impervious shoe covers.
- Clean blood and body fluid spills with sodium hydroxide (household bleach).
- Change gowns, gloves, suction tip(s), and ESU tip.
- Place tissue specimens into a specimen container, then place in a biohazard specimen bag (marked with the biohazard symbol) and labeled "CJD precautions."
- Per surgeon's order, clean the patient's head with 1 molar sodium hydroxide at the end of the procedure.

(continues)

TABLE 7-5 (continued)

Postoperative Case Management

- Reusable instruments: Place in impervious container, place in biohazard bags, label as "possible CJD," and handle according to hospital policy, which may include disposal.
- Body fluids and liquid waste: Collect, label, and bag in biohazard bags labeled "possible CJD"; keep separate from other waste bags and notify environmental services personnel to immediately collect and incinerate the bags.
- Disposable supplies: Place surgical attire, drapes, sponges, suction tip(s), etc. in biohazard bags labeled "possible CJD" and keep them separate from other red bags; notify environmental services personnel to immediately collect and incinerate the bags.
- Sharps: Place in separate sharps container labeled "possible CJD"; notify environmental services personnel to immediately collect and incinerate the container.

Environmental Cleaning

- Decontaminate all OR surfaces at the end of the procedure by wetting all exposed surfaces with 1 molar sodium hypochlorite for 60 minutes. Rinse with water and then clean in routine fashion.
- Surfaces contaminated with visible tissue or body fluids should be decontaminated with 1:10 dilution of 5.25% sodium hypochlorite, followed by routine cleansing with disinfectant according to hospital policy.

are pork tapeworms that can migrate out of the intestinal tract and travel to muscle and brain tissue, and the eyes. The cysticerci can cause palpable lumps in soft tissues, blurred vision and retinal detachment, and when located in the brain tissue cause seizures, ataxia, headaches, and possibly death. Helminths can also cause intestinal blockage and may rupture the intestinal wall if there is a large buildup of worms. Abdominal surgical procedures may be required to remove and repair the internal organs.

The groups of protozoa are amebas, flagellates, ciliates, coccidia, and microsporidia. Protozoa are unicellular eukaryotes that are responsible for causing human diseases such as malaria and chronic sleeping sickness (also called African sleeping sickness). Amebas move by extending pseudopods, flagellates move using flagella, and ciliates are propelled by the cilia that surround the cell. The intestinal protozoa are transmitted by the fecal-oral route. They are often responsible for infections in crowded environments such as day care centers and in underdeveloped countries where sanitary conditions are inadequate.

One of the more important protozoa from the standpoint of the surgical technologist is *Entamoeba histolytica*, the cause of amebic dysentery, an infection often found in patients who are scheduled to undergo a sigmoidoscopy or colonoscopy. The endoscope and other nondisposable instrumentation must be thoroughly decontaminated before use on the next surgical patient to prevent the spread of the organism. Additionally, the scope and instrumentation should be carefully handled during the procedure to prevent spread of the organism to other parts of the body, causing a secondary infection.

A common unicellular anaerobic protozoan is *Trichomonas vaginalis*. *T. vaginalis* is often part of the normal flora of the vagina and urethra. If the normal acidity of the vagina is upset, the protozoan population will grow and cause trichomoniasis. However, trichomoniasis is usually sexually transmitted.

Fungi

Mycology is the study of fungi. Fungi are eukaryotic organisms that are either unicellular yeasts or multicellular molds and mushrooms. Fungi reproduce either sexually or asexually by producing spores; a true spore is formed by either asexual cleavage or sexual meiosis. Fungal diseases are called *mycoses* (the plural of *mycosis*). The majority of fungi are opportunistic pathogens that cause disease when the host is immunocompromised. Opportunistic fungal infections are common in AIDS patients, and the increase in the number of fungal infections has paralleled the spread of HIV (Table 7-6).

TABLE 7-6 Common Fungal Infections

Microorganism	*Infections*
Candida albicans	Vaginal yeast infection Trench mouth (thrush) Immunocompromised patients prone to serious infections of the brain, meninges, and heart valves Patients intubated or who have indwelling venous catheter or other type long-term indwelling catheter should be monitored for infection
Blastomyces dermatitidis	Blastomycosis
Coccidioides immitis (Coccidiodes)	Coccidioidomycosis
Histoplasma capsulatum	Histoplasmosis
Pneumocystis jiroveci	*Pneumocystis* pneumonia

One particular fungus that merits brief discussion here is *zygomycosis*, caused by a common bread mold. The increase in the number of cases of zygomycosis has followed the increase in the number of organ transplants and the increased use of immunosuppressive drugs and antibiotics. One type of zygomycosis is the rapidly progressive, devastating, and destructive disease called rhinocerebral zygomycosis, which causes extensive damage to the bone and tissues of the face, including the loss of one or both eyes. If the organism enters the bloodstream and destroys the cranial bones, the brain tissue will be invaded. Patients may be scheduled for surgical irrigation and removal of infected bone tissue, and removal of one or both eyes if lost to the infection. Patients who recover may have to undergo extensive plastic and bone transplant surgery to repair the face.

METHODS OF TRANSMISSION

Any infection requires a primary agent, such as a bacterium, virus, fungus, or parasite. In the hospital setting, most infections are caused by bacteria and viruses, although fungi and parasites occasionally are involved in HAIs. Frequent handwashing helps to eliminate transient microbes from the skin, thereby reducing the risk of nococomial infection. See Technique: Basic Hand Washing.

Precautions

Transmission-based precautions are separate guidelines for infection control and prevention of cross-contamination of patients when the disease process has been diagnosed. The three types of precautions apply to the modes of transmission: contact (direct and indirect), airborne, and droplet. Modes of transmission are shown in Table 7-7. For example, disposable cover gowns and unsterile gloves should be worn by transporters of patients with known contact-transmissible diseases. Hospitals may have policies that require OR team members to change scrubs upon completion of methicillin-resistant *Staphylococcus aureus* (MRSA) or vancomycin-resistant enterococci (VRE) patient procedures.

Sources of Surgical Site Infections

Since most SSIs are acquired at the time of surgery, rather than at some point after surgery, the major sources of microbes causing these infections can be divided into two groups: environmental and endogenous. Environmental sources include personnel, the environment, and contaminated instrumentation. The other primary source is the patient's endogenous flora.

Personnel

The skin, hair, and nares of surgical personnel are reservoirs of bacteria, which may be discharged in particle form into the air and therefore pose a risk of SSI to the patient. Proper OR practice for the scrubbed members of the surgical team is to don OR attire, protective attire, and scrub attire prior to the procedure not only to protect the patient from any shed bacterial particles but to also protect personnel from contact with the patient's blood or body fluids (refer to Chapter 12).

Gowns and drapes cover the skin on areas of the body other than the hands. The primary purpose of wearing gowns, hair covers, and masks around the OR table is to provide a barrier to contamination, both from personnel to patient and from patient to personnel. Since a high percentage of individuals are carriers of *S. aureus*, the threat is considerable enough to warrant the use of hair covers and masks. Finally, personnel contribute to SSI through human error or lapses in sterile technique. When breaks in sterile technique occur, the patient is exposed to a preventable risk. Errors, therefore, should be noted, communicated, and corrected immediately; this practice is commonly termed surgical conscience.

TABLE 7-7 Modes of Transmission

Transmission Mode	*Examples*
Contact: Direct	Light handle drops into open wound; hypodermic needle-stick injury from two-handed recapping
Indirect	Bioburden on gloves contaminates equipment that is handled by ungloved person who rubs eyes
Droplet (>5 μm)	Infection spread through the air by droplets spread by sneezing, coughing, or talking
Airborne spread (<5 μm)	Infection spread through the air by sneeze droplets

TECHNIQUE

Basic Hand Washing

1. Turn on the faucet and adjust the water temperature.
2. Inspect hands and wrists.
3. Wet hands and wrists.
4. Apply soap; lather.
5. Use moderate friction and circular motions.
6. Interlace fingers to facilitate cleaning of the web spaces.
7. Continue washing for 30 seconds to 1 minute.
8. Rinse.
9. Turn off the water.
10. Dry hands and wrists.
11. Discard the towels.

Environment

A second source of microbial transmission is environmental, both from fomites and through the air. Fomites are inanimate objects that may contain infectious microorganisms including walls, floors, cabinets, furniture and equipment. A safe, clean, and spacious OR helps to provide a lower level of microbes in the environment. For example, ORs designed with a clean zone, filtered and controlled air systems, and the use of soil-resistant building materials have become routine in surgical services (see Chapter 5).

Surgical site infections have also been documented from such environmental sources as contaminated antiseptic solutions, contaminated wound dressings, and contaminated or improperly sterilized surgical instruments. The use of nonsterile medications also poses a risk of infection to the patient.

The Patient

The two primary sources of SSI risk to the patient are the endogenous flora encountered in contaminated procedures and the resident flora of the skin. This is certainly true for procedures in which the gastrointestinal tract or other contaminated areas are opened and exposed to the surgical wound. One common example is an SSI resulting from removal of the contaminated appendix through a skin incision during an appendectomy. Preoperative prophylaxis with antibiotics has been shown to reduce SSIs. Studies have shown that patients who are carriers of *S. aureus* are at particular risk for SSI, even in clean procedures. Carriers have colonies of these bacteria living in the deeper layers of their skin, making preoperative skin preparations less effective. As time passes after preoperative skin preparation, rebound growth of these resident bacteria reaches the surface, where they may be shed and contaminate the surgical incision. Use of antimicrobial-impregnated incise drapes may be helpful in preventing migration of these microbes into the surgical incision site. Patients who have infections at other body locations, such as patients with urinary tract infections, are also at increased risk for SSI, and nonemergent and elective procedures may be postponed until the infection has cleared.

FACTORS THAT INCREASE RISK OF SURGICAL SITE INFECTION

Patient-related factors that increase the risk of developing an SSI include:

- Age: Geriatric and pediatric patients have lower immunological defenses.
- Obesity: Diminished blood flow, larger wound sizes, and the difficulty of handling adipose tissue make these patients more susceptible to infection.
- General health: Patients in poor health or who have an inadequate nutritional intake generally have a predisposition to infection.
- Carriers of *S. aureus* or MRSA: These patients are at greater risk of infection from their own endogenous flora.
- Remote infections: Infections at other body sites increase the chance of SSI. Bacteria in the bloodstream enter and infect the surgical site.
- Preoperative hospitalization: Infection rates increase parallel to the duration of preoperative stay. Patients are exposed to higher numbers of antibiotic-resistant strains of bacteria within the hospital.
- Preexisting illness and related treatment: Infection rates are higher in patients with compromised immune systems from preexisting illness; patients who have been treated with certain medications, including steroids or chemotherapy agents; and patients who have recently undergone radiation therapy.

Other factors that may contribute to an increased likelihood of SSI include malnutrition, tobacco use, diabetes, malignancy, and immunosuppression.

Procedure-related risk factors that increase the danger of SSI include:

- Preoperative hair removal: Although hair removal has been a standard, studies have shown that hair removal is a risk factor for the development of SSI. The risk is greater when the preoperative shave is performed the day before surgery, and the use of razors carries a greater risk than the use of clippers. Razor blades leave many small cuts, nicks, and scrapes on the skin, allowing bacteria easier access for **colonization**. If the patient is not allergic, use of depilatory cream is less traumatic and is therefore a safer alternative. Hair removal by use of surgical clippers with disposable heads has replaced use of razors in most facilities.
- Type of procedure: Clean-contaminated (Class II), contaminated (Class III), and dirty (Class IV) cases carry a higher risk of infection (refer to Chapter11), as do cases that compromise blood flow to a particular area, such as coronary artery bypass procedures, where one or both internal mammary arteries are used.
- Duration of procedure: Longer anesthetic and operative times have an accompanying increase in time for bacterial contamination to occur, increased tissue damage, and greater immunosuppression. Surgical team members become more fatigued, which may lead to breaks in sterile technique.

Practice parameters of disease transmission in the perioperative environment are provided in Box 7-2.

Box 7-2 AST RECOMMENDED STANDARDS OF PRACTICE

The full text of each standard, including references, is located at www.ast.org.

Use of Eye Protection During Invasive Surgical Procedures

Standard I: Eye protection must be worn as part of personal protective equipment as a barrier to infectious material entering the eye as mandated by OSHA during all invasive surgical procedures, including endoscopic procedures, or in any situation where splash injury to the eyes could occur.
Standard II: Eye protection should be removed in an aseptic manner to minimize splashes of blood and body fluids to the mucous membrane, in particular the conjunctive to the eye.
Standard III: Disposable protective eyewear that is contaminated should be disposed of immediately. Contaminated nondisposable eyewear should be promptly decontaminated.
Standard IV: The proper type of goggles should be selected and worn in the operating room.
Standard V: The proper type of face shield should be selected and worn in the operating room.

Laundering of Scrub Attire

Standard I: It is the responsibility of each surgical department to follow recommended CDC and OSHA standards for OR attire.
Standard II: Surgical scrub attire can be a source of cross-contamination.
Standard III: Facility-controlled laundry or facility-approved and monitored commercial laundry reduces the risk of contamination from uncontrolled environments.
Standard IV: Clean, freshly laundered OR attire should be protected from contamination when transported from the health care facility laundry or facility-approved commercial laundry to the storage area.

Wearing Jewelry

Standard I: It is the responsibility of each surgical department to follow recommended CDC standards for recommended OR attire.
Standard II: Hand hygiene, including hand washing and surgical scrub, is vital in the prevention and transmission of harmful microorganisms.
Standard III: Jewelry may be a source of contamination and pose a risk of injury to the patient and surgical personnel.

Wearing the Lab Coat, Cover Gown, or Other Appropriate Cover Apparel

Standard I: Cover apparel, such as a lab coat, cover gown, or other appropriate clothing, should be worn when exiting the surgery department.

Hand Hygiene and Fingernails

Standard I: The surgical team members should practice on a daily basis effective hand and fingernail hygiene.
Standard II: Fingernails should be natural and polish-free. Fingernails should be short, debris free, and not extend past the tips of the fingers.
Standard III: The reinforcement of hand and fingernail hygiene should be constantly emphasized with surgical technology students and peers.

Head Covers in the Operating Room

Standard I: The surgical team members are responsible for preventing SSI by properly donning and wearing the appropriate head cover or hood.
Standard II: The surgical department should follow recommended OSHA and CDC standards for PPE.

Shoe Covers in the Perioperative Environment

Standard I: Health care workers (HCWs) should protect themselves from contact with blood and body fluids by wearing disposable shoe covers.
Standard II: HCWs should avoid tracking blood and body fluids, debris, and other gross contaminants throughout the surgical suite.
Standard III: HCWs should be aware of the hazards associated with workplace foot and toe injuries, and should protect themselves from injury by wearing the correct footwear.
Standard IV: Policies and procedures for surgical attire, including shoe covers, should be developed, written, and reviewed on a periodical base.

PART II: Disinfection, Decontamination, and Sterilization

CASE STUDY

A CST is setting up the back table and Mayo stand for a total hip arthroplasty. The supervisor of the CSPD enters the OR and informs the CST that the test steam BI turned yellow for the load in which the surgical instruments were processed through the steam sterilizer.

1. **What does the yellow color indicate to the CST?**
2. **How long was the steam biological monitor incubated?**
2. **At what temperature is the biological monitor incubated?**
4. **What other actions must the supervisor of the central sterile processing department take?**

INTRODUCTION

In this section of the chapter we discuss *decontamination, disinfection,* and *sterilization* and the appropriate uses of each. Proper cleaning, disinfection, and sterilization provide an environment and equipment that are conducive to the ability to follow the principles of **asepsis** and the practice of sterile technique.

BASIC TERMINOLOGY

The terminology related to the principles of aseptic technique is essential to all practices in the OR. Refer to Table 7-8 for a clear definition of terms related to asepsis and sterile techniques.

Three terms that must be understood by the surgical technologist and differentiated are disinfection, antisepsis, and sterilization.

- Disinfection refers to the process in which most but not all the microorganisms located on inanimate surfaces are destroyed. Decontamination is a category of disinfection.
- Antisepsis is a process in which most but not all microorganisms located on animate surfaces, such as the skin, are destroyed.
  - Antiseptic: name used to describe the solutions that are used by the sterile surgical team members to perform the surgical scrub and are used on the patient for skin preparation of the surgical site.
  - Sterilization: destruction of all microorganisms, including spores, on inanimate surfaces. Any item that will be used on and within the surgical wound must be sterile. Additionally, all items such as basins that are used within the **sterile field**, whether they come into contact with the patient's tissue or not, must be sterile.

TABLE 7-8 **Terminology of Asepsis and Sterile Technique**

Asepsis	Absence of pathogenic microorganisms
Aseptic principles	Principles applied through use of sterile techniques to prevent microbial contamination of the surgical environment
Bacteriocidal	Substance that destroys/kills bacteria
Bacteriostatic	Substance that inhibits the growth and reproduction of bacteria
Bioburden	The number of microbes or amount of organic debris on an object at any given time
Contamination	The presence of pathogenic materials
Cross-contamination	The contamination of a person or object by another
Decontamination	To reduce to an irreducible minimum the presence of pathogenic material

(continues)

TABLE 7-8 (continued)

Disinfectant	Chemical agent that kills most microbes, but usually not spores; usually used on inanimate objects because these compounds are too strong to be used on living tissues
Event-related sterility	Sterility determined by how a package is handled rather than time elapsed; a package is considered sterile until opened or the integrity of packaging material is damaged
Fomite	Inanimate object that harbors microorganisms
Fungicide	Agent that destroys fungus
Infection	Invasion of the human body or tissue by pathogenic microorganisms that reproduce and multiply, causing disease
Nosocomial	Infection acquired within a health care facility
Pathogen	Any microbe capable of causing disease
Resident flora	Microbes that normally reside below the skin surface or within the body
Sepsis	Infection, usually accompanied by fever, that results from the presence of pathogenic microorganisms
Spore	A resistant form of certain types of bacteria that are able to survive in adverse conditions
Sporicide	Substance that kills/destroys bacteria in the spore stage
Sterile	Having been rendered free of all living microorganisms, including spores
Sterile field	Specified area, usually the area immediately around the patient, that is considered free of microorganisms
Sterile technique	Techniques of creating a sterile field and performing within the sterile field to keep microbes at an irreducible minimum
Strike-through contamination	Contamination of a sterile field that occurs through the passage of fluid through, or a puncture in, a microbial barrier
Surgically clean	Mechanically cleaned and chemically disinfected but not sterile
Terminal disinfection	To render items safe to handle by high-level disinfection
Terminal sterilization	To render items safe to handle by sterilization
Transient flora	Microbes that reside on the skin surface and are easily removed
Vector	Living carrier that transmits disease
Virucide	Agent that destroys viruses

CLASSIFICATION OF PATIENT CARE ITEMS

The CDC and FDA utilize a classification system for patient care items and surgical devices. The system rates the degree of risk to patients for infection based on how and where the items will be used. The appropriate method of disinfection or sterilization corresponds to this risk assessment. The three classifications are:

- CRITICAL: Items that will be used for invasive procedures or vascular access and carry a high potential for causing SSIs include: surgical instruments, devices that enter the vascular or urinary systems (needles, catheters), implantable items (wires, screws, joint replacements, mesh, sutures), and any monitors or probes that enter deep tissue layers or cavities. These items should be sterilized.
- SEMI-CRITICAL: Items that come into contact with mucous membranes or non-intact skin carry a lesser risk of infection due to the properties of resistance of intact mucosal linings to many commonly encountered bacterial spores. Examples include: laryngoscopes, anesthesia and respiratory equipment, and some endoscopes. High-level disinfection should be used for items in this category.
- NON-CRITICAL: Items that come into contact with a patient's intact skin and clean environmental equipment items pose the least risk of infection. Examples include blood pressure cuffs, pulse oximeters, OR transport stretchers, and other furniture. These items require either intermediate-level or low-level disinfection.

AST RECOMMENDED STANDARDS OF PRACTICE APPLICABLE TO DECONTAMINATION AND STERILIZATION

AST reinforces decontamination and sterilization best practices through various recommended standards of practice. The following are the titles of the documents and links to their location on the AST web site:

- RSOP for the Decontamination of Instruments (http://www.ast.org/pdf/Standards_of_Practice/RSOP_Decontamination_%20Surgical%20Instruments_11.5.pdf)
- RSOP for Packaging Material and Preparing Items for Sterilization (http://www.ast.org/pdf/Standards_of_Practice/RSOP_Packaging_Materials_Preparing_Items.pdf)
- RSOP for Monitoring Sterility (http://www.ast.org/pdf/Standards_of_Practice/RSOP_Morintoring_Sterility.pdf)

DISINFECTION PRINCIPLES AND DISINFECTING AGENTS

This section provides an overview of disinfectant agents and their actions. Manufacturer directions should always be followed when using a disinfectant/sterilant agent. Additionally, the use of PPE may be necessary when handling the various chemicals. There are three levels of disinfection, as defined below.

- *Cleaning:* The physical removal of blood, body fluids, and/or gross debris **(bioburden)** from an inanimate object.
- *Disinfection:* Destruction of pathogenic microorganisms or their toxins or vectors by direct exposure to chemical or physical agents. Disinfection is discussed on three levels.
- *High-level disinfection:* Kills all microorganisms except spores and prions (CJD).
- ***Intermediate-level disinfection:*** Kills most microorganisms, including bacteria, most viruses and fungi. *M. tuberculosis* and HBV; ineffective against spores.
- *Low-level disinfection:* Kills some fungi and viruses, and most bacteria, but is not effective against spores and *M. tuberculosis.*
- *Sterilization:* Destruction of all microorganisms in or about an object with steam (flowing or pressurized), chemical agents (alcohol, phenol, heavy metals, or ethylene oxide gas), high-velocity electron bombardment, or ultraviolet radiation.

Disinfectant Efficiency

Certain disinfectant compounds also serve as sterilants when used in sterilization systems, such as peracetic acid, used in the Steris system, or when items are immersed and exposed to the liquid for a certain amount of time.

A number of factors influence the efficiency of disinfectants, including:

- Concentration level of the disinfectant solution
- Bioburden
- contact time
- Physical factors of the solution, including temperature of the solution, water hardness and pH level, and exposure time

While high concentrations of disinfectants increase the level of disinfection, the high concentration may then be too corrosive for use on certain items, such as rubber. Disinfecting solutions are strong chemical solutions and it is important to precisely follow the manufacturer's mixing instructions.

A direct relationship exists between the bioburden present on an item and the length of time necessary to achieve proper disinfection. The effectiveness of disinfection is decreased when blood, body fluids, or tissue are present on an item and prevent the disinfectant from making direct contact with the surface of the item. Therefore, it is important for contaminated items to be thoroughly cleaned prior to the decontamination process. Cleaning is accomplished with the use of a detergent mixed with water and mechanical action; this is a separate step from disinfection and sterilization. Because the number of microbes is reduced, less time is required for the disinfectant to kill the remaining microbes. Cleaning will be further discussed later in the chapter in relation to the decontamination and sterilization of surgical instruments.

For a disinfectant to be efficient, it must come into direct contact with all surface areas of the item and thus come into contact with the microorganisms present on the surface of the item. Instruments that have multiple parts must be disassembled. All ratchets and box locks must be opened to expose all surface areas. When disinfectants are being used in environmental settings (such as on OR furniture), all surfaces must be wiped with the disinfectant agent.

Disinfectants vary in their ability to kill microbes and the types of microbes that they can destroy. The selection of a disinfectant is based on the item to be disinfected and the category in which the item is classified (critical, semicritical, or noncritical). Twenty to 30 minutes of contact time is generally recommended for high-level disinfection. Intermediate and low levels of disinfection can be generally achieved in 10–15 minutes.

Before discussing the various types of disinfectants that are available, a general list of safety factors will be presented that should be followed when handling disinfectants. It must be remembered that disinfectants are solutions that contain strong chemicals that can damage skin and tissue. It also bears repeating that you should follow manufacturer's instructions and recommendations and, when necessary, review the Material Safety Data Sheet (MSDS).

Safety List

- The MSDSs should be kept in an easily accessible area.
- PPE, including gloves, mask (in some instances the use of respirators is recommended), cover gown or apron, and protective eyewear, should be worn when handling disinfectant solutions.
- Solution containers should be stored in a well-ventilated area where correct storage temperature can be maintained.
- The manufacturer's directions for diluting a solution must be followed and should not be altered unless the manufacturer is first consulted. To obtain the correct ratio of dilutant to disinfection solution, an appropriate measuring device should be used.
- Use the disinfection solution for the purpose for which it was developed.
- Do not mix disinfection solutions together; remember, these solutions are chemical compounds and the reaction that can occur by mixing solutions can be dangerous, creating a highly flammable solution that may also produce dangerous and toxic fumes.
- Expired solutions must be disposed of according to hospital policy, manufacturer's recommendations, and state laws.

High-Level Disinfectant Compounds

This section discusses high-level disinfectant solutions, including glutaraldehyde, which can also be used as a sterilant.

Glutaraldehyde

Glutaraldehyde is a high-level disinfectant. Its common commercial name is Cidex. Glutaraldehyde has been recognized as one of the best overall disinfectants/liquid sterilants available on the market.

Glutaraldehyde is used for devices that can withstand complete **immersion** in liquid. The liquid must contact all surface areas of the item, including lumens. A syringe filled with the solution should be used to inject any ports to remove trapped air and fill the lumens. Rigid and flexible **endoscopes** are two kinds of surgical instruments frequently decontaminated or sterilized using glutaraldehyde.

Glutaraldehyde has an established *shelf life*. Shelf life is defined as the period of time between activation of the disinfection solution (mixing of the alkaline buffer with the glutaraldehyde) or number of uses after which the efficiency is diminished. The shelf life for glutaraldehyde without a surfactant is 14 days; with a surfactant the shelf life increases to 28 days. The concentration of glutaraldehyde must be tested prior to each usage during the 14- or 28-day period to determine its strength. Commercially produced test strips are available to test the concentration and ensure it is at 2% strength by comparing the color change on the strip to the sample color strips on the test strip container. The person who has checked the concentration should place his or her initials next to the documented test results. If the concentration level has decreased, the solution should not be used, but should be disposed of, and a new solution should be mixed.

Prior to immersion, item(s) should be cleaned and rinsed; the item(s) should not be rinsed in close proximity to the glutaraldehyde soak basin to prevent inadvertent dilution. To avoid further dilution, all items should be dry before immersion in glutaraldehyde. Even small amounts of water from initial decontamination processes left on items submerged in glutaraldehyde over time will result in diluting its effectiveness.

All items disinfected with glutaraldehyde must be thoroughly rinsed with sterile water (do not use tap water since this will contaminate the item) before use on the patient to prevent the tissue of the patient from being chemically burned. For example, thoroughly rinse a cystoscope that is to be inserted into the urethra during a cystoscopy to prevent burning the tissue.

A minimum exposure of 20 minutes at room temperature is required for high-level disinfection. To render an item sterile it must be immersed for 10 hours.

Action

- Alkylation of cell protein

Advantages

- Dual-purpose solution: disinfectant or sterilant
- Used as a disinfectant it is bactericidal against gram-positive and gram-negative microbes, tuberculocidal, and virucidal.
- Sporicidal as a sterilant
- Noncorrosive to metals
- Noncorrosive to lensed and cemented items
- Noncorrosive to rubber and plastic

Disadvantages

- Noxious odor
- Vapors can cause irritation to the eyes and mucous membranes of the nose and respiratory tract.
- Unstable; shelf-life expiration date and variable use-life dependent on frequency of use and potential dilution
- Items to be disinfected must be cleaned and dried prior to immersion; solution weakens in the presence of organic matter or water.

Safety Considerations

- Must wear gloves and avoid placing unprotected hands in liquid.
- Avoid splashing.

- Must wear protective eyewear such as goggles.
- Use of a respirator to avoid inhalation of fumes is recommended. At the minimum a mask must be worn. Some health care facilities have installed fume hoods over the glutaraldehyde container to remove the vapors, but this does not negate need to wear a mask.
- Activated glutaraldehyde must be stored in a covered container in a well-ventilated room with a controlled room temperature.

Sodium Hypochlorite

Sodium hypochlorite (household bleach) is an effective disinfectant for surfaces, floors, and equipment. Sodium hypochlorite is such an effective and fast-acting solution, and the CDC recommends its use in cleaning blood and body fluid spills.

Action

- Disrupts cellular metabolism

Advantages

- Bactericidal, virucidal, tuberculocidal, effective against HIV, HBV, and other viruses
- Fast-acting solution
- Effective for cleaning surfaces, including floors and countertops

Disadvantages

- Corrosive to some metals, rubber, and plastics
- Rapidly loses effectiveness in presence of organic soil
- Noxious odor
- Harmful to the skin

Safety Considerations

- Must wear gloves and avoid splashing
- Must wear protective eyewear
- Wearing a protective gown or apron is recommended.
- Must wear a mask
- Solution needs to be stored in a well-ventilated room with a controlled room temperature.
- Do not mix or allow contact with formaldehyde; the result is the production of bis-chloromethyl ether, a highly carcinogenic solution.
- Never mix bleach with ammonia. A chlorine gas will result that is highly toxic, irritating to the lungs, and potentially fatal if inhaled.

Intermediate-Level Disinfectant Compounds

These disinfectants are not capable of killing spores or certain hydrophilic viruses; however, they do kill all bacteria, fungi, and non-hydrophilic viruses. Because these compounds are intermediate-level disinfectants, they are used to disinfect countertops, OR furniture, floors and other surfaces, and instruments that only come into contact with the skin of the patient.

PHENOL (CARBOLIC ACID)

Phenol is usually used as a concentrate with detergent additives and is diluted with tap water. Phenol is used to disinfect large areas such as floors and countertops and is used on a general basis as a health care facility cleaning agent.

Action

- Denatures enzymes and causes cell lyses

Advantages

- Economical choice for the OR because it is a highly concentrated solution that is easily diluted for use
- Particularly effective in eliminating fecal contamination

Disadvantages

- Highly irritating to the skin. Isopropyl alcohol should be used to neutralize the area of the skin on which phenol has made contact to prevent severe skin injury.
- Noxious odor
- Respiratory tract irritant
- Limited to disinfection of noncritical items

Safety Considerations

- Must wear PPE: gloves, eyewear protection, protective gown or apron, and mask
- Use of a respirator is recommended.
- Store solution in a well-ventilated room with a controlled room temperature.

Quaternary Ammonium Compounds

These compounds, commonly called *quats*, are bactericidal, fungicidal, and pseudomonacidal. They are not sporicidal, virucidal, or tuberculocidal. Common compounds include benzalkonium chloride and dimethyl benzyl ammonium chloride; however, newer and more effective compounds are available, such as dialkyl quats. Some facilities consider quats low-level disinfectants because of their inability to kill TB, spores, or viruses and their vulnerability to inactivation.

Action

- Cause leakage of the protoplasm in microbes

Advantages

- Low cost
- Easy to mix with water
- Odorless
- Noncorrosive; safe to use on metals

Disadvantages

- Kill limited number of classes of microbes
- Effectiveness easily reversed when solution contacts organic debris, tap water, or detergents
- Gauze or fabrics absorb the disinfectant ingredient, rendering the disinfection process ineffective, contraindicating the use of the solution for mopping or wiping surfaces

Safety Considerations

- Wear PPE, particularly gloves
- Store solution in a well-ventilated room with a controlled room temperature

Alcohol

Isopropyl and ethyl alcohol in a dilution of 60–70% alcohol concentration are tuberculocidal, bactericidal, virucidal, and fungicidal; they are not sporicidal. Alcohol is most useful in cleaning and disinfecting small noncritical surfaces. Recent studies show that these solutions may be as effective or more effective than other compounds for use in skin disinfection for surgical scrub and patient skin prep. Further studies are warranted.

Action

- Causes protein denaturation, lysis, and metabolic interruption of cells

Advantages

- Nontoxic to the skin, but can have drying effects with constant use
- Effectively reduces number of bacteria on the skin; often used as a step in the skin prep of the patient
- Good range of effectiveness against several types of microbes, including HIV

Disadvantages

- Slight odor
- Do not use in cleaning of surgical instruments; highly corrosive to stainless steel
- Do not use in cleaning of endoscopes; breaks down the cement
- Highly flammable

Safety Considerations

- Wear PPE, in particular gloves and mask.
- Avoid use if electrosurgery or lasers will be used. If used as part of the patient's skin prep, make sure skin is completely dry before applying the sterile drapes.
- Prevent pooling of the alcohol solution under the patient or under the grounding pad.
- Store solution in a well-ventilated room with a controlled room temperature.

ENVIRONMENTAL DECONTAMINATION

An important part of maintaining asepsis is minimizing microbial counts in the OR environment. The OR is designed to minimize contamination. Washable floors and walls and easily cleaned furniture are required in every OR. Effective sanitation and decontamination techniques and established procedures aid in preventing the intraoperative cross-infection of patients. These activities take place at the beginning of the day, between cases, weekly, monthly, and while the patient is in the OR. During a procedure any spills or contaminated items should be handled according to Standard Precautions. Environmental services personnel involved with OR decontamination must follow the guidelines for Standard Precautions and the use of PPE at all times. Additionally, the hospital exposure control plan, required by OSHA, should explain the protective measures needed to create a safe working environment. The following section discusses the decontamination of the OR and accessory areas of the OR, and the process of decontamination of surgical instruments.

Environmental Services

The following are guidelines for housekeeping, laundry, and regulated waste procedures.

- A routine schedule should be established for the cleaning and decontamination of OR surfaces, scrub sinks, cabinets, floors, walls, and ceilings.
- Contaminated work surfaces such as the OR floor should be decontaminated by the circulator with a disinfectant. When it is not possible to immediately decontaminate the floor while a surgery is in process (concurrent cleaning), this should be completed as soon as possible or at the end of the procedure.
- Reusable contaminated linens must be handled as little as possible to prevent airborne contamination. The contaminated linen should be placed and contained in a leakproof, red-colored biohazard bag that is clearly marked with the biohazard symbol.
- Contaminated linens must not be rinsed or sorted in the area of use.
- When handling contaminated linens, the surgical technologist must wear gloves and other PPE as deemed necessary.
- Regulated waste must be placed in leakproof bags that are either clearly marked with the biohazard symbol or are red in color. Only contaminated waste should be put in these designated bags because they are more costly to dispose of than common hospital waste.

Decontamination Practices in the OR: Prior to the First Procedure of the Day

Prior to the start of the first surgical procedure of the day the OR furniture, equipment, surfaces, and lights must be "damp-dusted" with a disinfectant solution using a lint-free cloth. Hospital policy will dictate the type of disinfectant solution to be used. The following cleaning actions should be accomplished:

- Clean all surfaces in the OR, paying particular attention to horizontal surfaces.
- Damp dusting should begin with the highest surface, such as the OR lights, to the lowest. This avoids the settling of dust on objects that have already been damp dusted.
- When cleaning the OR table, the pads should be removed in order to clean both sides of the pads and the surfaces and hinges of the OR table underneath the pads.
- The OR table should be unlocked and moved to one side to facilitate mopping the floor under the table. This also allows for the cleaning of the posts and casters on the OR table.
- If blood or body fluids are present on the OR walls, clean the area.
- Clean cabinet doors, paying attention to the track in which the door is opened and closed.
- Do not clean the surgical lights if they have not yet cooled off; the disinfectant solution, even though it is room temperature, may be too cold and the expensive light bulb could break upon contact with the solution.

Decontamination Practices in the OR: Intraoperative Decontamination

The following actions are accomplished by the surgical technologist during a surgical procedure. However, it must be noted that it may not always be possible to perform these activities in a timely manner due to the surgical technologist being busy throughout a procedure. These activities are secondary to paying close attention to the surgical procedure and working with the surgeon one-on-one where appropriate, such as during a minor procedure.

- A basin with sterile water should be available in the sterile field for the soaking and cleaning of instruments. Never use saline, as the salt in the solution can cause pitting and corrosion of the metal. Use a wet sponge such as a laparotomy sponge to wipe blood and body fluids from instruments between each use. Dried blood may cause instruments to become stiff, and subcutaneous fat may cause instruments to become slippery in the surgeon's hand.
- Instruments that are not easily cleaned with a sponge, such as orthopedic reamers and rasps, should be kept in the basin of sterile water to prevent the drying of blood, body fluids, and tissue on the instruments particularly if they will not be used again during the procedure.
- Instruments with a lumen should be periodically flushed with sterile water to prevent the lumen from becoming clogged.

The circulator is responsible for the following actions:

- Cleaning any blood or body fluids from the floor or other nonsterile surfaces as soon as possible.
- Changing suction containers when they are full to prevent spilling over. Wipe the outside of a full container and place it in a biohazard bag for disposal at the end of the procedure. Products that solidify regulated waste are available, such as Isolyser LTS-PLUS®, which is designed for encapsulation and antimicrobial treatment of medical waste. Canisters can then be disposed of in nonregulated trash in many states.
- Cleaning the outside of a specimen container before it is sent to the pathology department.
- Surgical instruments that become contaminated, such as by falling on the floor, should be retrieved by the circulator and placed in a basin that contains water or disinfectant solution, or, if the instrument is needed for the procedure, the circulator should clean it in the substerile room, after which it is immediate-use steam sterilized.
- The surgical technologist is responsible for dropping soiled sponges into the plastic-lined sponge or kick bucket. If there are several sponges, the circulator along with the surgical technologist can count the sponges in groups of 5 or 10, after which the circulator should immediately place the sponges in a clear plastic bag allowing for visible assessment of blood loss by the anesthesia provider. Sponges should not be lined up on the floor of the OR for purposes of counting.
- The circulator should be wearing PPE, including mask with face shield or mask with goggles, cover gown, and gloves.
- The circulator can use a device such as a sponge stick to transfer contaminated items such as soiled sponges, but the circulator should still wear gloves.

Decontamination Practices in the OR: Decontamination Between Procedures

The CDC recommends that all ORs be cleaned between procedures. This means removing all soiled linen and waste bags, wiping down the OR furniture and surgical lights, mopping the floor, and if necessary spot cleaning the walls. The surgical technologist, along with environmental services personnel, may be involved in the "turnover" of the room, which marks the preparation for the next procedure. Individuals should wear PPE when involved in the decontamination portion of the turnover. Besides these procedures, the following should also be accomplished:

- Suction containers must be disconnected from the suction unit, and the outside of the containers wiped down and disposed of according to hospital policy.
- The surgical technologist is responsible for disposing of the sharps by placing them into the puncture-proof sharps container. The container should not be allowed to overflow and should be immediately replaced when full.

- The linen and trash bags must be sealed and placed in the designated area for transfer by environmental services personnel for proper disposal.
- The surgical technologist is responsible for placing all instruments in a case cart or open cart or table that is covered with plastic for transfer to the decontamination room. Some ORs contain contaminated instruments in the same rigid containers used for sterilization. Care must be taken not to transfer bioburden to the exterior of the containers.

Most health care facilities have some type of case cart system in place (Figure 7-2). The case cart system is an efficient method for transporting surgical equipment, supplies, and instruments to the OR and back to the central sterile processing department (CSPD) for reprocessing. The CSPD may be adjacent to the surgical department or located on a separate floor. If the CSPD is located adjacent to the OR, the case cart can simply be transferred to the decontamination room. If the decontamination room is located on another floor, an elevator called a dumbwaiter may be used to transfer the cart to the CSPD. The typical case cart that is used is a stainless steel cart with doors on the front that swing open and shut; inside the cart may be one or two removable shelves. If the CSPD personnel are also responsible for "pulling" cases, the following is a typical process for the use of the case cart:

- At the end of the procedure the surgical technologist loads the case cart with the surgical instruments and equipment.
- The cart is transferred to the CSPD.

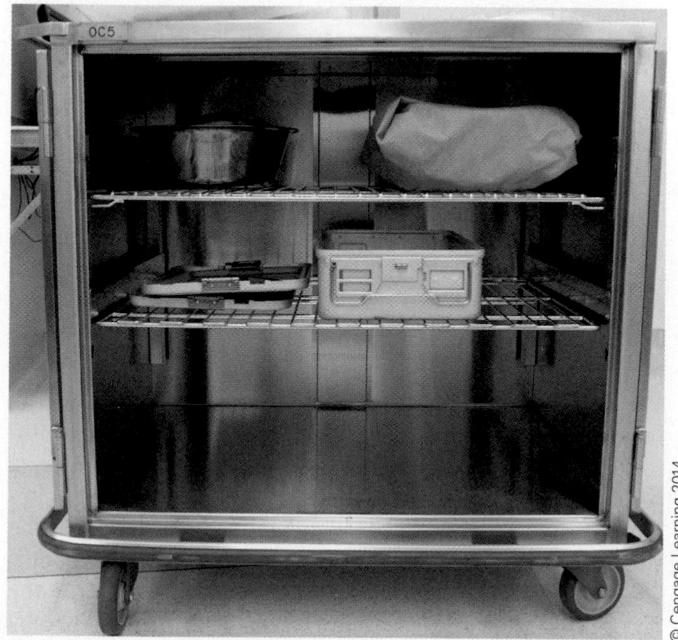

Figure 7-2 Case cart

- CSPD personnel clean, decontaminate, assemble, wrap, sterilize, and store the instrument trays and equipment. They are also responsible for decontaminating the case cart.
- CSPD personnel use a surgeon's preference card to "pull" the instruments, supplies, and equipment needed for a particular procedure and place them in a clean case cart. The personnel refer to the next day's surgical schedule to pull cases unless they have to pull for an emergency procedure.
- Once the case cart or carts are complete, they are transferred to the surgery department either that day or the morning of the next day.

Terminal Cleaning

Each health care facility designs its own end-of-day or "terminal cleaning" routine. This entails a more thorough cleaning of rooms and areas outside of the ORs after the last case of the day has been completed. The following are the activities that should be completed in each OR using a disinfectant solution:

- Ceilings and floors including surgical lights are wiped down. Ceilings and floors can be wiped down using a sponge mop.
- All furniture is wiped down, including the legs, casters, or wheels.
- The OR table is thoroughly wiped down, including the wheels. The pads should be removed and completely wiped down. Attachments used during procedures should be cleaned.
- All other equipment, including tables, stools, kick buckets, anesthesia machine, ESU, and suction unit should be completely cleaned.
- All other horizontal surfaces, such as cabinet shelves, cabinet doors, and handles, are cleaned.
- Once the above has been accomplished, the furniture and equipment (with the exception of the anesthesia machine) is moved to one side of the room and the OR floor is thoroughly wetted/flooded with a disinfectant solution and wet vacuumed.
  After the floor is dry, the furniture and equipment is placed back in its normal position.

Other areas of the surgical department that should be cleaned include the following:

- Substerile and storage rooms
- Stretchers used for transporting patients
- Scrub sinks, which demand particular attention due to their heavy use and the splashing of water and scrub solution that occurs
- Hallway floors should be cleaned similar to the floors in the OR; the floors should be thoroughly wetted/flooded with the disinfectant solution and wet vacuumed.

Particular attention should be paid to the scrub solution dispensers located at the scrub sinks. Gram-negative bacilli have been known to contaminate disinfectant solutions and soap dispensers in the OR, including the surgical scrub solution dispensers. This is usually due to the practice of refilling disinfectant dispensers when empty or topping them off with fresh solution without resterilizing them. This practice contaminates the solution inside. These containers should be sterilized before refilling and should not be topped off. Because the risk of this problem is higher with quaternary ammonium compounds, they should not be used for the surgical scrub. Many hospitals now purchase single-use, prepackaged sterile scrub brushes impregnated with antiseptic solution and/or single-use dispensers.

Weekly Cleaning

In addition to the case-by-case and daily cleaning routines, certain cleaning and disinfection practices are scheduled on a weekly basis by health care facilities. The following are the areas that are usually addressed in the weekly cleaning schedule policy of the facility:

- Ceilings, walls, and floor should be thoroughly cleaned inside and outside the ORs; this includes outside corridors.
- Mounted lighting tracks and fixtures should be cleaned.
- Air vents and heating duct grills must be vacuumed to remove dust laden with bacteria.
- Inside and outside of supply cabinets, including shelves, should be cleaned.
- Sterile and nonsterile supply rooms should be cleaned, including linen room.
- Housekeeping supply room should be cleaned.

Dirty Cases

Upon completion of a dirty case, the floor should be cleaned with a phenolic detergent and all equipment and furniture should be wiped down with 70% alcohol solution. Rubber and plastic tubing in the room should be replaced and if gross contamination of walls and ceilings has occurred, these should be wiped down with a disinfectant solution as well. Some health care facilities will attempt to schedule a dirty case as the last procedure of the day in an OR so a thorough terminal cleaning process will occur.

Surgical Instrument Decontamination Process

As previously mentioned, any critical patient item or instrument that will be used on open tissue or be placed in the sterile field must be sterilized to remove all microbes, including spores. Decontamination is the first step in the prevention of transmission of microbes from instruments to patient or from instruments to personnel and renders the instruments safe for handling by OR and CSPD personnel. The process begins in the decontamination room where the items are cleaned, disinfected, and lubricated if necessary; sorting, reassembling, wrapping, and sterilizing takes place in the clean, sterile processing area of the CSPD.

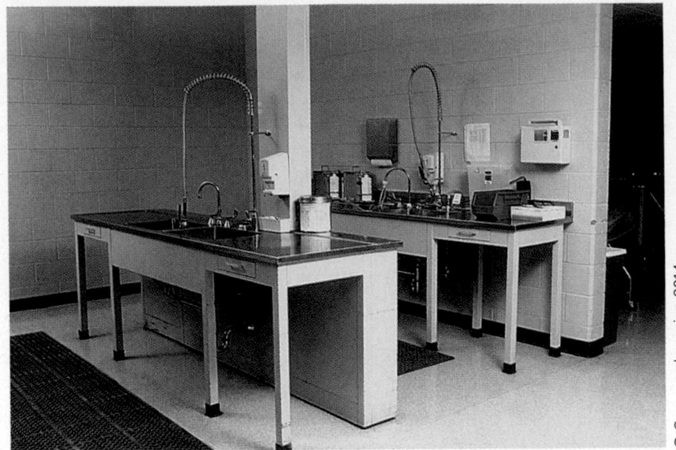

Figure 7-3 Decontamination room

The decontamination room is a separate area, usually in proximity to the clean sterile processing area (Figure 7-3). The design of the decontamination area environment should follow these principles:

- Filtered air is exhausted to the outside of the health care facility.
- The minimum air exchange rate is 10 times per hour.
- Temperature should be maintained between 64° and 70°F with a humidity of 35% to 72%.
- Negative air pressure is maintained.

When the design of the CSPD does not allow for the physical separation of the decontamination area and the clean work area into two rooms, the tasks of cleaning and assembly and preparation must be scheduled and performed at different times to prevent the potential depositing of contaminated droplets onto cleaned instruments ready for packaging. Personnel performing decontamination duties must don impervious gowns with open backs or vent holes to prevent overheating, long dishwashing-type gloves, hair cover, masks, safety eyewear, and shoe covers to prevent distribution of contaminated bioburden onto their skin or clothes and splash exposure to eyes or mucous membranes.

Cleaning

The first step in the decontamination process begins at the point of use. The surgical technologist is responsible for presoaking contaminated instruments to prevent the drying of organic matter. He or she is also responsible for the initial arrangement of the instruments when breaking down the sterile field at the end of a procedure and placing the items in some type of closed container for safe transport to the decontamination area. The following solutions may be used by the surgical technologist for soaking the instruments:

1. Sterile water; do not use saline. The salt will pit the metal on the instrument, permanently damaging the instrument and leading to the formation of rust.
2. Enzymatic solution
   a. Proteolytic enzymatic cleaner: Facilitates the removal of protein materials such as blood.
   b. Lipolytic enzymatic cleaner: Facilitates the removal of fatty material such as adipose tissue and bone marrow.
3. Detergent solutions

There are advantages and limitations to the use of each of these solutions (Table 7-9).

The surgical technologist should follow these recommendations when preparing the instruments for transport to the decontamination room:

- Place heavy instruments on the bottom of trays and not on top of smaller and/or delicate instruments.
- Instruments with ring handles should be unratcheted and strung using an instrument stringer that keeps the instruments open. String instruments keeping the curve of curved instruments facing the same direction and in a sequence of increasing size and length, e.g. mosquitoes, Kellys, Peans, etc.
- Instruments with multiple parts should be disassembled.
- Per hospital policy, an enzymatic foam can be sprayed over the instruments to aid in breaking down the proteinaceous debris on the instrument surfaces. Place the instrument tray or trays, along with all other items such as basins, into the case cart and transport them to the decontamination room.

Table 7-9 Advantages and Limitations of Presoaking Solutions

Solution	*Advantages*	*Limitations*
Sterile water	Keeps organic debris moist	Ineffective in softening or removing dried debris
Enzyme	Removes moistened and dried debris without the need for mechanical action	Efficiency depends on concentration of solution, temperature, and contact time
Detergent	Keeps organic debris moist while loosening dried-on debris	Mechanical action is necessary to completely remove soil

Cleaning is the first step when instruments arrive in the decontamination room. The purpose of cleaning is to physically remove debris that was not removed or softened during the presoak. Remember, disinfectant solutions are weakened or inactivated in the presence of organic soil; additionally, organic soil prevents the solution from making contact with the surface of the items. Thorough cleaning before disinfection cannot be overemphasized.

When cleaning instruments, remove organic and inorganic soil through one of the following methods, depending on the type of cleaning solution used:

- **Chelation**: The process of binding minerals, such as iron and magnesium, in the solution. This prevents their deposit on the surface of surgical instruments, which causes spotting.
- Enzymatic: Enzymes are catalysts that aid in breaking down organic soil such as blood and tissue into solution.
- Emulsification: The action of dispersing two liquids not capable of being mixed.
- Solubilization: The action by which the solubility of a substance is increased within a solution.

Table 7-10 shows the common types of chemical cleaners.

Table 7-10 Common Chemical Cleaners

Type	*Characteristics*
Enzymatic	Organic substance that aids in the chemical reaction of breaking down organic debris. As previously stated, enzymes are specific to the type of debris to be removed. Enzymes are usually used as a soaking solution. They require dilution and are more effective in warm water than cold because the temperature of the warm water increases the speed of the chemical reaction.
Ultrasonic	Cleaning solutions are manufactured specifically for use in ultrasonic cleaners. The solution may contain a surfactant (to enhance wetting ability) and chelating agents.
Manual detergent	Products usually used for hand cleaning of items and/or for presoaking. Some of the manual cleaners are high foaming and therefore should not be used in mechanical cleaning equipment. They must be diluted for use but are safe to use on most materials, including stainless steel. Mechanical action is required to assist in removing the soil. Surgical instruments must be thoroughly rinsed after being placed in the detergent.

(continues)

Table 7-10 (continued)

Washer-decontaminator	Liquid solution that is available in three different pH levels. *Neutral-pH product:* Least corrosive to surgical instruments but less effective at removing substantial amount of organic soil.
	Moderate-pH product: Low-level alkaline; may be combined with surfactants and chelating agents. Safe for use on stainless steel instruments but could be harmful to the chromium oxide layer that protects the instruments from corrosion.
	High-pH product: Most effective for removing heavy amounts of soil. Can be corrosive to stainless steel. If used, it must be neutralized by a neutralizing rinse to prevent damage to the instruments.

Ideally, a three-sink arrangement is utilized as follows:

- First sink: Wash sink with water and detergent solution
- Second sink: Intermediate rinse with distilled water
- Third sink: Final rinse with distilled water

The manual cleaning of instruments is a three-step process:

1. Instruments are immersed in a solution of lukewarm water, detergent, and/or enzymatic cleaner with a neutral pH. Hot water should not be used to initially rinse instruments to avoid blood and tissue from being set with heat on the metal surface. The manufacturer's instructions must be followed for correct dilution, temperature, and use of detergent solutions. The enzymatic cleaner aids in the removal of bioburden. Each instrument must be individually cleaned with a soft-bristled brush using friction to loosen the organic debris. The foundation of manual cleaning is friction. Friction will loosen the organic material to allow its removal during the rinsing process. When cleaning stainless steel instruments, a back-and-forth motion should be used to follow the grain of the instrument. Do not use a circular motion, which can scratch the surface of the item. The instrument and brush must be kept submerged in the solution during cleaning to prevent contaminated water droplets from aerosolizing. Particular attention must be directed toward serrations on jaws, ratchets, box locks, and teeth of instruments. Instruments with lumens may be cleaned with a tube brush, pipe cleaner, or handheld water pressure gun. The cleaning solution should be changed frequently to avoid buildup of microbes and soil.
2. The last step is to rinse the instruments in distilled water. Do not use tap water because it may contain minerals that can stain and form a film on the instruments when the tap water evaporates.
3. To avoid spotting the instruments, the items should be immediately dried after rinsing.

Decontamination

To protect individuals responsible for the decontamination of surgical instruments and equipment, most health care facilities have purchased mechanical cleaning equipment to eliminate manual cleaning. The types of cleaning equipment include washer-sterilizer, washer-decontaminator, and ultrasonic washer. The following recommendations should be followed when preparing instruments for decontamination in a machine:

- Instruments must be placed into a perforated or wire mesh tray to prevent interference with the cleaning action of the machine.
- Heavier instruments should be placed on the bottom of the tray to avoid damage to the lighter, more delicate instruments.
- Hinged instruments must be left in an open position to allow water, cleaning agent, and steam to contact the total surface area.
- Instruments with attachments must be disassembled.
- Instruments with concave surfaces should be placed upside down to allow proper cleaning, rinsing, steam contact, and drainage.

Washer-Decontaminator

The washer-decontaminator (WD) does not incorporate a sterilizing phase. The cycle of the WD is as follows:

1. Prerinse cycle: Some models allow the use of an enzymatic solution in this phase.
2. Cleaning cycle: Detergent solution is used in this cycle.
3. Final rinse: Hot water is used during this rinse. The water temperature is maintained at 180°–195°F.
4. Drying phase: High temperature is used to dry the instruments.

Some models add an ultrasonic cleaning phase after the cleaning cycle and/or a chemical disinfectant rinse. These units allow totally hands-off processing. Instruments that are placed in perforated or mesh-bottom trays can come directly from the point of use, such as the OR, and be placed in the WD without further handling or arranging of instruments by decontamination personnel.

At the conclusion of the cycle, items are considered clean and have been exposed to an intermediate level of disinfection. This makes the items safe for handling but not necessarily ready for immediate use.

Washer-Sterilizer

A majority of stainless steel surgical instruments and heat-tolerant items can be processed through the washer-sterilizer (WS) (Figure 7-4). After gross soil is removed, the items may be processed in the WS. Always consult the manufacturer's instructions for operating the WS and for arrangement of the instrument trays inside the machine. If the soil is not removed or instruments are improperly arranged, the remaining soil may not be removed during the wash phase and could be baked on during the sterilization phase, possibly damaging the stainless steel and making the removal of such baked-on materials difficult.

Stainless steel instruments should not be placed next to instruments made of other metals, such as brass or copper. (Some malleable retractors and uterine sounds are still made of copper.) An electrolytic conduction reaction can occur when two different metals come into contact in a wet, hot environment such as the WS chamber. The reaction causes one metal to fuse to the other and may permanently damage instruments.

A free-rinsing, low-sudsing detergent with a neutral pH should be used. High-sudsing detergent will leave residue on instruments and may cause overflow of detergent solution and decrease the efficiency of the pumps within the machine.

Some types of WS require the detergent to be added manually with each load; others are designed with a system that automatically adds the detergent when required. A typical WS cycle follows.

1. *Prerinse:* A continuous cool or tepid water spray rinse aids in removing organic and soil matter such as blood and tissue.
2. *Automatic detergent injection:* The machine injects a measured amount of detergent into the chamber.
3. *Fill phase:* The chamber is filled with water for total instrument immersion and cleaning.
4. *Wash phase:* Water is agitated inside the chamber for soil removal; the machine controls water temperature.
5. *Postrinse:* Loose soil and detergent film are rinsed off items.
6. *Sterilization phase:* Steam sterilization cycle—this is usually a gravity cycle.
7. *Lubrication* (milking)
8. *Drying phase*

Two types of WS machines are commercially available. The first type is a tunnel-like chamber with a door at each end and rotating sprayer arms that distribute the liquid detergent agent from multiple directions during the wash phase. The second type is the horizontal/cabinet type and has a door at one or both ends of the chamber. This design allows for the use of standard instrument trays that also allow easier and more efficient loading/unloading of the chamber. The chamber fills with water and detergent, not relying on rotating sprayer arms. Steam and air are injected through the solution, producing a turbulent action, which loosens the soil and produces the washing action. As the heated water expands and rises within the chamber, the loose soil overflows into the waste pipe line. The automatic program control activates the steam inlet valve to open and the water outlet valve to open. The steam enters at the top of the chamber, forcing the water out, and the sterilization cycle begins. The steam sterilization cycle is a gravity cycle at 270°F.

Although a steam sterilization cycle is the last step of the WS, items are not considered ready for use on patients but are safe for handling by CSPD personnel with bare hands. Because this is not a biologically monitored process, instruments must be organized into a standardized set, wrapped, and sterilized.

Ultrasonic Cleaner

After instruments have been processed through the WD or WS, they are placed in the **ultrasonic cleaner** (Figure 7-5). The ultrasonic cleaner removes small organic particles and soil from areas of instrumentation that manual or mechanical

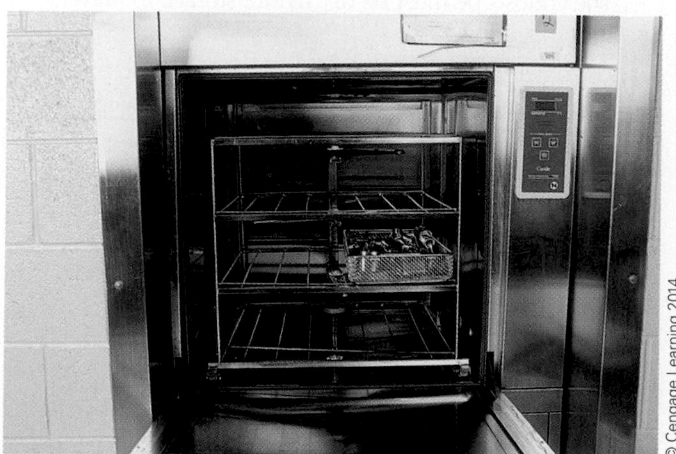

Figure 7-4 Washer-sterilizer

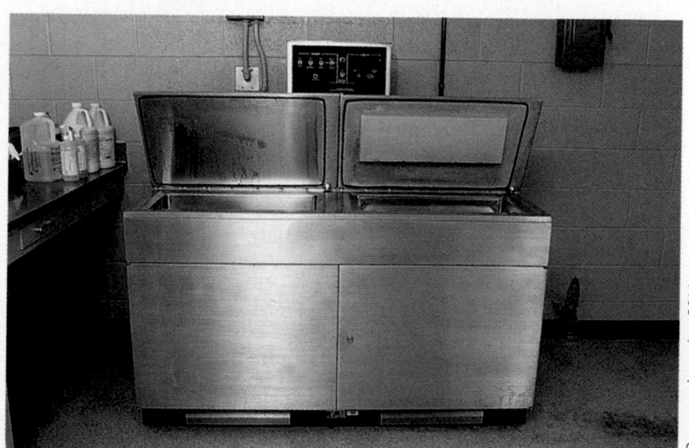

Figure 7-5 Ultrasonic cleaner

cleaning cannot reach. These areas include box locks, serrations, and ratchets. The ultrasonic cleaner utilizes the process of **cavitation** for cleaning instruments.

- The machine works by using high-frequency sound waves that are converted to vibrations in the solution.
- As the ultrasonic waves travel through the cleaning agent, the energy causes the molecules to be set in rapid motion, forming microscopic bubbles on the surface of the instruments.
- The bubbles enlarge, become unstable, and implode (collapse inward). The implosion creates a vacuum, dislodging minute particles of soil and organic material from the instruments.

Instruments processed through the ultrasonic cleaner are to be placed in a metal mesh tray. The tray is immersed in a solution of warm water and a low-sudsing, free-rinsing detergent with a neutral pH is used in the first chamber. When the solution is changed and the chamber refilled, it is necessary to run one empty cycle. Gas bubbles form during filling and absorb the ultrasonic energy generated by the machine, decreasing its cleaning effectiveness. Running an empty cycle degasses the chamber.

Ultrasonic cleaning is not considered a true disinfecting process but rather a method of cleaning instrumentation. The cleaning solution must be frequently changed due to the increase of bioburden with each use. The ultrasonic cleaning process creates fine aerosols that may contain microbes harmful to personnel. Whenever the ultrasonic cleaner is in operation the lid must be closed.

Various types of ultrasonic cleaners are available on the market. Models consist of one, two, or three chambers. For the three-chamber unit, the first chamber is for cleaning, the second chamber is for spray rinsing the instruments, and the third is for hot air drying. The rinse and dry cycles are combined in the second chamber in a two-chamber ultrasonic cleaner. Each cycle lasts approximately 4–5 minutes.

Instruments Requiring Special Care in Cleaning and Disinfection

Items with lumens such as trocar sheaths, nondisposable suction tips, and endoscopic instruments require special care to ensure adequate decontamination. Blood and tissue can be difficult to remove from lumens, especially if dried. Items may have to soak in an enzymatic solution for a period of time to loosen the debris. The lumen should be flushed until the fluid emerges clear. Hydrogen peroxide is an excellent flushing agent for ridding the lumen of blood. The peroxide reacts with the blood by producing foam, which disappears when the blood has been thoroughly rinsed away. The lumen must then be rinsed with distilled water to flush away the hydrogen peroxide.

Numerous surgical procedures, particularly orthopedic procedures, require the use of powered instruments such as saws and drills. Powered instruments must never be submerged in cleaning solution or placed in any type of mechanical decontaminating equipment. The manufacturer's instructions for cleaning must be followed. General instructions are as follows:

1. Leave the air hose attached to the power handle while cleaning. This will prevent any cleaning solution or rinsing water from entering into the cord or handle.
2. Wash off the cord with lukewarm water using a neutral detergent, cloth, or soft-bristled brush. Do not use alcohol to wipe down the hose; the alcohol will dry out the protective outside rubber, causing it to harden and crack. Hold the end of the cord not attached to the power handle downward to allow water to run off and prevent it from entering the hose.
3. Wipe down the handle using a cloth or soft-bristled brush, lukewarm water, and neutral detergent.
4. Rinse all components with distilled water and wipe them dry.
5. Powered instruments may require oiling to maintain optimum motor efficiency. The manufacturer's directions must be followed on the type of oil to be used and where to apply the drops of oil. The oil should be applied right after cleaning and prior to sterilization. The power tool may need to be run for 30–60 seconds after oiling.

There are two types of endoscopes: flexible and rigid. The following are general recommendations for the decontamination of both types.

Rigid Endoscopes

1. Channels, holes, and joints must be thoroughly cleaned and rinsed to remove blood and debris.
2. Soaking of the endoscope in an enzymatic solution is recommended.
3. Using a handheld water pressure gun for washing and compressed air for drying will aid in the cleaning process. The endoscope must be dry before storage to prevent bacterial growth.
4. Use a detergent recommended by the manufacturer.
5. Care should be taken to avoid damaging the delicate eyepiece and lens, which can easily be scratched.
6. Light fibers are situated within the endoscope. Denting the body of the endoscope will break the fibers. Hitting or crushing of the endoscope should be prevented.

Flexible Endoscopes

1. Flexible endoscopes have many channels that require cleaning. Examples include the suction, biopsy, and air/water channels. Cleaning brushes on the end of long, thin, flexible wires are available to clean the channels.

2. If recommended by the manufacturer, soaking the endoscope in an enzymatic solution with the channel ports open and flushing with the cleaning solution will help in the cleaning process.
3. The exterior of the endoscope should be cleaned with a neutral detergent and a soft brush or cloth.

Lubrication

As a last step before instruments are reassembled and prepared for sterilization, they are usually lubricated. Surgical instruments must be lubricated to maintain optimal function. Special surgical instrument lubricants are available and should be used to lubricate surfaces and box locks of instruments on a schedule developed by the facility. This process is commonly called milking, since the lubricant solution is usually white in color. The lubricating solution should be mixed according to the manufacturer's instructions. The instruments are immersed and left in the solution for a short period; again, consult the manufacturer's recommendations. The lubricant is penetrable by steam during the steam sterilization process, and therefore should not be wiped off the instruments prior to assembling, wrapping, and sterilization.

STERILIZATION PRINCIPLES AND PROCESSES

As previously discussed, sterility is the absence of all microbes, including spores. There is no grey area with sterility—an item is either sterile or it is not sterile. The tissues within the body are sterile; therefore, the items that come into contact with the tissues must be sterile. Using nonsterile or contaminated items could cause the patient to acquire a debilitating and life-threatening infection. In this section of the chapter instrument preparation, wrapping, and the various methods of sterilization will be discussed. Refer to Figure 7-6 for a diagram of the instrument processing cycle.

Instrument Preparation and Wrapping

Instruments must be checked for function and **integrity** and prepared for **sterilization**. This activity takes placed in a room located within the CSPD and designed for that purpose, commonly referred to as a clean room (Figure 7-7).

Packaging refers to the various types of materials available for the wrapping and enclosure of reusable items so they can be safely sterilized and stored until used. The federal Food,

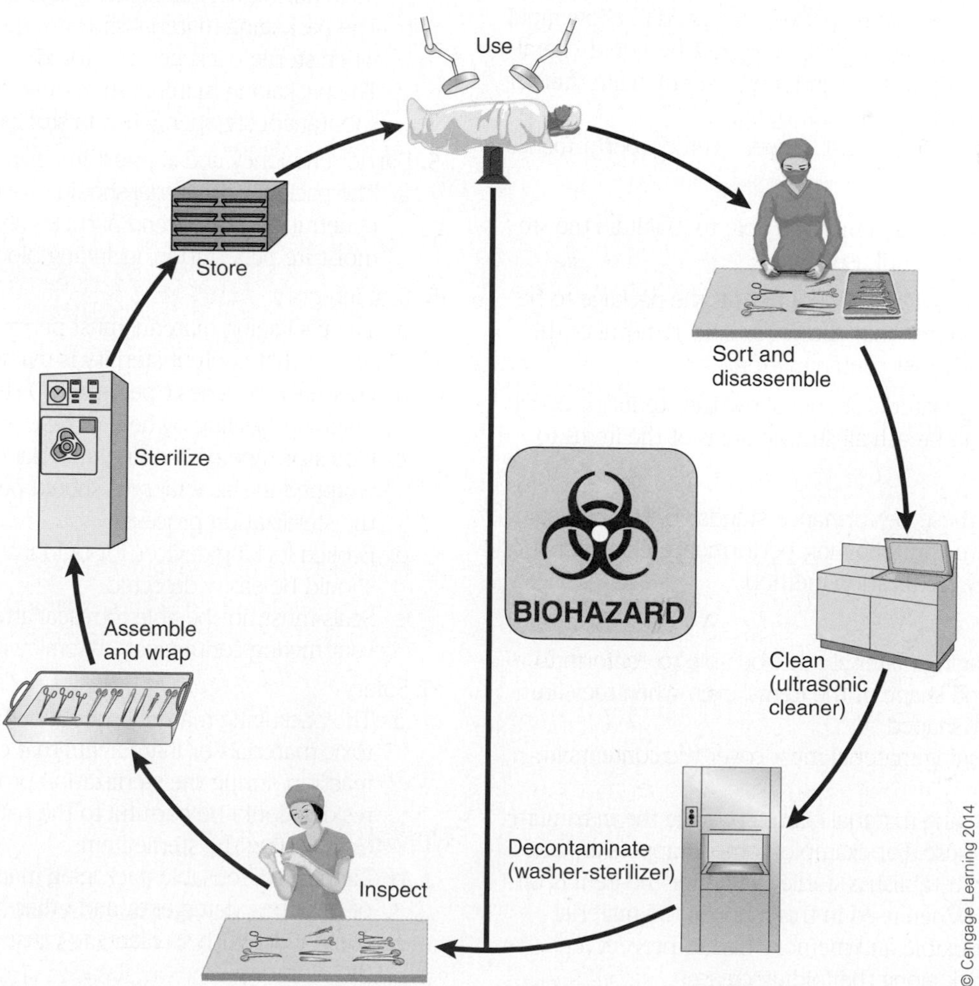

Figure 7-6 Instrument processing cycle

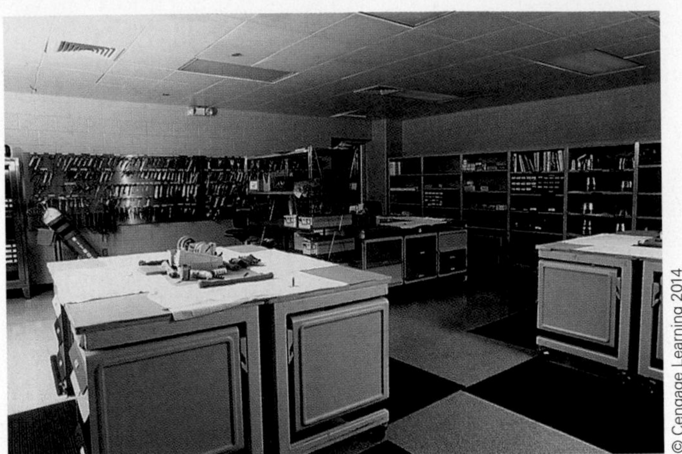

Figure 7-7 Clean processing area

Drug, and Cosmetic Act states that "the prime purpose and function of a packaging material (pack, sterilization wrapper, bag, or accessories) is to enclose a medical device that is to be sterilized by a health care provider. It is intended to allow sterilization of the enclosed device and also to maintain sterility of the device until it is used." This includes **immediate-use steam sterilization**, in which the item is placed in an open tray or covered rigid container that is specially designed to allow rapid steam penetration. Items that are sterilized by liquid chemical processes are not packaged and require immediate transfer from point of sterilization to point of use.

Packaging material must meet three performance standards:

- The packaging material must be able to maintain the sterility of the items until use.
- The packaging material should permit the package to be opened in a manner that allows for easy removal of the sterile items without contamination.
- The packaging material should allow the sterilizing agent to penetrate and reach all surface areas of the items to be sterilized.

Based upon these performance standards, the packaging material must have the following performance characteristics when used for any sterilization method:

1. Efficiency
   a. The packaging material must be able to conform to the size and shape of the items, even when they are irregularly shaped.
   b. The packaging material must cover the contents in entirety.
   c. The packaging material should provide the maximum amount of use. For example, some wrappers are also utilized to establish a sterile field after the item is unwrapped. When used in this manner, the material must be flexible and memory free to prevent any folding back along the folding creases.
2. Ease of opening
   a. The packaging material should allow the package to be easily opened and transferred to the sterile field or point of use while maintaining sterility.
3. Sterilization suitability
   a. The material must allow air to be completely removed from the package.
   b. The material must be able to withstand the physical conditions produced by the autoclave (moisture, pressure, and high temperatures).
   c. The material must allow for the escape of the sterilizing agent at the end of the sterilization cycle.
   d. The packaging material must allow the contents and material to dry after steam sterilization.
   e. The packaging material must allow the gas and moisture to escape during the aeration cycle after ethylene oxide sterilization.
   f. Packaging material must be compatible for the type of sterilizing agent used; for example, Tyvek® wrapper materials must be used with hydrogen peroxide gas plasma sterilizers.
4. Strength
   a. The packaging material should resist tears and punctures during normal handling and sterilization.
   b. The packaging material should not easily degrade when sterile packages are stored.
   c. The packaging material seals must not deteriorate and spontaneously open when in storage.
5. Barrier efficiency and support impermeability
   a. The packaging material should provide a barrier to the penetration of dust and particles and should resist moisture penetration, including blood and body fluids.
6. Seal integrity
   a. The packaging material must permit integrity of the seal so that content sterility is maintained.
   b. Peel-pack pouches ("peel-packs") should permit self-sealing or sealing by heat or tape.
   c. Indicator tape or banding material that secures items wrapped in flat wrappers should be able to withstand the sterilization process.
   d. Broken locking devices for rigid instrument containers should be easily detected.
   e. Seals must not be able to reseal after opening to prevent mixing contaminated items with sterile items.
7. Safety
   a. The packaging material should be free of dyes and toxic materials or ingredients that could produce a reaction during the sterilization process. This toxic residue could be harmful to the patient and individuals handling the sterile items.
   b. Laundered, reusable packaging materials must be free of bleaches, detergents, and other chemicals that could react with sterilants to cause instrument discoloration.

c. Rigid instrument containers must be rinsed free of cleaning detergents that could react with sterilants, causing discoloration of instruments.

8. Sterility maintenance
    a. The packaging material must maintain the sterility of the content until intentionally opened by a member of the surgical team (event-related).

Woven Textiles

- Made of cotton or blends of cotton with synthetic material such as polyester
- Reusable, meaning they must be laundered between uses. Over time, with repeated laundering, fibers are lost, increasing the space between the threads and reducing the microbial barrier. Eventually the wrapper will need to be discarded.
- After laundering and prior to re-use, wrapper must undergo lint removal and inspection process over a large illuminated table to detect holes, worn areas, and stains. Small holes can be repaired using heat-sealed patches, but must never be stitched closed since the needle and thread create another set of small holes that will allow microbes to enter.

Refer to Table 7-11 for advantages and disadvantages of woven materials.

Woven Textiles with Barrier Properties

- Made of cotton/polyester fiber blend
- Chemical treatment added to the fabric makes them moisture resistant
- 180, 240, 272, or 288 thread count (TC). TC is the number of threads per square inch. The higher the TC, the more it reduces the chances of bacterial and dust penetration.
- Manufactured as a single ply; two wrappers are required when wrapping an item, tray, or instrument set.
- Barrier fabrics do not absorb moisture; water droplets may be retained during steam sterilization. A towel is placed between the instrument tray and barrier wrap to absorb residual moisture.

Muslin

- Made of cotton
- 140 thread count
- Single or double ply (two muslin wraps sewn together)
- Double ply is the best choice to aid in preventing absorption of moisture, which can create a pathway for microbes to the inside of the sterile package through a wicking action.

Nonwoven Materials

Nonwoven materials are disposable wrappers that are designed for single use. They are commonly referred to as disposables. Nonwoven wraps are available in a variety of sizes to accommodate the various sizes and shapes of items to be sterilized. Nonwoven wrappers should be stored in a manner that eliminates folding. The advantages and disadvantages of nonwoven materials are listed in Table 7-12.

Paper is a type of single-use, nonwoven material, but has extreme memory characteristics and does not have the flexibility of other nonwoven materials. Paper is easily penetrated by steam, so it is particularly useful as a sterilization barrier. The advantages and disadvantages of paper materials are listed in Table 7-13.

TABLE 7-11 Woven Materials

Advantages	*Disadvantages*
Economical, reusable	The absorbent material may absorb moisture during steam sterilization, inhibiting necessary contact of the moisture with all surface areas of the items.
Easily penetrated by sterilants	Least effective at providing bacterial barrier when compared to other wrapping materials
	Not recommended for use with EtO
	Additional personnel required for laundering

TABLE 7-12 Nonwoven Materials

Advantages	*Disadvantages*
Excellent barrier properties	Cost, as they are single-use items
Lint free	Not as "memory-free" as woven materials
Impervious to moisture	
Tear resistant	

TABLE 7-13 Paper

Advantages	*Disadvantages*
Plentiful supply	Becomes brittle in dry conditions
Inexpensive	Easily torn, punctured, or ruptured
Porous	Not uniform in thickness

Two types of pouch packaging are generally used by health institutions:

- Paper–plastic combinations that are used for steam and EtO sterilization
- Tyvek–plastic combination used for EtO and Sterrad

Various polymers are used as sterilization barriers. The compatibility of the plastic with the chosen method of sterilization must be confirmed. Tyvek should only be used for EtO and Sterrad. Steam will melt or burn the material, creating a flammable hazard and damaging the contents of the package.

The most common type of pouch packing used in health care facilities is paper–plastic peel packs.

- One side of pouch is paper; the other side is plastic.
- Plastic layer must be a minimum of 2 mm and allow visualization of the contents.
- The side and bottom edges are heat sealed with an open end for placement of the item(s) to be sterilized. The bottom edge is designed for opening the peel pack for placement of the item(s) on the sterile field.
- Open end is heat-sealed or sealed with tape. Self-seal pouches are available with a strip of adhesive that is folded over to seal the pouch.
- Peel packs are available in a variety of precut sizes, including rolls that allow the user to cut the pouch to the desired length. After cutting a pouch, both open ends must then be sealed.
- Most heat-sealing machines have an internal timer that eliminates the need for holding the jaws closed during sealing and a dial to adjust the heat temperature.
- DO NOT use staples to close a peel pack; the staples cause small holes, creating an entry point for microbes.
- Do not use rubber bands, paper clips, or tape to "bind" package contents together. The binding material may prevent the contact of the sterilant with the surface of item(s).
- Place item(s) inside the peel pack so the end of the item to be grasped by the surgical technologist is presented. For example, because the end of the peel pack that was heat sealed by the manufacturer is used to open the peel pack, a clamp should be placed with the ring handles at the end. This makes the item easier for the surgical technologist to grasp when the peel pack is opened by the circulator and presented to the surgical technologist using aseptic technique. Instruments with box locks must be left unratcheted inside the pouch.
- The correct-size pouch must be selected. Pouches that are too small may not allow for adequate air removal, penetration of the sterilant, or drying. Additionally, the items may tear the peel pack if it is too small. Pouches that are too large allow for excessive movement of item(s), increasing the possibility of tears in the peel pack.
- If using a felt-tip marker to label the peel pack, write only on the plastic. Ink from the marker can seep through the paper, compromising the sterility of item(s). Items should be labeled prior to sterilization and never afterward.
- As much air as possible should be forced from the pouch before sealing to prevent the pouch from "bulging" outward during steam sterilization and thus rupturing the package.
- Sharp edges of items should be protected with sterilant-permeable tip protectors or foam sleeves to prevent the peel pack from being torn. Commercial tip protectors are available. Do not use latex tubing as a tip protector due to the sterilant-inhibiting property.
- Heavy item(s), items that have multiple pieces, or multiple items that must be kept together may be double peel packed. Items are placed in a peel pack that is subsequently placed in a larger peel pack that is sealed. The inner peel pack must not be sealed or folded to prevent the entrapment of air that can prevent penetration of the sterilant. The inner peel pack is considered sterile for transferring to the sterile field. The inner package should be placed with paper-to-paper and plastic-to-plastic for visualization of the item(s). Special package inserts that maintain instruments in the open position are commercially available.
- Peel packs are placed on their edge when placed in a sterilizer and positioned paper side to plastic side to ensure air removal, sterilant penetration, and drying. Perforated baskets with support pins are commercially available to maintain the position of the peel packs.

Rigid Instrument Containers

Reusable rigid instrument containers with locking lids have become popular with health care facilities. The containers are multipurpose and have the following characteristics:

- They provide containment of items during sterilization.
- The provide assurance of sterile package integrity because metal or plastic containers cannot be torn or compromised.
- They are easily opened and provide for excellent sterile presentation of contents.
- They can be used for returning contaminated items to the decontamination area.
- A disposable **chemical indicator** to verify exposure to sterilizing conditions may be incorporated within the lid or construction of the rigid instrument container.
- The containers are available in a variety of sizes and designs but always feature a removable lid that is sealable with some type of locking device. The containers are generally manufactured of a sturdy anodized aluminum, stainless steel, plastic, or a plastic-metal combination that allows the stacking of the containers in storage without damaging the containers or contents.

Sterilization recommendations when using rigid containers include:

- Rigid containers can be safely sterilized in the same load with other supplies. The containers should be placed on shelves beneath absorbent items to prevent the condensate from the containers from dripping onto the absorbent items.
- The drying phase should be increased to allow for the revaporization of moisture and condensation on the outside and inside of the container.
- Prevacuum sterilization should be used instead of gravity displacement because of the increased difficulty of adequate air removal.
- Gaskets should be inspected and replaced if torn, cracked, or nonpliable.
- Disposable filters should be replaced after every use.

General Principles of Packaging

A number of general packaging principles exist, including:

- After laundering, woven fabrics should be stored at a temperature of 68°–73°F (20°–23°C) and a humidity of 30–60% for at least 2 hours to rehydrate the fabrics.
- When using muslin wraps, the recommended maximum size of a linen pack is 12 in. high × 12 in. wide × 20 in. long. It must not weigh more than 12 pounds.

  According to the Association for the Advancement of Medical Instrumentation (AAMI), these recommendations are for muslin wraps only. They do not apply to the more commonly used wrapping products that are manufactured of very different materials. Instructions on pack preparation and parameters should be requested from the textile manufacturer.
- If linen packs are sterilized, they must be packaged loosely so that steam can make contact with all surface areas.
- Double, sequential wrapping is essential for proper bacterial barrier and sterile presentation of the contents if single-ply wraps are used. Double-ply wraps are commercially available, making it unnecessary to use two wraps.
- Any commercially or facility-sterilized package must be inspected for holes, tears, perforations, and seal integrity before opening.

After an item to be sterilized is prepared, it must be placed within a rigid container or wrapped in woven or nonwoven wraps. The outer wrapper is securely closed with chemical indicator tape and the tape is labeled to aid in identifying the contents.

It is important to choose the correct-size wrapper. Too large of wrapper can inhibit the penetration and release of the sterilant; too small of wrapper will not adequately cover the contents and could possibly tear at the corners. If the wrapper is to be used for the establishment of a sterile field, it should be large enough to extend to a minimum of 6 in. below the four sides of a table or basin ring stand. The wrapper must also be large enough to cover the hand of the individual opening it if the package is to be handed to the surgical technologist in a sterile manner or transferred onto a sterile field.

Before wrapping an item, it is advisable to place an absorbent towel between the bottom of the tray and the wrapper, especially if the wrapper is nonwoven material. If necessary, another towel may be placed on top of the instrument tray before wrapping. The towels cushion the sharp corners of the instrument trays and prevent tearing.

Density is a key factor for sterilizing an instrument set; the more densely packed the set, the greater the odds that the sterilant will not contact all surface areas and drying will not be adequate. ANSI/AAMI79: 2010 recommends that instrument sets should not exceed 25 pounds.

Protective plastic wraps that are 2–3 mm thick ("dust covers") can be used to cover a sterile package. These dust covers provide further barrier efficiency and aid in preventing contamination of the package. After sterilization, the package must be cooled to room temperature before being placed in the dust cover. The cover can be heat- or tape-sealed and should be clearly marked "dust cover" to prevent the mistake of using the cover as part of the sterile field.

Preparation of Instrument and Basin Sets

Preparation for sterilization of instruments begins after decontamination and involves the following steps:

1. Inspection
2. Reassembly
3. Preparation

The items to be sterilized must first be inspected for blood and soil remnants that may be left after decontamination. Scissors, hemostats, clamps, and forceps can be easily inspected under normal lighting. More complex devices, such as endoscopic instrumentation, contain areas that are more difficult to reach while cleaning and require thorough inspection.

Instrument function must be assessed for repair or replacement. The following are general guidelines to follow for functional testing:

1. The cutting edges of scissors should have no burs or cracks. The blades should close smoothly. Scissors should be sharp enough to cut two 4 × 4 sponges with little effort.
2. The ringed instrument's ratchet must be checked to ensure that it locks properly and will not spring open. If the instrument is tapped lightly in the palm of the hand and the ratchet remains closed, then the ratchet is working properly.
3. The jaws of clamps should close evenly with no gaps and the tips should be evenly lined. Needle holder jaws should be inspected for no gaps or wear.
4. Forceps should close evenly with tips evenly lined. Tissue forceps' teeth should fit smoothly in the groove of the opposite side.
5. Ratchets on self-retaining retractors should be checked to make sure they remain locked in the open position and release with little effort.

6. The points on nondisposable trocars should be inspected for burs, cracks, scratches, or bends. Dull or burred trocars make insertion difficult and cause tissue damage.
7. The manufacturer's instructions must be followed for proper inspection of powered instruments. An instrument may need to be lubricated and operated for a designated amount of time to ensure lubricant distribution. The power hose should be checked for cracks and cuts. The power hose should be coiled loosely to prevent kinking and damage.

Reassembly of instruments with more than one piece may be necessary before sterilizing. However, most surgical instruments, such as the Balfour retractor, should not be reassembled before sterilizing; this ensures that the sterilant can reach all surface areas.

Items must be properly prepared for effective sterilization. Proper preparation will ensure that:

- The sterilant comes into contact with all surface areas.
- The instruments are positioned in a protective manner until they are used.
- The instruments are evenly distributed.

Instruments should be placed in a mesh-bottom or wire mesh basket with an absorbent towel lining the bottom. A nonwoven disposable wrapper should not be used to line the tray because the water-repellent nature of the wrapper will cause moisture to pool at the bottom. The instruments should be evenly distributed within the basket for balance. Ringed instruments can be placed on a stringer or secured with clips and pins that can be used to maintain the instruments in an open, fixed position. Instruments of like size, shape, and function should be grouped together on the stringer to help the user quickly identify and retrieve the instruments needed for the surgical procedure.

Microsurgical instruments can be easily damaged if not properly arranged in preparation for sterilization. Special trays lined with molded plastic mats or pins and locking lids are commercially available to secure and protect these delicate instruments.

Instruments with lumens, such as a Frazier suction tip, require special preparation. Air trapped in the lumen may prevent steam from contacting the inner surface. To prevent this entrapment of air, a residual amount of distilled water should be left inside the lumen. The water will boil during sterilization, turning to steam and displacing the air within the lumen. This technique is especially important if gravity displacement steam sterilization is utilized.

Instruments with concave surfaces also warrant special preparation for sterilization. Examples include bone curettes, bone rongeurs, and gallstone scoops. To prevent moisture and air from being trapped within the concave surface, the instruments should be placed on their sides for sterilization.

Loose instruments are instruments that are not on a stringer but are arranged in the pan's bottom. They include forceps, retractors, knife handles, and suction tips. These instruments should not be tightly grouped together in a pile or grouped and packaged in peel packs. Instrument grouping and excessive metal contact will inhibit the ability of the sterilant to contact all surfaces and may allow condensate to collect.

Larger loose instruments, such as Deaver and Richardson retractors, and long forceps, should be arranged within the pan so that movement is minimized and should not be placed one upon the other. The heavier instruments should be placed on the bottom of the tray or at one end of the tray to avoid damaging other, more delicate instruments. In some instances, an absorbent towel can be used to separate layers of instruments within the tray to aid in absorbing moisture and drying. The two-basket system is ideal in that it not only evenly distributes the weight of the set but also increases the contact surface area. The instrument trays and/or containers should be laid flat on the shelves of the sterilizing cart.

Basin sets are conducive to the formation and retention of condensate due to their density. Basins that will be nested within each other or that may contain other metal items must have adequate air space between each item. An absorbent towel should be used to separate the basins and items.

The absorbent towel should be fully opened and placed between nested basins to absorb the condensate, to aid in air removal, and to create an adequate space for the penetration of steam. If other metal items are placed inside the basin, the towel should be used to separate the items from the bottom of the basin and from each other.

Sponges and woven fabrics should not be placed inside a basin because the material can deflect the steam, preventing proper surface contact. Hollow OR light handles should be placed into the basin with the handle down so that moisture can drain out of the handles when the basin is positioned on the sterilizing cart. Basins should be placed on the sterilizing cart with the fold down to aid in the removal of air and to prevent condensate accumulation. The weight of the wrapped basin sets should not be more than 7 pounds per ANSI/AAMI ST79:2010.

Surgical instruments may be prepared on trays that are designated for a specific procedure. Examples include cutdown trays, suture trays, and tracheotomy/tracheostomy trays. Only a few instruments are required for the assembly of these specialty trays, and most are assembled on a stainless steel, perforated tray. Procedural trays can be laid flat on the sterilizing cart because the trays are perforated. This also prevents the contents from scattering inside the tray.

Envelope and Square Folds for Wrapping

The two most common types of packaging methods are:

- The envelope, or diagonal fold, which is useful for smaller instrument trays and individual items
- The square fold, which is useful for large packs and instrument trays

Envelope Fold

1. The square wrapper is arranged diagonally on the table with a corner pointing toward the user.
2. The item to be sterilized is placed in the center of the wrapper using imaginary lines dividing the wrapper into quarters (Figure 7-8).

TECHNIQUE

Packaging (Envelope Fold)

(Figure 7-8 A–E)

1. Items to be wrapped are prepared for sterilization.
2. Assemble all necessary supplies (such as internal indicator, appropriate-size wrappers, external indicator, and labeling materials).
3. Place the wrapper diagonally on a flat surface.
4. Place the item to be wrapped in the center of the wrapper.
5. Place the internal indicator near the center of the package in a visible location.
6. The near corner of the wrapper is folded over the item.
7. A tab is created by folding 2–3 in. of the corner back onto itself.
8. One side of the wrapper is folded over the item as far as possible.
9. The corner is mitered, if necessary.
10. A tab is created by folding 2–3 in. of the corner back onto itself.
11. The opposite side of the wrapper is folded over the item as far as possible, overlapping the first side of the wrapper.
12. The corner is mitered, if necessary, and the tab is created.
13. The final flap is folded over the item, overlapping the wrapper sides.
14. The corners are mitered, if necessary.
15. If this is the first of two wrappers, the corner of the wrapper is tucked under the other three folds—the tab remains exposed. Otherwise, the corner of the wrapper is brought around the outside of the package and secured with the appropriate tape, which may also serve as the external indicator.
16. Repeat the process if a second wrapper is required.
17. Label the item according to facility policy.
18. The wrapped item is sterilized.

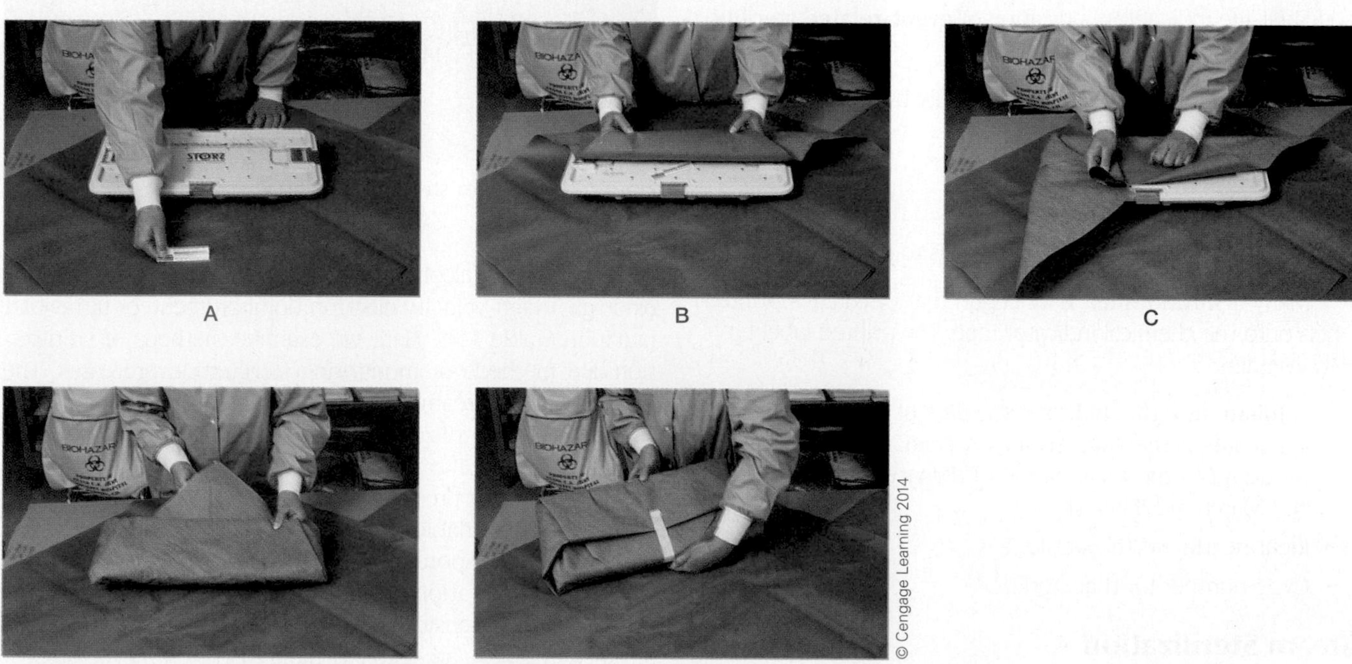

Figure 7-8 Packaging (envelope fold): (**A**) Placement of item on wrapper and addition of chemical indicator, (**B**) first fold with tab, (**C**) second fold with tab; repeat for third fold with tab, (**D**) final fold tucked, (**E**) package secured with chemical indicator tape

Square Fold

1. The square or rectangular wrappers are arranged squarely in front of the user.
2. The package is placed in the center of the wrappers.
3. The wrapper edge nearest the user is folded over the top of the item, covering the lower half of the item, and a cuff is formed.
4. The top section of the wrapper is folded down over the item and a cuff is formed that overlaps the first cuff.
5. The left section of the wrap is folded over the pack and a cuff is formed.
6. The right section of the wrap is folded over the pack overlapping the previous fold and a cuff is formed.
7. The second wrapper is applied in the same manner, except that the last cuff is folded under. The chemical indicator tape is then added.

Labeling

The user must be able to identify the contents of a package, especially when a woven or nonwoven wrap is used. Items within paper–plastic peel packs can be seen but should still be labeled. Items are also labeled for quality assurance, inventory control, and rotation of stock.

The packages should be labeled before being sterilized. Most facilities use a felt-tip, quick-dry marker for labeling. All the information can be recorded on the chemical indicator tape or on the plastic portion of the peel packs.

Written label information should include:

- Package contents
- Shelf-life indication (indication of **event-related sterility**)
- Date of sterilization
- Identification of the sterilizer (usually by number designation)
- Cycle number
- Initials of the employer who prepared the package
- Department to which the package is to be sent

Many institutions use a label gun that discharges printed labels onto the chemical indicator tape. The printed label typically contains:

- A **Julian date** that indicates the date of sterilization. The Julian date is the number of the calendar day (1-365/366); for example, the Julian date for February 27, 2013 is 58 and March 5, 2013 is 64.
- Identification of the sterilizer
- Cycle number for that sterilizer

Steam Sterilization

The destruction of all microorganisms in or about an object can be accomplished with the use of stream under pressure, chemical agents (alcohol, phenol, heavy metals, and ethylene oxide gas), high-velocity electron bombardment, or ultraviolet radiation (Table 7-14). Here we examine methods of sterilization and methods of monitoring sterilization processes. The focus is first on steam sterilization as a dependable, inexpensive method of sterilization (Figure 7-9).

Table 7-14 Items That Can Be Steam, Gas, or Chemically Sterilized

Thermal—Steam Dry Heat	*Gas—Ethylene Oxide, Gas Plasma*	*Chemical—Cidex, Peracetic Acid (Steris)*
Most metal surgical instruments	Powered instruments	Lensed instruments
Powered instruments (per manufacturer's instructions)	Delicate instruments	Fiber-optic instruments and cables
Microinstruments (per manufacturer's instructions)	Fiber-optic instruments, lensed instruments, plastic, rubber, porous instruments, moisture- or heat-sensitive instruments	Heat-sensitive instruments

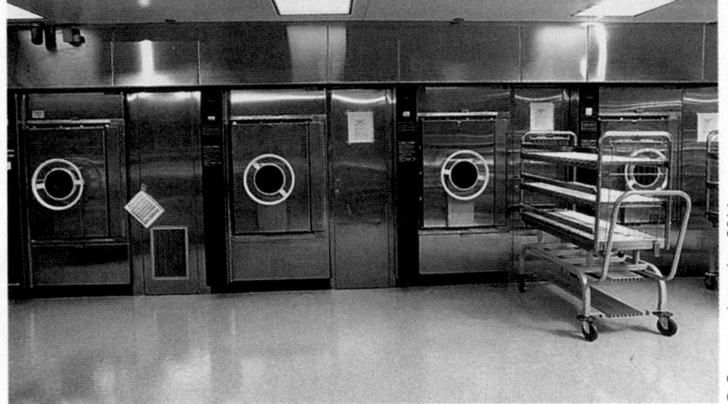

Figure 7-9 Steam sterilization area

Steam sterilization utilizes moist heat in the form of saturated steam under pressure within an enclosed environment. It is the most dependable method of sterilization in which all microbes, including spores, are destroyed. It is the recommended method of sterilization for items that are not heat-, moisture- or temperature-sensitive. Advantages and disadvantages of steam sterilization are listed in Table 7-15.

Microbes are killed by the combination of two factors: moisture and heat. Heat alone can destroy microbes, but the

Table 7-15 Advantages and Disadvantages of Steam Sterilization

Advantages	*Disadvantages*
Saturated steam is many times more effective in transferring thermal energy than hot air.	Not all items can be steam sterilized. Heat- and moisture-sensitive items must be sterilized by other methods.
Any type of resistant and protective outer layer of microorganisms is softened by steam, allowing the denaturation of protein within the microbe.	Human error is a factor that can contribute to sterilization failures.
It is the most economical and inexpensive sterilizing agent.	
It is the safest method of sterilization in comparison to other methods.	
The method is relatively quick.	
It is nontoxic and does not leave a toxic residue on items.	
Quality control/quality assurance methods are easy to control and maintain.	
Steam is readily available and easy to deliver to health care facilities.	

Table 7-16 Minimum Cycle Times: Gravity-Displacement Steam Sterilization

Contents	*250°F*	*270°F*	*Drying Times*
Instrument set, wrapped	30 minutes	15 minutes	15–30 minutes
Instrument set, unwrapped, no lumen instruments		3 minutes	0–1 minute
Instrument set, unwrapped, some instruments with lumens		10 minutes	0–1 minute

Table 7-17 Minimum Cycle Times: Dynamic-Air-Removal Steam Sterilization

Contents	*270°F*	*Drying Times*
Instrument set, wrapped	4 minutes	20–30 minutes
Instrument set, unwrapped, no lumen instruments	3 minutes	NA
Instrument set, unwrapped, some instruments with lumens	4 minutes	NA

process is accelerated with the addition of moisture and pressure. Pressure that is greater than that of the atmosphere is necessary to increase the temperature of the steam in order to cause the destruction of microbes. Therefore, when discussing steam sterilization it is important to consider five factors that are critical to the outcome of the sterilization process:

- Time: Length of time the sterilant must remain in contact with the items to render them sterile.
- Contact: The sterilant must have contact with all surfaces of the items being sterilized.
- Temperature: The temperature that must be achieved in order to kill all microbes, including spores.
- Moisture: The specific amount of moisture that must be present to aid in the destruction of microbes.
- Pressure: Pressure increases the temperature of steam to the level where it can destroy all microbes.

These five factors will be discussed in further detail in the following sections.

Time

The minimum time required for sterilization to occur depends on the temperature and type of cycle being used, e.g., gravity displacement or prevacuum. Not all microbes die at the same time when exposed to saturated steam at a constant temperature. Some microbes are more difficult to kill than others. Therefore, times and temperatures have been established, along with manufacturer's recommendations, to guarantee the sterility of items. Refer to Tables 7-16 and 7-17.

Contact

Just as with liquid disinfectant and sterilant solutions, steam must contact all surfaces of items in order to render them sterile. For that reason the principles of cleaning, decontamination, and proper packaging must be strictly followed. The most frequent reason for failures during the sterilization cycle is lack of contact between steam and surfaces of items to be sterilized, thereby allowing viable microbes to survive the sterilization cycle. The majority of sterilization failures may be traced to human error or mechanical malfunction. Reasons for failure include:

1. Strainer is obstructed. The strainer is located at the bottom front of the **autoclave** chamber. Its purpose is to prevent lint and objects from entering the exhaust line. If the strainer is not cleaned daily, it can become clogged and trap air in the chamber of the autoclave.
2. Containers are positioned incorrectly on the sterilization cart. Instrument trays, basins, and peel packs must be positioned to allow air to escape.
3. Items to be sterilized are inadequately cleaned. Soil and debris prevent the saturated steam from making direct contact with surface areas to kill microbes.
4. Wrapped packs are placed too close together on sterilizing cart. Packs should be loosely arranged on the autoclave cart to allow complete removal of trapped air and free circulation of steam.
5. Instrument trays, basins, and other wrapped items are wrapped too tightly. This also prevents the escape of air, which forms cool air pockets that prevent the temperature from increasing to the level needed to kill microbes and prevents saturated steam from reaching all surfaces.

Temperature, Pressure, Moisture, and Air

Steam is simply water vapor. When water is heated, the steam bubbles rise to the surface of the water, bursting and releasing the steam vapor. Steam is known as saturated steam when it contains the maximum amount of water vapor (97–100% relative humidity).

Moisture plays an important part in the steam sterilization of porous and nonporous items. The thermal destruction of microbes is the result of the denaturation and coagulation of protein within the cells. Moisture acts as a catalyst so coagulation can occur at lower temperatures as compared to the much higher temperatures required in the absence of moisture. In other words, moisture allows the use of a lower temperature than that normally required to denature proteins within the microbes. The role and importance of moisture are illustrated by a comparison. *Geobacillus stearothermophilus* spores are killed in 12 minutes at 250°F when saturated steam is used. However, the spores survived for more than 6 hours when dry heat was used at the same temperature. Pressure is used to raise the temperature of the steam to the temperature necessary to kill all microbes including spores, but has nothing to do with the microbial properties of the steam.

In the case of porous materials, such as woven linen towels, saturated steam heats the materials and permeates the porous material by the process of condensation. Only through condensation—the return of steam back to water—is the steam able to generate the heat needed for sterilization to occur. This explains why the correct arrangement of woven materials in a package to be sterilized is critical for steam to penetrate and sterilization to take place.

The same concepts apply to the sterilization of surgical instruments. Direct steam contact of all surface areas of the instruments must occur for an item to be rendered sterile; the objective is to heat and sterilize the surface. In this instance, condensation, which occurs due to moist heat contacting cold metal, heats the instrument to the temperature of the steam and sterilization occurs.

The quality of the steam should be at 97% with the remaining 3% being liquid water that is present in the autoclave. If water saturation levels are less than 3%, the steam in the chamber is known as dry steam. In these conditions the steam becomes superheated and there is a deficiency of heat transferred to the items, resulting in a sterilization failure. Steam that contains more than 3% liquid water can result in wet packs being removed from the autoclave. Such wetness contributes to strike-through contamination of the enclosed items, thus requiring reprocessing.

Air must be completely removed from the chamber if efficient sterilization of materials within is to occur. Unless the air is removed or steam displaces the air, the steam cannot make complete contact with the surface of items to be sterilized. Air and steam do not easily mix, resulting in temperature variations within the chamber and ineffective heat transfer and condensation on the surface of items. Air is removed either by gravity displacement or by a prevacuum cycle. Additional information is presented in this chapter on the processes of air removal.

Basic Components of an Autoclave Machine

The structure of an autoclave (steam sterilizer) is based on the chamber in which items are placed for sterilization. Autoclaves range in size from small tabletop units to large industrial-sized machines.

Some autoclaves generate their own steam, whereas others rely on steam from an outside source. When steam is supplied to the autoclave from an outside source, the walls of the chamber are preheated before the steam is allowed into the chamber. This is accomplished with a metal jacket that is built around the chamber. The space between the jacket and chamber is filled with steam to preheat the chamber walls when the machine is turned on. The steam remains there until the sterilizer is turned off. Preheating the chamber walls aids in maintaining a constant chamber temperature throughout the sterilization cycle and prevents the formation of condensation on the chamber walls when steam enters the chamber at the beginning of the cycle. Small sterilizers, such as tabletop models, usually do not rely on an external steam source, and the chamber walls must be heated for every load, increasing the total cycle time.

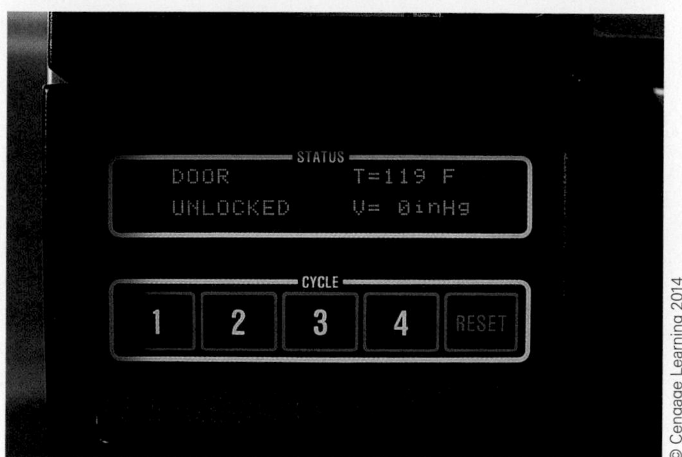

Figure 7-10 Steam sterilizer control panel

The system of pipes to the sterilizer is relatively simple. There are three main pipes:

1. A pipe to bring the steam to the sterilizer and the chamber
2. A drain pipe for steam, air, and water from the chamber
3. A pipe to deliver filtered air to the chamber at the end of a cycle

A series of filters is placed at intervals to prevent contaminants from entering the chamber and altering the quality of steam.

Last, each autoclave must have a control system. The electromechanical switches of older machines have been replaced by microprocessor systems that control the sterilization process and perform operation self-diagnoses (Figure 7-10).

Gravity Displacement Sterilizer

Gravity displacement sterilizers rely on gravity to passively remove air from the sterilization chamber. Steam enters at the top of the chamber and displaces the air. Air is heavier than steam, so as the steam occupies more space, the air is pushed out the drain at the bottom front of the chamber. During this stage of the cycle, the pressure in the chamber increases until the temperature of the steam reaches a preset temperature. Gravity displacement sterilizers are slower than prevacuum/dynamic-air-removal sterilizers because gravity is relied on to remove the air.

A general description of the cycle is as follows:

1. Condition: Steam inlet valve opens and steam enters into the chamber at the top rear opening. Air is displaced downward and exits through the drain at the front bottom of the chamber; pressure increases until preset temperature is reached; timing begins for exposure phase.
2. Exposure phase: The sterilizing temperature is maintained for the preset amount of time required to kill all microorganisms based on the types of items in the load. Periodically, cooled steam is removed through the bottom front drain and replaced with fresh steam from the inlet valve at the back top to maintain correct temperature.
3. Exhaust phase: When the timer signals the conclusion of the exposure phase, the steam inlet valve closes, the chamber drain opens, and the steam is removed from the chamber by displacement. Filtered air is reintroduced into the chamber and the chamber reaches atmospheric pressure. Newer model autoclaves will not allow chambers to be opened until atmospheric pressure has been achieved to prevent steam injuries to personnel.
4. Dry phase: Following the end of the exhaust phase, heated, fresh air and heat generated by the jacket slowly revaporize and remove moisture from the packs. At the end of this cycle, an audible signal indicates the door may be opened.

Prevacuum Steam Sterilizer

Prevacuum steam sterilizers, also called dynamic-air-removal autoclaves, are similar in construction to gravity sterilizers except that a vacuum pump is built into the system to remove air. Before the steam is injected into the sterilizer, air is removed from the chamber, reducing the total cycle time.

A typical cycle is as follows:

1. Prevacuum phase: Vacuum pump located in the chamber drain line in the bottom front of the sterilizer removes approximately 90% of the air from the chamber.
2. Conditioning phase: Steam is injected into the chamber from an inlet valve located at the top of the sterilizer to begin heating the load and aid in removing air.
3. Second prevacuum phase: Vacuum pump removes another 90% of the air. The combination of the two vacuum cycles removes 99% of the air.
4. Exposure phase: Steam inlet valve opens and steam enters the chamber. As with gravity, the temperature is held constant by the removal of cooler steam and replacement with fresh steam.
5. Exhaust phase: After the exposure phase is complete, an outlet drain opens and steam exits the chamber by activation of the vacuum pump.
6. Drying phase: Vacuum pump turns on again and draws a 90% vacuum. This vacuum is held during the drying phase and moisture is removed from packs by heat generated from the jacket. When the drying phase is complete, the vacuum is released as filtered air is allowed into the chamber. A signal indicates that the door can be opened when the chamber returns to atmospheric pressure.

Another version of the prevacuum cycle involves up to four or five vacuum phases instead of the two described above. Between each vacuum phase steam enters the chamber to aid in removing air and preconditions the load by penetrating the packages.

There are several advantages to the use of the prevacuum steam sterilizer:

1. Increases speed of operation and lowers total cycle time
2. More efficient at removing air than gravity sterilizers
3. Not as dependent on the positioning of load contents as gravity sterilizers
4. Condensate is produced during preconditioning phases, reducing cycle time

A test unique to the prevacuum sterilizer that must be performed is the **Bowie-Dick** test. The Bowie-Dick test derives its name from two English microbiologists who developed the test, J. H. Bowie and J. Dick. The test is used in the prevacuum sterilization cycle to check for air removal and entrapment and is conducted daily. The test is performed at the first run of the day before any loads are sterilized or after the sterilizer has undergone repairs. The test pack must be placed horizontally on an empty sterilizing cart on the front bottom shelf over the chamber drain in an empty prevacuum chamber.

Test packs may be commercially purchased or prepared in-house. Department-produced test packs consist of fan-folded absorbent towels with a Bowie-Dick test sheet placed in the center of the pack. The test sheet can be commercially purchased or three to four strips of steam autoclave chemical indicator tape can be placed in a criss-cross pattern on a plain sheet of paper. The in-house produced test pack consists of:

- Between 24 and 44 absorbent towels fan folded and placed in a stack that is 9 × 12 × 11 in.
- Bowie-Dick test sheet placed in the center of the pack
- Pack is single wrapped

The commercially available test is the Daily Air Removal Test (DART). This is a lightweight, compact, pre-assembled type of Bowie-Dick test.

All test sheets are filed as a permanent record for each sterilizer.

It must be emphasized that the Bowie-Dick test is not a sterilization test but rather a test of the vacuum system in a prevacuum sterilizer. It is never performed on gravity sterilizers since these sterilizers do not rely on a vacuum system. The result that is important to the Bowie-Dick test is not the intensity of the color change of the heat-sensitive ink but the uniformity of the color change. Any machine malfunctions causing air entrapment will result in uneven color changes of the chemical ink.

Immediate-Use Steam Sterilization

Immediate-use steam sterilization, formerly referred to as "flash" sterilization, is the process of sterilizing unwrapped items, such as instruments that have been dropped during a surgical procedure. Immediate-use steam sterilization has become a necessity in the OR but in some instances has been misused to compensate for an inadequate inventory of surgical instruments. It is recommended that immediate-use steam sterilization be avoided for the routine sterilization of instrument sets and its use be reserved for sterilizing items that are immediately needed.

Items to be immediate-use steam sterilized must be decontaminated and cleaned with detergent and water. The composition of the item to be immediate-use steam sterilized, not its size or shape, determines the exposure time.

Immediate-use steam sterilization is accomplished with the item unwrapped and placed in a perforated instrument tray. Immediate-use steam sterilization containers that contain the instrument in its entirety are commercially available. Immediate-use steam sterilization of implantables should not be practiced by any health care facility.

Immediate-use steam sterilization can be performed in gravity or prevacuum sterilizers. Refer to Tables 7-16 and 7-17 for sterilization times and temperature.

General Safety Precautions

Safety considerations to remember include:

- Caution must be used with jacketed sterilizers. After the steam enters the jacket, the chamber walls are hot and can cause burns if skin contacts them.
- Make sure the door is tightly closed before starting the sterilizer.
- The door is to be opened only when the exhaust valve indicates zero pressure. To avoid hot steam, stand behind the door when opening.
- Do not touch the sterilizing cart until it is sufficiently cool.

Steam Sterilization Minimum Exposure Temperatures, Pressures, and Times

The most common temperatures and pressures required for gravity sterilizers are 250°–275°F (121–135°C) at 15–17 psi. For prevacuum sterilizers the temperature is 270°–275°F (132–135°C) at 27–30 psi. Again, refer to Tables 7-16 and 7-17 for additional details pertaining to time and temperature standards.

Mechanical Monitoring of the Steam Sterilization Process

Quality assurance is an essential component of any type of sterilization process. Methods must be used to confirm the sterility of items and proper operation of the sterilizers. Three methods of monitoring the sterilization process exist:

1. Mechanical
2. Chemical
3. Biological

Autoclaves are equipped with recorders and gauges that allow the operator to monitor the progress of the machine during the sterilization cycle. The monitors also aid the operator in confirming that sterilization parameters for time, temperature, and pressure have been met, assuring the machine is properly working.

A permanent record of the temperature of some autoclaves is attained through the use of a cycle tracing on a chart recorder. The autoclave contains a standard electrically driven clock mechanism that slowly revolves a 6-in. recording chart once over a 24-hour period. Each sterilization cycle temperature is recorded on the chart by a tracing pen. After 24 hours, the chart must be changed.

Older autoclaves use needle gauges to display the pressure. Pressure gauges reveal the performance of the sterilizer during every load. Sterilizers use two main gauges, jacket steam pressure and chamber steam pressure.

Newer autoclaves utilize digital recorders that are much easier to read. Also, a printout is produced by the machine, providing detailed information on the performance of the machine. The operator initials the printout, verifying the cycle parameters were achieved and maintained, and the printout is filed for record-keeping purposes. This record is considered information that can be reviewed in a court of law.

Chemical Methods of Monitoring the Steam Sterilization Process

Chemical indicators are used externally and internally to verify that item(s) have been exposed to sterilizing conditions. It must be emphasized that chemical indicators only validate the contents of the package were exposed to a specific temperature, humidity, and sterilant; they do not verify the sterility of the item(s). Chemical indicators aid in detecting potential sterilization failures that may result from:

- Machine malfunction, including entrapment of air
- Incorrect assembly or wrapping of the package
- Incorrect loading of the sterilizer cart or basket

Chemical indicators are assigned a class designation based on the specific information that the device indicates.

- Class 1: Process indicators—external indicators that provide a visual indication of exposure of the package/item to the sterilizing agent.
- Class 2: Indicators for use in specific tests—assessment of a specific function of the steam sterilizer (e.g., Bowie-Dick test).
- Class 3: Single-variable indicators—determine if a single parameter is being met, such as a sterilizer reaching the preset temperature.
- Class 4: Multi-variable indicators—designed to react to two or more of the parameters of the sterilizing process (e.g., temperature and exposure to sterilant).
- Class 5: Integrating indicators—designed to react to all sterilization parameters. Most accurate of the internal chemical indicators and used as pack control monitoring. They can be used to release loads that do not include implants. An example is a challenge test pack.
- Class 6: Emulating indicators—designed to react to all sterilization parameters of a specific sterilization cycle.

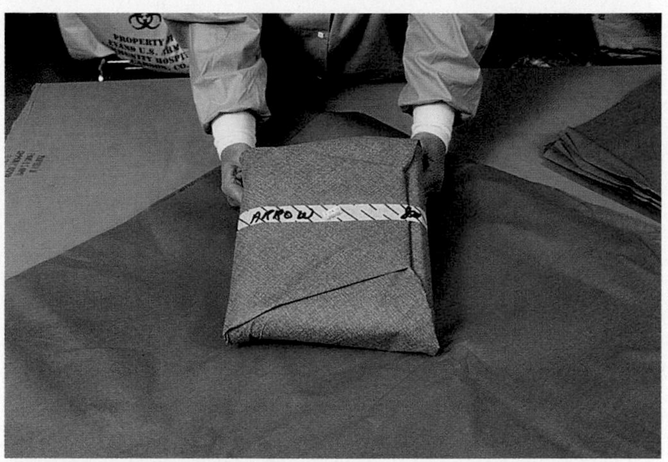

Figure 7-11 Indicator tape showing color change appropriate for exposure to the steam sterilization process

Chemical indicators consist of paper that has been impregnated with a dye that changes color in the presence of temperature and sterilant. The most popular type of external chemical indicator is autoclave tape (Figure 7-11). The tape is used as a package closure to keep CSR wraps in place. Prior to exposure to the steam sterilization process the autoclave tape is cream-colored with light diagonal lines of ink. Following sterilization the lines change to a uniform black color to provide a visual indication of exposure to the sterilant.

Internal steam chemical indicators are placed inside packages, peel packs, and instrument trays to indicate the contents have been exposed to the conditions of sterilization. Internal indicators are available as commercial strips of paper impregnated with ink. The indicators should be placed in the area of the package or tray where the greatest challenge exists for penetration of steam and air removal. The internal indicator is read when the package or tray is opened at time of use. If the indicator or tape has not uniformly changed to black, the contents of the package may not have been exposed to the correct sterilizing temperature, or other conditions such as lack of air removal prevented sterilant exposure and the contents should be considered nonsterile.

Locking devices for rigid instrument containers may have a chemical indicator "dot" that changes to black during the steam sterilization process. Paper load cards on the outside of rigid containers also contain a strip of chemical indicator that turns black with exposure to the sterilant. Filter paper placed on the bottom of the container and lid may have a chemical indicator "dot" that changes color during sterilization. Peel packs are also available with the ink impregnated into one of the paper's edges.

Biological Methods of Monitoring the Steam Sterilization Process

A **biological indicator** (BI) is a device that contains a specific type of microorganism that is killed when exposed to the sterilizing conditions. The microbe is in the spore stage and therefore is difficult to kill. The BI is the only test that guarantees items are sterile and the conditions necessary for sterilization have been met.

The BI for steam sterilization contains the bacterial spore *Geobacillus stearothermophilus*. This microbe has been determined to be highly resistant to being killed by steam sterilization, but is harmless to humans.

Most institutions purchase commercial test packs that contain a vial of the microorganism in the spore stage impregnated on a disk. Test packs can be produced in-house based on standards established by AAMI, but constructing the packs is time consuming and consistency is difficult to maintain. Therefore, the commercial test packs offer many advantages over the in-house produced packs.

A steam biological test pack produced in-house consists of:

- Sixteen absorbent towels approximately 16 × 26 in. in size, each folded to approximately 9 × 9 in.
- Towels are stacked with the BI vial placed in the center.
- The pack is taped together and should weigh approximately 3 pounds.

The test pack is placed in the area of the sterilizer that is most difficult for the sterilant to reach. This represents the "coldest" area of the sterilizer where air entrapment is most likely to occur. For steam sterilization the coldest point is on the bottom front of the sterilizing cart over the chamber drain. After the sterilization cycle is complete, the test pack is removed and the BI vial is taken out to be incubated. The vial is "crushed" by gently squeezing on the sides of the vial, thus releasing the growth medium that covers the spore-impregnated disk. The nutrient broth is red in color; after incubation, if the liquid remains red, the results are considered negative, meaning the spores have been killed. However, if the broth turns yellow in color, the results are positive, meaning the conditions for sterilization were not met, the spores were not killed, and the items in the load must be considered nonsterile. The items in the load must be immediately recalled and reprocessed. Additionally, the sterilizing machine must be checked for possible malfunctioning and repaired if necessary.

Steam BIs are incubated for 24 hours before the reading is recorded. The steam BI is incubated at 131°–140°F (55°–55°C). The steam BI that was put through the sterilization process is incubated with a control vial that was not put through the process in order to validate the results of the test vial. If the control vial that was not autoclaved shows no growth after incubation, the batch of vials must be considered compromised and a new box opened and tested.

The recommended frequency of BI monitoring varies. Various organizations such as AAMI, American Hospital Association (AHA), AORN, CDC, and The Joint Commission vary in their recommendations. For steam sterilization, the recommended frequency varies from every load to one load per week. At a minimum, steam sterilization should be monitored as least weekly. All test results are filed as a permanent record for each steam sterilizer. Only two recommendations are agreed on by all five organizations:

1. Loads containing implantables must always be monitored and the BI must be read before the implantables are used. The implantables must be quarantined and not released for distribution until the BI indicates negative results.
2. The placement of the test pack on the bottom front of the sterilizing cart for steam loads

Troubleshooting Steam Sterilization

A wet pack or instrument set, whether the moisture occurs on the outside or within, must be considered **contaminated**. Moisture creates a pathway for microorganisms from the outside to the inside of a package through wicking action and strike-through.

If packs are consistently wet, the cause must be identified and corrective actions performed. Various reasons exist for moisture found on the outside and/or inside of packages:

- Condensate dripping from the shelves and/or railings of the sterilizing cart
- Condensate buildup in steam lines
- Metal items on upper shelf of cart dripping condensate onto items below

Moisture on the inside of packs may result if:

- Too many instruments are placed in the tray, producing more condensate than can be revaporized.
- Instrument and basin sets are assembled without absorbent towels, which soak up moisture and are an aid to efficient drying.
- Woven textile packs, such as towels, are wrapped too tightly and retain moisture.
- Trays and items are improperly loaded on sterilizer cart and moisture is unable to escape from the package.

The steam that enters the sterilizer must be as pure as possible and free of contaminants. Hospital maintenance of the sterilizer, including examining the pipes that transport the steam to the autoclave, should be performed at least once a year and documented. Even though a series of filters are in place to filter the water used during steam sterilization, small contaminants can still penetrate the filters and contaminate the water and thus the steam. If instrument trays contain brown or orange water or instruments are spotted, this could indicate that the purity of the steam has significantly decreased. Hospital maintenance personnel should be notified in order that they can run a diagnostic check of the purity of the steam and inspect the pipes and filters.

Ethylene Oxide

Gas sterilization is used to process materials that cannot be processed using steam sterilization, such as heat- or moisture-sensitive materials. Ethylene oxide (EtO) has been the predominant chemical used in this sterilization process and has long been used to sterilize plastics, rubber, and other materials that would be damaged by the high steam temperatures. It is effective against all forms of microbes and is sporicidal. It does not corrode metal and passes through woven materials just like steam.

The FDA, EPA, and OSHA have strict guidelines regarding the use of EtO because of the real and potential risks to patients, health care personnel, and the environment. Exposure to EtO is a risk for employees. It is very expensive, and the sterilization process can take up to 16 hours, because sterilized packages must be aerated, or "aired out," before use. This presents a disadvantage in situations where supplies are limited and quick turnover time is necessary or where an instrument may be needed in an emergency situation. The gas is flammable and very toxic, with effects ranging from skin irritation to respiratory difficulty, headaches, and nausea. The CDC has stated that EtO has been linked to cancer, reproductive difficulties, and chromosomal alteration. EtO produces chlorofluorocarbons (CFCs), which are considered damaging to the earth's ozone layer. All of these issues have caused health care providers to search for other technologies to replace EtO sterilization.

Because of the dangers presented by EtO gas, sterilization is performed in a closed room specifically designed for EtO sterilization. This room is designed with the ability to vent extra gas at the end of the sterilization process without releasing it into the atmosphere. Several factors are required for proper EtO sterilization:

- EtO gas concentration: The gas comes in cylinders, which are attached per the manufacturer's instructions to the sterilization machine at the beginning of the cycle. The machine withdraws air from the chamber and replaces it with pressurized EtO gas.
- Temperature: The temperatures used in the EtO sterilization process increase the **permeability** of cell walls. Gas sterilizers, however, are designed to work at lower temperatures than steam sterilizers, and most operate at temperatures between 85° and 145°F.
- Humidity: Moisture hydrates spores and bacteria that would otherwise be resistant to the gas alone. Humidity is kept between 30 and 80% during the EtO sterilization process.
- Time: EtO sterilization is a lengthy process. Instruments must be clean, dry, and free of all lubricants for the EtO process to be effective. The gas cannot penetrate lubricating oils. If water is present in tubing or **lumen** of instruments, EtO will bind with water to create the toxic substance ethylene glycol.

The EtO sterilizer consists of a sterilization machine within a separate vented chamber. These machines have vacuum pumps to evacuate air from the chambers and humidifiers to maintain the proper humidity levels. The most favorable setup is a combination of a sterilization machine and an aerator, which aerates the materials after sterilization. If this setup is not available, materials are removed from the sterilizer after the sterilization process and placed on shelves within the chamber for aeration. Personnel moving EtO loads from sterilizer to aeration area must take care to pull carts instead of pushing them to avoid the possibility of being "downwind" of residual fumes that may vent from packs on the load cart. Special respirator masks or hoods are available for personnel to reduce their exposure to EtO gas.

The EPA has voiced concern over the effects of EtO on personnel and the environment. CFCs are used to reduce the flammability of EtO but are damaging to the ozone layer, and many countries have eliminated the use of CFCs. This, combined with the danger to personnel, has led to the search for safer, quicker methods of sterilization for sensitive instruments. OSHA has developed strict permissible exposure limits (PELs). The advantages and disadvantages of EtO are listed in Table 7-18.

Mechanical and Chemical Monitoring of EtO

EtO autoclaves utilize electronic digital recorders to produce a printout of the performance of the machine. Chemical indicators are also used for EtO. The tape is usually green in color with diagonal lines of evenly spaced ink. When the ink has been exposed to EtO, it changes to a uniform brown color. Commercially available internal indicators are also available that turn color upon exposure to EtO. The indicators should also be placed in the area of the package where there is the greatest chance of the EtO not reaching the item(s). If the tape or internal indicator has not uniformly changed to the proper

TABLE 7-18 Advantages and Disadvantages of Gas Sterilization

Advantages	*Disadvantages*
Can be used to sterilize materials too heat sensitive for steam sterilization	Aeration times required with the EtO sterilization process can be extraordinarily lengthy—up to 21 days with internal pacemakers
In some cases, these processes are significantly less corrosive to metals	Personnel hazards are created by the use of EtO gas
Less damaging to sensitive plastic and rubber materials	The EtO sterilization process is damaging to certain materials, requiring the availability of more than one alternative process

color, the contents of the package may not have been exposed to the correct sterilizing temperature or some other condition was not met.

Biological Monitoring of EtO

The BI for EtO contains the spore *Bacillus atrophaeus*. This microbe has been determined to be the most resistant to EtO but harmless to humans.

Just as with steam BIs, most institutions purchase commercial test packs that contain a vial of the microorganisms in the spore stage impregnated on a disk. In-house test packs can be produced as follows:

- One biological indicator is placed in a 20- or 30-mL syringe so that the plunger does not touch the vial when inserted into the syringe. The needle end of the syringe must be open with the tip guard removed.
- The syringes and chemical indicator strip are placed within the folds of an absorbent towel.
- The towel is placed in a peel pack and sealed.

The test pack is placed in the part of the sterilizer that is most difficult for the EtO to reach, which is the center of the load. The test pack is placed on its side. The same process is followed for EtO as is followed for steam BIs: upon completion of the sterilization cycle, the vial is removed, squeezed to release the growth medium, and incubated with a control vial. EtO BIs are incubated for 48 hours even through they can be read after 24 hours. The BI is incubated at 95°–98.6°F (30.5°–37°C).

EtO sterilization is monitored more frequently than steam sterilization due to the more complex process. It is recommended that every EtO load be monitored. All test results for each EtO sterilizer and load are filed as a permanent record.

Hydrogen Peroxide Gas Plasma

Hydrogen peroxide gas plasma (HPGP) sterilization, commercially referred to as Sterrad,™ uses gas at low temperature to sterilize heat- and/or moisture-sensitive items. This method of sterilization is safer than EtO and in many health care facilities is replacing it. The most commonly used plasma sterilization system uses hydrogen peroxide in plasma form. The process involves diffusion of the hydrogen peroxide gaseous state, then a strong electrical field is created by radiofrequency and passed through the gas, causing a cloud of plasma to be produced. Hydrogen peroxide is a highly reactive molecule that must penetrate all packaging materials and reach all surfaces prior to its reaction then conversion to water and oxygen. The plasma creates free radicals (hydroxyl and hydroperoxyl), inactivating all microbial life. The biological indicator is *Bacillus atrophaeus*.

HPGP use with narrow-lumen or channeled instruments has been limited because of the challenge of the sterilant reaching the innermost surfaces. This problem has been addressed outside of the United States by use of a diffusion enhancer; however, at this time the FDA has not approved this device for health care facility use.

Packaging materials must be made of nonwoven polypropylene or other synthetic, non-cellulose, nonwoven material. Peel packages made of Tyvek are appropriate for use. Any paper/cellulose or linen materials will absorb the sterilant, causing the cycle to fail and the process to abort. Indicator tape is light blue in color with diagonal lines that are dark blue prior to exposure and turn to light pink upon exposure.

Sterilizer units vary in size; however, the chambers must be loaded with adequate space between items to allow for penetration of the sterilant to all surfaces quickly as it reacts and converts easily back to its basic components of oxygen and water. Premixed, multi-pack cartridges are loaded into the sterilizer for multiple cycles. The cycle time ranges from 28 to 38 minutes and does not require aeration, drying or cooling at the completion of the cycle. An automatic paper readout demonstrating cycle parameters is generated for administrative record keeping and quality control.

Liquid Chemical Sterilization Processes

Liquid chemical sterilization is an alternative to steam under pressure and EtO, appropriate for items that are heat sensitive but moisture stable. These chemical sterilants, which can also be used as high-level disinfectants, have been discussed in this chapter in the section on disinfectant solutions. The two primary liquid chemical sterilization compounds are peracetic acid, used in the tabletop Steris System™, and glutaraldehyde (Cidex™). Refer to the sectioni on disinfection for further information on glutaraldehyde.

In 2009 the FDA issued a warning statement regarding the Steris System 1™ peracetic acid sterilizer. Health care facilities were given an 18-month timeline for replacing the system with an alternative option due to concerns about the efficacy of the process as well as marketing practices outlined in the Federal Food, Drug and Cosmetic Act. Resolution of the issues resulted in the development of the new Steris System 1E™ sterilizer. The following is a discussion of the use of peracetic liquid chemical sterilization.

Health care facilities seek to maintain a lower instrument inventory, particularly for endoscopic instruments, and search for methods that provide for a fast and efficient reprocessing of items between cases. Prior to the widespread use of this system, hospitals had to maintain a higher inventory of endoscopic equipment because of the longer sterilizing process required with the use of glutaraldehyde. Most endoscopic instruments are incompatible with the high heat of steam sterilization. The Steris System 1E™ performs a 23-minute cycle that is safe for semi-critical and critical patient care items that are heat sensitive and moisture stable. The cycle phases are:

- 1–2 minutes: Water enters the processor through a three-step treatment process.
- 2–4 minutes: Treated water mixes with a peracetic acid germicide, creating a solution to process the items.
- 4–10 minutes: 6-minute exposure phase destroys all microbial life on items.
- 10–12 minutes: Solution rinses safely down the drain.

- 12–18 minutes: Two rinse phases remove chemical residue.
- 18–23 minutes: Automated filter integrity test confirms that the filter operated successfully.
- 23rd minute: Validated items are ready for immediate use.

Peracetic acid is a strong sterilant and should be handled carefully; studies have shown this compound promotes skin tumors in mice. As mentioned, this sterilant is used with the Steris™ machine, which heats the sterilant to 122°F (50°C) and can be used to sterilize flexible and rigid endoscopes. Because the sterilant can only be used for a single sterilization cycle, this method of sterilization is expensive, but it is useful for instruments that would be difficult to sterilize otherwise. Products sterilized with this system cannot be stored because they are sterilized within the system cassette itself. Therefore, items sterilized in this fashion are for immediate use only (Figure 7-12).

The BI *Geobacillus stearothermophilus* has been used with peracetic acid sterilizers; however, there is no consensus regarding the efficacy of using an impregnated strip submerged in the chamber with possible spore "wash-off" causing less valid monitoring. Chemical strips that detect that the active ingredient is present in greater than 1500 parts per million (ppm) are available for routine monitoring of concentration levels during sterilization cycles.

Ionizing Radiation

Ionizing radiation is used by industrial manufacturers to sterilize prepackaged products for use in the OR and hospital environment. It uses a process of irradiation to produce thermal and chemical energy, which causes the death of all microbes and spores by disrupting their DNA. These sterilization methods primarily use gamma rays or beta particles to sterilize products. Sterilization times vary depending on the source of radiation used. The manufacturer usually does not use chemical indicators and the package integrity is the primary method for determining sterility.

Alternative Sterilization Methods

Ozone gas sterilization oxidizes bacteria, thus destroying them. Like plasma sterilization, its use is limited by the products suitable for sterilization and in the types of containers and wrappers that can be used. Ozone is destructive to rubber and plastics and corrodes some metals. This method cannot be used for long cannulated instruments.

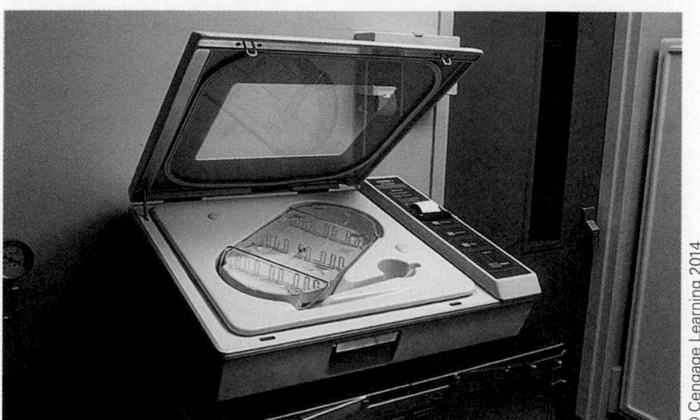

Figure 7-12 Peracetic acid (Steris™) sterilization system

In this process, a generator converts oxygen into ozone. Ozone has the ability to penetrate cell membranes and cause them to explode. These machines use a vacuum pump to increase penetration of ozone. At the end of the sterilization cycle, the chamber is purged of ozone, which is replaced with oxygen. These machines have a cycle time of up to 60 minutes and can be used with metals. This method leaves no residue and aeration is not required.

Vaporized hydrogen peroxide (VHP) uses hydrogen peroxide in gas form. At concentrations of 30% in vapor phase, hydrogen peroxide sterilizes in less than 30 minutes and requires no aeration. However, VHP cannot be used with paper wrappers. Nylon and rubber products become brittle and it is corrosive to certain metals. VHP has not been cleared by the FDA for sterilization of medical devices in any health care facilities.

Chlorine dioxide gas sterilizes rapidly at temperatures from 77°F to 86°F (25°C to 30°C). The sterilization machine generates the gas for each cycle and the gas is exhausted at the end of the cycle. The gas is generated by the reaction of chlorine gas with sodium chlorite, a simple and inexpensive process. This method is corrosive to some metals and may not penetrate paper wrappers well. Studies are ongoing as to the effects of exposure to this substance on personnel. This method has not yet received FDA approval for use.

Administrative Controls of Sterilization Processes

Administrative controls include all test results that are filed as a permanent record for each sterilizer. In health care, documentation is key and the relevant philosophy is "If it isn't documented, it didn't happen." All scheduled preventative maintenance measures as well as any mechanically generated printouts must be kept on file. Additionally, the results of BIs following incubation and the Bowie-Dick tests for prevacuum autoclaves must be filed for each sterilizer. Infection control officers investigating a patient's SSI will track all possible points of system failure, including the documented results of quality control measures. The Joint Commission inspectors frequently examine administrative sterilization process logs to assess compliance with record-keeping requirements. For example, the mechanical printouts of the immediate-use steam sterilization cycles for a randomly selected day must correlate to the written documentation of what items were immediate-use steam sterilized, patient's name, surgical team member that ran the immediate-use steam sterilizer, and CI results for that load.

Upon completion of sterilizing a load, the operator should verify the cycle parameters were achieved and maintained, initial the printout, and file for record-keeping purposes. This record is considered information that can be reviewed by a court of law.

EVENT-RELATED STERILITY

Event-related sterility is a concept that has replaced the older time-related system. The concept of event-related sterility means that the sterility of an item is determined by how it is handled and that contamination is "event related" rather than "time related." For years, expiration dating was used to indicate that at the end of a prescribed number of days microbes invade a sterile package and render the item(s) nonsterile; now a specific expiration date is not required.

With improved packaging materials and a better understanding of the factors that affect sterility, AAMI and The Joint Commission have changed their standards to reflect the premise that contamination is event related and items will remain sterile indefinitely until the package becomes wet or torn or the seal is broken and package opened. Some manufacturer-sterilized items (e.g., absorbable sutures, graft materials) may still have an expiration date due to the potential for degradation over time. These items must not be used beyond their imprinted expiration date.

The adoption of the practice of event-related sterility is economical for the health care facility. Previous use of expiration dating meant that on a weekly basis "out-dates" had to be checked and the expired items pulled from the shelf. The items had to be reprocessed, which was labor intensive and costly due to the waste of disposable wrapping materials. Event-related sterility eliminates this practice, as well as many steps in the sterility assurance process, while continuing to provide the necessary sterility of items for use in the sterile field.

PART III: Unifying Principles of Sterile Technique

CASE STUDY

DIRECTIONS

Read the following scenario and list the breaks in aseptic technique.

After performing the scrub and donning sterile gown and gloves, a CST proceeds to set up the back table and Mayo stand for a breast biopsy. The CST adjusts the sterile back table cover by moving it toward the back of the table. The CST notices that the table is a little too close to the wall and moves the table by grabbing the front edge of the table and moving it forward a few inches. As the CST begins setting up the back table, the circulator wishes to pour 1% xylocaine into a medicine cup. The CST turns her back to the back table while holding the medicine cup and the circulator pours the xylocaine. While setting up, the CST observes a portion of the suction tube hanging below the table edge; the CST retrieves the tubing and recoils it on the back table. When the back table and Mayo stand have been set up the CST is told there will be a slight delay in the procedure; therefore the CST sits down on a stool and folds her arms with hands in the axillary region in order to be comfortable.

The patient is brought into the room and positioned, and the surgeon gowned and gloved. The CST stands across from the surgeon, hands the green towels across the OR table for the surgeon to square off the incision, and then places the sterile drape. The CST brings the suction tubing and Bovie up onto the sterile field and clamps them in place using a perforating towel clip. However, the CST does not like the placement of the cords in relation to where the surgeon is standing, so the CST removes the towel clip and repositions the cords using the towel clip.

SURGICAL CONSCIENCE

Surgical conscience is the basis for the practice of strict adherence to **sterile technique** by all surgical team members. It involves a level of honesty and moral integrity that every surgical technologist must uphold in order to deliver quality patient care. Surgical conscience is a responsibility toward the patient and oneself that seeks to ensure consistent delivery of quality care to the patient.

The surgical technologist must be conscientious enough to be able to recognize and correct breaks in sterile technique, whether they were committed in the presence of others or alone. There should be no reluctance on the part of the surgical technologist or any member of the surgical team to admit a break in technique. The surgical technologist who hesitates or cannot carry through with this duty has no place in the OR. *There can be no compromise of sterile technique.* Surgical conscience requires practices that put the safety and well-being of the patient first, avoiding any lapse in technique that puts the patient at risk of immediate physical harm or future SSI.

The safety of the patient depends on strict adherence to the practice of sterile technique by the surgical team to prevent postoperative SSI. The surgical technologist must not only practice sterile technique, he or she must also be constantly aware of the sterile technique of other members of the sterile surgical team to identify breaks in technique as well as monitor the position and activities of nonsterile team members within the OR. Adherence to the principles of asepsis reflects the surgical technologist's surgical conscience and his or her ability to aid in preventing SSI.

Armed with an understanding of microbiology, disease transmission, and processes to prevent cross-contamination, as well as disinfection and sterilization processes, the surgical technology student should understand the difference between principles and practice to fully understand the order of the presentation of the following information. Principles are fundamental rules that serve as the basis for action and guide those actions. Therefore, the practice of principles is synonymous with action. As applied to the profession of surgical technology, three aseptic principles are presented. Underneath each principle are several bulleted practices or actions that support the application of the principle in the surgical environment. The principles and practices are designed to protect the sterile field from contamination and keep the microbial counts to an irreducible minimum, thus protecting the patient from an SSI.

The AST Recommended Standards of Practice for the Surgical Technologist and Surgical Assistant© are applicable to the principles of aseptic technique and support the practices through evidence-based research and literature review. See Box 7-3.

Box 7-3 AST RECOMMENDED STANDARDS OF PRACTICE RELATED TO STERILE TECHNIQUE

The full text of each standard, including references, is located at www.ast.org.

AST Recommended Standards of Practice for Creating the Sterile Field

Standard I: To provide for a safe and uneventful surgical procedure, the Certified Surgical Technologist (CST) should have all the necessary instruments, supplies, and equipment needed to prepare the sterile field for the surgical procedure.

Standard II: The OR furniture and equipment should be grouped and positioned prior to opening the sterile items.

Standard III: Sterile technique must be strictly adhered to by the surgical team members when opening sterile instrument sets, packages, and peel packs.

Standard IV: Traffic in and out of the OR should be monitored and controlled when the surgical team begins to open sterile items.

Standard V: Sterile supplies should be opened as close to the time of surgery as possible and for one surgery only.

Standard VI: To contribute to the efficiency of surgical patient care, the CST in the first scrub role should implement the principles of economy of motion when completing the setup of the sterile field.

AST Recommended Standards of Practice for Bowel Technique

Standard I: The principles of bowel technique should be utilized by the surgical team in order to avoid cross-contamination and reduce the risk of surgical site infection to the patient.

AST Recommended Standards of Practice for Sterility of the Underside of the Mayo Stand

Standard I: A principle of aseptic technique states that only sterile items should be placed within, or moved within, a sterile field—in other words, sterile to sterile.

AST Recommended Standards of Practice for Surgical Drapes

Standard I: Only sterile drapes should be used within the sterile field.

Standard II: A compromise in the integrity of the microbial barrier results in contamination.

Standard III: Drapes should be resistant to fluid penetration.

Standard IV: Drapes should be lint free.

Standard VII: Drapes made of reusable woven fabric should have the same barrier characteristics as single-use nonwoven disposable fabrics.

Recommended Standards of Practice for Gowning and Gloving

Standard I: All sterile surgical team members are required to don a sterile surgical gown prior to entering the sterile field to aid in preventing surgical site infection (SSI).

Standard II: A compromise in the integrity of the microbial barrier results in contamination.

Standard IX: All sterile surgical team members are required to don sterile gloves prior to entering the sterile field to aid in preventing SSI.

Standard XI: Double gloving is recommended for all surgical procedures.

PRINCIPLE 1: A STERILE FIELD IS CREATED FOR EACH SURGICAL PROCEDURE

The primary method through which microbes are kept to an irreducible minimum in the OR is through the creation of a sterile field for each procedure. The sterile field is a separate, sterile area that consists of the surgical site itself, the draped portions of the patient and OR table, the sterile portions of the gowns and gloves of the sterile team members, and the draped ring stands, Mayo stand, and back table. Within this sterile field are the sterile instruments, sutures, and equipment to be used during the procedure (Figure 7-13).

- **If in doubt about the sterility of an item, consider it nonsterile and do not use.** "If in doubt, throw it out."
- **The sterile field should be created as close as possible to the time of use and be monitored at all times.** As time passes, the likelihood that a sterile field has become contaminated by error or airborne contamination increases. After the sterile supplies have been opened, the room must be constantly monitored to prevent unintentional contamination by personnel; monitoring the room also is required if a case is delayed.
- **If a case is switched to another OR, and the sterile supplies and instruments have already been opened and the sterile field created in the originally assigned OR, the sterile field should never be covered with a sterile drape to be moved to the other OR because it is impossible to remove the drape without contaminating the sterile supplies and instruments.** Sterile supplies and instruments should be obtained for the procedure in the newly assigned OR.
- **The surgical technologist must check the chemical indicators to ensure the instruments have been exposed to the sterilization process.** If the CIs have not changed to the proper color, the instruments should be considered nonsterile, passed off the field, and not used on the patient.
- **Instruments and sharps, such as scalpel blades, that come into contact with the skin of the patient should not be reused.** The items should be returned to a designated area of the Mayo stand or back table by the surgical technologist to prevent further use on deeper tissue.
- **For clean-contaminated and contaminated procedures, such as cases where the bowel is opened, separate setups should be used for the clean and dirty portions of the procedure.** Personnel should not reuse the instruments used during the open bowel or dirty portion of the procedure and should regown and reglove before returning to the use of sterile instruments from the clean setup.
- **When removing contents from the autoclave, the surgical technologist must not touch the edge of the sterilizer with the instruments, instrument tray, gown, or gloves.** Sterile transfer handles may be used by the surgical technologist, or, if the sterile items are within a tray, the circulator can remove the tray using the transfer handles and the surgical technologist can remove the items inside the tray.
- **The inner edge of a heat-sealed peel pack is considered the line between sterile and nonsterile.** The flaps of the peel pack should be pulled back when opening with no tears in the pack itself. The contents should then be transferred onto the sterile field or the surgical technologist should grasp only the edge of the inner contents without touching the peel pack, lifting upward. The contents must never be allowed to slide over the edge of the peel pack when delivered to the sterile field.
- **The inside of paper wrappers containing linens or other sterile items is considered sterile except for a 1-inch perimeter around the outside edge of the wrapper.** Sterile items must not be placed within this 1-inch border. If the paper wrap has been opened on a table, the surgical technologist must remove the sterile item without touching the 1-inch border.
- **The circulator is responsible for opening a sterile package using aseptic technique to prevent contamination of the enclosed sterile item(s).** When opening a sterile package, the circulator opens the top flap away from the body, grasping it in the hand holding the package. The side flaps are then opened downward, securing them in the same hand, and the last flap is pulled toward the body, exposing the sterile contents while covering the nonsterile hand. The item is then transferred onto the sterile field (refer to Chapter 12) or is taken from the package by the surgical technologist.

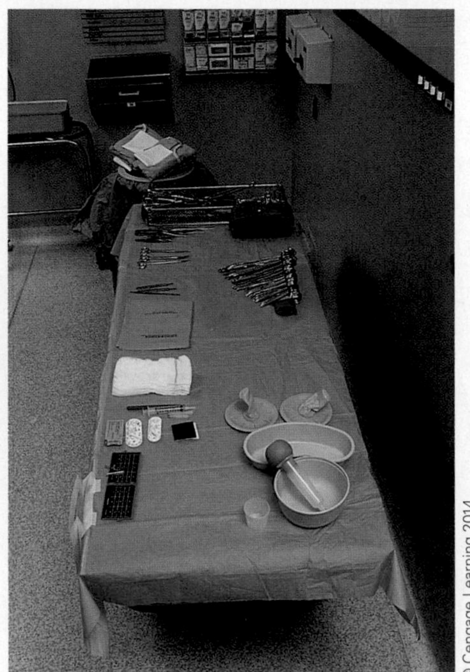

Figure 7-13 Sterile back table

- **The top of a sterile, draped table is the only portion that is considered sterile.** Any part of the drape extending below the top of the table is considered nonsterile.
- **Any item extending or falling below the table edge is considered nonsterile.** Examples are suction tubing or the cord to a power instrument hanging below the table edge. The portion hanging below the table edge must not be brought onto the sterile field.
- **Once sterile drapes have been placed, they should not be repositioned.** The portion of the drape that falls below the table edge is considered nonsterile and repositioning the drape exposes the sterile field to contaminated portions of the drape.
- **The integrity of sterile packages must be checked before opening.** There must be no evidence of strike-through, tears, or punctures; all seals must be intact; and CIs must have turned color to indicate exposure to sterilizing conditions.
- **Sterile packages found in storage areas commonly used for storage of nonsterile items must not be used.** The package should be opened and if it contains resusable items, they should be taken to the CSPD for repackaging and sterilization.
- **If a sterile package that is wrapped in a pervious woven material drops to the floor, this can allow for the implosion of air into the package.** The dropped package is considered contaminated. If the wrapper is impervious and the floor or area of contact is dry, the item can be transferred to the sterile field for use, but should not be placed back in sterile storage.
- **Punctures, tears, or strike-through compromises the sterility of drapes.** Destruction of the integrity of microbial barriers by puncture, tear, or strike-through results in contamination.
- **If a permeable drape covers a table or sterile field and any liquid penetrates the drape either from above or below, the drape must be considered contaminated.** The drape must be removed and replaced with a new sterile drape.
- **Sterile packages and drapes should be stored on smooth, clean, dry surfaces to prevent damage to packaging materials.** Sterile packages should be stored in a designated sterile supply storage area. Sterile packages should be handled only with clean, dry hands.
- **Unnecessary pressure should not be placed on sterile packs to prevent forcing out air and allowing air to be pulled inward.** Peel packs should be stored on their sides to prevent pressure that can rupture the sealed sides and violate the integrity of the package.
- **If towel clips used on the sterile field puncture any draping material, the tips of the instrument must be considered contaminated and should be left in place until the end of the procedure.** Preferably the surgical technologist should use nonperforating towel clips to hold draping material and any cords and tubing, such as the suction tubing and ESU cord, in place. If a penetrating towel clip is removed, the surgical technologist should pass the instrument to the circulator without touching the tips and cover the area with a sterile drape or towel.

PRINCIPLE 2: STERILE TEAM MEMBERS MUST BE APPROPRIATELY ATTIRED PRIOR TO ENTERING THE STERILE FIELD

Sterile team members must be appropriately attired prior to entering the sterile field. The attire worn by sterile individuals, including gown, gloves, mask, hair cover, and shoe covers, aids in preventing SSI.

- **The surgical gown is considered sterile in front 2 inches below the neckline to table level; bilaterally; and sterile gloved hands to 2 inches above elbows.** The upper chest area on the front of the gown is considered nonsterile because it cannot be directly viewed by the wearer and because of the possibility of the chin coming into contact with this part of the gown.
- **When the team member is standing at a table, the gown should be considered sterile to the top of the operating table or the back table's top surface.** Areas below this level may contact nonsterile surfaces and should be considered contaminated.
- **The arms should not be folded with the hands in the axillary region.** This region is considered nonsterile because it cannot be viewed by the wearer and because strike-through contamination from perspiration can occur in this area.
- **Hands should never be allowed to fall below the waist or table level.** The team member should avoid raising the hands above the mid-chest line or over the head to prevent contamination. A few exceptions exist, such as reaching for sterile light handles to adjust OR lights. This should be done at the beginning of the case and should not be repeated unless absolutely necessary.
- **The back of the sterile gown is considered nonsterile.** When wearing a sterile gown, the nonsterile back should never be turned toward the operative field or back table. The surgical technologist should not position the back table behind himself or herself, but rather at an angle.
- **A separate sterile surface should be used for gowning and gloving to avoid contamination of the back table.** The gown and gloves for the surgical technologist should be opened on a separate Mayo stand or small table prior to the surgical scrub.

- **The stockinette cuffs of the surgical gown are considered nonsterile and should be covered by the cuff of the sterile gloves at all times.** When the team member is self-gowning, the hands should not extend beyond the cuffs and should remain covered by the sleeve of the gown.
- **Members of the surgical team should sit only when the entire surgical procedure will be performed sitting down.** While seated, the hands must not be allowed to fall into the lap.
- **If a member of the sterile team must stand on a platform, the platform should be positioned before the individual approaches the field.** Members of the team should avoid to the extent possible changing levels at the sterile field. Moving from a lower position to a higher position within the field exposes contaminated areas of the gown to the field.

PRINCIPLE 3: MOVEMENT IN AND AROUND THE STERILE FIELD MUST NOT COMPROMISE THE STERILE FIELD

Sterile to Sterile

- **Only sterile items and sterilely attired individuals may contact sterile areas.** Only sterile items may be placed within or moved within a sterile field.
- **Only sterile members of the surgical team may touch sterile surfaces and items.** Contamination occurs when the sterile person touches or makes contact with a nonsterile surface or item.
- **The circulator and other nonsterile personnel must not touch or come into contact with sterile surfaces or items and should never walk between two sterile areas.** Contamination of a sterile surface occurs when a nonsterile surface contacts a sterile surface. If a nonsterile person walks between two sterile areas the chances of contamination greatly increase.
- **Scrubbed personnel should stay close to the sterile field throughout the procedure.** The surgical technologist must always face the sterile field or area to avoid contamination. In some situations, such as procedures that involve a large sterile setup and/or the participation of many sterile team members, sterile members may be required to move about. However, this increases the risk of contamination.
- **Movement within the sterile field should be kept to a minimum to avoid airborne contamination.** Movement by nonsterile and sterile team members should be kept to a minimum. This includes keeping traffic in and out of the surgical suite to a minimum, because opening the door(s) to the OR causes air currents to disturb dust and other particles, creating airborne contaminants that can settle into a surgical wound. Drapes and linens should be handled as little as possible by the sterile team members to prevent the airborne release of dust particles and lint, which can settle into a surgical wound or promote airborne transmission of bacteria.
- **Sterile surgical team members should either pass while facing one another or pass back to back by rotating 360 degrees.** The surgical technologist should turn her or his back to a nonsterile individual or area when walking past.
- **Talking, especially within the sterile field, should be kept to a minimum to prevent contamination from airborne moisture droplets.** Surgical masks should be properly worn to prevent the release of contaminated airborne moisture, and should completely cover the mouth and nose.
- **A nonsterile individual must maintain a minimum distance of 12 inches from any sterile item, area, or field to prevent contamination.** Additionally, equipment and furniture that is not covered by a sterile drape must not be included in the sterile field and must be kept a minimum of 12 in. away from a sterile surface or item. The surgical technologist must be conscious of these nonsterile items and personnel and maintain the 12-in. distance.

Nonsterile to Nonsterile

- **Nonsterile items and individuals may only contact nonsterile areas.** Sterile items should be opened by the nonsterile individual using sterile technique and transferred onto the back table. Nonsterile individuals must never extend over a sterile field to transfer sterile items to a sterile individual. Extending the hands over a sterile area could lead to contamination of that area by skin fallout.
- **To avoid reaching over a sterile basin, the circulator should hold only the lip of a bottle over the sterile basin or container and should maintain a 12- to 18-in. distance above the sterile container while pouring.** Sterile fluid bottles should never be recapped and reused; replacing the cap contaminates the fluids within the bottle.
- **The surgical technologist must place basins and/or medicine cups to be filled near the edge of the sterile table to allow the circulator to pour fluids without extending over the table.** It is also acceptable practice for the surgical technologist to hold the medicine cup while the circulator, maintaining proper distance, pours the medicine into the cup.
- **When draping a nonsterile table to create a sterile field, the nonsterile individual should cuff the hands in the underside folds of the drape or table cover to avoid contaminating the top surface.** The drape should be opened away from the body toward the far side of the table first and then toward the body to avoid contamination.

CASE STUDY Early one morning, Lucy is setting up a case in OR 3. The patient has been brought into the room and is on the OR table. The anesthesia provider is about to induce general anesthesia. After confirming that the steam indicator changed color, Lucy moves her basin set from the sterile ring stand to the back table and begins to remove items from the basin and place them in the appropriate positions on the table. Just before anesthesia is induced, the circulator notices water on the paper in which the basin set had been wrapped.

1. **Should the anesthesia provider go ahead with the induction of anesthesia?**
2. **What action should be taken by the surgical technologist in this instance to alleviate the danger of contaminating the patient?**
3. **Would the basin set still be considered sterile, since the indicator inside showed that it has been sterilized?**
4. **May the surgical technologist simply replace the basin set if it is determined to be nonsterile, or must the entire back table be replaced?**
5. **Should an incident report be filed?**

QUESTIONS FOR FURTHER STUDY

1. What different information about sterility comes from a chemical indicator and a biological indicator?
2. What conditions are necessary to guarantee sterility via steam sterilization?
3. What steps are required to verify both contact with the sterilant and sterilization of an instrument set?
4. What is a prion and why is it a concern in the operating room environment?
5. What safety guidelines apply when utilizing EtO as a sterilant?

BIBLIOGRAPHY

Allen, D. (1998). Packaging for the surgical suite. *Pharmaceutical & Medical Packaging News, 6*, 21–23.

Association for the Advancement of Medical Instrumentation. (1996). *ANSI/AAMI ST33:1996 Guidelines for the selection and use of reusable rigid container systems for ethylene oxide sterilization and steam sterilization in health care facilities.* Arlington, VA: Author.

Association for the Advancement of Medical Instrumentation. (2006). *ANSI/AAMI ST77: 2006 Containment devices for reusable medical device sterilization.* Arlington, VA: Author.

Association for the Advancement of Medical Instrumentation. (2008). *ANSI/AAMI ST41: 2008 Ethylene oxide sterilization in health care facilities: Safety and effectiveness.* Arlington, VA: Author.

Association for the Advancement of Medical Instrumentation. (2010). *ANSI/AAMI ST79: 2010 & A1:2010 Comprehensive guide to steam sterilization and sterility assurance in health care facilities.* Arlington, VA: Author.

Association for the Advancement of Medical Instrumentation. (2011). *Statement endorses guidelines for sterilization process.* Retrieved from http://www.aami/org/publications/AAMINews/Mar2011/sterilization.html

Association of Surgical Technologists. (2011). *Core curriculum for surgical technology* (6th ed.). Littleton, CO: Author.

Bennett, J. V., & Brachman, P. S. (1992). *Hospital infections* (3rd ed.). Boston: Little, Brown.

Donaldson, J. (1998). *An overview of the process of sterilization.* Retrieved from http://www.nurseceu.com/cpul.htm

Fraise, A., Lambert, P. A., & Maillard, J. (Eds.). (2004). *Principles and practice of disinfection, preservation & sterilization* (4th ed.). Hoboken, NJ: Wiley-Blackwell.

Gruendemann, B. J., & Mangum, S. S. (2001). *Infection prevention in surgical settings.* Philadelphia: W.B. Saunders.

International Association of Healthcare Central Service Materiel Management. (2009). *CRCST lesson plans.*

Retrieved from http://iahcsmm.org/Recertification/LessonPlans/CRCST_lessonPlans/CRCST_Lessons/CRCST_107.html

Mangram, A. J., Horan, T. C., Pearson, M. L., Silver, L. C., & Jarvis, W. R. (1999). Guideline for prevention of surgical site infection, 1999. *Infection Control and Hospital Epidemiology, 27,* 97–134.

Perkins, J. J. (1983). *Principles and methods of sterilization in health sciences* (2nd ed.). Springfield, IL: Charles C Thomas.

Phillips, N. (2007). *Berry & Kohn's operating room technique* (11th ed.). St. Louis. MO: Mosby.

Reichert, M., & Schultz, J. (2001). CJD instrument processing. *OR Manager, 17*(7), 21–22.

Rieu, E. V. (Ed.) (2003). *The odyssey*. New York: Penguin Group (USA).

Ross, T. A. (2002). Cruetzfeldt-Jakob disease. *The Surgical Technologist, 34*(4), 10–18.

Rutala, W., & Weber, D. (2001). Creutzfeldt-Jakob disease: Recommendations for disinfection and sterilization. *Clinical Infectious Diseases, 32,* 1348–1356.

U.S. Food and Drug Administration. (2004). *Federal Food, Drug, and Cosmetic Act*. Retrieved from http://www.fda.gov/opacom/laws/fdcact/fdctoc.htm

CHAPTER

8

Hemostasis, Emergency Situations, and All-Hazards Preparation

CASE STUDY Mary is an 82-year-old woman who suffers from rheumatoid arthritis. Today, she fell and hit her head. She was alert when she arrived at the emergency department but quickly lost consciousness. The physician thinks she has a probable left ventricular myocardial infarction. She is scheduled to be taken to the OR for coronary artery bypass surgery.

1. The patient's blood is typed and cross-matched to confirm she is a universal recipient. What is her blood type?
2. The patient's own blood will not be able to be used for transfusion purposes. What blood product will be used?
3. What other blood factor must be identified when typing and cross-matching is completed?

OBJECTIVES

After studying this chapter, the reader should be able to:

C 1. Compare and contrast methods of hemostasis and blood replacement and demonstrate the preparation and use of appropriate agents or devices.

A 2. Recognize developing emergency situations, initiate appropriate action, and assist in the treatment of the patient.

R 3. Apply knowledge of radiological and chemical injuries and biological warfare to the treatment of the patient.

E 4. Discuss nature-, human-, and nature/human-caused types of disasters.

5. Explain the various components of personal, health care facility, and national disaster planning.
6. Describe the initial response and steps taken when an all-hazards event occurs.
7. Discuss the various roles the surgical technologist can fulfill during an all-hazards event.

Select Key Terms

autologous	hemolysis	hyperthermia
cardiac dysrhythmia	hemostasis	Rh (Rhesus) factor
Compress	hemostat	suction
CPR	homologous	

HEMOSTASIS AND BLOOD REPLACEMENT

Because surgery is invasive, it is almost a given that some blood and fluid loss is expected. In most surgical procedures, blood loss is negligible; however, major blood loss must be anticipated. **Hemostasis** is stopping the loss of blood (hemorrhage). This may be accomplished by clot formation or vessel spasm, or surgically by mechanical pressure, ligation, or the application of hemostatic agents. Intraoperative hemostasis may also be achieved thermally. Some patients in need of surgery have congenital or acquired clotting disorders, making the maintenance of hemostasis more difficult.

Blood usually flows smoothly through the vascular system without cellular adherence to the vessel walls. When vascular injury occurs following trauma or in certain vessel diseases or surgery, the endothelial cells interact with platelets and clotting factors to form a blood clot at the site of injury.

When a blood vessel is injured, such as by being incised during surgery, the hemostatic process begins in order to stop the flow of blood. The body uses the process of *coagulation* to achieve hemostasis. As soon as a vessel is injured, a period of vasoconstriction begins, in which the muscular walls of the vessel constrict to help slow the flow of blood. This constriction of the vessel only lasts for a short time and slows but does not stop the bleeding. After the vasoconstriction of the vessel, platelets begin to adhere to the sides of the injured vessel walls, clumping together to form a plug at the cut end of the injured vessel. Once the platelets adhere to the vessel walls, they begin to release their contents, including epinephrine, serotonin, and, most important, adenosine diphosphate (ADP). The release of ADP causes more platelets to clump on the first layer, resulting in an initial *thrombus*. In small vessels, this initial thrombus formation may be enough to stop the flow of blood. In larger vessels, however, a second, permanent thrombus must be formed. After the initial white cell thrombus formation, reaction between plasma and fibrin from the connective tissue of the cells activates clotting factors that cause another set of reactions. Prothrombin reacts with thromboplastin to form thrombin. Thrombin then reacts with fibrinogen and forms fibrin, which has an ability to stabilize blood clots. If any of these factors are deficient, bleeding may continue. Over time, fibrin strands form a matrix through the clot to form a stronger, more solid plug that can withstand the pressure of blood within the vessel.

The phases of the clotting process are as follows:

1. Platelets adhere to subendothelium of vessel walls.
2. Platelets release ADP.
3. Release of ADP causes further layers of platelets to adhere.
4. Platelet aggregate forms a thrombus.
5. Permanent thrombus forms after clotting factor reaction.

Factors Affecting Hemostasis

Congenital hemostatic defects and acquired hemostatic disorders affect the ability of the patient's body to form blood clots naturally.

Congenital Hemostatic Defects

Some patients have congenital bleeding disorders that will affect bleeding during the surgical procedure. Hemophilia is the most common of these and manifests itself as a clotting deficiency. Preoperative testing is useful in determining whether these conditions exist.

Acquired Hemostatic Disorders

More commonly seen in the operating room (OR) are bleeding disorders caused by an outside source, called *acquired bleeding disorders*. Among these are liver disease, anticoagulant therapy with heparin or warfarin sodium, and aplastic anemia. Drug-therapy–induced platelet dysfunctions also affect hemostasis in the OR. Patients may be requested not to take aspirin for 1 week prior to surgery because of its anticoagulant properties.

Mechanical Methods

Mechanical hemostasis can be achieved with the use of several types of devices to control bleeding until a clot forms.

Clamps

Clamps are used to **compress** the walls of vessels and to grasp tissue. Most commonly used is the **hemostat** that is available with either straight or curved jaws. Special hemostatic clamps are available for different situations, such as vascular clamps designed to be atraumatic so they cause little damage to delicate vessels. Over the years, the hemostat clamp has taken on a variety of names, such as snap, clamp, stat, crile; much of this is dependent upon the region or where the surgeon may have trained during his or her residency.

Ligature

Ligatures, or ties (referred to as "stick ties" when a needle is attached), are strands of suture material used to tie off blood vessels. Ligatures are made of either natural or synthetic material and are designed either to dissolve over a period of time or to remain in the body tissue permanently (see Chapter 11 for information on suture material). Vessels are ligated using a ligature of the smallest possible diameter in order to reduce tissue reaction and are often placed at the base of a hemostat that has been used to clamp the end of a vessel. The hemostat may then be removed, the ligature tightened and tied, and the ends cut as close to the knot as possible, yet not so close as to allow a knot to come undone, dependent upon the type of suture material being used. Thus, when the material used to tie off a bleeding vessel is of a monofilament type, the tails of the suture should be left approximately 1/8 inch long from the knot. This will enhance the knot's security.

Clips

Ligating clips are often used in place of suture ligatures when many small vessels need to be ligated in a short period of time. These clips are made of a nonreactive metal, such as titanium or stainless steel, or plastic material and come in various sizes as well as absorbable or permanent varieties. They are applied either from a manually loaded applicator or from any of several preloaded disposable applicators.

When placed near the cut end of a vessel and squeezed shut, these clips occlude the vessel and stop the bleeding or clips are placed and the vessel divided.

Sponges

Sponges are used to apply pressure on bleeding areas or vessels and to absorb excess blood or body fluids. The various types of sponges include the following:

- Raytec, also called 4 × 4's (the size of the sponge)
- Laparotomy sponges, also referred to as lap sponges or "tape" sponges due to the radiopaque strand or tape that hangs from the sponge
- Tonsil sponges (round sponges)
- Patties (cottonoids) are smaller compressed radiopaque sponges used for neurosurgical procedures
- Kitners and peanuts, also referred to as dissecting sponges, which consist of small pieces of tightly rolled gauze (See Chapter 10 for detailed information on sponges.)

Pledgets

When bleeding occurs through needle holes in vessel anastomosis, small squares of Teflon® called *pledgets* are used as buttresses over the suture line. Using suture, these are sewn over the hole in the vessel and exert outside pressure over the small needle holes to prevent bleeding and promote clotting. These are often used in peripheral vascular and cardiovascular surgery.

Bone Wax

Bone wax, made of refined and sterilized beeswax, is used on cut edges of bone as a mechanical barrier to seal off oozing blood (see Chapter 9 for detailed information about bone wax).

Suction

Suction is the intraoperative aspiration of blood and body fluids by mechanical means to keep the surgical site clear. Several different styles of suction tips are available for different types of procedures, and most are disposable. It is important that suction always be available during surgery and until the patient has left the room, in case of an emergent bleeding situation. It is also vitally important that anesthesia personnel have suction available for them at the beginning and end of every surgical procedure when the patient is intubated and extubated. (See Chapter 10 for detailed information about the suction apparatus.)

Drains

Drains are used postoperatively to remove blood and body fluids from the operative site to prevent edema and hematoma formation, and aid in removing air in order to prevent dead spaces within the surgical wound. Several different types of drains are available, each with a specific use (see Chapter 10 for detailed information about drains).

Pressure Devices

The application of external pressure to a vessel, as with the use of a tourniquet, occludes the flow of blood until a clot has time to form. Prophylactically, pressure devices, such as sequential stockings, may also be used to prevent venous stasis and deep venous thrombosis.

Tourniquets

Tourniquets are often used on extremities to keep the operative site free of blood. The provision of a bloodless field makes visualization easier and reduces the operative time. Bleeding must be controlled prior to removal of the tourniquet, however, because the use of a tourniquet alone does not achieve hemostasis (see Chapter 10 for detailed information on tourniquets).

Thermal Hemostasis

One of the most common means of obtaining hemostasis during a surgical procedure is with the use of heat. Several different types of devices are available for achieving thermal hemostasis.

Electrosurgery

Electrosurgery is the most commonly used thermal hemostatic device. The components of electrosurgery are the active electrode or Bovie pencil, electrosurgical or generator unit (ESU), and inactive or dispersive electrode, also called the grounding pad (see Chapter 6 for detailed information about electrosurgery).

Lasers

The laser provides an intense and concentrated beam of light that is able to cut and coagulate tissue at the same time with very little surrounding tissue destruction. Several types of lasers are available, each with a specific surgical use (see Chapter 6 for details on lasers).

Argon Plasma Coagulation

Argon plasma coagulation involves the use of argon gas in combination with monopolar electrical energy in the form of a noncontact, white light beam. The argon beam coagulator provides rapid hemostasis that travels from a generator to a pencil-like handpiece. There is little to no tissue adherence since the handpiece does not come in direct contact with the tissue that is bleeding. There is less charring of the tissue compared to the ESU.

Ultrasonic (Harmonic) Scalpel

The ultrasonic scalpel consists of a single-use titanium blade attached to a handpiece and a portable generator. The generator converts the electrical energy into mechanical energy, thus causing the blade to move by rapid ultrasonic motion that simultaneously cuts and coagulates tissue. The vibrations of the blade denature protein molecules within the tissue, producing a sticky coagulum that seals the vessels. Additionally, the continuous denaturing of protein produces heat within the tissue to produce deeper coagulation. This continuous action does not cause a significant increase in temperature and therefore does not cause charring of the tissue or produce a smoke plume. Damage to adjacent tissue is minimal. Since electricity is not required to produce the cutting and coagulation effects on the tissue, a grounding pad is not necessary.

Pharmacological Agents

Several pharmacological agents that aid in hemostasis are available, with more being developed each year. Each has its own method of action and preferred usage, and manufacturer's instructions should be carefully followed. The following is a list of pharmacological hemostatic agents; see Chapter 9 for detailed information about each agent.

- Absorbable gelatin (Gelfoam®)
- Collagen (Avitene®)
- Oxidized cellulose (Nu-Knit®; Surgi-Cel®)
- Silver nitrate
- Epinephrine
- Thrombin

Blood Loss

Blood loss is monitored by several means intraoperatively to aid the surgeon and anesthesia provider in making decisions regarding the patient's status and potential need for transfusion or autotransfusion. Blood loss is charted by the circulator and reported to the surgeon upon request or immediately in extreme-loss situations.

Calibrated suction devices (canisters) are used between the suction tubing and the vacuum source to collect and monitor the amount of blood and body fluids suctioned from the field. The surgical technologist should keep close track of the amount of irrigation fluids used; the amount of irrigation fluid used is subtracted from the total volume of fluid in the canister to give a more accurate measurement of blood loss.

In addition, the circulator may weigh sponges removed from the field to provide an estimate of blood. The circulator may use a scale and a predetermined sponge weight formula; alternatively, some hospitals have a bloody-sponge weight estimate that is used and multiplied by the number of sponges removed from the field. The sponges must be weighed wet as the formula is based on the dry and wet weights of the sponges. This is not an exact method but provides the surgeon and anesthesia provider with a fairly reliable estimate of blood loss.

Blood Replacement

When blood loss is too great to be controlled by intraoperative hemostatic techniques alone, blood replacement therapies are in order. The estimated blood loss (EBL) is reported to and monitored by the anesthesia provider, who will make the determination in consultation with the surgeon if blood replacement is necessary. Some types of surgery, such as cardiovascular or prostate surgery, will often call for blood replacement due to the high volume of blood loss. Blood replacement involves the administration of whole blood or blood components such as plasma, packed red blood cells, or platelets via an intravenous (IV) line. This is used to increase the circulating blood volume, to increase the number of red blood cells, and to provide plasma-clotting factors. Blood products may be **homologous** (donated by another person) or **autologous** (donated previously by the patient and stored, or obtained through autotransfusion). Autotransfusion is the use of the patient's own blood, which has been processed for reinfusion. When homologous banked blood is used, blood typing and cross-matching are essential to prevent transfusion reactions.

Blood Types and Groups

The four main blood types are A, B, O, and AB, based on the presence or absence of A and B red cell antigens. In addition, the blood contains agglutinins, which are antibodies that work against the A and B antigens. Individuals with type A blood naturally produce anti-B agglutinins and individuals with type B blood naturally produce anti-A agglutinins. An individual with type O blood, however, naturally produces both A and B agglutinins, making the O individual a universal donor. Type AB individuals produce neither antibody, and therefore type AB individuals may receive any type and are called universal recipients. If mismatched blood is transfused, a transfusion reaction occurs and may range from a mild reaction to anaphylactic shock.

Also to be taken into consideration in blood matching is the **Rh (Rhesus) factor**, which is an antigenic substance found in the erythrocytes in most people. Individuals with the factor are termed Rh positive, whereas individuals lacking the factor are termed Rh negative. If blood given to an Rh-negative individual is Rh positive, **hemolysis** occurs, leading to anemia.

Due to these factors, blood is carefully typed and crossmatched prior to being administered.

Handling of Blood Replacement Components

Blood products are usually obtained from the blood bank by a responsible individual, signed for, and brought to the OR. If the products are not to be used immediately, they should be stored in a refrigerator at a temperature between 1° and 6°C (33.8°–42.8°F). Prior to administration, blood products must be carefully identified as to the proper product and patient. Two individuals should perform this identification; individuals who can perform the identification are the surgical technologist, registered nurse, surgeon, and anesthesia provider. One individual reads aloud while the other checks and verifies the information. The information for blood group, Rh type, and unit number must match the tag on the blood bag, the patient's armband, and the patient's chart, and these should be checked by the two-individual verbal method listed above. The physician's order should also be double-checked, as should the expiration date on the blood bag. Finally, the product itself should be inspected for clots. If clots are present or any of the information does not match correctly, the blood must not be administered and is returned to the blood bank. In addition, the patient's armband should be checked for final verification of identification. In some instances due to the patient position and draping, the armboard cannot be accessed and the chart should be checked.

Autotransfusion

Autotransfusion is the reinfusion of the patient's own blood, whether donated prior to surgery or collected and reinfused perioperatively. This process is preferable to the use of homologous blood because it uses the patient's own blood, eliminating the danger of a compatibility mismatch or disease transmission. Blood may either be donated prior to surgery or recovered during surgery and reinfused. In the latter case, blood is suctioned directly from the wound into a cell saver or cell salvager machine that filters and anticoagulates the blood and reinfuses it intravenously with little or no damage to the red blood cells. Several machines are available for intraoperative use and all work on the same principle. Some are designed for more rapid reinfusion in emergency situations. In addition to suctioned blood, blood may be drained from bloody sponges into a basin of saline, and then aspirated into the autotransfusion machine. Blood that has been exposed to collagen hemostatic agents and certain antibiotics cannot be used with these devices, as blood may coagulate in the system. If the procedure involves blood exposed to gastric or enteric contents or amniotic fluid, it may not be salvaged, and blood may not be used when the patient has a known local or systemic infection. Additionally, if cancer cells are suspected or known to be present, the blood will not be used as the cell saver cannot wash or remove the cancer cells.

When a cell-salvaging machine is not available, blood may be collected in a salvage collection bag containing an anticoagulant and reinfused through a blood filter. Another available method is the use of a sterile blood collection canister into which blood can be suctioned. There, it collects in a reservoir. When the canister reaches capacity, it is emptied and the contents are washed in a red cell washer and reinfused. In many hospitals, this equipment is located in the blood bank and the blood must leave the OR for washing, so this method takes more time than the two previously outlined.

Hemolytic Transfusion Reactions

If blood is not properly matched including Rh factor prior to transfusion, a hemolytic transfusion reaction may develop. This may result from Rh incompatibility from mismatched blood transfusions. Severe hemolytic reactions can be fatal and must be treated immediately.

The conscious patient may exhibit fatigue and complain of lack of energy. The patient may experience rapid pulse, shortness of breath, and pounding of the heart. The skin may appear jaundiced and pallor may be exhibited, especially in the palms of the hands.

The patient under general anesthesia will not show these signs, and the only signs noted may be a generalized loss of blood and a lowered blood oxygen saturation level due to the inability of the red blood cells to carry oxygen.

If a hemolytic transfusion reaction is suspected, the transfusion should be immediately stopped and a blood sample sent to the blood bank to rule out the mismatch. Appropriate drug therapies, usually including steroid therapy, should be begun as quickly as possible. Urine output is monitored closely in these patients, as hypovolemia may hinder kidney function. In some cases, the patient will need to undergo dialysis, which will aid in the systemic removal of the mismatched blood.

INDICATIONS OF EMERGENCY SITUATIONS

The surgical technologist is frequently called on to work in emergency surgery situations or to react appropriately when an elective surgery becomes an emergency. The surgical technologist must be able to anticipate emergency situations and prepare for them in advance. This skill improves with experience, but the entry-level surgical technologist should be able to recognize an emergency situation when it occurs. Such indicators as rapidly dropping blood pressure, **cardiac dysrhythmia**, and any vital sign out of the normal range provide the surgical team with information about impending emergent situations. In addition, some emergencies, such as rapid hemorrhaging, occur suddenly, with little or no warning, and must be immediately acted upon. It is extremely important that the entire surgical team react in a calm and quick fashion in these circumstances. Prior to surgery, the surgeon or anesthesia provider should be notified immediately if any of these indicators of an emergency situation arise:

- Difficulty breathing
- Chest pain
- Changes in skin color
- Changes in vital signs
- Open bleeding wounds or visible punctures not indicated on the patient's chart
- Inability to move an extremity
- Misshapen/misaligned body part
- Disorientation or confusion

The surgeon and/or anesthesia provider will assess the situation in these cases and provide the surgical team with instructions on how they should respond.

OBJECTIVES AND PRIORITIES IN EMERGENCY SITUATIONS

The objectives of emergency care and emergency and trauma surgery are to preserve life, to prevent further deterioration of patient condition, and then to provide whatever care necessary to restore the patient to his or her previous lifestyle.

When providing emergency care, treatment should be prioritized to fit the objectives. As soon as an emergency patient situation is identified, the health care provider (HCP) in the field or the surgical team member should signal for assistance. Treatment will then follow a pattern of priorities of care. The first priority in any emergency situation is to check for and provide a patent airway to ensure or restore respiratory status and breathing. Second, cardiovascular status should be maintained or restored and hemostasis should be provided to maintain circulatory status. Following these first two priorities, treatment is provided for the following:

- Chest injuries
- Shock
- Wound protection/closure
- Fractures
- Vital sign monitoring
- Provision of reassurance and comfort for the patient

The following section covers some of the most commonly seen emergencies in the OR.

CARDIOPULMONARY RESUSCITATION

Every health care professional should be familiar with the techniques of cardiopulmonary resuscitation (**CPR**), a technique of manually providing chest compression and ventilations to patients in cardiac arrest in an effort to provide oxygenated blood to the brain and vital organs and reverse the processes that lead to death. The best way for the surgical technologist to learn this technique is to obtain certification in CPR or Basic Life Support (BLS), offered in classes available in hospitals and from such organizations as the American Red Cross and the American Heart Association (AHA). Hospital employees should attend the training seminar every 2 years to renew their CPR/BLS certification.

Coronary heart disease (CHD) is estimated to be responsible for approximately 330,000 out-of-hospital and emergency department deaths in the United States each year. Many of the individuals that experience sudden cardiac arrest (SCA) exhibit ventricular fibrillation (VF) at some point during the arrest. Treatment of VF SCA demands early CPR and defibrillation. CPR that is delivered in the correct manner can highly increase the survival rates from SCA. However, survival for out-of-hospital SCA victims is very low in the United States and Canada. One major reason for this low rate is the fact that fewer than one-third of SCA victims receive bystander CPR and the CPR that is delivered is not high quality.

CPR must be started as quickly as possible, as time is of the essence in cardiac arrest. Clinical death begins the moment heart action and breathing stop; the patient has only 4–6 minutes before the cells of the brain begin to deteriorate. Therefore, it is very important that breathing and circulation be restored within this time frame to prevent biological death from occurring.

There are several warning signs of impending cardiac arrest, and the surgical technologist should be able to recognize these in order to anticipate emergent needs of the patient. A patient who exhibits any of the following may be in danger of cardiac arrest:

- Chest pain (in the awake patient)
- Unstable blood pressure
- Tachycardia
- Cardiac dysrhythmias
- Respiratory changes
- Hypovolemia
- Laryngospasm

A *chain-of-survival* concept applied to both in-hospital and out-of-hospital arrests addresses the ABCs—airway, breathing, and circulation—as well as providing the "D," definitive treatment. Successful resuscitation requires:

- Early recognition of cardiac arrest
- Early activation of trained responders

- Early CPR
- Early defibrillation
- Early Advanced Cardiac Life Support (ACLS)

To provide these early interventions, the hospital develops written policies and procedures that the HCP must be familiar with. In the OR, the surgical technologist's primary function is to protect the sterile field; however, circumstances may require the surgical technologist to use CPR skills in the OR. Additionally, the surgical technologist may encounter an out-of-hospital situation.

In 2010 the AHA published the revised "Guidelines for Cardiopulmonary Resuscitation and Emergency Cardiovascular Care" that includes significant changes from the 2005 version. The following information is a synopsis of the 2010 guidelines with an emphasis on the HCP. (**Important:** This review is meant only to highlight some of the more important 2010 guidelines and revisions that have occurred since 2005; the surgical technology student will still need to complete a formal comprehensive course in CPR that includes hands-on training and maintain CPR certification when employed):

1. A change in the sequence of BLS from A-B-C (airway, breathing, chest compressions) to C-A-B (chest compressions, airway, breathing) for adults, adolescents, and infants (excludes newborns).
   a. The guidelines now emphasize a "chain of survival" that includes:
      (1) Immediate recognition of cardiac arrest and activation of the emergency response system (ERS)
      (2) Early CPR that emphasizes chest compressions
      (3) Rapid defibrillation
      (4) Effective advanced life support
      (5) Integrated post–cardiac arrest care

2. "Look, Listen, and Feel" has been eliminated due to the inconsistency in the performance of these steps and their time consumption, thus delaying the start of chest compressions.
   a. The 2010 guidelines stress immediate activation of the ERS and starting chest compressions. Once the HCP recognizes the victim is unresponsive with no breathing or displays an abnormal breathing pattern such as gasping, she or he should immediately activate the ERS and begin chest compressions.
   b. Early recognition of SCA is based on assessing responsiveness and abnormal or no breathing. HCPs should be aware that the cardiac arrest victim may display abnormal agonal breathing patterns such as gasping. HCPs should be trained in recognizing unusual breathing presentations of SCA.
   c. The HCP can check for responsiveness and breathing simultaneously. However, the HCP should no longer shake the victim, but rather tap the shoulder and shout, "Are you all right?"

3. A change with the 2010 guidelines is to immediately start chest compressions before giving rescue breaths (C-A-B rather than A-B-C).
   a. There is an increase in the focus on delivering high-quality chest compressions at the appropriate rate and depth, including complete recoil of the chest after each compression. Additionally, there is focus on preventing any pauses in compressions as well as avoiding excessive ventilation; defibrillation should be incorporated in a way that minimizes the interruption of chest compressions. Minimizing the interruption of chest compressions cannot be overemphasized until the return-of-spontaneous circulation (ROSC) or termination of resuscitation efforts. Interruptions in chest compressions, including longer-than-necessary delays in giving rescue breaths, decreases the effectiveness of CPR.
   b. Positioning the head, attaining a tight seal in mouth-to-mouth rescue breathing, or obtaining and assembling a device such as a bag-mask device all take precious time.
   c. Beginning chest compressions immediately rather than giving two rescue breaths prevents delay in giving the first compression and getting the circulation moving.
   d. The ratio of chest compressions to rescue breaths for infants, adolescents, and adults is still 30:2.
   e. The new concept of "push hard, push fast" is to be applied to CPR. The recommendation is at least 100 compressions per minute. The depth of compression for adults has changed from a depth of 1½ inches to 2 inches to a consistent depth of 2 inches. The HCP should place the heel of one hand on the middle of the victim's chest (lower half of sternum) and the heel of other hand on top of first in parallel fashion, push down 2 inches, and allow chest to completely recoil after each compression. Studies suggest that lifting the heel of the hand slightly, but completely, off the chest can promote chest recoil.
   f. Hospital beds are not firm and therefore some of the force of chest compressions can be lost. The use of a backboard is recommended as long as placement avoids a delay in initiating CPR or minimizes interruptions in CPR. Air-filled mattresses should be deflated.
   g. HCP fatigue is a factor in the delivery of quality chest compressions. When two or more rescuers are available, it is recommended to switch chest compressors every 2 minutes or about every five cycles of compressions and ventilations. The switch should be made in less than 5 seconds.

4. A new emphasis of the guidelines is that airway maneuvers should be performed quickly and efficiently and minimize the interruption of chest compressions.
   a. In the absence of evidence of head or neck trauma, the HCP should use the head tilt–chin lift maneuver to open the airway. If a spine injury is suspected, the airway should be opened using a jaw thrust without head movement.

   b. The breath should be delivered over 1 second and product a visible rise in the chest.
   c. When an advanced airway is in place during two-person CPR, one breath is given every 6 to 8 seconds without attempting to synchronize between chest compressions (this works out to 8 to 10 breaths per minute). There should be no pause in chest compressions in order to provide ventilations.
   d. Excessive ventilation must be prevented in order to avoid the complications including regurgitation and aspiration.

5. Rapid defibrillation has been shown to be a highly important factor in the survival of the VF SCA patient. Reducing the interval in the use of the automated external defibrillator (AED) in out-of-hospital settings or in-hospital defibrillator setting greatly improves the potential for patient survival.
   a. After activating the ERS, the HCP should obtain an AED (if nearby and accessible) and upon return to the victim use the AED, and then begin chest compressions.
   b. When two HCPs are present, one should begin chest compressions while the second activates the ERS and obtains the AED.
   c. The AED should be used as soon as possible.
6. HCP training is emphasizing building the team as each provider arrives and quickly delegating roles. Many tasks, including chest compressions, airway management, rescue breathing, rhythm detection, defibrillation, and administration of emergency drugs, are performed concurrently and not in a stepwise fashion. Some resuscitation may start with a lone provider who activates the emergency response system, resulting in other HCPs arriving to the scene. As the additional providers arrive, duties may be delegated to a team of providers who can perform them simultaneously in order to have an integrated team of highly trained rescuers in attempt to achieve the best patient outcome possible.
7. The 2010 guidelines deemphasize the importance of checking the pulse by HCPs. Detection of a pulse can be difficult, especially in an emergency situation when the HCP is in a hurry, and therefore HCPs often incorrectly assess the absence or presence of a pulse. HCPs should take no more than 10 seconds to check if a pulse is present.
8. The majority of pediatric cardiac arrests are asphyxial; resuscitation should be a combination of ventilation and chest compressions. The depth of compression for infants is approximately 1½ inches and 2 inches in adolescents.
9. The A-B-C sequence for neonatal arrests is still retained since cardiac arrests are nearly always asphyxia. The ratio for chest compressions to rescue breaths for newborns is still 3:1. If the arrest is due to a cardiac etiology, the ratio should be 15:2.

One last consideration is the trauma patient in cardiac arrest. For these patients, it has been shown that cardiac arrest is usually caused by exsanguinations or a critical thoracic injury. When treating these patients, the head tilt should not be used to open the airway if any suspicion of cervical spine injury exists. In trauma patients, it has been shown that chest compressions usually are not adequate to reverse the cardiac arrest and that the more critical factor is the restoration of circulating blood volume. Many of these patients will require resuscitative thoracotomy.

CPR is not performed without danger of injury to the patient. The technique must be performed with great care. Careful attention to proper technique helps minimize injury to the patient. Certification in CPR/BLS and renewal of the certification help ensure that the HCP has an adequate working knowledge of the technique.

Cardiac Arrest in the Surgical Setting

In the surgical setting, the "D" of the C-A-Bs of cardiac arrest is undertaken when the physician begins to provide definitive treatment. This will include control of dysrhythmias by cardiac defibrillation or the use of IV drugs and postresuscitation care. Arterial lines are used to monitor blood pressure and blood gases. The role of the surgical technologist in this situation is to protect the sterile field from contamination during the resuscitation efforts. In some cases, the surgical technologist may be required to assist by providing artificial respiration ("bagging the patient") or providing chest compressions. In most cases, roles are well defined by facility policy and each team member will have a specific function. In the OR, anesthesia personnel are available to manage the cardiopulmonary arrest situation or "code." They provide IV access and arterial pressure and blood gas monitoring as well as airway management and respiratory and cardiac support, including defibrillation. The circulating nurse is available to provide support to the patient and physicians and to bring necessary supplies, including the "crash cart" when necessary.

MALIGNANT HYPERTHERMIA

Malignant **hyperthermia** (MH) is a life-threatening, acute pharmacogenic disorder, developing during or after anesthesia. MH is usually triggered by an anesthetic agent, such as halothane, enflurane, or isoflurane, and may be triggered by muscle relaxants such as succinylcholine. MH is characterized by a rapid increase in body temperature, unexplained tachycardia, unstable blood pressure, muscle rigidity, tachypnea, and cyanosis. See Chapter 9 for detailed information about MH.

DISSEMINATED INTRAVASCULAR COAGULATION

Disseminated intravascular coagulation (DIC) is a pathological process in the body that occurs when blood begins to coagulate within the body. The body's blood clotting mechanisms are activated throughout the body instead of being localized to a specific area of injury. This leads to the consumption of coagulation factors and platelets, and the overstimulation of fibrinolytic degradation products that act as anticoagulants. Therefore, the initial hypercoagulation is replaced by a deficiency in clotting factors, leading to hypocoagulability and internal hemorrhaging.

DIC may result in clotting symptoms or, more often, in bleeding due to the depletion of the body's blood clotting mechanisms. The bleeding associated with DIC is usually severe and life threatening. DIC may be stimulated by the following factors:

- Infection of the blood by bacteria or fungus
- Severe tissue trauma, e.g., head injury, shock, or burns
- Leukemia or cancer
- Severe liver disease
- Recent blood transfusion reactions
- Obstetric complications

The treatment for DIC involves determining the underlying cause of the disorder and providing appropriate measures. The patient with DIC may receive a transfusion of fresh-frozen plasma to replace the coagulation factors. Cryoprecipitate may be initiated if fibrinogen is extremely low. Additionally, heparin (used to prevent thrombosis) is sometimes prescribed in combination with replacement therapy. The prognosis for patients is often poor and depends on the underlying cause of the disorder.

ANAPHYLACTIC REACTIONS

Anaphylactic reaction is an exaggerated allergic reaction to a substance or protein. Among the substances most likely to cause anaphylactic reaction are drugs such as local anesthetics, codeine, antibiotics, animal-derived drugs such as insulin, contrast media, and in some cases the latex found in many surgical supplies.

A patient suffering an anaphylactic attack generally first shows only mild inflammatory symptoms such as itching, swelling, and, in some cases, difficulty breathing. Hives or urticaria may be present on the skin with severe itching. These symptoms may cause apprehension in the patient and should not be ignored, as these symptoms can rapidly escalate to a systemic anaphylactic attack. As the reaction progresses, the patient experiences further difficulty breathing due to bronchospasm and laryngeal edema. At the same time that these respiratory symptoms are occurring, another chain of events takes place that causes vascular collapse due to shifts in body fluid. This presents with hypotension, tachycardia, and diminished urine output.

During an anaphylactic reaction, the surgical team must maintain the airway and provide supplemental oxygen or the patient may die of respiratory failure. The symptoms of vascular collapse and shock must also be treated to prevent death from cardiovascular failure. Epinephrine is the first-line drug in the treatment of a severe anaphylactic reaction. Epinephrine causes bronchodilation, reduces laryngeal spasm, and raises blood pressure. After the administration of epinephrine, steroids are administered to stabilize mast cells and slow or stop the chain of events that caused the reaction. Intravenous fluids and plasma may also be utilized to restore fluid volume, and vasopressor agents such as Levophed are given to increase blood pressure.

Because an anaphylactic reaction occurs so quickly and can often lead to death, it is important that it be avoided altogether in the clinical setting by identifying patients with known allergies and making this information available to the entire surgical team. Allergies should be clearly identified on the chart and preferably on the patient identification band, and any prior history of reactions should be carefully noted in the chart. If suspicion of reactivity exists, skin testing prior to surgery can help determine what drugs should be used intraoperatively.

ALL-HAZARDS PREPARATION

The term "all-hazards preparation" is an all-encompassing term that refers to the many different emergencies. "Emergencies" are defined as those that require the emergency response of outside assistance, which may be at the local, county, state, or federal levels. "Emergency preparedness" is an older term used to define the action taken by individuals, governments, and health care facilities and systems to be prepared for an emergency. Emergency planning tends to focus on the events that could occur locally or regionally; therefore, it is "individualized." For example, people that live near the Mississippi Delta probably have emergency plans in place for flooding but not for blizzards.

However, when an emergency or disaster situation occurs, there are many similarities that exist, such as the systems that are in place to respond to the emergency, procedures for communication and evacuation, response to caring for special needs patients, and so forth. Due to these similarities, the term "all-hazards preparation" is used, which provides a template for generalized training and emergency preparation that can be applied to all disaster situations rather than training that is focused on a limited number of local or regional types of emergencies.

Due to the number of disasters that have occurred over the last few years, manmade and natural, the roles and duties of allied health professionals have received increasing emphasis since they make up the majority of the health care workforce. During a disaster situation, the allied health professional's roles and duties may expand, and the individual is asked to fill many roles typically not performed on a daily basis. However, due to the allied health professional's knowledge and skills of providing care to sick and/or injured patients, it is imperative that she or he is able to respond to this workforce need to fill important roles during an emergency response. The following information is meant to familiarize the entry-level surgical technologist with the basic principles of all-hazards preparation. Further training will be provided by the workplace that may include a simulated disaster with hands-on training.

Natural Disasters

Natural disasters are unfortunately the most commonly occurring type of disasters that can affect large populations. As previously mentioned, the type of natural disaster is often unique to the area where it occurs, and the severity can vary. Throughout the Rocky Mountain region of the United States, avalanches are a concern and the types of avalanches include snow during the winter season and rock slides during the spring and summer seasons. Winter sport enthusiasts who head into the mountains must be ever cognizant of the conditions that are conducive to the occurrence of a snow avalanche, which can block highways, cause major destruction, and take lives by burying someone under several feet of packed snow. HCPs should be ready to treat the victim for asphyxiation, fractures, and hypothermia.

Rockslides and landslides are also usually weather-related occurrence. Hard rains can loosen the rocks and/or land, which begin to tumble, gathering speed as well as larger rocks (boulders), dirt, bushes, and trees. Rock slides in the Rocky Mountain region are often due to heavy snow pack and/or "spring run-off," the melting of the snow pack. Vehicles on highways can be suddenly caught in a rockslide and/or landslide, causing serious injuries or death.

Winter storms are often not thought of as a natural disaster. The storms bring life-threatening cold temperatures, low visibility, and dangerous driving conditions. Usually the National Weather Service can predict a winter storm, including where it will hit and how soon, in order for communities to prepare. However, predicting weather is not an exact science, as seen with the back-to-back snowstorms that hit Colorado in December 2006 that almost brought everything to a halt, including grocery stores running out of food. Transportation can be brought to a standstill; emergency vehicles such as ambulances will experience delays in reaching victims as well as transporting to an emergency department. People stuck in cars on barren highways or mountain passes are exposed to hypothermia and frostbite; carbon dioxide poisoning can occur if they leave the vehicle running for heat, especially if the tail pipe becomes jammed with snow.

Opposite of winter storms are heat waves, which also are often not thought of as creating a disaster situation by the general public except for the HCPs who are caught up in treating the large number of affected patients. A heat wave is defined as an extended period of abnormally hot weather that may be accompanied by high humidity. It is caused by an air mass that becomes stationary over a region. Heat waves are dangerous because the heat taxes the human body beyond its normal abilities. In 2003, a heat wave that struck five European countries was responsible for between 22,000 and 35,000 deaths. Infants, adolescents, and elderly, obese, or chronically ill people have the highest percentage of being victims of a heat wave. Additionally, males are at a higher risk for heat-related illnesses due to sweating more than females. Obviously, the number one heat-related complication is dehydration; however, other serious heat-related illnesses include severe sunburn, heat cramps, heat exhaustion, and heat stroke (also called sunstroke) (see Table 8-1). Another consequence of individuals exposed to extended periods of heat is the psychological effects. Excessive heat causes psychological stress, which can affect the performance of individuals, ranging from chronic malaise to an increase in tempers; increases in violent crimes are associated with heat waves.

Table 8-1 Terms Related to Heat Wave

- **Heat index:** Number in degrees Fahrenheit that tells how hot is feels when relative humidity is added to the air temperature. Exposure to full sunshine can increase the heat index by 15°F.
- **Heat cramps:** Muscular pains and spasms due to activity; often first sign/reaction by the body to the heat.
- **Heat exhaustion:** Due to exercising or working for a period of time in a hot, humid place and body fluids are lost at a great rate through sweating without replacement. Mild form of shock because the body increases the blood flow to the skin, thus reducing blood flow to the vital organs.
- **Heat stroke:** A life-threatening condition where the patient's internal temperature control system stops working. The body temperature can rapidly increase, causing neurological damage as well as leading to death if not immediately treated.

A consequence of heat waves can be wildfires. During the 2003 European heat wave, wildfires raged throughout the countryside, causing major devastation to agricultural land while destroying hundreds of buildings. Wildfires quickly spread especially if weather conditions are windy and dry, and there is a large amount of fuel such as a forest that has not been cleared of dead and dry vegetation. Major wildfires and/or multiple fires can lead to local or regional government health agencies issuing warnings about the dangers of smoke-related complications due to the accumulation of smoke over a large area that is spread by winds. Respiratory and cardiovascular conditions can be worsened by the smoke. Additionally, people who do not evacuate from a wildfire scene are at risk for burns, as are firefighters. Wildfires will leave an area devoid of vegetation that usually holds the soil in place; heavy rains can cause landslides to occur.

One of the more powerful natural disasters are earthquakes that produce an incredible amount of energy when two portions of the earth's crust slide by one another (one portion on top and the other below) along a fault line. The energy travels outward from the epicenter in seismic waves, causing a violent shaking of the ground. Strong earthquakes cause damage

TABLE 8-2 **Richter Scale**

<3.5	Earthquake may be felt, but not recorded by a seismograph
3.5–5.4	Earthquake felt; rarely causes damage
<6.0	Slight damage to well-designed, earthquake-resistant buildings; major damage to poorly constructed buildings
6.1–6.9	Heavy damage and destruction up to 62 miles from the epicenter
7.0–7.9	Major earthquake that causes heavy damage and destruction over a very large area
8 or greater	Strongest of earthquakes, with serious damage and destruction for hundreds of miles

to buildings and bridges, in some instances causing them to collapse, which can lead to fires due to broken gas lines and downing of electrical wires. Earthquakes are measured on the Richter scale; see Table 8-2.

Varying factors will contribute to the effect an earthquake will have on the population, including how powerful the earthquake was (Richter scale measurement), whether it occurred in a populated or rural area, the types of building and housing construction affected, and when it occurred. The injuries the HCP will encounter include lacerations, fractures, serious head injuries, eye injuries, and crushing injuries due to falling debris, collapse of houses and buildings, and collapse of sidewalks, streets, and bridges. People can become trapped under collapsed structures, sometimes for hours or days, with injuries and dehydration becoming life threatening. The infrastructure of towns and cities can be seriously disrupted (e.g., hospitals destroyed, no electricity for several days, clean water supply disrupted, highways destroyed, etc.).

A serious earthquake can cause the formation of a tsunami (also called tidal wave). A tsunami is an immense wave of incredible force that can travel for many miles before dissipating. It is usually of extremely long length generated by disturbances such as an earthquake that occurs below or near the ocean floor. The wave height can range from a few feet to over 200 feet or more and reach speeds exceeding 500 miles per hour. The coastal areas of countries are most vulnerable to a tsunami; in the United States, the states that border the Pacific Ocean are vulnerable. As mentioned, a tsunami has a terrible force when it hits land, causing major devastation, injuries, and death. The wave of water can travel several miles inward and becomes congested with large pieces of debris and vehicles that contribute to causing additional damage.

Tsunamis can also be caused by the underwater eruption of a volcano. By definition, volcanos are an opening in the earth's crust that allows poisonous gases and magma (melted rock) to escape. The magma and gases build up in the earth's interior, creating an enormous amount of pressure, and eventually explode outward, releasing the poisonous gases and flow of lava (Figure 8-1). Additionally, a large plume or cloud of super-heated volcanic ash is released into the atmosphere that can affect a large population of people (Figure 8-2). The volcanic ash can cause respiratory complications and damage the lungs as well as cause serious burns. The volcanic ash can

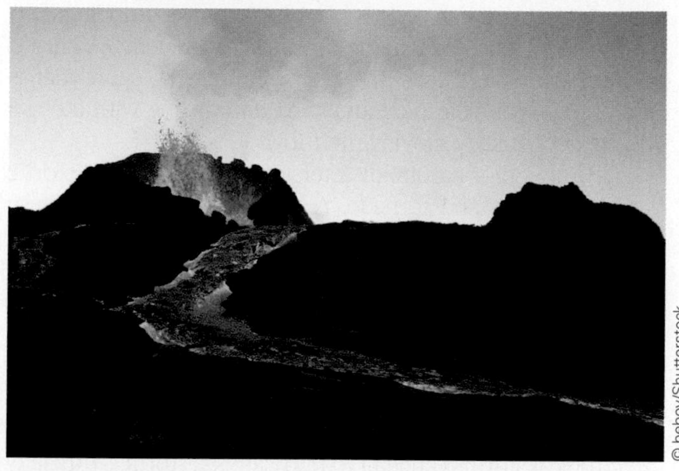

Figure 8-1 Lava flow

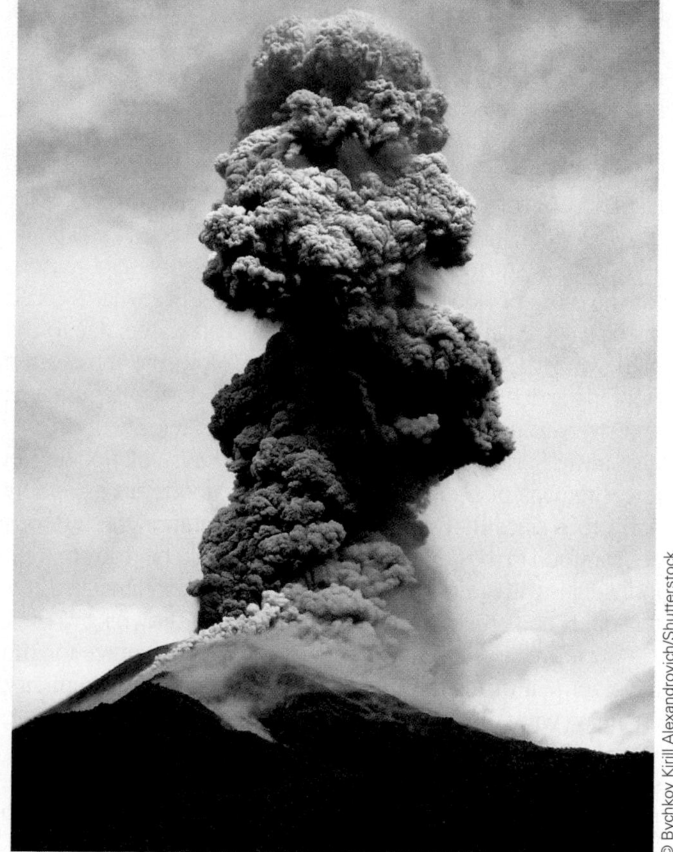

Figure 8-2 Karimsky volcano eruption

be so thick that it causes loss of visibility, making driving conditions dangerous and leading to vehicular accidents. A hazard of volcanos is mudflows; the heat will melt the snow that is often present on volcanic mountains, and mixing with the ash will create a quickly moving mudflow.

The next four natural disasters are related: tropical storm, hurricane, flood, and tornado. A tropical storm is an intense thunderstorm accompanied by sustained high wind speeds, but not as high as a hurricane; to be classified as a tropical storm the winds must be between 39 and 73 miles per hour (mph). Tropical storms can cause damage to houses and buildings but usually not as extensive as what is seen with a hurricane. People are advised to take precautions and seek proper shelter to avoid injuries (see earthquake section for types of injuries).

Tropical storms can lead to hurricanes; a storm is officially classified as a hurricane when the sustained wind speed is 74 mph (see Table 8-3). Hurricanes are large storms that produce heavy amounts of rain, storm surges, and high winds. Hurricanes can affect a large geographical region; for example, it may strike the Caribbean Islands, move onward and hit Florida, and possibly move into the Gulf of Mexico to strike the regions along the coast. HCPs will be treating fractures, lacerations, and head and eye injuries due to falling trees, flying debris, and collapse of structures; burns and electrical shock due to fallen electrical wires; and providing resuscitation efforts for drowned individuals.

Tropical storms and hurricanes are one of several reasons for the cause of floods. Hurricanes often produce what is called a storm surge, an abnormal rise of the ocean waters due to the high winds that sweep forward inland. However, most often flooding is due to a large amount of rainfall that causes streams and rivers to overflow their banks, or causes a levee or dam to give away. Spring snow melt often is the cause of flooding in lower regions of the United States. Flash floods are extremely dangerous since they rarely allow any preparation; flash floods are common in the desert regions. HCPs should be ready to treat individuals with gastrointestinal illness due to contaminated water supply and provide resuscitation efforts for drowning victims.

Tropical storms and hurricanes can be one source for the development of tornadoes further inland due to the humidity, changing wind directions, and wind speed, which all contribute to the formation of a funnel. However, we most commonly associate tornadoes with severe thunderstorms. HCPs should be prepared to treat fractures; head, spine, and eye injuries due to

TABLE 8-3 Hurricane Categories

•Category 1	Sustained winds 74–95 mph
•Category 2	Sustained winds 96–110 mph
•Category 3	Sustained winds 111–130 mph
•Category 4	Sustained winds 131–155 mph
•Category 5	Sustained winds >155 mph

flying debris or collapse of a structure; or a person who was picked up and thrown a distance by the high winds. Electrical power to a community can be out, causing complications for the chronically ill.

Associated with many of these natural disasters are infectious diseases. Infectious diseases can quickly spread among a large gathering of displaced people who must stay in a crowded shelter or remain in a temporary outdoor shelter (tent camp) that may have poor sanitation infrastructure and little to no access to health care services. However, an infectious disease by itself can become a natural disaster, turning into an epidemic or pandemic event. The recent worldwide preparations for the H1N1 flu brought the seriousness of a pandemic event to the forefront. An epidemic or pandemic event can quickly overwhelm the health care systems and create a shortage of HCPs who themselves become ill. Additionally, there are secondary complications to many diseases that will need to be treated; for example influenza can lead to respiratory complications and pneumonia, and the HCPs could run short of ventilation equipment.

Man-made Disasters

Man-made disasters refer to disasters caused by people, such as transportation accidents and acts of terrorism or industrial incidents. Natural disasters can become a combination natural disaster—man-made disaster; for example, an earthquake can break gas lines and the escaping gas catches fire or, as seen in the recent Japan earthquake in March 2011, a nuclear power plant can be affected, with resulting radioactive emissions into the atmosphere. The man-made disasters that will be discussed are chemical release, explosion, infrastructure incidents, transportation accidents, radiation release, and terrorism.

Chemical release accidents are a life-threatening event that can cause severe damage to the environment. The use of chemical weapons is still a reality based on modern-day incidents such as the domestic terrorism that occurred in Japan when sarin gas was released in several subways by a group of individuals and when chemical weapons were used on the Kurd population by the Iraqi government in the town of Halabja in March 1988 (Table 8-4). Chemicals can be flammable, toxic, and/or caustic. Chemicals can cause permanent respiratory tract damage, skin burns, and diseases and permanently damage the eyes.

There are a myriad number of ways explosions occur, such as bombs and other weapons of mass destruction, various types of factory explosions, gas tank explosions, and explosions inside mines. Explosions have the potential to injure all body parts, challenging HCPs in determining the injuries that require immediate treatment to preserve the life of the patient (life over limb). There will be injuries that are common to many explosions, such as penetrating wounds, blast soft tissue injuries (liver, spleen, and lungs), fractures, and burns, but there will also be injuries unique to the disaster. It is recommended that HCPs be familiar with the factors that exist in their local and regional area that can contribute to the occurrence of an

Table 8-4 Specific Chemical Agents

Type of Agent	*General Information*	*Mechanism of Action*	*Signs and Symptoms*
Nerve agent	Most toxic of known chemical agents; often cause death in minutes due to respiratory obstruction and cardiac failure.	Bind with acetylcholinesterase, thus not allowing it to act on the myoneural junction of muscles, causing paralysis of the muscles.	Rhinorrhea, extreme difficulty breathing, apnea, seizure, paralysis, loss of consciousness
Vesicants	"Blister agents," commonly known as mustard gas.	Necrosis of the epidermis, severe conjunctivitis, and if inhaled, injury to the mucosal tissues of the larynx and tracheobronchial tree.	Skin blisters and burning of the skin and eyes, airway injury causing difficulty in breathing, conjunctivitis that varies in severity
Choking agents	Most common agents are phosgene and diphosgene. Cause severe irritation of the upper and lower respiratory tracts.	Absorbed by inhalation. Reactions occur at the level of the alveolar–capillary membrane.	Pulmonary edema; eye, nose, and throat irritations; choking; coughing; tightness in the chest; development of fatal pulmonary edema during 2- to 24-hour period

explosion, such as types of factories and industries, and the injuries that may be seen if an incident occurs.

Infrastructure incidents include the collapse of roads, bridges, and structures. The incidents can be caused by a natural disaster such as an earthquake, flood, tornado, hurricane, or avalanche or be due to poor maintenance or poor construction. It has been recognized that the infrastructure of the United States is rapidly deteriorating and must be addressed. The collapse of the I-35W bridge in Minneapolis and the failure of the New Orleans levee system highlight the deterioration that is occurring (Figure 8-3). Infrastructure incidents primarily cause crushing injuries and severe lacerations.

Transportation accidents are infrequent but tend to remain in the minds of people due to their large scope of injuries and fatalities. Transportation accidents include wrecks that involve multiple vehicles, such as the 34 vehicles involved in a pile-up in November 2010 on I-25 in Colorado due to icy conditions, and airplane and train accidents. HCPs will be treating severe lacerations, fractures, crushing injuries, burns, and eye injuries.

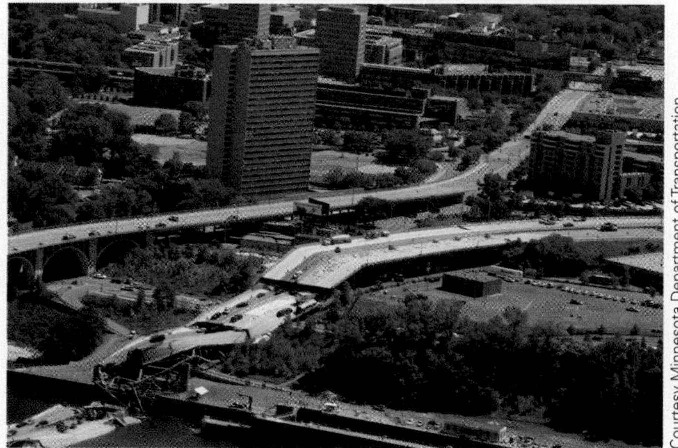

Figure 8-3 Collapse of I35W bridge, Aug. 1, 2007

Radiological injuries in the civilian population will most likely occur due to the detonation of an improvised nuclear device or radiological dispersal device referred to as a "dirty bomb" or because of a nuclear power plant accident. The primary injuries related to exploded nuclear devices that occur are blast injuries, thermal/flash burns, and ionizing radiation injuries. Additionally, flash blindness may occur as a result of peripheral vision of the intense light energy that is produced by a blast. Retinal burns may occur, resulting in scarring, permanent altered vision, or blindness. Many patients will suffer a combination of these injuries. Radiation exposure because of a nuclear power plant leakage can cause mutations to occur in the cells of the body, resulting in various types of cancer. Radiological injuries greatly decrease the body's hematopoietic and immune systems, contributing to the morbidity and mortality of patients who cannot fight off bacterial and viral infections.

Terrorism is defined by the U.S. Department of Defense *Dictionary of Military and Associated Terms* as "the unlawful use of violence or threat of violence to instill fear and coerce governments or societies. Terrorism is often motivated by religious, political, or other ideological beliefs and committed in the pursuit of goals that are usually political" (Department of Defense, 2010). Terrorists use many of types of weapons to strike at the populace, including chemical, biological, radiological, and nuclear (CBRN).

Bioterrorism is the intentional use of infectious agents, or germs, to cause illness. Bioterrorism preparedness has been made a priority by the state and federal government agencies. Health care facilities may be the initial site for recognition and response to bioterrorism evens. It is imperative that all HCPs become familiar with their health care facility's Bioterrorism Readiness Plan (BRP) in preparation for a suspected or real bioterrorism attack. Bioterrorism may occur as a covert event where individuals are unknowingly exposed and an outbreak is only suspected after unusual disease clusters or symptoms are recognized. The first indication of an attack is usually when large numbers of patients present with the same set of signs and symptoms.

Biological agents can enter the body through the respiratory tract or can be absorbed through the mucous membranes, eyes, skin, or open wounds. The Centers for Disease Control and Prevention (CDC) has identified the following biological diseases as posing the highest risk to nations: anthrax, botulism, plague, smallpox, tularemia, and viral hemorrhagic fevers. Of those six, anthrax and smallpox are identified by the CDC as the two most likely biological agents to be uses as bioweapons. Patients with these diseases will probably not be surgical patients except for unusual and extenuating circumstances, such as a patient with anthrax who experiences appendicitis. But this does not mean the surgical technologist should not have knowledge of these agents and how to treat patients; given the likelihood of an epidemic combined with the national crisis, surgical technologists along with all other HCPs will be called upon to mobilize and care for patients.

Personal Disaster Planning

When a disaster situation occurs, the first question that comes to the mind of most individuals, "Is my family okay?" In many instances, until this question can be resolved, the HCP may not respond to the event or report to work, or will not be able to fully concentrate on providing care to patients. Response to a disaster begins with personal and family preparations. The following are steps to take in personal and family preparation:

- Research, identify, and familiarize yourself and family with the local and regional emergencies that could occur.
  - Research the recommended emergency procedures provided by local disaster management and public health agencies.
- Create a family emergency plan for each type of emergency.
  - Confirm children know the purpose of 911 and when to use it.
  - Adults should be familiar with health care insurance, disability insurance, life insurance, and homeowners' insurance plans.
  - Family members who are old enough should obtain certification in BLS/CPR (infant, adolescent, and adult) and first aid.
  - Communication: Be prepared that all technology will not be available, including cell phone service. Families should designate a familiar meeting place such as a nearby bus stop, parking lot, park, etc.
  - Establish an out-of-town relative and/or friend as a "communication center" if family members become separated. Every family member should know the designated person, home address, phone numbers, and e-mail address. Family members should have a prepaid phone card to call the designated person. If the family must evacuate the town or city, the designated person should be notified as soon as possible to let the person know where the family is going to relocate.
  - Family members should have the cell phone number and e-mail address of each other.
  - All emergency contact information should be kept by family members at all times in a wallet, briefcase, or backpack.
  - Practice, Practice, Practice the emergency plan.
- Family should prepare emergency supplies.
  - A "go bag" should be packed that can be quickly grabbed in the event of an evacuation that includes bottled water and nonperishable foods; cash; flashlight and batteries; battery-powered radio; battery-powered walkie-talkies; medications (make sure to replace when they expire); first-aid kit; emergency contact information of family members and the "communication center"; copies of documents; and pet supplies.
- Family should prepare essential in-home emergency supplies that include the same items as listed for the go-bag but with extra water and nonperishable foods, including pet supplies; water purification tablets; waterproof matches; camping mess kits; tools and small foldable shovel; sleeping bags; tarps with duct tape (to create a shelter outdoors if necessary); and garbage bags.

Local/Community/Regional Response

The response to a disaster situation is divided into the local and federal responses. Local governments bear the burden of primary responsibility of responding to an emergency. As seen with recent disasters, the federal government rarely becomes involved.

Overtime, the establishment of emergency response agencies has become standardized along with standardization of the "language" that is used so first-line responders and HCPs are all on the same page. Initially, all the various titles and acronyms may seem overwhelming, but as the HCP becomes familiar with the emergency response procedures, the use of the acronyms becomes second nature. The following is a summary of local response agencies, chains of command, and how a local emergency operations plan (EOP) is developed.

- National Incident Management System (NIMS)
  - All local government and nongovernment agencies must follow these federal guidelines; the NIMS must be used in order to receive federal money for all-hazards preparation.
  - Provides a national model for coordinating the emergency response of governments, public health sector, private agencies, and nongovernmental organizations to any type and size of disaster.

  - NIMS establishes: common standards so every responder has the knowledge and skills in understanding how communities take action; standard procedures for coordinating the use of resources including responders; a plan that can be adapted to any all-hazards situation no matter the size.
  - Local agencies such as the Local Emergency Management Agency (LEMA) and its components are developed under the auspices of NIMS.
- Local Emergency Management Agency (LEMA): Community agency that has the lead management and coordinating authority in response to an emergency.
  - Lead responsibility for coordinating all local agencies' (e.g., fire department, EMS, police, public health department) response to an emergency.
  - Reports to the city manager, city council, or mayor.
  - A small community's public safety department supervisor, police official, or fire department supervisor may be head of LEMA; large cities often have an Office of Emergency Management.
  - LEMA develops the local EOP; the purpose of the EOP is to designate who is in charge of what, including who will coordinate the actions of public and private agencies, including the health care sector. The plan includes maintaining an inventory of emergency response equipment and supplies, personnel training, and list of first responders including all community HCPs and their medical specialties.
    - A large part of the EOP is the all-hazards plan. The plan should be developed in such a manner that it can be applied to the response of all types of disaster and emergency situations, rather than several separate plans for each type of disaster (remember during previous discussion that disasters have similarities that can be responded to in a uniform manner).
  - Emergency Operations Center (EOC): When the appropriate local authority, such as the head of LEMA, determines a disaster situation could occur, she or he will activate the EOC. A predesignated location for establishing the EOC will have been addressed in the EOP; personnel from all responding agencies will meet at the EOC to implement the EOP and coordinate the local response.
- Incident Command System (ICS): Management system set up by LEMA to coordinate the response to a disaster; ensures all responders know their roles and duties, and whom to report to.
  - The ICS has a chain-of-command structure in order to prevent confusion and establish a single person who is in charge and gets things done through others by making assignments. The charge person is the Incident Commander (IC).
  - However, if a disaster situation is complicated and requires the input of individuals with varying skills and knowledge, a Unified Command (UC) may be established to direct the emergency response as a group effort. Each person will be in charge of a specific workforce and/or agency that will work together in implementing the EOP.
    - The UC leaders are broken down into five groups:
      - Command: Led by the IC; establishes the goals of the emergency response through the use of the EOP. The following four groups report to the IC:
        - Operations Group: Carries out the orders to achieve the EOP objectives (e.g., provide treatment to the victims at the scene of a tornado)
        - Planning Group: Gathers and documents continual updates and information on the emergency operations response and provides reports to the IC (e.g., how well are things going or not going)
        - Logistics Group: Establishes the emergency response infrastructure (e.g., transportation, supplies, food, communications, equipment including maintenance, electricity for ICS)
        - Finance and Administration Group: Records costs

Federal Emergency Response

Federal assistance must be requested through formal channels by the local and state governments. If the federal government approves the request, the ICS is still responsible for coordinating the personnel, supplies, and equipment sent to the emergency scene. When the request is made, the local and state officials should not expect federal assistance for up to 3 days or possibly longer.

- LEMA initially requests federal assistance through the state government. The governor forwards the request to the president that a federal disaster be declared, which is called a presidential declaration.
- Federal Emergency Management Agency (FEMA): division of the U.S. Department of Homeland Security (DHS). FEMA is the lead federal agency during a nationally declared emergency and coordinates providing treatment to victims and food and shelter at the emergency scene.
  - FEMA makes the decision if the emergency is eligible for federal assistance. The assistance can come in the form of prior to an anticipated disaster to ensure supplies and responders are in a position to immediately respond or after the disaster event.
- National Response Framework (NRF): Developed by the DHS; guide for coordinating the disaster relief activities by government agencies, private sector, and nongovernment agencies when a presidential declaration has been made. The guide is flexible and scalable (able to quickly adapt to a change in the size of the emergency response).
- National Disaster Medical System (NDMS): Enacts the NRF; responsible for sending medical equipment, supplies, and teams to the disaster scene. Also assists with

the transportation needs (e.g., transport injured and sick patients to hospitals). NDMS has over 100 medical teams across the United States as well as over 1,000 hospitals that are NDMS registered to which patients can be transported. Three of the more well-known specialty teams are:

- Disaster Medical Assistance Teams (DMATs): Specialized teams that can be rapidly deployed to the emergency scene to supplement the local HCPs in caring for victims. Surgical technologists are members of many DMATs. The surgical technologist who has completed additional training in preparing and applying first aid dressings, splints, starting IV lines, etc. is used on a DMAT. Additionally, the surgical technologist may be a member of a DMAT specialty surgical team such as the burn team or orthopedic team.
- Disaster Mortuary Operations Response Team (DMORT): Team members include medical examiners, pathologists, radiographers, and dental assistants who aid in recording the identification of victims.
- National Pharmacy Response Teams (NPRTs): Team members are pharmacists and pharmacy technicians who dispense drugs and provide vaccinations to the population within the disaster area.

Health Care Facility Emergency Response

Health care facilities, including hospitals, private and public clinics, long-term care facilities, and ambulatory surgery centers, have an emergency action plan (EAP—similar to an EOP) that follows state and federal emergency response guidelines as required by The Joint Commission and in order to continue to receive Medicare funding. The Joint Commission requires health care facilities to practice their EAP at least twice a year; if the health care facility has an emergency department, one of the drills must have volunteer patients in the department in order to provide hands-on training. (Additionally, the U.S. Occupational Safety and Health Administration [OSHA] requires all businesses, including health care facilities, that have more than 10 employees to have a written EAP.)

- The EAP must be scalable in order to adjust from dealing with emergencies that are relatively small (e.g., three-car accident) to large community disasters. The EAP must also address the following components of comprehensive emergency management (local, state, federal government agencies, private organizations, nongovernment agencies, and health care facilities all participate in comprehensive emergency management; therefore they are in all four components):
  - Mitigation: Identification of hazards located in the community and plans to prevent emergencies as well as reduce the dangers; for example, families that live in forested areas are advised to clear a large area of vegetation to create a zone around their house to possibly prevent it from being burned down during a wildfire.
  - Preparedness: Includes development of an EAP and establishing the health care facility EOC.
  - Response: Preparations before the emergency event and actions during and after the event; includes all first responders and health care facilities.
  - Recovery: Activities performed to aid the community in returning to as normal as possible, such as rebuilding structures and homes, rebuilding the infrastructure, and restoring the local and regional health care system. In some instances, full recovery may not be achievable, such as in the case of Hurricane Katrina; New Orleans still does not have the same level of health care services compared to pre-Katrina conditions.
- Hospital Incident Command System (HICS): The Joint Commission and federal standards require health care facilities to establish an HICS. The HICS mirrors the local ICS; it has a chain of command that specifies the roles of HCPs. The written responsibilities of HCPs are established during the preparedness phase through job action sheets. Usually the CEO of the facility is the IC. HICS allows the health care facility to work efficiently with other health facilities and responding agencies since everyone will be using the same terminology and guidelines.
- HCP responsibilities: The HCP should be familiar with the following:
  - Personal responsibilities in responding to an emergency
  - Departmental role in the health care facility
  - Chain of command
  - Knowledge of the health care facility's signals and codes to indicate there is an emergency and the type of emergency and signals/codes used during the emergency
  - Procedure for how supervisors will communicate to HCPs that the EAP is activated
  - Communication procedures with HICS and between health care facility departments
- Evacuation of patients is a serious decision due to the logistics, costs, and risks involved. However, if the decision is made not to evacuate, the consequences can be devastating, such as in the case of New Orleans during Hurricane Katrina, where several hundred people in hospitals and nursing homes died due to the decision of administrators not to evacuate.
  - Health care facility EAPs should outline an evacuation plan, including sheltering-in-place, which is moving patients to the area of the facility that has been identified as the most secure.
  - Logistical factors to consider during an evacuation include:
    - Transportation of medications, blood, and blood products
      - Challenge in preserving medications, solutions, blood, and blood products that require refrigeration. As part of the EAP, the health care facility should have an inventory of items that require refrigeration.

- Availability of backup gas-powered generators in order to keep electrical equipment running in case health care facility electrical backup generators do not work due to damage.
- HCPs should consult the pharmacist for those medications that are refrigerated but may be usable for a short period of time, such as Phenergan.
- Saving, protecting, and transporting patient medical records is of utmost importance. Hurricane Katrina brought to the forefront the challenges when chronically ill home-bound patients and hospital patients are displaced as far away as to other states, and their medical records have been destroyed.
  - It is essential in this age of advanced technology that medical records be stored electronically off-site in remote backup systems.
  - Laptops should be available to use at a medical facility in case the electricity goes out and the backup generators are damaged; laptops have batteries that allow them to be used for a short period of time.
  - Evacuation plans should include the procedures for the transportation of medical records. In the instance of an impending disaster, medical records can be stored on USB/thumb drives, DVDs, or electronic devices such as the iPad®.
- The EAP should include memorandums of understanding (MOUs) that are agreements with other health care facilities to receive patients during an evacuation situation.
  - The health care facility should take into consideration the distance to the receiving facility.
  - The health care facility should take into consideration, when approaching a facility about an MOU, whether that facility can care for the types of patients at the health care facility (e.g., facility has open heart surgery patients and receiving facility must have capacity to care for those patients).
- Factors to consider when evacuating patients:
  - Account for all health care facility staff and patients at the evacuation site.
    - The evacuation plan should include the safest location or area where patients will be moved from their health care facility room to where they will wait to be transported to the next receiving facility; this is called the staging area.
    - The evacuation plan must include the use of a form for tracking the location of patients; this is especially important if the patient is transferred or relocated more than once. The form should include health care facility patient identification number, time patient was transported, where the patient was transported, medications and equipment sent with the patient, medical record sent with patient or where it can be located, nearest relative or friend notified of transfer including the person's name and contact information, and primary physician notified of the patient's transfer.
  - Health status of the patient:
    - Chronically ill
    - Recently had surgery or possibly the day of the evacuation
    - Equipment to be moved with the patient, in particular ventilator support
    - Mobility of the patient—able to walk on his or her own or need to be transported by wheelchair or stretcher. Even if the patient can walk, he or she should be closely observed at all times by an HCP.
    - Disabilities—limb prostheses, visual or hearing impaired, arthritis, neurologically impaired
  - Surgical technologists can play a valuable role in the evacuation and transportation of patients due to their knowledge of patient positioning, transporting, and patient factors to be taken into consideration.

Medical Office EAP

The EAP should be developed based on the community emergency response plans and coordinated with the local and regional health care system.

- The medical office EAP should address the following items:
  - Procedures for notifying employees of an emergency
  - Procedures for evacuating the medical office building, to include a common central meeting place in order to account for all the staff and patients that were in the building; transporting patients with disabilities and/or limited range of motion; shutting off gas and oxygen and other critical systems.
  - Some medical offices are sophisticated enough that they can serve as a limited receiving facility of patients being evacuated from other facilities, patients transported to the office, or walk-ins from the scene of an emergency.

Immediate Response to an All-Hazards Event

The following information is based on the immediate response of first responders to the scene of a disaster.

- First and foremost, health care responders should not enter the scene of a disaster without ensuring it is safe in order to mitigate the potential for additional casualties.
  - It may be necessary to first allow industry specialists such as electricians, firefighters, and public safety individuals to enter the scene to remove hazards such as downed electrical wires or put out fires. Additionally, health care responders should not enter a home or other building that has sustained damage until it has been declared structurally safe and sound.
  - If the emergency is a CBRN disaster, health care responders trained in those specific disasters will be deployed (e.g., trained in patient decontamination procedures, including removal and proper disposing of

contaminated clothing, and handling of chemicals used to decontaminate the skin).
    - Health care responders will need to create a safe zone as soon as possible for setting up the triage and initial treatment area. Law enforcement personnel should be employed to protect the safe zone and prevent admittance by the general public.
    - By the time a safe zone is created and health care responders have arrived at the disaster scene, LEMA will have been activated as well as the establishment of an EOC. Some type of communication system will need to be established between the safe zone and the EOC.
- Standard Precautions and personal protective equipment (PPE): To the extent possible, health care responders should follow Standard Precautions guidelines to prevent cross-contamination. Just as in the health care facility, health care responders should assume all disaster victims are potentially infectious. There are four levels of PPE: A through D; the IC determines the level. Level A indicates the highest level of protection, such as when a chemical spill occurs and the responders are wearing the fully enclosed space suit, and Level D indicates the wearing of basic PPE (medical mask, eye protection, and medical mask). Hand washing, handling of sharps, and wearing of PPE should be followed by all health care responders.
    - PPE includes: protective clothing (gowns, aprons); eye and face protection (mask with attached face shield, goggles); hand protection (latex or nonlatex examination gloves); and medical masks that cover the mouth and nose.
    - Respirators are part of the PPE; they must be worn at the disaster scene when the airborne contamination exceeds the OSHA permissible exposure limit (PEL). Each individual must be fit-tested to make sure the respirator forms a firm seal.
    - In the field, the health care responder will most likely not have access to a hand-wash station. However, the hands need to be cleaned between treating patients; therefore, waterless solutions are available, such as alcohol-based foams, hand sanitizers, or wipes.
- Patient decontamination area: Decontamination of patients is particularly important when it is a radiological or chemical disaster.
    - A separate shelter from the main treatment area should be set up that includes separate rooms for males and females.
    - Uninjured non–health care individual(s) who came to the aid of contaminated victim(s) to transport to the treatment area must also undergo the decontamination procedure.
    - The decontamination process will vary with the type of disaster:
        - Radiological decontamination procedure: Clothing should be removed as soon as possible; up to 90% of the radiological contamination will be eliminated with removal of the clothing, which should be placed in a sealed waterproof and vapor-resistant bag. If the victim has any wounds, those should be first addressed by thoroughly irrigating with normal saline. Intact skin and hair should be decontaminated with warm water and soap. Injured patients or patients who feel ill from the radiological exposure may be brought into the decontamination area on a stretcher and health care responders will need to perform the decontamination procedure.
        - Chemical decontamination procedure: The initial treatment of the patient contaminated with a chemical agent is removal of the clothing. The skin and wounds are decontaminated with 0.5% sodium hypochlorite (household bleach; one part bleach mixed with nine parts water) and thoroughly irrigated with normal saline. The solution is contraindicated for use on brain and spinal cord wounds, the eyes, and the peritoneal cavity.
    - Disposable sponges and towels should be used.
    - Gowns or other clothing should be available to provide to the victim to prevent hypothermia and for the non–health care uninjured.
- Triage of victims: Triage is the process of sorting victims according to their injuries and physiological status in order to maximize the medical resources that are available. The goal is to provide treatment to as many patients as possible while spreading out and making the most of the medical resources.
    - Individuals who usually have the most training in triage are emergency medical technicians and emergency medicine physicians.
    - Surgical technologists may complete training in performing triage and/or serve in support roles such as providing BLS/CPR, first aid treatment, and transporting patients.
    - A separate triage area should be established in the treatment area. However, triage can occur in several locations; for example, if a building collapses during an earthquake, the initial triage will most likely occur at the scene. Once the victims arrive at a health care facility, they may be triaged a second time.
    - Patients should be tagged if possible to indicate the triage category (further information on categories is given later).
    - A separate ambulance loading area should be established. A team should be assigned to the loading area, with one person who is assigned to coordinate the actions of the team as well as remain in communication with the IC and receiving health care facilities to make the decisions on where patients should be transported.
    - The individual performing the triage of patients should follow some basic guidelines:
        - She or he does not provide patient care; if he or she did so, the other patients would be delayed in being triaged and provided care by the treatment teams.

- Assessment of each patient should take no longer than 1 minute; the person should move quickly from patient to patient.
- Patients will need to be constantly reassessed; for example, a patient may have injuries that are not deemed to be life threatening, but his or her physiological condition deteriorates, requiring re-categorization.
- The triage person will have difficult decisions to make based on the goal of providing quality treatment to as many patients as possible while using medical supplies and manpower in an economic fashion. Patients who would normally be provided a good amount of individual attention and a large number of medical supplies used may only receive basic first aid treatment and be transported as soon as possible.

- A popular system of triage is "Simple Triage and Rapid Treatment" (START). START uses four categories in which to place patients: DIME (Delayed, Immediate, Minimal, Expectant). See Table 8-5.
  - A triage tag is attached to the patient and treatment is based on the color of and information written on the tag.

TABLE 8-5 DIME Triage Categories

Minor—Green Tag
- "Walking wounded"
- Minor injuries—sprains, minor cuts
- Self-care
- Physiologically stable and will remain so

Delayed—Yellow Tag
- Airway is patent
- Bleeding has been treated and controlled
- Patient is physiologically stable
- Injuries may be serious, but transport can be delayed

Immediate—Red Tag
- Quick, short immediate treatment intervention can stabilize the patient, such as establishing an airway and treating bleeding
- Treatment must be given during the "golden hour" (within 1 hour) in order for victim to survive
- Once stabilized, the patient may be re-categorized to delayed depending on extent of injuries; if it involves head or spine injury, penetrating wound, or fracture(s), patient should be transported as soon as possible

Expectant—Black Tag
- Injuries are so extensive patient is not expected to survive; use of medical resources is not advisable in order to use for the other three categories of patients
- Victim is made as comfortable as possible and pain relief given

- Triage of chemical and nuclear disaster victims requires a separate system of triage in order to contain the contamination. The patients are triaged three times:
  - Hot zone: Central area where the disaster occurred. Level A PPE should be worn. Patient is quickly assessed for airway patency and severe hemorrhage.
  - Warm zone: Triage zone 300 feet or more from the hot zone. Patients are quickly triaged into the four categories.
  - Cold zone: Triage zone near the warm zone where patients are evaluated for injuries secondary to severe injuries and transported to a facility.

- Point of Distribution (POD) site: A POD is a temporary site for providing vaccines and medicines to a large population, called mass prophylaxis.
  - Strategic National Stockpile (SNS): Centers for Disease Control and Prevention (CDC) storage of medications and vaccines that are divided into push packs; push packs are containers with the medications and vaccines that can be quickly shipped to the disaster scene. The local EOP addresses the establishment of PODs and receiving and distribution of medications and vaccines.
  - Two phases of delivering of push packs: First phase—the push packs do not include medications for chronic diseases such as diabetes; second phase—the ICS has been able to evaluate specific medications that are needed and the estimated amount and communicate this to the federal government, which has contracted with the pharmacy manufacturers, called vendor-managed inventory.
  - National Pharmacy Response Team will be present at the push-pack arrival site and will inventory the packs, repackage them, and distribute to the PODs.
  - Distribution is achieved by "pull" and "push": Pull—patients come to the PODs; push—medications and vaccines are delivered to people at their homes.
- Risk communication with the public: This is communicating information to the public in as timely and accurate of manner as possible about the disaster.
  - Questions from the media and public should be referred to the appointed spokesperson, who usually is the public information officer (PIO).
  - When a disaster occurs, methods of communication can be destroyed; therefore unique strategies for communicating with the public will need to be established.
    - Normal communication methods will include television, e-mail to laptops and cell phones, reverse phone call service, radios, and newspapers.
    - Disaster communication methods include disseminating written information that includes where the

PIO will be conducting briefings; law enforcement, EMS, and fire department personnel going from door to door; and neighborhood watch groups assisting in going from door to door.
    - Barriers to communication include language barriers, elderly who do not understand, hearing impairment, and young children.
- Moral, ethical, and legal issues associated with providing care during a disaster
  - During a disaster situation, HCPs must make quick decisions on how to treat a patient and carry forward with the treatment plan. However, as previously mentioned, HCPs will be faced with difficult decisions based on limited medical resources and supplies and using those resources to benefit the largest number of people possible.
    - For example, a patient with a severe head injury who is not responding may have to be triaged as expectant, whereas the individual who can be quickly stabilized by just establishing an airway will receive the most immediate attention. There will not be time to debate moral and ethical issues of preservation of life and dying and death at the scene of a disaster.
    - Another example is the distribution of a limited number of ventilators. Questions to consider ahead of time on who will receive ventilation support include whether it should be based on age, health status (patient with no secondary illnesses compared to the patient with comorbid illnesses), and/or economic status.
  - Hurricane Katrina brought forth many legal aspects of treating disaster victims. The post-Katrina lawsuits highlighted the vulnerability of HCPs during a disaster situation. For example, there are legal issues that state and federal governments are trying to resolve as related to health care responders who are from out of state to ensure they are protected under the state's medical laws. Additionally, there is debate as to whether health care responders to a disaster scene should be protected from being sued due to the difficult, quick treatment decisions that must be made.
  - Another issue during a disaster situation that HCPs must remember is that medical care life goes on—meaning that not only must the disaster victims be treated, but patients from all of the population will continue to need health care treatment and surgery. Women will still come to the hospital needing emergency cesarean sections; people will still have heart attacks not related to the disaster situation; people with chronic illnesses will still need treatment.
- Emergency System for the Advanced Registration of Volunteer Health Professionals (ESAR-VHP) and Community Emergency Response Team (CERT):
  - ESAR-VHP: Each state as an ESAR-VHP system to preregister health professional volunteers who can respond to an emergency within their state and out of state. The volunteers are deployed through the Emergency Management Assistance Compact (EMAC), an interstate agreement to coordinate the deployment of medical supplies and equipment, and health care volunteers.
  - CERT: Individuals who wish to be a member of CERT complete training through an agency such as the fire or police department; they are trained in all-hazards preparation and basic response such as fire safety, basic first aid, and search and rescue. The nearest program can be found on the CERT web site, www.citizencorps.gov.

CASE STUDY A female patient is undergoing a breast biopsy. The surgeon has injected the incision site with 1% xylocaine. A few minutes into the operation, the patient reports to the anesthesia provider that she is feeling an overall itching sensation. The anesthesia provider confirms that the patient's skin has broken out into hives. Within seconds the patient is experiencing difficulty in breathing and slight hypotension and tachycardia.

1. **Based on these signs and symptoms, what is the patient experiencing?**
2. **What is the first priority of the surgical team?**
3. **What is the first drug that will be administered to the patient, and what are the actions of the drug?**
4. **What drug is given to slow the chain of events that caused the reaction to occur?**

Questions for Further Study

1. What are three signs of malignant hyperthermia?
2. What can be used to prevent bleeding through suture needle holes when repairing or anastomosing vessels?
3. What pharmacological agent is often added to xylocaine and other types of local anesthetic agents to lengthen the time of effectiveness?
4. When a patient experiencing a sudden cardiac arrest has an advanced airway in place, how many breaths should be provided to the patient?
5. What solution is used to decontaminate the skin and superficial wounds of patients who have been exposed to chemical agents?

BIBLIOGRAPHY

Association of Surgical Technologists. (2011). *Core curriculum for surgical technology* (6th ed.). Littleton, CO: Author.

Berg, R. A., Hemphill, R., Abella, B. S., et al. (2010). Part 5: Adult basic life support: 2010 American Heart Association guidelines for cardiopulmonary resuscitation and emergency cardiovascular care. *Circulation, 122*(suppl 3), S685-S705.

Bowen, D. R. (2009). Intraoperative thermoregulation. In J. J. Naglehout & K. L. Zaglinicny (Eds.), *Nurse anesthesia* (4th ed.). Philadelphia: W. B. Saunders.

Centers for Disease Control and Prevention. (2002). *Anthrax.* Retrieved from http://www.cdc.gov/nczved/divisions/dfbmd/diseases/anthrax/

Centers for Disease Control and Prevention. (2002). *Facts about botulism.* Retrieved from http://www.bt.cdc.gov/agent/botulism/factsheet.asp

Cieslak, T. J., & Eitzen, E. M. (2002, July–August). Clinical and epidemiological principles of anthrax. *Emerging Infectious Diseases, 5*(4). Retrieved from http://www.cdc.gov/ncidod/EID/vol5no4/cieslak.htm

Department of the Army. (2004). *Emergency war surgery* (3rd ed.). Washington, DC: Government Printing Office.

Field, J. M., Hazinski, M. F., Sayre, M. R., et al. (2010). Part I: Executive summary: 2010 American Heart Association guidelines for cardiopulmonary resuscitation and emergency cardiovascular care. *Circulation, 122*(Suppl 3), S640-S656.

Lawrence, P. (2005). *Essentials of general surgery* (4th ed.). Baltimore: Williams & Wilkins.

O'Toole, M. (Ed.). (2005). *Miller-Keane encyclopedia & dictionary of medicine, nursing, & allied health* (7th ed.). Philadelphia: W.B. Saunders.

Phillips, N. F. (2007). *Berry & Kohn's operating room technique* (11th ed.). St. Louis: Mosby.

RXmed. (n.d.). *Gelfoam.* Retrieved from http://www.rxmed.com/b.main/b2.pharmaceutical/b2.prescribe.html.

Siemens Health care Diagnostics Hemostasis Technical Services. (2011). *Hemostasis basics programmed learner, part I. Dade Behring online.* Available from http://www.dadebehring.com/education/hemostasis/tutorial.htm

U.S. Department of Defense. (2010). *Joint publication 1-02, DOD dictionary of military and associated terms.* Retrieved from http://www/dtic.mil/doctrine/dod_dictionary/

Veach, L. M., & Heller, M. (2008). *Clinical medical assisting: A professional, field smart approach to the workplace.* Clifton Park, NY: Delmar Cengage Learning.

Way, L. (2002). *Current surgical diagnosis & treatment* (11th ed.). New York: McGraw-Hill.

Chapter

9

Surgical Pharmacology and Anesthesia

Case Study Amber has been scheduled for insertion of a venous access device for chemotherapy to treat right breast cancer. This procedure will be performed under local anesthesia with monitored anesthesia care supplementation. The following medications are listed on the surgeon's preference card:

a. Xylocaine 1% plain in a 10-cc vial

b. Heparin sodium 5,000 units per mL—3 mL

c. Heparin sodium 5,000 units in 500 mL saline for injection

d. Normal saline for irrigation—500 mL

1. Which one of these medications will be used to prevent Amber from feeling pain during the port insertion?
2. What are the three areas of a medication label that need to be verified when accepting medications onto the sterile field?
3. Which medication would be considered the "dilute" heparin solution? What is the concentration of this solution (units per mL)?
4. Which of these solutions would be used as the "final flush" to assure that the port and its catheter do not become occluded by a blood clot between uses? What is the total amount of heparin (in units) in this solution?
5. Which medication is used to counteract the effects of heparin sodium if too much is administered or the effects of heparin sodium are no longer desired?

Objectives

After studying this chapter, the reader should be able to:

1. Assess the action, uses, and modes of administration of drugs and anesthetic agents used in the care of the surgical patient.
2. Convert equivalents from one system to another and accurately identify, mix, and measure drugs for patient use.
3. (C) Recognize general terminology and abbreviations associated with pharmacology and anesthesia.
4. (A) Demonstrate safe practice in transferring drugs and solutions from the nonsterile area to the sterile field.
5. Demonstrate the procedure for identifying a drug or solution on the sterile field.
6. (R) Recognize the side effects and contraindications for the use of various drugs and anesthetic drugs.
7. Interpret the factors that influence anesthesia selection for individual patients.
8. List the equipment used during anesthesia administration.
9. (E) Demonstrate the precautions when identifying drugs and solutions in the operating room.
10. Interpret the principles and demonstrate the measurement and recording of vital signs.
11. Analyze how sterile technique is used in relation to anesthesia procedures.
12. Compare and contrast the roles of the surgical technologist and circulator during the administration of anesthesia.

Select Key Terms

agonist	BSS	hypnosis	pharmacodynamics
amnesia	biotechnology	indication	pharmacokinetics
anaphylaxis	buccal	induction	pharmacology
anesthesia	contraindication	intra-articular	retrobulbar
antagonist	Doppler	laryngospasm	sedative
antimuscarinic/anticholingergic	drug	NPO	topical
apical pulse	generic	PACU	volatile agents
aspiration	homeostasis	parenteral	

PHARMACOLOGY

Pharmacology is the study of medications and their actions, including drug origins, properties, and uses. A **drug** is defined as a substance used for the diagnosis, treatment, cure, mitigation, or prevention (prophylaxis) of disease or a condition. Humans have been aware of the therapeutic value of natural substances since the beginning of time. Modern pharmacology is a progressive, exact science that constantly seeks new drugs for the treatment of specific problems. Most of the drugs available on the market today have been standardized and approved for safety, dosage accuracy, and effectiveness by the U.S. Federal Drug Administration (FDA) after undergoing several phases of formal, independent testing.

Drug Sources

Drugs are derived from five primary sources. These sources are summarized in Table 9-1.

DRUG PROPERTIES

When studying pharmacology and medications, the learner must understand the major concepts that guide medication use and dosage selection. These concepts involve the properties

Table 9-1 Drug Sources

Source	*Examples*	*Additional Information*
Plants	morphine sulfate digitalis	At one time, the majority of drugs originated from plants; a number of plant-based medications still in use today
Animals	heparin sodium thrombin	Nonsynthetic hormones are derived from animal sources, including human sources; drugs obtained from cows are referred to as *bovine* and those from pigs as *porcine*
Minerals	calcium iron magnesium zinc	Derived from the earth, minerals, and mineral salts
Laboratory synthesis	meperidine sulfate (Demerol) aminoglycoside antibiotics	The majority of drugs used today are manufactured in the laboratory; laboratory synthesis is accomplished by two methods: • Synthetic drugs—manufactured totally from laboratory chemicals • Semi-synthetic drugs—natural substances that are chemically altered
Biotechnology	hepatitis B vaccine	The newest source of drugs from the laboratory; results from a process known as genetic engineering or *recombinant DNA technology* artificially constructed by introducing foreign DNA into the DNA of a specific organism; the two types of DNA combine and the new DNA and its specific protein are replicated in the daughter cells of the organism.

of pharmacologic agents, including **pharmacodynamics** and **pharmacokinetics.**

Pharmacodynamics

Pharmacodynamics involves the study of the interaction of drug molecules with the target cells of living tissue. Types of drug interactions include inhibition or destruction of foreign organisms or malignant cells; protection of cells from foreign agents; supplementation or replacement of specific hormones, vitamins, or enzymes; and increasing or decreasing the speed of a physiologic function. Certain variables, such as the type of drug, dosage, route of administration, and patient condition, affect various aspects of pharmacodynamics.

MEDICATION ACTION

Medications can interact with patient tissues and with other medications in several ways. Drug interaction can occur when two substances are prescribed concurrently, causing a modification of the action of one or both drugs. Drug interaction may be intentional (beneficial) or undesirable (detrimental).

Agonists

An agonistic interaction occurs when a drug potentiates or enhances the effect of another substance. The agonistic medication binds to a specific receptor site in the body, producing an alteration in biological function. Synergists and additives are two examples of agonists.

Synergistic Agents

Synergists act in combination to produce a stronger or more powerful effect than would be demonstrated if each agent was administered individually. In a synergistic relationship, the action of one agent increases the action of the other agent when delivered together. As a result, each agent can be given in a lower, sometimes safer dose while obtaining the same desired effect. The use of midazolam (a **sedative**) and fentanyl (a narcotic analgesic) permits the use of lower concentrations of volatile gases during the administration of general inhalation **anesthesia**.

Additive Agents

Medication additives alter some aspect of the action of the original agent. An example of an additive is the addition of epinephrine to the local anesthetic lidocaine to prolong the anesthetic action.

Antagonists

An **antagonist** binds to the agonist's receptor site, preventing the **agonist** from binding there and causing its desired effect. This results in an absence of the agonist's action, referred to as agonist reversal. This interaction is demonstrated when flumazinil (Mazicon®) is given to reverse the sedative effects of midazolam HCl (Versed®).

THERAPEUTIC ACTION

The therapeutic action of a medication describes the application or situation for which the medication is used and the timing of the effects commonly associated with a given medication and dosage. Terms associated with the therapeutic action of medications include:

- **Indication**: The indication is a listing of the medical conditions that the medication is known to treat. The dosage for each indication, as well as the delivery form, may vary according to the patient's medical condition, weight, and age.
- **Contraindications**: The contraindications are a list of circumstances or medical conditions under which the medication should not be used. Depending on the medication and how it is metabolized in the body, common contraindications for medication use include pregnancy, liver failure, or renal failure.
- Onset: The onset of a medication is the period of time required for the effects of the medication to begin to be demonstrated in the patient.
- Peak Effect: The peak effect time is the period of time when the maximum effect(s) of the medication are demonstrated in the patient.
- Duration: The duration is the overall period of time when the effects of a medication are demonstrated in the patient.

The timing of medication administration will depend on the time of onset, peak effect, and duration of action.

MEDICATION EFFECTS

The goal of medication administration is to provide the patient with chemical preparations designed to assist in the treatment of illness or disease. When the correct dosage is appropriately applied, medications are able to affect illness or disease by preventing, improving, or treating the medical conditions. Improper dosages of medications can have little or no effect, or can be harmful, or even toxic, to the patient. Medication effects include:

- Therapeutic effect: The concentration or dose of a medication used to produce the desired result without producing harmful effects.
- Side effect: An expected, undesirable, but tolerable effect of a medication. These can include symptoms such as dry mouth, constipation, diarrhea, dizziness or drowsiness.
- Adverse effect: An undesirable and potentially harmful effect of a medication that can lead to organ damage or failure. Susceptible organs include the brain, liver, kidney, and cardiovascular system. Some predictable adverse reactions can be avoided or altered by considering certain factors such as patient age and weight, and the timing of drug administration. A common adverse reaction is hypersensitivity or allergic reaction, which can range from mild skin irritation to **anaphylaxis**.
- Toxic effect: An undesirable and unacceptable effect of a medication. The effect can include the promotion of growth of cancerous tumors (carcinogens) or the development of birth defects (teratogens).
- Tolerance: A reduction in the effect of a medication given at the same dose over a period of time. The dosage of the medication must be increased in order to achieve the desired effect.
- Addiction: A physical or psychological dependency on the effect of a medication.

PHARMACOKINETICS

Pharmacokinetics is the term used to describe the metabolic processing of a drug within the body. The processes of *pharmacokinesis* involve absorption, distribution, biotransformation, and excretion.

Absorption

A drug must be absorbed to produce an effect. Absorption occurs at the site of administration, where the substance is eventually taken into the bloodstream by the capillaries. This process is referred to as *passive transport*. The drug is transferred from an area of higher concentration to an area of lower concentration until the concentration on both sides of the cell membrane is equal. Passive transport requires no energy. Most drugs are transported in this manner.

Active transport is required for a limited number of drugs. An energy source in the form of a cation, such as sodium, is required to carry the substance from an area of lower concentration to one of higher concentration.

The rate of absorption affects the final action of a substance. Absorption is influenced by several factors that include the type of drug preparation, dosage, route of administration, and the patient's condition. For example, a liquid that has been injected will be absorbed more quickly than an ingested tablet that must dissolve prior to being absorbed. Rapid absorption is not always desirable. A drug intended for local use must remain at the site of administration to be effective. The vasoconstrictor epinephrine can be added to a drug preparation to slow absorption.

Distribution

Distribution involves the transport of a medication within the body once it enters the circulatory system. Medication is distributed to the target cells for action, to the liver for biotransformation, and to the liver or kidneys for elimination.

Table 9-2 Drug Administration Routes

Categories	Routes	Definitions
Enteral: Through the gastrointestinal tract		
	Oral (PO, meaning *per os* or by mouth)	Placed in the mouth and swallowed
	Rectal	Placed into the rectum
Parenteral: Other than through the gastrointestinal tract; by injection		
	Intradermal	Placed between the layers of the skin
	Subcutaneous (SC or SQ)	Placed into the adipose (fat) tissue layer under the skin
	Intramuscular (IM)	Placed within a muscle
	Intravenous (IV)	Placed directly into a vein
	Intra-articular	Placed within a joint
	Intrathecal	Placed into the subarachnoid space
	Intracardiac	Placed into the heart
Topical: Applied to the skin or mucous membrane to provide a localized or systemic effect		
	Buccal	Placed between the cheek and the teeth/gums until it is dissolved and/or absorbed
	Sublingual	Placed under the tongue until it is dissolved and/or absorbed
	Instillation	Placed in a hollow or cavity, such as the conjunctival fold or bladder
	Inhalation	Directly administered to the respiratory tract, usually as a gas or aerosol

The distribution of medication is affected by the rate of absorption, systemic circulation (cardiovascular function), and regional blood flow to the target organ or tissue. The medication is transported not only to the intended target tissue, but also to all parts of the body, where effects other than those that are intended may be noted. The distribution of a medication is also affected or limited by plasma protein binding, tissue binding, and certain barriers established by the body, such as the placental barrier and the blood–brain barrier.

Biotransformation

Biotransformation or metabolism of a drug most often occurs in the liver, but other tissues, including the intestinal mucosa, lungs, kidneys, and blood plasma, may be involved. Several medications are converted to an active substance by the liver, but the main function of the liver in drug metabolism is to break down the drug molecules in preparation for excretion. The products of metabolic breakdown are called *metabolites*. They are smaller, inactive substances.

Excretion

The effect of medication in the body continues until it is biotransformed and/or excreted. Medications are physiologically removed from the target organ or tissue via the circulatory system in either an intact or biotransformed (changed or inactivated) state. The kidneys are primarily responsible for the filtration of medications from the blood and elimination of medications and metabolites as part of urine formation and excretion. Some medications and metabolites may be eliminated fecally, via sweat or saliva, or exhaled. Some medications are also eliminated in breast milk, which may affect the breastfed baby.

ROUTES OF ADMINISTRATION

The route of administration is the method used to deliver the medication into the body. Some drugs are formulated in several different ways to allow administration via several routes. The most common routes of administration for medications in the operating room (OR) are **parenteral**, with intravenous (IV) administration being the most common. Drug administration routes, found in Table 9-2, include enteral, parenteral, and **topical**.

DRUG STANDARDS

Medications for use in the United States are required to undergo review and approval by the FDA. Listings of approved drugs and formulas are found in several publications noted in Table 9-3.

TABLE 9-3 Drug Publications

Publication Name	*Type of Drug Information*
National Formulary	Contains information on single drugs and the formulas for drug mixtures; includes drug testing and purity information; lists drugs using generic names; lists medications no longer included in the USP
Pharmacopeia of the United States (USP)	Contains information on medications used in current medical practice; lists drugs using generic names; includes the medication source, properties, category/classification, dosage range, and therapeutic dosages
American Hospital Formulary Service Index	Presents medical information arranged in therapeutic or pharmacological classes according to generic name
Physician's Desk Reference (PDR)	Not an official pharmacological listing, but commonly used by physicians for referencing medications for prescription; medications are listed alphabetically by manufacturer using their brand names
The Joint Commission National Patient Safety Goals	The National Patient Safety Goals include policies on "Look-alike/sound-alike medications" and the "Official Do Not Use" abbreviation list

TABLE 9-4 Forms of Drug Preparation

Category	*Subcategory*	*Types*	*Definition/Example*
Gas			Oxygen and nitrous oxide are included in this category
Liquid			Two primary types of liquid preparations: solution and suspension
	Solution		Drug (solute) is dissolved in a liquid (solvent)
		Aqueous	Solution prepared with water
		Syrup	Sweetened aqueous solution
		Tincture	Solution prepared with alcohol
		Elixir	Sweetened alcohol solution
	Suspension		Solid particles are suspended in a liquid—particles may settle and must be redistributed by shaking prior to administration of a suspension
	Emulsion		Combination of two liquids that cannot mix—droplets of one liquid are dispersed (suspended) throughout the other
Solid			Powder is considered a solid form of a drug—it may be in the powdered state, contained within a capsule, or compressed into tablet form—some powders must have liquid added (called reconstitution) prior to use—troches or lozenges also fall into this category
Semisolid			Creams, foams, gels, lotions, ointments, and suppositories

DRUG FORMS

Drugs are prepared for administration in several different forms. The type of preparation or form in which the drug is available will determine its route of administration as well as the pharmacodynamics and pharmacokinetics of the medication. The forms in which drugs are prepared for administration are found in Table 9-4.

LEGAL DRUG CLASSIFICATIONS

The two legal drug classifications most commonly used are prescribed medications and over-the-counter medications. To better understand the two classifications, the related term "controlled substances" is also discussed.

TABLE 9-5 **Controlled Substances Act**

Schedule Or Class	Description	Examples
I	Includes substances for which there is a high abuse potential and no current approved medical use	heroin, marijuana, LSD, other hallucinogens, and certain opiates and opium derivatives
II	Includes substances that have a high abuse potential and a high ability to produce physical and/or psychological dependence and for which there is a current approved or acceptable medical use	morphine sulfate, oxycodone, hydromorphone, meperidine, codeine, anabolic steroids
III	Includes substances for which there is less potential for abuse than drugs in Schedule II and for which there is a current approved medical use	hydrocodone, codeine, and others in combination with other drugs
IV	Includes drugs for which there is a relatively low abuse potential and for which there is a current approved medical use	benzodiazepines (Valium, Ativan)
V	Drugs in this category consist mainly of preparations containing limited amounts of certain narcotic drugs for use to treat coughing and diarrhea. (Federal law provides that limited quantities of these drugs may be bought without a prescription by an individual at least 18 years of age. The product must be purchased from a pharmacist, who must keep appropriate records; however, state laws vary, and in many states, such products require a prescription.)	cough syrups with codeine; diphenoxylate (Lomotil)

Controlled Substances

Controlled substances are those drugs with a high potential to cause psychological and/or physical dependence and abuse. The Controlled Substances Act of 1970 designates certain drugs as controlled substances, classifying these substances according to their level of addictiveness and therapeutic potential. The classification ranges from Class I, with a high potential for abuse and low therapeutic indication, to Class V, with a low potential for abuse and known positive therapeutic applications. This information is summarized in Table 9-5. The labeling of these substances includes the symbol "C" with the schedule number (I–V) included next to the letter.

TABLE 9-6 **Commonly Used Alternative Medications**

Fish Oil/Omega 3/DHA	Ginseng
Glucosamine combined with chondroitin	Vitamins E and C
Echinacea	Calcium
Flaxseed oil	B-complex vitamins
Gingko biloba	Aloe vera

Prescribed Medications

Prescription medications are those medications that, if used inappropriately, could cause significant harm to the patient. A prescription is a written order for the preparation and dispensing of a medication. The prescription includes the name, dose, quantity, and timing of a medication. The licensed health care provider is responsible for prescribing the medication and the registered pharmacist is responsible for preparing the medication according to the directions on the prescription and dispensing it to the patient for use.

Over-the-Counter Medications

Over-the-counter (OTC) medications are pharmacologic agents that are prepared in a dosage that are safe to administer without the direction of a physician. Some prescription medications can be sold OTC in lower doses. Examples include ibuprofen (Motrin, Advil); 200-mg tablets are sold OTC, but ibuprophen (Motrin) 800-mg tablets require a prescription.

Alternative Medications

Alternative medication use is becoming more predominant in today's society. Dietary supplements include nutritional supplements, herbal medicines (also known as botanicals), probiotics, vitamins, minerals, and other natural products. Some of the common alternative medications in use today are listed in Table 9-6.

These products are commonly sold "over-the-counter" and often have undergone only limited studies to determine the safety and effectiveness of these therapies, resulting in a limited understanding as to why they enhance more traditional Western medicine practices or provide treatment in and of themselves; many of the products are not U.S. FDA approved. Alternative medication supplements may interact with traditional medications, producing side effects, and may include ingredients that can be harmful, especially to pregnant women, children, and the elderly. Additionally, alternative medications may react with anesthetic drugs, causing serious reactions such as respiratory difficulties and cardiac dysrhythmias. Patients should notify their health care practitioners of all medications—prescription, OTC, and alternative medications—being used on a routine basis.

TABLE 9-7 **Example of Drug Names**

Trade Name	*Generic Name*	*Chemical Name*
Marcaine®	bupivicaine hydrochloride	2-piperidinecarboxamide, 1-butyl-N-(2,6-dimethylphenyl), monohydrochloride,
Sensorcaine®		monohydrate

MEDICATION INFORMATION

Surgical technologists are responsible for understanding basic information regarding the medications they handle on the sterile field. This information includes the names, classifications, actions, indications, uses in the surgical setting, and dosages for use in the surgical setting.

Names

Three different names are assigned to each drug. They are as follows:

- Trade, brand, or proprietary name: the name assigned to a medication and copyrighted by the manufacturer for marketing (proprietary) purposes; may include a reference to the intended use. The trade name of the medication is capitalized and may be followed by the ® symbol, indicating that the name and chemical formula used by the specific company have been registered with the federal government. There may be slight differences in the chemical preparation used by each manufacturer, making the preparation under each trade name slightly different. The trade name is prominently displayed on the medication label.
- **Generic** name: the nonproprietary name for a drug. It is often a shortened version of the chemical name. The generic name is often selected by the original developer and is written using all lowercase letters. Generic medications may be produced by several manufacturers. The generic name is prominently displayed on the medication label.
- Chemical name: the precise chemical composition and molecular structure of the medication. The chemical name is complex and difficult to use. The chemical name is not included on the medication label, but is included in the package insert that accompanies the medication from the manufacturer (Table 9-7).

Use of the generic name is advocated in the health care setting to avoid confusion between medications with similar-sounding trade names, such as oxytocin (Pitocin) and vasopressin (Pitressin). The Joint Commission publishes a "Look-alike/sound-alike" list of medications. Care should be taken to verify the generic name of the medication to reduce the potential for medication errors.

Classifications

Drugs are classified in many ways for a variety of reasons; each classification may have several subclassifications. This can be confusing, as some of the classifications overlap and a specific drug may be cross-referenced in several categories.

Drugs are classified according to their principal action, e.g., barbiturate; the organ or body system affected, e.g., neurologic agent; the physiological action produced by the drug, e.g., central nervous system depressant; or its therapeutic action, e.g., anticonvulsant. Phenobarbital is an example of a medication that fits into each of these categories.

Actions

Drug actions define the effects of the substance at the target site. Three main theories have been developed to explain the ways that a drug produces its effect(s). The theory of drug–receptor interaction states that the active substance in the drug has an affinity for a specific chemical constituent of a cell. The interaction occurs on a molecular level with a specific receptor on the cell surface or within the cell to produce the pharmacological response. The theory of drug–enzyme interaction states that a drug may combine with a specific enzyme to inhibit the action of the enzyme or alter the cellular response to the enzyme. A third type of interaction, nonspecific drug interaction, is related to a drug that does not act by either of the two previously described methods and is considered nonspecific in its interaction.

Indications

The indication is a listing of common medical conditions that a particular medication is used to treat. While any given medication may have multiple indications, the surgical technologist should be familiar with the indication(s) for use that are related to applications in the OR.

Dosage

The medication dose is the amount of medication delivered to the patient in order to achieve the desired therapeutic effect. The dose will depend on several factors, including the patient's age, weight, and overall medical condition. Other factors affecting dosage include the delivery route of the medication and recommended maximum dosage. A medication dosage is commonly expressed in a ratio of medication concentration per kilograms of patient body weight (mg/kg). An example of dosage for the use of dantrolene sodium, given to treat malignant hyperthermia, includes different dosages for the loading dose and the maintenance dose. The loading dose for dantrolene sodium is 2.5 mg/kg. The maintenance dose for dantrolene sodium is 1 mg/kg, with a maximum dose of up to 30 mg/kg. It is important for the surgical technologist to be able to perform medication calculations to determine the amount of medication to be administered as well as to accurately track and document the amount of medication delivered to the patient intraoperatively. The next section provides information and examples for performing medication calculations.

MEDICATION CALCULATIONS

Many medications used in today's OR setting are prepared in the pharmacy and transferred to the sterile field in a ready-to-use form. In some facilities and in emergency situations, medications are prepared in the OR by the surgical team. Surgical technologists must understand the concentration, therapeutic dose, and application for each and every medication on the sterile field as they actively participate in the various steps of medication administration.

Concentration

The concentration of the medication is the ratio of *solute* to *solvent*, the two components of a solution. This concentration can vary, depending on the strength of the solute and the amount of solvent added to create a solution. The concentration of medication is found on the medication label and should be checked carefully for accuracy. For medications in a powdered form that need to be reconstituted into a liquid form for administration, the manufacturer's directions on the label and in the package insert list the amount and type of solvent, commonly 0.9% sodium chloride for injection, required to create a solution with the concentration indicated on the label. An example of this is cefotetan disodium. Cefotetan disodium (Cefotan) comes in 1-gram (g) or 2-g powdered form that must be reconstituted. If given intravenously, 1 g of cefotetan disodium is reconstituted using 10 mL of sodium chloride 0.9% for injection, resulting in a concentration of 100 mg/mL, but when used for intraoperative wound irrigation, 1 g (1,000 mg) is commonly added to 500 mL of sodium chloride 0.9% for irrigation, resulting in a concentration of 2 mg/mL.

Medications can also come in a concentrated liquid form that may be used in the concentrated form or diluted for use in a less concentrated form. An example of this is heparin sodium. Heparin sodium is available in several concentrations, including 500 units per milliliter, 1,000 units per milliliter, and 10,000 units per milliliter. Normal saline for injection can be added to any of these heparin concentrations to make a dilute concentration.

Dose

The dose is the overall amount of medication delivered to the patient. The dose or dosage is documented in the patient's record as part of the "sixth right" of medication administration. On occasion, several different concentrations of the same medication are used during the same procedure. The cumulative dose of the medication should be documented.

Heparin sodium can be used in different concentrations during insertion of a venous access device. Dilute heparin solution, 10 units per milliliter, is used to irrigate the device and its catheter during placement. Concentrated heparin, 5,000 units per milliliter, is used at the "final flush" to maintain patency of the device and catheter while not in active use.

Application

The application is the medication's use in the surgical setting. Consideration should also be given to any contraindications for use, such as patient sensitivity/allergy, seen with penicillin use in the penicillin-sensitive patient, or when administering vasopressin to a patient who is hypertensive, which could lead to a hypertensive crisis.

Some medications have differing uses within the surgical setting. Lidocaine HCl is commonly used as a local anesthetic; however, lidocaine HCl can also be used as an antiarrhythmic to decrease abnormal heartbeats. The surgical technologist should be aware of how and under which situation each medication on the sterile field is used and delivered. Epinephrine, in concentrations of less than 1:100,000, can be injected as a vasoconstrictor, but in concentrations of 1:1,000, it should only be used topically to prevent serious patient complications, including death.

CALCULATING MEDICATION DOSAGES

In order to calculate medication dosages on the sterile field, the surgical technologist needs to understand two basic concepts: concentration and cumulative dose. There are two basic formulas that will assist in calculating these amounts.

Concentration

In order to calculate concentration, you need to convert the solution into units of medications per one unit of fluid; in other words, solute to solvent. This is accomplished using the following formula:

$$A : B = C : D$$

Example: If the label reads 500 milligrams per 5 milliliters:

$500 : 5 = X : 1$ (multiply the means and extremes)

$500 = 5X$

Reduce the fraction by dividing both sides by "5"

$100 = X$

When diluting a medication by adding more solvent to the solute, the concentration changes. For example, when

1 milliliter of heparin sodium 10,000 units per mL is added to 1,000 milliliters of normal saline for injection, the concentration of this medication is 10,000 units per 1,000 mL and needs to be converted using the previous formula:

10,000 : 1,000 = X : 1 (multiply the means by extremes)

10,000 = 1,000X

Reduce the fraction by dividing both sides by "1,000"

10 = X or 10 units per mL

Cumulative Dose and Conversion

The cumulative dose, the total amount of medication given to the patient, is calculated by taking the amount of solution delivered and multiplying it by the amount of solute from the previous ratio. Based on the previous example, if the surgeon used 250 milliliters of heparinized saline solution during a procedure, the patient would have received 2,500 units of heparin sodium (10 units per milliliter = × per 250 milliliter).

Another calculation commonly used in the OR setting is the conversion of patient weight between the more familiar apothecary system of pounds to the more accurate metric system. This conversion uses the formula 2.2 pounds = 1 kilogram. To convert pounds to kilograms, divide the number of pounds by 2.2. Therefore, a 185-pound patient would weigh approximately 84.1 kilograms (185 ÷ 2.2 = 84.1). In an emergency situation, weight can be estimated by dividing the pounds in half, then subtracting the first digit of the answer from the answer, e.g., 185/2 = 93 − 9 = 84.

PERCENTAGES

A percentage represents a fraction in which the denominator is always 100, but percentages are typically expressed as a whole number followed by the percent symbol, %. Percentages can also be expressed as a decimal by moving the decimal point two places to the left of the written number to indicate hundredths. Examples of converting between fractions and percentages are as follows:

75% = 0.75 or 75/100

Examples of percentage calculations:

- 15 is what percentage of 30?

  15/30 = 0.50 or 50%

- What is 20% of 80?

  Change the 20% to a decimal and multiply by 80:

  20% = 0.20 × 80 = 16

CONVERSION OF TEMPERATURE

Two scales commonly used to measure temperature include the Fahrenheit scale and Celsius scale. The monitoring of body temperature of the surgical patient is important for the following reasons:

- Preoperatively, if the patient's body temperature is not within a normal range, the surgical procedure may be delayed or canceled to determine the nature of the disorder resulting in the body temperature change. Postoperatively, a rise in temperature could indicate the possibility of a surgical site infection.
- Intraoperatively, the patient's temperature is constantly monitored by the anesthesia care provider. Hyperthermia and hypothermia affect the homeostasis of the patient's body by changing metabolic rate, blood pressure, heart rate, or circulation. Hyperthermia can be a precursor to malignant hyperthermia.
- Certain anesthetic agents affect the thermoregulatory centers in the brain, leading to the body's inability to adapt to temperature changes.

Several temperature reference points are frequently referenced, including the freezing point of water, which is 32°F or 0°C; the boiling point of water, which is 212°F or 100°C; and normal body temperature, which is 98.6°F or 37°C.

The conversion formulas for converting between Fahrenheit and Celsius scales are as follows:

(°F − 32) 5/9 = °C

(°C x 9/5) + 32 = °F

UNITS OF MEASURE

Surgical technologists may be required to calculate medication dosages and perform conversions when two or more drugs on the sterile back table need to be properly mixed. Therefore it is important to have an understanding of the metric and apothecary systems of measurement in order to perform simple calculations.

Metric System

The metric system, also referred to as the International System of Units, is based on powers or multiples of 10 and the value of numbers is established by the use and placement of a decimal point to indicate whole numbers versus fractions. Each position to the left or right of the decimal point represents a lower or higher power of 10. Table 9-8 illustrates the values of each position.

Metric, Household, and Apothecary Systems of Measurement

The metric system is the primary system of measurement used in the health care field, in particular in the measurement of drug dosages, and is the measurement system that health care providers should be most familiar with in the workplace. However, there are two other measurement systems the surgical technologist should be familiar with: the household and apothecary measurement systems.

The measurements in the metric system are based on the following units of measure:

- Length: meter (m)
- Weight: gram (g)
- Volume: liter (l)

Table 9-8 Decimal Values

15,878.674914		
1	ten thousands	10^4
5	thousands	10^3
8	hundreds	10^2
7	tens	10^1
8	ones	10^0
Decimal Point		
6	tenths	10^{-1}
7	hundredths	10^{-2}
4	thousandths	10^{-3}
9	ten thousandths	10^{-4}
1	hundred thousandths	10^{-5}
4	millionths	10^{-6}

The abbreviations used in the metric system are as follows:

- Length
  - Meter = m
  - Centimeter = cm
  - Millimeter = mm
- Weight
  - Kilogram = Kg or kg
  - Gram = g
  - Milligram = mg
  - Microgram = mcg
- Volume
  - Kiloliter = kl
  - Liter = l
  - Cubic centimeter = cc
  - Milliliter = mL or ml

Table 9 illustrates common metric conversions.

Even though the household and apothecary systems of measurement are rarely used in the medical field, it is still important for the surgical technologist to have a basic idea of the two systems. Pharmacists sometimes use the apothecary system, and therefore it is important to know the basics of the measurement system. The following abbreviations are for the household measurement system.

- Teaspoon = tsp
- Length
  - Yard = yd
  - Foot = ft
  - Inch = in
- Volume
  - Teaspoon = tsp
  - Tablespoon = tbsp

Table 9-9 Metric Conversions

Length	*Weight*	*Volume*
1 meter = 100 centimeters	1 kilogram = 1,000 grams	1 kiloliter = 1,000 liters
1 meter = 1,000 millimeters	1 gram = 1,000 milligrams	1 liter = 1,000 milliliters
1 meter = 1,000,000 microns	1 gram = 1,000,000 micrograms	
1 millimeter = 1,000 microns	1 milligram = 1,000 micrograms	

  - Ounce = oz
  - Pint = pt
  - Quart = qt
  - Gallon = gal
- Weight
  - Pound = lb

The *apothecary* system is based on the weight of a grain of wheat. In this system, 12 ounces (rather than the more commonly known 16 ounces) equals one pound. The units of measure are the *minim* for volume and the *grain* for weight. The following are the abbreviations for the apothecary system.

- Volume
  - Minim = m
  - Dram = dr
  - Drop = gtt
  - Ounce = oz
  - Pint = pt
- Weight
  - Grain = gr
  - Pound = lb

Table 9-10 provides the most common equivalents among the three measurement systems.

ABBREVIATIONS RELATED TO MEDICATION ADMINISTRATION

In recent years, a number of medication errors have been attributed to the use of abbreviations related to physician's orders and prescriptions due the similarity of certain abbreviations. The Joint Commission cautions practitioners against using abbreviations that can easily be misinterpreted. The Joint Commission recommends that the medication abbreviations in Table 9-11 no longer be used by practitioners.

TABLE 9-10 Measurement Equivalents

Length
• 1 meter = approximately 1 yard or 36.37 inches
• 2.54 centimeters = 1 inch
Volume
• 1 milliliter = 1 cubic centimeter
• 1 fluid ounce = 30 milliliters
• 1 gallon = 4 liters or 4000 milliliters
• 1 quart = 1,000 milliliters or 1 liter
• 1 pint = 500 milliliters
Weight
• 1 kilogram = 2.2 pounds
• 30 grams = 1 ounce
• 60 milligrams = 1 grain

TABLE 9-11 The Joint Commission—Offical "Do Not Use" List

Do Not Use	*Use Instead*
U (unit)	Write "unit"
IU (international unit)	Write "international unit"
Q.D., QD, q.d., qd (daily)	Write "daily"
Q.O.D., QOD, q.o.d., qod (every other day)	Write "every other day"
Trailing zero (X.0 mg)	Write X mg
Lack of leading zero (.X mg)	Write 0.X mg
MS	Write "morphine sulfate"
MSO_4 and $MgSO_4$	Write "magnesium"
Possible Future Inclusion in "Do Not Use" List	*Use Instead*
> (greater than)	Write "greater than"
< (less than)	Write "less than"
Abbreviations for drug names	Write drug names in full
Apothecary units	Use metric units
@	Write "at"
cc	Write "mL," "ml," or "millilieters"
µg	Write "mcg" or "micrograms"

TABLE 9-12 The Six "Rights" of Medication Administration

- The "right" patient
- The "right" drug
- The "right" dose
- The "right" route of administration
- The "right" time and frequency
- The "right" documentation, including labeling

DRUG-HANDLING TECHNIQUES

Drug safety is of utmost concern to all involved. Medication errors can be minimized by following some basic safety guidelines:

- Know the pertinent state and federal laws
- Know the policies and procedures of the health care facility

There are six basic "rights" for correct drug handling, as noted in Table 9-12. These six items are all components of the physician's medication order, whether written or verbal. In the OR, the list of medications commonly used for a specific procedure is found on the surgeon's preference card. The medication order for each surgical patient is finalized verbally. The surgical technologist and circulator are responsible for preparing and recording the name, amount, and delivery method used for every medication managed within the sterile field and administered to the patient, other than those given by the anesthesia care provider. Everyone on the team is responsible for making certain that these six "rights" are utilized each time a medication is administered.

MEDICATION IDENTIFICATION

Medications used in the OR are available from the manufacturer in many types of packaging, including glass, plastic, and metal containers. Each type of container requires different techniques for access or use. Common types of containers include the following:

- *Ampule:* Glass container that requires the top to be broken off to access the contents—usually contains liquid medication. Extra caution must be used when handling glass ampules to ensure that glass does not contaminate the medication upon opening the ampule (Figure 9-1).

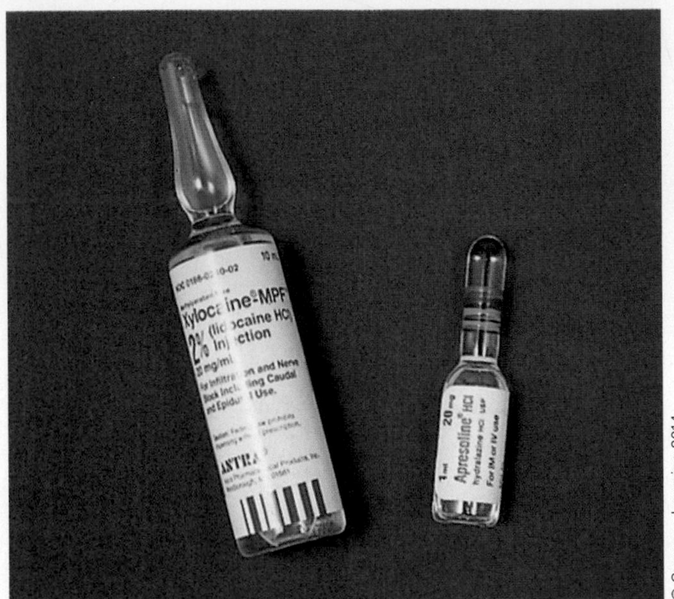

Figure 9-1 Ampules

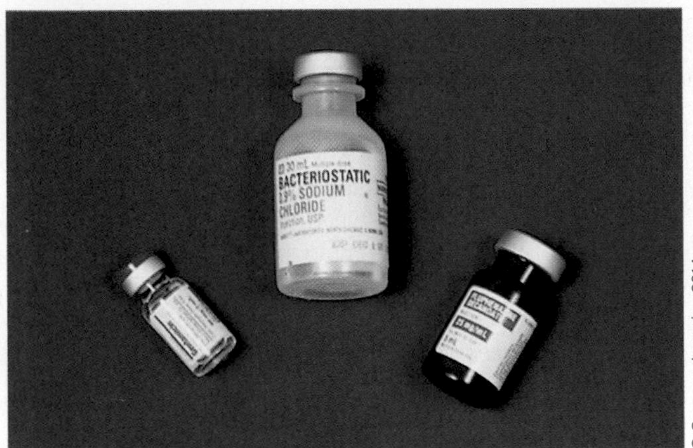

Figure 9-2 Vials

- *Vial:* Plastic or glass container that has a rubber stopper at the top that is held in place with a metal retaining ring—may contain liquid, powder, or compressed powder (Figure 9-2).
- *Preloaded syringe:* Usually contains liquid medication.
- *Tube:* Metal or plastic—may contain medication in cream, gel, or ointment forms.

No matter the type of packaging used, all drugs must be labeled by the manufacturer and the label must contain the following information:

- Drug name (trade and generic)
- Manufacturer
- Strength

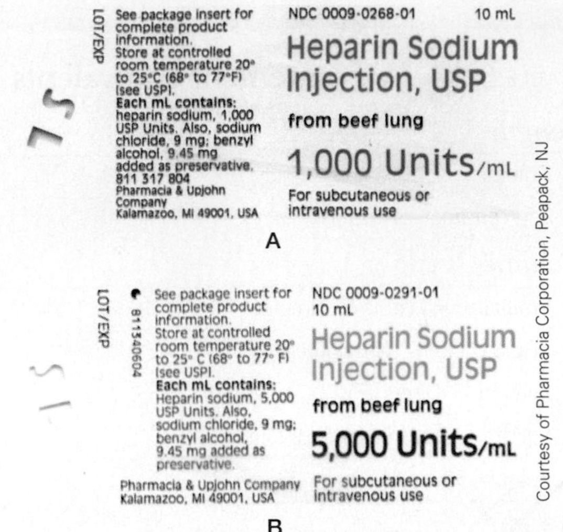

Figure 9-3 Medication label

- Amount
- Expiration date
- Route of administration
- Lot number
- Handling/storage precautions and warnings
- Instructions for reconstitution (if applicable)
- Controlled substances classification (if applicable)

Examples of medication labels are found in Figure 9-3.

The following is an example of the steps taken and the interaction that occurs between the circulator and the surgical technologist during transfer of a medication. Note that the medication name, strength, amount, and expiration date should be verified a minimum of three times prior to administration.

1. The circulator and surgical technologist check all medications and supplies prior to the start of the case (first identification/verification).
2. The surgical technologist or circulator may initiate the request to transfer a medication to the sterile field.
3. The circulator approaches the sterile field with the medication.
4. The circulator will hold the medication container so that both individuals can see the label. The circulator will read out loud the the name of the drug, strength of the drug, and expiration date (second identification/verification).
5. The medication is transferred to the sterile field using the appropriate method of transfer. The following is detailed information related to transfer of medications.
   - Various supplies are used for the reconstitution, transfer, and administration of different medications. Medications requiring reconstitution are usually mixed

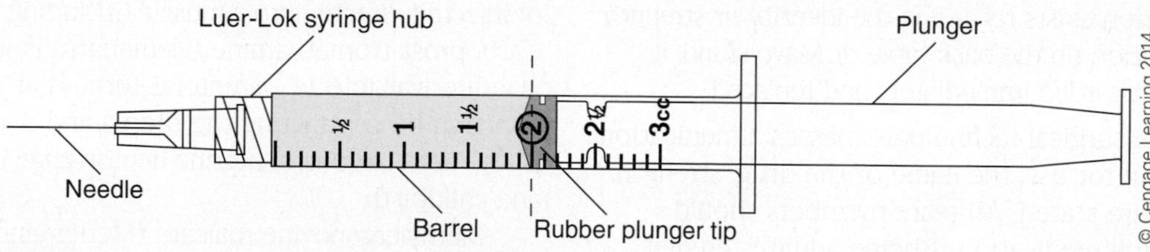

Figure 9-4 Syringe

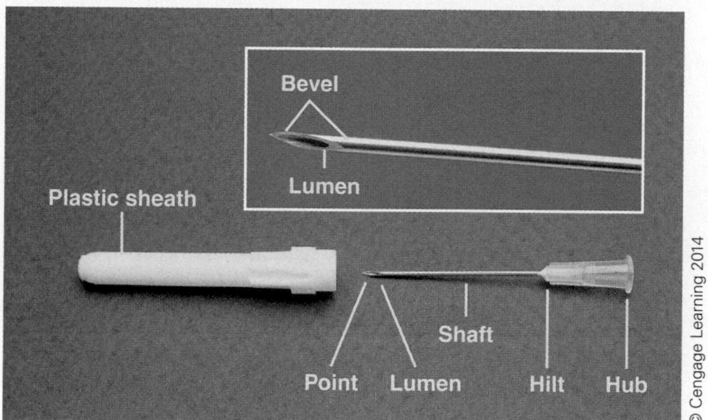

Figure 9-5 Needle

by the circulator and transferred to the sterile field. Medications are transferred to the sterile field by pouring or squeezing into a medicine cup or small basin on the sterile back table. A syringe (Figure 9-4) and hypodermic needle (Figure 9-5) are frequently used by the surgeon to inject medications. A graduated pitcher and/or Asepto syringe are use for the administration of irrigating fluids, in particular into a body cavity. Irrigation fluids commonly include an antibiotic. Occasionally, a medication is applied directly from a dropper or a tube, such as into the ear canal.

- Medications from a vial may be transferred by one of four methods:
  - Circulator cleans the stopper at the top of the vial using an alcohol wipe and holds the vial at an angle while the surgical technologist inserts a hypodermic needle attached to the syringe through the stopper and withdraws the medication.
  - Circulator inserts a sterile medication vial transfer device (a long straw-like device with a spiked end) into the vial stopper and pours the medication into a container on the back table.
  - Circulator cleans the stopper, draws the medication into a syringe using the hypodermic needle, and ejects the mediation into the container on the back table.
  - Circulator removes the metal retaining ring and rubber stopper and pours the medication into the container on the back table.
- Medications from an ampule may be transferred using one of two methods:
  - Circulator removes the top of the ampule, draws the medication into a syringe using the hypodermic needle, and ejects the medication into the container on the back table.
  - Circulator removes the top of the ampule and holds it at a slight angle while the surgical technologist withdraws the medication into a syringe via hypodermic needle.
- Medications from a tube are squeezed by the circulator onto a towel, into a small cup or directly onto a sterile dressing material on the back table.
- Some medications are provided in sterile packages by the manufacturer, allowing the contents (ampule, vial, tube, spray bottle) to be opened directly onto the back table.
- All medication containers are to remain visible for the duration of the surgical procedure for re-verification of the medication.

6. Once the medication is delivered to the sterile field, the circulator will hold the medication container so that both individuals can see the label. The surgical technologist will read out loud the name of the drug, strength of the drug, and expiration date (third identification/verification).
7. The drug(s) is/are immediately labeled with the medication name and concentration on the sterile field. Many individual and commercial techniques for labeling are available, including:
   - Sterile preprinted drug labels
   - Sterile preprinted reusable drug labels
   - Surgical-technologist-crafted labels using a sterile marking pen and a blank sterile label. If blank labels are not available, a sterile skin closure tape (Steri-Strip™) is a possible alternative.
   - It may be necessary to have the same medication in two locations on the sterile field. For example, lidocaine HCl has been drawn into a syringe that is placed on the Mayo stand and additional lidocaine HCl is in a medicine cup on the back table. The syringe and medicine cup must be clearly labeled.
   - When placing medication labels on syringes, make sure the calibrations for medication measurement on the syringe barrel are not covered.

- If any question exists regarding the identity or strength of a medication on the back table or Mayo stand, it **MUST** be discarded immediately and replaced.

8. *Every time* the surgical technologist passes a medication to the surgeon for use, the name of the drug, strength, and amount are stated. All team members should be aware that a medication is being administered; it may be particularly important for the anesthesia provider to be informed that a drug (e.g., epinephrine) is in use.

Finally, before the administration of any medication, *verify that the patient is not allergic to the medication.* It is important to note not only the patient's allergy status to medications, but to foods and other substances as well (e.g., a shellfish allergy could be indicative of an iodine allergy or an allergy to beets could indicate an allergy to dextrose that may be manufactured with beet sugar). Verification of patient allergies is performed as one component of the "time-out" preoperative verification protocol recommended by the World Health Organization (WHO) and Association of Surgical Technologists and included in The Joint Commission's Universal Protocol, which is focused on reducing patient errors in the health care setting.

MEDICATIONS IN THE OPERATING ROOM

Table 9-13 identifies some of the common pharmacologic agents used in the OR setting. Note that some agents have more than one classification, action, and use in the surgical setting. Medications used principally by the anesthesia care provider as part of the anesthesia delivery are listed in Table 9-20.

MEDICATIONS FOR USE WITH SPECIFIC SURGICAL SPECIALTIES

Obstetric and Gynecologic Surgery

Three classifications of drugs are associated with surgical interventions of the female reproductive tract—oxytocics, vasopressin, and immunoglobin. Oxytocic drugs are used to induce labor and control uterine hemorrhage associated with pregnancy and childbirth. Oxytocin (Pitocin, Syntocinon) is used to induce or continue labor, contract the uterus following vaginal or cesarean birth, and as an adjunct in the treatment of incomplete or spontaneous abortion, planned abortion, and to control uterine bleeding following an abortion. In the OR, oxytocin is most commonly used in the parenteral form, given intravenously by the anesthesia care provider or injected directly into a muscle (including the myometrium). Carboprost tromethamine (Hemabate) is a synthetic prostaglandin available in parenteral form that is used to induce abortion by contracting the uterus and dilating the cervix. It is also used to control uterine hemorrhage following abortion and childbirth.

Methylergonovine maleate (Methergine) is an ergot alkaloid that is used following abortion or delivery to control hemorrhage by causing uterine muscle contraction. It is available in oral and parenteral preparations. Ergot alkaloids are known to pass into the breast milk and may cause serious neonatal effects such as vomiting, decreased circulation to the extremities, diarrhea, weak pulse, unstable blood pressure, and convulsions. Side effects of oxytocic drugs include an increased risk of uterine rupture, irregular heartbeat (maternal), an increase in post-partum bleeding in the mother and jaundice in the neonate. The presence of certain medical conditions such as heart disease, hypertension, kidney disease, and jaundice may affect the use of oxytocics.

Vasopressin (Pitressin) is the second medication used in gynecologic surgery involving the cervix. Vasopressin is injected around the cervix during a vaginal hysterectomy, cervical conization, or into a uterine fibroid during myomectomy to reduce intraoperative bleeding.

A third medication is sometimes administered in the OR. RhoGam, an immunoglobin, is administered to Rh-negative women who are pregnant to prevent sensitization of the maternal immune system when pregnant with an Rh-positive fetus. Once sensitized, maternal Rh antibodies can cross the placenta during subsequent pregnancies, where the antibodies destroy fetal circulating red blood cells. This condition is known as erythroblastosis fetalis, hemolytic disease of the newborn, and results in newborn anemia, edema, and jaundice, which can lead to severe brain damage in the newborn or even death.

Orthopedic Surgery

Routine pharmacological supplies used in orthopedics include antibiotics, hemostatic agents, and steroids. Antibiotics are used intravenously and mixed with irrigation solutions. Polymixin, bacitracin, and cephalosporin antibiotics are mixed with irrigation solutions or injected into the bags of solution used during irrigation and/or pulsed lavage of the surgical wound.

Hemostatic agents used in orthopedic surgery include absorbable gelatin sponge (Gelfoam), microfibrillary collagen (Avitene), thrombin (Thrombinar), and bone wax (see section "Chemical Methods of Hemostasis" for further information).

Steroids are used for their anti-inflammatory action. Dexamethasone (Decadron), a short-acting corticosteroid; dexamethasone long-acting (Decadron LA); or betamethasone (Celestone), a long-acting corticosteroid, may be administered to reduce inflammation in a joint area caused by trauma, given therapeutically to treat the inflammation, or administered perioperatively to aid in reducing tissue inflammation resulting from the surgical intervention.

TABLE 9-13 **Medications Used in the Surgical Setting**

Category	Generic Name	Trade Name	Action	Indication	Surgical Use	Dosage
Adrenergics	epinephrine	Adrenalin Chloride	Causes vasoconstriction, resulting in reduced blood flow	Superficial bleeding; prolongs the effect of local anesthetics	Topical hemostasis; added to local anesthesia to prolong effect	Topical: solution of 1:1,000 applied with Kittner sponge or neurosurgical cottonoid to bleeding area—NEVER INJECTED! In local anesthesia: concentrations of 1:500,000 to 1:50,000, with most common being 1:100,000 and 1:200,000
	phenylephrine hydrochloride (HCl)	Neosynephrine	Stimulates alpha adrenergic receptors, causing vasoconstriction	Shrink mucous membranes before nasal surgery; treat malignant hypotension; pupil dilation before cataract surgery	Treatment of spinal-anesthesia-induced hypotension; shrinks nasal mucous membranes; paralyzes the iris sphincter, resulting in mydriasis—pupil dilation	100–180 mcg/minute then maintenance at 40–60 mcg/minute; 1–2 sprays of 0.5% solution; 10% solution for ophthalmic use—mydriasis
Analgesics (narcotic analgesics)	fentanyl citrate	Sublimaze	Stimulates the opioid receptors in the CNS, resulting in pain relief	Moderate to severe pain	Adjunct to general or regional anesthesia	0.5–1 mcg/kg IV over several minutes
	meperidine hydrochloride (HCl)	Demerol	Stimulates the opioid receptors in the CNS, resulting in pain relief	Moderate to severe pain	Adjunct to general or regional anesthesia	Repeated slow IV injection of 10 mg/ mL or 1 mg/mL IV infusion titrated to patient needs
	morphine sulfate	Morphine	Stimulates the opioid receptors in the CNS, resulting in pain relief	Severe pain	Adjunct to general or regional anesthesia	2.5–15 mg IV every 4 hours as needed; intrathecal injection of 0.2–1 mg for 24-hour pain relief
Analgesic—antipyretic–nonsteroidal anti-inflammatory (NSAID) agents	tromethamine	Toradol	NSAID that provides pain relief	Short-term moderately severe pain management	Postoperative pain management	60 mg IM or 30 mg IV
Antianxiety—Sedative/Tranquilizer	midazolam hydrochloride (HCl)	Versed	Depresses CNS by potentiating the effects of GABA	Sedation; reduce anxiety related to surgery	Preoperative and intraoperative sedation	0.07–0.08 mg/kg; 0.5 mg IV over a 2-minute period

(continues)

TABLE 9-13 **(continued)**

Category	Generic Name	Trade Name	Action	Indication	Surgical Use	Dosage
	diazepam	Valium	Depresses CNS by potentiating the effects of GABA	Sedation; reduce anxiety related to surgery	Preoperative and intraoperative sedation	Up to 10 mg IM or IV
	lorazepam	Ativan	Depresses CNS by potentiating the effects of GABA	Sedation; reduce anxiety related to surgery	Preoperative and intraoperative sedation	1–2 mg PO preoperative
Anti-arrhythmics	lidocaine hydrochloride (HCl)	Xylocaine, Lignocaine	Decreases depolarization and excitement of the Purkinje fibers of the heart	Ventricular arrhythmias	Emergency medication used during cardiac arrest or ventricular tachycardia/fibrillation	1–1.5 mg/kg IV bolus, not to exceed 300 mg in a 1-hour period
	procainamide hydrochloride (HCl)	Pronestyl	Decreases excitability and conduction velocity in the heart conduction pathway	Ventricular arrhythmias	Emergency medication used during cardiac arrest or ventricular tachycardia/fibrillation	50–100 mg IV push slowly over a 5-minute period; not to exceed 500 mg
Antibiotics/Anti-infective Agents						
Aminoglycosides	gentamycin sulfate	Garamycin	Inhibits protein synthesis, causing cell death—bacteriocidal	Treatment of infection caused by GI microbes	Preop prophylaxis for bowel or GU surgery; endocarditis prophylaxis	3 mg/kg/day IM or IV divided into three doses
	neomycin sulfate	Neosulf				50 mg/kg/day divided into four doses
Penicillins	—	Penicillin G	Inhibits cell wall synthesis during multiplication	Moderate to severe systemic infection	Sepsis	1.2–24 million units/day IM or IV in divided doses
Cephalosporins	cefazolin sodium cephalexin monohydrate	Ancef, Kefzol Keflex	1st-generation cephalosporin; inhibits cell wall synthesis	Treatment of infection of respiratory, biliary, and GU tracts; skin, soft tissue, or bone/joint infection; septicemia	Surgical prophylaxis; sepsis	250 mg to 1.5 g IM or IV every 6–8 hours
	cefuroxime sodium	Ceftin, Zinacef	2nd-generation cephalosporin; inhibits cell wall synthesis	Treatment of serious urinary and respiratory, gynecologic, skin, abdominal, and bone/joint infections	Surgical prophylaxis; sepsis	750 mg to 1.5 g IM or IV every 8 hours

	cefoxitin	Mefoxin				1–2 g IV or IM every 8 hours
	cefotetan disodium	Cefotan				1–2 g IV or IM every 12 hours
	cefamandole	Mandol				0.5–1 g IM or IV every 12 hours
	ceftriaxone sodium	Rocephin	3rd-generation cephalosporin; inhibits cell wall synthesis	Treatment of serious urinary and respiratory, gynecologic, skin, abdominal, and bone/joint infections	Surgical prophylaxis; sepsis	1–2 g once per day
	ceftazidime	Claforan				1–2 g IV or IM every 8–12 hours
	cefoperazone	Cefobid				1–2 g IM or IV every 12 hours
	cefepime HCl	Maxipime	4th-generation cephalosporin; inhibits cell wall synthesis	Treatment of serious urinary and respiratory, gynecologic, skin, abdominal, and bone/joint infections	Surgical prophylaxis; sepsis	1–2 g IM or IV every 12 hours
Antiamebicide / Antiprotozoal	metronidazole	Flagyl	Enters cells, inhibiting synthesis, causing cell death	Bacterial infections caused by anaerobic microbes and protozoa	Prevents infection from GI microbes	15 mg/kg IV
Miscellaneous antibiotics	bacitracin	Bacitracin	Hinders cell wall synthesis, damaging the cell	Staphylococcus infections	Prophylactic orthopedic/GU irrigation	50,000 units per 1,000 mL irrigation fluid
	neomycin, polymixin, bacitracin	Neosporin	Hinders cell wall synthesis, damaging the cell	Staphylococcus infections	Topical ointment to prevent postoperative wound infection	Ointment (ung); as indicated
	neomycin, polymixin, hydrocortisone	Cortisporin	Hinders cell wall synthesis, damaging the cell; steroidal anti-inflammatory	Staphylococcus infections	Antibiotic and steroid to prevent infection and reduce inflammation	Drops (gtts) or ointment (ung)—applied as indicated
	vancomycin hydrochloride (HCl)	Vancocin	Hinders cell wall synthesis and inhibits RNA synthesis	Severe infections; methacillin-resistant infections	Severe infections; methacillin-resistant infections	1–1.5 g IV every 12 hours
	polymixin B sulfate	Aerosporin	Alters the osmotic barrier of the cell membrane	Eye, pseudomonas, or gram-negative infections	Prophylactic orthopedic irrigation	500,000 units per 1,000 mL irrigation
	quinupristin-dalfopristin	Synercid	Interferes with protein synthesis, inhibiting reproduction	Vancomycin-resistant bacteremia	Vancomycin-resistant infections	7.5 mg/kg IV every 8 hours
	linezolid	Zyvox	Interferes with protein synthesis, inhibiting reproduction	Vancomycin-resistant bacteremia	Vancomycin-resistant infections	600 mg IV every 12 hours

(continues)

TABLE 9-13 **(continued)**

Category	Generic Name	Trade Name	Action	Indication	Surgical Use	Dosage
Fluoroquinolones	ciprofloxacin	Cipro	Inhibits DNA synthesis; bacteriocidal	Urinary tract infections (UTIs); respiratory and skin infections; bone/joint infections	Severe orthopedic or abdominal infections; sinusitis	400 mg every 12 hours
Sulfomamides	silver sulfadiazine	Silvadene	Acts on the cell wall and cell membrane to kill gram-positive and gram-negative microbes	Prevents infections in open burns	Treatment of skin burns	Cream: apply 1/16-inch thickness to clean, debrided burns once or twice per day
Anticoagulants	heparin sodium	Heparin	Prevents conversion of prothrombin into thrombin, prevents clot formation	Treatment/prevention of DVT, thrombosis, pulmonary embolus	Prevents blood clot formation during vascular procedures or during placement of intravascular devices	150–300 units/kg IV; 10–100 units IV for filling vascular access devices
Anticoagulant antagonist	protamine sulfate	Protamine Sulfate	An anticoagulant by itself; binds with heparin to inactivate heparin's effect	Heparin reversal	Reverses the effects of heparin sodium	1 mg for each 90–115 units of heparin given; not to exceed 50 mg
Anticonvulsants		Phenobarbital	Central nervous system (CNS) depressant; barbituate	Treatment of generalized tonic-clonic seizures	Decrease brain activity during neurosurgical procedures; treat seizures	50–100 mg 2–3 times per day with a loading does of 15–20 mg/kg
Antiemetics	droperidol	Inapsine	Action unknown: produces sedation and reduces nausea and vomiting	Intraoperative sedation; perioperative and postoperative nausea and vomiting (PONV) management	Anesthesia adjunct to reduce anxiety and PONV	0.22–0.275 mg/kg IV
	metoclopramide	Reglan	Blocks dopamine receptors to reduce nausea and vomiting	Treatment/prevention of PONV	Perioperative PONV	1–2 mg/kg IV; 10–20 mg IM
	ondansetron hydrochloride (HCl)	Zofran	Blocks serotonin receptors on the vagus nerve	Treatment/prevention of PONV	Perioperative PONV	4 mg IV over 2–5 minutes
	granisetron hydrochloride (HCl)	Kytril	Blocks serotonin receptors on the vagus nerve	Treatment/prevention of PONV	Perioperative PONV	10 mcg/kg IV over 5 minutes
	dolasetron mesylate	Anzemet	Blocks serotonin receptors on the vagus nerve	Treatment/prevention of PONV	Perioperative PONV	12.5 mg IV

Antihistamine	diphenhydramine	Benadryl	Competes with histamine for receptor sites	Hypersensitivity reaction	Not commonly used in the OR setting	25–50 mg IM
Antihypertensive	nitroprusside sodium	Nitropress; Nipride	Relaxes smooth muscles of blood vessels	Hypertensive crisis	Control hypertensive episodes intraoperatively	0.25–0.3 mcg/kg/minute IV
Cardiac agents	isoproterenol hydrochloride (HCl)	Isuprel	Stabilizes heart rate and strengthens heart contractions	Heart block; ventricular arrhythmias	Emergency medication used during cardiac arrest or ventricular tachycardia/ fibrillation	0.02–0.06 mg IV then 5 mcg/ minute
	labetalol	Normodyne	Reduces peripheral vascular resistance	Hypertensive crisis	Hypertensive crisis	200 mg diluted in 160 mL of D5W, infused at 2 mg/minute
	digoxin	Lanoxin	Strengthens cardiac contractions	Heart failure, supraventricular tachycardia, atrial fibrillation	Emergency medication used during cardiac arrest or heart failure	0.5–1 mg IV over 24 hours with a maintenance dose of 0.125–0.5 mg IV daily
Cholinergic	neostigmine bromide	Prostigmin	Inhibits acetyl-cholinesterase production	Myasthenia gravis; residual neuromuscular blockade	Residual neuromuscular blockade; given with atropine or glycopyrrolate to prevent bradycardia	0.5–2.5 mg IV slowly
Coagulant	vitamin K	AquaMephyton	Increases the synthesis of prothrombin in the liver to promote clot formation	Hypoprothrombinemia	Promote clot formation	2.5–10 mg IM up to 50 mg
Contrast media	diatrizoate meglumine; diatrizoate sodium; hypaque meglumine	Cystografin; Hypaque; Renografin	Block full penetration of ionizing radiation (X-ray, fluoroscopy)	Outline hollow structures for visualization during radiologic examinations	Outline structures during biliary or urinary surgical interventions	May be used full strength or diluted; dose depends on structure and number of radiographic images
	iodipamide	Cholografin Meglumine	Block full penetration of ionizing radiation (X-ray, fluoroscopy)	Outline hollow structures for visualization during radiologic examinations	Outline structures during biliary or urinary surgical interventions	May be used full strength or diluted; dose depends on structure and number of radiographic images
	iothalamate meglumine barium sulfate iopamidol ioversol	Angio-Conray; Conray Barium Isovue Optiray	Block full penetration of ionizing radiation (X-ray, fluoroscopy)	Outline hollow structures for visualization during radiologic examinations	Outlines structures during biliary, urinary and cardiovascular surgical interventions.	May be used full strength or diluted; dose depends on structure and number of radiographic images
Coronary artery dilator	nitroglycerine	—	Decreases cardiac preload and systemic vascular resistance; increases coronary artery blood flow	Myocardial ischemia; angina pectoris	Hypertension and heart failure due to myocardial infarction	5–20 mcg/minute every 3–5 minutes

(continues)

Table 9-13 (continued)

Category	Generic Name	Trade Name	Action	Indication	Surgical Use	Dosage
Diuretics	furosemide	Lasix	Loop diuretic that prevents reabsorption of sodium and water in the kidney	Pulmonary edema, hypertension	Maintain urinary output intraoperatively; fluid overload	40 mg IV
	mannitol	Osmitrol	Osmotic diuretic that inhibits reabsorption of water and electrolytes	Generalized edema, oligouria; impaired renal function	Decrease intracranial pressure (ICP), intraocular pressure (IOP), or generalized fluid retention/ edema	1.5–2 g/kg IV over 30–60 minutes
Dyes	brilliant green	—	Leaves a visible tract by staining an area of tissue	Skin marking, tattooing, following a tract	Stains tissue	As indicated
	gentian violet	—	Leaves a visible tract by staining an area of tissue	Skin marking, tattooing, following a tract	Stains tissue	As indicated
	indigo carmine	—	Leaves a visible tract by staining an area of tissue	Skin marking, tattooing, following a tract	Stains tissue	As indicated
	methylene blue	—	Leaves a visible tract by staining an area of tissue	Skin marking, tattooing, following a tract	Stains tissue; mild GU antiseptic	As indicated
	isosulfan blue	Lymphazurine	Binds to interstitial proteins, delineating lymphatic vessels and glands	Used to identify lymph pathways and lymphadenopathy	Used to identify sentinel lymph nodes	3 mL of 1% solution
Fibrinolytic	streptokinase	Streptase	Activates plasminogen to cause fibrinolysis of thrombus	Lysis of thrombi in acute myocardial infarction	Lysis of arteriovenous cannula occlusion; arterial thrombosis	250,000 – 100,000 IU/hr over 24 – 72 hours
Hemostatic agents	absorbable gelatin sponge	Gelfoam; Gelfilm	Serves as a mechanical plug over open vessels to promote clot formation	Promote clot formation	Topical hemostasis	Various sizes
	microfibrillar collagen	Avitene	Attracts platelets, promoting clot formation	Promote clot formation	Topical hemostasis	Various sizes
	oxidized cellulose	Oxycel; Surgicel	Swells to become a gelatinous mass that stimulates clotting	Promote clot formation	Topical hemostasis	Various sizes

	absorbable collagen sponge	Collastat; Hemopad	Attracts platelets, promoting clot formation	Promote clot formation	Topical hemostasis	Various sizes
	thrombin	Thrombinar	Speeds the conversion of fibrogen to fibrin to promote clot formation	Promote clot formation	Topical hemostasis	1,000 units/mL
	fibrin sealants	Tisseel	Forms a fibrin seal over areas of oozing to promote clot formation	Not for intravascular injection; must be thawed prior to use	Topical hemostasis	Prepackaged for delivery using a duploject syringe system
	gelatin matrix/ thrombin	Floseal	Speeds the conversion of fibrogen to fibrin to promote clot formation	Not for intravascular injection or ophthalmic use	Topical hemostasis	Prepackaged for reconstitution
Histamine 2 (H2) blockers	cimetidine	Tagamet	Inhibits hydrochloric acid secretion in the stomach	Gastric/duodenal ulcers, Gastroesophageal reflux disease (GERD)	Prevention of gastric ulcer formation/gastritis	300 mg IV
	ranitidine	Zantac	Inhibits hydrochloric acid secretion in the stomach	Gastric/duodenal ulcers, gastroesophageal reflux disease (GERD)	Prevention of gastric ulcer formation/gastritis	50 mg IV every 6–8 hours
	famotidine	Pepcid	Inhibits hydrochloric acid secretion in the stomach	Gastric/duodenal ulcers, gastroesophageal reflux disease (GERD)	Prevention of gastric ulcer formation/gastritis	20 mg IV every 12 hours
	sodium citrate	Bi-Citra	Neutralizes stomach acid	Neutralizes gastric acid preoperatively	Neutralizes gastric acid preoperatively	15–30 mL PO
Hormones	glucagon	GlucaGen	Raises blood glucose level by promoting conversion of glycogen to glucose	Hypoglycemia; diagnostic aid for assessment of the biliary tree	Dilation of sphincter of Oddi for cannulation during ERCP	1–2 mg IV
	insulin		Controls glucose movement into cells	Regulates blood glucose levels; pancreatic insulin insufficiency	Management of blood glucose levels intraoperatively	As indicated, based on blood glucose levels; short-acting insulin used in the OR setting
	medroxy-progetersone acetate	Depo-Provera	Suppresses ovulation and follicular maturation; decreases endometrial proliferation	Menorrhea, menorrhagia, endometriosis	Controls abnormal uterine bleeding	400–1,000 mg IM

(continues)

TABLE 9-13 (continued)

Category	Generic Name	Trade Name	Action	Indication	Surgical Use	Dosage
Immunoglobin		RhoGam	Prevention of Rh immunization	Prevent Rh immunization in an Rh-negative mother whose fetus is Rh positive during pregnancy and following delivery or abortion	Treats Rh sensitization in the Rh-negative mother	300 micrograms IM given to the mother; IM use only
MH antagonist	dantrolene sodium	Dantrium	Interferes with calcium transportation in skeletal muscle, reducing contraction	Malignant hyperthermia	Management of malignant hyperthermia (MH)	2.5 mg/kg initial dose; max dose 10–30 mg/kg as indicated by patient condition
Narcotic antagonist	naloxone hydrochloride (HCl)	Narcan	Displacement of narcotics from CNS receptor sites	Narcotic overdose	Reverse narcotic analgesics	0.4–2 mg IV every 2–3 minutes
	nalmefene	Revex	Displacement of narcotics from CNS receptor sites	Narcotic overdose	Reverse narcotic analgesics	0.5–1.5 mg/kg
Oxytocic	oxytocin	Pitocin	Stimulates uterine and mammary gland smooth muscle	Stimulation of labor	Contraction of the uterus during/following childbirth or abortion	10–40 units IV in 500 mL solution at 20–40 milliunits per minute
	carboprost tromethamine	Hemabate	A synthetic prostaglandin that stimulates uterine smooth muscle	Used to control uterine hemorrhage following abortion and childbirth	Contraction of the uterus during/following childbirth or abortion	250 micrograms IM every 15–90 minutes, not to exceed 2 mg
	methylergonovine maleate	Methergine	An ergot alkaloid that stimulates uterine smooth muscle	Used to control uterine hemorrhage following abortion and childbirth	Contraction of the uterus during/following childbirth or abortion	0.2 mg IM every 2–4 hours after delivery
Stains	Lugol's solution	—			Stain cervical mucosa during conization	Topical agent
	Schiller's solution	—			Stain cervical mucosa during conization	Topical agent

Steroids	dexamethasone	Decadron	Decreases inflammation by suppressing the immune response	Cerebral edema, adrenocortical insufficiency	Decrease postoperative edema related to surgery trauma; adjunct for the treatment of postoperative nausea and vomiting (PONV)	40 mg IV every 2–6 hours
	hydrocortisone sodium succinate	Solu-Cortef	Decreases inflammation by suppressing the immune response	Inflammation; adrenal insufficiency	Maintenance of cortisone levels for patients with insufficiency during the stressors of surgery	100–500 mg IV as indicated
	methyl- prednisolone acetate	Solu-Medrol	Decreases inflammation by suppressing the immune response	Inflammation or immunosuppression	Shock, maintenance of adrenal hormone levels for patients with insufficiency during the stressors of surgery	30 mg/kg IV every 4–6 hours
	betamethasone, sodium phosphate and betamethasone acetate	Celestone	Decreases inflammation by suppressing the immune response	Inflammation or immunosuppression	Decrease inflammation and edema related to surgical trauma	Administered topically or IM only; 0.5–9 mg IM
Vasoconstrictor	vasopressin	Pitressin	Causes blood vessels to constrict, increasing blood pressure and decreasing bleeding	Vasoconstrictor	Injected into the cervix or uterine myometrium to decrease intraoperative bleeding	20 units in 30 mL saline for injection
Vasodilator	papaverine hydrochloride (HCl)	Papaverine	Causes smooth muscle relaxation	Vasodilator	Used to dilate arteries during cardiac and peripheral vascular procedures	30–120 mg in irrigation solution
Electrolyte replacement	sodium bicarbonate	—	Alkalinizer for treatment of acidosis	Metabolic acidosis	Cardiac arrest; neutralize the pH of local anesthetic agents	1 mEq/kg IV of 7.5% or 8.4% solution, followed by 0.5 m Eq/kg IV every 10 minutes
Irrigation solution	sterile distilled water for irrigation				Used to soak debris from instrumentation intraoperatively; may be used to irrigate the surgical wound or cavities, such as the bladder, in certain specific situations	1,000-mL and 3,000-mL containers or bags; not for injection
		Normal saline (0.9%) for irrigation			Used to irrigate the surgical wound to reduce contamination	500-mL, 1,000-mL, 3,000-mL containers; not for injection

(continues)

Table 9-13 (continued)

Category	Generic Name	Trade Name	Action	Indication	Surgical Use	Dosage
Intravenous solution		Dextrose 5% in water	Water and sugar		Used to correct hypoglycemia and replace water lost during normal metabolism	500-mL and 1,000-mL bags
		Lactated Ringer's solution	Physiological salt solution containing electrolytes		Serves as a glucose source for body metabolism, to correct fluid and electrolyte deficits, and to treat mild acidosis when blood or blood products are being administered	500-mL and 1,000-mL bags
		Normal saline (0.9%) for injection	Physiological salt solution			250-mL, 500-mL, 1,000-mL bags; 10-mL and 30-mL vials for mixing powdered medications (saline for injection)
		Sterile water for injection	Sterile distilled water for intravenous use		Used for mixing medications	30-mL vials for mixing powdered medications (sterile water for injection)
Blood volume expander		Dextran	Large sugar molecules that do not diffuse from the intravascular space; may prevent clotting for short period of time	Hypovolemia; hypovolemic shock	Hypovolemia when blood products cannot be given	Dextran 40 and Dextran 70–25 mL per hour
Plasma expander	hetastarch	Hespan	Expands plasma volume and provides fluid replacement	Hypovolemia; hypovolemic shock	Replaces blood volume for patients who decline blood transfusion or when blood replacement is not available	500–1,000 mL IV; not to exceed 1,500 mL
Other agents	acetic acid				Cleanses the mucous membrane of the vagina during laser surgery	5% solution; as indicated

Cardiovascular Surgery

Heparinized saline solution for intravascular irrigation is commonly used during cardiac and peripheral vascular procedures. Dilute and concentrated heparin solutions may be required for use during the same procedure, and the surgical technologist should clearly label and separate these solutions to prevent medication errors. Additional medications used during vascular procedures include contrast media for arteriography, topical papaverine HCl (Papaverine) for dilating blood vessels when working with small-diameter vessels, lidocaine HCl for local anesthesia, and oxidized cellulose (Oxicel, Surgicel) for hemostasis.

Neurosurgery

Drugs and solutions used during neurosurgical procedures include antibiotics in warm saline for irrigation, heparinized saline solution for intravascular irrigation, contrast media for cerebral arteriography, topical papaverine HCl (Papaverine) for dilating blood vessels during procedures involving cerebral vasculature, lidocaine HCl injection or absorbable gelatin sponge soaked in thrombin for hemostasis, and the use of polifeprosan 20 with carmustine implants (Gliadel Wafers) for topical placement onto the post-resection tumor bed for the treatment of glioblastoma multiforme.

Ophthalmic Surgery

Various drugs are used in ophthalmic surgery to facilitate diagnosis and treatment of pathological conditions of the eye. The surgical technologist must be aware that many of the drugs used in ophthalmic surgery are the same drugs used in other surgical specialties, with one significant exception—all medications used during eye surgery should be labeled "for ophthalmic use," as these medications are more pure than those delivered for systemic use and the concentration of the medication is usually more potent than the concentrations used in other specialties. A summary of medications used in ophthalmic surgery is listed in Table 9-14.

Mydriatics and cycloplegic agents cause the iris to contract, resulting in dilation of the pupil referred to as mydriasis. While both categories of agents results in mydriasis, each have a different effect within the eye. Mydriatics primarily paralyze the iris sphincter, without affecting the lens' ability to focus light rays on the retina. Cycloplegics paralyze the ciliary muscles, resulting in both pupil dilation and the inability of the ciliary process to focus the lens of the eye. In surgery, these agents are used to optimize exposure and removal of a cataract lens. The commonly used mydriatic agent is phenylephrine HCl (Neo-Synephrine). Commonly used cycloplegic agents include tropicamide (Mydriacyl), cyclopentolate (Cyclogyl), and atropine sulfate (Atropisol)

Miotic agents act on the iris, resulting in iris relaxation and, therefore, pupil constriction. Miotic agents include pilocarpine HCl (Pilocar, Isopto Carpine) and carbachol (Miostat). They may be administered by instillation into the anterior chamber of the eye. These drugs also facilitate the drainage of aqueous humor through the trabecular meshwork of the canal of Schlemm, thus decreasing intraocular pressure (IOP), making them useful for the treatment of increased IOP due to glaucoma. Miotics are used intraoperatively when pupil constriction is necessary, as in laser iridectomy or following placement of an intraocular lens (IOL) implant.

Viscoelastic/viscosurgical agents are used to expand the anterior chamber and prevent injury to the corneal endothelium and surrounding tissues during cataract extraction. These agents can also be used as a replacement for vitreous humor. Chondroitin sulfate-sodium hyaluronate (Viscoat) and sodium hyaluronate (Healon, Amvisc) are commonly used viscoelastic agents.

Hyperosmotic drugs are diuretics that are used perioperatively to shrink the vitreous body, thus reducing IOP. They are also used intraoperatively to aid scleral closure during retinal detachment repair. Agents commonly used include IV mannitol (Osmitrol) and oral acetazolamide (Diamox).

Anti-inflammatory agents include steroids and nonsteroidal anti-inflammatory drugs (NSAIDs). Steroids and NSAIDs are used in traumatic eye injuries to suppress the inflammatory response and to control postoperative inflammation. Common steroids include prednisolone acetate (PredForte), dexamethasone (OcuDex), and betamethasone (Celestone Suspension).

Ophthalmic antibiotic ointments, used for the treatment or prevention of ocular infections, include the aminoglycosides gentamycin (Genoptic), erythromycin (Ilotycin), tobramycin (Tobramycin Ophthalmic), and ciprofloxan (Ciloxan). These agents are commonly delivered as liquid medication injected into the subconjunctival space, or in drop form or as an ointment placed in the subconjunctival sac. Antibiotics for ophthalmic use are commonly combined with a steroid, such as tobramycin and dexamethasone (Tobradex).

Many ophthalmic procedures are performed under local anesthesia. Tetracaine (Pontocaine) and proparacaine (Ophthaine) are the most commonly used topical anesthetics. **Retrobulbar** anesthesia may be necessary for some procedures to block both sensory and motor nerve function. Retrobulbar anesthesia is accomplished by injecting the area around the optic nerve with a combination of lidocaine HCl and bupivacaine, both without epinephrine. Hyaluronidase (Wydase) is added to aid in distribution of local anesthetic agent(s), or epinephrine may be added to the solution to decrease bleeding during procedures of the eyelid

Irrigating solutions are necessary during ophthalmic surgery to keep the cornea from drying out. Balanced Salt Solution (**BSS**), a sterile, physiologically balanced irrigating fluid, is the solution most frequently employed. The surgical technologist will use a droptainer bottle of 15 or 30 mL, with an olive-tipped cannula, for irrigating the exposed cornea during the procedure. BSS Plus, balanced salt solution enhanced with bicarbonate, dextrose, and glutathione, is used for intraocular irrigation during extracapsular lens extraction, vitrectomy, and anterior segment procedures.

Table 9-14 Medications Used in Ophthalmic Surgery

Category	Generic Name	Trade Name	Action	Indication	Surgical Use	Dosage
Mydriatics	phenylephrine HCl	Neo-Synephrine	Pupil dilation by paralyzing the iris sphincter—does not affect the ability to focus	Cataract extraction and vitrectomy—permits access to the posterior chamber of the anterior cavity	Preoperative mydriasis	10% drops—1 drop every 5–15 minutes until sufficient pupil dilation achieved
Cycloplegics	tropicamide cyclopentolate atropine sulfate	Mydriacyl Cyclogyl Atropisol	Pupil dilation with inability to focus	Cataract extraction and vitrectomy—permits access to the posterior chamber of the anterior cavity	Preoperative mydriasis and cycloplegia	1% drops—1 drop every 5–15 minutes until sufficient pupil dilation achieved
Miotics	pilocarpine HCl	Pilocar	Pupil constriction	Cataract extraction—assists in holding the intraocular lens (IOL) in place and promotes the flow of aqueous humor	Postoperative miosis; treatment of glaucoma	1%–4%—used as postoperative drops
	acetylcholine HCl	Miochol	Pupil constriction	Cataract extraction—assists in holding the intraocular lens (IOL) in place and promotes the flow of aqueous humor	Intraoperative miosis	20 mg/2 mL—instillation into the anterior segment of the anterior chamber of the eye
	carbochol	Miostat	Pupil constriction	Cataract extraction—assists in holding the IOL in place and promotes the flow of aqueous humor	Intraoperative miosis	0.01%—instillation into the anterior segment of the anterior chamber of the eye
Ophthalmic viscoelastic/ viscosurgical agents	sodium hyaluronate chondroitin sulfate-sodium hyaluronat	Healon, Amvisc Viscoat	Intraocular lubricant	Expands the anterior chamber of the eye and protects the corneal endothelium during cataract extraction and lens placement	Intraocular lubrication	Prepackaged

Steroids	prednisolone acetate	PredForte	Anti-inflammatory	Reduces inflammation	Postoperative inflammation	1–2 drops instilled in the subconjunctival sac every 6–12 hours
	dexamethasone sodium phosphate	OcuDex, Decadron	Anti-inflammatory	Reduces inflammation	Postoperative inflammation	0.1%—1–2 drops instilled in the subconjunctival sac every 4–6 hours
	betamethasone sodium phosphate and betamethasone acetate	Celestone	Anti-inflammatory	Reduces inflammation	Postoperative inflammation	0.1%—1–2 drops injected in the subconjunctival space at the end of the surgical procedure
Nonsteroidal anti-inflammatory drugs (NSAIDs)	ketorolac tromethamine	Acular	Anti-inflammatory	Reduces inflammation	Postoperative inflammation	1 drop every 6 hours
Antibiotics	gentamycin erythromycin	Genoptic Ilotycin	Antibiotic	Prevents/treats infection	Prevent/treats postoperative infection	1–2 drops instilled in the subconjunctival sac every 4–6 hours
	tobramycin	Tobramycin Ophthalmic	Antibiotic	Prevents/treats infection	Prevent/treats postoperative infection	1–2 drops instilled in the subconjunctival sac every 4–6 hours
	ofloxacin	Ocuflox	Antibiotic	Prevents/treats infection	Prevent/treats postoperative infection	1–2 drops instilled in the subconjunctival sac every 4–6 hours
	ciprofloxan	Ciloxan	Antibiotic	Prevents/treats infection	Prevent/treats postoperative infection	1–2 drops instilled in the subconjunctival sac every 4–6 hours
Antibiotic and anti-inflammatory combinations	tobramycin and dexamethasone	Tobradex	Antibiotic and anti-inflammatory combination	Prevents infection and reduces inflammation	Post-op prevention of infection and inflammation	1–2 drops instilled in the subconjunctival sac every 4–6 hours
	neomycin, polymixin B and dexamethasone	Maxitrol	Antibiotic and anti-inflammatory combination	Prevents infection and reduces inflammation	Post-op prevention of infection and inflammation	1–2 drops instilled in the subconjunctival sac every 4–6 hours

(continues)

Table 9-14 **(continued)**

Category	*Generic Name*	*Trade Name*	*Action*	*Indication*	*Surgical Use*	*Dosage*
Hyperosmotic Agents	mannitol	Mannitol Injection	Osmotic diuretic, decreases IOP	Hinders reabsorption of water by the kidneys	Osmotic diuretic, decreases IOP	25% IV
	acetazolamide	Diamox	Carbonic anhydrase inhibitor	Decreases the secretion of aqueous humor, resulting in decreased IOP	Decreases IOP	250 mg PO every 8–12 hours
Dyes	fluoresceine sodium		Dye	Stains tissues	Detect alterations in anatomical structures, such as corneal abrasions and patent nasolacrimal ducts	Mixed with BSS solution for irrigation or 1–2 drops onto cornea
Irrigants		Balanced Salt Solution (BSS)	Intra- and extraocular irrigating solution	Replacement for physiological tears or aqueous humor	Corneal moistening and intraocular irrigation	1–2 drops on the conjunctiva periodically during the surgical procedure to maintain corneal moisture; instilled into the anterior chamber intraoperatively to maintain chamber shape following extraction of the viscoelastic agent; 250 mL BSS Plus with epinephrine added for intraocular irrigation during cataract extraction
Zonulysis agents	alpha chymotrypsin	Alpha-Chymar	Zonulysis agent	Dissolves zonules holding the capsule of the lens in place during intracapsular lens extraction	Intracapsular lens extraction	50 units/mL; 1–2 mL instilled into the posterior chamber
Anesthetic agents	propericaine HCl	Alcaine	Local anesthetic	Blocks nerve conduction	Topical anesthesia	0.5% drops applied topically to the conjunctiva
	tetracaine HCl	Pontocaine				

	lidocaine HCl	Xylocaine	Local anesthetic	Blocks nerve conduction	Topical or retrobulbar anesthesia	1-4%—with or without epi—injected
	bupivicaine HCl	Marcaine	Local anesthetic	Blocks nerve conduction	Retrobulbar anesthesia	0.25%–0.75%—injected
	hyaluronidase	Wydase	Enzyme	Aids in distribution of the local anesthetic agent(s)	Retrobulbar anesthesia	150 units/mL; 1 mL added to local anesthetic solution
Glaucoma agents (not commonly used in the OR setting)	levobunolol	Betagan	Beta-adrenergic blocker	Decreases the production of aqueous humor	Decreases IOP, treats glaucoma, not commonly used in the OR	1–2 drops daily
	betaxolol HCl	Betoptic				1 drop every 12 hours
	timolol	Timoptic				1 drop every 12 hours
	metipranolol	Optipranolol				1 drop every 12 hours
	dorzolamide	Trusopt	Carbonic anhydrase inhibitors	Decreases the production of aqueous humor	Decreases IOP, treats glaucoma, not commonly used in the OR	1 drop every 8 hours
	demecarium bromide	Humorsol	Miotic	Decreases the production of aqueous humor	Decreases IOP, treats glaucoma, not commonly used in the OR	1–2 drops per day titrated to 1–2 drops per week
	Latanoprost	Xalatan	Prostaglandin analog	Decreases the production of aqueous humor	Decreases IOP, treats glaucoma, not commonly used in the OR	1 drop daily

HEMOSTASIS AND BLOOD REPLACEMENT

Because surgery is invasive, it is almost a given that some blood and fluid loss is expected. It is the goal of every surgeon to minimize blood loss and to anticipate any major blood loss. The term *hemostasis* refers to techniques and practices that control and minimize the loss of blood during a surgical procedure. Hemostasis involves the use of physical, mechanical, or chemical processes to control bleeding.

Factors Affecting Hemostasis

Preexisting hemostatic defects and acquired hemostatic disorders affect the ability of the patient's body to form blood clots naturally (Table 9-15).

Control of Bleeding During Surgery

Patients undergoing a scheduled surgical procedure usually enter the OR hemodynamically normal. However, 50% of postoperative bleeding is due to poor hemostasis during surgery. If a patient enters the OR bleeding from a traumatic injury or other source, it is the goal of the surgical team to control bleeding and achieve hemostasis. While intraoperative bleeding from cut vessels is the most obvious and immediately treated, oozing from denuded surfaces and smaller vessels can eventually lead to a large-volume blood loss and must also be controlled. In addition, certain procedures, such as the use of cardiopulmonary bypass and liver transplant surgery, are commonly associated with large blood losses that may require the administration of blood and blood products in order to achieve hemostasis.

Table 9-15 Hemostatic Disorders Leading to Increased Intraoperative Bleeding

Type	*Examples*
Preexisting hemostatic defects	Clotting factor deficiencies—hemophilia, von Willebrand disease
Acquired hemostatic disorders	Liver disease Anticoagulant therapy—heparin sodium, warfarin sodium (Coumadin) Antiplatelet therapy—clopidogrel (Plavix), ticlopidine (Ticlid), acetylsalicylic acid (aspirin) Aplastic anemia Acoholic-induced liver failure

Intraoperative methods of hemostasis are classified as mechanical, thermal, and chemical methods. Mechanical and thermal methods are discussed in Chapter 10.

Chemical Methods of Hemostasis

Chemical methods have individual actions and the manufacturer's instructions for preparation and use should be carefully followed.

Bone Wax

Bone wax is a sterile mixture of beeswax applied to the cut edges of bone as a mechanical barrier to seal off oozing blood. This method should always be used sparingly because the body recognizes bone wax as a foreign body, and this may cause tissue reaction and rejection. Bone wax is only minimally absorbed by the body. Bone wax is used in thoracic surgery when the sternum is split, in neurosurgical procedures when a craniotomy is performed, and for orthopedic and otorhinolaryngologic (ENT) procedures. The surgical technologist should soften the bone wax by kneading prior to use; it is then rolled small balls that are then applied to the wound site with the back of a flat instrument, such as a Freer elevator.

Absorbable Gelatin Sponge

Absorbable gelatin sponge is composed of collagen, a structural protein found in connective tissues. It is available in either powder form or a foam pad (Gelfoam, Gelfilm) that comes in a variety of sizes that can be cut. When the absorbable gelatin is placed over an area of bleeding, fibrin is deposited, initiating clot formation. In addition, the sponge may be applied dry, soaked in saline to increase its pliability, soaked in thrombin (Thrombinar) to enhance clot formation, or soaked in epinephrine to enhance vasoconstriction. The absorbable gelatin may be left in the wound postoperatively, because it will be absorbed by the body in approximately 30 days.

Microfibrillar Collagen

Microfibrillar collagen (Avitene) assists in activating the coagulation process. Microfibrillar collagen is a powder available in preloaded applicators or via a powered dispenser. It must be kept dry or it becomes extremely sticky and difficult to use; it should therefore be applied directly to the surface such as bone using only dry forceps and gloves. A dry 4 × 4 sponge is used to apply pressure over the microfibrillar collagen to ensure it adheres to the wound surface. The collagen is soluble, and as hemostasis occurs, it is absorbed and eliminated from the body.

Oxidized Cellulose

Absorbable oxidized cellulose products are available in the form of pads (Nu-Knit, Fibrillar, and SNoW) or fabric (Surgicel—Original). Blood clots rapidly form in the presence of oxidized cellulose, and these products form a gel, which aids in hemostasis as it becomes soaked with blood. These products are applied directly to the bleeding surface and held in place until bleeding stops.

Silver Nitrate

Silver nitrate is often used to control cervical or nasal bleeding. It is applied either in stick form as a caustic pencil or in solutions of 0.01% to 10% silver nitrate.

Epinephrine

Epinephrine is a potent vasoconstrictor and is often combined with local anesthetic agents or with Gelfoam to aid in local hemostasis. It is absorbed rapidly by the body but provides good localized hemostasis.

Thrombin

Part of the blood-clotting mechanism, thrombin is an enzyme that results from the activation of prothrombin. Thrombin of bovine origin is used as a topical hemostatic (never injected). Thrombin is available in liquid or powder and may be poured, sprayed, or applied directly onto a bleeding site. Thrombin kits can include a spray bottle for applying the thrombin or delivered using a 4 × 4 or Gelfoam sponge. A Gelfoam pad, collagen sponge, or cottonoid sponge may be soaked in thrombin. Thrombin should be discarded if not used within several hours, because it loses potency.

Blood Loss

Blood loss is monitored intraoperatively by several means to aid the surgeon and anesthesia care provider in assessing the patient's hemodynamic status.

Calibrated suction devices (canisters) are used between the suction tubing and the vacuum source to collect and monitor the amount of blood and body fluids suctioned from the field. The surgical technologist should keep close track of the amount of irrigation fluids used; the amount is subtracted from the total volume in the canister to give a more accurate measurement of blood loss.

In addition, the circulator may weigh sponges removed from the field to provide an estimate of blood loss contained in used surgical sponges.. The circulator may use a scale and a predetermined sponge weight formula; alternatively, some hospitals have a bloody-sponge weight estimate that is used and multiplied by the number of sponges removed from the field. The sponges must be weighed wet as the formula is based on the dry and wet weights of the sponges. While not an exact method, weighing used sponges provides the surgeon and anesthesia care provider with a fairly reliable estimated blood loss (EBL).

EBL is reported to and monitored by the anesthesia care provider who, in consultation with the surgeon, will determine if blood replacement therapy is indicated.

Blood Components

The most common type of homologous blood replacement therapy used in the operating room is the administration of packed red blood cells (PRBCs). Other blood products administered in the OR setting are included in Table 9-16.

Handling of Blood Replacement Components

Blood products are usually obtained from the blood bank by a responsible individual, signed for, and brought to the OR. If the products are not to be used immediately, they should be stored in a refrigerator at a temperature between 1° and 6°F (33.8–42.8°C). Most hospitals have a refrigerator placed in a convenient location for use by several ORs at one time. Prior to administration, blood products must be carefully identified and verbally verified by two licensed personnel to assure the correct blood product is administered to the correct patient. Information verified includes the blood group, Rh type, unit number, and expiration date and time, if applicable. All information should match the documentation on the blood bag, the patient's armband, and the patient's chart. The product itself should be inspected for clots. If clots are present or any of the information does not match correctly, the blood should not be administered and should be returned to the blood bank.

TABLE 9-16 Common Blood Components

Blood Component	*Contents*	*Use*
Whole blood	All components of blood—not commonly used	Used to treat trauma-induced hemorrhage
Packed red blood cells (PRBCs)	Red blood cell (RBCs) from 1 unit of whole blood after most of plasma is removed	To restore oxygen-carrying capacity
Fresh-frozen plasma (FFP)	The fluid component of blood containing clotting factors removed from 1 unit of whole blood	Restores clotting factors; usually 1 unit of FFP is given for every 4 units of PRBCs
Platelets	Platelets removed from 1 unit of whole blood	Enhances blood's clotting ability when platelet count is low—less commonly used

Autotransfusion

Blood replacement therapy involves the administration of whole blood or blood components such as plasma, PRBCs, fresh-frozen plasma (FFP), or platelets via an IV line. This is used to increase the circulating blood volume, to increase the number of red blood cells, to increase the number of circulating platelets for clotting, or to provide clotting factors that have been depleted during surgery. Blood products are obtained through homologous sources (donated by another person) or autologous methods (donated prior to surgery by the patient and stored in the blood bank or obtained through autotransfusion).

Autotransfusion involves the use of the patient's own blood that has been processed for reinfusion. During procedures where blood loss is anticipated to be significant, as in cardiovascular, prostate, and major orthopedic procedures, suctioned fluids containing blood may be collected in an autologous blood retrieval system (Cell Saver®) for use in autotransfusion. An autologous blood retrieval system suctions blood, mixed with heparinzed saline, directly from the wound into a sterile canister attached to a filter to remove debris and a chamber for separating red blood cells from excess fluids with little or no damage to the red blood cells. The blood is then pumped into a separate reinfusion bag, attached to the patient's IV line. When homologous banked blood is used, blood typing and cross-matching are essential to prevent transfusion reactions based on incompatibility. The use of autologous blood is preferable to the use of homologous blood because using the patient's own blood eliminates the danger of incompatibility or disease transmission.

Blood that has been exposed to cancer cells, gastric or intestinal contents, amniotic fluid, collagen hemostatic agents, or certain antibiotics cannot be retrieved for autotransfusion.

METHODS AND TECHNIQUES OF ANESTHETIC ADMINISTRATION

Anesthetic agents have developed significantly from the days where the use of opium and alcohol was the common method of pain relief during a surgical intervention. Newer, safer, and better agents are constantly replacing the myriad of anesthetic agents available in an attempt to find the "ideal" anesthetic. Optimal balanced anesthesia is achieved when all of the following components are addressed:

- *Hypnosis:* **Hypnosis** results from an altered state of consciousness related to the patient's perception of the surgical environment and the surgical procedure. Many patients fear "being awake" during surgical intervention. Today's pharmaceutical agents permit varying levels of hypnosis to be achieved, from the light, more natural sleep of sedation to the fully unconscious state associated with general anesthesia.
- *Anesthesia:* Freedom from pain is the major focus of anesthesia practice. A patient's concern for proper and consistent pain management lies second only to the fear of anesthesia-related death. Today's anesthesia practices deliver pain-free surgery in a variety of ways using topical, local, regional, and general agents.
- *Amnesia*: Amnestic agents provide a lack of recall of perioperative events and permit the use of safer, less toxic anesthetic agents and techniques while providing a calm and cooperative surgical patient.
- *Muscle relaxation:* Neuromuscular blocking agents, used in combination with inhalation agents, are capable of producing profound muscle relaxation, facilitating endotracheal intubation and the development of new surgical interventions and techniques. Since a muscle layer overlies most surgical areas, a means of relaxing these muscles facilitates retraction and exposure of underlying organs and tissues.
- *Optimal patient positioning:* Advances in surgical procedures demand advantageous access to the surgical site. General anesthesia, patient physiological monitoring, and control of essential life processes must function in harmony to provide for an optimal patient outcome. Patient positioning must allow for surgical site access while maintaining physiological **homeostasis**.
- *Continued homeostasis of vital functions:* It is said that general anesthesia is intentionally capable of inducing a state close to death and requires maintenance of the patient at this level for the duration of the surgical procedure. This makes anesthesia administration the most dangerous component of any surgical intervention. Today's use of invasive and noninvasive monitoring devices to track the patient's critical physiological processes, as well as the use of safer anesthetic agents, assists the anesthesia care provider in maintaining the patient in a state of optimal "physiological balance" during the entire surgical experience.

Anesthetic agents are administered primarily in two ways: via the use of inhalation agents (gas) or via the use of injectable agents. General anesthesia focuses on altering the patient's level of consciousness, thereby minimizing pain and awareness of the surgical environment. Regional anesthesia involves the prevention of sensory nerve impulse transmission in a specific location of the body, allowing the patient to remain conscious but not "feel" the pain of the procedure. Many of today's anesthetic administrations involve components of both methods.

The choice of anesthetic methods, agents, and techniques is made on a case-by-case basis. The goals of maximum patient safety and optimal surgical outcomes include consideration of multiple factors, including:

- Anticipated procedure and estimated duration
- Intraoperative patient positioning
- Individual patient considerations, including:
  - Age, height, and weight of the patient
  - Physical, mental, and emotional status of the patient
  - Co-morbid conditions—diabetes, hypertension, heart disease
  - Current medications
  - Patient medication and food allergies
  - Patient history of substance abuse
  - Emergency conditions
- Surgeon, anesthesia care provider, and patient preference

The American Society of Anesthesiologists (ASA) uses a physical status classification system for assessing patient anesthetic risk, as indicated in Table 9-17.

GENERAL ANESTHESIA

General anesthesia involves an alteration in patients' perception of their environment through alterations in their level of consciousness. This is accomplished using three techniques: agent inhalation, agent injection, and, less commonly, agent instillation. When several agent delivery methods are used in combination during general anesthesia administration, the technique is referred to as *balanced anesthesia.*

Agent inhalation involves the delivery of gases across the lung's alveolar membrane where the agent enters the vascular system and is transported to the brain, where it is able to cross the blood–brain barrier, affecting CNS function. Medication delivery relies on an adequately functioning respiratory and circulatory system. These agents are delivered via a closed anesthesia circuit connected to a vaporizer.

Agent injection during general anesthesia involves the intravenous administration of medications directly into the bloodstream. This is accomplished by use of a venous access device, usually a peripheral intravenous catheter or a central venous delivery system. Medication effect does not rely on adequate respiratory function for distribution, only on circulatory function. Occasionally, a medication is injected intramuscularly (e.g., Ketamine).

Agent instillation involves the administration of medication into an area such as the rectum, where the agent is absorbed via the mucous membranes and transported to the CNS by the circulatory system. This method can be used in selected cases where patient cooperation is less than optimal.

TABLE 9-17 ASA Physical Status Classification

Class	*Description*
1	A patient without organic, physiological, biochemical, or psychiatric disturbances
2	A patient with mild to moderate systemic disease disturbance: controlled hypertension, history of asthma, anemia, smoker, controlled diabetes, mild obesity, age less than 1 or greater than 70
3	A patient with severe systemic disturbance or disease: angina, post-myocardial infarction (MI), poorly controlled hypertension, symptomatic respiratory disease, massive obesity
4	A patient with severe systemic disease, disorders that are life threatening: unstable angina, congestive heart failure, debilitating respiratory disease, hepatorenal failure
5	A patient who is near death and is not expected to survive with or without the surgical procedure
6	Brain-dead patient on life support for the purposes of organ procurement
Emergency modifier (E)	Applied when doing emergency surgery

Depth of General Anesthesia

There are four stages to describe the depth of general anesthesia, as indicated in Table 9-18.

Phases of General Anesthesia

The period prior to the start of general anesthesia is sometimes referred to as the *preinduction period.* It begins when premedication agents are administered and ends when the induction of anesthesia is begun. The patient may receive supplemental oxygen during this period.

There are four phases of general anesthesia: induction, maintenance, emergence, and recovery.

Induction phase: Induction involves altering the patient's level of consciousness from the conscious state to the unconscious state. During induction, loss of consciousness occurs and may be associated with depressed reflexes, respiratory depression, and an inadequate airway. Induction may be carried out in two ways: the use of an IV induction agent or the inhalation of gaseous vapors. Management and maintenance of the patient's airway is critical and may involve the use of an oral or nasal airway, face mask, laryngeal mask airway (LMA), or endotracheal tube. The patient's hearing is the last sense to be suppressed by the induction agent(s) and may even become more acute during this phase of anesthesia; therefore, environmental noise

TABLE 9-18 **Stages of General Anesthesia**

Stage	*Name*	*Characteristics*
I	Amnesia stage	Begins with the initial administration of an anesthetic agent to loss of consciousness
II	Excitement or delirium stage	Consists of the period from the loss of consciousness to the return of regular breathing and loss of the eyelid reflex • Uninhibited patient movements demonstrated • Vomiting, **laryngospasm**, hypertension, and tachycardia may be seen during this stage • The activities of this stage may be reduced or passed through rapidly by the administration of an IV **induction** agent, which rapidly brings the patient from Stage I to Stage III.
III	Surgical anesthesia stage	Consists of the period between the onset of regular breathing and loss of eyelid reflex to the cessation of breathing • The patient is unresponsive to painful stimuli and sensation, with the sense of hearing being the last sense to be blunted • This stage is often divided into four planes, with planes 2–3 considered to be the optimum level of anesthesia for surgical intervention
IV	Overdose stage	Dilated and nonreactive pupils are noted, the cessation of respiration and marked hypotension lead to circulatory failure; if uncorrected, this stage leads to patient death

should be kept to an absolute minimum. The surgical technologist should stop setting up the back table and Mayo stand to avoid making noise until the patient fully unconscious.

Maintenance phase: The surgical intervention takes place during the maintenance phase of anesthesia. Anesthesia administration is most dynamic during this period. The anesthesia care provider monitors the patient closely for changes in oxygen saturation, blood loss, muscle relaxation status, and cardiac status. Surgical manipulation may quickly change any of these parameters, and it is the responsibility of the anesthesia care provider to adjust anesthetic levels accordingly.

Emergence phase: Emergence occurs as the surgical intervention is being completed. The goal of emergence is to have the patient as awake as possible at the end of the surgical intervention. The primary focus of activities during this period is the monitoring of adequate and independent respiratory rate and function, with the restoration of the gag reflex. Extubation, if indicated, will be performed during this phase. Residual, undesired neuromuscular blockade may require the administration of a neuromuscular blockade reversal agent. As the state of consciousness increases, the patient is at risk for developing laryngospasm. Patients may also experience thermoregulatory changes due to the effects of the anesthetic agents and exposure of the viscera. It is common to see patient rigidity and/or tremors late in the emergence period.

Recovery phase: Recovery is that period of time during which the patient returns to the optimum level of consciousness and well-being. It usually begins in the OR suite, continues through the patient's stay in the postanesthesia care unit (**PACU**) and is completed following the patient's discharge and initial healing stages.

Advantages of General Anesthesia

The use of general anesthesia has several advantages:

- The patient is usually unaware of the activities and noises associated with the operative intervention.
- Once an adequate airway has been secured, the depth and rate of respiration can be controlled and the pulmonary tree is usually protected from **aspiration**.
- Medication dosages can be easily titrated to control the depth of anesthesia.
- Muscle relaxation for intubation and exposure of the surgical site is easily achieved.

Risks and Complications Associated with General Anesthesia

The risks and complications associated with general anesthesia administration are many. Fortunately, current monitoring techniques and improved pharmacological agents have lowered the morbidity associated with anesthesia administration and reduced the risk of mortality to less than one death per 200,000 anesthetics administered. Complications of anesthetic administration may occur even during "routine" surgery and must always be anticipated.

TABLE 9-19 ASA Fasting Recommendations to Reduce the Risk of Pulmonary Aspiration (Healthy Patient, Elective Procedures)

Fasting Period (Minimum)	*Ingested Item*
2 hours	Clear liquids
4 hours	Breast milk
6 hours	Infant formula/nonhuman milk/light meal
8 hours or longer	Solids (meat, fried or fatty foods)

Note: The standard "rule" is NPO after midnight.

Aspiration (inhaling foreign fluid or solids into the lungs) of secretions or gastric contents may occur in patients where inadequate time for gastric emptying has elapsed, such as trauma patients with a full stomach. The risk of aspiration is greatest during the induction and emergence phases of general anesthesia. Induction agents and neuromuscular blockade both permit relaxation of the cardioesophageal sphincter, allowing gastric contents to enter the esophagus. Without adequate protection of the trachea by a functioning "gag reflex," the application of cricoid pressure, use of an LMA, or use of a cuffed endotracheal tube, the gastric contents or secretions may be aspirated into the airway, resulting in a chemical pneumonitis that can lead to development of a bacterial lung infection. This is referred to as *aspiration pneumonia*. Table 9-19 lists the ASA fasting recommendations for reducing the risk of pulmonary aspiration of gastric contents.

The term **NPO** is from the Latin *non per os* or *nil per os*, meaning "nothing by mouth." If this is not possible, the application of cricoid pressure can reduce the risk of aspiration. Suction apparatus should be available at all times.

Cricoid Pressure

Sellick's maneuver, the application of cricoid pressure, is performed to reduce the risk of aspiration (Figure 9-6). This maneuver is designed to prevent the stomach contents released into the esophagus from entering the laryngopharynx, thereby reducing the risk of aspiration into the respiratory tract.

Firm pressure is applied with the thumb and index finger forming a V to the cricoid cartilage, located inferior to the prominence of the thyroid cartilage. The external pressure causes occlusion of the esophagus between the cricoid ring and the body of the sixth cervical vertebrae. Cricoid pressure must be applied prior to the induction of anesthesia and continued until the endotracheal tube is placed, the correct position of the tube is verified, and the cuff of the endotracheal tube is inflated. The individual applying cricoid pressure does not release the compression until directed to do so by the anesthesia care provider controlling the airway.

A

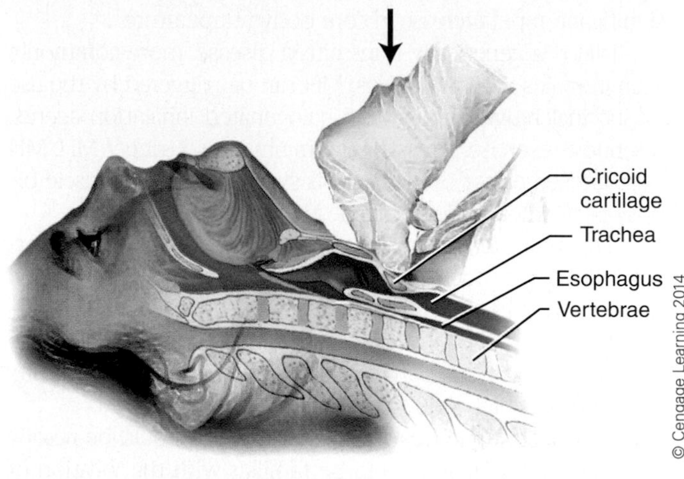

Figure 9-6 Cricoid pressure: (A) Application technique, (B) compression mechanism

Cricoid pressure is employed in situations when the patient requires emergency surgery shortly after eating, the NPO status of the patient cannot be verified, or the patient is experiencing gastrointestinal (GI) bleeding. Cricoid pressure may also be applied during basic life-support settings as needed.

Laryngospasm and Bronchospasm

Laryngospasm and bronchospasm are reactions demonstrated by the lightly anesthetized patient. A slight trigger of the "gag" reflex results in a spasm or rigidity of the upper respiratory tract, resulting in an inability of the patient and/or anesthesia care provider to move air and waste gases in and out of the lungs.

Laryngospasm and bronchospasm may be triggered by saliva in the back of the throat, stimulation of the lightly anesthetized surgical patient, or inflammation due to endotracheal tube placement. Laryngospasm and bronchospasm may occur during induction of or emergence from anesthesia and can lead to total airway obstruction, which is treated with positive-pressure breathing. If this does not provide relief, the patient will be given an ultra-rapid-acting neuromuscular blocker, preferably succinylcholine, to relax the spasm. The patient will need artificial respiratory support and monitoring until independent respiratory ability returns.

Malignant Hyperthermia

Malignant hyperthermia (MH) is a potentially fatal hypermetabolic state of muscle activity resulting from a defect in calcium transportation within the muscle fibers of skeletal muscles. During MH crisis, the striated skeletal muscles are stimulated to contract, but due to an abnormal release of calcium within the muscle cells, the muscles cannot relax, resulting in rigidity, heat generation, and a buildup of lactic acid and carbon dioxide. An MH crisis is characterized by increased production of carbon dioxide, tachycardia, muscle rigidity, and, finally, a significant, rapid increase in core body temperature.

MH is a genetically transmitted disease, more commonly seen in males than in females. MH can be triggered by the use of succinylcholine, curare, and halogenated inhalation agents. Strenuous exercise, stress, or trauma may also trigger MH. MH is diagnosed either by acute crisis symptoms or by muscle biopsy performed under local anesthesia.

The first sign of an MH crisis is unexplained tachycardia followed by tachypnea and an increased level of carbon dioxide. Shortly thereafter, an unstable blood pressure, perspiration, muscle contraction, and cyanotic, mottled skin are demonstrated. A late sign of MH crisis is a rise in temperature, sometimes as high as 107°F.

Supplies for the treatment of MH crisis should be readily available, and all staff should be familiar with the location of the supplies and the treatment protocol. The treatment interventions for a patient in MH crisis include the discontinuation of anesthesia administration and the oxygenation of the patient with 100% oxygen. A nontriggering anesthetic agent may be given. Dantrolene sodium (Dantrium) is the pharmacological agent administered specifically for the direct treatment of MH crisis. It is reconstituted using sterile injectable water and is given IV. A loading dose of 2.5 mg/kg is given, followed by a dose of 1 mg/kg every 5 minutes until a maximum dose of 10 to 30 mg/kg is reached. Additional interventions include the administration of chilled IV fluids of normal saline or dextrose in water.

Chilled saline lavage of body cavities is also performed, including the rectum, stomach, and peritoneum, if exposed. The bladder is not irrigated, to permit accurate monitoring of urinary output. The patient is also packed with ice along heat transfer points, including the axilla, base of skull, and groin area. Care needs to be taken that, as the crisis diminishes, the patient does not become hypothermic.

Other treatment interventions during MH crisis include the administration of sodium bicarbonate to assist in metabolic and respiratory acidosis regulation, dextrose and insulin to provide available glucose to the cells to maintain cellular metabolism, furosemide or mannitol to promote renal clearance of waste products, and heparin to prevent intravascular clot formation. An indwelling Foley catheter, attached to an urimeter, is inserted into the urinary bladder to monitor urinary output.

Pseudocholinesterase Deficiency Syndrome

Pseudocholinesterase deficiency syndrome is a genetically transmitted trait that decreases the amount of acetylcholinesterase available in the neuromuscular junction to break down acetylcholine during muscle stimulation. Acetylcholine remains effective in the neuromuscular junction, permitting prolonged effect of depolarizing neuromuscular blockade agents. This prolonged effect can last for several hours after agent administration. There is no direct treatment for pseudocholinesterase deficiency beyond respiratory support of the patient until the body eliminates the neuromuscular blockade. Prophylactic treatment includes avoiding the administration of depolarizing neuromuscular blocking agents and notifying the anesthesia care provider of the syndrome prior to future anesthesia administration.

Allergic Reaction

An allergic reaction is the result of histamine release in response to exposure to an allergen, a triggering protein. An allergic reaction may be mild, such as skin irritation, or a life-threatening anaphylactic reaction. Anaphylaxis is an immediate hypersensitive reaction resulting in respiratory distress that leads to vascular collapse and shock. The patient's history should include any prior allergic reactions, and those substances should be avoided if possible. The treatment for an allergy will vary according to the severity of the reaction, ranging from the use of diphenhydramine to the use of pressors, such as ephedrine, to maintain blood pressure and steroids to reduce the immune response to the antigen.

Shock

Shock is an abnormal physiological state indicated by the presence of reduced cardiac output, tachycardia, hypotension, and diminished urinary output. This state may be induced secondary to severe tissue damage, significant blood loss, infection, or anesthetic agent administration.

The goal in the treatment of shock is to promote optimal circulatory volume and function. This may be accomplished by pharmacological treatment, including cardiotonic agents to increase the contractility and output of the heart in the treatment of cardiogenic shock; IV fluids; colloids; plasma expanders and blood products to treat hypovolemic shock; and antibiotics and IV fluids to treat septic shock. The treatment of shock may also involve a surgical intervention to limit blood loss or treat infection.

Cardiac Dysrhythmias

Cardiac dysrhythmias involve abnormal heart rate or rhythm, evidenced by electrocardiogram monitoring. The dysrhythmias may be atrial or ventricular in origin and some may be deadly, if untreated. Dysrhythmias can also be triggered by the combination of anesthetic agents administered to the patient.

Life-threatening dysrhythmias include ventricular tachycardia and ventricular fibrillation. The treatment for cardiac dysrhythmia includes the IV administration of lidocaine HCl. Additionally, defibrillation and pacemaker insertion may be necessary.

Cardiac Arrest

Cardiac arrest involves the cessation of heart pumping action and blood circulation. This, in turn, prevents the delivery of oxygen and glucose to cells for metabolism and the removal of wastes, resulting in metabolic and respiratory acidosis. The initial treatment for cardiac arrest is CPR, followed by advanced cardiac life support (ACLS).

ANESTHETIC AGENTS

Anesthetic agents are divided into three categories: inhalation agents, intravenous agents, and local/regional agents. The patient is provided supportive oxygen therapy during the use of these agents. A summary table of anesthetic agents is found in Table 9-20.

Inhalation Agents

Anesthetic agents that are inhaled and pass into the bloodstream via the respiratory system are called inhalation agents. These agents are delivered to the lungs in a gaseous state, where they cross the alveolar membrane and enter the circulatory system for delivery to the brain. Any exhaled inhalation

TABLE 9-20 Anesthesia Medications

Category	*Generic Name*	*Trade Name*	*Action/Indication*
Inhalation agents	nitrous oxide		Adjunct agent to other anesthetic gases that reduces the concentration of more hazardous inhalation agents
	sevoflurane	Ultane	Volatile liquid inhalation anesthetic; maintains unconsciousness
	desflurane	Suprane	
	isoflurane	Forane	
	enflurane	Ethrane	
	fluothane	Halothane	
Induction agents	propofol	Diprivan	Sedative/hypnotic for IV sedation and/or anesthesia induction
	thiopental sodium	Sodium Pentothal	CNS depressant that induces hypnosis and anesthesia but not analgesia
	metohexital sodium	Brevital	Short-acting barbiturate-anesthetic
Dissociative agent	ketamine hydrochloride (HCl)	Ketalar	Selectively disrupts the associative pathways of the brain
Opiate/narcotic analgesics	fentanyl citrate	Sublimaze	Short-acting barbiturate for pain relief
	sufentanil citrate	Sufenta	
	alfentanil citrate	Alfenta	
Opiate/narcotic analgesics	remifentanyl hydrochloride (HCl)	Ultiva	Ultra-short-acting barbiturate for pain relief
Sedative/tranquilizer	midazolam hydrochloride (HCl)	Versed	Preoperative sedation
	diazepam	Valium	Preoperative sedation
	lorazepam	Ativan	Preoperative sedation
Narcotic antagonist	naloxone hydrochloride (HCl)	Narcan	Binds to opioid receptor sites in the CNS to reverse the effects of narcotic analgesics
	nalmefene	Revex	

(continues)

TABLE 9-20 **(continued)**

Category	*Generic Name*	*Trade Name*	*Action/Indication*
Benzodiazapine antagonist	flumazenil	Mazicon	Binds to benzodiazepine receptor sites in the CNS to reverse the effects of agents such as Versed
Neuroleptoanalgesic	droperidol	Inapsine	Sedative/tranquilizer; aides in management of PONV; may be used in combination with fentanyl citrate
Neuromuscular blockade agents—nondepolarizing	rocuronium bromide	Zemuron	Bind to receptor sites on the nerve side of the neuromuscular junction to prevent muscle contraction
	vercuronium	Norcuron	
	mivacurium chloride	Mivacron	
	atricurium	Tracrium	
	pancuronium bromide	Pavulon	
	tubocurarine chloride	Curare	
Neuromuscular blockade agents—depolarizing	succinylcholine	Anectine	Rapid-acting agent that binds to receptor sites on the muscle side of the neuromuscular junction to prevent muscle contraction
Neuromuscular blockade reversal	endrophonium	Tensilon	Increase production of acetylcholine at the neuromuscular junction
	neostigmine bromide	Prostigmin	
Antimuscarinic/ anticholinergic	glycopyrrolate	Robinul	Block the cholinergic effects of acetylcholine and vagus nerve stimulation; increase heart rate; decrease bronchial and gastric secretions
	atropine sulfate	Atropine	
Nerve blockades—amides	lidocaine hydrochloride (HCl)	Xylocaine; Lignocaine	Block nerve conduction
	bupivicaine hydrochloride (HCl)	Marcaine; Sensorcaine	
	mepivicaine hydrochloride (HCl)	Carbocaine	
	cocaine hydrochloride (HCl)	Cocaine	
	etidocaine hydrochloride (HCl)	Duranest	
	ropivicaine hydrochloride (HCl)	Naropin	
Nerve blockades—esters	tetracaine hydrochloride (HCl)	Pontocaine; Cetacaine	Block nerve conduction
	procaine hydrochloride (HCl)	Novocaine	
Vasoconstrictor	ephedrine sulfate	Ephedrine	Relaxes smooth muscles of the bronchi and stimulates contraction of peripheral blood vessel wall muscles

agents or excess gas in the anesthesia circuit, referred to as waste gas, is captured with a scavenging system for removal from the OR environment, and filtered prior to being vented to the outside air to prevent occupational exposure to these gasses by health care workers.

Oxygen

Although oxygen is not classified as an anesthetic agent, it is a component of most anesthetic administration. In its pure form, oxygen provides the gas essential to the survival of the patient by promoting cellular function.

Nitrous Oxide

Nitrous oxide is a clear, colorless gas with a subtle fruity odor and is the only true gas still in use. It interacts with the cellular membrane of the CNS to produce analgesia with some amnesia. It is not sufficiently potent to be used alone for general anesthesia, but may be used in conjunction with other anesthetic agents to reduce the use of high concentrations of other more potent and dangerous inhalation agents. Nitrous oxide freely diffuses into closed spaces, such as the middle ear, the bowel, and the pleural space, causing increased pressure within those spaces, contraindicating its use during segments of some surgical interventions such as following graft placement during tympanoplasty. Nitrous oxide is eliminated by exhalation. Recent studies indicate that nitrous oxide use may contribute to postoperative nausea and vomiting (PONV).

Volatile Agents

The **volatile agents** consist of a group of liquids whose potent vapors, when inhaled, produce general anesthesia through CNS depression and decreased electroencephalogram (EEG) activity. They also produce generalized myocardial and respiratory depression. Muscle tone is generally decreased, enhancing the ease of exposure to the surgical site. The volatile agents are delivered from a vaporizer, a component of the anesthesia machine, to the patient via a series of tubings called the anesthesia circuit. Agents commonly in use today include sevoflurane, desflurane, and isoflurane. Less commonly used agents include enflurane and halothane.

Sevoflurane (Ultane) is an odorless inhalation agent that does not cause irritation to the respiratory tract. It has a rapid and smooth onset and recovery, making it an ideal agent for both adult and pediatric patients. Sevoflurane causes bradycardia, hypotension, and cardiac dysrhythmias and reduces cardiac output. It may also produce PONV. Sevoflurane does not cause liver damage, but may cause mild to moderate renal complications. Its use potentiates the action of neuromuscular blocking agents and can be a triggering agent for MH. Despite the fact that the agent is significantly more expensive to use than other agents on the market, sevoflurane is becoming the agent of choice for inhalation anesthesia for appropriate patient populations.

Desflurane (Suprane) has a pungent aroma, contraindicating its use during inhalation induction. It provides a rapid onset and recovery. Because it is not biotransformed in the liver, desflurane is safe to use for patients with hepatic insufficiency. Desflurane is less costly to use than is sevoflurane, and studies indicate that it equals sevoflurane in causing PONV and overall length of recovery.

Isoflurane (Forane) is a halogenated inhalation agent that provides a moderately rapid induction and recovery. It is a profound respiratory depressant and may cause hypotension, which is reversed with surgical stimulation. Isoflurane markedly enhances the effects of neuromuscular blockade. It also increases intracranial pressure (ICP), which is reversible with hyperventilation.

Enflurane (Ethrane) and halothane (Fluothane) are less commonly used inhalation agents. Both agents have a pleasant, nonirritating aroma and are rapid acting. Enflurane can cause alteration in renal function. Halothane produces profound muscle relaxation and bronchial dilation, but may induce hepatitis in the adult surgical patient. Halothane is a potent uterine muscle relaxant and therefore should never be used on the pregnant female.

INTRAVENOUS AGENTS

Intravenous (IV) agents delivered directly into the bloodstream act quickly. IV access is commonly achieved by placement of a catheter in a peripheral vein of the upper extremity. IV agents are removed from the body through redistribution and biotransformation in the liver and excretion by the kidneys. The safety of IV agents is directly related to their ease of metabolism and is dependent on the patient's overall level of hepatic and/or renal function. IV agents are grouped into induction, dissociative, opioids, sedatives/tranquilizers, neuromuscular blocking, **antimuscarinic/anticholingergic**, and adjunctive.

Induction Agents

The IV induction agents are those medications used to permit a rapid transition from a state of consciousness (Stage I) to unconsciousness (Stage III) by causing the patient to quickly pass through the excitement or delirium stage (Stage II). While induction agents do not provide pain relief or motor-impulse blockade, they do produce marked sedation and amnesia. Hypotension and respiratory depression are common side effects of induction agent administration, requiring the availability of supportive and resuscitative equipment when these agents are used. Some induction agents may also be used during maintenance of general anesthesia.

Propofol (Diprivan) is a sedative-hypnotic agent. Due to its milky appearance, the drug has been nicknamed the "milk of amnesia." Propofol is a soy-oil-in-water emulsion capable of supporting microbial growth. Strict sterile technique is used during its preparation and administration. Induction doses produce unconsciousness, but lower doses produce conscious sedation. Because of its alkaline nature, propofol is irritating to the vein and may cause patient discomfort at the IV site during administration. Lidocaine HCl given IV just prior to propofol injection may ease the discomfort of this side effect. Propofol provides a rapid induction and emergence without the prolonged "hangover" effect of other agents. It is the induction agent of choice for many surgical interventions and procedures. Because it causes increased ICP and marked hypotension, propofol is contraindicated for those patients with unstable hemodynamics and/or head trauma.

Etomidate (Amidate) is a nonbarbiturate hypnotic agent used for anesthesia induction. Similar to propofol in the time of induction and emergence, etomidate does not produce analgesia. Because it produces minimal cardiovascular system effects, etomidate is the preferred agent of choice for anesthesia induction with the hemodynamically unstable patient. PONV and adrenal suppression are seen more frequently in patients given etomidate.

Thiopental sodium (Pentothal Sodium) is a short-acting, potent barbiturate that does not provide anesthesia or muscle relaxation but does have hypnotic, amnesic, and sedative effects. Repeated administration of thiopental sodium during the surgical intervention has a cumulative effect, as the medication is stored in lipid-based tissues and slowly released. While less expensive to administer than propofol, thiopental sodium leaves the patient with a residual "hangover" effect that can prolong the patient's emergence and recovery phases. The advantages of thiopental sodium use include nonflammability, nonirritable to the respiratory tract, and lack of salivary stimulation. Thiopental sodium in combination with nitrous oxide and opioids has a synergistic effect, permitting lower and safer doses of these potent agents to be used. Disadvantages of thiopental sodium use include laryngospasm, resulting from minor patient stimulation during the lighter stages of anesthesia administration, and the alkaline nature of the drug, which may be locally irritating to the vein, and respiratory and circulatory depression immediately following injection.

Methohexital sodium (Brevital) is similar in action to propofol and thiopental sodium. Methohexital sodium has an ultrashort onset and duration of action, making it the agent of choice for achieving short-term loss of consciousness during regional blockade for ophthalmologic cases.

Dissociative Agents

The dissociative agents selectively interrupt the associative pathways of the brain. Patients may appear wide awake, yet they are unaware of their surroundings. Dissociative agents also produce amnesia and profound analgesia.

Ketamine HCl (Ketalar) is the most commonly used dissociative agent and it is administered either IM or IV. It produces a rapid induction of the dissociated and amnesic state, which may be accelerated by the concurrent use of other narcotics and/or barbiturates. Ketamine HCl by itself does not produce relaxation or reduce the patient's reflexes, in particular the "gag" reflex. Muscle tone is generally increased. It also increases ICP, IOP, blood pressure, and salivation. The major disadvantage of ketamine HCl use is the production of vivid imagery and morbid hallucinations during administration and recovery. Documented cases of "flashbacks" limit this agent's use to children 2–10 years of age.

Opiate/Opioids

The opiate/opioids are a group of narcotics classified as analgesics, which also produce sedation. They act by binding to CNS and spinal cord receptors, producing a decrease in pain impulse transmission. Euphoria or a feeling of happiness and well-being may also be experienced, thereby also reducing surgery-related anxiety. High doses of these agents may lead to a loss of consciousness and respiratory depression. Opioids do not produce muscle relaxation, but rather they tend to increase overall muscle tone. Opioids are commonly used as an adjunct to general anesthesia agents, permitting the use of lower, safer concentrations of inhalation agents. Occasionally, opioids are used as the sole anesthetic agent, as is sometimes used during cardiac surgery. They are biotransformed primarily in the liver and eliminated in urine. All opiates/opioids are controlled substances regulated by the FDA and include meperidine (Demerol), fentanyl (Sublimaze), sufentanil (Sufenta), alfentanil (Alfenta), and remifentanil (Ultiva).

Morphine sulfate is used for the control of severe pain. It is given IM or IV as a preoperative sedative/analgesic or postoperative analgesic, IV as an anesthetic agent, or intrathecally via spinal administration for intraoperative and postoperative pain control. The use of morphine sulfate permits a reduction in dosage and/or concentration of more potent agents. Side effects include bradycardia, hypotension, vasodilation, nausea and vomiting, confusion, and respiratory depression.

Meperidine (Demerol) is similar in action to morphine. Used to treat moderate to severe pain, meperidine may be administered IM but is given IV when used as an anesthetic adjunct. In addition to respiratory depression, side effects include increased ICP, tachycardia, and vasodilation.

Fentanyl citrate (Sublimaze) action is inhibiting CNS pain pathway stimulation, resulting in an alteration in pain perception and an increased pain threshold. Given IV, fentanyl citrate has a rapid onset and short duration of action. Adverse reactions include bradycardia, laryngospasm, and cardiorespiratory arrest. Its use is contraindicated in patients with myasthenia gravis, a pathological condition characterized by debilitating muscle weakness, especially in the face and throat.

Sufentanil citrate (Sufenta) is similar in nature to fentanyl but is five times more potent. Sufentanil citrate produces analgesia with sedation and euphoria. Sufentanil citrate is a respiratory depressant and has a rapid onset of action when given IV. It has a short duration of activity and is rapidly eliminated.

Alfentanil HCl (Alfenta) is similar in action and usage to fentanyl citrate and sufentanil citrate but acts on pain receptors of the limbic system, thalamus, midbrain, and hypothalamus, altering pain perception and response. It is a short-acting analgesic, but the induced respiratory depression may outlast the analgesic effect.

Remifentanil HCl (Ultiva) is an ultra-short-acting synthetic opioid metabolized in blood and muscle tissue. It has a short duration of action, approximately 5–10 minutes. Its potency and action are similar to those of the other synthetic opioids. Remifentanil may cause respiratory depression, bradycardia, hypotension, and muscle rigidity. The advantage over other opioids is that its short duration of action allows more accurate dose titration.

NARCOTIC ANTAGONISTS

The effects of opioids can be reversed by the administration of naloxone HCl (Narcan), which works by competing for CNS receptor sites, preventing opioid binding. Naloxone

HCl given IV leads to an abrupt onset of pain, as the opioid previously administered no longer provides pain relief. This may cause tachycardia and hypertension. Because the effects of naloxone HCl usually last 15 to 30 minutes, which is usually shorter than the effects of the opioid, patients should be closely monitored for opioid-induced rebound respiratory depression.

Benzodiazepines

Benzodiazepines are sedative/tranquilizers used in anesthesia in two ways: to reduce the anxiety and apprehension of the preoperative patient and as an adjunct to general anesthesia to reduce the amount and concentration of other more potent agents. Sedatives do not produce analgesia. The most commonly used sedatives come from the benzodiazepine group and are used for their ability to produce amnestic, anticonvulsive, hypnotic, sedative, and muscle relaxation effects. Hypotensive changes and respiratory depression may occur, especially when benzodiazepines are administered with an opioid agent. The two most commonly used benzodiazepines are diazepam (Valium) and midazolam HCl (Versed).

Diazepam (Valium) is a Class IV controlled substance. Its primary use related to anesthesia administration is to reduce anxiety and provide some skeletal muscle relaxation. It also provides retrograde amnesia of short duration. Given IV, diazepam has a rapid onset of action and is metabolized in the liver for renal excretion.

Midazolam HCl (Versed) is also a Class IV controlled substance. It is a rapid-onset and short-acting benzodiazepine, making it an ideal agent for patients undergoing outpatient procedures. Its action is similar to diazepam, but its memory impairment is of shorter duration. Since midazolam is twice as potent as diazepam, the IV dosage is commonly diluted with injectable dextrose/water or saline for administration.

Droperidol (Inapsine) produces sedation and amnesia with a long duration of action. Droperidol provides the additional benefit of acting as an antiemetic. Innovar® is a mixture of fentanyl citrate and droperidol providing a combination of sedation and analgesia.

Benzodiazepine Antagonists

The effects of benzodiazepines may be reversed by the administration of flumazenil (Mazicon). Flumazenil works by competing for benzodiazepine inhibitory receptor sites. Flumazenil has a rapid onset of action that reverses the sedative effects but may not reverse the amnesia effects. Convulsions may also occur with flumazenil administration. Patients need to be assessed and monitored for rebound sedation and/or respiratory depression.

Neuromuscular Blockade

Skeletal muscle relaxants, or neuromuscular blockers (NMBs), interfere with the passage of impulses from motor nerves to skeletal muscles, resulting in muscle weakness and paralysis. Jaw relaxation is achieved to facilitate endotracheal intubation, the muscles of respiration are affected, allowing for mechanical ventilation, and the musculature at the surgical site is relaxed to allow tissue retraction for surgical exposure. Administered IV, NMBs serve as an adjunct to other general anesthesia agents, permitting a decrease in dosage and concentration of other more potent agents. Depending on the agent's onset and duration, NMBs are commonly readministered throughout the surgical procedure. The blockade effect is monitored by the use of a peripheral nerve stimulator. Neuromuscular blockade must be naturally or pharmacologically reversed prior to extubation to reverse the respiratory muscle paralysis.

NMBs are divided into two major categories: nondepolarizing agents and depolarizing agents (see Table 9-20).

Nondepolarizing Agents

Nondepolarizing agents work by competing for postsynaptic receptor sites at the neuromuscular junction. This competition prevents acetylcholine from being able to stimulate muscle contraction. Spontaneous recovery of neuromuscular blockade may occur as the agent diffuses from the receptor sites into the synapse. Nondepolarizing agents may also be reversed by the administration of agents that inhibit acetylcholinesterase, the enzyme that breaks down acetylcholine.

Mivacurium chloride (Mivacron) is a short-acting nondepolarizing muscle relaxant with intermediate length of onset. It should be used with caution in patients with a familial history of pseudocholinesterase deficiency and in patients with hepatic or renal insufficiency.

Vecuronium bromide (Norcuron) is a short-acting nondepolarizing muscle relaxant with an intermediate onset. The use of succinylcholine for intubation prior to administering vecuronium for maintenance may prolong the effects of neuromuscular blockade.

Rocuronium bromide (Zemuron) is a short-acting nondepolarizing muscle relaxant with a rapid onset. It may be given by IV bolus for induction or by continuous IV drip for maintenance. It provides a rapid, spontaneous recovery, similar to succinylcholine, without the side effects of depolarizing blocker usage. Because rocuronium is metabolized by the liver, it should be used with caution in patients with hepatic insufficiency.

Atracurium besylate (Tracrium) is an intermediate-acting nondepolarizing muscle relaxant with a short onset. It provides a rapid recovery from NMB effect.

Cisatracurium besylate (Nimbex) is an intermediate-acting nondepolarizing muscle relaxant with an intermediate duration of action. It is two to three times more potent than atracurium besylate.

Tubocurarine chloride (Curare) is a long-acting nondepolarizing muscle relaxant with a rapid onset of action. It causes histamine release and may induce bronchospasm and hemodynamic changes.

Pancuronium bromide (Pavulon) is a long-acting nondepolarizing muscle relaxant with an intermediate onset. The action of pancuronium is enhanced by inhalation agents, requiring a reduction in dosage. It may cause an elevation of blood pressure and heart rate. It is eliminated in urine, and therefore care should be used when administering this agent to patients with renal disease.

Depolarizing Agents

Depolarizing agents work by mimicking a release of acetylcholine across the neuromuscular junction. The agent binds to the postsynaptic receptors, causing muscle contraction to occur, which is followed by a period of muscle fatigue. The contraction/relaxation cycle in the muscle is strong enough to be visible; the action is referred to as *fasciculation* and the patient may experience postoperative muscle ache because of the strength of the fasciculation. The effects of depolarizing agents cannot be pharmacologically reversed.

The main depolarizing agent in use today is succinylcholine (Anectine), an ultra-short-acting agent. It has a rapid onset and is useful in producing rapid neuromuscular blockade for intubation. It causes an increase in both IOP and ICP. Succinylcholine may be given as an IV bolus or in a continuous IV drip for neuromuscular blockade maintenance. A mild nondepolarizing agent may be given just prior to succinylcholine administration to reduce or eliminate fasciculation. Succinylcholine is also a known triggering agent for MH.

Neuromuscular Blockade Antagonism

The reversal or antagonism of nondepolarizing neuromuscular agents can be produced through the use of one of two drugs: edrophonium chloride (Tensilon) and neostigmine (Prostigmin). These are two cholinergic drugs that prevent the destruction of acetylcholine (ACh). The increase in the ACh restores the transmission of impulses from the nerves to the skeletal muscles. To prevent a cholinergic crisis, these agents are usually given in conjunction with an antimuscarinic agent such as atropine sulfate or glycopyrrolate (Robinul).

OTHER AGENTS COMMONLY USED DURING ANESTHESIA ADMINISTRATION

Antimuscarinic Agents

Antimuscarinic (formerly known as *anticholinergic*) agents act to block the cholinergic effects of certain drugs or stimulation of the parasympathetic nervous system, including excessive salivation and bradycardia. The two most commonly used agents are atropine sulfate and glycopyrrolate (Robinul).

Nonsteroidal Anti-inflammatory Drugs

Ketorolac (Toradol) is an NSAID used for moderate pain control. This agent is given IM to aid in pain management during emergence and recovery.

Gastric Acid Management

Histamine (H_2) antagonists and antacids are agents used to alter the pH of gastric secretions and reduce gastric volume. They are given during the preoperative or intraoperative period. Included in this group are the oral agent citric acid (Bicitra) and the IV agents cimetidine (Tagamet) and ranitidine (Zantac). Metoclopramide (Reglan), a cholinergic agent, can also be used to promote pyloric emptying.

Lubricants

Lubricants are used to protect the cornea when the eye is unable to close or when natural lubrication of the eye is impaired. Lubricants such as Lacri-lube or Duratears are used when general anesthesia is administered, to prevent corneal drying.

Antiemetics

Antiemetic agents are used to prevent post-operative nausea and vomiting (POVN). Droperidol (Inapsine), metoclopramide (Reglan), ondansetron HCl (Zofran), granisetron HCl (Kytril), and dolasetron mesylate (Anzemet) have antiemetic properties and are usually given by intravenous injection.

SOLUTIONS USED IN THE OPERATING ROOM SETTING

Many pharmacologic agents used during anesthesia administration are delivered directly into the bloodstream. Access to the vascular system during a surgical intervention is maintained through the use of a peripheral or central venous catheter. Patency of the vascular catheter is maintained using an infusion of intravenous solution. These solutions include:

- *Ringer's solution:* Ringer's solution is a water-based solution for injection that contains essential serum electrolytes in the forms of sodium chloride, potassium chloride, and calcium chloride and is physiologically similar to plasma.
- *Lactated Ringer's (LR) solution:* LR has sodium lactate added in addition to the electrolytes, which enables it to serve as a glucose source for body metabolism. Both Ringer's solution and LR are used to correct fluid and electrolyte deficits and mild acidosis.
- *5% dextrose solution (D5W):* D5W is a solution of water with a 5% concentration of dextrose monohydrate added that serves as a source of glucose, a sugar normally obtained by eating. D5W is used to correct hypoglycemia and replace water lost during normal metabolism.
- *0.9% saline solution (normal saline):* Normal saline (NS) is a solution of water with the addition of sodium chloride. NS is used to correct deficits of sodium and chloride and treat metabolic alkalosis. It is used in the OR when blood or blood products are being administered.

ADJUNCTS TO GENERAL ANESTHESIA

Several types of supplemental treatments are now incorporated into balanced anesthesia to enhance the safety and effectiveness of the medications previously discussed.

Induced Hypothermia

Induced hypothermia involves the artificial, deliberate lowering of the body's core temperature below normal limits. The resulting lower temperature causes an overall reduction in body metabolism along with a reduction in oxygen and glucose consumption and waste production. Induced hypothermia permits the use of lower dosages of inhalation and IV agents, providing a safer level of anesthetic agent administration.

There are four levels of cooling involved with induced hypothermia. Light hypothermia, where the core body temperature is brought to a range between 98.6° and 89.6°F, results in an altered or reduced level of consciousness. A core body temperature ranging from 89.6° to 78.8°F is classified as moderate hypothermia. A core body temperature between 78.8° and 68°F is classified as deep hypothermia. Profound hypothermia occurs when the core temperature drops below 68°F.

Hypothermic levels are induced by several methods, including body surface cooling, internal cavity cooling, and systemic blood circulation cooling. Induced hypothermia is indicated as an adjunctive therapy for use during open-heart surgery, following cardiopulmonary resuscitation, as a treatment for MH, and during a hypertensive crisis, organ transplantation, and periods of decreased blood flow to the brain.

Induced Hypotension

Induced hypotension involves a controlled decrease of blood pressure during anesthetic administration. Hypotension results in a decrease in bleeding while increasing visibility within the surgical field. Induced hypotension is an adjunctive therapy technique used as one of the "bloodless surgery" protocols for those patients who do not desire to receive a blood transfusion.

Neuroleptanalgesia and Neuroleptanesthesia

Neuroleptanalgesia uses high doses of neuroleptics (tranquilizers) and narcotic analgesic agents to induce a state of diminished anxiety, sedation, and amnesia, allowing the patient to retain the ability to respond to commands. Two medications commonly used to induce neuroleptanalgesia are fentanyl citrate and meperidine HCl. Neuroleptanesthesia uses neuroleptanalgesia techniques supplemented with an inhalation agent.

NERVE CONDUCTION BLOCKADE

Nerve conduction blockade anesthesia, commonly referred to as local or regional anesthesia, involves the use of pharmaceutical agents to prevent the transmission of sensory nerve impulses. The conduction blocking agent is absorbed by the nerve sheath, decreasing nerve impulse conduction to a point where sensory impulses are unable to be transmitted. Motor impulse transmission may or may not be affected, depending on the function of the blocked nerve. A variety of techniques are used for nerve conduction blockade, as listed in Table 9-21.

TABLE 9-21 Nerve Blockade Techniques

Name	Description
Topical anesthesia	Agent applied to mucous membrane, conjunctiva, or skin
Local anesthesia	Agent is injected at the site of the surgical procedure
Regional anesthesia	Agent is injected to provide anesthesia to a specific area of the body, e.g., foot, arm, lower extremities
Nerve plexus block	Agent is injected in the tissues surrounding a major nerve plexus, such as the brachial (axillary), cervical (neck), caudal (sacrum), or lumbar (lower back) plexus
Spinal (intrathecal) block	Agent is injected into the cerebrospinal fluid within the subarachnoid space
Epidural block	Agent is injected into the space above the dura
Bier block (intravenous)	Agent is injected into a vein in the arm that has been drained of blood following placement of a tourniquet

Nerve Conduction Blocking Agents

Nerve conduction blocking agents are used in low concentrations (0.25%–4%), with the exception of topical cocaine HCl, which is commonly used in slightly higher concentrations (up to 10%). The agents are divided into two groups: the amino amides and the amino esters (Table 9-22).

Amino Amide Group

Drugs in the amino amide group are metabolized in the liver and excreted by the kidneys; toxicity may occur in patients with liver disease. Drugs in this group include lidocaine HCl (Xylocaine, Lignocaine), mepivacaine HCl (Carbocaine), bupivacaine HCl (Marcaine, Sensorcaine), and etidocaine HCl (Duranest).

Lidocaine HCl is a widely used local anesthetic agent with a rapid onset of action with moderate duration. Lidocaine HCl can be administered topically for application on mucous membranes, injected locally for peripheral nerve block, or injected into the tissues surrounding a major nerve root to provide regional blockade. Available in concentrations ranging from 0.5% to 5%, lidocaine HCl is prepackaged with or without

TABLE 9-22 Commonly Used Nerve Conduction Blocking Agents

Type	*Name*	*Brand Name(s)*
Amino amides	lidocaine HCl	Xylocaine, Lignocaine
	mepivacaine HCl	Carbocaine
	bupivacaine HCl	Marcaine, Sensorcaine
	etidocaine HCl	Duranest
	ropivicaine HCl	Naropin
Amino esters	cocaine HCl	Cocaine
	procaine HCl	Novocaine
	tetracaine HCl	Pontocaine, Cetacaine

epinephrine. (*Note:* Lidocaine HCl is also used to treat heart arrhythmias.)

Mepivacaine HCl (Carbocaine) is similar in action to lidocaine HCl but has a longer duration. It is commonly used for patients who are hypertensive, since a significant rise in blood pressure upon administration does not occur.

Bupivacaine HCl (Marcaine, Sensorcaine) is four times more potent than lidocaine HCl. It has a longer onset of action and a longer duration. It is commonly administered by local injection for regional blockade, and is used for both intraoperative and postoperative pain management. Used in concentrations of less than 1%, bupivacaine HCl comes prepackaged without or with epinephrine. Concentrations of 0.75% bupivacaine HCl produce complete motor and sensory blockade; lesser concentrations may only produce sensory blockade. Lidocaine HCl and bupivacaine HCl may be combined to provide an agent that has a rapid onset of anesthesia with prolonged duration.

Etidocaine HCl (Duranest) has a long onset and duration of action. Used in concentrations of less than 2%, etidocaine HCl is used as a topical agent in surgical wounds, minimizing postoperative surgical site discomfort. The drug is highly toxic; therefore, its use is contraindicated in children younger than 12 years of age.

Ropivacaine HCl (Naropin) is slightly less potent than bupivicaine HCl but has less overall toxicity. Like bupivicaine HCl, ropivacaine HCl has a long onset and duration of action. It is used in concentrations of 1% or less. Ropivicaine HCl is not combined with epinephrine, as this does not prolong the duration of its effect. It is commonly used for major nerve conduction blocks, epidural anesthesia in labor and delivery, and for postoperative pain management, especially following major abdominal, cardiac, and thoracic surgery. It is not commonly used for local or spinal anesthesia.

Amino Ester Group

Drugs in the amino ester group include cocaine HCl (Cocaine), procaine HCl (Novocaine), and tetracaine HCl (Pontocaine, Cetacaine).

Cocaine HCl, a CNS stimulant, is used only as a topical agent on the mucosa of the upper aerodigestive tract due to its high toxicity. It is classified as a controlled substance. In concentrations of 4% to 10%, cocaine HCl produces localized anesthesia and vasoconstriction, with shrinkage of mucous membranes. Cocaine is metabolized in the liver and excreted by the kidneys.

Tetracaine HCl (Cetacaine, Pontocaine) is an agent with a slow onset of action but prolonged duration. Its primary uses are as a topical anesthetic on oropharyngeal mucous membranes and ocular conjunctiva, or for intrathecal injection during spinal anesthesia administration. It is not used for local injection or peripheral nerve block.

Adjunctive Agents to Nerve Conduction Blockade

Two adjunctive agents associated with nerve conduction blockade agents that influence the onset and duration of action of these agents are hyaluronidase (Wydase) and epinephrine.

Hyaluronidase (Wydase) is an agent added to local anesthetic agents to assist in medication distribution within the subcutaneous tissues for contact with the peripheral nerves. This is especially useful during retrobulbar ocular block.

Epinephrine, commonly referred to as "epi.," is a potent vasoconstrictor. Because of its vasoconstrictive properties, the use of epinephrine as an adjunctive agent to nerve conduction blocking agents provides two main benefits.. First, the area's blood flow is reduced, decreasing intraoperative bleeding; second, because the blood flow to the area is reduced, the body is unable to redistribute the anesthetic agent effectively, prolonging the overall anesthetic effect.

Caution must be exercised in administering epinephrine to patients with hypertension or cardiac disease, and its use should be limited during administration of a digital or penile block, for use in tissue with preexisting vascular compromise, and in children because of its vasoconstrictive properties.

As a convenience, epinephrine is available premixed by the manufacturer with lidocaine HCl or bupivacaine HCl. The label of these premixed agents is usually color-coded red to indicate the addition of epinephrine.

TOPICAL ANESTHESIA

Topical anesthesia involves the placement of a nerve conduction blocking agent onto the skin or mucous membrane. This method is used to provide anesthesia on mucous membranes of the upper aerodigestive tract, urethra, vagina, rectum, eye, and skin. The tissue effect is limited to the area in contact with the topical anesthetic, onset is rapid, and duration of action is usually related to the specific agent and dose used. Topical anesthesia can be administered by the anesthesia care provider or the surgeon and is achieved with either the use of cryoanesthesia and/or a pharmacological agent.

Cryoanesthesia involves the reduction of nerve conduction/transmission by localized cooling. This may be accomplished with ice or the use of a cryoanesthesia machine to produce the cooling action, or the reduced skin temperature may be a result of a pharmaceutical agent sprayed onto the skin, such as ethyl chloride. The result is a localized "freezing" of the skin and superficial nerve endings, blocking nerve impulse transmission and therefore eliminating pain.

Pharmacological agents applied directly to the skin are absorbed and come in contact with the peripheral nerve endings, providing anesthesia by preventing the initiation of the nerve impulse. Lidocaine HCl and cocaine HCl are examples of agents typically used for topical anesthesia.

LOCAL ANESTHESIA

Local infiltration involves the injection of a nerve conduction-blocking agent into the tissues surrounding a peripheral nerve or nerves that serve only the tissue at the site of surgical intervention. The onset, depending on the agent used, occurs within 5–15 minutes. The surgeon usually administers the local anesthetic, and readministration may be necessary as the surgical site is expanded or additional tissue layers are exposed.

Monitored Anesthesia Care

Monitored anesthesia care (MAC) involves the use of a combination of nerve conduction blockade supplemented with analgesics, sedatives, or amnesics. It is indicated for use in patients with complex medical problems or as a supplement to local anesthesia to provide amnesia. The surgeon commonly performs nerve conduction blockade with patient monitoring and IV sedation/analgesia performed by the anesthesia care provider.

REGIONAL ANESTHESIA

Regional blockade involves the administration of an anesthetic along a major nerve tract by the anesthesia care provider. This technique blocks nerve impulse conduction from all tissues distal to the injection site. Onset of action is slower than with local infiltration, and the duration is agent dependent. Common types of regional blockade include the nerve plexus block, Bier block, spinal block, and epidural block.

Nerve Plexus Block

The nerve plexus block has surgical, diagnostic, and therapeutic applications. It is accomplished with the injection of an anesthetic solution in an area of a major nerve plexus, such as the brachial plexus or at the base of a structure. The resulting anesthesia includes all tissue innervated by the plexus. Commonly used in conjunction with IV sedation, plexus blockade permits analgesia to continue through the immediate postoperative/recovery phase.

Bier Block

Bier block provides anesthesia to the distal portion of the upper extremity by injecting a large volume of low-concentration anesthetic agent, usually 50 mL of 0.5% lidocaine HCl without epinephrine, into a vein at a level below a tourniquet. A double-cuffed tourniquet is placed on the upper arm, and venous access is obtained by the placement of a catheter close to the intended site of surgical intervention. The limb is then exsanguinated with the use of an Esmarch bandage, and the proximal cuff of the tourniquet is inflated to a level approximately 100 mm Hg above the systolic blood pressure. The inflated cuff confines the agent in the limb while providing a bloodless surgical field. Once the agent has been injected via the IV catheter, the catheter is removed. The agent is absorbed into the surrounding tissues through the vein walls. The tourniquet remains inflated for the duration of desired anesthesia, preventing normal circulation from redistributing the anesthetic agent. Should the patient experience discomfort related to pressure from the tourniquet cuff, the distal cuff may be inflated after limb anesthesia has been established and the proximal cuff released. Bier block is used on interventions of the extremity of 1-hour duration or less. At the conclusion of the surgical intervention, the tourniquet is slowly released, permitting the agent to circulate throughout the body. Inadvertent systemic delivery of the anesthetic agent could occur due to tourniquet failure, or when releasing the tourniquet soon after agent administration, resulting in potentially adverse cardiovascular or CNS effects.

Spinal Block

Spinal anesthesia, also referred to as intrathecal block, involves injection of an anesthetic agent into the cerebrospinal fluid (CSF) within the subarachnoid space between the pia mater and arachnoid mater (meningeal layers), resulting in loss of sensation to the entire body below the level of the diaphragm. The procedure for spinal administration is found in Table 9-23.

Spinal anesthesia lasts approximately 1–1½ hours, depending on the agent used. Additives to the anesthetic solution may prolong the action of the agent. (*Note:* The procedure for obtaining spinal fluid for analysis is similar, but instead of injecting an anesthetic, spinal fluid is withdrawn. This is commonly called a *spinal tap*.)

Several factors can influence the effect of the spinal anesthetic:

- *Patient cooperation:* Patient cooperation is critical to the successful administration of spinal anesthesia. Patients are commonly sedated prior to needle placement to reduce anxiety and promote cooperation.
- *Patient Position:* The patient is usually positioned in the lateral or sitting position, depending on the anesthesia care provider's preference, the patient's primary and/or secondary medical conditions, and the patient's ability to cooperate. It is possible to administer a spinal anesthetic with the patient in the prone position, but this is rarely done. Regardless of the position used, the goal is to expand the intervertebral space(s) to allow for needle placement (Figure 9-7).

Table 9-23 Procedure for Spinal Anesthesia Administration

1. The circulator assists the patient into the desired position (sitting or side-lying) and assists the patient in maintaining the position and provides emotional support.
2. The lower lumbar area is cleansed (prepped) and draped with a fenestrated sheet.
3. Prior to placement of the spinal needle, a small amount of local anesthetic is placed into the subcutaneous tissues along the intended needle path to maximize patient comfort and cooperation.
4. Access to the subarachnoid space is achieved by the insertion of a fine-gauge, 3-in. spinal needle through the tissues of the L2–3 or L3–4 disk spaces of the vertebral column.
5. Correct needle placement is confirmed by the presence of CSF in the needle hub when the needle stylet is removed.
6. The syringe containing the anesthetic is gently connected to the spinal needle, ensuring that air is not allowed to enter the system.
7. The agent is then slowly injected, and the needle is removed. A dressing may be applied. Onset of effect is seen within 3–10 minutes.
8. The patient is repositioned for the intended procedure.

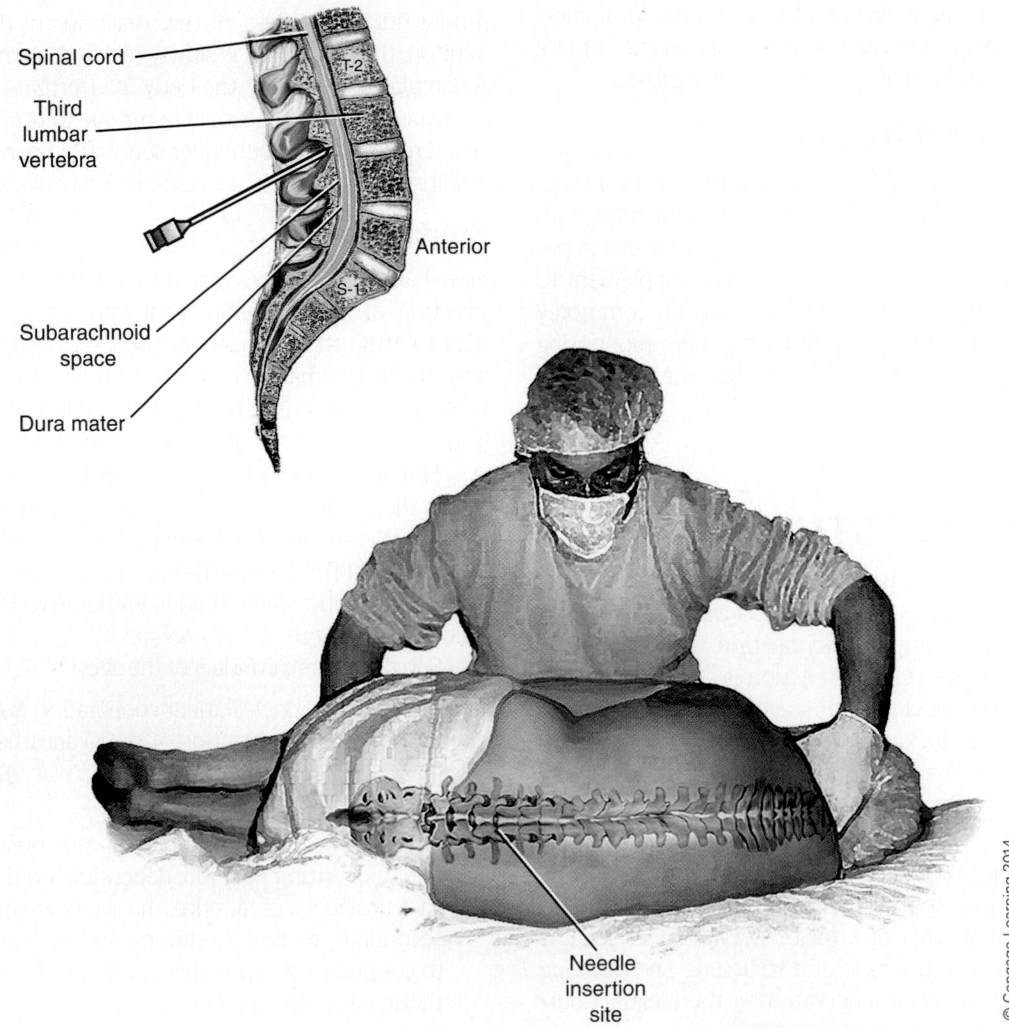

Figure 9-7 Positioning for spinal anesthesia

- *Agent baricity: Baricity,* in spinal anesthesia, refers to the specific gravity of the anesthetic solution in comparison to CSF. Solutions with high specific gravity are referred to as hyperbaric solutions and tend to settle toward gravity. Inversely, a solution with low specific gravity is referred to as a hypobaric solution and tends to "float" or move away from gravity. Isobaric solutions are solutions with the same specific gravity as CSF.

Prior to administration, the anesthetic agent may be combined with sterile injectable water or sterile injectable dextrose solution to create one of the three solution baricities previously described. These, in conjunction with the patient's position following agent administration, are the principal determinants of agent effect.

The most common baricity used is the hyperbaric spinal. The patient is positioned with the operative side in the dependent position. Following agent administration, the patient will remain in this position while the agent "settles" and affects the nerve roots of the dependent area.

A hypobaric spinal is used for patients undergoing procedures in the prone or jackknife positions. The patient is positioned immediately following agent administration, permitting the agent to "settle" around the nerve roots of the sacral and caudal areas.

- *Rate of injection:* The rate of agent injection will affect the agent's placement. Rapid injection will promote turbulence as the medication combines with CSF. This may cause the agent to spread over a larger area, increasing the area of effect.
- *Increased CSF pressure:* An increase in CSF pressure may result from the position of the operating table, coughing, straining, or muscle contraction. This can occur in the patient who has a uterine contraction immediately following agent placement, or it may occur during patient repositioning following agent placement. An increase in pressure may result in migration of the anesthetic agent and unintended contact with nerve roots controlling major body functions. Spinal anesthesia may cause a loss in the sensations associated with breathing or may, in fact, cause loss of sensory and/or motor function of the diaphragm. Should this occur, respiratory assistance is necessary until function is restored.

Spinal Anesthetic Agents and Additives

The most commonly used agent for spinal anesthesia administration is tetracaine HCl. Other agents for use in spinal anesthesia administration include lidocaine HCl and procaine HCl.

Duration of the anesthetic may be enhanced with the addition of epinephrine to the anesthetic solution, preventing rapid redistribution of the agent. Postoperative pain management may also be performed during the same injection by the addition of an intrathecal opioid, such as preservative-free morphine sulfate (Duramorph).

Advantages and Disadvantages of Spinal Anesthesia

The patient remains conscious during spinal anesthesia, permitting the patient to remain in control of the airway. Many patients choose not to be fully aware of the surgical environment, and spinal anesthesia is easily supplemented with IV sedation.

Spinal anesthesia is nonirritating to the respiratory tract. Patients do not experience the discomfort of endotracheal intubation or the irritation sometimes caused to mucous membranes of the upper respiratory tract from exposure to inhalation agents.

Spinal anesthesia blockade of the sympathetic and parasympathetic nervous system produces bowel contraction, facilitating exposure within the abdominal cavity during surgical interventions of the abdomen or pelvis.

Spinal anesthesia is also an excellent muscle relaxant, permitting ease of retraction of the abdominal wall without additional pharmacological intervention.

Spinal anesthesia also has several disadvantages and complications.

Following agent administration, blood vessels innervated by the blocked pathways dilate, resulting in pooling of blood. This results in the hypotension commonly seen immediately following injection. It may continue for a period of time until the body's homeostatic mechanisms can adjust. Blood pressure can drop significantly, leading to ischemic-related issues such as angina or myocardial infarction or cerebrovascular accident in patients who are predisposed to these conditions.

Hypotension is treated in several ways. Patients undergoing spinal anesthesia administration are pretreated with a bolus dose of IV fluids during the immediate preoperative period. This provides a readily available source of fluid support to the circulatory system to counteract venous pooling. Higher-than-normal-volume fluid delivery is continued postinjection for those patients able to tolerate increased fluid loads.

Following spinal anesthesia agent administration, hypotensive episodes are detected with close monitoring of blood pressure and mean arterial pressure. If a hypotensive crisis is detected, the patient is treated with IV ephedrine administration. Ephedrine is a potent vasoconstrictor, resulting in a rise in blood pressure. When this treatment does not result in significant blood pressure stabilization, the patient may be treated with phenylephrine HCl (Neo-Synephrine).

Nausea or vomiting may be induced by the administration of spinal anesthesia. Hypotensive episodes cause the body to shunt blood away from the gastrointestinal organs. Cerebral ischemia and rapid gastric emptying occur in response to reduced blood flow, resulting in nausea and, commonly, vomiting. Vomiting may also be induced by traction on visceral organs of the abdominal cavity during interventions involving the gastrointestinal tract or pelvis.

Dosage control presents another potential problem. The agent, once delivered to the patient, cannot be titrated or adjusted. The anesthesia care provider must use methods other than titration and dose adjustment to manage the side effects and complications of the agent's effects.

Spinal headache is a less frequent complication of spinal anesthesia. Spinal headache results from meningeal layer irritation resulting from a decrease in CSF pressure. This commonly occurs as a result of fluid leaking through the dural puncture site. Primary treatment for "spinal headache" includes bedrest, lying in a horizontal position (prone position is the best choice, but sometimes impractical), and the administration of increased fluids, either by mouth or parenterally (IV). For persistent fluid leakage, a blood patch may be performed. A blood patch involves the creation of a clot over the dural puncture site by the injection of the patient's blood at the site of leakage.

The potential exists for patients to develop temporary or permanent paraesthesia or paralysis related to spinal anesthesia administration. This may be due to inadvertent patient movement during needle placement, inadvertent injection directly into a nerve, or sepsis related to break in sterile technique during administration.

Epidural Anesthesia

Epidural anesthesia involves the administration of an anesthetic agent into the tissues directly above the dura mater, through which the agent is then absorbed into the CSF. An epidural can be administered using a single injection to provide anesthesia of short duration. More commonly, a lumbar approach is used to place an indwelling catheter. The catheter is secured and left in place, permitting titration of the agent's effect by permitting re-administration of additional agent as the patient's condition warrants. When no longer necessary, the catheter is removed.

The rate and volume of agent delivered influence the level or area of anesthesia. The more rapidly a bolus of medication is delivered and the larger the volume given in an injection, the more likely the agent is to spread through the tissue, causing an effect on a larger number of nerve fibers. Patient position and baricity of the anesthetic solution have no effect on the level of anesthesia obtained.

NONTRADITIONAL ANESTHESIA OPTIONS

Several options for nontraditional anesthesia therapy are in use today. These may be used individually or may supplement more traditional Western medicine approaches to anesthesia delivery.

Hypnoanesthesia is an adjunctive therapy useful in altering the patient's level of consciousness and awareness of the surgical environment. The patient must be totally compliant and the hypnotherapist must accompany the patient throughout the procedure. On a more practical level, hypnotherapy is particularly useful during the induction stages of general anesthesia for children undergoing mask induction, focusing the child's attention on a familiar or predetermined thought or activity, making the child less aware of the induction agent and mask aromas. The anesthesia care provider often implements this type of hypnosis.

Acupuncture involves the intense electrical stimulation of specific body sites to alter the perception of pain at the surgical site by the release of endorphins. While a common principal method of intraoperative pain control in Eastern medicine practices, acupuncture is used as an adjunctive therapy in the United States.

ANESTHESIA EQUIPMENT

The primary goal during anesthesia is to maintain homeostasis throughout the perioperative period. The following equipment and devices allow the surgical team to identify physiological changes and implement interventions for many conditions prior to their becoming life threatening.

Anesthesia Machine

Today's anesthesia machine provides a combination of inhalation agent delivery systems, including vaporizers, respiratory support equipment, and sophisticated monitoring devices (Figure 9-8). The inhalation gases and respiratory support

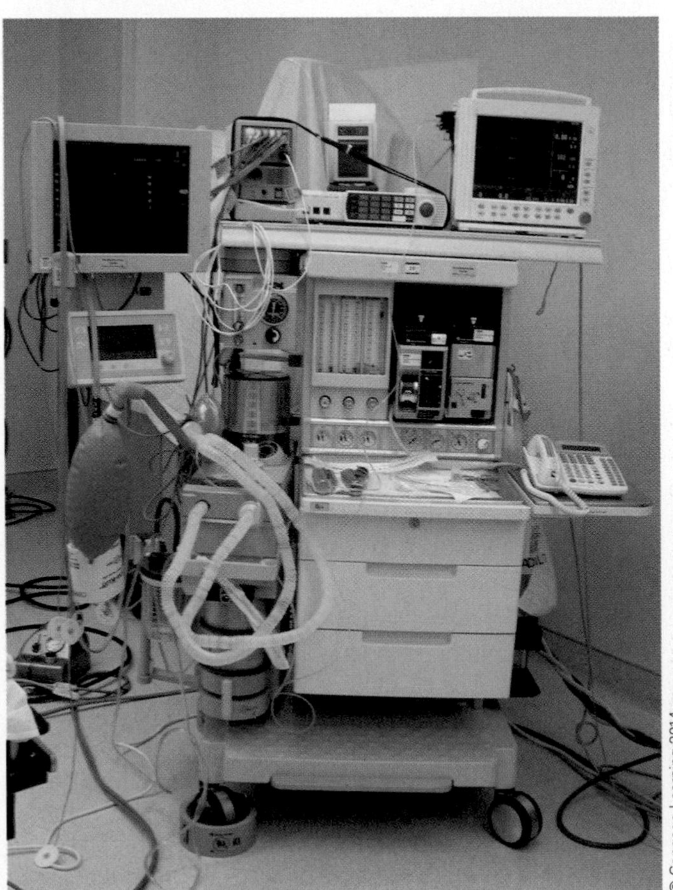

Figure 9-8 Anesthesia machine

are provided to the patient through a series of tubing that is referred to as the anesthesia circuit. Many machines also incorporate an integrated system for patient monitoring and documentation.

Airway Delivery/Maintenance Devices

Ventilators are commonly used in conjunction with neuromuscular blockade during general anesthesia. Mechanical ventilation permits the anesthesia care provider to control the rate and volume of respiration during the surgical intervention. Ventilators are equipped with disconnect alarms and spirometers with built-in high and low alarms. An overpressure "pop-off" valve is included.

Endotracheal (ET) tubes are devices placed through the patient's nose or mouth, between the vocal cords, and into the trachea to provide a patent airway intraoperatively or during ventilatory support (Figure 9-9). A laryngoscope is used to facilitate tube placement. Tubes are commonly made of polyvinylchloride (PVC) but may also be made of rubber or silicone impregnated with metal particles for use in oropharyngeal and laryngeal laser procedures. ET tubes are available in many diameters and configurations. Adult- and pediatric-size tubes include inflatable cuffs (ballooned), permitting the creation of a closed airway system when the cuff is inflated. The ET tube is connected to the anesthesia machine by the anesthesia circuit.

A *stylet* is used to modify the curve of an ET tube or support (stiffen) an ET tube during placement. A stylet is made of malleable metal or stiff plastic and is placed within the lumen of the ET tube. The distal tip should not protrude beyond the end of the ET tube, and the proximal end should be severely bent to prevent accidental retention. The stylet is removed from the ET tube following tube placement into the trachea.

McGill forceps are used to aid and facilitate the placement of endotracheal, nasotracheal, and nasogastric tubes or to insert pharyngeal packing. They are used transorally to grasp the tube or packing material and direct the item to the appropriate area for placement.

The laryngoscope (Figure 9-10) is a device used to expose the glottis to facilitate endotracheal intubation. The rigid laryngoscope consists of a handle and interchangeable blades. The handle contains batteries, which provide current to the small light bulb or fiberoptic bundle found on the distal aspect of the blade. Laryngoscope blades come in two basic shapes: straight and curved. Several variations are available to adjust to the shape and size of the patient. The flexible fiber-optic laryngoscope aids in visualization and performance of difficult intubations. The ET tube is placed over the insertion tube of the scope. The scope is then passed into the laryngopharynx. Once the vocal cords are visualized through the tip of the scope, the ET tube is advanced into position. The scope is then removed.

The laryngeal mask airway (LMA) (Figure 9-11) is a device with an inflated cuff placed into the laryngopharynx through the mouth to form a low-pressure seal around the laryngeal inlet, while providing minimal stimulation to the airway. It provides a simple and effective way of establishing a patent airway without the dangers and complications of endotracheal intubation. Constructed of silicone rubber, the reusable airway has three openings to allow for ventilation in the distal flanged area. The mask is connected to a tube, exiting the patient's mouth which is connected to the anesthesia circuit for the delivery of inhalation agents.

The face mask is used to cover the nose and mouth area of the patient and permit the delivery of anesthetic gases and/or oxygen to the patient. The mask is made of plastic with a molded or balloon-like cuff to facilitate the creation of an airtight seal. Some face masks are manufactured of clear plastic to allow the anesthesia care provider to observe the nose and mouth for secretions or vomitus.

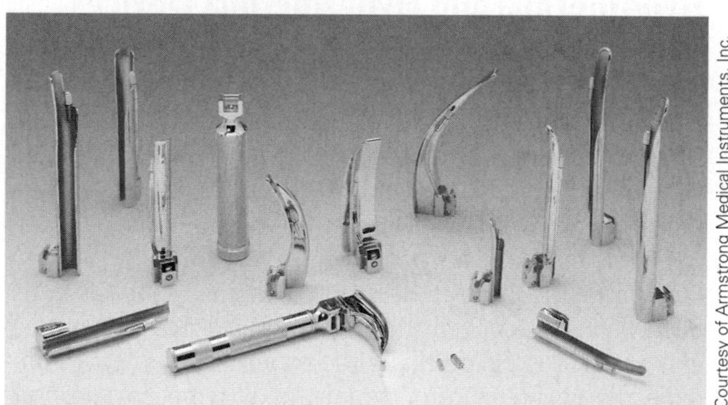

Courtesy of Armstrong Medical Instruments, Inc.

Figure 9-10 Laryngoscope and various blade attachments

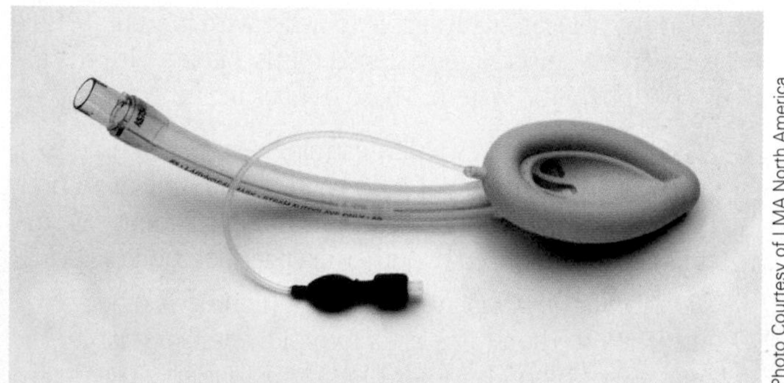

Photo Courtesy of LMA North America

Figure 9-11 Laryngeal mask airway—classic (LMA Classic™)

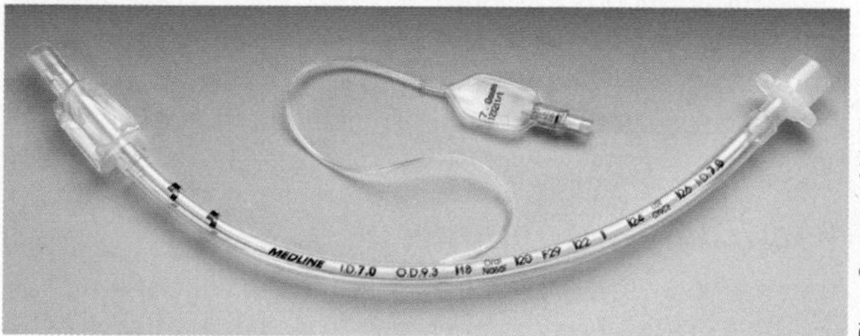

Photo Courtesy of Medline Industries, Inc.

Figure 9-9 Endotracheal tube

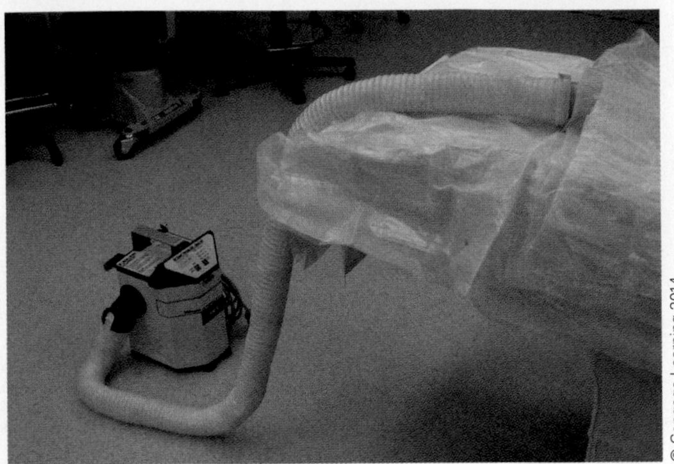

Figure 9-12 Bair Hugger surgical access blanket

Oropharyngeal airways and nasal airways are devices used to provide a passageway around the relaxed tongue, establishing an unobstructed airway for normal respiration. Oropharyngeal airways, placed through the mouth, are rigid plastic, with a preformed curve, which lifts the tongue forward. Nasopharyngeal airways, placed through the nostril, are soft, hollow tubes with a flanged end to prevent aspiration of the tube. The airway lifts the soft palate away from the back of the oropharynx.

Hypothermia and Hyperthermia Devices

The Bair Hugger® is a patient-warming device that utilizes warm air blown into a special blanket that is placed over the patient (Figure 9-12). The blankets come in a variety of sizes and configurations to meet the needs of the surgical patient and surgical procedure. The blanket may be secured to the patient's skin with an adhesive strip and/or restraining ties to prevent blanket migration.

Warming/cooling devices utilize warmed or cooled, distilled water or isopropyl alcohol, which circulates through coils in a pad that is placed under the patient. These devices promote the maintenance of optimal body temperature during surgical intervention. Alternatively, the body temperature can also be manipulated for therapeutic reasons, as when induced hypothermia is used in conjunction with general anesthesia or to cool a febrile patient.

Various devices are available to assist with patient IV fluid delivery. These devices are designed for use along with the patient's peripheral IV system. These devices include:

- *Fluid-warming devices:* Fluid-warming devices are used to raise the temperature of blood and other IV fluids to body temperature just prior to infusion into the patient. Warming prevents induced hypothermia and metabolic acidosis.
- *Rapid infusion pump:* A rapid infusion pump is a device attached to the IV line used to rapidly deliver a large volume of blood or other fluid to the patient. The device may be a complex computerized machine or as simple as a pressurized cuff wrapped around the outside of the fluid administration bag to exert external force. The device may also incorporate a fluid-warming device, eliminating the need for a second piece of equipment.
- *Infusion control devices:* Infusion control devices are mechanical devices that regulate the delivery of IV fluids and medications. They may involve the attachment of a monitoring device to the external surface of the IV tubing drip chamber or may hold a syringe of medication that is delivered in a prescribed and controlled manner.

MONITORING DEVICES

The surgical patient is monitored continuously prior to induction and throughout the perioperative period. Monitoring devices of various types are used to accomplish this task.

Electrocardiogram

The electrocardiogram is a noninvasive method used to monitor the rate, rhythm, and electrical conduction of the heart, indicating cardiac function. Detection, identification, and treatment of any dysrhythmia or arrhythmia are critical. Electrodes are placed on the patient's skin and are connected to the monitor with a series of leads.

Blood Pressure Monitor

Blood pressure monitoring is used to evaluate the patient's cardiac output and vascular status. Blood pressure measurement is commonly performed using noninvasive techniques but may also be monitored invasively with the insertion of an arterial line. Systolic, diastolic, and mean arterial pressures are monitored and tracked for trends indicating any changes. Automatic devices with adjustable time interval settings perform most blood pressure monitoring in the OR.

Arterial and Venous Catheterization

Pulmonary artery catheters are invasive monitoring devices placed into the pulmonary artery via subclavian or jugular vein access. The catheter is then threaded through the right side of the heart, with the ballooned tip "wedged" in the pulmonary artery. The catheter is connected via sterile tubing to a monitor, providing information in a digital format. The catheter permits monitoring of cardiac output from the right side of the heart, an indicator of overall cardiac function and fluid status. The reading is referred to as the pulmonary wedge pressure.

Central venous pressure (CVP) catheters are invasive monitoring devices placed into the right atrium via subclavian or jugular access. The catheter is placed to monitor blood pressure in the vena cava and right atrium, indicating the patient's fluid status.

Temperature Monitors

Noninvasive or invasive temperature monitors are used to assess the patient's body temperature. A common form of temperature monitor, the surface monitor, is commonly placed on the patient's forehead. The ear monitor is often used for general patient care but less practical in the OR setting. Other more invasive monitors of body core temperature include esophageal, bladder, and rectal probes, all of which are better suited for intraoperative use. Monitoring of patient body temperature is helpful in assessing intentional changes in the patient's temperature or for identifying hypothermia (which can lead to metabolic acidosis) and hyperthermia (an indicator of sepsis or MH).

Pulse Oximeter

Pulse oximetry involves noninvasive assessment of the blood oxygenation levels in arterial blood. A small sensor is commonly placed on the fingertip, but it can also be placed on the toe, earlobe, and the bridge of the nose. The sensor is motion sensitive, giving a false reading or no reading during patient motion. Some substances, such as dyes (nail polish), methemoglobin, and carbon monoxide, may affect accurate monitoring.

Bispectral Index™ (BIS) Monitor

The BIS monitor assists anesthesia care providers in monitoring the patient's level of anesthesia during the surgical intervention. A noninvasive sensor is placed on the patient's forehead and attached by a cable to the monitor, which continuously monitors the patient's brain waves, computing them into a number ranging from 0 to 100. The number correlates with the patient's level of consciousness, with a recording of 100 when the patient is wide awake and under 60 when the patient is unconscious. As the numbers change, the dose of anesthetic is titrated or adjusted, providing the patient with an optimal level of surgical anesthesia.

SARA

The System for Anesthetic and Respiratory Analysis (SARA) is a monitoring device incorporated into the anesthesia machine and is used to monitor the patient's physiological respiratory and anesthetic gas levels. This device is capable of several monitoring functions, including:

- *Capnography:* provides breath-by-breath analysis of expired carbon dioxide (end-tidal CO_2).
- *Spirometry:* provides information regarding the pulmonary status by monitoring ventilatory flow, volume, and pressure. This information allows for calculations pertaining to lung compliance and resistance, providing information that could indicate emphysema or adult respiratory distress syndrome (ARDS), which can influence the administration of inhalation anesthetic agents.
- *Oxygen analyzer:* Confirms the delivery of oxygen to the patient and that the concentration of oxygen is adequate.

Stethoscope

The stethoscope is used for auscultation during anesthetic delivery. Assessment of proper ET tube placement by auscultating the lung fields, assessing lung sounds, verifying placement of nasogastric tubes, and checking the stomach for inadvertent esophageal placement of the endotracheal tube are all uses of the stethoscope in the surgical setting. An internal stethoscope is available in the form of an esophageal probe; a thermometer is often included with this device.

Doppler

The **Doppler** is an ultrasonic device used to identify and assess vascular status of peripheral arteries and veins by magnifying the sound of the blood moving through the vessel. This may assist in the identification of structures for cannulation/venous catheterization and/or locating obstructions. A sterile probe is available for use within the sterile field.

Peripheral Nerve Stimulator

The peripheral nerve stimulator is a battery-operated device used to assess the level of neuromuscular blockade by causing muscle contractions. The most common site for stimulation is the ulnar nerve, with the noninvasive electrodes placed over the medial aspect of the wrist, causing the muscles of the hand and fingers to contract upon stimulation when neuromuscular blockade agents are not affecting nerve impulse conduction.

Arterial Blood Gases

Arterial blood gases (ABGs) involve invasive monitoring of pH, oxygen saturation, and carbon dioxide levels. ABGs are commonly obtained by accessing the radial artery or by placement of a monitoring line into the radial artery (arterial line or a-line). Direct blood pressure monitoring may also be performed via the a-line.

VITAL SIGNS

The measurement of vital signs involves the mechanical or automated measurement of essential life indicators such as body temperature, pulse, respirations (TPR), and blood pressure. Baseline vital signs, including patient height and weight, are determined when the patient's history and physical is completed. This information provides the basis by which to determine and monitor homeostatic changes in the surgical patient. Prior to the administration of pre-operative medications, the anesthesia care provider will apply monitoring equipment to assess and record the patient's vital signs throughout the perioperative period. Vital signs measurements are recorded to help protect the hospital and surgical team against potential liability.

Temperature

Human body temperature is regulated by the *hypothalamus,* which monitors the processes of heat production and heat loss. When the hypothalamus senses a lowered body temperature, it signals the body to increase heat production through muscle contractions and increased cellular metabolism (Table 9-24).

Increases in core body temperature can be triggered by any of several outside factors, including infection, increased physical exertion, exposure to environmental heat, pregnancy, medication administration, stress, and age. Core body temperature decreases can result from viral infections, decreased physical activity, depressed emotional state, exposure to environmental cold, metabolism-decreasing drugs including anesthetic agents, and age. The elderly tend to have a slightly decreased core body temperature. Core body temperature is also affected by the time of day, with core body temperature at its lowest early in the morning. In the OR setting, core body temperature can be affected by such outside factors as cold prep solutions, exposure, and anesthesia administration.

When core body temperature rises above the baseline preoperative level, the patient is said to be febrile (have a fever). Fever may indicate infection, drug reaction, or even the late stages of malignant hyperthermia.

In the OR, patient body temperature is closely monitored by automatic monitoring devices controlled by the anesthesia care provider. It is important to monitor patient temperature to avoid undesirable hypothermia or hyperthermia. The methods for temperature monitoring are listed in Table 9-25.

Pulse

The pulse is composed of two phases of heart action (systole and diastole) and is assessed by palpation of an artery, usually the radial artery (Table 9-26). If the pulse is being monitored electronically, a pulse oximeter monitor is used to assess pulse and blood oxygen saturation levels simultaneously. The pulse is also measured by the electrocardiogram (ECG or EKG) machine used to assess cardiac electrical conduction. Blood under pressure moves through the artery and expands the arterial wall. When the heart ventricles relax, the intra-arterial pressure decreases. Each heartbeat consists of one contraction phase and one relaxation phase, felt as a pulsation of the artery wall.

The pulse may be felt in any point of the body that has near-surface arteries and bony understructures. These sites include the temporal, carotid, brachial, radial, femoral, popliteal, and dorsalis pedis arteries. The pulse may also be monitored at the apex of the heart, referred to as the **apical pulse**, by use a stethoscope to listen between the fifth and sixth ribs just to the left of the sternum and just below the nipple. The most commonly utilized pulse point is the radial artery, located about 1 in. proximally to the base of the thumb. In addition to heart rate, several other pulse characteristics are monitored, including rhythm (regularity of the beats), volume, and strength (strong = bounding pulse; weak = thready pulse). To measure the pulse rate, the number of pulsations is counted for one minute. The number of beats is noted as the pulse, or heart rate. The pulse may also be measured for 15 seconds, and the number is multiplied by 4 to obtain the heart rate. The rate will vary with age, level of activity, pain, medication administration, and emotional condition. Patients entering the OR will sometimes have an elevated pulse rate due to anxiety.

Common pulse abnormalities include bradycardia (pulse rate less than 60) and tachycardia (pulse rate over 100) (Table 9-27). An arrhythmia or dysrhythmia is an irregular heartbeat and may indicate heart disease. Premature ventricular contractions (PVCs) are a commonly noted arrhythmia that is felt as a pulse beat earlier than expected. It can occasionally occur due to stress or may be caused by caffeine, nicotine, or alcohol intake or by sleep deprivation. Ventricular fibrillation is a serious arrhythmia resulting in the ventricle of the heart "quivering" rather than contracting, which does not permit blood to be pumped into the circulatory system and can rapidly lead to patient death. Any pulse abnormalities should be noted and the surgeon or anesthesia care provider should be alerted.

Respiration

The normal respiratory rate is called eupnea and varies with age, emotions, activity level, and medication administration. Normal respiration consists of one respiration for every four heartbeats, or a 1:4 ratio (Table 9-28).

TABLE 9-24 Normal Temperature Values

Oral	98.6°F (37°C)
Rectal	99.6°F (37.6°C)
Axillary	97.6°F (36.4°C)

TABLE 9-25 Temperature-Monitoring Methods in the Operating Room

Noninvasive	Liquid crystal adhesive skin thermometer
	Tympanic membrane thermometer
Invasive	Oral thermometer
	Rectal thermometer
	Esophageal thermometer (esophageal probe—combines temperature probe and stethoscope)

TABLE 9-26 Normal Pulse Values

Birth	130–160 bpm*
Infants	110–130 bpm
Children (1–7 years)	80–120 bpm
Children (over 7)	80–90 bpm
Adults	60–80 bpm

*bpm = beats per minute.

When monitoring respiration, the rate, rhythm, and depth are noted. The rhythm of respiration is a measure of the pattern of breathing. This will vary with age, with adults having a regular pattern and infants having an irregular one. The depth of respiration is the amount of air inhaled and exhaled with each respiration, an amount that is easily measured by anesthesia equipment in the OR. Manually, it is assessed by watching the rise and fall of the chest. The respiratory rate is recorded, along with whether respirations are shallow or deep (Table 9-29).

Blood Pressure

Blood pressure is the force that blood exerts against the walls of the blood vessels as the heart contracts (systole) and relaxes (diastole). It is affected by several different factors, including the pumping action of the heart, the resistance of the arteries to the flow of blood in the body, and the thickness of the blood. The extracellular fluid volume also affects blood pressure. The pumping action of the heart is a measure of the strength of ventricular contracture, cardiac output, and how

TABLE 9-27 Pulse Abnormalities

Type	*Rate*	*Causes*
Normal	60–80 bpm	• Age, activity level, and gender variations (refer to Table 9-25)
Tachycardia	Greater than 100 bpm	• Stimulation of the sympathetic nervous system by stress or drugs • Exercise • Congestive heart failure, anemia
Bradycardia	Less than 60 bpm	• Very fit athlete • Stimulation of the parasympathetic nervous system by certain drugs • Physical problems such as cerebral hemorrhage and heart blockage
Arrhythmia—irregular heartbeat	Uneven beat intervals	• Cardiac irritability or hypoxia • Chemical or drug issues such as potassium imbalance • If premature beats are frequent, this condition may indicate a serious arrhythmia

TABLE 9-28 Normal Respiration Rates

Infants	30–60 respirations per minute
Children (1–7 years)	18–30 per minute
Adults	12–20 per minute

TABLE 9-29 Breathing Patterns

Name	*Description*	*Cause*
Eupnea	Normal breathing	Normal CO_2 level feedback to the respiratory center of the brain
Apnea	No breathing	Obstructed airway occurs due to blockage Disruption or damage to lateral medulla oblongata (breathing center) Can occur on temporary or long-term basis with administration of some anesthetic agents
Bradypnea	Slow, even respirations	Normal during sleep Depression of respiratory center of the brain
Cheyne-Stokes	Fast, deep breaths for a period of time, followed by 20–60 seconds of apnea	Increased intracranial pressure (ICP) Congestive heart failure (CHF) Renal failure Cerebral anoxia
Dyspnea	Difficulty breathing and may be painful	Intense physical exercise Heart disease Lung disease Asthma
Kussmaul's	Fast, deep, labored breaths over 20 per minute	Blood pressure systolic 140–160, diastolic 70–90
Tachypnea	Rapid breathing accompanied by a rise in core body temperature	Pneumonia Respiratory insufficiency Respiratory center lesions Respiratory acidosis as body attempts to rid itself of excess CO_2 High fever as body attempts to rid itself of excess body heat

Source: Data from Mednet (www.sermed.com).

efficiently and effectively blood is moved from the left side of the heart into the circulatory system.

Blood pressure is usually expressed as two numbers, the systolic number and the diastolic number (Table 9-30). *Systole* refers to the contraction of the heart, which forces the blood through the arteries. The relaxation phase of the heartbeat is referred to as *diastole*. As the heart contracts and blood is forced into the aorta, the walls of the aorta and major arteries are forced to expand by the pressure of the blood being pumped through the artery lumen. As the heart relaxes between beats, the aortic valve closes, preventing blood from flowing back into the chambers of the heart. The arterial walls spring back from the expansion that took place during the contraction of the heart, forcing the blood throughout the body between contractions of the heart. These actions produce two separate pressure readings—the higher number recorded during ventricular contraction and a lower number during ventricular relaxation. These two pressure measurements are referred to as the systolic blood pressure and diastolic blood pressure.

In the OR, blood pressure is most commonly assessed using an automated, electronic blood pressure monitor. To obtain an accurate blood pressure reading, an appropriately sized blood pressure cuff is selected and applied, usually around the upper portion of the patient's arm. As air is pumped into the cuff through an inflation device, the cuff pressure increases and the arterial blood flow is momentarily stopped. The cuff is slowly released and the monitoring device determines the systolic and diastolic pressure readings.

When blood pressure is assessed manually, the health care practitioner uses a cuff with a manual inflation device, a sphygmomanometer, and a stethoscope to auscultate for Korotkoff's sounds, which will be heard as a tapping sound that gradually increases in intensity as the cuff is deflated (Table 9-31). These sounds take place in five distinct phases, which must be recognized for proper blood pressure measurement.

Blood pressure is recorded in a fraction format on the patient's chart, including the location of the measurement and the position of the patient (e.g., "120/80, left arm, supine"). In children and patients where the blood pressure sounds can still be heard at zero, the beginning of phase IV and zero should both be recorded (e.g., "120/90/0").

In some critically ill patients, and especially in the OR, blood pressure can be monitored via intra-arterial blood pressure monitoring, also referred to as an "art-line" or "a-line," which provides constant, accurate blood pressure data. A catheter is inserted into an artery and attached to a

Table 9-30 Normal Blood Pressure Values and Classifications of Abnormal Blood Pressure

	Children	
	Newborn	50–52 systolic/25–30 diastolic
	Child (under 6)	95/62
	Child (to 10 years)	100/65
	Adolescent	118/75
	Adults	
Category	*Systolic (mm Hg)*	*Diastolic (mm Hg)*
Normal†	Less than 120	Less than 80
Prehypertension	120–139	80–89
Hypertension‡		
Stage 1 (mild)	140–159	90–99
Stage 2 (moderate)	At or greater than 160	At or greater than 100

†Optimal blood pressure with respect to cardiovascular risk is systolic less than 120 and diastolic less than 80. However, unusually low readings should be evaluated for clinical significance.
‡Based on the average of two or more readings taken at each of two or more visits following an initial screening. Thus, a reading in the OR of 140–159 would not necessarily classify a patient as clinically chronically hypertensive.
Source: From the Fifth Report of the Joint National Committee on Detection, Evaluation, and Treatment of High Blood Pressure, Oct. 30, 1992.

Table 9-31 Korotkoff's Sounds

Phases	*Sounds*
Phase I	On hearing two initial tapping sounds, the sphygmomanometer is read and the number is recorded as the systolic blood pressure
Phase II	Soft swishing sound as more blood passes through the vessels while the cuff is being deflated
Phase III	Rhythmic tapping sound returns as more blood passes through the vessels while the pressure is slowly being released in the cuff (Note: if phases I and II are missed, phase III may be improperly recorded as the systolic pressure)
Phase IV	Muffled, fading, tapping sounds heard as the cuff is deflated further
Phase V	Sounds disappear altogether—the point at which these sounds disappear is recorded as the diastolic blood pressure

TECHNIQUE

Temperature Assessment (Manual Technique)

1. Wash your hands.
2. Assemble equipment and supplies.
   - Watch or clock with second hand
   - Thermometer of choice, including accessories
   - Gloves and lubricant, if necessary (*Note:* The patient's condition may require the use of gloves.)
   - Appropriate waste receptacle
3. Prepare equipment.
   - Apply gloves, if necessary.
   - Cover or remove thermometer from package, as needed.
   - Place thermometer in ready mode, if electronic.
   - Apply lubricant, if necessary.
4. Introduce yourself, identify the patient, and explain the procedure, if necessary.
5. Position the patient, if necessary.
6. Place the thermometer according to site location.
7. Keep the thermometer in position for the prescribed length of time.
8. Support the thermometer, if necessary.
9. Carefully remove the thermometer according to protocol for site location.
10. Read the thermometer.
11. Wash your hands.
12. Record or report findings.
13. Care for the equipment as needed.

TECHNIQUE

Pulse Assessment (Manual Technique)

1. Wash your hands.
2. Assemble equipment and supplies.
   - Watch or clock with second hand
   - Stethoscope, if checking apical or fetal pulse
   - Gloves, if warranted by the patient's condition
3. Introduce yourself, identify the patient, and explain the procedure, if necessary.
4. Position the patient, if necessary.
5. Locate the site by gently palpating with the first two or three fingertips (don't use the thumb)
6. Gently compress the artery or listen with the stethoscope.
7. Note the time. Note: For accuracy, the pulse rate should be counted for one full minute.
8. Count the pulse rate and note the rhythm, volume, and condition of the arterial wall.
9. Wash your hands.
10. Record or report findings.
11. Care for equipment as needed.

TECHNIQUE

Respiration Assessment (Manual Technique)

1. Wash your hands.
2. Assemble the equipment and supplies.
   - Watch or clock with second hand
   - Stethoscope, if necessary
   - Gloves, if warranted by the patient's condition
3. Introduce yourself, identify the patient, and explain the procedure, if necessary.
4. Position the patient, if necessary.
5. Note the time. *Note:* For accuracy, the respiratory rate should be counted for one full minute.
6. Obtain respiratory rate, depth, rhythm, and breath sounds.
7. Wash your hands.
8. Record or report findings.
9. Care for the equipment as needed.

TECHNIQUE

Blood Pressure Assessment (Manual Technique)

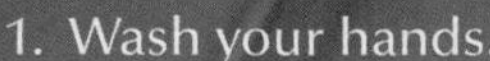

1. Wash your hands.
2. Assemble the equipment and supplies.
   - Sphygmomanometer
   - Stethoscope, if necessary
   - Gloves, if warranted by the patient's condition
3. Introduce yourself, identify the patient, and explain the procedure, if necessary.
4. Position the patient and expose the site, if necessary. *Note:* Left upper extremity is preferred.
5. Apply the appropriate size blood pressure cuff.
6. Place the stethoscope.
   - Stethoscope is placed over the brachial artery.
   - Stethoscope is secured with fingers only (not the thumb).
7. Inflate the blood pressure cuff to the desired pressure.
8. Deflate the blood pressure cuff slowly, while listening for Korotkoff's sounds.
   - Listen for Korotkoff phase I; note systolic blood pressure.
   - Continue to listen for sequential Korotkoff phases.
   - Note diastolic blood pressure; listen for Korotkoff phase V.
9. Continue deflation of blood pressure cuff and note ausculatory gap, if present.
10. Continue deflation of blood pressure cuff and remove it.
11. Wash your hands.
12. Record or report findings.
13. Care for the equipment as needed.

catheter-monitor-transducer system. The catheter is usually inserted and monitored by the anesthesia care provider with the pressure readings displayed on a monitor attached to the anesthesia machine.

TEAM MEMBER ROLES DURING ANESTHESIA ADMINISTRATION

Every surgical team member has a responsibility to the patient during anesthesia administration. All patient care related to the delivery of anesthesia care is documented by the anesthesia care provider on a separate "anesthesia record." Figure 9-13 is an example of an intraoperative anesthesia record.

Tables 9-32 through 9-36 list those responsibilities with respect to each type of anesthesia. These are typical examples of the chain of events starting in the preoperative holding area through admission to the PACU. General and spinal anesthetic scenarios will be used as illustrative procedures.

PREOPERATIVE VISITS

In most circumstances, the patient is visited in the preoperative holding area by the anesthesia care provider and the circulator (Table 9-32). This interview may be conducted separately or jointly as much of the same information is obtained or verified by both team members. This is also an opportunity for patient education. The surgeon will often visit to answer any final questions and offer emotional support.

PREOPERATIVE ROUTINE—ALL TYPES OF ANESTHESIA

Each team member contributes to preoperative care in different ways. These roles are summarized in Table 9-33.

Team Member Duties During General Anesthesia

Each team member also contributes during the induction of anesthesia and the anesthetized state. Some common contributions are listed in Table 9-34.

Team Member Duties During Spinal Anesthesia

Spinal anesthesia requires a variation in routines. These are summarized in Table 9-35.

POSTANESTHESIA CARE

Following the surgical procedure, duties change relative to termination of the anesthetized state or for patients who will remain intubated, transferral of the patient to the PACU or ICU, and initiation of postoperative care. These duties are summarized in Table 9-36.

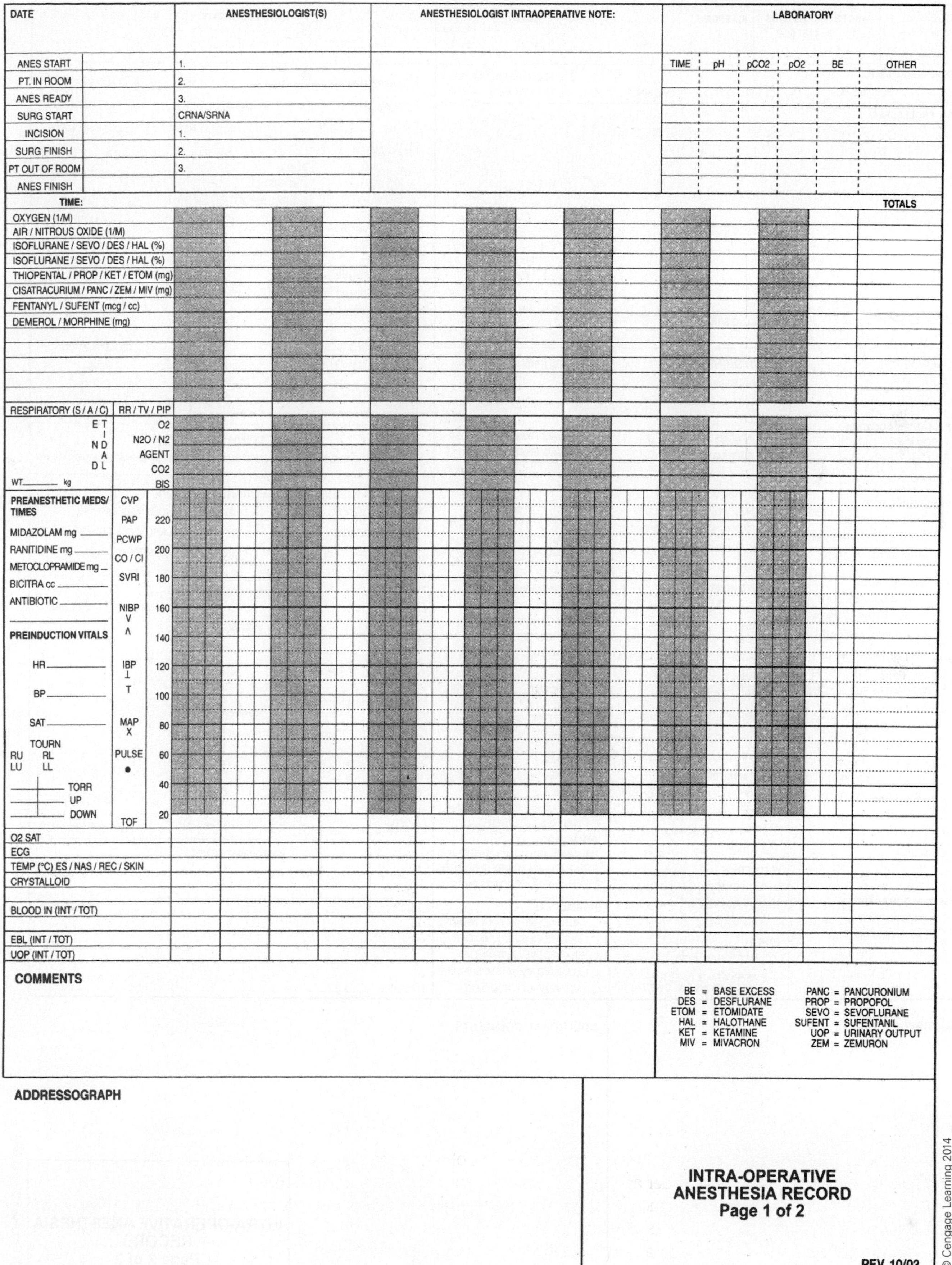

DATE	ANESTHESIOLOGIST(S)	ANESTHESIOLOGIST INTRAOPERATIVE NOTE:	LABORATORY

ANES START		1.
PT. IN ROOM		2.
ANES READY		3.
SURG START		CRNA/SRNA
INCISION		1.
SURG FINISH		2.
PT OUT OF ROOM		3.
ANES FINISH		

TIME	pH	pCO2	pO2	BE	OTHER

TIME:

TOTALS

OXYGEN (1/M)
AIR / NITROUS OXIDE (1/M)
ISOFLURANE / SEVO / DES / HAL (%)
ISOFLURANE / SEVO / DES / HAL (%)
THIOPENTAL / PROP / KET / ETOM (mg)
CISATRACURIUM / PANC / ZEM / MIV (mg)
FENTANYL / SUFENT (mcg / cc)
DEMEROL / MORPHINE (mg)

RESPIRATORY (S / A / C) RR / TV / PIP
E T I N D A D L — O2, N2O / N2, AGENT, CO2, BIS
WT._______ kg

PREANESTHETIC MEDS/ TIMES
MIDAZOLAM mg ______
RANITIDINE mg ______
METOCLOPRAMIDE mg ___
BICITRA cc ______
ANTIBIOTIC ______

PREINDUCTION VITALS
HR______
BP______
SAT______
TOURN
RU RL
LU LL
TORR
UP
DOWN

CVP
PAP
PCWP
CO / CI
SVRI
NIBP V Λ
IBP ⊥ T
MAP X
PULSE •
TOF

220
200
180
160
140
120
100
80
60
40
20

O2 SAT
ECG
TEMP (°C) ES / NAS / REC / SKIN
CRYSTALLOID
BLOOD IN (INT / TOT)
EBL (INT / TOT)
UOP (INT / TOT)

COMMENTS

BE = BASE EXCESS
DES = DESFLURANE
ETOM = ETOMIDATE
HAL = HALOTHANE
KET = KETAMINE
MIV = MIVACRON
PANC = PANCURONIUM
PROP = PROPOFOL
SEVO = SEVOFLURANE
SUFENT = SUFENTANIL
UOP = URINARY OUTPUT
ZEM = ZEMURON

ADDRESSOGRAPH

INTRA-OPERATIVE ANESTHESIA RECORD
Page 1 of 2

REV. 10/03

Figure 9-13 Anesthesia Intraoperative record

DATE

ASA PHYSICAL STATUS 1 2 3 4 5 6 E

ALLERGIES

WEIGHT kg

ORAL INTAKE STATUS
☐ NPO FOR SOLIDS SINCE ____ ☐ NPO FOR CLEAR FLUIDS SINCE ____ ☐ PO STATUS UNCONFIRMED ☐ FULL STOMACH

ALL PROCEDURES

PATIENT IDENTIFICATION
☐ BY PATIENT
☐ BY BAND
☐ OTHER ____

ATTENDING SURGEON(S)

PROCEDURE LOCATION
ROOM # ____
OR OB RAD ENDO MRI
OTHER ____

CASE DISPOSITION
☐ CANCELLED PREOP
☐ CANCELLED AFTER INDUCTION
☐ INTRAOPERATIVE DEATH

MACHINE CHECKLIST
☐ UNUSED CONTROLS OFF
☐ CYLINDER PRESSURES OK
☐ 02 FAILURE ALARM OK*
☐ PIPELINE GAS PRESS OK
☐ GAS FLOW CONTROLS OFF
☐ VAPORIZERS FULL AND OFF
☐ MACHINE LEAK TEST OK
☐ 02 MONITOR OK*
☐ ABSORBER OK
☐ CIRCUIT OK*
☐ VENTILATOR & MONITORS OK
☐ SCAVENGING SYSTEM ON
☐ SUCTION OK*
☐ ALARMS OK
*SECONDARY

SPECIAL EQUIPMENT
☐ FLUID WARMER
☐ LEVEL 1 INFUSER
☐ ACT

MONITORING

NON-INVASIVE MONITORS
☐ PULSE OXIMETER
☐ ECG ☐ NIBP
☐ CAPNOMETER
☐ TEMPERATURE
☐ NERVE STIMULATOR
☐ 02 ANALYZER
☐ PRECORDIAL STETHOSCOPE
☐ ESOPHAGEAL STETHOSCOPE
☐ PC DOPPLER
☐ BIS

INVASIVE MONITORS

	NUM. ANES. PLACED	NUM. MON.
ARTERIAL LINE	____	____
LOCATION	____	____
CENTRAL LINE (NOT PAC)	____	____
LOCATION	____	____
PAC	____	____
LOCATION	____	____

OTHER MONITORS
TEE BY: ☐ ANES. ☐ CARD.
☐ ICP
☐ EVOKED POTENTIALS
☐ OTHER ____

IV ACCESS
____ GUAGE L / R / ARM / LEG
____ GUAGE L / R / ARM / LEG
____ GUAGE L / R / ARM / LEG

OTHER
☐ NGT / OGT PLACED
☐ APPROPRIATE INFECTION PRECAUTIONS FOLLOWED

ANESTHETIC CARE INFORMATION
☐ GENERAL INDUCTION ☐ RAPID SEQ.
☐ IV ☐ INHALATION
☐ SMOOTH ☐ PREOXYGENATED
☐ CHANGE FROM LOCAL / REGIONAL
☐ CHANGE FROM MAC
☐ REGIONAL ☐ ANKLE BLOCK
☐ SPINAL ☐ ____
☐ EPIDURAL ☐ CAUDAL
☐ AXILLARY BLOCK ☐ INTERSCALENE
☐ SUPRA-CLAVICULAR ☐ IV REGIONAL
☐ MAC

SPECIAL TECHNIQUES
☐ INDUCED HYPOTHERMIA
☐ INDUCED HYPOTENSION
☐ FIELD AVOIDANCE
☐ CP BYPASS

EYE CARE
☐ LUBRICATED ☐ SCLERAL SHIELD
☐ TAPED ☐ WET GAUZE
☐ SEWN ☐ GOGGLES
☐ OTHER ____

POSITIONING
☐ SUPINE ☐ LAT. DECUBITUS L/R
☐ PRONE ☐ LITHOTOMY
☐ SITTING ☐ TBURG / RTBURG
☐ LUD/RUD ☐ OTHER ____
ARM POSITION
L: TUCKED ARM BOARD SUSPENDED
R: TUCKED ARM BOARD SUSPENDED
☐ ALL PRESSURE POINTS PADDED

THERMAL CARE
☐ ROUTINE PASSIVE BODY WARMING
☐ PASSIVE CIRCUIT HUMIDIFIER
☐ CONVECTIVE AIR WARMER
☐ ELEVATED ROOM TEMPERATURE
☐ ACTIVE HEATED HUMIDIFIER

AIRWAY INFORMATION

☐ SUPPLEMENTAL OXYGEN ONLY ☐ NC ☐ FACEMASK
☐ MASK ONLY AIRWAY: ☐ ORAL ☐ EASY MASK
☐ LMA ____ SIZE ☐ NASAL ☐ DIFFICULT MASK
☐ INTUBATED ☐ N/A
☐ ORAL ☐ BLIND ☐ DIRECT LARYNG
☐ NASAL ☐ FIBEROPTIC
☐ TRACH ☐ LIGHTED STYLET MILLER #: ____ ☐ EASY
☐ ARRIVED INTUBATED ☐ BULLARD MAC #: ____ ☐ MOD. DIFF.
☐ AWAKE ☐ JET VENT ☐ DIFFICULT
____ ☐ IMPOSSIBLE

☐ ET TUBE TYPE
☐ STANDARD # ATTEMPTS: ____ ☐ ATRAUMATIC
☐ PREFORMED ☐ TRAUMATIC
☐ LASER
☐ REINFORCED CONFIRMATION:
☐ DBL. LUMEN ____ SIZE ☐ EBBS
☐ STYLET ☐ ET–CO2
☐ UNCUFFED ☐ VISUAL

EMERGENCE
☐ SMOOTH ☐ REVERSED ☐ SUCTIONED ☐ EXTUBATED W/ADEQUATE STRENGTH

IMMEDIATE POST-ANESTHESIA NOTE
PATIENT DISPOSITION: ☐ PACU ☐ ICU ☐ HOLDING ROOM / ASU
TRANSPORTED: ☐ AWAKE ☐ SEDATED ☐ UNCONSCIOUS/ANESTHETIZED
☐ MASK/NC ☐ SUPPLEMENTAL OXYGEN
☐ INTUBATED ☐ T-PIECE ☐ AMBU. BAG
☐ TRANSPORT MONITOR

VITAL SIGNS
PACU / ICU
HR ____ BP ____/____ SAT ____
TEMP ____ RR ____

COMMENTS

SIGNATURE ____
☐ I's & O's TOTALED ☐ DRUGS TOTALED ☐ REPORT GIVEN ☐ PHARMACY FORM COMPLETED

POSTOPERATIVE NOTE
☐ GAG REFLEX INTACT/CYANOSIS ABSENT ☐ NO APPARENT ANESTHETIC COMPLICATION
HR ____ BP ____/____ RR ____
☐ OTHER ____

SIGNATURE ____ DATE ____ TIME ____

ADDRESSOGRAPH

ADDITIONAL COMMENTS

INTRA-OPERATIVE ANESTHESIA RECORD
Page 2 of 2

Figure 9-13 (continued)

TABLE 9-32 Preoperative Visit in the Waiting/Holding Area

Role Responsibility	*Circulator*	*Anesthesia Care Provider*
Assure patient privacy. Introduce self and state purpose for visit.	X	X
Identify patient and verify biographic information (e.g., age, gender, social history).	X	X
Review patient chart for completeness (e.g., history and physical, consent[s], reports of diagnostic studies).	X	X
Note physical findings (e.g., height, weight, allergies, NPO status, vital signs, medication history, level of consciousness, presence of any physical or sensory defects, presence of pain, existing wounds).	X	X
Note mental and emotional status (determine that the patient has an accurate understanding of events about to occur).	X	X
Read surgeon's orders and be sure that all preoperative orders have been completed (e.g., bowel preparation, preoperative medications administered, including prophylactic antibiotics).	X	X
Provide basic orientation information to the patient pertaining to the OR and PACU experiences.	X	X
Allow the patient (and family or significant others, if appropriate) an opportunity to express concerns and ask questions.	X	X
Provide emotional support as needed and answer any questions. Questions may be redirected to the surgeon, if applicable.	X	X
Order additional diagnostic studies and/or consultations with other physicians (e.g., cardiologist) regarding patient's condition.		X
Order or administer premedication if necessary.		X
Assign patient risk status according to ASA guidelines.		X
Ensure all preoperative protocols have been carried out (e.g., patient appropriately attired, IV inserted and patent, jewelry removed, necessary prosthesis removed, surgical site marked, if indicated).	X	
Formulate a plan of care specific to the patient's needs.	X	X
Transport patient to OR. (The staff responsible for patient transport to the O.R. varies at each facility.)	X	X

TABLE 9-33 Routine Preoperative Tasks

Anesthesia Care Provider	*Circulator*	*Surgical Technologist*	*Surgeon*
Transports patient to operating room	Transports patient to operating room	Greets patient; introduces self	
	Assist patient transfer to operating table; ensures safety and comfort	Makes a mental assessment of the patient's size and condition to anticipate specialized items that may be required for the procedure	
Introduces and applies monitoring devices (e.g., temperature, blood pressure, ECG, pulse oximeter)	Applies monitoring devices as needed; secures arms on armboards; protects ulnar nerves Ensures suction is readily available and activated	Keeps conversation and preparatory noise to a minimum (e.g., clanking of instruments, limits use of negative "triggering" terms—needle, knife, etc.)	
Begins induction of anesthesia	Resuscitation devices should be readily available as needed		Is available to assist during anesthesia induction as needed

Table 9-34 Tasks During General Anesthesia Induction and Maintenance

Anesthesia Care Provider	*Circulator*	*Surgical Technologist*	*Surgeon*
May preoxygenate patient	Stays at patient's side to provide emotional support for the patient and assistance for the anesthesia care provider	Maintains quiet environment while completing preparatory tasks	Is available to assist as needed
Induction begins with IV or inhalation agents	Has suctioning equipment readily available	Absolute quiet may be requested at this time; preparatory activities may be halted temporarily	
Provides oxygen support as needed	Observes and monitors patient for any change; reports as necessary		
Intubates patient if required	Assists with intubation by providing suctioning, passing instrumentation and supplies as needed; is prepared to apply cricoid pressure	The possibility of an emergency tracheotomy exists if severe airway problems arise	
Verifies ET tube placement and secures endotracheal tube	Assists with ET tube stabilization until the tube is secured	Observes and monitors patient for any change; reports as necessary	
Gives permission for other preoperative activities to begin or continue	Final preparations are completed (e.g., Foley catheter insertion, application of antiembolic stockings, final positioning, shave, skin prep)	Consults with surgeon as needed; variations specific to the patient may be made regarding suture or medication requirements	Confers with OR team about any specific patient variances in the procedure; assists with patient preparation and positioning; scrubs for entry into the sterile field
Monitors patient and records necessary information; titrates and administers anesthetic agents and IV fluids, as indicated	Observes patient for any significant homeostatic changes and reports as indicated; assists sterile team members with entry into and establishment of the sterile field (gowning and gloving, draping, etc.	Assists other team members to don sterile attire; assists with draping the patient for the procedure	Enters the sterile field and prepares for procedure
Maintains optimal patient homeostasis; reports any significant changes in patient's condition to the surgeon	Receives and connects tubings/cords from the sterile field; activates surgical lights and equipment; positions furniture for procedure; assists the anesthesia care provider, as indicated; monitors the sterile field; records operative events on appropriate forms; performs counts with STSR; transfers medications and additional supplies to sterile field	Passes tubings/cords to circulator to be connected to appropriate devices; positions sterile furniture for use; provides instruments and supplies for surgeon as needed; monitors the sterile field; performs counts with circulator	Initiates incision and performs necessary surgical maneuvers; reports any significant changes in operative plan or patient's condition to anesthesia care provider
Facilitates emergence from anesthetic agents	Performs closing counts; provides dressing material	Provides suture and supplies for closing and accomplishes closing counts	Completes surgery; notes accuracy of counts
Patient is extubated, if planned	Stays at patient's side; has suctioning equipment available; notifies PACU staff that patient will be arriving (gives estimated time, if possible) and advises of any special condition or equipment that will be necessary; requests next patient to be transported to the OR holding area	Applies dressings; removes drapes; cleans the operative and surrounding patient sites	Leaves the sterile field to write postoperative orders and dictate operative report
Helps transfer patient to gurney or bed and transports to PACU	Assists with transfer and transport	Maintains sterile field until patient has left the OR or per hospital protocol; may assist with patient transfer	Assists with transfer and transport as needed

TABLE 9-35 **Duties During Spinal Anesthesia**

Anesthesia Care Provider	*Circulator*	*Surgical Technologist*	*Surgeon*
Indicates preference for patient position	Prepares necessary positioning supplies	Maintains quiet environment while completing preparatory tasks	Is available to assist as indicated
May provide oxygen support and sedation	Assists with oxygen apparatus as needed		
Assists patient with positioning and verifies that position is accurate	Assists with patient positioning and remains at patient's side to provide emotional support and to help the patient maintain the position		
Opens sterile supplies; dons sterile gloves; preps patient's skin	Continues to assist patient in maintenance of the position; informs patient of what to expect (e.g., prep solution may be cold)		
Administers local anesthetic and introduces spinal needle	Encourages patient to remain still	Anesthesia care provider may insist on quiet during insertion of the spinal needle	
Verifies needle placement and introduces anesthetic	Patient must remain still and not strain	Observes patient and monitors for any change; reports as indicated	
Gives permission for patient to be repositioned	Assists patient to operative position; ensures safety and comfort		Assists with patient positioning if needed
Gives permission for other preoperative activities to begin	Final preparations are completed (e.g., Foley catheter insertion, application of antiembolic stockings, skin prep); performs counts with STSR	Remembers that patient is and will remain awake for the entire procedure; consults with surgeon as needed; variations specific to the patient may be made regarding suture or medication requirements	Confers with OR team about any specific patient variances in the procedure; assists with patient preparation and positioning; scrubs for entry into the sterile field
Monitors patient and records information; introduces supplementary sedation as needed	Observes patient for any significant homeostatic changes and reports as indicated; assists sterile team members with entry into and establishment of the sterile field (gowning and gloving, draping, etc.)	Assists other team members to don sterile attire; assists with draping the patient for the procedure	Enters the sterile field and prepares for procedure
Provides airway support, if indicated; maintains optimal patient homeostasis; reports any significant changes in patient's condition to the surgeon	Receives and connects tubings/cords from the sterile field; activates surgical lights and equipment; positions furniture for procedure; assists the anesthesia care provider, as indicated; monitors the sterile field; records operative events on appropriate forms; performs counts with STSR; transfers medications and additional supplies to sterile field	Passes tubings/cords to circulator to be connected to appropriate devices; positions sterile furniture for use; provides instruments and supplies for surgeon as needed; monitors the sterile field; performs counts with circulator	Initiates incision and performs necessary surgical maneuvers; reports any significant changes in operative plan or patient's condition to anesthesia care provider

(continues)

TABLE 9-35 **(continued)**

Anesthesia Care Provider	*Circulator*	*Surgical Technologist*	*Surgeon*
Anesthesia care provider may request (or the surgeon may desire) to test the operative site prior to making the incision to be sure that the anesthesia is complete	Available to provide support if indicated	Provides device necessary for test; often a needle or tissue forceps with teeth is used	Ensures that the anesthesia is effective
Maintains optimal patient homeostasis; reports any significant changes in patient's condition to the surgeon	Receives and connects tubings/cords from the sterile field; activates surgical lights and equipment; positions furniture for procedure; assists the anesthesia care provider, as indicated; monitors the sterile field; records operative events on appropriate forms; performs counts with STSR; transfers medications and additional supplies to sterile field	Passes tubings/cords to circulator to be connected to appropriate devices; positions sterile furniture for use; provides instruments and supplies for surgeon as needed; monitors the sterile field; performs counts with circulator	Caution is used when discussing the patient's condition or requesting instruments so that the patient does not become alarmed (e.g., the surgeon may use hand signals when requesting scalpels, scissors, needles, or other sharps or use "nontriggering" names for items); initiates incision and performs necessary surgical maneuvers; reports any significant changes in operative plan or patient's condition to anesthesia care provider
Raises patient's level of consciousness as needed	Performs closing counts; provides dressing material; notifies PACU staff that patient will be arriving (give estimated time, if possible) and advises of any special condition or equipment that will be necessary; requests next patient to be transported to the OR holding area	Provides suture and supplies for closing and accomplishes closing counts; applies dressings; removes drapes	Completes surgery; notes accuracy of counts; leaves the sterile field to write postoperative orders and dictate operative report
Helps transfer the patient to gurney or bed and transports to PACU	Assists with transfer and transport	Maintains sterile field until patient has left the OR or per hospital protocol; may assist with patient transfer	Assists with transfer and transport as needed

Table 9-36 Postanesthesia Duties

Anesthesia Care Provider	*Circulator*	*PACU Caregiver*	*Surgeon*
Main responsibility during transport is airway maintenance and patient ventilation	Guides and propels transport device to PACU	Directs OR team with patient to proper cubicle; has suction and monitoring equipment ready	Completes written postoperative orders; accompanies patient to PACU
Gives verbal patient status report to PACU staff	Locks transport device in place; assists PACU caregiver with attaching monitoring devices; provides verbal operative report to PACU staff	Assesses and maintains airway as indicated; applies monitoring devices; listens to verbal reports from anesthesia care provider circulator	Gives verbal orders as needed; is available for assistance as indicated
Ensures patency of airway	Gives verbal patient status report to PACU staff	Obtains baseline vital signs and reports to surgeon and anesthesia care provider and documents results	Once the patient is stable, the surgeon speaks with the patient's family or significant others
May leave the immediate area when patient is stable but should remain available for unexpected events and patient discharge	Transfers patient care to PACU staff	Assesses patient vital signs, provides airway support as indicated; administers medications and fluids as ordered; monitors and maintains dressings and drainage (catheter, drains); provides emotional support as required	May leave the immediate area when patient is stable, but should remain available for unexpected events
Discharges patient from PACU when discharge criteria are met		Patient usually remains in PACU for a minimum of 1 hour, longer if necessary; patient is discharged when specific predetermined criteria are met and on the order of a physician	Writes orders for post-PACU care

Case Study Jamal is a healthy 19-year-old athlete at the local college. He has been admitted to the hospital for out-patient surgery, an arthroscopic examination of his right knee. Shortly after the administration of the general anesthetic agent, the anesthesia care provider notices that Jamal is breathing rapidly and producing a high amount of carbon dioxide; his muscles appear rigid; and the monitor shows tachycardia and an increase in body temperature.

1. What condition is likely affecting Jamal? Is it dangerous?
2. What are the steps that the surgical technologist needs to take during the treatment of this condition? The anesthesia care provider? The circulator?
3. What medication is routinely administered to specifically treat this condition? Which intravenous solution is used to reconstitute this medication?
4. What two medications will be given simultaneously to ensure that the body has enough basic energy for cell metabolism? What is the purpose of each medication?
5. What medication will be given to ensure that waste products are efficiently removed from Jamal's system?

Case Study Glenda is scheduled to undergo laparoscopic cholecystectomy with intraoperative cholangiography. The patient is MRSA positive. Due to unexpected bleeding in the liver bed, the procedure converts to an open cholecystectomy intraoperatively.

1. Which category of medications will be used during the "intraoperative cholangiography" segment of the procedure? Name three medications included in this category.
2. The surgeon requests half-strength diatrizoate sodium solution. You have 30 mL of diatrizoate sodium on the sterile field and a 50-cc syringe. How much diatrizoate sodium and how much normal saline is added to the syringe to prepare the medication as requested by the surgeon?
3. The surgeon requests an antibiotic irrigation for use during wound closure at the end of the procedure. Which antibiotic would be requested for use, considering the patient's medical history? What information should be included on the label secured to the basin containing the requested irrigation? Which surgical supply would be used to deliver the irrigation to the surgical wound?
4. Name three medications that might be used to control bleeding in the liver bed intraoperatively.
5. The surgeon is concerned that Glenda may have inflammation of the liver bed from manipulating the tissues while trying to control the bleeding and that she might have postoperativeerative nausea and vomiting from manipulating the abdominal organs. Which single medication would the surgeon ask the anesthesia care provider to give intraoperatively to treat both of these conditions?

Questions for Further Study

1. What is Sellick's Maneuver, when is it used, and how is it performed?
2. Why might bupivacaine HCl be a better choice for local anesthesia during an inguinal herniorrhaphy than lidocaine HCl?
3. Describe Korotkoff's sounds and their implications in measuring blood pressure. How many sounds are commonly heard and which are of significance?
4. What is the primary difference between spinal and epidural anesthesia?
5. Is the placental barrier effective in protecting the fetal environment from the effects of general anesthetics? Why or why not?

BIBLIOGRAPHY

Alternative Medicine Homepage. Available from http://www.pitt.edu/~cbw/altm.htm

American Society of Anesthesiologists. Available from http://www.asahq.org

Asperheim, M. K. (2008). *Pharmacology: An introductory text* (11th ed.). Philadelphia: W.B. Saunders.

Association of Surgical Technologists. (2011). *Core curriculum for surgical technology* (6th ed.). Littleton, CO: Authors.

Bispectral Index™ monitoring. Available from http://www.aspectms.com

Division of Anaesthesiology & Intensive Care of the University of Queensland. Available from http://gasbone.herston.uq.edu.au/gasbone.html

Drug Enforcement Agency. *Controlled Substances Act.* Available from http://www.usdoj.gov/dea/pubs/csa.htm

Egan, T. *Remifentanil: An esterase-metabolized opioid.* Available from http://web2.searchbank.com

Evans, T. J. *The unusual history of "ether."* Available from http://www.anesthesia-nursing.com/ether.html

Fearnley, S. *Pulse oximetry.* Nuffield Department of Anaesthetics University of Oxford. Available from http://www.nda.ox.ac.uk

Feix, J. (2006). *Pharmacology handbook for the surgical technologist.* Clifton Park, NY: Thomson Delmar Learning.

FloSeal. Available from http://www.baxter.com/products/biopharmaceuticals/downloads/FloSeal_PI.pdf

Greater Houston Anesthesiology. Available from *GHAMD@chooseGHA.com*

Higashide, T., & Sugiyama, K. *Use of visoelastic substance in ophthalmic surgery—focus on sodium hyaluronate.* Available from http://www.ncbi.nlm.gov/pmc/articles/PMC2698691/

Hurford, W., Bailin, M., Davison, J., Haspel, K., & Rosow, C. (2006). *Clinical anesthesia procedures of the Massachusetts General Hospital* (7th ed.). Philadelphia: Lippincott-Raven.

Joint Commission, The. *Look-alike/sound-alike list of medications.* Available from http://www.jointcommission.org/NR/rdonlyres/C92AAB3F-A9BD-431C-8628-11DD2D1D53CC/0LASA.pdf

Joint Commission, The. *National patient safety goals.* Available from http://www.jointcommission.org/PatientSafety/NationalPatientSafetyGoals

Joint Commission, The. *The official "Do Not Use" list of abbreviations.* Available from http://www.jointcommission.org/Do_Not_Use_List_of_Abbreviations/

Joint Commission, The. *Universal protocol.* Available from http://www.jointcommission.org/standards_information/up.aspx

Lewis, S. (2007). *Medical-surgical nursing: Assessment and management of clinical problems* (7th ed.). St. Louis, MO: Mosby-Year Book.

Macario, A., Dexter, F., & Lubarsky, D. (2005). Meta-analysis of trials comparing postoperative recovery after anesthesia with sevoflurane or desflurane. *American Journal of Health-System Pharmacy, 62*(1), 63–68.

Malignant Hyperthermia Association of the United States (MHAUS). Available from http://www.mhaus.org/whatismh.html

Miller, R. (2006). *Anesthesia* (5th ed.). New York: Churchill Livingstone.

National Center for Complementary and Alternative Medicine. Available from http://nccam.nih.gov/

Nursing 2011 Drug Handbook (31st ed.). (2011). Philadelphia: Lippincott Williams & Wilkins.

O'Campo, V. V., & Foster, C. S. *Cataract, senile: Treatment and medication.* Available from http://emedicine.medscape.com/article/1210914-treatment

Pinosky, M. *Laryngeal mask airway: Uses in anesthesiology.* Southern Medical Association. Available from http://www.sma.org

Rai, J. *Cervical ripening.* Available from http://emedicine.medscape.com/article/263322-overview

RxList. (n.d.). Retrieved February 6, 2006, from http://www.rxlist.com

RxMed. (n.d.). *Naropin*, *astra, ropivacaine HCl, local anesthetic.* Retrieved March 12, 2006, from http://www.rxmed.com/b.main/b2.pharmaceutical/b2.1.monographs/CPS-%20Monographs/CPS-%20 (General%20Monographs-%20N)/NAROPIN.html

Snyder, K., & Keegan, C. (2006). *Pharmacology for the surgical technologist* (2nd ed.). Philadelphia: W.B. Saunders.

Spratto, G. R., & Woods, A. L. *Delmar's A-Z NDR—98.* Clifton Park. NY: Delmar Learning.

Tissell. Available from http://www.baxter.com/products/biopharmaceuticals/downloads/Tisseel_PI.pdf

University of Michigan. (2004). *Table of blood products.* Retrieved March 12, 2006, from http://www.pathology.med.umich.edu/bloodbank/BLOODTABle82004.pdf#search='blood%20products%20%20description'

Warner, M. A. *Practice guide for preoperative fasting and the use of pharmacologic agents to reduce the risk of pulmonary aspiration: Application to healthy patients undergoing elective procedures.* Available from http://www.ottawa-anesthesia.org/paureading/asa_fasting.pdf

Yale Medical School. Managing malignant hyperthermia. Available from http://gasnet.med.yale.edu/gta/mh/clinicalupdate.html

CHAPTER

10

Instrumentation, Equipment, and Supplies

CASE STUDY Maria is a surgical technology student working a rotation in the sterile processing department. She has been asked to gather instrumentation and supplies for an emergency procedure involving a gunshot wound to the chest. The patient has just arrived in the emergency department (ED), and the ED nurse has advised the OR team that the patient will be stabilized and on the way to the OR soon.

1. **What equipment should be in the room for this procedure?**
2. **What supplies should be gathered?**
3. **What instrument sets should be gathered?**
4. **With limited time, what supplies should be opened first, and what supplies should be opened later?**

OBJECTIVES

After studying this chapter, the reader should be able to:

C 1. Explain the relationship between instrumentation, equipment, and supplies and with quality patient care in the operating room (OR).

A 2. Explain the relationship between instruments, equipment, and supplies and the OR environment with safety concepts.

R 3. Indicate items that require sterilization prior to use in the sterile field.

4. Recognize basic instruments by type, function, and name.

5. Demonstrate proper care, handling, and assembly of instruments.

6. Differentiate the types of special equipment utilized in OR practice and demonstrate proper care, handling techniques, and safety precautions.

7. Cite the names and functions of accessory equipment and demonstrate proper care, handling, and assembly.

E 8. Collect and prepare supplies used in the OR.

Select Key Terms

aperture
bipolar electrosurgery
capillary action
catheter
cottonoid
cryo
drain
fenestration
insufflation
irrigation
magnification
monopolar cautery
pneumatic
resistance
retract
scalpel
serrations
stainless steel
teeth
ureteral
urethral

INSTRUMENTATION

Most modern surgical instruments are made of **stainless steel**, which is a combination of carbon, chromium, iron, and a few other metals (alloys). This combination of metals adds strength to the instrument and resistance to corrosion during repeated sterilization. Chromium increases **resistance** to corrosion. Titanium is stronger and lighter in weight than stainless steel. Titanium is nonmagnetic and is more resistant to corrosion than stainless steel. Titanium instruments generally have a blue finish of titanium oxide, which is designed to reduce glare during the surgical procedure.

Manufacturers of surgical instruments also add one of three other types of finish during fabrication. A highly polished, bright finish increases resistance to corrosion but can be distracting to the surgical team because of its tendency to reflect light. A satin (dull) finish is less reflective and reduces glare. An ebonized (black chromium) finish is nonreflective and virtually eliminates glare. This type of finish is recommended for procedures involving a laser because it prevents deflection of the laser beam.

CLASSIFICATIONS

Instruments are classified as cutting/dissecting, grasping/holding, clamping/occluding, retracting/viewing, probing, dilating, suturing, and suctioning. Other instruments that do not fit easily into these classifications are referred to as accessory instruments. These include the ring forceps, used to grasp a folded radiopaque 4-in. × 4-in. sponge for sponging or retraction deep within a wound (with the sponge, it is referred to as a sponge stick); curved ring forceps, which may be used to create tunnels for placement of catheters or arterial grafts; and towel clips, used to hold folded towels together during square-draping and occasionally to grasp, hold, and reduce small fractured bones.

Cutting/Dissecting

Instruments with one or more sharp edges that are used for incision, sharp dissection, or excision of tissue are classified as cutting/dissecting instruments. These typically include knives, scalpels, scissors, and bone-cutting instruments (osteotomes, curettes, chisels, gouges, and rongeurs). Saws, drills, biopsy punches, adenotomes, and dermatomes may also be classified as cutting instruments. *Note:* The suffix *-tome* refers to an instrument for cutting. The base word generally describes the type of tissue to be cut. For example, an *osteotome* is an instrument designed to cut bone.

Scalpels

The terms *knife* and **scalpel** are often used interchangeably, although scalpels typically have a detachable disposable blade and nondisposable handle, and, generally, knives have a nondisposable handle and blade as a single unit (e.g., amputation knife or cataract knife).

Some organizations have converted to safety scalpels, which are single-use, disposable knife blades that include a safety shield. The safety scalpels may include a disposable or nondisposable knife handle depending upon the manufacturer. The OSHA Bloodborne Pathogen Standard as well as the frequency of employee sharps injuries has driven many organizations to convert to safety scalpels.

Scalpel handle sizes include #3, #4, #7, and #9. The #3 and #4 standard handles are 5 in. in length, and the #7 handle is slightly longer (Figure 10-1). The #3 knife handle is also available as a long handle, marked 3L at the end of the handle, and is used in deep wounds. The end of a #3 knife handle, either standard or long, may be angled where the blade is fitted to aid the surgeon in reaching difficult areas. The #4 knife handle is also available as a long handle and is marked 4L at the end of the handle. Other types of knife handles include the miniature blade handle with chuck (device used to tighten the blade onto the handle), used for procedures that require very small

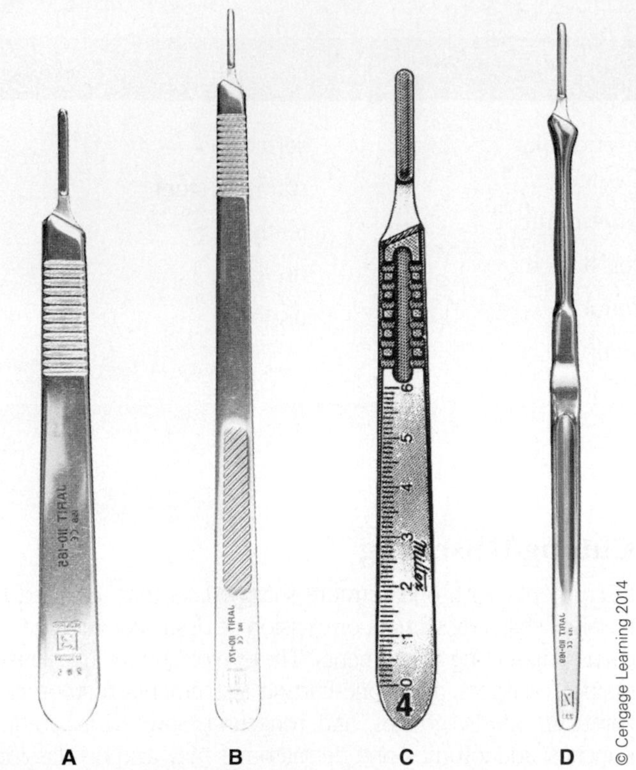

Figure 10-1 Scalpel handles: (A) #3, (B) #3L, (C) #4, (D) #7

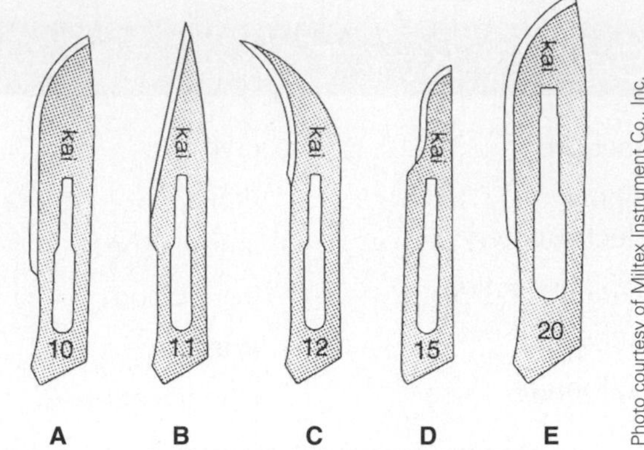

Figure 10-2 Scalpel blades: (A) #10, (B) #11, (C) #12, (D) #15, (E) #20

incisions, such as eye procedures, and the Beaver handle, which is specifically designed to hold the small Beaver blades.

Disposable blades are made from carbon steel and slide into a groove on the end of the scalpel handle, although some scalpel handles have a locking mechanism instead of a groove for easy loading (Figure 10-2). The blades must be loaded onto and removed from the handle with an instrument, typically a needle holder, and never with the fingers. The blades fit specific handles:

- Blades #10, #11, #12, and #15 fit #3, #7, and #9 handles.
- Blades #20–#25 fit a #4 handle.

Any size Beaver blade will fit a Beaver blade handle. The most frequently used Beaver blade is a #69.

The #10 is the blade most frequently used and is typically loaded onto the #3 handle. The #11, #12, and #15 blades are usually loaded onto the #7 handle, although the #15 blade is frequently used with the #3 handle for superficial procedures requiring a small incision, such as plastic or hand procedures or the #3L handle for use in deep surgical wounds. The #12 blade is used almost exclusively for tonsillectomy. The #20 blade is occasionally used for long and deep abdominal incisions.

Scissors

Scissors used during a surgical procedure may be tissue scissors, suture scissors, wire scissors, or bandage/dressing scissors. In general, tissue scissors should never be used to cut anything other than tissue because it will dull the blades. Wire scissors are only used for cutting wire, but straight Mayo suture scissors are occasionally used for cutting dressings, drapes, drains, and other nonsuture items.

Tissue scissors may be of heavy construction for tough tissue, medium construction for tissue that is neither tough nor delicate, or light construction for thin, friable tissue. Tips may be pointed or blunt, and blades may be straight or curved. The blades of tissue scissors have sharp cutting edges and are available in varying lengths (in general, the deeper the wound, the longer the scissors needed) and degrees of blade curves. Most tissue scissors blades are curved so that the tips can be seen by the surgeon and can reach around structures. In addition to cutting tissue (sharp dissection), scissors can be used to spread and open tissue planes (blunt dissection). Curved Mayo scissors are often the scissors of choice for heavy tissue; straight Mayo scissors are always used to cut suture and rarely used to cut tissue; and curved Metzenbaum scissors are used for medium to fine tissue. Delicate tissue is frequently dissected with curved iris, Jamison, Westcott, Stephen's tenotomy, or Potts-Smith scissors (Figure 10-3). Other scissors used for cutting suture include straight iris scissors, frequently used to cut fine sutures during ophthalmic or plastic procedures, and curved Metzenbaum scissors, preferred by some cardiovascular surgeons for cutting polypropylene suture.

Examples of specialized scissors include Potts-Smith scissors for incisions into ducts, veins, or arteries; Jorgenson scissors for hysterectomy; Cushing scissors for dural incision; and Castroviejo scissors for microsurgery. Scissors for eye procedures include strabismus, iris, and corneal scissors.

Grasping/Holding

Grasping/holding instruments are designed to manipulate tissue to facilitate dissection or suturing or to reduce and stabilize fractured bone during internal fixation. These instruments may or may not have a ratcheted locking mechanism. *Tissue forceps*, also referred to as *pick-ups* or *thumb forceps*, do not have ratchets and are constructed with a flattened spring handle. Tissue

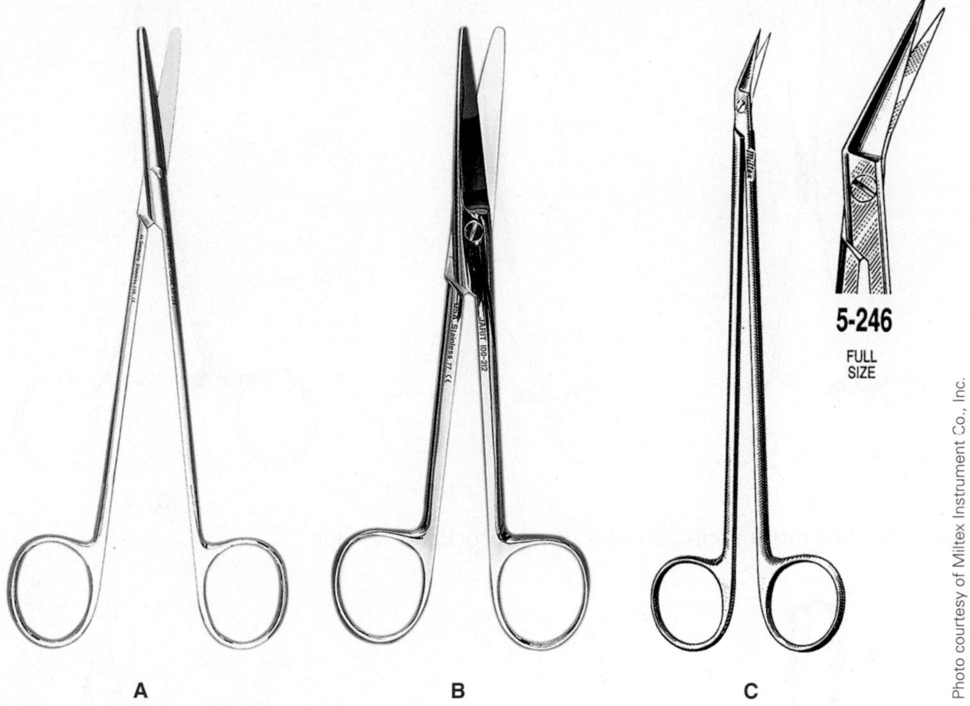

Figure 10-3 Scissors: (A) Metzenbaum, (B) curved Mayo, (C) Potts-Smith

forceps are usually used in the nondominant hand to grasp and hold tissue when suturing or dissecting. Tissue forceps may have **teeth, serrations**, or may be smooth and vary greatly in length and type. Common examples include Adson (with and without teeth), Ferris-Smith, DeBakey, Brown, Russian, Gerald (with and without teeth), and Cushing bayonet forceps (with and without teeth) (Figure 10-4). Ratcheted grasping/holding instruments include Allis, Babcock, and Kocher (Ochsner) (Figure 10-5). A tenaculum is another example of a ratcheted grasping/holding instrument. The tenaculum can contain one of more teeth and can be used to hold fibrous tissue during dissection and removal.

Bone-holding clamps are typically ratcheted and are designed to hold a bone in place for eventual pinning or plating. Smaller bone-holding forceps for bones of the hand or foot may resemble the Backhaus towel clamp, but larger bone-holding forceps have working ends that are designed to either encircle a large or medium bone or firmly grasp and hold it with multiple serrated edges. Examples include Lane, Kern, Lowman, and Lewin (Figure 10-6).

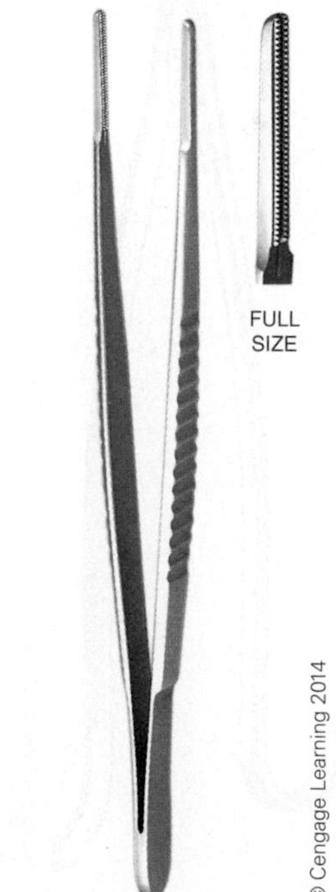

Figure 10-4 DeBakey tissue forceps and detail of tip

Clamping/Occluding

Clamping/occluding instruments are designed to occlude or constrict tissue and are constructed with opposing ring handles for fingers, interlocking ratchets located just below the ringed handles to lock the instrument in place, and two shanks that connect the ringed handles to the box lock, or hinge joint of the clamp. The box lock controls the opposing jaws of the instrument. The instrument may be straight or curved in varying degrees, and the tips may be pointed or rounded. Additionally, the jaws of the clamp may be bent at a 90° angle to facilitate placement on vessels such as arteries or organs such as the colon. Jaw serrations may be horizontal, longitudinal, or cross-hatched for better traction on tissue (Figure 10-7).

Most vascular and intestinal clamps have atraumatic serrations that run along the length of the jaws and permit the partial

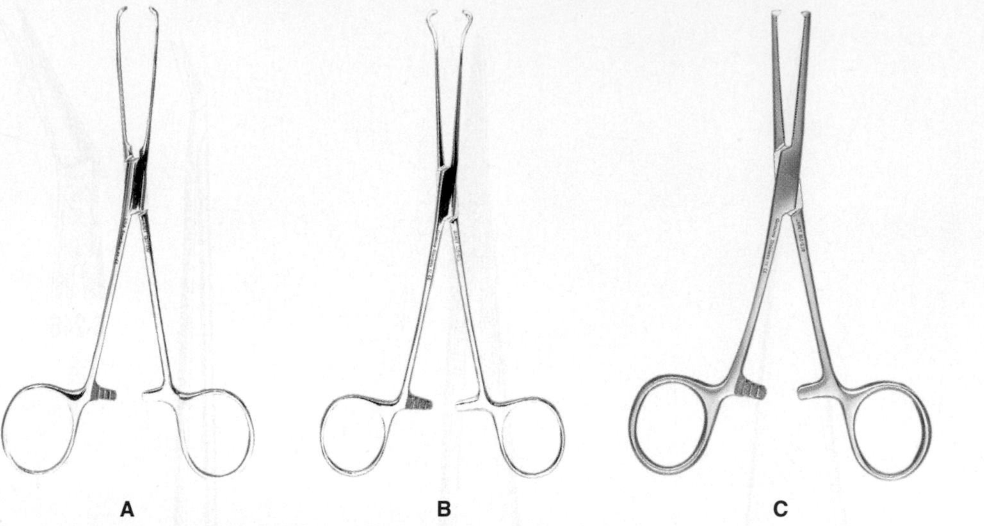

Figure 10-5 Grasping/holding instruments: (A) Allis, (B) Babcock, (C) Kocher

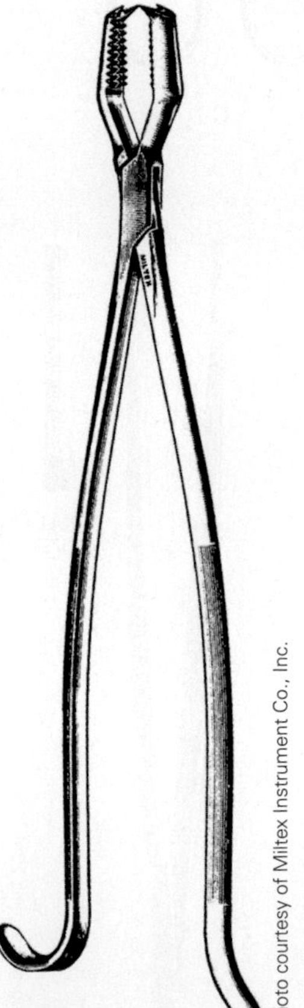

Figure 10-6 Lane bone-holding forceps

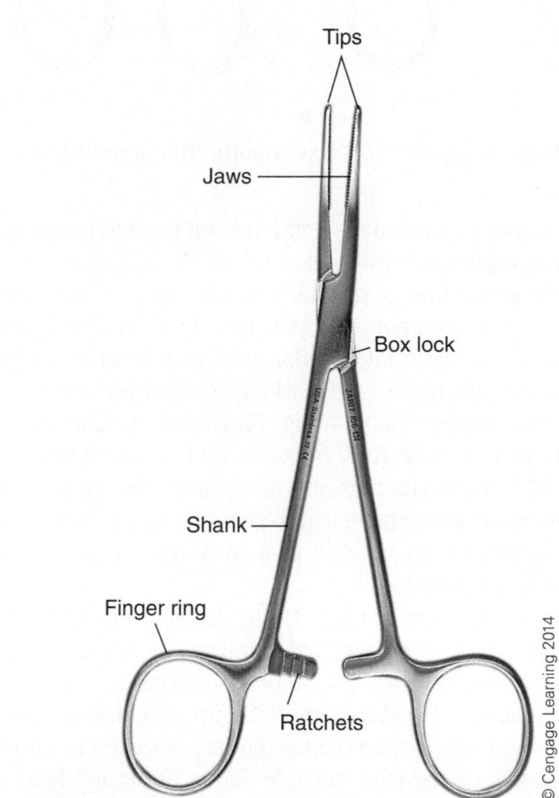

Figure 10-7 Instrument anatomy

or total occlusion of vessels or the colon without damage to the delicate tissue. Vascular clamps are also constructed with long, flexible jaws for increased vessel protection during occlusion. Some vascular clamps, such as the Fogarty Hydro-grip, protect the vessel with disposable, protective plastic inserts that slide on each jaw of the instrument. Bulldog vascular clamps are small, spring-loaded devices with atraumatic serrations.

Hemostatic clamps are designed to occlude bleeding vessels until they can be ligated, occluded with stainless steel or titanium ligaclips, or coagulated. Hemostats are typically curved, although straight hemostats are frequently utilized for "tagging" sutures; "tagging" is performed when a suture strand is not immediately cut. The straight hemostat is placed on the end of the suture strand to keep it secured and out of the surgical wound until the surgeon is ready to tie the suture (Figure 10-8).

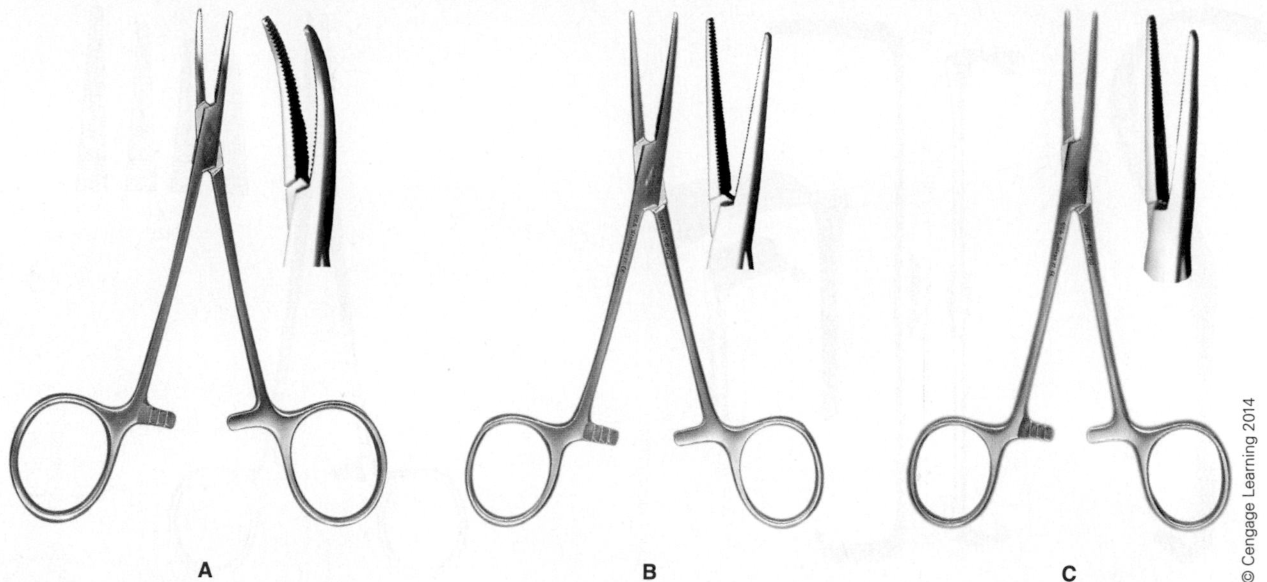

Figure 10-8 Clamping/occluding instruments: (A) Mosquito and detail of tip, (B) Crile and detail of tip, (C) Kelly and detail of tip

Retracting/Viewing

Instruments designed for the exposure of the operative site are called *retractors*. Retractors may be handheld or self-retaining and are constructed in a variety of sizes and designs. Many handheld retractors are double ended, with a slight variation of size on each end, and are frequently used in pairs on opposite sides of the incision. Self-retaining retractors, such as the Weitlaner, Gelpi, Bookwalter, O'Connor–O'Sullivan, and Balfour retractors, remain in place by mechanical means; the Bookwalter, O'Connor–O'Sullivan, and Balfour have interchangeable blades for varying wound depths and tissue types. Self-retaining retractors for abdominal or brain procedures may attach to the OR table for stabilization, for example, the Thompson retractor and the Greenberg retractor. (Figure 10-9).

Handheld retractors with a blunt edge are typically used to **retract** the abdominal wall or abdominal and thoracic organs (Figure 10-10). Sharp rake-like retractors are used for retraction of nonvital structures, such as fat or skin. Single-hook or double-hook retractors are utilized for the retraction of skin during plastic procedures. Flat malleable retractors (for example, the Ribbon retractor) may be bent into desired positions for various retraction duties. Brain spoons are an example of a malleable retractor that can be handheld or applied to a self-retaining retractor for retraction of brain tissue.

Viewing instruments may provide retraction; however, their main function is to allow visualization of a structure. For example, a nasal speculum is used to spread the nares, allowing visualization of the internal nose. Specula and endoscopes are examples of viewing instruments.

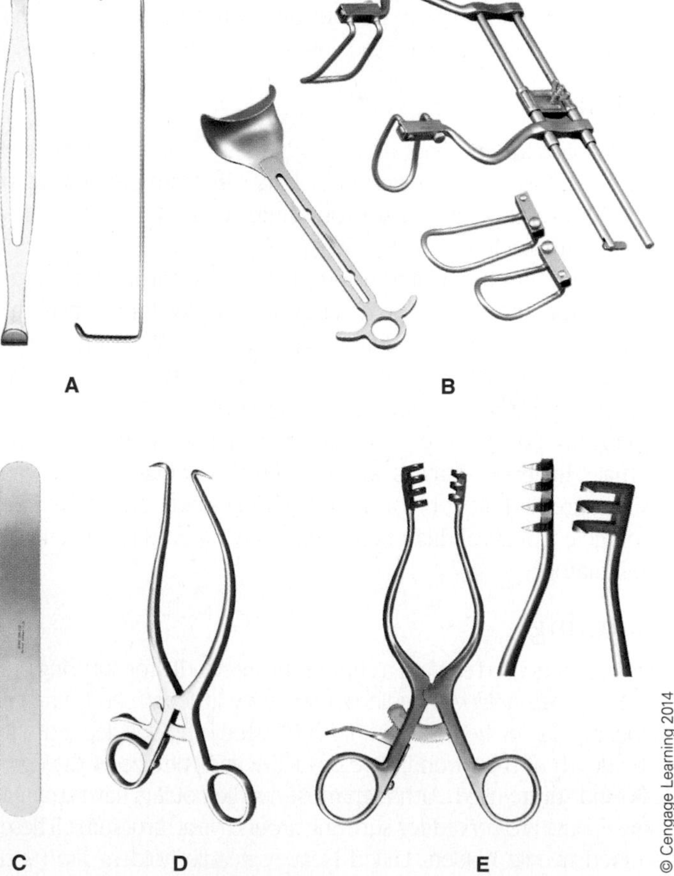

Figure 10-9 Retracting/viewing instruments: (A) U.S. Army retractor, (B) Balfour with blades, (C) ribbon-malleable, (D) Gelpi, (E) Weitlaner and detail

Probing

Malleable, wire-like instruments for the exploration of a structure such as a fistula, duct, or vessel are called *probes*. Probes

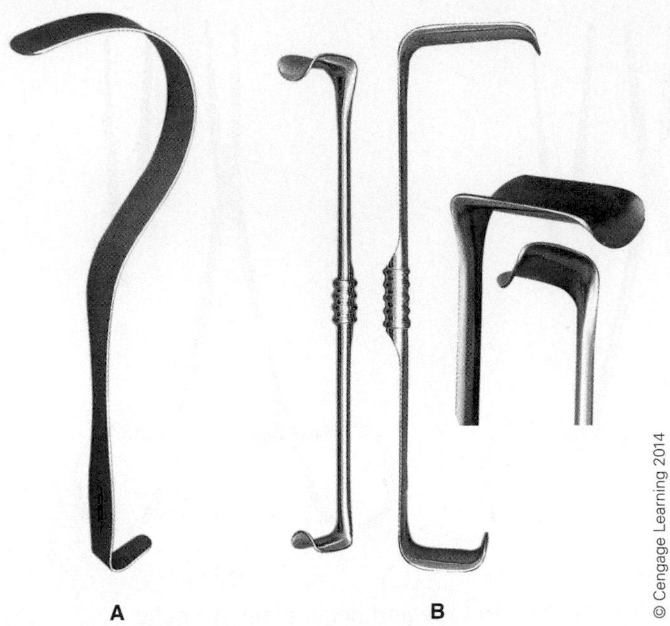

Figure 10-10 Retracting/viewing instruments: (A) Deaver, (B) Richardson

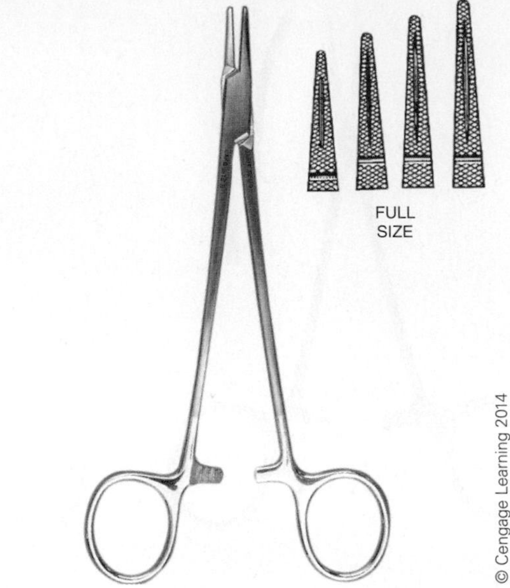

Figure 10-11 Needle holder and detail of tips

are typically found in abdominal, gallbladder, or rectal instrument sets and are often used with guides called *grooved directors*. Probes for coronary arteries are small and malleable and can also be used to dilate the coronary artery.

Dilating

Dilators are instruments used to gradually dilate an orifice or duct to allow for introduction of larger instrumentation or to open a stricture. Vessels are sometimes dilated during cardiovascular procedures.

Structures are dilated using the smallest through the largest dilators, so these instruments are usually found in numbered sets. Dilators gradually taper to the distal end from the wider, proximal end where it is held by the surgeon. The Heaney and Hegar cervical dilators are double ended, with the opposite end one size up or down in diameter. Single-ended female **urethral** dilators are shorter than single-ended Van Buren urethral dilators for men. The long single-ended flexible Bougie esophageal dilators are gradually tapered to the end of the dilator.

Suturing

Instruments used to hold a curved suture needle for suturing are called *needle holders*. Needle holders vary in length and may be fine, regular, or heavy. The choice of needle holder depends on the depth of the wound, type of tissue, and the size of the needle and suture used. Although most needle holders have straight jaws, some are curved for suturing around vital structures. These curved needle holders, called Heaney needle holders, are used during certain genitourinary and gynecological procedures.

The jaws of a needle holder are designed to prevent the needle from moving during suturing. Jaws with tungsten carbide inserts with cross-hatched serrations are usually effective for needle immobilization.

Most needle holders are constructed as clamps; that is, they are designed with ringed handles, ratchets, shanks, box locks, and jaws (Figure 10-11). Needle holders for microsurgical, ophthalmic, and certain vascular procedures, however, have a spring action with a single ratchet that protects the small, delicate suture needle and allows the surgeon to use more subtle maneuvers when suturing. Castroviejo needle holders used for plastic and ophthalmic procedures have a locking device to hold the needle in place.

Suctioning

The removal of blood and body fluids from an operative site to provide better visualization is accomplished with a suction tip that is connected by plastic tubing to a suction canister or other suction device such as the Neptune. The suction canister is in turn connected to a vacuum device. Suction tips may be nondisposable or disposable and vary in size and design, depending on the procedure and the amount of fluid to be suctioned.

Neurosurgeons prefer an angled suction tip with a proximal thumbhole that allows for variability in suction strength. This feature prevents neural tissue from being damaged when fluids are aspirated. Because these small-diameter suction tips have a tendency to become obstructed, they are furnished with a flexible stylet that is inserted through the lumen to facilitate cleaning. The Frazier and Baron suction tips are examples of this type and are also used by plastic and orthopedic surgeons. These suction tips are numbered according to size (Figure 10-12).

Commonly used for aspiration of abdominal fluids are the Yankauer and Poole abdominal suction tips. The angled Yankauer suction tip was designed for pharyngeal suctioning

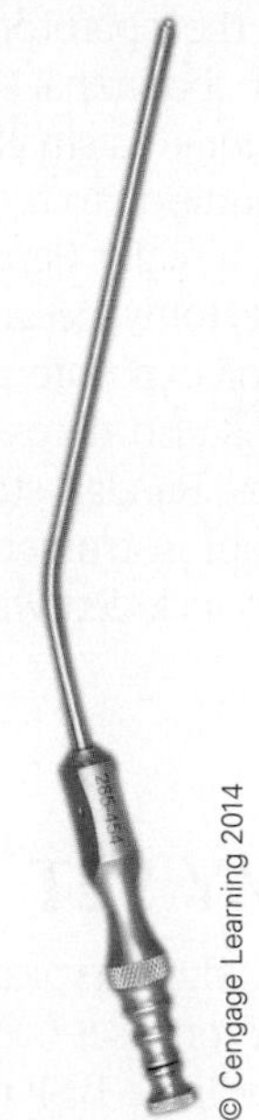

Figure 10-12 Frazier suction tip

during tonsillectomy but is frequently used for abdominal procedures. The straight Poole abdominal suction tip has a removable guard with multiple holes that allows the surgeon to rapidly aspirate large amounts of fluid, usually **irrigation** fluid, from the abdominal cavity without interference from abdominal viscera. Occasionally, to further aid in preventing damage to abdominal viscera, the surgeon will wrap the tip with a sponge. The irrigation fluid is suctioned through the sponge, preventing the tissue from being sucked up against the tip. The guard can be removed for more precise suctioning (Figure 10-13).

Some disposable suction tips have an attached active electrode that allows for simultaneous suctioning and coagulation. These special devices are frequently used by ENT surgeons during tonsillectomy. Other specialty suction tips include long straight metal devices used during rigid laryngoscopy, esophagoscopy, mediastinoscopy, and bronchoscopy procedures. The Rosen suction tip resembles a large, bent hypodermic needle and is included with an adapter for suction tubing attachment. The Rosen suction tip is available in a variety of sizes and is typically used for ear procedures.

A *trocar* is an instrument with a sharp point and cutting edges that allow for penetration of a body cavity for the drainage of fluid or the introduction of an endoscope. The trocar fits inside a hollow cannula that is left in place after tissue penetration. After removal of the trocar, suction tubing can be attached to the cannula, and the contents of the cavity aspirated. Trocar/cannula assemblies are frequently used to **drain** sinuses or the gallbladder.

Microinstrumentation

Instruments that are used to perform microsurgery are very small, delicate, and precise devices that, when used in conjunction with an operating microscope, allow the

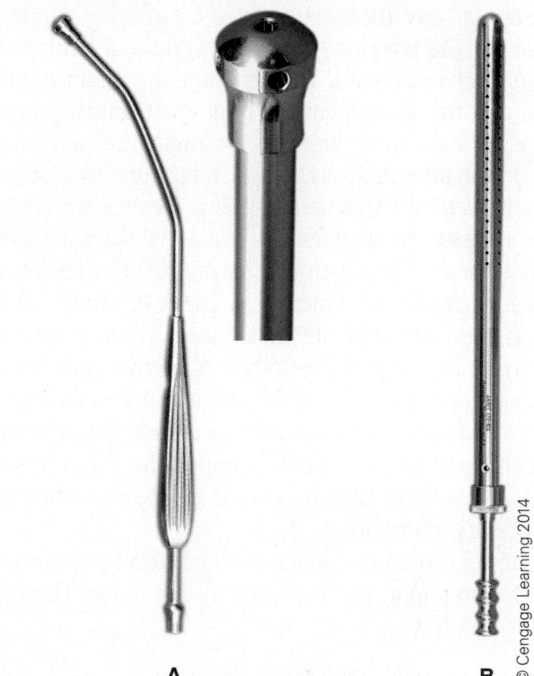

Figure 10-13 Suction tips: (A) Yankauer and detail of tip, (B) Poole

manipulation and repair of very small structures or tissue. These instruments are typically made of titanium or stainless steel, but titanium is preferred because it is stronger yet lighter in weight. The finish is dull so that light from the operating microscope is not reflected into the eyes of the operating team.

Microinstruments are designed to be held with the thumb and forefinger, allowing for more subtle movements than are allowed with finger rings. Scissors and needle holders are typically spring loaded, with a locking device for the needle holder. Scalpels for microsurgery are usually of the Beaver type; the arachnoid knife, a delicate knife with an angled tip, is frequently used for neurosurgery. Microdissectors and nerve hooks are used for blunt dissection, and spring-loaded vascular or aneurysm clips are used to occlude small vessels. Forceps for microsurgery may have fine teeth or may be smooth. Forceps may also be curved or straight. The tips of the forceps must be protected because they are easily bent or thrown out of alignment. Bipolar forceps are frequently used for coagulation of tissue during microsurgery.

INSTRUMENT CARE AND HANDLING

The handling of instruments, like all tasks related to the surgical procedure, has three phases: preoperative, intraoperative, and postoperative tasks. The combination of these three phases is referred to as the *instrument cycle*.

Preoperatively, the instrument set and other supplies are gathered for the planned surgical procedure according to the surgeon's preference card. The instrument container must be opened, and the instrument set removed from the container. Instruments, and other supplies, are organized and prepared for use on the back table and Mayo stand (refer to Chapter 12).

Intraoperative instrument handling involves a complex set of critical thinking and interactive tasks. The surgical technologist must be able to anticipate, or predict, the needs of the patient and surgical team members. The A POSitive CARE Approach is used to anticipate these needs through knowledge of normal anatomy and physiology, operative pathology, and the planned operative procedure, and an understanding of any variations that may be necessary to accommodate the specific patient (refer to Chapter 12). It is imperative that the surgical technologist observe the progression of the procedure to obtain necessary information.

Postoperative instrument handling involves all of the steps related to preparing the instruments for reuse. These steps include:

- Cleaning and decontamination
- Inspection and maintenance
- Reassembly of the instrument set
- Preparation for sterilization
- Sterilization
- Storage

Additional information about the postoperative phase of the instrument cycle is found in Chapter 7.

All surgical instruments must be handled with great care during all phases of the instrument cycle. This helps to (1) prevent injury to the patient or surgical team members, (2) extend the life of the instrument, and (3) allow the instrument to perform correctly and consistently. Some instruments may be complex and expensive to replace. Delicate instruments, such as microinstrumentation, may require special handling. Instruments are occasionally used for purposes other than intended; this practice is not recommended because damage to the instrument may result.

TYPES OF INSTRUMENT SETS

Instruments are typically assembled into sets, sterilized, and stored for later use. The instruments within each type of set are standardized according to the type of procedure for which they will be used and the needs of the facility. An instrument list or *count sheet* is used to ensure that all necessary instruments are included in the set (Figure 10-14). Generally, some instruments from each category are included in the set. Names for similar instrument sets may vary from one facility to another. For example, the laparotomy set may be alternately referred to as a major or abdominal set.

Some procedures require a smaller, secondary set of specialized instruments in addition to the larger, primary set of instruments. For example, a major (laparotomy) set is necessary to perform a cholecystectomy because it contains all of the basic instrumentation for exposure and closure of the abdomen. A gallbladder set is also necessary for its common bile duct dilators and scoops, Randall stone forceps, Mixter right angles, and cholangiogram instrumentation. Other specialized instruments that are not included with any set would have to be opened separately.

LAPAROTOMY SET

General abdominal procedures typically require a major laparotomy or a minor laparotomy set (also called a major or minor procedures set). Refer to Table 10-1 for a suggested list of the instrumentation in a basic laparotomy set. The self-retaining Balfour retractor with additional blades for exposure of abdominal contents is occasionally opened separately. Some institutions require a separate bowel resection set for removal of any portion of the bowel. Rectal procedures will require a rectal set in addition to a minor procedures set. Some institutions have a separate hemorrhoid set for hemorrhoidectomy.

Laparoscopic sets, used with increasing frequency for abdominal procedures, are equipped with one set of basic laparoscopic instruments and electrosurgical cords that can be steam sterilized and another set that has the camera, light cord, insufflator hose, and laparoscope that must be sterilized via an alternative method (e.g., Steris) that will not cause damage to the delicate lenses and fiber optics. Other types of instrument sets include bowel resection/intestinal; rectal; peripheral vascular; cardiothoracic; craniotomy; major orthopedic; cataract; major genitourinary.

Instrument List/Count Sheet

As instrument sets are assembled, an instrument list, or count sheet, with the type and number of instruments is referred to by the assembler to minimize errors (Figure 10-14). After assembly, this list is signed by the assembler and placed into the instrument pan before wrapping. The signature assures that any mistakes in assembly can be traced to the proper source. During the setup for the surgical procedure, the surgical technologist hands the instrument list to the circulator; together they perform a visual and verbal instrument count by referring to the sheet. As each instrument is confirmed by the surgical technologist, the circulator writes the correct number next to the printed instrument name on the count sheet. During the various phases of wound closure, the counting process is repeated.

Instrument List/Count Sheet — Minor Set

Instrument Name	*Quantity*	*Set Assembly*	*Initial Count*	*First Count*	*Final Count*
Halsted mosquito straight 5″	4				
Halsted mosquito curved 5″	8				
Crile curved 5½″	4				
Crile straight 5½″	2				
Rochester-Pean 6¼″	2				
Allis 6″	2				
Babcock 6¼″	2				
Mayo-Hegar needle holder 7″	2				
Crile-Wood needle holder 6″	1				
Mayo scissors straight 5½″	1				
Mayo scissors curved 5½″	1				
Metzenbaum scissors curved 7″	1				
Metzenbaum scissors curved 5½″	1				
Foerster sponge forceps straight 9½″	2				
Backhaus perforating towel clamp 5¼″	4				
Lorna nonperforating towel clamp 5¼″	2				
Senn sharp	2				
Volkman 3 prong sharp	2				
U.S. Army retractor	2				
Richardson-Eastman medium/large	2				
Yankauer suction tip	1				
Frazier suction tip 9 French with stylet	1				
Probe with eye 5½″	1				
Grooved director 5½″	1				
Tissue forceps without teeth 5½″	1				
Tissue forceps with teeth 5½″	1				
Adson tissue forceps with teeth 4¾″	2				
Knife handle #3	2				

Signature of individual preparing set: ______________________________

Figure 10-14 Sample instrument list

TABLE 10-1 **Basic Laparotomy Set**

Yankauer suction tip	1 ea.	Mayo-Hegar needle holder, 6 in.	2 ea.
Poole suction tip	1 ea.	Mayo-Hegar needle holder, 7 in.	2 ea.
8-, 10-, and 12-in. DeBakey forceps	1 ea.	Mayo-Hegar needle holder, 8 in.	2 ea.
#3, #4, and #7 knife handles	1 ea.	Mayo-Hegar needle holder, 10½ in.	2 ea.
Mayo scissors straight	1 ea.	Goelet retractor	2 ea.
Mayo scissors curved	1 ea.	U.S. Army retractor	2 ea.
7- and 9-in. Metzenbaum scissors	1 ea.	Ribbon retractor, ¾ in.	1 ea.
Ferris-Smith forceps	2 ea.	Ribbon retractor, 1¼ in.	1 ea.
Adson tissue forceps with teeth	2 ea.	Deaver retractor, 1 in.	1 ea.
Russian tissue forceps	2 ea.	Deaver retractor, 2 in.	2 ea.
Cushing tissue forceps	2 ea.	Richardson retractor, large	1 ea.
Halsted mosquito forceps curved	6 ea.	Kelly retractor, 2½ in.	1 ea.
Crile forceps, 5½ in. curved	12 ea.	Balfour retractor and blades	1 ea.
Rochester-Pean forceps, 8 in.	6 ea.	Lahey gall duct forceps, 7½ in.	2 ea.
Rochester-Ochsner forceps, 6¼ in.	4 ea.	Allis tissue forceps, 6 in.	2 ea.
Mixter forceps, 7¼ in. curved	1 ea.	Allis tissue forceps, 10 in.	2 ea.
Mixter forceps, 9 in.	1 ea.	Babcock tissue forceps, 6¼ in.	2 ea.
Baby Mixter forceps, 5¼ in. curved	1 ea.	Babcock tissue forceps, 9¼ in.	2 ea.
Backhaus towel clamp	8 ea.	Stainless steel ruler	2 ea.
Foerster sponge forceps	2 ea.		

If a count is waived for the procedure due to an emergency, the surgical technologist can confirm that the instrument set is complete by referring to the instrument list afterward. The health care facility will have a policy and procedure that addresses the other steps to take if an instrument, sharps, or sponge count is waived due to emergency.

SPECIALTY EQUIPMENT

Every OR contains a certain amount of standard equipment. However, as technology affects operative practice, an increased amount of specialized equipment is required.

Endoscopes

Endoscopes are used for diagnosis, biopsy, visualization, and/or repair of a structure within a body cavity or the interior of a hollow organ (Figure 10-15). Because the endoscope is introduced either through a body opening, such as the urethra, or through a small skin incision, hospital stays are shortened and recovery time is less than for a major surgical procedure. Many endoscopic procedures can be done on an out-patient basis.

Advances in fiber-optic technology have allowed routine endoscopic access to areas that were once considered beyond reach, such as the ventricles of the brain. Lumbar discectomy can now be performed through an endoscope, as can many abdominal and thoracic procedures.

Endoscopes with or without cameras can be inserted into body cavities or joint spaces through trocar/cannula assemblies for diagnostic purposes or surgical repair. These include arthroscopes, laparoscopes, and thoracoscopes.

Endoscopes can also be inserted through body orifices for viewing, repairing, or biopsy of tissue. They may also be used for hemorrhage control or retrieval of a foreign body. These include bronchoscopes, laryngoscopes, colonoscopes, gastroscopes, hysteroscopes, sigmoidoscopes, proctoscopes, sinuscopes, otoscopes, cystoscopes, and resectoscopes.

Many modern fiber-optic endoscopes are flexible with a maneuverable tip and channels for the introduction of flexible instruments, suction, and fluid injection. Rigid scopes may be hollow or constructed with a telescopic lens system and eyepiece. Examples of rigid scopes are those typically used for cystoscopy, laparoscopy, thoracoscopy, proctoscopy, sigmoidoscopy, and arthroscopy. Rigid bronchoscopy is preferred for retrieval of a foreign body from a bronchus, but flexible bronchoscopes are most often used for diagnostic purposes.

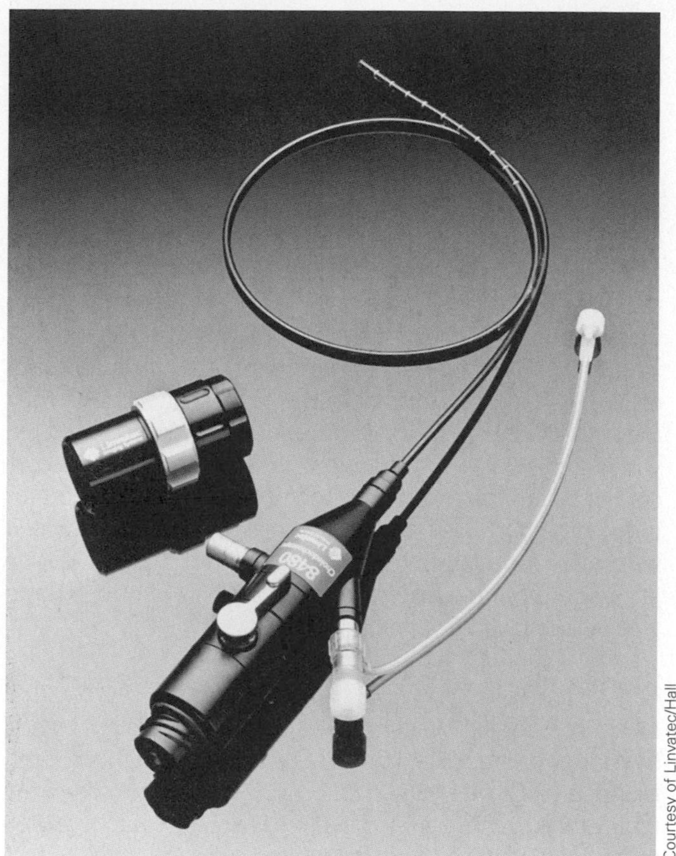
Courtesy of Linvatec/Hall

Figure 10-15 Flexible endoscope

Endoscopes can be attached to a camera that produces an image on a monitor for viewing by the surgical team. A light cord that has one end attached to the endoscope and the other attached to an electrical light source produces the illumination necessary for viewing.

Specialty endoscopes include:

- Choledochoscopes, for exploration of the biliary system
- Mediastinoscopes, for visualization and biopsy of the structures of the mediastinum
- Ureteroscopes, for exploration of the ureters
- Angioscopes, for visualization of the heart and major vessels, or vascular endoscopes for the interior of smaller vessels
- Ventriculoscopes, for exploration of the brain's ventricular system
- Fetoscopes, for visualization of a fetus *in utero*

Endoscopes can be used with electrosurgical devices for coagulation or tissue dissection. The resectoscope uses a monopolar electric current to shave hypertrophied prostate tissue from within the proximal urethra, and instruments with **monopolar cautery** and **bipolar electrosurgery** active electrodes are commonly used during laparoscopy for tissue coagulation and dissection.

Powered Instruments

Instruments used in the OR that are powered by compressed air, nitrogen, electricity, or battery are called *powered instruments.* Powered instruments have many uses, including:

- Drill holes into the skull and connect the holes to turn a bone flap for access to the brain
- Ream the central shaft of a long bone for rod placement
- Drill holes for screws to secure a plate on a fractured bone
- Saw the femoral or humeral head for joint replacement
- Saw through the sternum for access to the heart
- Reshape bone for plastic/reconstructive procedures
- Drive pins to reduce and stabilize fractured bone
- Cut skin, usually for skin grafting
- Sand the skin for dermabrasion

Power saws have either a reciprocating (back-and-forth) or oscillating (side-to-side) action for cutting bone, and the blades for these power instruments are available in a variety of sizes and shapes (Figure 10-16). The blade of a craniotome cuts through the cranium with a rotary motion, and the delicate tissue underneath is protected by a dural guard at the foot of the instrument.

Drills utilize a rapid rotary motion for carving bone with burs or drilling holes for wire, pins, or screws. Drivers also utilize a rapid rotary motion for inserting, or "driving," sharp pins to reduce a bone fracture or guide a driven nail. Reamers utilize a slower rotary motion for reaming the shaft of a long bone to insert a nail or rod. Cranial perforators use a rotary motion to drill holes in the cranium and are designed to stop before penetrating the brain.

Nitrogen for power instruments is supplied from a tank or is piped in from outside the surgery department. The tank is mobile, allowing for easier hookup for power hoses. Adapters

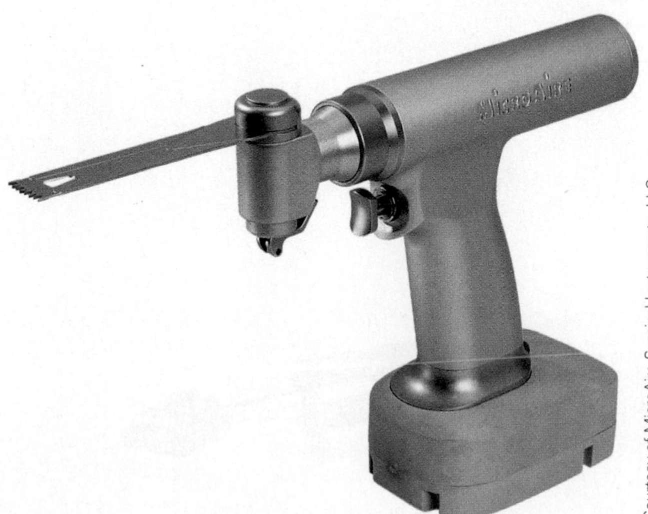
Courtesy of MicroAire Surgical Instruments, LLC

Figure 10-16 Oscillating power saw

are fitted to the tank for the connection of two power hoses. Pressure gauges on the regulator are set by the OR team at the specifications of the manufacturer of the power equipment and should be followed closely to prevent damage to the instrument and its hose or injury to the patient.

Larger power equipment is frequently powered by battery or nitrogen, while delicate bone work may require a faster air-powered instrument for greater precision and reduction of heat and vibration. Many older dermatomes for skin grafts are electric powered, but the newer dermatomes and high-speed dermabraders are powered by compressed nitrogen.

Microscopes

The compound operating microscope is a binocular apparatus that uses bent light waves for variable **magnification** of tissues during microsurgery. It may be suspended from the ceiling or mounted on a mobile frame with locking casters. The operating microscope consists of the optical lens system, magnification and focus controls, the illumination system, a mounting system for stability, an electrical system, and accessories (Figure 10-17). The eyepieces and objective lenses are interchangeable according to the needs of the surgeon.

Magnification

The optical lens system provides the magnification and resolving power necessary to do the surgical work. The *resolving power* of the microscope refers to the ability of the optical system to filter out adjacent images and to clarify detail. The optical system is composed of the objective lens and eyepieces (referred to as *oculars*). The focal length of the objective lens ranges from 100 to 400 mm, signifying the distance of the lens from the target tissue. This distance is referred to as the working distance. The binoculars serve as magnifiers of the actual image provided by the objective lens. Achromatic capabilities of the oculars sharpen the image in the actual colors of the target tissues. A second set of binoculars for an assistant is attached to the body of the microscope. A beam splitter allows the second set of oculars to match the original set's field of view. The microscope can be adapted for attachment to a laser or a camera can be attached to the beam splitter for viewing the target tissues on a monitor. The microscope can be covered with a sterile drape by the surgical technologist, or sterile covers can be attached to the focusing knobs by the surgeon for minor procedures. Most operating microscopes are equipped with a zoom lens operated by a foot control that can quickly increase or decrease magnification. Focusing is controlled by a foot pedal and/or hand control.

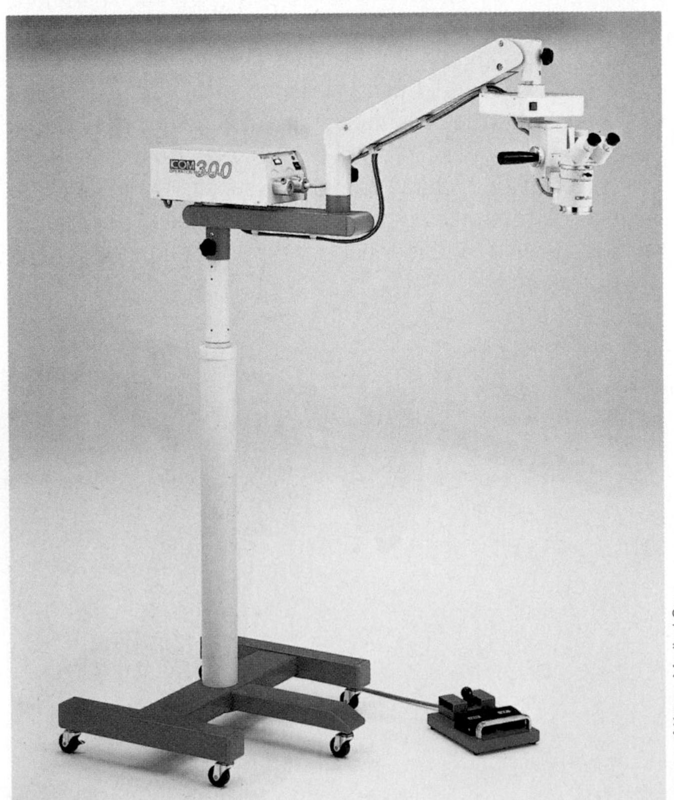

Courtesy of Konan Medical Corp.

Figure 10-17 Operating microscope

Illumination

Light waves for illumination of the operative field are provided by paraxial or coaxial illuminators. Paraxial illuminators contain tungsten or halogen bulbs and focusing lenses mounted to the body of the microscope. This type of illuminator can be angled inward to illuminate the operative site and is equipped with a diaphragm to narrow the beam. Coaxial illuminators use fiber optics to transmit light waves through the microscope's optical system. The light transmitted by this type of illuminator is cool to protect tissues from excessive heat. Light intensity is controlled by a switch on the support arm.

Video Monitors, Recorders, and Cameras

Video cameras can be attached to microscopes or endoscopes so that the procedure can be viewed on a video monitor and recorded for documentation. Still images can be taken with the camera and printed with a microcomputer imaging system for later study. Video cameras should be sterilized according to the manufacturer's recommendations.

Fiber-Optic Headlamps and Light Sources

Fiber-optic headlamps are worn by surgeons for additional lighting of the operative site. These devices are worn on the head of the surgeon to focus an intense light beam of small diameter in body cavities that are poorly illuminated by the overhead operating lights. The light cable from the headlamp is connected to an electrical light source that is situated on a mobile cart. Although every specialty makes use of the fiber-optic headlamp, it is most frequently worn by neuro-, cardiovascular and otorhinolaryngology surgeons (Figure 10-18).

A fiber-optic light cable may be attached to an illuminator fixed to a retractor for illumination of deep pockets or cavities

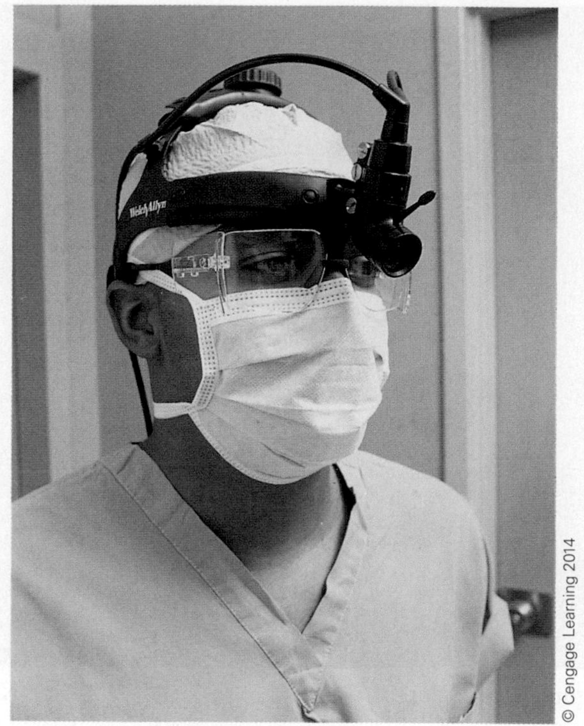

© Cengage Learning 2014

Figure 10-18 Fiber-optic headlamp

that are not easily reached with the beam of the overhead OR lights. These types of retractors are frequently used for breast augmentation or mastectomy.

To illuminate the interior of the body during endoscopic procedures, a fiber-optic light cord is connected to an electric light source at one end and to the endoscope to the other end. The light cord should be sterilized according to the manufacturer's instructions.

Pulse Lavage Irrigator

A pulse lavage irrigator powered by nitrogen, battery, or electricity is utilized to thoroughly irrigate a traumatic, infected, or surgical wound. It is often used during orthopedic procedures to irrigate contaminated fractures to clean out the debris and in total joint arthroplasties. The surgical team must be protected from the splattered fluids, so a circular shield is often placed on the hand control.

Phaco-Emulsifier and Irrigation/ Aspiration Units

Diseased eye lenses may be fragmented and removed with a Phaco-Emulsifier, a machine that uses ultrasonic energy (cavitation) to fragment the lens, and an irrigator/aspirator (I/A) to remove the fragments. IA flow is automatically adjusted for pressures within the anterior chamber of the eye. The newer piezoelectric machine uses electric impulses to generate heat and is cooled by air or fluid that flows through the power cord. Aspirant flows through transparent tubes away from the operative site.

Cryotherapy Units

A **cryo** therapy unit uses liquid nitrogen, Freon, or carbon dioxide (CO_2) gas to deliver extreme cold through an insulated probe to diseased tissues, creating necrosis without damage to adjacent tissues. The diseased tissue can then be removed under hemostatic conditions. Because cryotherapy preserves neighboring tissue and removes diseased tissue without significant hemorrhage, it is useful for the removal of vascular tumors, brain tumors, and the prostate gland. Cryotherapy is also utilized to repair retinal detachments and extract cataracts.

Insufflators

Laparoscopic procedures cannot be performed unless CO_2 gas is infused into the abdominal cavity through either a Verres **insufflation** needle or a Hasson blunt trocar. The machine that infuses the CO_2 gas into the abdominal cavity is called an *insufflator.* Expansion of the abdominal cavity with CO_2 gas, referred to as insufflation, creates a space for viewing an endoscope and for work within the cavity through cannulas inserted at strategic points through the abdominal wall. The machine may have a warmer and/or humidifier attached to warm and humidify the CO_2 gas in order to aid in maintaining the internal body temperature of the patient.

Nerve Stimulators

Nerve stimulators produce very small electric currents that, when applied to tissue, help to identify and preserve essential nerves for cranial, facial, neck, or hand reconstructive procedures. The nerve stimulator is especially useful for identification of the seventh cranial (facial) nerve during acoustic neuroma removal and to identify the facial, acoustic, cochlear, and vestibular nerve branches during otological procedures. Anesthesia providers may use the nerve stimulator to assess the actions of neuromuscular blockers administered during anesthesia.

To operate the intraoperative nerve stimulator, the needle that is attached by wire to the locator probe is inserted into adjacent, nonessential tissue. The structure in question is touched with the probe and the electric current is delivered to the structure. If a nerve is nearby, the surrounding tissue will move slightly, or the tissues that the nerve innervates will respond with movement. The nerve stimulator used by the anesthesia care provider is an external device that is a small rectangular box with two short antenna-like prongs on one end. The prongs are gently placed against the temple of the patient and a button is pushed to elicit the nerve response.

ACCESSORY EQUIPMENT

An assortment of equipment is needed for surgical procedures routinely. This equipment is referred to as accessory equipment.

Suction Systems

Suction apparatus utilizes a vacuum to remove fluids from the surgical site and patient's airway. A minimum of two suction units is required in each operating room. One unit must be available at all times to assist the anesthesia care provider with airway maintenance and the other is used within the surgical field. The components of the suction system include:

- *Vacuum source*—May be portable or centralized. The centralized vacuum source is accessed via outlets located in each operating room (OR).
- *Vacuum source tubing*—Connects the vacuum source with the collection unit.
- *Collection unit*—May be reusable or contain a disposable liner. The collection unit may have incremental markings to allow estimation of the amount of fluid contained within.
- *Tubing*—Connects the collection unit to the suction tip. Is usually disposable and may be sterile or nonsterile according to the situation.
- *Suction tip*—Removes the fluid from the source. May be sterile or nonsterile, disposable or reusable, and one of a variety of styles (see previous discussion on surgical instruments for information about the Yankauer and Poole suction tips).

The sterile suction tubing and tip are opened onto the sterile field in preparation for the procedure. The surgical technologist will connect the suction tip to the tubing and set the apparatus aside for placement on the sterile field following drape application. Once the patient has been draped, the suction tubing is secured to the drape with a nonpenetrating towel clamp. The end with the suction tip applied remains on the sterile field and the opposite end is passed from the sterile field to the circulator for attachment to the collection device. Once connected, the vacuum is turned on and adjusted by the circulator.

Lights

Good lighting is necessary for any surgical procedure. White fluorescent overhead lights provide general illumination for the room. Ceiling-mounted overhead operating lights provide the focused lighting necessary for precision illumination during the surgical procedure. Most ORs are equipped with two overhead operating lights, although ORs equipped for open-heart procedures usually have four, as will some trauma and neurosurgical rooms (Figure 10-19).

Overhead operating lights are freely adjustable to any angle desired and provide an intense light appropriate for the size of the incision. The diameter and focus of the light pattern can be adjusted with a control mounted on the light fixture. The beam should generally be set at a 10- to 12-in. depth of focus so that the intensity of the beam is relatively equal at the surface and depth of the incision.

The light beam from the overhead OR light produces no shadows and minimal heat and is near the blue/white color of daylight. The light fixtures and suspension-mounted tracks or central mount are built so that they are easily cleaned and do not retain dust.

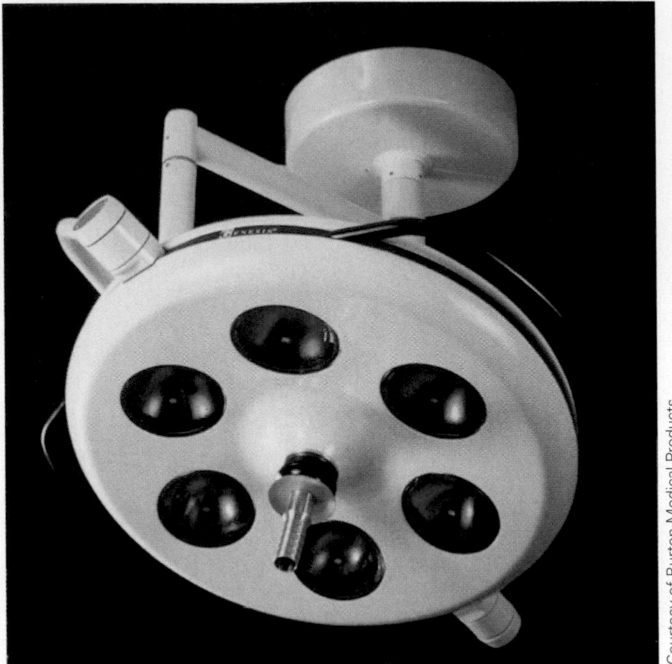

Courtesy of Burton Medical Products

Figure 10-19 Surgical lights

Light fixtures are equipped with a screw or clip device within the center of the fixture for attachment of sterile handles. These autoclavable handles are used by the operative team to manipulate illumination for the operative site. The handles may be left permanently attached to the fixture and covered with disposable sterile plastic covers for each sterile procedure.

Light intensity from overhead operating lights is controlled by a wall-mounted fixture with a dimmer and on/off switch. The OR light should never be turned off unless the dimmer has been turned down. This prevents expensive light bulbs from blowing out.

Pneumatic Tourniquets

Tourniquet use is necessary during some procedures on the extremities to restrict blood flow to the surgical site. The tourniquet serves two main purposes:

1. The amount of blood lost by the patient is minimized.
2. Visualization of the surgical site for the sterile team members is improved.

The patient may suffer neurovascular damage from incorrect cuff placement, excessive tourniquet pressure, and/or prolonged inflation. Improper application of the tourniquet cuff may also lead to blistering, bruising, pinching, or necrosis of the skin.

The electrically operated **pneumatic** tourniquet consists of the following components (Figure 10-20):

- *Cuff*—Consists of a rubber bladder contained within a fabric or plastic covering, similar to a blood pressure cuff

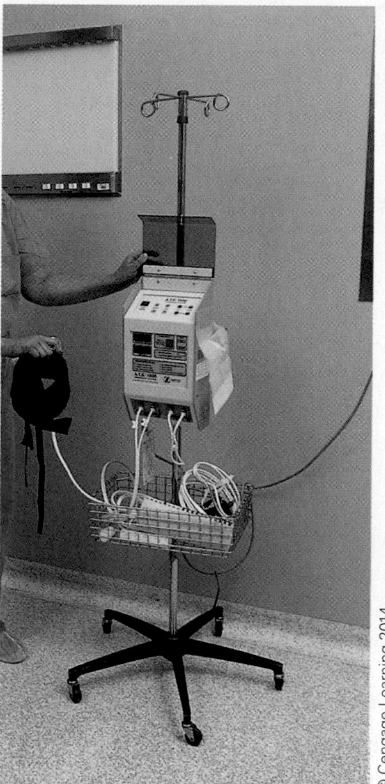

Figure 10-20 Pneumatic tourniquet system

and may house a single or double chamber. The double-chamber tourniquet is used for intravenous regional (Bier) blocks (refer to Chapter 9).

- *Tubing*—Connects the cuff to the pressure source.
- *Pressure device*—Consists of an air compressor, pressure controls, pressure gauge, and timer.
- *Power source*—The compressor is run by electricity. The unit is usually plugged in to a wall outlet; however, some units also have a battery that is capable of operating the compressor for a short time. This is useful in case of a power failure and for patient transport from the emergency department to the OR. (Compressed air may also be piped into the OR or may be obtained from a portable tank.)

The technique for tourniquet preparation, application, and use is as follows. *Note:* The surgeon may request a sterile cuff and tubing, requiring a variation of this procedure.

Placement of the cuff is determined by the physician. As a rule, the cuff is placed as far proximally on the extremity as possible. Variations may occur according to the patient's specific situation.

Tourniquet pressure is determined by the surgeon and/or anesthesia provider according to the patient's systolic blood pressure and any other related medical conditions(s). Generally, the tourniquet pressure for the lower extremity is higher than the systolic blood pressure by one-half the value. The

TECHNIQUE

Tourniquet Application

1. All equipment is checked for accuracy, function, integrity, and cleanliness.
2. Preset the pressure according to the physician's order.
3. Padding, such as stockinette or rolled cotton sheeting, is applied circumferentially to the patient's skin.
4. The appropriate-size cuff is snugly applied and secured over the padding.
5. The tubing is connected securely to the cuff.
6. If necessary, a protective covering is applied to the cuff.
7. The patient is prepped and draped.
8. The extremity is exsanguinated with the use of gravity and/or an Esmarch bandage.
9. The tourniquet is inflated to the correct pressure and the timer started.
10. The tourniquet is deflated and the time noted.
11. Presence, type, and thickness of padding, size and location of the cuff, inflation pressure, duration of inflation, and condition of the skin prior to and following tourniquet use are documented in the patient's operative record.

tourniquet pressure for the upper extremity is approximately 30–70 mm Hg higher than the patient's systolic blood pressure. During a lengthy procedure (duration greater than one hour), it is recommended that the tourniquet be temporarily deflated periodically to permit limb reperfusion. The inflation and deflation times are documented within the patient's intraoperative record.

Sequential Compression Devices

The *sequential compression device (SCD)* consists of a compressor that is electrically operated, connecting tubing, and one or more sleeves that enclose that patient's limb(s). The sleeves house a series of chambers that are filled with fluid or air when the device is activated. Fluid or air is pumped into the distal portion of the sleeve causing any fluid (e.g., blood, lymph) within the limb to move proximally. Once the chambers have filled, they are emptied (decompressed) and the cycle repeats. The pressure and frequency of the compressions can be adjusted according to the physician's order.

In the OR, SCDs are applied to the patient's legs to prevent venous stasis, thereby reducing the risk of development of deep vein thrombosis that can lead to pulmonary embolism. Use of the device may be extended to the postoperative period. SCDs are also used to treat edema and may be applied to the patient's upper extremity following an axillary lymph node dissection. Battery-operated portable devices are available.

SUPPLIES

Supplies refers to a large variety of sterile and nonsterile goods. These include drapes; sponges and dressings; catheters; tubes and drains; and irrigators and syringes.

Drapes

Surgical drapes are used by the surgical team to serve as a barrier to isolate and protect the operative site from contaminants and microbes that can cause a surgical site infection (SSI).

Effective drape materials should be:

- Lint free to prevent airborne particles from entering the surgical wound
- Fluid resistant to prevent strike-through contamination
- Antistatic to prevent sparking that could ignite the drapes or flammable gases
- Tear and puncture resistant
- Free of toxic residue
- Porous enough so that body heat is not retained, resulting in hyperthermia
- Finished with a color that does not reflect the operating lights
- Flame retardant so that they do not ignite if exposed to the beam of a laser or spark from an electrosurgical unit

Drape Materials

Various materials have been used for surgical draping over the years. Drape materials may be nonwoven textile fabrics, woven textile fabrics, or plastic.

Nonwoven Fabrics

Nonwoven fabric drapes are disposable and are typically made from compressed synthetic fibers, such as nylon or polyester bonded with cellulose. Aluminum-coated materials are preferred during laser procedures for their flame-retardant properties. Nonwoven drapes are light, yet strong, and offer the advantage of disposability. They need not be washed, folded, repaired, or sterilized by OR personnel, and contact with contaminants is minimized.

Disposable drapes have reinforced layers of material surrounding the **fenestration** (opening) of the drape. Some may have a plastic cover with a central slit over a rounded fenestration for snug fits around extremities. They are also equipped with special tags for attachment of suction tubing, electrosurgical cords, or power cords to the drape. A built-in, antimicrobial incise drape across the fenestration is also available for certain specialty drapes.

Woven Textile Fabrics

Reusable drapes are popular with hospitals because they are cheaper to use than disposable drapes. The cotton fibers of the material swell when they become wet, making the material impermeable to liquids. The material is also treated with a fluorochemical finish to further increase its fluid-repellent action.

Reusable drapes have certain disadvantages: They must be laundered, folded, inspected for wear, and sterilized after each use. Frequent washings cause the fibers of the material to wear down, requiring heat-seal patches. Small holes may be missed, compromising the integrity of the barrier. Because they are reusable, the handlers' risk of exposure to contaminants is increased.

Plastic Adhesive Drapes

Plastic adhesive drapes are made of a thin, clear, plastic material that has an adhesive backing and can be applied to the skin without blocking vision.

Incise Drapes. *Incise drapes* have an adhesive backing that may be impregnated with an antimicrobial iodine agent that is slowly released after application to destroy bacteria from the patient's skin during the surgical procedure. Incise drapes are applied to the patient's skin after four towels have been placed "squaring off" the incision site. The prepped skin should be allowed to sufficiently dry so that the incise drape sticks properly. The incision is made through the drape.

Aperture Drapes. Aperture drapes are small, clear plastic drapes with openings that are surrounded by an adhesive backing. They are used to drape eyes and ears. These types of drapes allow the surgeon to view landmarks that would normally be covered.

Isolation aperture drapes are large, clear plastic drapes with an adhesive backing surrounding the fenestration and are frequently utilized as drapes for hip pinning. The isolation drapes are used to drape a patient who has been positioned on a fracture table that maintains traction of the affected extremity. Isolation drapes allow the surgeon to visualize the patient and the C-arm during fluoroscopy.

Drape Types

Drapes may be fenestrated, meaning that they have openings for exposure of the area to be incised, or they may be nonfenestrated. Each fenestrated drape has openings specific to the area to be exposed. For example, a laparotomy drape has a large, longitudinal fenestration within the center of the sheet because it is used to expose longitudinal incisions of the abdomen. A thyroid sheet has a small, transverse fenestration at the top of the sheet because it is used to expose transverse incisions of the thyroid. The remainder of any drape should always be sufficient to cover the feet and anesthesia screen. For tall patients, a nonfenestrated, reinforced three-quarter sheet may be added to sufficiently cover the feet.

Fenestrated drapes are used for the following procedures:

- Laparotomy or "lap sheet": Abdomen
- Pediatric or "pedi" sheet: Pediatric abdomen
- Transverse lap sheet: Thorax and kidney
- Thyroid sheet: Neck, especially the thyroid
- Extremity sheet: Extremities
- Hip sheet: Hip
- Perineal sheet: Perineum
- Craniotomy sheet: Cranium

Nonfenestrated sheets may be used to "square off" the surgical incision site, or to cover unaffected body parts that are not completely covered by the primary drape sheet. "Flat" sheets are square or rectangular sheets that may be placed under an extremity as a base for further draping. They are also used to cover arms on armboards or as a shield for the anesthesia provider. Flat sheets include the minor, medium, and reinforced three-quarter sheets.

Nonfenestrated drapes are also custom designed to cover specific areas. For example, the four-piece perineal sheet is designed to cover a patient in lithotomy position. The opening for the perineum is created by two leg coverings (leg pockets), an under-buttocks drape, and an abdominal drape.

Nonfenestrated split sheets are used to create an opening for a surgical site or to drape an extremity. One end of the split sheet is open down the center, creating a U shape. The free ends of the drape are referred to as the "tails" of the drape. The tails of two split sheets can be overlapped to create a fenestration of desired size, or the tails of one split sheet can be brought around a stockinette-covered extremity.

Stockinettes are stretchable gauze tubes to cover extremities. One end of the tube is closed to encase the distal portion of the extremity. The other is open for the proximal end. The stockinette is packaged in a roll and is unrolled over the extremity while the extremity is held aloft. Some stockinettes are covered with plastic to be fluid impermeable. These are frequently used to cover extremities for coronary bypass or hip replacement procedures.

Sterile Packs

Sterile packs are the first item opened for a surgical procedure and are placed onto the back table to serve as the initial sterile field. Most basic sterile packs contain a Mayo stand cover, two gowns, a suture bag, four sticky paper drapes for square draping, and two paper towels for hand drying. Some sterile packs are packaged and sterilized by the facility with reusable items.

Sterile packs have become highly specialized over the years. Most surgical specialties have one or more specific sterile packs; examples include:

- General surgery: laparotomy pack; thyroidectomy pack
- Gynecological surgery: vaginal hysterectomy pack; laparoscopy pack
- Orthopedic surgery: arthroscopic pack; total hip pack
- GU surgery: TURP pack
- ENT surgery: ear pack
- Neurosurgery: craniotomy pack
- Cardiovascular surgery: CABG pack

Each specialized pack contains supplies and drapes that are specific to the specialty or the surgical procedure.

Sponges and Dressings

Surgical sponges are used by the operative team to absorb blood and tissue fluids, blunt dissection of tissues, and protect important structures during the surgical procedure. Surgical sponges are soft and lint free and contain a radiopaque strip so that they can be located by X-ray if left within a wound. They are counted for most surgical procedures.

Laparotomy sponges are the largest and most absorbent of the surgical sponges and are available in several sizes, including small pediatric size. These sponges are used on procedures requiring large incisions, such as laparotomy or thoracotomy. They are often moistened with saline prior to use. When operating on the abdomen the general surgeon will use lap sponges as "packs" to retract and protect nonoperative viscera. Laparotomy sponges are also referred to as *laps*, *tapes*, or *packs* and are assembled five per package.

Radiopaque four-by-fours are smaller and less absorbent than laparotomy sponges. Referred to as *Raytec sponges*, they are used for procedures requiring smaller incisions. Raytec sponges can be folded and clamped by sponge/ring forceps to make sponge sticks for sponging and retracting within an abdominal wound. Loose Raytec sponges are not permitted on the operative field during an open laparotomy procedure because they can be easily lost within the wound. As a rule, Raytec sponges are removed from the operative field and replaced with laparotomy sponges and stick sponges as soon as the peritoneum is entered. Raytec sponges are assembled as 10 sponges per package (Figure 10-21).

Neurosurgical sponges are referred to as *patties* or **cottonoids**. They are used to protect delicate neural tissue when suctioning and to assist with hemostasis during neurosurgical procedures. By placing a moistened neurosurgical sponge onto bleeding neural tissue, suction can be applied without damage to the underlying tissue. Neurosurgical sponges have a radiopaque string attached to the sponge for easy location within the wound. The sponge is moistened with saline before use. These sponges are assembled 10 per package.

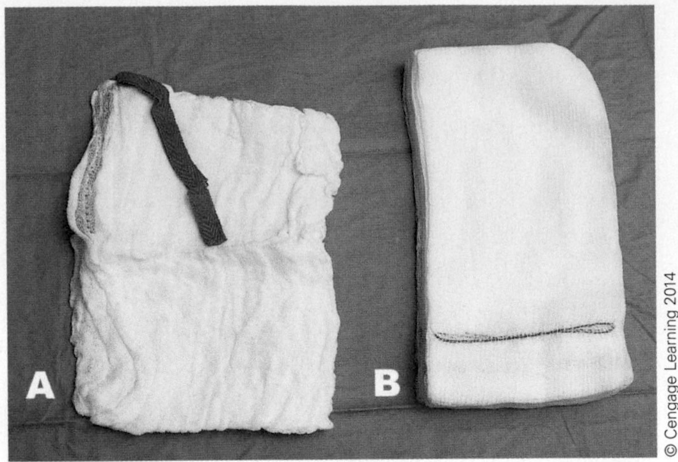

Figure 10-21 Surgical sponges: (A) Laparotomy, (B) X-ray detectable 4-in. × 4-in. (Ray-tec)

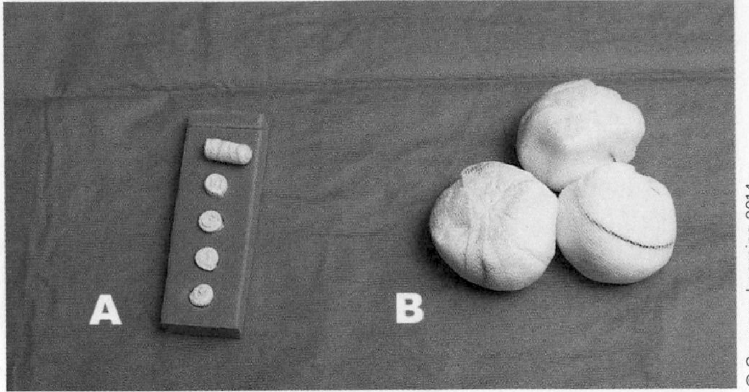

Figure 10-22 Surgical sponges: (A) Kitner, (B) tonsil

Tonsil sponges are cotton-filled gauzes with a string attached. These sponges are used during tonsillectomy to pack the bed after tonsil removal and are typically loaded and passed on a Schnidt (tonsil) clamp. These sponges are assembled in packages of five.

Kitner dissecting sponges are small rolls of cotton tape that are used to aid the surgeon in blunt dissection of tissues. They are always loaded onto a clamp, such as a Rochester-Pean, for use. These sponges are assembled in packages of five, and the surgical technologist should always have one loaded onto an instrument and four within the carrier (Figure 10-22).

Peanut sponges are small gauze sponges used for blunt dissection or fluid absorption. These sponges are also loaded onto a clamp for use.

Surgical Dressings

A surgical dressing is applied to most wounds (traumatic or surgical) to serve the following functions:

- Protect the wound from trauma
- Protect the wound from microbial contamination
- Absorb drainage and secretions
- Support the incision
- Provide pressure to reduce or eliminate dead space, reduce or prevent edema, assist in maintaining hemostasis, and prevent hematoma formation
- Maintain an environment that allows for preservation of new epithelial tissue and destruction of microbes
- Conceal the wound aesthetically

Prior to application of any type of dressing, the incision and surrounding skin must be clean and dry. A skin preparation material such as tincture of benzoin or Mastisol may be applied prior to application of the dressing. The functional dressing must be of appropriate size and type for the specific wound, secure, and relatively comfortable for the patient.

In the OR, dressing application is considered the final step of the surgical procedure and must be applied using sterile technique. Dressing changes are also considered a sterile procedure. The first scrub surgical technologist should remove the outer soiled sterile gloves before handling the dressing material by passing to the surgeon or placing on the patient. Dressing changes are occasionally scheduled in the OR and to allow the patient to be anesthetized if the procedure is expected to be painful (e.g., burn patient) or the patient is not cooperative (e.g., infant).

Some dressing materials are referred to as *sponges*. Use caution not to confuse dressing sponges and surgical sponges. Dressing sponges do not contain radiopaque markers, the exception being certain types of packing material that could potentially be inadvertently retained within a body space or cavity (e.g., vaginal pack). To avoid confusion, dressing sponges are not opened onto the sterile field by the circulator until the final count is complete and the body cavity is closed.

Note: Some types of back-table specialty procedure packs may contain the dressings specific to that procedure. In this situation, the dressings are to remain in their original packaging until the final count is complete.

Dressing Types

The type of dressing to be applied is determined by several factors, including:

- Type, size, and location of the wound
- Amount of drainage expected
- Surgeon preference
- Age and size of the patient
- Underlying medical conditions (including known allergies)
- Condition of the surrounding skin
- Comfort of the patient

Dry sterile dressings are most often applied to closed surgical wounds. The surgeon may desire to place an antiseptic or antibiotic ointment on the wound prior to dressing application.

Biologic Dressings. Biologic dressings or biosynthetic skin substitutes are used for temporary coverage of open wounds due to trauma, burns, or skin ulcers. Examples of biologic dressings include Integra,™ Dermagraft,® and Apligraf.® Biologic dressings can protect wounds, can prevent wound contamination, and can reduce fluid (serum) loss. Specific biologic dressings may also provide matrix proteins and growth factors to the wound site. This process is designed to provide an optimal wound-healing environment.

Skin Grafts. A skin graft (autologous) is a graft that is surgically taken from a specific area of the patient's own body. Skin grafts may come from another source such as from another person or may be obtained from a cadaver (homografts). Xenografts or heterografts involve tissue that is transplanted from one species to another (for example pigs [porcine] to humans). Skin grafts are applied to deepithelialized areas following traumatic injury or thermal injury, or are applied to areas of extensive skin loss. Skin grafts can be classified by graft type and are: split-thickness grafts (STSG), full-thickness grafts (FTSG), and composite grafts. Skin grafts and related procedures are discussed in **Chapter 19, Plastic and Reconstructive Surgery.**

One-Layer Dressing. A one-layer dressing is used to cover a small incision from which drainage is expected to be minimal (e.g., endoscopic incision). These dressings are also frequently used to cover the site of intravenous access. A one-layer dressing consists of transparent polyurethane film with an adhesive backing. Examples of brand-name products used as one-layer dressings include Op-site and Bioclusive. Additionally, liquid *collodion* (a type of liquid chemical dressing) may be applied to the wound and allowed to dry, forming a seal over the incision; it is often used on pediatric patients. Collodion is flammable and may not be permitted in some health care facilities. Other examples of one-layer dressings include aerosol adhesive sprays, foams, gels, hydrocolloids, and skin closure tapes. *Note:* Skin closure tapes are used to maintain approximation of the wound edges and may be used alone or in conjunction with another type of dressing (e.g. Steri Strips). Benzoin spray may be used to aid in keeping the skin closure tapes in place; the benzoin is applied to each side of the incision.

Dermabond is a liquid skin adhesive applied by surgeons to close wounds. This strong, flexible agent supports many wounds and incisions with needle-free wound closure. Dermabond may not be appropriate for all wounds or skin surfaces.

Three-Layer Dressing. A three-layer dressing is used to cover any size incision from which drainage (light, moderate, or heavy) is expected. A three-layer dressing consists of the following components: the inner (contact) layer, the intermediate (absorbent) layer, and the outer (securing) layer. The layers of a three-layer dressing may also be referred to as the primary, secondary, and tertiary layers. A three-layer dressing may be as simple as an elastic adhesive bandage (e.g., Band-Aid) or very complex.

The inner contact layer covers the wound completely and remains in direct contact with the wound. The wicking action of the contact layer allows passage of the drainage or secretions away from the healing wound into the intermediate absorbent layer. The contact layer will be one of three types with these purposes:

1. *Nonpermeable (occlusive)*—A nonpermeable dressing is a fine mesh gauze that has been impregnated with an emulsion (e.g., Vaseline Gauze, Xeroform Gauze). The occlusive dressing is used to create an airtight and watertight seal. It is nonadherent and allows passage of drainage to the absorbent layer. A nonpermeable dressing may be placed around an exit wound for a chest tube or wound drainage device to prevent air from reentering the pleural space.
2. *Semipermeable (semi-occlusive)*—A semipermeable dressing is a hydrocolloid (e.g., ExuDerm, Tegasorb) or hydrogel (e.g., Nu-Gel, AQUA-GEL). The semiocclusive dressing is used to create a mechanical surface and allow for passage of air and fluids. A hydrocolloid dressing may be used on a chronic wound such as a burn or decubitus ulcer.
3. *Permeable (nonocclusive)*—A permeable dressing is a nonadherent material (e.g., Telfa, Adaptic) used to draw secretions from the wound (called *wicking action*) and allow passage of air and fluid. The nonadherent material should allow "painless" removal of the dressing.

The intermediate (absorbent) layer is placed over the contact layer to absorb any drainage or secretions. The thickness of the absorbent layer will vary according to the amount of drainage that is expected. Examples of absorbent dressings include 2-in. × 2-in. gauze sponges, 4-in. × 4-in. gauze sponges (e.g., Toppers, Sof-Wick), fluffed gauze sponges (Kerlix), and abdominal pad (also referred to as an ABD pad or combine pad) dressings (e.g., Surgipad, Tendersorb).

The outer (securing) layer is used to secure the contact and absorbent layers in position. Several options are available for securing the dressing:

- *Tape* (e.g., paper, silk, adhesive, cloth, foam)—Some patients may be allergic to some types of tape.
- *Wrap* (e.g., elastic bandage), Ace; *adhesive crinkled gauze*, Coban; *rolled gauze*, Kling; *fluffed rolled gauze*, Kerlix—Used to secure a dressing or a splint to an extremity, provide pressure and support, conform to body contours, or secure a thoracic dressing while allowing for movement of the chest wall during respiration. The wrap may contain a self-adhesive (e.g., Velcro) or may be secured with tape. A wrap (rolled cotton sheeting, Webril) may be applied as padding under a cast. *Note:* Neurovascular damage may result if a wrap is applied too tightly.
- *Stockinette*—Used prior to splint or cast application
- *Tube gauze*—Used on a digit
- *Montgomery straps*—Used in situations that may require frequent wound inspections or dressing changes

Pressure Dressing. A pressure dressing is a type of three-layer dressing to which additional material is added to the intermediate layer or one that is tightly secured to cause compression of the surgical wound. Tissue compression influences wound-healing dynamics and may promote wound healing; however, a dressing applied too tightly may cause neurovascular compromise that will negatively influence the wound-healing process. The pressure dressing may serve one or more of the following purposes:

- Immobilization of an area
- Support
- Absorption of excessive drainage
- Even pressure distribution
- Elimination of dead space
- Reduced edema
- Reduced hematoma formation

Bulky Dressing. A bulky dressing is a type of three-layer dressing to which additional material is added to the intermediate layer. The bulky dressing is used to immobilize an area, provide additional support to the wound, and absorb excessive drainage.

Rigid Dressings. Casts and splints are examples of rigid dressings applied following a closed traumatic injury (e.g., simple fracture) or surgery to provide support and/or to prevent movement. They are made of plaster or a lightweight synthetic such as fiberglass. Some types of splints may be manufactured of molded plastic or a metal (e.g., aluminum finger splint).

A splint is applied to one side of a structure to provide support and prevent unidirectional movement. For example, a finger splint may be applied after tendon surgery to prevent flexion.

A cast encircles a body part to provide support or prevent any type of movement. A cast is applied to immobilize the bone proximal and distal to the affected area. The most widely used type of cast is the cylindrical cast that is applied to an extremity.

Other common types of cast include these:

- *Body jacket*—Extends from the axillae to the hips to immobilize the lower thoracic and lumbar vertebrae
- *Walking cast*—Cylindrical cast of the lower extremity that has a polyurethane sole or rubber heel added to allow for ambulation
- *Spica cast*—Secured to the torso to support the hip or shoulder in the desired position
- *Minerva jacket*—Extends from the head (incorporating the mandible while exposing the face) to the hips to immobilize the cervical and upper thoracic vertebrae

Because each cast is custom made, a number of other types of cast may be fashioned to suit the patient's individual situation.

Specialty Dressings. Certain types of dressings have been designed for specific applications or uses. Examples of the specialty dressings include bolster dressing, wet-to-dry dressing, wet-to-wet dressing, thyroid collar, ostomy bag, drain dressing, tracheotomy dressing, eye pads and shields, and the perineal pad:

- *Bolster dressing*—Dressing that is sutured into position. The bolster dressing may also be referred to as a "stent dressing" or a tie-over dressing. The bolster dressing is often placed over a skin graft recipient site to apply even pressure and prevent fluid from accumulating under the graft or to secure a dressing to an area that is contoured, such as the face, neck, or nose. Long sutures are placed lateral to the wound edges and the suture ends are tied over the dressing to secure it.
- *Wet-to-dry dressing*—Wet gauze (soaked in the liquid of the surgeon's choice; e.g., normal saline, antibiotic solution, Dakin's solution) is applied to the wound and allowed to dry. The dried dressing is removed along with any tissue that has adhered to the dressing. This form of mechanical wound debridement is often performed on burn wounds and may be performed under anesthesia in the OR to provide patient comfort.
- *Wet-to-wet dressing*—Wet gauze is applied to the wound and is changed before it dries. Removal of the dressing while it is still wet provides minimal wound debridement and causes the patient less pain than the wet-to-dry dressing.
- *Thyroid collar (Queen Anne's collar)*—Circumferential neck wrap applied to secure the dressing over a thyroid incision. The thyroid collar may be manufactured or fashioned from a surgical towel. Ensure that the collar is not applied too tightly.
- *Ostomy bag*—Applied over an intestinal stoma to contain excretions. The bag is attached to the patient's skin with an adhesive that is incorporated around the edges of the bag.
- *Drain dressing*—Gauze sponge that is manufactured (e.g., Sof-Wick drain sponge) or fashioned with a scissors (usually a slit or "Y" shape) to accommodate a wound that contains a drain.
- *Tracheotomy dressing*—A drain dressing is placed around a tracheotomy tube, and the tube itself is secured with wide umbilical tape that is tied around the patient's neck. Straps manufactured with Velcro fasteners are also available for this purpose.
- *Eye pad*—Oval-shaped gauze applied over the eyelid to retain medication and keep the lid closed.
- *Eye shield*—Rigid oval shield applied over the eye pad to protect the eye from pressure or trauma.
- *Perineal (peri) pad*—Used to absorb vaginal or perineal drainage (e.g., sanitary napkin). May require the use of a belt or underpants to keep in position.

Packing Material. Packing material is used to assist with hemostasis, provide pressure, support a wound, and/or eliminate dead space. Packing material may be placed in the nose, rectum, vagina, or in an open wound. Packing material is typically a long strip (e.g., 1 yard, 5 feet, 8 feet) of gauze and is available in a variety of widths (e.g., ¼, ½, or 1 in.) The gauze may be plain (e.g., NuGauze Packing Strip-Plain), impregnated with an antiseptic (e.g., NuGauze Packing Strip with Iodoform 5%), or contain a radiopaque marker.

CATHETERS, TUBES, AND DRAINS

A variety of **catheters**, tubes, and drains are available to serve many patient care functions. They are placed within surgical wounds, tubular structures, and hollow organs in order to assist with diagnosis, restore function, promote healing, or prevent complications. Typically, these are hollow, cylindrical-shaped objects that are not easily categorized. For example, a "chest tube" is used to provide drainage of the thoracic cavity; therefore, it can be considered both a tube and a drain. It is imperative that the surgical technologist learn the names and understand the functions of these devices.

Catheters

Catheters are used to remove fluid or other objects, such as thrombi and stones, from the body (Figure 10-23). They are also used to monitor body functions and for the instillation of fluids, including contrast media and medications. Soft, flexible catheters are manufactured of polyvinyl chloride, Teflon, silicone, latex, polyethylene, and polyurethane.

Urinary Catheters

Urinary catheters are typically used to drain urine, but may have other applications as well. For example, the Robinson catheter may also be used to provide irrigation fluid within a duct or is threaded through the nasal cavity into the oral cavity and used to retract the uvula when a tonsillectomy is performed. Urinary catheters are classified as urethral, **ureteral**, and suprapubic according to the method for placement, and further classified as nonretaining and self-retaining. Urinary catheters use the French scale for sizing; catheters are available as small as 5Fr. for infants and pediatric patients and up to the largest size 30Fr. Most catheter types are available in a variety of sizes. The catheter may possess one or more openings or "eyes" in the tip to allow for drainage. The procedure for insertion of a urethral catheter is described in Chapter 8.

Nonretaining catheters are temporarily inserted through the urethra into the bladder to obtain a urine specimen, decompress the bladder, or maneuver around an obstruction. Examples of the nonretaining urethral catheter include the Robinson, which has a straight, plain tip (may also be referred to as a "red rubber" or "straight cath"), and the Coudé catheter, which has a rigid curved tip. Nonretaining urethral catheters do not require the use of a drainage bag.

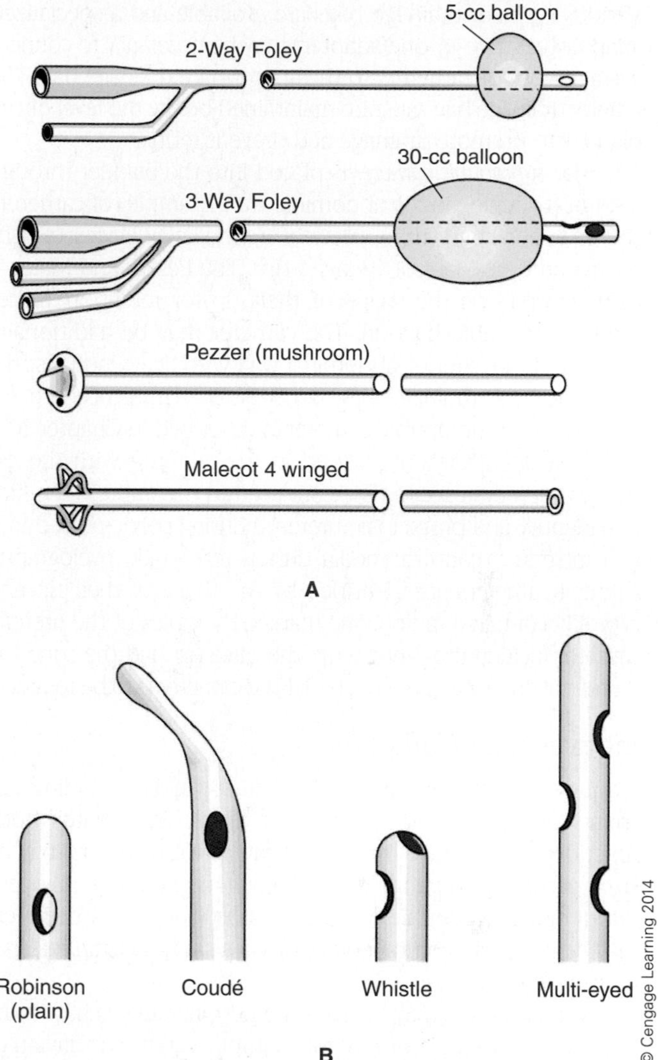

Figure 10-23 Catheter types: (A) Self-retaining, (B) nonretaining

Self-retaining or indwelling urethral catheters are called Foley catheters. *Foley catheters* are used to measure urinary output over an extended period or provide bladder decompression. The Foley catheter uses a balloon to retain the catheter within the bladder, allowing for continuous drainage of urine. The balloon may have a 5- or 30-cc capacity. A syringe is used to inflate the balloon with sterile water. Sterile water, rather than normal saline, is used for balloon inflation to prevent erosion of the balloon wall. Typically, 8–10 cc of water is placed within the syringe used to fill a 5-cc balloon to compensate for the water that remains in the catheter lumen between the syringe port and the balloon. The two-way Foley has two ports that allow for balloon inflation and drainage of urine. The three-way Foley has an additional port that allows for instillation of irrigation fluid or medications into the bladder. Some Foley catheters contain a thermometer in the tip that is used to measure the patient's core temperature. Self-retaining urinary catheters require the use of a gravity drainage bag (e.g., Urimeter).

Various types of drainage bags are available and a specialized adapter (e.g., five-in-one adapter) may be necessary to connect certain types of catheters to the appropriate drainage bag. The gravity drainage bag must be maintained below the level of the bladder to promote drainage and prevent reflux.

The *suprapubic catheter* is placed into the bladder through a surgical opening in the abdominal wall. Examples of catheters that may be placed suprapubically are the Foley, Pezzer (mushroom), and the Malecot (winged tip). The Pezzer and Malecot catheters rely on the shape of their tip for retention, rather than an inflatable balloon. The catheter may be additionally secured to the exterior abdominal wall with heavy nonabsorbable suture. A drainage bag is necessary. The procedure for insertion of a suprapubic catheter is described in Chapter 20.

Ureteral catheters are placed in the ureter(s) with the assistance of a cystoscope. They are used to decompress the kidney, identify and protect the ureter(s) during pelvic procedures, and introduce contrast media during retrograde pyelography. Ureteral catheters are identified by the shape of their tip and typically contain a radiopaque marker. Examples of the ureteral catheter include the whistle tip, the olive tip, and the cone tip. A ureteral drainage bag is needed if the catheter is to be retained.

Intravascular Catheters

Intravascular catheters are used to infuse fluids (including nutrients and medications), obtain a diagnosis, monitor body functions, and remove thrombi. Intravascular catheters may be sized according to gauge or the French method and may contain a single or double lumen. Intravascular access catheters may be inserted percutaneously or via a small incision referred to as a *cut-down*.

Venous access may be achieved peripherally, usually in the upper extremity, or centrally, for example, via the subclavian or jugular vein. The Angio-Cath is an example of a vascular catheter used to provide peripheral access, and the Groshong is one of the more common central vein catheters.

Arterial catheters may be inserted temporarily to draw arterial blood for laboratory study or may be indwelling to provide information about the patient's physiological condition (e.g., arterial blood pressure). Arterial catheters are also used to perform diagnostic studies and various procedures such as coronary artery angioplasty.

A Fogarty is a balloon-tipped catheter. The catheter is passed beyond an obstruction within the lumen of a vein, artery, or duct. The balloon is then inflated, and the catheter is withdrawn along with the obstruction (e.g., thrombus or stone). A variation of the Fogarty catheter is used for irrigation of the biliary system.

Specialty Catheters

Some of the more common types of catheters are discussed below. Keep in mind that a number of specialty catheters such as the cholangiocatheter, the Swan-Ganz catheter, and the Tenckhoff catheter are also available. The cholangiocatheter is a plastic catheter with a small lumen and a port for attaching a Luer-Lok syringe. The syringe will contain a dye such as Hypaque or Renografin. The end of the catheter is inserted into the common bile duct, dye is slowly injected, and intraoperative X-rays are taken to detect the presence of calculi.

Central venous pressure is monitored with a single-lumen or multilumen radiopaque catheter. The double- or triple-lumen Broviac or Hickman catheters are the most frequently used. The Swan-Ganz pulmonary artery catheter is also used to monitor the CVP. The catheter is inserted through the subclavian vein into the superior vena cava or right atrium under fluoroscopy. Once in place the free end of the catheter is attached to a monitor.

For intermittent or continuous peritoneal dialysis, the Tenckhoff silicone catheter is placed into the peritoneal cavity to infuse dialysis fluid into the cavity so that waste can be filtered from the blood. The catheter has one or more synthetic cuffs to hold it in place in the subcutaneous tissue layer.

Tubes

Tubes are used to remove air and fluids from the body for the purpose of decompression. Tubes are also used to maintain the patency of a lumen and for the administration of oxygen, anesthetic gases, medications, and fluids, including nutrition supplements.

Gastrointestinal Tubes

Gastrointestinal tubes are used to aspirate air and fluids from the gastrointestinal tract. The gastrointestinal tube may be passed through the nose or mouth into the stomach or intestine, through the rectum into the intestine, or may be inserted surgically. Gastrostomy (feeding) tubes are also considered gastrointestinal tubes. Many gastrointestinal tubes employ the sump design. The term *sump* refers to a dual-lumen tube in which one lumen is used for evacuation of fluid and the second allows air to enter for equalizing the pressure within the structure, reducing the risk of damage to delicate tissues by preventing constant negative pressure.

Airway Tubes

Airway tubes are used to maintain patency of the upper respiratory tract. Airway tubes include:

- *Endotracheal (ET) tube*—Available in adult and pediatric sizes as well as cuffed and uncuffed styles. The ET tube is passed through the nose or mouth, between the vocal cords, and into the trachea of the unconscious patient.
- *Oral airway*—Inserted through the mouth to separate the jaws and depress the tongue.
- *Nasal airway*—Inserted through the nose to prevent obstruction of the airway due to relaxation of the soft palate. Sometimes referred to as a nasal "trumpet" because of its shape.
- *Tracheotomy tube*—Placed directly into the trachea via an incision in the neck. The tracheotomy tube has three components: (1) outer cannula (may be cuffed, uncuffed, or fenestrated), (2) inner cannula, and (3) obturator.

Chest Tubes

Chest tubes are inserted percutaneously through a "stab" wound to treat pneumothorax or following cardiothoracic surgical procedures to evacuate air and fluid from the pleural space. If two chest tubes are inserted ipsilaterally, one is placed in the upper portion of the thoracic cavity to allow evacuation of air and the second is placed in the lower portion for evacuation of fluids. The chest tube is secured to the exterior wall of the thorax with heavy nonabsorbable suture. The chest tube is connected to a closed water-seal drainage system (Figure 10-24). Two chest tubes may be connected to the same collection device with the use of a "Y" connector. The water-seal drainage system uses water in the collection unit to prevent air from reentering the pleural space, thereby maintaining the negative pressure necessary for effective respiration. The collection unit must be maintained below the level of the thoracic cavity to promote gravity drainage and prevent reflux. Prior to connecting the water-seal drainage system to the chest tube(s), it must be prepared according to the manufacturer's instructions. It may be necessary to use an adapter to connect the chest tube to the drainage system. Suction may be applied to some types of drainage systems to facilitate evacuation of air and fluid from the thoracic cavity (Figure 10-24).

Drains

Drains are used to evacuate air and fluids from a surgical or traumatic wound. Drains function passively or actively.

Passive Drains

Passive drains allow a pathway for fluid or air to move from an area of high pressure to one of lower pressure. A passive drain may be connected to a gravity collection device or the drainage may be contained within an absorbent dressing. Examples of passive drains include:

- *Penrose drain*—Latex tubing that is placed partially within the wound, allowing fluid to move out of the wound into the dressing by **capillary action**.
- *Cigarette drain*—Penrose drain with gauze inside encourages fluid to move out of the wound into the dressing by wicking action.
- *T-tube*—Placed within the biliary system, it drains bile via gravity into a specialized collection unit called a *bile bag*.
- *Gastrostomy tube*—Inserted through the abdominal wall into the stomach; removes gastric contents or provides instillation of nourishment ("tube feeding").
- *Cystostomy tube*—Inserted through the abdominal wall into the urinary bladder; removes urine.
- *Nephrostomy tube*—Inserted percutaneously into the kidney; removes urine.

Active Drains

Active drains make use of negative pressure (Figure 10-25). Negative pressure is created by removing air from the collection device manually or mechanically. An electric or battery-operated pump or the facility's vacuum system may be used to provide mechanical evacuation. Active drains are connected to a collection device. The chest tube and water-seal drainage system is an example of an active drainage system. Additional examples include:

- *Hemovac*—Typically used following orthopedic procedures when a moderate amount of drainage is expected.
- *Jackson-Pratt*—Typically used following abdominal procedures when a moderate amount of drainage is expected. Also used in neurosurgery and other general surgery procedures such as a mammoplasty.
- *Stryker*—Typically used following orthopedic procedures. Effective in reducing dead space due to the strength of the battery-operated evacuation pump.

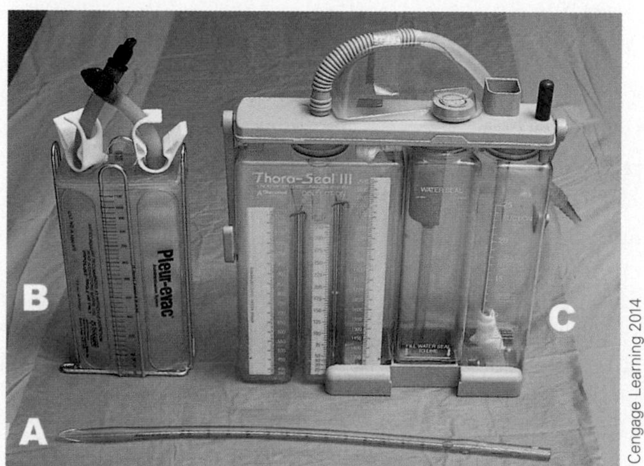

Figure 10-24 Chest drainage systems: (A) Chest tube, (B) Pleurevac auto transfusion system, (C) Thora-seal (water-seal) system

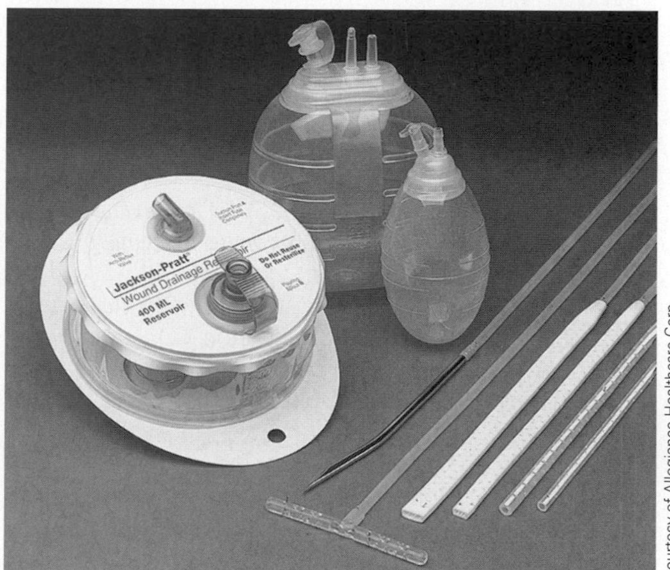

Figure 10-25 Closed-wound drainage systems

IRRIGATORS AND SYRINGES

A syringe consists of a tip that may be plain (Luer-Slip) or locking (Luer-Lok). The plain tip accepts needles that simply slip over the syringe tip. This connection is not nearly as secure as the Luer-Lok tip, which locks the needle onto the syringe tip with a twisting motion. *Syringes* may be made of plastic or glass and are used to irrigate wounds, aspirate fluids, or inject medications.

Syringes vary in size, containing from 1 to 60 cc of fluid. Syringes are calibrated in milliliters and/or cubic centimeters, while insulin syringes are calculated in units. Tuberculin syringes are calculated in tenths or hundredths of a cubic centimeter. Tuberculin syringes contain up to 1 cc of fluid. The 10-cc syringe is the most commonly used standard syringe.

The 10-cc syringe used for injecting local anesthetics may have finger and thumb holes for better control. These syringes are referred to as *three-ring* or *control* syringes.

Irrigating syringes may be bulb or bulb/barrel syringes or larger syringes with a heparin needle attached for intra-arterial irrigation. The irrigating bulb/barrel syringe for most procedures is the bulb Asepto syringe, which holds approximately 120 cc. The ear syringe does not have a barrel and is used to irrigate smaller incisions and structures such as the ear and to remove fluids from the nose and mouth of an infant.

CASE STUDY Chang is a surgical technology student in a clinical rotation. The assignment for the day is to work with the central sterile supply team preparing instruments and instrument sets for sterilization. Chang has been asked to prepare a dilatation and curettage set.

1. How will Chang know what instruments the hospital routinely places in this set?
2. What categories of instruments will be represented in this set?

QUESTIONS FOR FURTHER STUDY

1. What are the strengths and weaknesses of each type of material used for drapes?
2. Why are some instrument finishes dull or black?
3. In what situation(s) is a water-seal drainage system used?
4. What is the purpose of a Tenckhoff catheter?
5. Explain the difference between a scalpel and a knife. List one or more examples of each.

BIBLIOGRAPHY

Ansell Healthcare Products, Inc. (2006). *Understanding the relationship between surgical gloves and electrosurgery* [CE Module]. Redbank, NJ: Author.

Association of Surgical Technologists. (2011). *Core curriculum for surgical technology* (6th ed.). Littleton, CO: Author.

Deitch, E. A. (1997). *Tools of the trade and rules of the road: A surgical guide.* Philadelphia: Lippincott Williams & Wilkins.

Goldman, M. A. (2007). *Pocket guide to the operating room* (3rd ed.). Philadelphia: F. A. Davis.

Miltex, Inc. (2010). *Miltex surgical instruments.* York, PA: Author.

Phillips, N. (2007). *Berry & Kohn's operating room technique* (11th ed.). St. Louis: Mosby.

Rothrock, J. C. (2010). *Alexander's care of the patient in surgery* (14th ed.). St. Louis: Mosby.

Smith, M. F., & Stehn, J. L. (1993). *Basic surgical instrumentation.* Philadelphia: W. B. Saunders.

Stoker, R. (2008, May). Scalpel safety: Protecting patients and clinicians. *Managing Infection Control,* 24–30.

Tighe, S. M. (2007). *Instrumentation for the operating room: A photographic Manual* (7th ed.). St. Louis: Mosby.

Valleylab. (2006). *Principles of electrosurgery.* Retrieved November 16, 2006, from http://www.valleylab.com

Chapter

11

Wound Healing, Sutures, Needles, and Stapling Devices

Case Study Frances, a 63-year-old woman, has been suffering from right upper quadrant pain. Diagnostic tests have confirmed the presence of gallstones. Her physician has scheduled her for an open cholecystectomy with a common bile duct exploration. Frances also has diabetes and is obese.

1. **What is the surgical wound classification expected to be?**
2. **What considerations should be made during closure because of Frances' underlying conditions?**
3. **By what method is Frances' wound expected to heal?**

Objectives

After studying this chapter, the reader should be able to:

C 1. Indicate terms relevant to wound healing.
2. Summarize the possible complications of wound healing.
A 3. Recognize the classifications of surgical wounds.
4. Indicate and give examples of types of traumatic wounds.
5. Analyze the factors that influence healing and recognize the manner in which they affect the healing process.
R 6. Recognize the characteristics of inflammation.
7. Cite and interpret common suture terms.
8. Classify and differentiate suture materials and stapling devices and their usage.
9. Recognize the types, characteristics, and uses of natural and synthetic absorbable suture materials.
10. Compare and recognize the common natural and synthetic nonabsorbable sutures, stating their sources, common trade names, and uses.
11. Demonstrate application of recommended preparation and handling techniques for suturing and stapling devices and provide rationale for choice.
12. Cite and interpret common suture techniques.
13. Summarize the basic uses and advantages of stapling instruments.

14. Distinguish, describe the use of, and demonstrate proper handling of the various types of surgical needles.
15. Assess the types of injuries that cause damage to tissues.
16. Recognize the characteristics of the types of healing.
17. Recognize the stages/phases of wound healing.

Select Key Terms

Adhesion	Dehiscence	inflammation	second intention
anastomosis	Evisceration	laceration	secondary suture line
approximated	first intention	ligated	swaged
Chromic gut	French-eyed needle	monofilament	tensile strength
Chronic wounds	friable	packing	third intention
cicatrix	herniation	primary suture line	vessel loops
dead space	immunosuppressed patient	PTFE	
debridement			

INTRODUCTION

The surgical technologist must have an understanding of the various types of wounds—surgical (intentional) and traumatic (accidental)—and the processes involved in tissue repair and wound healing. Incision choice, tissue-handling techniques, wound closure options, and possible complications all influence wound healing. Ideal wound healing involves restoration of continuity, strength, function, and appearance to the tissue.

TYPES OF WOUNDS

The word *wound* is described as any tissue that has been damaged by surgical or traumatic means.

Surgical Wounds

Surgical wounds are incisional or excisional. An *incision* is an intentional cut through intact tissue for the purpose of exposing underlying structures. Once an incision is made the surgeon may perform an excision, such as a splenectomy (removal of the spleen) or hemicolectomy (removal of a portion of the colon).

Classification of Surgical Wounds

Surgical wounds are classified into four categories according to the degree of microbial contamination and are referred to in the patient record by Roman numeral (Table 11-1). The Centers for Disease Control and Prevention (CDC) wound classification categories are as follows:

Class I: Clean

- Incision made under ideal surgical conditions
- No break in sterile technique during procedure
- Primary closure
- No inflammation is encountered
- Closed wound drainage device if necessary
- No entry to aerodigestive or genitourinary tract

Class II: Clean Contaminated

- Primary closure
- Open/mechanical drainage
- Minor break in sterile technique occurred
- Controlled entry to aerodigestive (includes biliary tract) or genitourinary tract

Class III: Contaminated

- Open traumatic wound (less than 4 hours old) with retained necrotic tissue
- Major break in sterile technique occurred
- Acute **inflammation** present
- Entry to aerodigestive (includes biliary tract) or genitourinary tract with spillage

Class IV: Dirty/Infected

- Open traumatic wound (more than 4 hours old)

TABLE 11-1 Wound Classification

Classification	*Definition*	*Examples*
Clean (Class I)	Uninfected, uninflamed operative wound in which the respiratory, alimentary, genital, or uninfected urinary tracts are not entered	Coronary artery bypass graft, total hip, breast biopsy, craniotomy
Clean contaminated (Class II)	Uninfected operative wound; respiratory, alimentary, genital, or urinary tract is entered under controlled circumstances without unusual contamination	Appendectomy, cholecystectomy, tonsillectomy
Contaminated (Class III)	Acute, nonpurulent, inflamed operative wound or open, fresh wound, or any surgical procedure with major breaks in sterile technique or gross spillage from the gastrointestinal (GI) tract	Open fracture, colon resection with gross spillage of GI contents, penetrating trauma
Dirty (Class IV)	Clinically infected operative wound or perforated viscera or old, traumatic wounds with retained necrotic tissue	Resection of ruptured appendix

- Microbial contamination prior to procedure
- Perforated viscus

Surgical wound classification is subject to change during the procedure according to the situation. The final wound classification is assigned at the end of the procedure and is included in the intraoperative documentation.

Traumatic Wounds

Traumatic wounds are classified in several different ways according to severity. A single wound may fall into more that one category. The classifications are:

- *Closed wound:* The skin remains intact, but underlying tissues suffer damage.
- Open wound: The integrity of the skin is damaged.
  - Simple wound: The integrity of the skin is compromised. There is no loss or destruction of tissue and there is no foreign body in the wound.
  - Complicated wound: Tissue is lost or destroyed, or a foreign body remains in the wound.
  - Clean wound: Wound edges can be **approximated** and secured. A clean wound is expected to heal by **first intention**.
  - Contaminated wound: Contamination occurs when a dirty object damages the integrity of the skin. A contaminated wound can become infected within a short period of time. **Debridement** of infected and/or necrosed tissue may be necessary, followed by thorough irrigation of the wound to further clean and wash out the contaminants, a procedure commonly referred to as an irrigation and debridement (I and D).

Another method of classifying traumatic wounds is by the mechanism of injury. Some examples are:

- *Abrasion:* Scrape
- *Contusion:* Bruise
- ***Laceration***: Cut or tear
- *Puncture:* Penetration
- *Thermal:* Heat or cold (can be chemical)

Chronic Wounds

Chronic wounds are those that persist for an extended period of time. A chronic wound may develop because of an underlying physical condition that the patient suffers, for example, from pressure sores and decubitus ulcers. A chronic wound may also be due to infection.

INFLAMMATORY PROCESS

Inflammation is the body's protective response to injury or tissue destruction. The inflammatory process serves to destroy, dilute, or wall off the injured tissue. The classic signs of inflammation are:

- Pain
- Heat
- Redness
- Swelling
- Loss of function

An inflammatory reaction occurs when injured tissues release histamine from the damaged cells. The histamine causes the small blood vessels in the area to dilate, increasing the blood flow to the area, resulting in heat, redness, and swelling.

TYPES OF WOUND HEALING

Three types of wound healing are identified. They are listed as first intention (primary union), **second intention** (granulation), and **third intention** (delayed primary closure).

The type of wound healing will be determined by the type and condition of the tissue.

First Intention (Primary Union)

First intention healing occurs with a primary union that is typical of an incision opened under ideal conditions. Healing occurs from side to side in a sterile wound in which **dead space** has been eliminated and the wound edges have been accurately approximated. Wounds heal rapidly with no separation of the edges and minimal scarring. Wound **tensile strength** plateaus at the third month at 70–80% of original strength. Healing by first intention occurs in three distinct phases (Figure 11-1).

Phases of Wound Healing by First Intention

Phase 1: Lag Phase or Inflammatory Response Phase

This stage begins within minutes of injury and lasts approximately 3–5 days. It is defined by the physiological changes associated with inflammation manifested as heat, redness, swelling, pain, and loss of function. The warmth and redness associated with inflammation are a result of the arterial dilatation that increases blood flow to the area. This stage of repair controls bleeding through platelet aggregation, delivers blood to the injured site through vessel dilation, and forms epithelial cells for repair. A scab forms on the surface to seal the wound, preventing serous leakage and microbial invasion. Increased capillary permeability triggered by chemicals released by injured cells permits leakage of protein-rich fluid into the extravascular fluid compartment, resulting in edema and localized pain.

Leukocytes move to the endothelial lining of the small vessels within hours after the injury, eventually moving through the endothelial spaces outside of the vessels. Once in the extravascular space, they are drawn to the site of the injury. The neutrophils and macrophages begin to neutralize foreign particles by phagocytosis.

Basal cells migrate across the skin edges, closing the surface of the wound. Fibroblasts in the deeper tissue begin the reconstruction of the nonepithelial tissue. The wound does not gain tensile strength during this phase.

Phase 2: Proliferation Phase

This stage begins on approximately the 3rd postoperative day and continues for up to 20 days. Fibroblasts multiply and bridge the wound edges. The fibroblasts secrete collagen that forms into fibers that give the wound approximately 25–30% of its original tensile strength. New networks are formed from existing capillaries by the 5th to 8th day and lymphatic networks are reformed by the 10th day, many of which diminish during the final phase of wound healing.

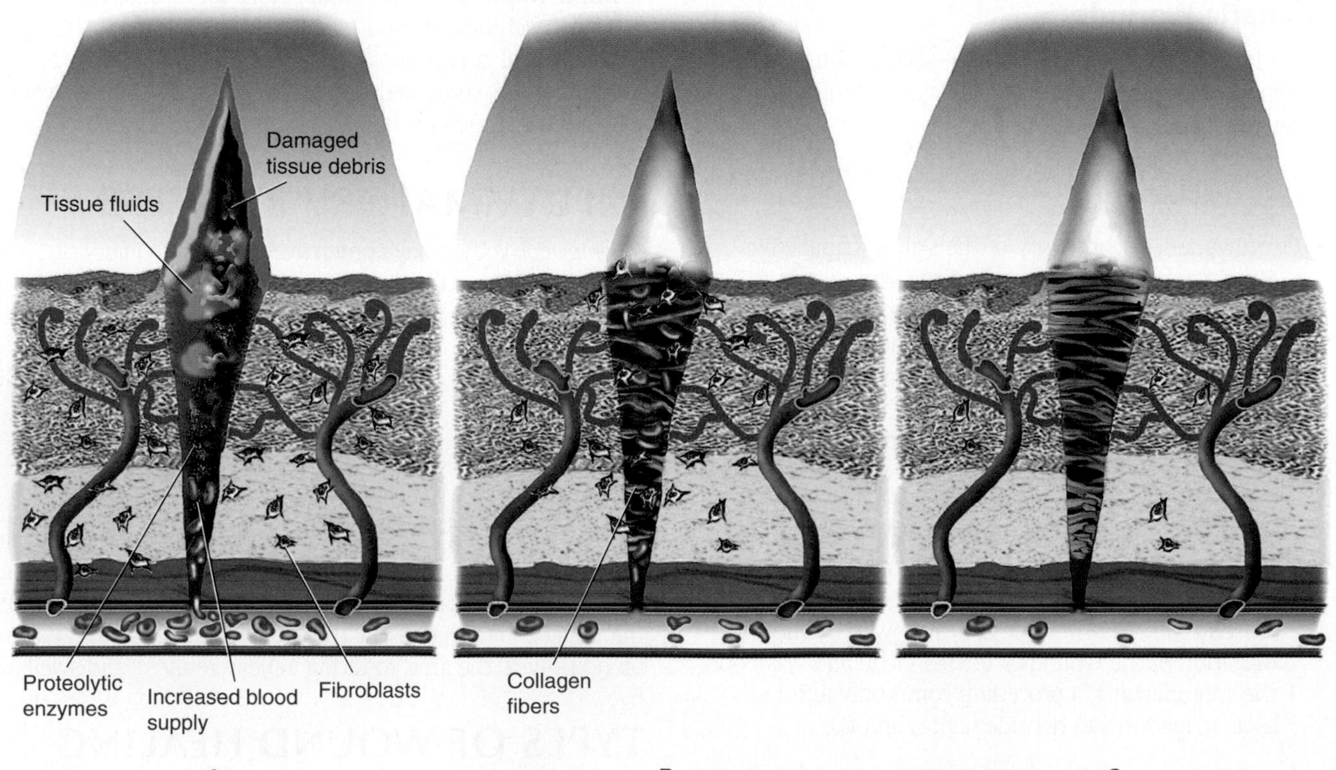

Figure 11-1 Tissue response to injury: (A) Phase 1, inflammatory response and debridement process, (B) Phase 2, collagen formation (scar tissue), (C) Phase 3, sufficient collagen laid down

Phase 3: Maturation or Differentiation Phase

This stage begins on the 14th postoperative day and lasts until the wound is completely healed (up to 12 months). During this phase, the wound undergoes a slow, sustained increase in tissue tensile strength with an interweaving of the collagen fibers. Wound contraction resulting from the work of dermal and subcutaneous myofibroblasts is completed in approximately 21 days. Collagen density increases and formation of new blood vessels decreases, causing the scar tissue to pale. A small, white, mature surface scar, called a **cicatrix**, appears during the maturation phase.

Second Intention (Granulation)

Second intention healing occurs when a wound fails to heal by primary union. It generally occurs in large wounds that cannot be directly approximated or in which infection has caused breakdown of a sutured wound. It also occurs in a wound in which primary wound closure would result in infection. Second intention healing may be allowed following the removal of necrotic tissue or after a wide debridement. The wound is left open and allowed to heal from the inner layer to the outside surface. Granulation tissue that contains myofibroblasts forms in the wound, causing closure by contraction.

As the wound heals, large gaps in tissue fill, from the bottom upward, with granulation tissue, leaving a weak union and a wide, irregular scar that may result in **herniation**. Excessive granulation tissue, sometimes referred to as "proud flesh," may protrude above the defect margins and block re-epithelialization.

Third Intention (Delayed Primary Closure)

Third intention healing, or delayed primary closure, occurs when two granulated surfaces are approximated. The traumatic (Class III or Class IV) surgical wound is debrided and purposely left open to heal by second intention (granulation) for approximately 4 to 6 days. The patient may be treated with systemic antibiotics and special wound care techniques may be used to treat or prevent infection, such as packing the wound with antibiotic-impregnated fine mesh gauze. The infection-free wound is then closed and allowed to finish the healing process through first intention (primary closure). The result is a wound that heals by contraction, granulation, and connective tissue repair with intermediate tensile strength and scarring. This method of repair works well for contaminated or dirty wounds.

FACTORS INFLUENCING WOUND HEALING

Three main factors influence the rate at which wound healing occurs, the strength of the healed wound, and the risk of infection.

The first consideration is the physical condition of the patient, which includes:

- *Age:* Pediatric and geriatric patients may have decreased vascularity or poor muscle tone.
- *Nutritional status:* Dietary deficiencies can alter the healing process.
- *Obesity:* The weight and pressure of adipose tissue may make it difficult to achieve a secure wound closure and contribute to incisional hernia. Adipose tissue also has a poor blood supply contributing to slow healing.
- *Disease (chronic or acute):* Metabolic disease, cardiovascular or respiratory insufficiency, malignancy, and infection all negatively impact wound healing.
- *Smoking:* Smoking causes vasoconstriction, diminishes oxygenation, and causes coughing that can put stress on a healing wound.
- *Radiation exposure:* Patients undergoing radiation treatment in large doses may experience a decrease in blood supply to the irradiated tissue.
- *Immunocompromised or* **immunosuppressed patients**: The patient's immune system may be deficient due to congenital or acquired conditions.

The second consideration is intraoperative tissue handling, which includes:

- Length and direction of the incision
- Dissection technique (sharp or blunt)
- Duration of surgery
- Amount of tissue handling (tissue should be handled as little and as gently as possible)
- Achievement of hemostasis
- Precise tissue approximation
- Elimination of dead space
- Secure wound closure

The third consideration is the application of the principles of asepsis through the use of sterile technique:

- Any microbial contamination of the wound could lead to an infection, causing an increase in morbidity or mortality.

COMPLICATIONS OF WOUND HEALING

Tissue disruption, whether intentional or accidental, leaves the patient vulnerable to infection and other complications. Meticulous application of sterile technique alone will not ensure that the patient will remain complication free. Many factors influence wound healing:

- ***Dehiscence***: Dehiscence is the partial or total separation of a layer or layers of tissue after closure. Dehiscence frequently occurs between the 5th and 10th postoperative day and is seen most often in debilitated patients with **friable** (easily torn) tissue. However, dehiscence can also be caused by abdominal distention, too much tension on the wound, inappropriate type or strength of suture material, or improper suturing technique. The patient often reports a "popping" or tearing sensation associated with coughing, vomiting, or straining. Dehiscence can result in retrograde infection (infection that travels backwards or inwards into the abdominal cavity), peritonitis, or evisceration if an abdominal incision is involved. Surgery may be required to correct the defect, depending on the severity of the separation. Table 11-2 lists factors in preventing dehiscence.

- ***Evisceration***: Evisceration is protrusion of the viscera through the edges of a totally separated wound. Evisceration is an emergency situation that requires immediate surgical intervention to replace the viscera and close the wound.
- *Hemorrhage:* Hemorrhage may be concealed or evident and occurs most frequently in the first few postoperative hours. Hemorrhage can result in postoperative shock. Surgery is frequently required to achieve hemostasis.
- *Infection:* Infection of a wound occurs when microbial contamination overrides the resistance of the host. It results in increased morbidity and mortality. In addition to antibiotic therapy, additional surgery may be required as part of the treatment regimen. Table 11-3 lists factors in preventing infection.
- ***Adhesion***: An adhesion is an abnormal attachment of two surfaces or structures that are normally separate. Fibrous tissue can develop within the peritoneal cavity because of previous surgery, infection, improper tissue handling, or the presence of a foreign body (lint or glove powder granule). The fibrous tissue that develops can cause abnormal attachments of the abdominal viscera that may cause pain and/or bowel obstruction.
- *Herniation:* Herniation is a result of wound dehiscence and occurs most often in lower abdominal incisions. A hernia is usually discovered 2–3 months postoperatively and could result in bowel incarceration. Surgery may be required to correct this condition.
- *Fistula:* A fistula is an abnormal tract between two epithelium-lined surfaces that is open at both ends. It occurs most often after bladder, bowel, and pelvic procedures. Abnormal drainage is a prevalent sign. Surgery is required for correction.

Table 11-2 Factors in Preventing Dehiscence

Factor	*Response*
Long paramedian incisions	Avoid when possible. Provide careful closure.
Adequacy of closure	Provide careful closure. Use interrupted, nonabsorbable suture on fascia.
Intra-abdominal pressure	Use special closing techniques. Use interrupted, nonabsorbable suture on fascia. Use retention suture; secondary suture line.
Deficient wound healing	Provide for local tissue perfusion. Treat systemic problems. Use interrupted, nonabsorbable suture on fascia. Use retention suture.
Infection (already present)	Use scrupulous sterile technique. Irrigate wound (antibiotic solution may be used). Close dead spaces. Leave wound open to heal by second intention when necessary. Use monofilament suture.

Table 11-3 Factors in Preventing Infection

Factor	*Response*
Degree of contamination	Use scrupulous sterile technique. Irrigate wound. Close dead spaces. Leave wound open to heal by second intention if necessary.
Virulence of organism	Respond proactively to probable infective agents.
Amount of nonviable tissue	Debride nonviable tissue. Handle tissue carefully.
Adequacy of local blood supply	Use hemostatic agents cautiously.
Presence of dead space	Close all dead spaces or leave open for healing by second intention or delayed primary closure. Drain wound appropriately.
Presence of coagulated blood	Irrigate wound. Drain wound appropriately.
Presence of excessive suture	Use proper suturing technique. Use monofilament suture.
Presence of undrained serum	Drain wound appropriately. Leave wound open.
Presence of foreign material	Remove gross material. Irrigate wound, if possible, with use of antibiotic solution.

- *Sinus tract:* A sinus is an abnormal tract between two epithelium-lined surfaces that is open at one end only. Its occurrence is highest in bladder, bowel, and pelvic procedures. Abnormal drainage is a common sign. Surgery is often required to correct this condition.
- *Suture complications:* Suture complications occur because of either a failure to properly absorb the suture material or an irritation caused by the suture that results in inflammation. It occurs most frequently with silk and is characterized by an evisceration (referred to as "spitting") of the suture material from the wound or sinus tract formation.
- *Keloid scar:* Keloid formation is a hypertrophic scar formation and occurs most frequently in dark-skinned individuals. Corticoid injections and use of pressure dressings can help reduce the size of the scar, but plastic surgery may be required for correction.
- *Dead space:* Separation of wound layers that have not been closely approximated or air that has become trapped between tissue layers (Figure 11-2). The space may allow for serum or blood to collect and provide a medium for microbial growth, resulting in a wound infection. Dead space is eliminated by use of proper suturing techniques, wound drains, and/or pressure dressings.

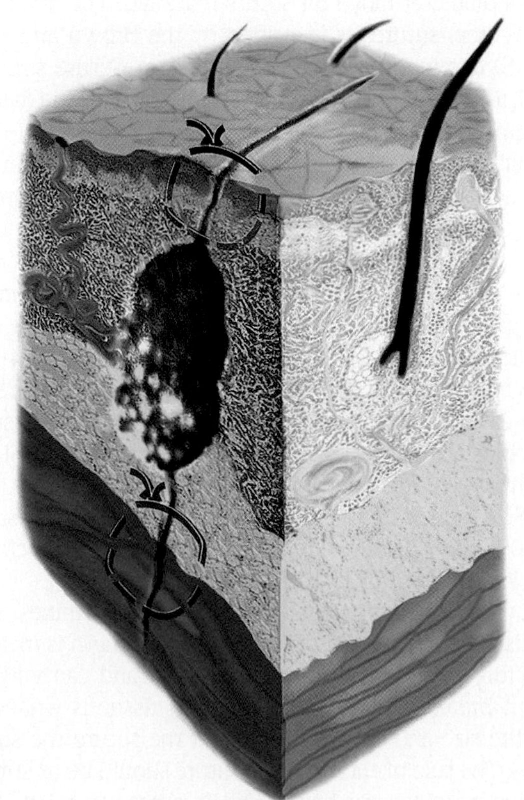

Figure 11-2 Dead space in a wound

POSTOPERATIVE WOUND CARE

The goal of postoperative wound care is prevention of infection and other complications. Postoperative wound care may include the use of drains and protection of the wound with different types of dressings.

Wound Drains

Drains are devices that have been designed to remove unwanted fluids or gases from the body. Drainage can occur preoperatively, intraoperatively, and postoperatively. Not every drain is necessarily a "wound" drain. A patient may need more than one type of drainage system as part of the postoperative care. Refer to Chapter 10 for a complete description of the types of drains and how they work.

Dressings

Dressings are an important part of postoperative wound care and the surgical technologist should be familiar with the types of dressings (refer to Chapter 10) and the uses for each. This knowledge should include proper application using sterile technique and awareness of potential complications. The type of dressing applied varies with the type of procedure, specialty, surgeon preference, and patient status.

Dressings are applied using sterile technique in the OR as the final step of the procedure. The purpose of the dressing is to provide an optimal physiological environment to promote wound healing. If a dressing must be changed within 48 hours of initial application, or if the wound is open, sterile technique and Standard Precautions must be employed. Dressings are removed or changed if they become wet or soiled or if the patient shows signs of infection. They are generally removed after 48 hours for closed nonchronic wounds. Stomas or areas affected by incontinence may require the use of special products to provide safe drainage, such as a stoma bag.

For a contaminated wound the skin and subcutaneous tissues are generally left open and packed loosely with fine mesh gauze, such as Iodoform. **Packing** is removed after 4–5 days and, if no infection is present, the wound may be closed at that time. If the wound is still infected, it is allowed to heal by second intention. For this type of healing the wound should be repacked twice daily with wet-to-dry dressings (refer to Chapter 10 for a description of this type of dressing).

Sutures

The surgical technologist is knowledgeable about sutures and basic suturing techniques. The surgical technologist should be aware of the factors that directly affect suture choice and technique. The surgeon selects the best suture for the particular task and patient plus the wound closure technique that provides optimal patient recovery. Factors that influence the choice of suture and technique include the health of the patient and whether preexisting conditions, such as diabetes, are present that can affect the wound-healing process.

The surgical technologist should acquire the same understanding and knowledge of suture as the surgeon.

Types of Suture Material

Suture material may be classified as *absorbable*, meaning it is capable of being absorbed by tissue within a given period of time, or *nonabsorbable*, meaning that it resists enzymatic digestion or absorption by tissue. Suture material can also be classified as **monofilament**, made of a single thread-like structure, or *multifilament*, consisting of multiple thread-like structures braided or twisted into a single strand.

Sutures are designed to support healing tissues as well as hold tissue edges together until they heal. Sutures should have a certain amount of elasticity to accommodate tissue swelling and strains placed on the wound by coughing or body movements. With the exception of some inert suture materials such as surgical steel, sutures are treated as foreign material by the body and the longer they dwell within tissues, the more likely the tissues will react negatively and impair the healing process. Ideally, the absorbable sutures should be completely absorbed by the time the tissue no longer requires them for stability. Therefore, suture absorption time should closely coincide with the time that it takes the tissue to heal.

Monofilament sutures are relatively inert and do not readily harbor bacteria. They glide through tissues more easily than multifilament sutures, resulting in minimal tissue damage because they encounter little resistance within the tissue. Monofilament sutures, however, do not hold knots as well as multifilament sutures and are relatively difficult to handle.

Multifilament sutures exhibit a characteristic called *capillarity*, which is the capability to harbor bacteria and retain tissue fluids that can be communicated along the length of the strand. For this reason, multifilament sutures should not be used in the presence of infection. Multifilament sutures handle well and hold knots securely. Their multistrand configuration affords them greater tensile strength, pliability, and flexibility. Many brands are coated for enhanced handling capability and easier passage through tissues.

Suture material may be natural, meaning that it is made from naturally occurring substances, such as cellulose, an animal product, or tissue; or synthetic, consisting of polymers from petroleum-based products. Natural absorbable sutures are digested by body enzymes that attack the suture strand, eventually destroying it. Synthetic absorbable sutures are hydrolyzed by the body. Water within the tissue penetrates the strand and breaks down the synthetic fiber's polymer chain, resulting in minimal tissue reaction.

Suture Sizes and Tensile Strength

Size indicates the diameter of the suture material. The suture diameter is referred to as the *gauge* of the suture. The surgeon will try to use the smallest-diameter suture that will support the tissue wound closure. This serves two purposes: (1) minimizes tissue trauma as the suture passes through tissues; (2) contributes to minimizing the amount of foreign material implanted in the body. The United States Pharmacopeia (USP) specifies diameter range for suture materials. The diameter of stainless steel sutures is identified by the Brown and Sharpe (B and S) commercial wire gauge numbers. Suture size is numerical; as the number of 0's increase, the smaller the diameter. For example, 3-0 or 000 is smaller in diameter than 1-0 or 0. The smaller the size, the less tensile strength of the suture. The largest available suture for use in surgery is #5; it is approximately the size of commercial string. The progression downward in size is listed in Table 11-4.

TABLE 11-4 Comparison of Suture Gauges

USP	*B and S*	*Metric*
#5	20 g	7
#4	22 g	6
#3	23 g	6
#2	24 g	5
#1	25 g	4
0	26 g	3.5
2-0	28 g	3
3-0	30 g	2
4-0	32 g	1.5
5-0	35 g	1
6-0	40 g	0.7
7-0		
8-0		
9-0		
10-0		
11-0 (smallest)		

USP suture sizes #1 through 4-0 are the most commonly used. Sizes #1 and #0 are used frequently for closure of orthopedic wounds and abdominal fascia. Suture sizes 4-0 and 5-0 are typically used for aortic **anastomosis**, whereas suture sizes 6-0 through 7-0 are used for smaller vessel anastomoses, such as those on the coronary or carotid arteries. Size 8-0 through 11-0 sutures are used for microvascular and eye procedures. Size 4-0 sutures are used to close dural incisions; size 3-0 and 4-0 sutures are used for most subcuticular skin closures. Suture lengths range 5 in. to 59 in.

However, an important factor that determines suture choice is *knot tensile strength*. Knot tensile strength is measured by the force in pounds that the suture strand can withstand before it breaks. The tensile strength of tissue is what determines the size and tensile strength of the suture the surgeon chooses. The rule of thumb is the suture should be as strong as the tissue on which it is being used; in other words, the suture tensile strength should equal the tissue tensile strength.

General Factors Affecting Choice of Suture

Factors that must be considered when choosing suture material are the type of procedure, the condition of the patient's tissue, the nature of the disease process, the surgeon's preference, suture availability, and cost. The choice of suture is often a matter of opinion. The surgeon typically sticks to what he or she learned during surgical training.

The surgeon must decide what size suture to use for each particular type of tissue encountered and if the suture should be monofilament or multifilament, absorbable or nonabsorbable.

Absorbable sutures are often the first choice for tissue that does not need continued support. Nonabsorbable sutures are used where continued strength is necessary, for instance, to close abnormal openings in the heart. They are typically used to close the dura over the brain or spinal cord and for fascia and skin closure; for example, silk sutures are commonly used for ligating vessels. Absorbable sutures may be used for fascia and nonabsorbable sutures used for the mucosal layer of the intestine and skin; however, as with many instances in surgery, surgeon's preference will always dictate the suture to be used during a procedure.

The condition of the patient's tissue is an important factor in suture choice. Not all tissues are alike. Some tissues are stronger than others and some heal faster. Fascia and skin are strong but heal slowly. Gastrointestinal tissue is relatively weak but heals quickly. The normal strength and healing characteristics of a tissue are modified by the condition of that tissue in each patient. Some factors modifying the normal condition of tissue are as follows:

- Age of the patient
- Weight of the patient
- Metabolic factors
- Carbohydrates
- Proteins
- Vitamins
- Dehydration
- Vascularization
- Thickness of tissue at a given time
- Edema or induration (hardening and thickening of tissue)
- Incision relative to fiber direction
- Amount of devitalized tissue within wound
- Radiation therapy

The nature of the disease process is also important to consider in suture choice because disease affects the patient's metabolic processes, which in turn modify the condition of the tissues as noted above. Wound healing and suture selection are affected by these factors. Some individual disease processes affecting suture choice that the surgical technologist should be aware of are:

- Diabetes mellitus
- Immune system diseases
- Pituitary gland dysfunction
- Localized infection
- Systemic infection

Characteristics of Common Sutures

Suture materials have distinguishing characteristics that can be compared. Physical characteristics include configuration, capillarity, ability to absorb fluid, size (diameter), tensile strength, knot strength, elasticity, and memory. Sutures may vary in pliability, how easily they pass through tissue, how easily they tie, and knot security. Each suture has a certain predictable effect on the tissue in which it is used. Table 11-5 provides the key information the surgical technologist should remember.

PACKAGING OF SUTURE

Suture dispenser boxes contain one to three dozen suture packets and provide clear product identification through color coding, bold graphics, and descriptive symbols. The most important information that the surgical technologist should learn to look for on the box is suture size and material and the type and size of needle. Other important information displayed on the suture box includes:

- Surgical application
- Product code number
- Suture length and color
- Metric diameter equivalent of suture size and length
- Shape and quantity of needles (shown in silhouette)
- Needle point geometry
- Lot number
- Expiration date, if necessary

The primary suture packet is color coded and identifies the product code, number, material, size (USP and metric), and needle type and number. A suture strand with only one needle is represented by a single, actual-sized needle silhouette on the packet. A double-armed (two-needle) suture is represented by two needle silhouettes. Any needle number greater than 2 is represented by a single needle silhouette and the number of needles is written in red. Rapid release needles, also referred to as controlled release (CR), are designed to "pop off" the suture strand after a single suture has been placed.

The primary suture packet is sterile and contained within an outer wrapper similar to a peel pack. The contents of the wrap are sterile; however, the outside of the package is not.

LIGATURES

Ligatures, also referred to as *ties*, are used to occlude vessels for hemorrhage control or for organ or extremity removal. For example, the occlusion of the femoral artery is necessary to

TABLE 11-5 Sutures

Suture Name	Absorption Rate	Tensile Strength	Tissue Reaction	Coating	General Usage	Suture Color	Other Information
Absorbable Natural Monofilament							
Plain gut: Collagen from serosa of beef intestine or submucosa of sheep intestine	• Enzymatic digestive process • Complete within 70 days	Maintained 7–10 days	Moderate	None	• Ligating superficial blood vessels • Subcutaneous	Yellow	• Not used on tissues under stress • Not for use in CV and neurology • Packaged in alcohol; avoid opening near surgical wound
Chromic gut	Complete within 90 days	Maintained 10–14 days	Moderate, but less than plain gut	None	Same as plain gut	Beige/tan	• Plain gut treated with chromium salt solution to prolong absorption rate • Not used on tissues under stress; CV or neurology • Packaged in alcohol
Absorbable Synthetic Monofilament							
Polydioxanone (PDS II): Polyester polymer	• Slow hydrolysis • Minimal until 90th day • Complete within 6 mo	• 70% at 2 weeks • 50% at 4 weeks • 25% at 6 weeks	Minimal reaction	None	All types of soft tissue approximation, including orthopedics, gynecology, eye, plastic, digestive, and pediatric CV	Clear, blue, violet	• Not for use on neural and adult CV tissue; microsurgery • Should not be used with prosthetic devices, e.g., heart valves • Exhibits low affinity for microbes • Good pliability • Little memory
PDS Plus Antibacterial	• Hydrolysis • 183–238 days	• 60–80% at 2 weeks • 40–70% at 4 weeks • 35–60% at 6 weeks	Minimal reaction	None	Same as PDSII, except no contact with cornea and sclera	Undyed, violet	• Chemical impregnated in suture kills bacteria and inhibits colonization of suture • Same information as PDS II

poliglecaprone *25 (Monocryl):* Copolymer of glycolide and epsilon-caprolactone	• Hydrolysis • 91–119 days	• Undyed: All strength lost by 21 days • Dyed: All strength lost by 28 days	Minimal reaction	None	Soft tissue approximation and/or ligation	Undyed, violet	• Undyed: Should not be used on fascia • Should not be used on neural, CV, eye tissues; microsurgical • Good knot security • Good pliability
Monocryl Plus Antibacterial	• Hydrolysis • 91–119 days	Wound support for about 14 days	Minimal reaction	None	Same as Monocryl	Undyed, violet	• Chemical impregnated in suture kills bacteria and inhibits colonization of suture • Same as Monocryl
Polyglyconate (Maxon): copolymer of glycolic acid and trimethylene carbonate	• Hydrolysis • Complete within 6 mo	• 75% at 2 weeks • 65% at 3 weeks • 50% at 4 weeks	Minimal reaction	None	Soft tissue approximation; pediatric CV tissue; PV tissue	Undyed, green	Should not be used on adult CV, eye, neural tissues, or microsurgical
Biosyn by Syneture: synthetic polyester consists of glycolide, dioxanone, trimethylene	• Hydrolysis • 90–110 days	• 75% at 2 weeks • 40% at 3 weeks	Minimal reaction	None	Soft tissue approximation and ligation; eye surgery	Undyed, violet	• Good knot security • Minimal memory • Gradual encapsulation by fibrous connective tissue • Not for use in CV and neurologic surgery
Caprosyn by Syneture: polyglytone 621	• Hydrolysis • 56 days	• 50–60% at 5 days • 20–30% at 10 days • None by 21 days	Minimal reaction	None	Soft tissue approximation and ligation	Undyed, violet	• Good knot security • Rapid absorption • Not for use in eye, CV, neurourgery; microsurgery
Absorbable Synthetic Multifilament							
Polyglactin 910 (Vicryl): copolymer of glycolide and lactic acid	• Hydrolysis • Minimal for 40 days • Complete in about 50–60 days	• 6-0 and larger: 75% at 2 weeks; 50% at 3 weeks • 7-0 and smaller: 40% at 3 weeks	Minimal reaction	See below	Tissue that requires long-term tensile strength, but absorbable suture desired; soft tissue approximation and/or ligation	Violet	• Uncoated monofilament available for use in eye surgery • Good knot security • No memory

(continues)

Table 11-5 (continued)

Suture Name	Absorption Rate	Tensile Strength	Tissue Reaction	Coating	General Usage	Suture Color	Other Information
Polyglactin 910, coated (Coated Vicryl): copolymer of glycolide and lactic acid	• Hydrolysis • Minimal for 40 days • Complete between 56 and 70 days including coating	• 75% at 2 weeks • 6-0 and larger: 50% at 3 weeks • 7-0 and smaller: 40% at 3 weeks	Minimal reaction	Yes; polyglactin 370 and calcium stearate; absorbable, adherent, nonflaking lubricant	• Soft tissue approximation and/or ligation • Eye procedures	Undyed, violet	• Also available in monofilament • Can be used in presence of infection • Should not be used on CV and neural tissues • Conjunctival sutures should be removed within 7 days to avoid local irritation
Vicryl Plus Suture	• Hydrolysis • 56–70 days	Wound support for about 4 weeks	Minimal reaction	Yes	Same as Vicryl, except not for use in eye, CV, and neurologic surgery	Undyed, violet	• Same as Vicryl • Braided
Polyglycolic acid (Dexon): homopolymer of glycolic acid	Complete within 30 days	50% at 21 days	Minimal reaction	Coated and uncoated available	• Tissues that require long-term tensile strength, but absorbable suture desired • General soft tissue approximation and/or ligation, including eyes	Beige, green	• Available monofilament and braided • Braided not for use in CV and neural tissue
Polysorb by Syneture: copolymer of glycolide and lactide	• Hydrolysis • 56–70 days	• 80% at 2 weeks • 30% at 3 weeks	Minimal reaction	Yes; mixture of caprolactone/glycolide copolymer and calcium stearoyl lactylate	• Soft tissue approximation and ligation • Eye surgery	Undyed, violet	• Braided • Good knot security • Gradual encapsulation by fibrous connective tissue • Not for use in CV and neurologic surgery
Nonabsorbable Synthetic Monofilament							
Nylon (Ethilon by Ethicon; Dermalon and Monosof by Syneture): synthetic fiber polyamide polymer of coal, air, water	Nonabsorbable	Degrades at rate of 15–20% per year	Minimal reaction	None	General soft tissue approximation and/or ligation, including eye, CV, and neural tissues; microsurgery	Undyed, black, blue, green	• Very low tissue reactivity—inert • "Memory" of suture strand requires more throws in the knot • More pliable and easier to handle when damp • Gradual encapsulation by fibrous connective tissue

Supramid (nylon) by S.Jackson, Inc.	Nonabsorbable	Good tensile strength	Minimal reacation	None	• Soft tissue approximation • Skin suture • Plastic surgery	Undyed, black	• Good knot security • Good handling qualities • *Supramid Extra:* cable-type suture made of many fine inner nylon fibers enclosed in smooth nylon outer shell
Polybutester (Novafil): copolymers glycol and butylene	Nonabsorbable	Excellent	Minimal reaction	None	Tissue that requires long-term tensile strength; running subcutaneous closure; blood vessel anastomosis	Undyed, blue	Has the greatest ability to stretch in response to a given load
Polypropylene (Prolene): synthetic fiber from polymerized propylene	Nonabsorbable	Excellent	Least reactive of all synthetic materials	None	• Frequently used in general, orthopedic, plastic, CV, and neurologic surgery • Suture of choice for vascular anastomosis	Clear, Blue	• Especially useful in contaminated wounds and in presence of infection • Does not adhere to tissues; advantage as a pull-out suture • Commonly used as mesh for tissue reinforcement (herniorraphy)
Polytetrafluoro-ethylene	Nonabsorbable	Excellent	Minimal reaction	None	Soft tissue approximation; bone grafting; soft tissue implants; plastic surgery	White	• Good knot security • Excellent handling characteristics • No memory
Stainless Steel: 316L stainless steel–chromium and nickel alloys	Nonabsorbable	Indefinite	Minimal reaction	None	Abdominal wound closure; hernia repair; sternal closure; cerclage; tendon repair; bone repair; retention sutures; respiratory tract	Silver	• Most inert of all suture materials • Can be used in presence of infection • Must not be used in presence of other types of metal prostheses or implants • May be braided • May be twisted with wire twisters rather than tied • Cut with wire cutters • Should not be used in patients with allergies to 316L stainless steel, chromium, and/or nickel

(continues)

TABLE 11-5 (continued)

Suture Name	*Absorption Rate*	*Tensile Strength*	*Tissue Reaction*	*Coating*	*General Usage*	*Suture Color*	*Other Information*
GORE-TEX by Gore Medical Products: Expanded PTFE (ePTFE)	Nonabsorbable	Excellent	Minimal reaction	None	Anastomosis of vascular grafts; mitral valve repair; chordae tendineae repair; carotid endarterectomy; hernia repairs; pelvic floor repair; robotic surgery	White	• Microporous • Offers benefits of monofilament and multifilament sutures • Excellent handling characteristics • Good knot security • No memory • Sizing is different from USP; sizing is prefix "CV" with number, CV-8 is smallest and CV-0 is largest
Nonabsorbable Natural Multifilament							
Surgical Silk: Natural fiber from silkworm cocoons	Listed as nonabsorbable by USP, but it is actually a very slow absorbing suture–not detected in tissue after 2 years	Loses most tensile strength in 1 year	Less than plain or chromic gut, but more than synthetics	Ethicon coats its silk suture product with waxes or silicone	Serosa of GI tract; fascia; frequently used for suture ligatures	Undyed, black	• Available braided or twisted • Should not be used in presence of infection • No memory • Must be used dry; loses tensile strength if wet
Nonabsorbable Synthetic Multifilament							
Nylon (Nurolon by Ethicon; Surgilon by Syneture)	Nonabsorbable	Excellent tensile strength, but gradual loss occurs over time	Minimal reaction	Polybuti-late; PTFE; and silicone coatings to reduce tissue drag	General soft tissue approximation when continual strength is needed; commonly used for neurologic closures; used in eye and CV surgery	Undyed, black, green	• Knot security excellent • Gradual encapsulation by fibrous connective tissue
Bralon by Covidien: nylon	Nonabsorbable	Excellent	Minimal reaction	Polybutylene	Used with Endo Stitch™ for a variety of laparoscopic MIS procedures	Undyed, black	• Braided
Polyethylene terephthalate (Mersilene): polyester fibers	Nonabsorbable	Excellent—no significant change known to occur	Minimal reaction	None	General soft tissue approximation and/or ligation; eye, CV, and neurologic surgery; respiratory tract	Undyed, green	• Braided • Gradual encapsulation by fibrous connective tissue • Knot security excellent • 10-0 and 11-0 monofilament for eye surgery

Polyethylene terephthalate coated with polybutilate (Ethibond by Ethicon) polyester fibers	Nonabsorbable	Excellent	Minimal reaction	Polybutilate	General soft tissue approximation and/or ligation; commonly used to close incisions of the heart; tendon repair; eye and neurologic surgery	Undyed, green	• Braided • Gradual encapsulation by fibrous connective tissue
Dacron: polyester fibers	Nonabsorbable	Excellent	Minimal reaction	Uncoated or coated	Soft tissue approximation and ligation; especially useful in respiratory tract and some CV procedures	Undyed, green	• Good knot security • Pliable and easy to handle • Braided • Uncoated drags through tissue with tearing effect
Ti-Cron: polyethylene terephthalate	Nonabsorbable	Tensile strength retained indefinitely	Minimal reaction	• Uncoated • Coated with silicone	Soft tissue approximation and ligation; eye, CV, and neurologic surgery	White, blue	• Braided • Excellent security with prosthetic implants • Good knot security • No contraindications for use • Gradual encapsulation by fibrous connective tissue
Tevdek by Deknatel: polyester	Nonabsorbable	Excellent	Minimal reaction	Heavy coat of PTFE	Soft tissue approximation and ligation; eye, orthopedic, CV, and neurologic surgery	White, green	• Virtually inert • Good knot security • Easy handling characteristics
Polydek by Deknatel: polyester	Nonabsorbable	Excellent	Minimal reaction	Light coat of PTFE	Soft tissue approximation and ligation; eye, orthopedic, CV, and neurologic surgery	White, green	• Virtually inert • Good knot security • Easy handling characteristics
Fiberwire	Nonabsorbable	Excellent	Minimal reaction	Silicone	Orthopedic surgery: soft tissue repairs such as tendon and rotator cuff repairs; of the most commonly used high-tensile strength sutures used in orthopedic surgery	Black	• Braided • Good knot security • Good handling characteristics

prevent hemorrhage when amputating the leg. Typically, vessels that are not coagulated or occluded with stainless steel clips are **ligated** with suture. Ties are available as full-length or precut suture strands in a package, or wound onto radiopaque reels for superficial bleeders.

Standard lengths for nonneedled suture material are 54 in. for absorbable material and 60 in. for nonabsorbable material. These strands may be cut in half-, third-, or quarter-lengths by the surgical technologist. Single-strand ligating material is available in precut lengths of 18-, 24-, and 30-in. strands. Superficial bleeders will usually require ligatures no more than 18 in. in length. Deep bleeders require a suture length of between 18 and 30 in.

Ligating Methods

Ligating methods include the free-tie, ligature reel, instrument tie (tie-on-a-pass), and suture ligature (stick tie).

Free-Tie

Ligating material may be used as either single-strand ties or as continuous ties from a reel or other device (see Figure 11-3). Precut ties that are removed as single strands from the package or were cut to length by the surgical technologist and placed into the opened hand of the surgeon for use as ligatures are referred to as *free-ties*. This type of tie is not on a reel and is not loaded onto an instrument. The ligatures may be placed around a hemostatic clamp that has been affixed to a bleeding vessel. After the first knot is thrown, the surgical assistant removes the clamp and the ligature is secured with a surgeon's knot. The assistant then cuts the excess suture. Monofilament sutures, because the knots can slide, are typically cut leaving ¼-in. ends. Multifilament sutures can be cut closer to the knot (⅛-in.) because they do not slide as readily as monofilament sutures.

Ligature Reel

Ligature reels may be wound with absorbable or nonabsorbable sutures and are typically used to occlude superficial bleeders. Reels with absorbable suture material are frequently used on superficial bleeders of subcutaneous tissue just after the incision is made. The most commonly used ligature reels are chromic, plain, or polyglactin 910 sutures. Silk ligature reels are still available for use, as well.

Ligature reels are radiopaque and are included in the count in many institutions because they can easily be lost within a wound. The most commonly used sizes are 2-0, 3-0, and 4-0. The size of the material is indicated by the number of holes visible on the side of the reel. The surgical technologist should prepare the reel by unhooking the end of the suture strand and pulling it 2–3 in. away from the reel so that the surgeon can grasp the suture without struggling to find the end.

Instrument Tie (Tie-on-a-Pass)

Deep bleeding vessels that have been occluded with a hemostat clamp may be inaccessible for a free-hand ligature. Therefore, a suture is loaded onto an instrument, usually a Crile hemostat, Schnidt tonsil clamp, Mixter clamp, Adson clamp, or Sarot clamp, for easier placement around the tip of the occluding hemostatic clamp.

Suture Ligature (Stick Tie)

Large vessels are typically occluded with *suture ligatures*, or *stick ties*, to prevent suture slippage that can lead to uncontrolled hemorrhage. Stick ties are sutures with a **swaged** atraumatic needle loaded onto a needle holder for placement through the center of a large vessel after a hemostat clamp has been applied. The ends of the suture are brought around the clamp so that the vessel is doubly ligated (Figure 11-4). For superficial

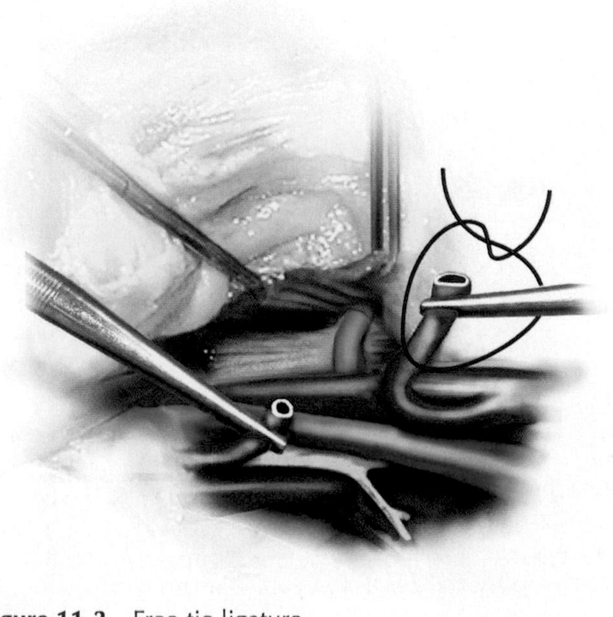

Courtesy of Ethicon, Inc.

Figure 11-3 Free-tie ligature

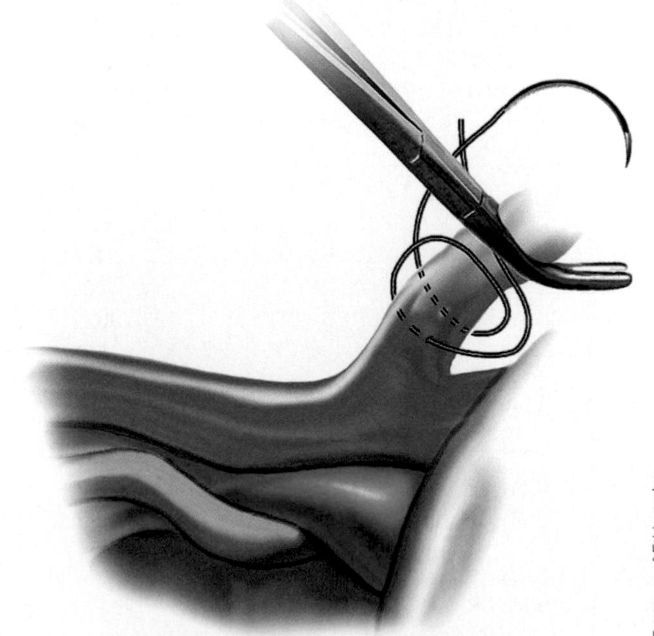

Courtesy of Ethicon, Inc.

Figure 11-4 Stick-tie ligature

bleeders, 18-in. stick ties are used and 27-in. stick ties are used for deeper vessels. Sizes 2-0 and 3-0 are the most commonly used stick-tie sizes and silk is the preferred suture material. In theory, however, any suture material can be used as a stick-tie ligature; it depends on the tissue to be sutured.

Suture for the Procedure

To determine what sutures will be necessary for a particular surgical procedure the surgical technologist should consult the surgeon's preference card and gather the sutures accordingly. Preference cards contain the surgeon's suture "routine," suture sizes, needles, and product code numbers for specific procedures. The surgical technologist should consult with the surgeon to find out if any sutures from the preference card can be excluded or if any need to be added, or if the patient's size or condition requires modification of the suture routine.

The surgical technologist should open only as many suture packets as are necessary because leftover sutures cannot be resterilized and must be discarded. Inexperienced surgical technologists tend to overcompensate for lack of suture knowledge by opening too many packets. However, if too few packets are opened, the surgical procedure may be prolonged unnecessarily while the circulator retrieves the additional sutures. Good communication between the surgical technologist and the surgeon, in addition to regularly updated preference cards, can minimize waste and keep supply costs down.

After the suture packets have been opened onto the sterile field and counted, the surgical technologist can arrange the sutures in the order in which they will be used during the procedure. Ligature reels should be removed from their packets and placed onto the Mayo stand with the strand end extended slightly. Free-ties should be opened at the end of the packet and placed on the Mayo stand with the suture strands protruding for easy access. Longer free-ties can be removed from their packets completely and placed into a rolled or folded towel. If hemorrhage is anticipated, stick ties should be loaded onto needle holders in advance of need and placed within reach and ties-on-passes should also be loaded and ready. For routine procedures, such as coronary bypass, sutures can be loaded onto needle holders and arranged in the order in which they will be used. Otherwise, the suture packets are left unopened on the sterile field until they are needed with the exception of packets that contain multiple needles. In order to avoid having to count the needles intraoperatively, the surgical technologist will often open the packet and count the needles during the preoperative count with the circulator.

Suture needs can be anticipated by the surgical technologist by paying close attention to the course of the procedure and listening to the comments of the surgeon and assistants. Additionally, the surgical technologist should thoroughly know the procedure in order to know the suture sequence.

Placement on Field

The sterile suture package is transferred to the sterile field using one of the two techniques used for opening any type of peel-packed item (refer to Chapter 12). It may be placed onto the sterile field or secured by the surgical technologist (Figure 11-5).

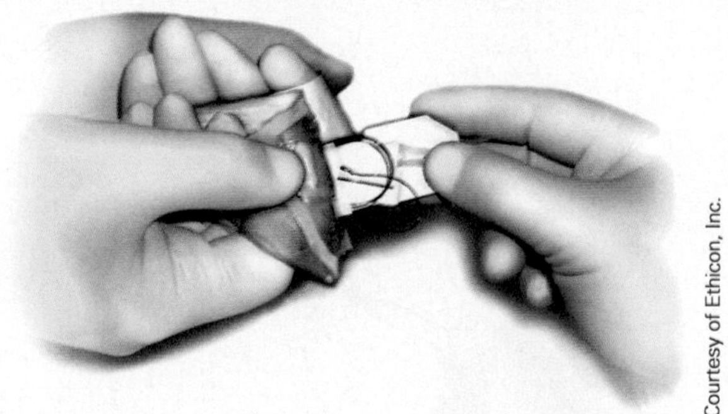
Courtesy of Ethicon, Inc.

Figure 11-5 Sterile suture transfer to the surgical technologist

Loading the Suture

Suture with a needle attached is prepared for use in the following manner (Figure 11-6). The surgical technologist chooses an appropriate needle holder based on the size of the suture needle to be used, the surgeon's preference, and the depth of the surgical wound. The needle holder is clamped approximately one-third of the distance from the swaged end of the needle to the needle point. Tougher tissue may require the needle holder to be moved to the half-point of the needle. The swaged area of the needle (that part of the needle in which the suture enters the needle) should never be clamped; that is the weakest section of the suture/needle. Modern suture packets allow the surgical technologist to load the needle without touching it.

After loading the suture onto the needle holder, depending on the type of suture, the surgical technologist should straighten the suture with a gentle pull. Other handling tips include:

- Do not attempt to pull or stretch plain or chromic gut. Excessive handling with rubber gloves can weaken and fray these sutures. Nylon sutures should be drawn between gloved fingers to remove memory. Care should be taken when straightening controlled-release (pop-off) suture so as not to remove the needle and waste the suture.
- Do not place any tension on the needle suture attachment (swage).
- Avoid crushing or crimping sutures with instruments.
- Keep surgical gut away from heat.
- Never soak plain or chromic gut in saline or water, which will cause it to deteriorate.
- Do not wet rapidly absorbing sutures.
- Keep silk dry.
- Do not bend stainless steel wire.

The surgeon should receive the needle holder and suture with the needle pointed toward the surgeon's chest. The surgical technologist should control the trailing end of the suture to prevent snagging or dropping off the sterile field. After use, the surgeon should place the needle holder onto a neutral zone (see Chapter 5). The surgical technologist should not attempt to remove the armed needle holder from the surgeon's hands.

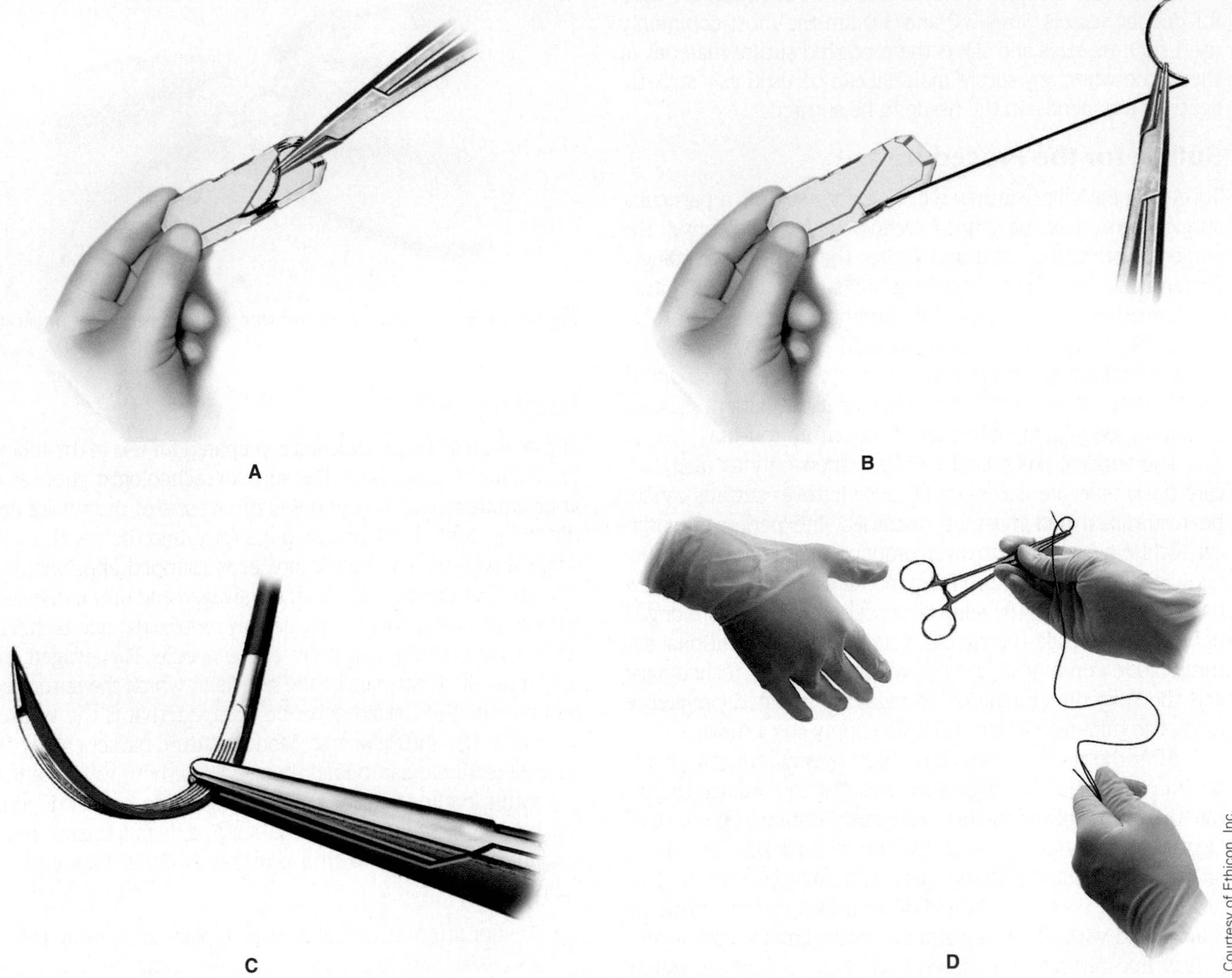

Figure 11-6 Loading the suture: (A) Needle holder is clamped onto the needle approximately one-third the distance from the swage. (B) Suture is removed from the package without placing tension on the swage. (C) Needle is correctly armed on needle holder (close-up). (D) The armed needle holder is placed in the surgeon's hand.

Cutting Suture

Suture is usually cut by the surgical technologist. The act of cutting suture may sound simple, but requires practice and developing a "feel" for the act of cutting. Suture is usually cut close to the knot unless directed by the surgeon to leave a longer "tail" than usual. The following serve as guides for cutting suture:

1. Using the dominant hand, the surgical technologist should place the index finger on the screw joint to stabilize the suture scissors (straight Mayo scissors).
2. The scissors should be slightly opened and blades angled; the tip of one blade is placed gently against the suture and slid downward to where the knot is felt and is then cut. The tips should be used to cut the suture.
3. Ideally, the surgical technologist should be able to visualize the suture strand and knot in order to avoid cutting other adjacent tissue. However, there may be times when the surgical technologist will need to slide the scissors into a wound in which visualization is not possible (surgeon and surgical assistant are busy and cannot move to allow visualization). The surgical technologist will need to get a feel for sliding the scissors downward, feeling the knot, and cutting the suture without cutting the knot.

NEEDLES

Surgical needles are used to insert suture material into tissue and are available in a wide variety of sizes and shapes. However, only a few types are used consistently. They are made of

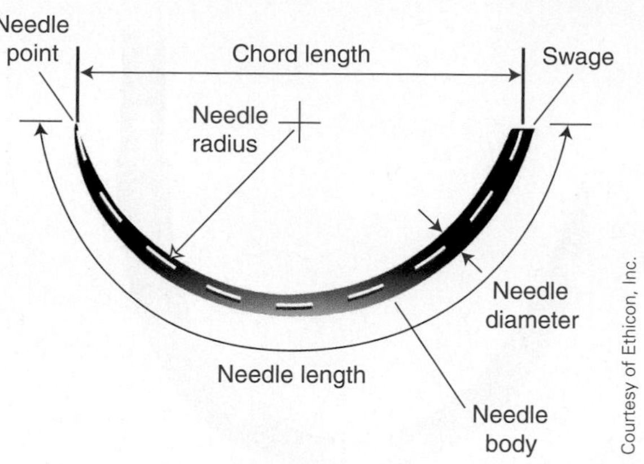

Figure 11-7 Needle anatomy

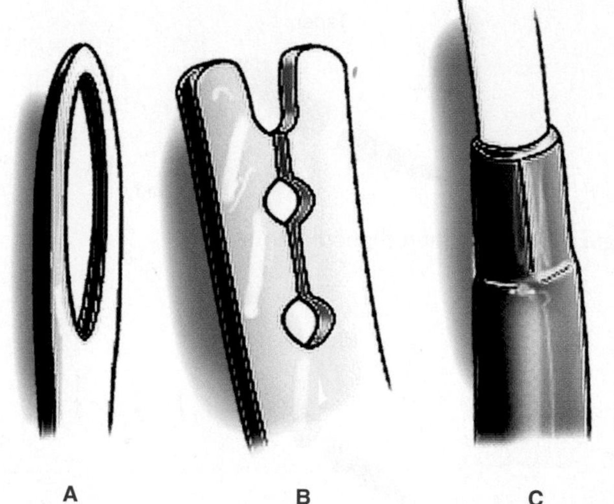

Figure 11-8 Types of needle eyes: (A) Closed, (B) French, (C) swaged

steel and should be strong enough so that they do not bend or break during suturing.

Needles can be described in terms of the following characteristics: eye, point, body, and shape (Figure 11-7).

Needle Eyes

The *eye* is the portion of the needle where the suture strand is attached. Surgical needles may be closed-eyed, French-eyed, or eyeless (swaged) (Figure 11-8).

Closed-eyed needles may have round or square holes and are loaded by inserting the end of the suture material through the hole. The eyed needle allows the use of a wide variety of sutures with a wide variety of needles. Loading the eyed needle with the suture strand can be a cumbersome process when wearing gloves or if the needle is small. The eyed needle causes more tissue damage than the eyeless (swaged) needle because the suture strand is not continuous with the needle.

The **French-eyed needle** is loaded by pulling the taut strand into a V-shaped area just above the eye. This type of needle is loaded more quickly than a closed-eyed needle, but still results in more tissue damage than the eyeless needle.

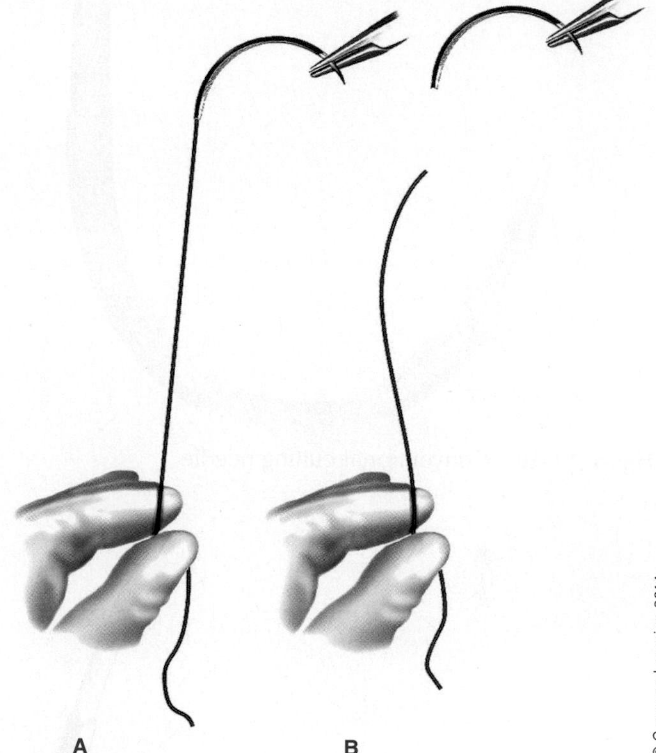

Figure 11-9 Rapid-release needle technique: (A) Hold the needle securely in the needle holder. The suture should be grasped securely and pulled straight and taut. (B) Release needle with a straight tug on the needle holder.

Needles that are manufactured with suture strands inserted into one end are referred to as *eyeless* or *swaged needles*. These needles are continuous with the suture strand, and the hole created in the tissue by the needle should be completely filled by the suture strand when suturing.

Eyeless needles may have a single-arm attachment or a double-arm attachment. The single-arm attachment is a single needle swaged to the suture strand. These may by used for interrupted or continuous suturing.

The double-arm attachment involves a needle swaged to each end of the suture strand. These are commonly used for anastomosis of vessels, allowing the center of the suture to be sewn to the center of the vessel with one suture end sewn to the left and the other to the right. The stitches meet in the middle on the opposite side of the vessel.

Eyeless needles may have the suture strand permanently attached or, as previously discussed, may be a controlled-release needle used for rapid, efficient placement of interrupted sutures (Figure 11-9).

Needle Points

Needle points may be cutting, tapered, or blunt and the needle itself straight or curved. Cutting needles are used for tough

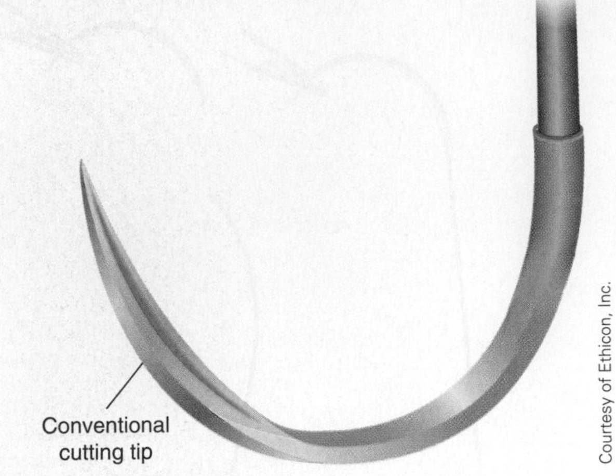

Figure 11-10 Conventional cutting needle

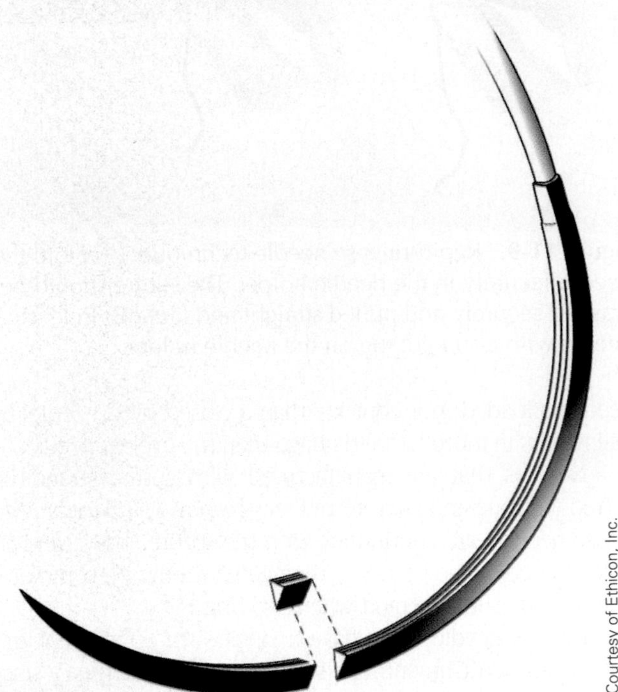

Figure 11-11 Reverse cutting needle

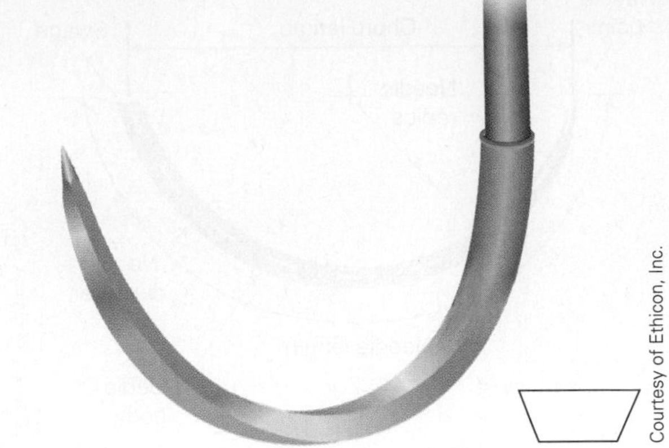

Figure 11-12 Side-cutting (spatula) needle

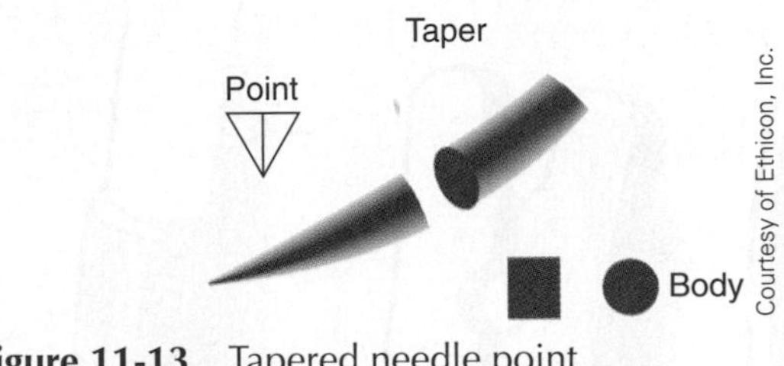

Figure 11-13 Tapered needle point

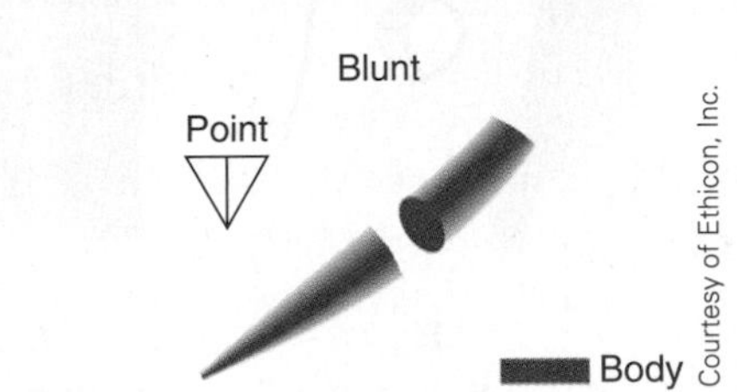

Figure 11-14 Blunt needle point

tissue that is difficult to penetrate. The sharp edges of this type of point actually cut the tissue as they penetrate it. Cutting needles are typically used for the sclera of the eye, tendons, or skin.

Conventional cutting needles (Figure 11-10) consist of three cutting edges that are directed along the inner curve of the needle. These needles place a small cut in the direction of the pull of the suture.

Reverse cutting needles (Figure 11-11) consist of opposing cutting edges in a triangular configuration that extend into the full length of the shaft. They are used for the skin because they have a flat edge in the direction of the pull. This results in less tearing of tissue.

Side cutting needles (Figure 11-12) are used primarily for ophthalmic procedures because they will not penetrate into deeper tissues and separate the tissue layers during placement.

Tapered point needles (Figure 11-13) have a round shaft without a cutting edge, so they penetrate tissue without cutting it. These points are used for delicate tissues, such as the tissue of the gastrointestinal tract.

Blunt points (Figure 11-14) have a round shaft that ends in a blunt tip. These points are used primarily for the kidney or liver due to the tissue being so friable or weak.

Prosthetic grafts sewn onto vessels require the use of a needle that is sharp enough to penetrate the graft but delicate enough to prevent damage to the vessel. The *ground point wire needle* has a point with sharp edges, but the round body of a tapered needle that permits easy passage through the graft without damage to the vessel.

Needle Bodies

The shaft, or body, of the needle is located between the suture strand and the point. Its size and shape are variable and

CODE	MEANING
BB	Blue Baby
BIF	Intraocular Fixation
BN	Bunnell
BP	Blunt Point
BV	Blood Vessel
BVH	Blood Vessel Half
C	Cardiovascular
CC	Calcified Cornary
CCS	Conventional Cutting Sternotomy
CE	Cutting Edge
CFS	Conventional for Skin
CIF	Cutting Intraocular Fixation
CP	Cutting Point
CPS	Conventional Plastic Surgery
CPX	Cutting Point Extra Large
CS	Corneal-Scleral
CSB	Corneal-Scleral Bi-Curve
CSC	Corneal-Scleral Compound Curve
CT	Circle Taper
CTB	Circle Taper Blunt
CTX	Circle Taper Extra Large
CTXB	Circle Taper Extra Large Blunt
CV	Cardiovascular
DC	Dura Closure
DP	Double Point
EN	Endoscopic Needle
EST	Eyed Straight Taper
FN	For Tonsil
FS	For Skin
FSL	For Skin Large

CODE	MEANING
FSLX	For Skin Extra Large
G	Greishaber
GS	Greishaber Spatula
J	Conjunctive
KS	Keith Straight
LH	Large Half
LR	Larger Retention
LS	Large Sternotomy
M	Muscle
MF	Modified Fergusan
MH	Medium Half (circle)
MO	Mayo
MOB	Mayo Blunt
OPS	Ocular Plastic Surgery
OS	Orthopaedic Surgery
P	Plastic
PC	Precision Cosmetic
PS	Plastic Surgery
RB	Renal (artery) Bypass
RD	Retinal Detachment
RH	Round Half (circle)
RV	Retinal-Vitreous
S	Spatula
SC	Straight Cutting
SFS	Spatulated for Skin
SH	Small Half (circle)
SIF	Ski Intraocular Fixation
SKS	Sternotomy Keith Straight
SM	Spatulated Module
ST	Straight Taper

CODE	MEANING
STB	Straight Blunt
STC	Straight Cutting
STP	Straight Taper Point
TE	Three-Eighths
TF	Tetralogy of Fallot
TG	Transverse Ground
TGW	Transverse Ground Wide
TN	Trocar Needle
TP	Taper Pericostal / Point
TPB	Taper Pericostal / Point Blunt
TS	Tendon Straight
TQ	Twisty Q
UCL	5/8 Circle Colateral Ligament
UR	Urology
URB	Urology Blunt
V	TAPERCUT Surgical Needle
VAS	Vas Deferens
X or P	Exodontal (dental)
XLH	Extra Large Half (circle)
XXLH	Extra Extra Large Half (circle)

Courtesy of Ethicon, Inc.

Figure 11-15 Ethicon needle codes and their meanings

choice depends on the type of tissue to be sutured. Typically, the heavier the tissue, the heavier the body. Length is determined by the depth of the "bite" of the tissue to be sutured. The shape of the body may be straight (Keith needle), ¼ circle, ⅜ circle, ½ circle, or ⅝ circle. Microsurgical needles and retention suture needles are usually ⅜ circle, as are needles for skin closure (Figure 11-15).

NONSUTURE NEEDLES

Nonsuture needles, such as hypodermic, arterial, intravenous, irrigation, biopsy, insufflation, and spinal needles, are commonly utilized during surgical procedures.

Hypodermic needles are used to inject medications into tissues or intravenous tubing. The surgical technologist uses them to withdraw medications into a syringe from a vial held by a circulator. Hypodermic needles may also be used to withdraw fluids from tissues. They are produced in varying sizes and lengths. Needle lengths range in size from ½ to 4 in., and gauge sizes range from 12 to 30, with smaller needles having the larger gauge number.

Arterial or *venous/cannula needle* assemblies employ a needle to introduce a plastic indwelling catheter into a vessel (commonly called an IV in order to deliver IV fluids, blood, and/or blood products into the circulatory system). Arterial needle/cannula assemblies are used to obtain arterial blood gases or are attached to a line leading to a transducer to directly monitor arterial blood pressure. Intravenous cannula/needle assemblies, such as the Angio-Cath, are attached to IV lines for the introduction of fluids and/or medications into the patient's system.

Arterial needles, such as the Potts-Cournand needle/cannula assembly, are used to introduce diagnostic or angioplasty guiding catheters over guiding wires into the arterial system.

Venous needles with an aspirating syringe are used to puncture large veins for the introduction of monitoring catheters, such as the Swan-Ganz. *Heparin needles* attached to syringes are used during open cardiovascular procedures to irrigate open arteries with a saline-heparin solution.

Irrigation needles actually are not needles but a small-diameter cannulated tube attached to a plastic needle hub for placement on a syringe. The irrigation needles are available straight and angled, disposable or nondisposable, and in various lengths. They are commonly used during eye and microsurgery procedures.

When laparoscopic procedures are performed the abdomen must be distended or insufflated with CO_2. A Veress needle that is attached to the CO_2 tubing is introduced percutaneously into the abdomen to facilitate the delivery of the gas. See laparoscopic appendectomy or basic laparoscopy sections for additional details.

Large percutaneous *biopsy needles* are used to obtain tissue samples from within the body for biopsy. This type of biopsy is sometimes guided with the aid of CT scan or fluoroscopy. Examples of this type of needle include the Dorsey cannulated needle for biopsy of cerebral tissue through a burr hole, the Chiba biopsy needle for biopsy of lung tissue through the chest wall, the Franklin-Silverman cannulated biopsy needle with a "trap door" tip for biopsy of the liver and other internal organs, and the Tru-cut biopsy needle. The Tru-cut biopsy needle has a sharp cutting cannula to facilitate insertion into the tissue and cutting the tissue; a removable stylet allows for multiple biopsies to be taken. Some brands of the Tru-cut allow a luer slip syringe to be placed on the end for aspiration when the stylet has been removed. The Tru-cut needle is usually either 14 or 18 gauge and ranges in length from 3 to 6 inches. Bone marrow trocars introduced through cortical bone may be used to obtain bone marrow.

Biopsy needles attached to syringes may be used to aspirate fluid from a cyst or abscess. Very small biopsy needles can obtain cells from breast lesions, lymph nodes, or other shallow tissues.

Spinal needle/cannula assemblies are 3–4 in. long with a sharp, beveled stylet within the metal cannula. These needles are typically employed to introduce anesthetic agents into the epidural or subdural space or to obtain cerebral spinal fluid for diagnostic purposes.

LAYER CLOSURE

Abdominal wounds are closed in layers. From inner to outer, these layers include the peritoneum, fascia, muscle, subcutaneous, subcuticular, and skin layers (Figure 11-16).

Peritoneum

The peritoneum, a fast-healing, thin membrane lining the abdominal cavity, lying beneath the posterior fascia, may not require suturing if the posterior fascia is closed properly. If the surgeon chooses to close the peritoneum, a continuous 3-0 absorbable suture is frequently utilized.

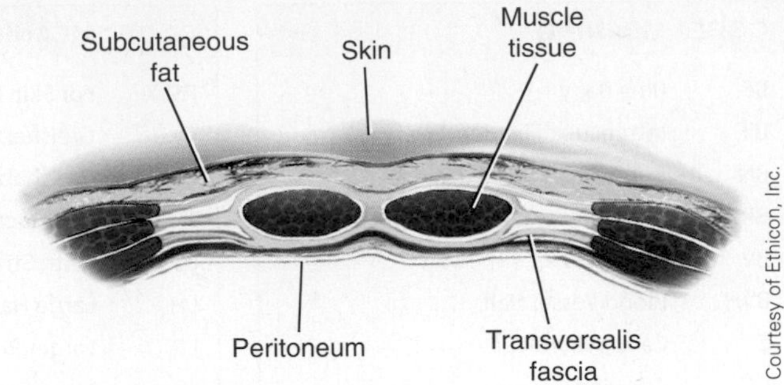

Figure 11-16 The abdominal wall

Fascia

The fascia is a layer of tough connective tissue covering the body's muscles. It is the primary supportive soft tissue structure of the body and great care must be taken to close the abdominal fascia layer securely. This layer heals slowly and must endure the brunt of wound stress; therefore, interrupted, heavy-gauge, nonabsorbable multifilament suture is preferred for added strength. If an absorbable suture material is used, it should be slow absorbing and have high tensile strength. If the fascial layer is weak, polypropylene surgical mesh may be sutured in with polypropylene sutures for structural support.

Muscle

Muscles are typically not closed with suture because they do not tolerate suture material well. Muscles are usually separated or retracted and therefore do not need to be closed (Figure 11-17). If they are incised, however, they should be loosely approximated with interrupted absorbable sutures.

Subcutaneous

Like muscle, subcutaneous tissue does not tolerate sutures well. Many surgeons prefer to place a few interrupted sutures into this layer to prevent dead space, especially for obese patients. Plain gut is often the preferred suture material for subcutaneous closure.

Subcuticular

The subcuticular layer is an area of tough connective tissue just beneath the skin and just above the subcutaneous layer. A subcuticular closure is often utilized to minimize scarring. Short lateral stitches are placed in a continuous or interrupted fashion just under the epithelial layer of the skin, in a line parallel to the wound (Figure 11-18). Absorbable sutures are preferred as opposed to nonabsorbable sutures because the surgeon need not remove them. Small-gauge sutures can be utilized for subcuticular closure because the fascia endures the brunt of tension for the healing wound.

Skin

Skin may be closed with interrupted or continuous monofilament, nonabsorbable sutures on a cutting needle or with

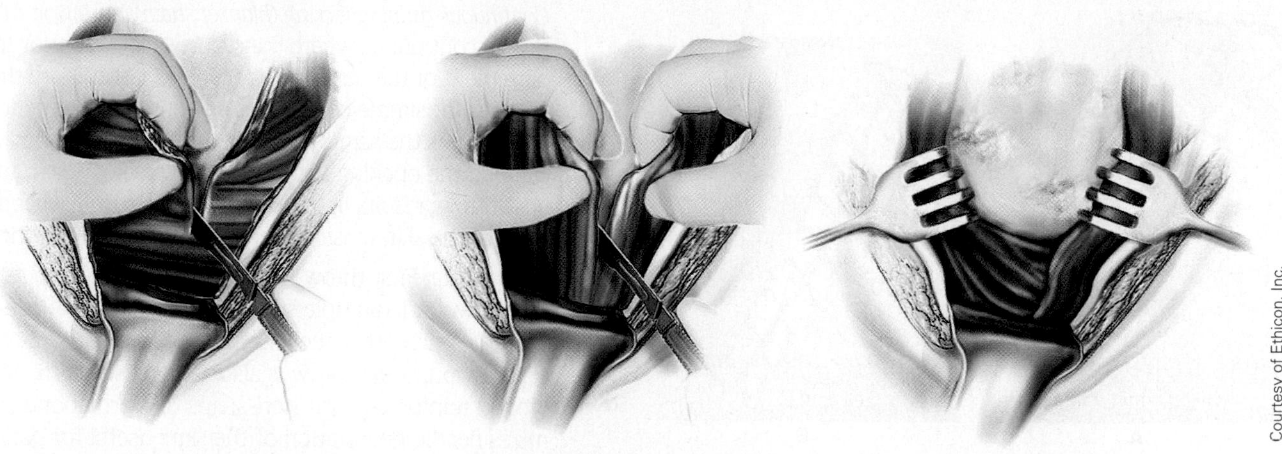

Courtesy of Ethicon, Inc.

Figure 11-17 Muscle separation: (A) Cutting, (B) splitting, (C) retracting

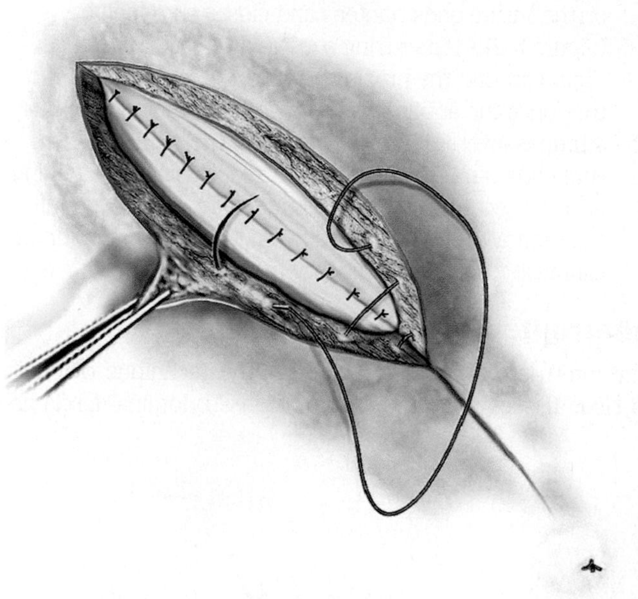

Courtesy of Ethicon, Inc.

Figure 11-18 Subcutaneous sutures

stainless steel staples (skin stapler). Polypropylene or nylon are the preferred suture materials; however, stainless steel staples result in less tissue reaction. The drawback to skin closure is that the wound scars more than with a subcuticular closure and sutures must eventually be removed. If subcuticular closure is performed, the skin will be approximated with skin closure tapes.

SUTURING TECHNIQUES

Suturing techniques include the various methods for proper closure of wounds under any conditions. All wounds are not the same and one technique for closure may not be applicable in all situations. The **primary suture line** refers to the sutures that approximate wound edges for first intention healing. These sutures are placed in either an interrupted or continuous fashion. Other types of primary sutures include buried, purse-string, and subcuticular, which are used for specific purposes.

Continuous Suturing Techniques

The *continuous*, or *running*, *suture* is a primary suture line consisting of a single strand of suture placed as a series of stitches often used for closure of long incisions. The strand is tied after the first stitch is placed at one end and tied again after the last stitch is placed at the other end. Evenly distributed tension along the suture line is a hallmark of the continuous suture closure (Figure 11-19). The surgical assistant "follows" or "runs" the suture by holding the lower quarter of the suture taut and away from the area of closure. This process keeps the proper amount of tension on the suture line and keeps the suture strand out of the surgeon's line of view.

The drawback to this type of closure is that if any segment of the continuous strand breaks, the entire suture line is jeopardized, resulting in dehiscence or evisceration. For this reason, continuous sutures should not be used to close tissues that are under a lot of tension. The use of a continuous suture technique is contraindicated in the presence of infection; bacteria and tissue fluids can travel along the length of a wound by way of a continuous suture strand, referred to as wicking. The following are brief descriptions of the various continuous suturing techniques:

Simple Continuous: Used for long straight incisions when the wound edges easily evert. Simple suture is placed at one end and tied off; suture is placed at equal distances along the wound; final throw is not pulled all the way through since the tie is done with the loop end of the suture. The surgical technologist keeps gentle tension on the suture behind the next throw to keep the suture material out of the way of the surgeon as well as to prevent the previous throws from loosening.

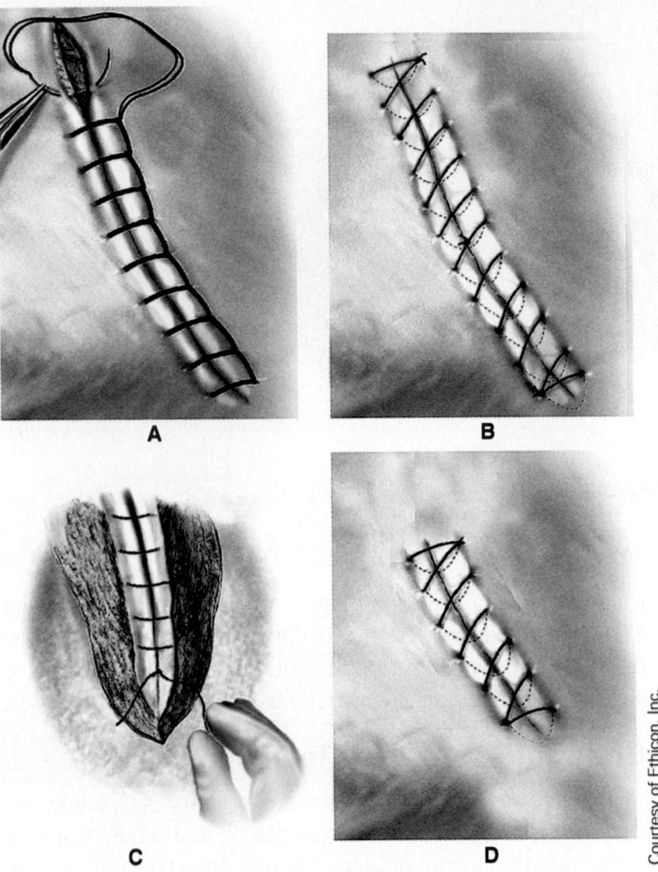

Figure 11-19 Continuous suturing techniques: (A) Interlocking stitch, knotted at each end, (B) two strands, knotted at each end and in the middle, (C) looped suture, tied to itself, (D) over-and-over running stitch

Continuous running/locking (blanket stitch): Variation of the simple continuous where the suture is locked prior to placement of the next throw; first and last ties are the same as for simple continuous and suture placement in the tissue is the same; however, the suture is looped through the opening and pulled into place prior to the next throw; results in increased wound edge eversion and reduces the skin tension more than the simple continuous.

Subcuticular: First throw is a single suture technique at end of wound; multiple subcuticular bites are made opposite each other the length of the wound; opposite end of wound the throw is also a single suture technique; wound reinforced with steri-strips or Dermabond™; minimizes needle penetration of the skin; useful for patients prone to developing keloids where needle holes in the skin promote excessive cicatrix formation.

Pursestring: A drawstring suture is placed in a circular fashion around a structure in such a way that pulling on the suture ends tightens and closes an opening (Figure 11-21). Pursestring sutures are placed into the cecum around the proximal portion of the appendix so that once the appendix is removed and the appendiceal stump is inverted into the lumen of the cecum, the suture ends can be tightened and tied, closing the opening into the cecum. Pursestring sutures are also placed into the right atrium and ascending aorta for introduction of cannulae for cardiopulmonary bypass.

Interrupted Suturing Techniques

The interrupted suture technique is the technique of choice to close tissues that are under tension. Abdominal fascia and

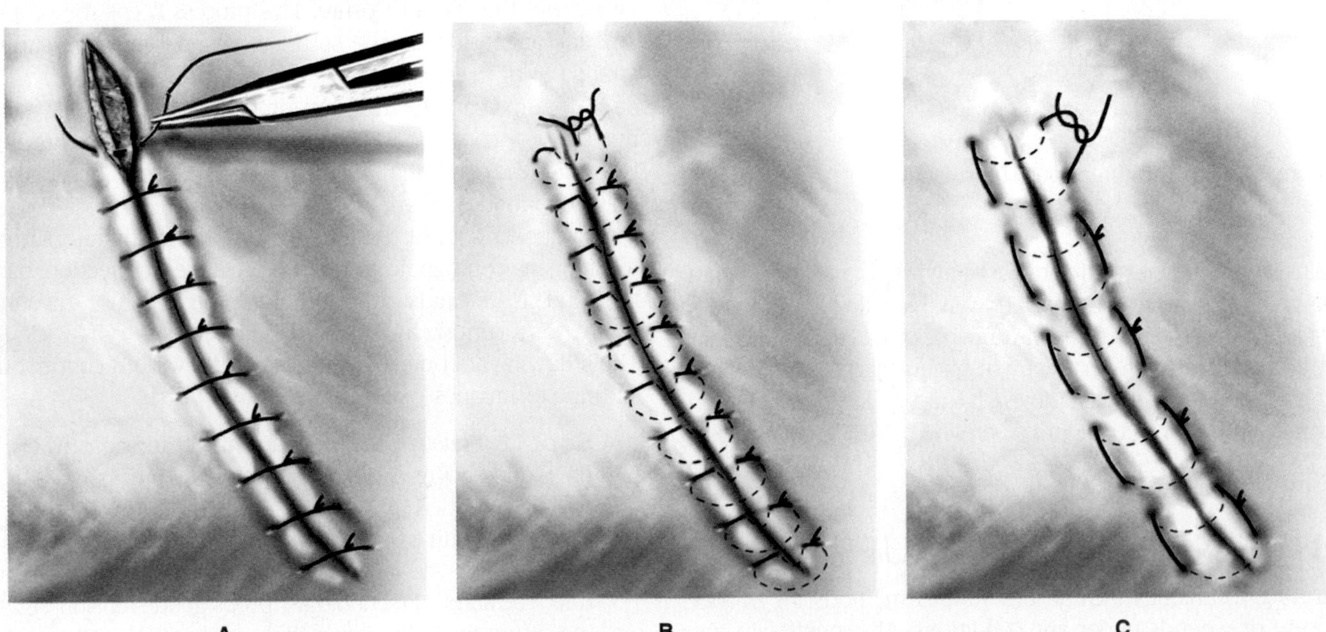

Figure 11-20 Interrupted suturing techniques: (A) Simple interrupted, (B) interrupted vertical mattress, (C) interrupted horizontal mattress

tendons are examples of tissue that are closed by interrupted suture technique. The *interrupted suture line* is also the suture technique of choice to close infected tissues. The interrupted suture "interrupts" the pathway of the bacteria, localizing the area of infection to a smaller area of the wound (Figure 11-20). For these and other reasons, Dr. Halsted condoned the use of small-gauge, interrupted sutures for wound closure; see Box 11-1 for the historical Halsted's principles of suture technique. The following are brief descriptions of the various interrupted suturing techniques:

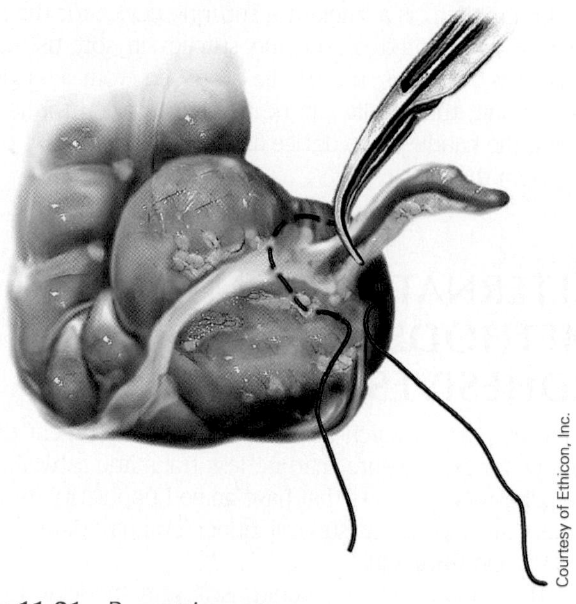

Figure 11-21 Pursestring suture

Simple interrupted: Each stitch is individually placed, tied, and cut for the length of the wound; wound edges are approximated and everted.

Interrupted horizontal mattress: Two-bite suture technique; the two stitches are placed parallel to each other on each side of the wound; first bite is a simple suture; second bite is placed parallel to the first bite and travels back across the wound edge to end on the same side as the first bite; each suture placement substitutes for two simple interrupted stitches.

Interrupted vertical mattress: Two-bite suture technique; first small bite is placed close to the wound edge; second bite is placed slightly behind the first bite and deeper in the tissue; the needle comes out the side where the first bite was placed; used for deep wounds; provides excellent eversion and skin approximation.

Figure-of-8 Stick Tie: Tissue or vessel to be tied is held in a hemostat; first throw is a surgeon's knot; suture is then passed back and forth through the tissue around the two sides of the clamp in a figure-8 fashion and the suture is tied.

Buried: Sutures are placed so the knot is located under the layer to be closed and is not projecting outward.

HALSTED'S PRINCIPLES OF SUTURE TECHNIQUE

Dr. William Halsted was a famous surgeon who was the professor of surgery at Johns Hopkins Hospital from 1893 to 1922. Notable contributions include development of the Penrose drain and introduction of the use of the surgical glove and use of hemostats for clamping bleeding vessels. However, he is well known for his principles of tissue handling and suturing techniques. The following are Halsted's suture technique principles. It should be understood these principles were based on the only two suture materials that were available for use in that time period; with the development of improved synthetic suture materials, wound closure can be performed by the surgeon using various techniques with few complications.

1. Interrupted sutures should be used to promote greater strength along the wound; each suture should be tied separately. If one knot slips or breaks, all other knots will hold.
2. Interrupted sutures are a barrier to infection, preventing microbes from traveling along a continuous suture strand.
3. Sutures are as fine as is consistent with security. A suture stronger than the tissue in which it is placed in is unnecessary.
4. Sutures should be cut close to the knots. Long ends can increase tissue inflammation and irritation.
5. A separate needle should be used for each skin stitch.
6. Dead space in the wound is prevented and eliminated.
7. Two fine sutures are used instead of one large suture.
8. Silk material should not be used in the presence of infection.
9. Undue tension should not be placed on the tissue by the suture to avoid strangulation of the blood supply.

Traction Sutures

Traction sutures are used to retract a structure that may not be easily retracted with a conventional retractor instrument. A nonabsorbable suture is placed into or around the structure and the suture ends are clamped with a hemostatic clamp. The structure is then pulled to the side of the operative site. Examples of traction sutures are those placed into the sclera of the eye, the myocardium of the heart, or the tongue.

Secondary Suture Line

A **secondary suture line** is useful for support of the primary suture line. It helps to ease tension on the primary suture line, thus reinforcing the wound closure and obliterating any dead spaces. Retention sutures are an example of a secondary suture line.

Retention

Retention sutures are large-gauge, interrupted, nonabsorbable sutures placed lateral to a primary suture line for wound reinforcement. These sutures may be placed through all layers of the tissue. They are used when the surgeon suspects that the wound will not heal properly or will heal slowly due to immunosuppression, obesity, diabetes, or other compromising factors. Retention sutures can also prevent wound disruption that may result from sudden increases in abdominal pressure created by postoperative vomiting or coughing (Figure 11-22).

Endoscopic Suturing

There are two methods of endoscopic suturing: extracorporal and intracorporeal. The extracorporeal method actually refers to creating the knot outside the body prior to instrument transfer through the trocar cannula to the tissue site. A common method is forming extracorporeal slip locking knots with subsequent transfer of the knot to the tissue site. The intracorporeal method simply refers to the surgeon using instruments inserted through the trocar cannula to facilitate the internal suturing of tissues and knot tying. There are also various devices available for intracorporeal placement of suture and knots, including Endoloop® and Endo Stitch™. The Endoloop® ligature is used to ligate tissue pedicles during endoscopic procedures. A suture is inserted through a long, thin plastic tube, which is formed into a loop with a knot. When ligature is in position, the tube is pulled upward to tighten the loop and knot.

Endo Stitch™ is a single-use suturing device for the placement of interrupted or running stitches in soft tissue. The device has two jaws; the needle is loaded from a single-use loading unit; the needle can be passed between the jaws by closing the handles. The device also serves as the knot pusher to tighten the knot.

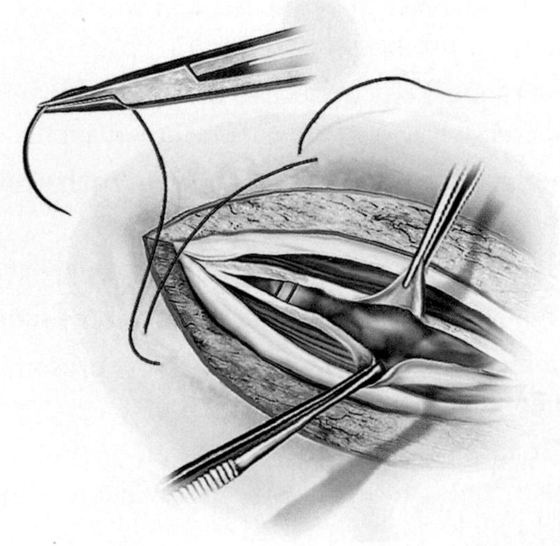

Courtesy of Ethicon, Inc.

Figure 11-22 Retention suture

ALTERNATIVE SKIN CLOSURE METHODS AND TISSUE ADHESIVES

In recent years research has lead to the development of new options for skin closure that are less traumatic as well as tissue adhesives. Products that have gained popularity for use in surgery are the wound/surgical zipper, cyanoacrylate (Dermabond™), and fibrin glue.

The wound zipper is a noninvasive, atraumetic device used for skin closure. It combines a zipper and two lateral adhesive strips. After surgery the adhesive strips are placed on each side of the surgical skin incision; the surgical technologist should make sure the skin has been cleaned and is dry prior to placement. The surgical team may want to don clean gloves prior to handling the wound zipper. As the zipper is closed it approximates the edges of the wound, providing a secure closure. It is recommended that the zipper be 3–4 cm longer than the surgical wound. Advantages include elimination of needle holes in the skin, elimination of the possibility of sharp injuries from suture needles when skin closure is being performed, and that it is faster than suturing.

Cyanoacrylate is a synthetic adhesive used for skin closure; two commercial names are Dermabond™ (Ethicon product) and Indermil™ (Syneture product). A pencil-like device is held and a button on the side is pushed to deliver the chemical liquid glue. A small brush on the end is used to apply the glue, which dries in approximately 2 minutes. The glue provides a strong, flexible wound closure and naturally wears off in 7 to 10 days. Uses include ob-gyn surgical procedures such as cesarean sections; general surgery procedures; peripheral vascular procedures that involve incisions in the arm or leg; plastic surgery; and facial surgery, as long as the incision is not too close to the eyes. It is contraindicated for use in the presence of infection and patients who are allergic to cyanoacrylate or formaldehyde.

Fibrin glue is a biologic adhesive and hemostatic agent. Fibrin glue consists of fibrinogen, cryoprecipitate derived from human plasma, calcium chloride, and thrombin. The surgical technologist mixes the calcium chloride and thrombin in a specimen cup on the back table and draws the solution into a syringe and attaches a 14-gauge IV catheter. The cryoprecipitate is drawn into the second syringe that also has a 14-gauge IV catheter. The surgeon is handed one syringe and discharges the solution onto the tissue at the same time the surgical technologist discharges the other syringe. The thrombin immediately converts fibrinogen to fibrin to produce a clot.

Uses of fibrin glue include deep tissues as a liquid or spray to control bleeding and approximate wound edges of tissues that are difficult to suture; fixation of ocular implants and middle ear reconstructive procedures; and microsurgical anastomoses of nerves and blood vessels.

A type of fibrin glue is autologous or homologous plasma. Plasma is collected from a patient (autologous donor) or a single donor (homologous) and manufactured into a cryoprecipitate that contains clotting factor XIII to produce fibrinogen. The autologous or homologous fibrinogen must be warmed to 98.6°F right before use. Thrombin is reconstituted to 1000 units/mL. The solutions are drawn up separately in two syringes and applied simultaneously to the tissue.

Another type of fibrin glue is pooled-donor plasma. It is manufactured from multiple donors, but the fibrinogen must undergo cleansing and destruction of viruses to prevent the transmission of blood-borne pathogens to the patient. It is used in Europe but has not been approved by the U.S. Food and Drug Administration (FDA) for use in the United States.

ACCESSORY DEVICES

Accessory devices for wound closure include bolsters and bridges, buttons, lead shots, and adhesive skin closure tapes. Although **vessel loops** and umbilical tapes are not used for closure of a wound, they are described here.

Bridges and Bolsters

Various devices are employed to keep retention sutures from cutting into the skin. *Bridges* are plastic devices that "bridge" the closed incision. Retention suture ends are brought up through holes on each end of the bridge and tied at the middle. A circular tightening device on the bridge allows tension to be adjusted on the retention sutures (Figure 11-23).

Bolsters are pieces of plastic or rubber tubing threaded over the retention suture ends before the ends are tied. Once

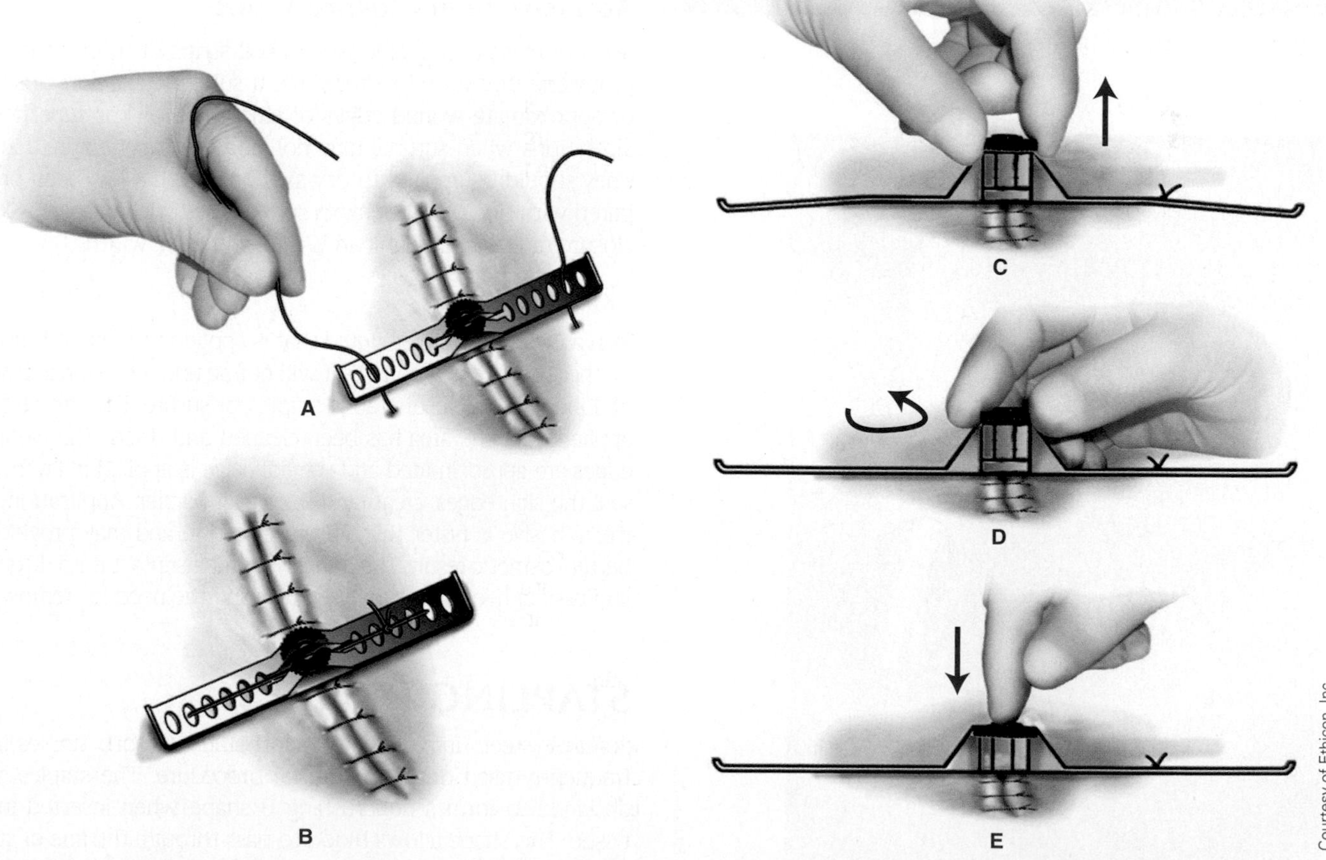

Figure 11-23 Adjustment of retention suture bridge: (A) Pass the retention suture through the appropriate holes in the bridge, (B) place the suture with tension over the slit in the capstan and tie, (C) to adjust tension, lift capstan, (D) rotate capstan until desired tension is attained (E) to lock, press capstan down into bridge.

tied, the bolsters cover the retention sutures and prevent them from cutting into the skin (Figure 11-24).

Buttons and Lead Shots

Tendon sutures may be pulled through *buttonholes* and tied over a button to prevent tissue damage (Figure 11-25). *Split lead shots* may be clamped onto the ends of subcuticular sutures after skin closure.

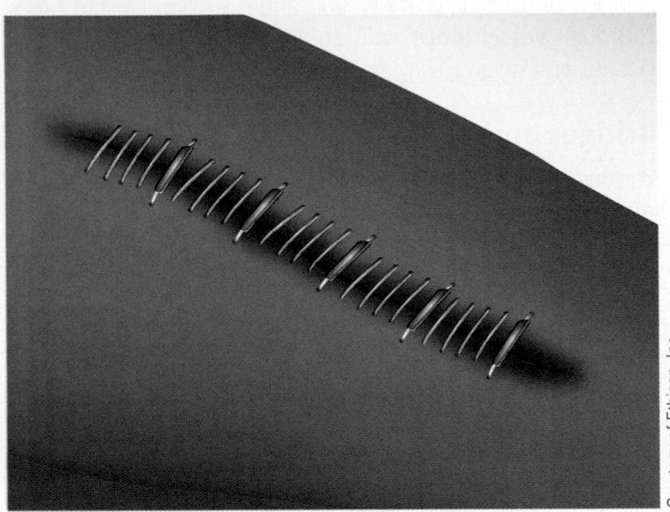

Figure 11-24 Suture bolster

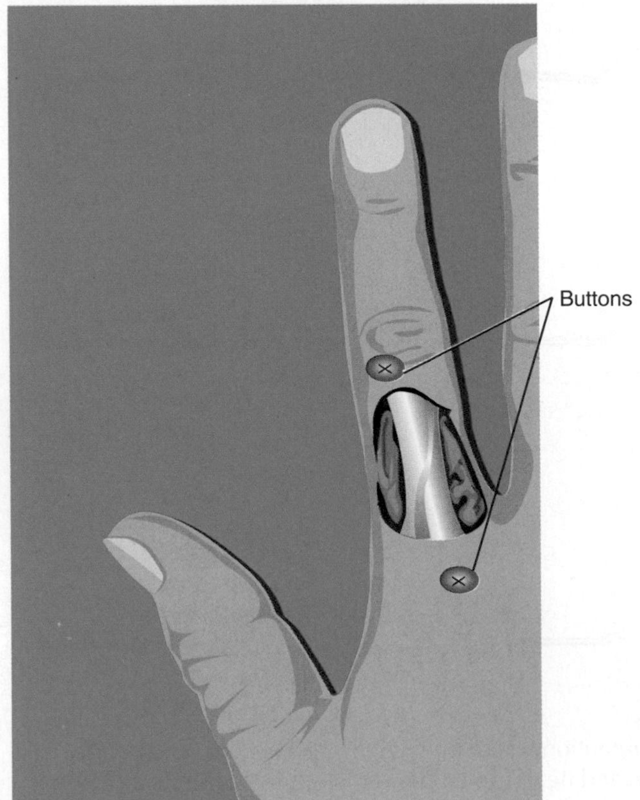

Figure 11-25 Buttons

Umbilical Tape

Cotton *umbilical tape* was once used to ligate the severed ends of the umbilical cord after childbirth. It is used in the OR as a retraction and isolation device for bowel, nerves, vessels, or ducts. Umbilical tape is usually packaged with two strands in a pink packet and is best used moistened with saline and loaded onto a hemostat.

Vessel Loops

Silicone *vessel loops* have, for the most part, replaced umbilical tape as isolation/retraction devices for vessels, nerves, or ducts. The elasticity of the vessel loops makes them ideal for retraction of delicate structures or for temporary occlusion of a vessel. Vessel loops are colored for easy identification of different adjacent structures. Typically, white and yellow loops are for nerves or ducts, red loops are for arteries, and blue loops are for veins. They are packaged in pairs.

Suture Anchors

Suture anchors are used in orthopedic surgery for fixing tendons and ligaments to bone. The device consists of the anchor, such as a screw made of metal or absorbable material, that is inserted into the bone and an eyelet through which the suture passes. The anchor inserts into the bone and this facilitates the suture attaching to the tendon and thus fixing the tendon to the bone.

Adhesive Skin Closure Tapes

Skin closure tapes are adhesive-backed strips of nylon or polypropylene tapes used to reinforce a subcuticular skin closure or approximate wound edges of small incisions or superficial lacerations when sutures may not be necessary (Figure 11-26). They should be applied to dry skin or skin that has been prepared with tincture of benzoin so that they stick properly. Skin closure tapes are available in ⅛-, ¼-, and ½-in. widths.

Skin Adhesive

Skin adhesive is a sterile liquid that is applied topically. It is used on the surface of a wound that will not be under tension in place of adhesive skin closure tapes, staples, or suture. The adhesive is applied after the area has been cleaned and dried. The wound edges are approximated and the adhesive is applied in layers to seal the skin edges, creating a microbial barrier. Application of the adhesive is faster than suture insertion and may provide a better cosmetic result. The adhesive remains intact for 5–10 days and is sloughed off naturally, eliminating the need for removal.

STAPLING DEVICES

Stainless steel, titanium, and absorbable polysorb staples are frequently used during a surgical procedure. The staples are designed to form a noncrushing B shape when inserted into tissue. This shape allows blood to pass through the line of staples, preventing tissue necrosis and promoting healing.

Staplers may be disposable or nondisposable with disposable color-coded staple cartridges. Nondisposable staplers must be assembled by the surgical technologist during case setup.

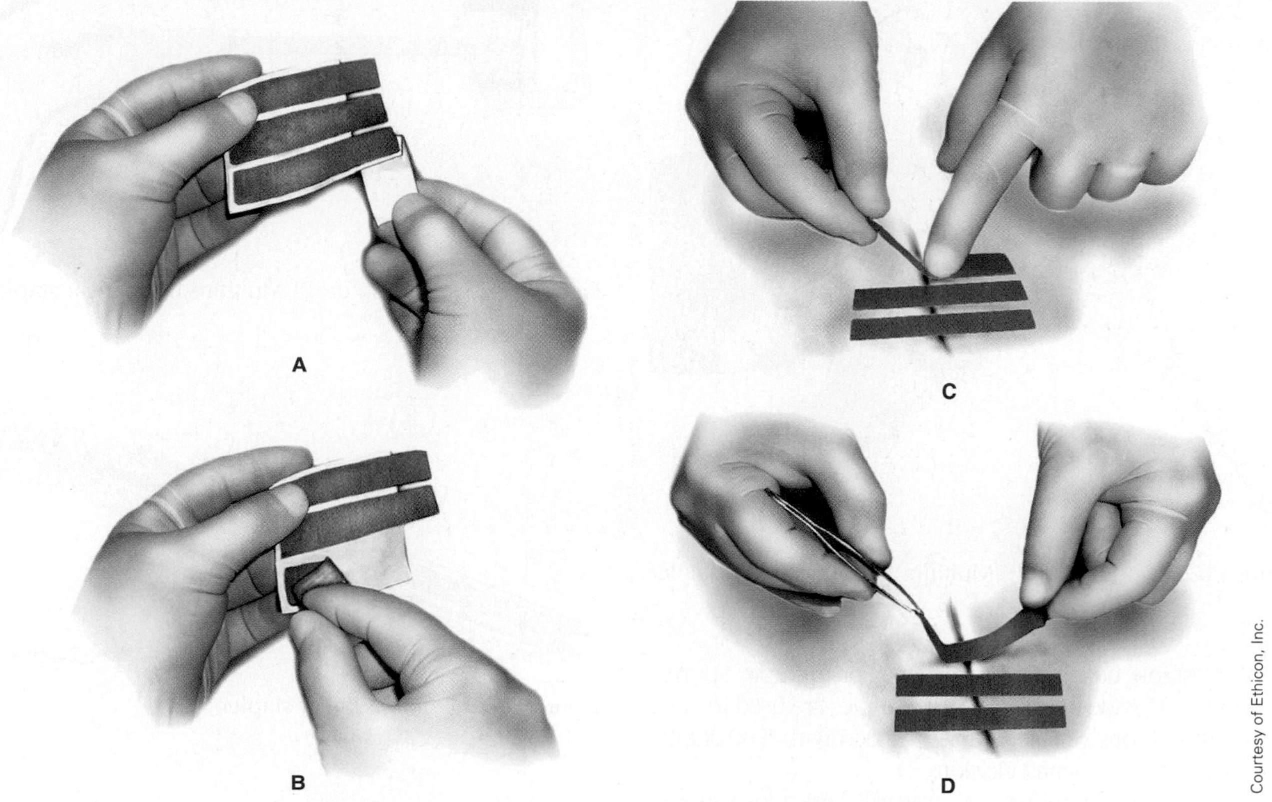

Figure 11-26 Application of skin closure tapes: (A) Using sterile technique, remove card from sleeve and tear off tab, (B) peel off tapes as needed in a diagonal direction, (C) apply tapes at 1/8-in. internals as needed to complete apposition (make sure the skin surface is dry before applying each tape), (D) when healing is judged to be adequate, remove each tape by peeling off each half from the outside toward the wound margin. Then, gently lift the tape away from the wound surface.

Disposable staplers are preassembled, packaged, and sterilized by the manufacturer and are discarded after use. Disposable staplers also have removable, disposable cartridges so that a new stapler is not required each time the stapler is fired.

Stapling offers the following advantages over suturing:

- *Less tissue reaction:* Stainless steel is the least reactive of all wound closure materials.
- *Accelerated wound healing:* Tissues are not handled as much as they would be with suturing, increasing the odds that the wound will heal without incidence. The B shape of the staples allows nutrients to pass through the staple line to the tissue edges.
- *Less operating and anesthesia time:* Stapling takes less time to perform than suturing, resulting in less blood loss during the procedure.
- *Efficiency:* Staples create an airtight and leak-proof anastomosis or closure.

The disadvantages of staple use include:

- *Increased cost.*
- *Staples must be precisely placed:* Errors in technique for linear or circular stapling are much more difficult to correct than suturing errors.

A variety of stapling devices are available to perform the following applications:

- Anastomosis
- Biopsy
- Closure of organs
- Division of tissue
- Fascial closure
- Ligation
- Resection
- Skin closure

TYPES OF STAPLERS

Stapling devices include skin, linear (stapling and cutting), ligating, and intraluminal types. Stapler styles are available to accommodate open and endoscopic procedures.

Skin

Skin staplers are used to approximate skin edges during skin closure (Figure 11-27). These disposable devices dispense a single staple with each activation and they are supplied in a

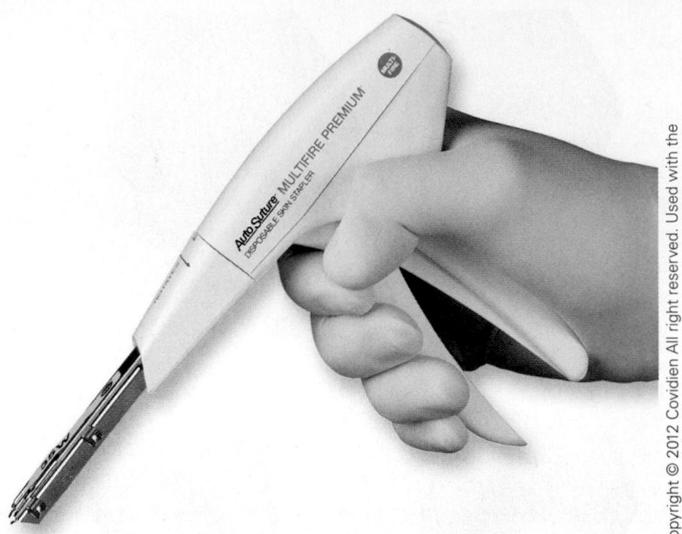

Figure 11-27 AutoSuture™ Multifire™ Premium skin stapler

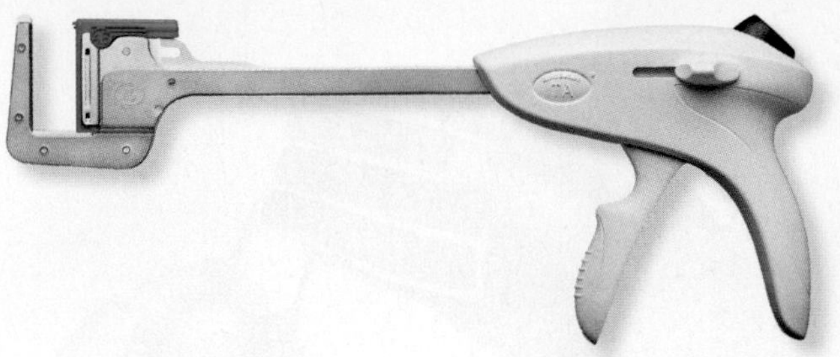

Figure 11-28 AutoSuture™ Multifire TA™ linear stapler

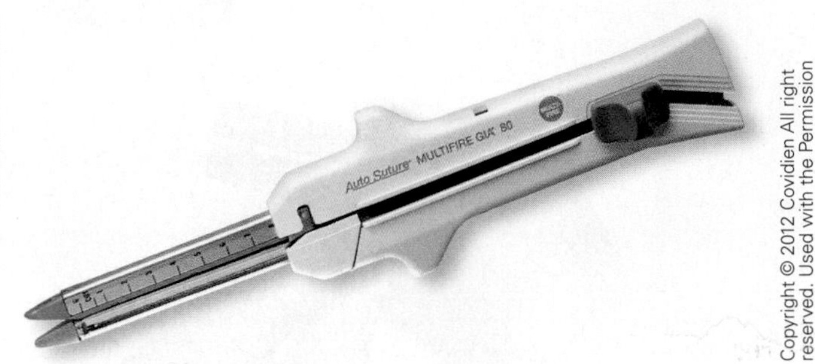

Figure 11-29 GIA™ linear stapler

variety of staple quantities and widths. For example, staplers loaded with 35 wide or regular-width staples are used to close most long incisions. Smaller staplers loaded with 5–10 staples are available to close small incisions.

The surgeon everts (turns outward) and approximates the skin edges with Adson tissue forceps with teeth and the operator positions the stapler at the approximated edges with the aid of an arrow located on the stapler head. A single squeeze and release of the mechanism positions the staple.

Individual staples can also be used to close the tough tissue of the abdominal fascia. This layer is thick and heals slowly. The nonreactive nature of metallic staples makes them an ideal choice for fascia.

Fascia

Fascia staplers are not much different from skin staplers. They are a disposable stapler shaped like a gun and discharge a single wide stainless steel staple by squeezing the handle. The staple first penetrates the fascia and then is formed to approximate the fascia. It is frequently used in abdominal, gynecological, and orthopedic surgery.

Linear Staplers

Linear staplers are used to insert two straight, staggered, evenly spaced, parallel rows of staples into tissue (Figure 11-28). Linear staplers are typically used to staple tissue to be transected within the alimentary tract or thoracic cavity, although they have many other surgical applications as well. The linear stapler is available in various lengths.

To operate the linear stapler, the tissue is placed within the jaws of the stapler at the level of transection. The stapler is closed, compressing the tissue. The safety mechanism is removed and the stapler is activated.

Linear Cutters

The *linear cutter* is used to staple and transect the tissue (Figure 11-29). Linear cutters deliver *two* double staple lines (similar to the one produced by the linear stapler) and contain a knife blade that passes between the two staple lines, dividing the tissue. The linear cutter is especially useful during gastrointestinal procedures.

A variation of the linear cutter is available for endoscopic procedures and is especially useful during gynecological procedures (Figure 11-30).

Ligating Clips

A *ligating clip* is used to occlude a single small structure, such as a blood vessel or a duct. A structure to be divided must have at least two individual clips placed (one or more proximally and one or more distally). The structure is then divided with a scissors or a scalpel. The stainless steel, titanium, tantalum, or absorbable clips are available in an automated disposable applier (Figure 11-31) or may be manually loaded onto a reusable device. A variation of the automated disposable applier is available for endoscopic procedures and is especially useful during cholecystectomy.

Linear Dissecting Stapler

The *linear dissecting stapler* ejects two ligating clips side by side and then divides the tissue between the clips with a single activation. It is especially useful during gastrointestinal procedures for division of the greater omentum.

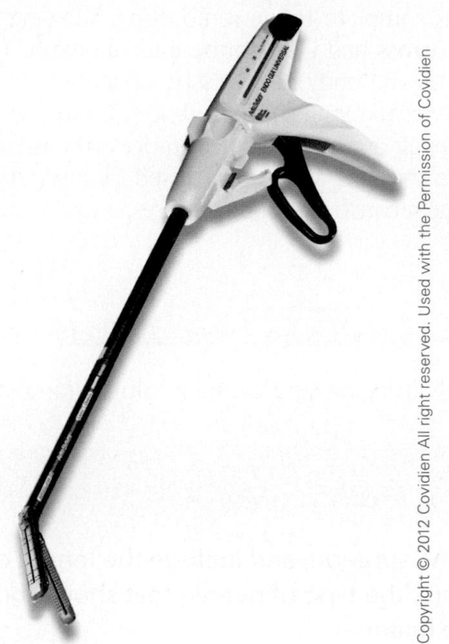

Figure 11-30 Endo GIA™ Universal linear cutter for endoscopic procedures

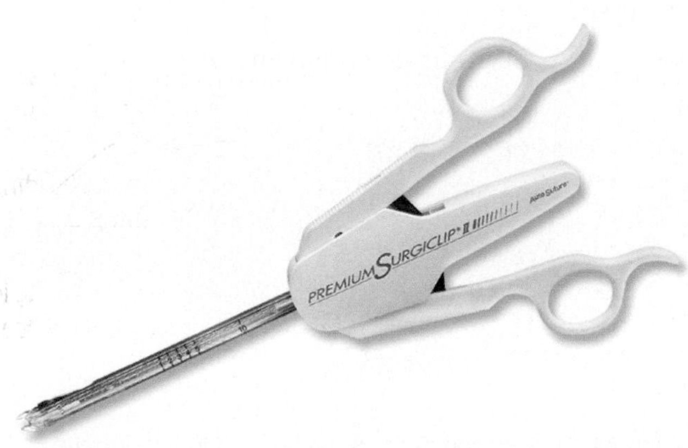

Figure 11-31 Premium Surgiclip™ ligating clip applier

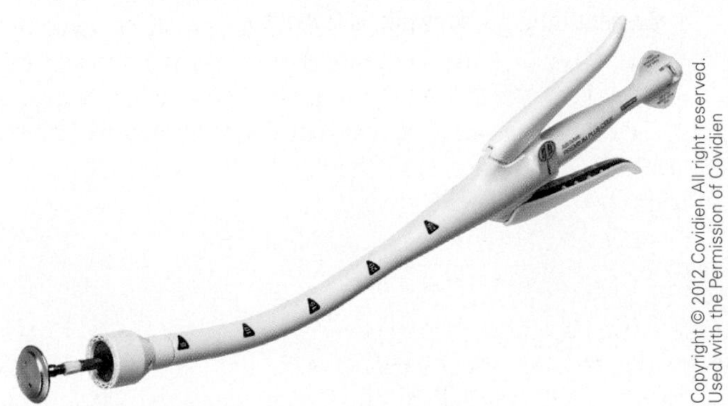

Figure 11-32 EEA™ open intraluminal stapler

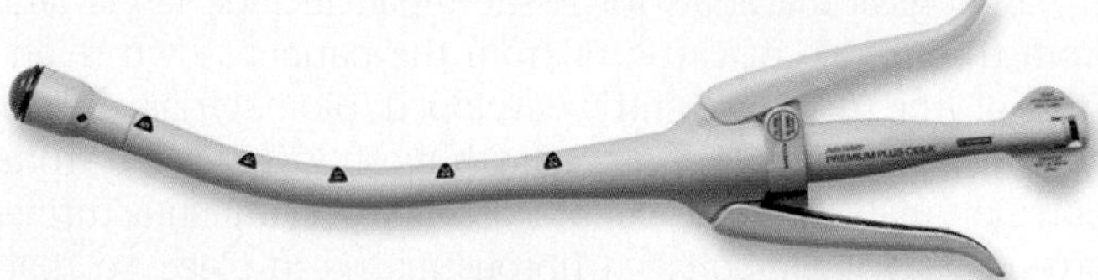

Figure 11-33 EEA™ closed intraluminal stapler

Intraluminal Staplers

Intraluminal (circular) staples are used to anastomose tubular structures within the gastrointestinal tract (Figures 11-32 and 11-33). This stapler fires a double row of circular staples and then trims the lumen with a knife located within the head of the stapler. These staplers are commonly used during resection and reanastomosis of the distal colon or rectum.

MESHES OR FABRICS

Synthetic materials can be used as a bridge for tissues that cannot be brought together without placing a great deal of tension on the tissues. They may also be used as a reinforcement for fascia defects. Surgeons often make use of meshes to strengthen the damaged fascia during hernia repair. Advantages of synthetic meshes include:

- Pliable (except for stainless steel mesh)
- Easy to cut to create the correct size to be implanted
- Easy to suture into place in open or endoscopic procedures
- Porous: Pores in mesh allow fibrous tissue to grow through the mesh, strengthening the tissues

Examples of synthetic meshes include:

- *Polypropylene mesh:* This is a relatively inert material that can be used in the presence of infection. It has excellent elasticity and high tensile strength.
- *Polyglactin 910 mesh:* This is an absorbable material that provides temporary support during healing.
- *Polytetrafluoroethylene (**PTFE**) mesh:* This is a soft, flexible material that is not absorbable and should not be used in the presence of infection.
- *Stainless steel mesh:* This material is rigid and hard to apply, resulting in discomfort for the patient. It is, however, the most inert of the mesh materials and can be used in the presence of infection or during second intention healing.
- *Polyester fiber mesh:* The least inert of the synthetic meshes, it should never be used in the presence of infection because its multifilament fiber construction can harbor bacteria.

Biological materials for tissue repair include fascia lata from the muscle of cattle or from the patient's own thigh. One of the more recently developed biomaterials is in-growth mesh (Surgisis™). In-growth mesh is harvested from porcine small intestine submucosa and the manufacturing process leaves the collagen fibrous matrix in place, so that it is porous to allow for new tissue in-growth. The mesh facilitates complete tissue remodeling, allowing new tissue to grow across and incorporate into the mesh. The mesh is replaced by the body's own tissue, creating a permanent repair without the long-term presence of a foreign body. During the repair and tissue growth process the mesh maintains its tensile strength. The mesh is used for a variety of general soft tissue reconstruction procedures.

CASE STUDY A surgeon working deep within the abdomen suddenly asks the surgical technologist for a stick tie.

1. **Describe what should be passed to the surgeon, and include the length of the needle holder, the length of the suture, the type of needle that should be used, and the type and gauge of the suture material.**

QUESTIONS FOR FURTHER STUDY

1. During what situations would a controlled-release needle be used?
2. What type and gauge of suture would be used to anastomose a synthetic aortic graft onto an aorta during an abdominal aortic aneurysmectomy?
3. Under what conditions are retention sutures used?
4. What are the classic signs of systemic inflammation?
5. How does phagocytosis contribute to wound healing?

BIBLIOGRAPHY

Association of Surgical Technologists. (2006). *Core curriculum for surgical assisting* (2nd ed.). Littleton, CO: Author.

Ethicon, Inc. (2007). *Wound closure manual.* Somerville, NJ: Author.

Fortunato, P. N. (2007). *Berry and Kohn's operating room technique* (11th ed.). St. Louis, MO: Mosby.

Huerk, C. A., & Van Way, C. W., III. (1986). *Pocket manual of basic surgical skills.* St. Louis, MO: Mosby.

Miller, B. F. (2003). *Encyclopedia and dictionary of medicine, nursing, and allied health* (7th ed.). Philadelphia: W. B. Saunders.

Ravitch, M. M., Steichen, F. M., & Welter, R. (1991). *Current practice of surgical stapling.* Philadelphia: Lea & Febiger.

Rothrock, J. C. (2007). *Alexander's care of the patient in surgery* (13th ed.). St. Louis, MO: Mosby Elsevier.

United States Surgical Corporation. (1974). *Stapling techniques in general surgery.* Norwalk, CT: Author.

CHAPTER

12

Surgical Case Management

CASE STUDY During a lumbar discectomy procedure, the surgical technologist removed a specimen from the jaws of a pituitary rongeur. She looked at the specimen and said to the neurosurgeon, "I think you should stop and look at this specimen. It does not look like disc material to me." "How so?" the surgeon asked. "It has a lumen," she said. The surgeon looked at the tissue, had the circulator call a genitourinary specialist, completed the procedure, and assisted on the repair of the ureter.

1. **What did the surgical technologist have to know in order to make this important observation?**
2. **What is the relationship between anatomical and physiological knowledge and practical application in the OR?**
3. **Did the surgical technologist handle the situation well? Explain your response.**

OBJECTIVES

After studying this chapter, the reader should be able to:

C 1. Analyze the role of the surgical technologist in caring for the surgical patient.
2. Verify the preoperative routines that must be completed.
3. Demonstrate the transportation of the surgical patient.
4. Apply the principles of surgical positioning.

A 5. Demonstrate techniques of opening and preparing supplies and instruments needed for any operative procedure with the maintenance of sterile technique at all times.
6. Summarize the methods of preparation of the operative site for surgery.
7. Demonstrate the application of thermoregulatory devices.

R 8. Interpret the principles and demonstrate the taking and recording of vital signs.
9. Interpret the principles of urinary catheterization and demonstrate the procedure.
10. Analyze how the principles of operative site preparation and urinary catheterization are related both to patient care and to the principles of asepsis.

E 11. Demonstrate the proper techniques for the surgical hand scrub, gowning, gloving, and assisting team members.
12. Demonstrate the proper technique for preparing supplies and instruments on a sterile field.
13. Demonstrate and explain in detail the procedure for counting instruments, sponges, needles, and other items on the sterile field.
14. Demonstrate the initial steps for starting a procedure.
15. Demonstrate intraoperative handling of sterile equipment and supplies.
16. Summarize and demonstrate postoperative routines.

SELECT KEY TERMS

adhesive
anticipate
antimicrobial
apical pulse
biohazard
catheterization
circumferentially
count
craniotomy
cylindrical
donning
dyspnea
hand wash
indicator
lap sponge
mask
neutral zone
pathology
PPE
prep
prone
resident organisms
sedation
sterile attire
sterile team members
supine
surgeon's preference card
surgical scrub
transient organisms
vital signs
wraparound-style gown

INTRODUCTION

The surgical technologist provides surgical case management during the perioperative phase. The three phases of case management are the preoperative, intraoperative, and postoperative phases. The surgical technologist normally performs the first scrub role during the surgical procedure, but also performs many nonsterile assisting circulator duties.

1. The preoperative case management phase occurs prior to the skin incision or insertion of an endoscope. Some of the duties of the surgical technologist during the preoperative case management phase are:
   - Don operating room (OR) attire and personal protective equipment (**PPE**).
   - Prepare the OR.
   - Gather the necessary instrumentation, equipment, and supplies for the planned procedure.
   - Scrub and don **sterile attire**.
   - Prepare, organize, and maintain the sterile field.
   - **Count** sponges, sharps, and instruments.
   - Gown and glove sterile team members for entry to the sterile field.
   - Assist with draping the patient.
2. The intraoperative case management phase is the time during which the surgical procedure is being performed. Some of the duties of the surgical technologist during the intraoperative case management phase are:
   - Maintain and continually monitor the sterile field.
   - Pass instrumentation, equipment, and supplies to the surgeon and surgical assistant(s) as needed.
   - Anticipate the needs of the patient and surgeon and provide the necessary items in order of need.
   - Prepare and handle medications.
   - Count sponges, sharps, and instruments.
   - Care for the specimen(s).
   - Apply sterile dressings.
3. The postoperative case management phase begins when the sterile dressing is applied or with extraction of the endoscope. Some of the duties of the surgical technologist during the postoperative case management phase are:
   - Maintain the sterile field until the patient is transported to the postanesthesia care unit (PACU) or critical/intensive care unit (CCU or ICU; health care facilities will use either term).
   - Remove used instrumentation, equipment, and supplies from the OR.
   - Care for and maintain instrumentation, equipment, and supplies following use.
   - Prepare the OR for the next patient.

ANTICIPATION

The ability to **anticipate**, or predict, the needs of the surgeon during case management is one of the most important skills of the surgical technologist. Information gathered during the preoperative phase of case management (from sources such as the **surgeon's preference card** or communication with surgical team members) is integrated into the procedure as needed. Additional information is obtained during the intraoperative case management phase by observing the progression of the procedure, processing the information, and providing any necessary items before they are needed.

Anticipatory skills can be very basic for the novice surgical technologist and they may become more refined as the surgical technologist gains more experience within the surgical suite. Experience is gained by working with a variety of surgeons and by first scrubbing an array of surgical procedures.

Early on in the surgical technologist's training, he or she will learn to employ basic anticipatory skills, such as when the surgeon requests pick-ups, the surgical technologist should be ready with forceps. For example, the surgical technologist who is participating in an appendectomy, using the traditional approach on an adult patient, will expect the surgeon to initiate a McBurney's incision. To make the incision, the surgeon will require a No. 10 scalpel blade loaded onto a No. 3 scalpel handle. Immediately after the incision is made, the wound will most likely bleed. The surgical technologist will be prepared to assist in achieving hemostasis by offering the surgeon the electrosurgical pencil or hemostats, such as curved Criles. It will then be necessary to separate the wound edges for the dissection to continue. Due to the small size of the McBurney's incision and its location in the abdominal wall, the surgical technologist should predict that the surgical assistant will want to use a pair of U.S. Army or small Richardson retractors. Alternatively, if a surgical assistant is unavailable, the surgeon may prefer to use a small self-retaining retractor such as a Weitlaner.

Notice that the sequence of events described above applies not only to the appendectomy procedure but to virtually any surgical procedure. The surgical technologist can predict, or anticipate, that for most procedures an incision will be made, hemostasis achieved, and exposure provided.

PART I: Preoperative Case Management

The preoperative case management phase typically begins at the start of the workday and may be repeated several times throughout the day according to the caseload. A basic preoperative routine and the related concepts and technical skills are presented later in this chapter. The situation described is "ideal"; keep in mind that variations in this routine can occur for a variety of reasons, such as product differences or facility policy. The first portion of this section will discuss preoperative patient routines and then address the specifics of the surgical technologist in preparing the case.

PREOPERATIVE PATIENT ROUTINES

Preoperative preparation includes the psychological and physiological preparation of the patient before surgical intervention. No two patients are exactly the same and each has his or her own specific set of psychological and physiological needs. Providing for the safety of the patient requires knowledge not only of the procedure to be performed but also of any special needs, such as physical limitations or allergies. Every effort should be made to make the patient as mentally and physically comfortable with the process as possible. For the safety of the patient as well as the hospital, all protocols must be followed. Knowledge of the proper techniques of patient identification, transport, and chart documentation are essential in preparing the patient for surgery, as are proper techniques of positioning and emergency procedures.

In the past, almost all surgical patients were admitted several days before surgery for all required laboratory work and surgical preparation. The nurse in the physician's office completed presurgical patient education and the postsurgical stay in the hospital ranged from a few days to weeks of in-hospital recovery. In today's "managed care" environment, patients are usually admitted the day of surgery to a same-day surgery unit, where final laboratory work and preoperative teaching are performed by the hospital's staff nurses. Patients with special medical conditions such as diabetes mellitus or heart disease may be admitted earlier so that these conditions can be monitored and controlled as much as possible throughout the process.

Prior to surgery, certain information and studies must be compiled into the patient's chart or record. Common items found in a patient's chart include the following:

- Laboratory results
- Radiology reports
- Consent for treatment
- Surgical consent form
- Anesthesia consent form
- Preoperative checklist
- Special consent form(s), such as a consent to sterilization (if applicable)

- Previous **pathology** reports
- Nurse's notes
- History and physical report (H & P)
- Identification of patient allergies, handicaps, or other limitations

The records kept in the chart provide both information for the surgical team and an accurate record of patient care. Special needs of the patient may be easily identified from the information available in the chart. The surgical technologist should review the surgical consent form. The history and physical form will give important background on the patient that may help the team member anticipate necessary equipment and possible intraoperative complications. For instance, the patient with arthritis will need special care to avoid pain prior to anesthesia induction and special care during positioning to prevent joint damage. It is especially important that the surgical technologist as well as other members of the team note any pharmacologic or food allergies. These are written in bold letters on a bright colored label affixed to the outside of the chart to minimize danger of administration of drugs to which a patient may have an allergic reaction.

Currently, many health care facilities are implementing an electronic medical record (EMR). An EMR is a computerized version of the patient's medical record. EMRs provide accessibility across health care systems, remove safety concerns of poor legibility, can be continuously updated to reflect the most current patient information, and allow for off-site storage to facilitate access during an all-hazards situation. The surgical technologist should defer to the current patient documentation process within his or her clinical setting.

Preoperative Education

The patient facing surgery has many decisions to make, any of which may produce anxiety. Being given the opportunity to talk with supportive individuals who will be directly involved with the procedure at hand helps to alleviate this anxiety and has been shown to promote better postoperative outcomes. Studies have shown that patient education has a positive effect on postoperative recovery, including improvement in patients' ventilatory status and a decreased need for postoperative analgesic medications. In addition, patients who have received preoperative education have shorter hospital stays, some by as much as 1.3 days.

Increasingly, preoperative education is being done in the physician's office prior to admission. The advent of short-stay and same-day surgery has increased the percentages of admissions on the morning of surgery, bringing about the need for in-office patient education. In some cases, educational pamphlets, CDs, or DVDs are used. The amount of information presented preoperatively should be based on the background of the patient, as well as the interest and anxiety level of the patient. Most patients will find information relating to preoperative tests and procedures and postoperative expectations helpful. The patient should also be informed about what pains and discomforts he or she may expect to experience postoperatively, along with the proper use of any prescribed postoperative medications or other pain management therapies. The patient will also be educated at this point about how to deal with any body changes, immobilizations, or permanent disabilities.

Certain preoperative procedures will be scheduled the evening or morning before surgery. If the patient is being admitted on a same-day basis, some of these procedures will be explained in the office to the patient, and the patient will be expected to complete these procedures at home, such as preoperative bathing, bowel **prep**, or specific hair removal guidelines.

Patients may benefit from information about sensations they may have in the OR, such as the environment of the OR or feelings of drowsiness from preoperative medications. It is helpful to reassure the patient that little or no discomfort is to be expected prior to anesthesia, other than a small needle stick for IV insertion, and that warm blankets will be provided for comfort if desired.

Many patients are taught specific activities to help alleviate preoperative anxiety. These include deep-breathing exercises and positive imagery. One recent approach is the use of music therapy both preoperatively and in the OR.

In the process of preoperative patient education, the need, type, and extent of the surgery should be explained to the patient and to his or her significant others. The patient's understanding should be clarified and explanations should be given about any preoperative tests. The patient should be given the opportunity to express his or her feelings and concerns about the surgery, and significant others who may offer support should be identified.

Patient Possessions

The patient should be instructed to leave valuables at home. Prior to surgery, any remaining valuables and possessions should be collected and either given to a family member or significant other or locked in the hospital's safe or patient unit lockers for security purposes. The patient should be reassured that his or her possessions are safe and that they will be returned after surgery. If the patient is permitted to wear a wedding ring, it should be taped or otherwise secured to the hand to prevent loss. Generally, all jewelry should be removed prior to surgery. Dentures, prostheses, and removable implants must be removed prior to surgery, labeled, and placed in safekeeping with the rest of the patient's possessions. Dentures must be removed because of the danger that they will fall into the pharynx and cause respiratory obstruction when the jaw relaxes under anesthesia. Some anesthesia providers prefer that the patient leave the dentures in until the moment of intubation, as the shape of the dentures allows for a better fit for the face mask. Wigs and hairpins must be removed, because hairpins may become dislodged and injure the scalp and wigs may be lost. If the patient utilizes a hearing aid, it may be left in place. This will facilitate verbal communication with the surgical team in the OR.

A common admissions process for the surgical patient is as follows:

1. Patient arrives at hospital the evening before or morning of surgery.
2. Required paperwork is completed, including all operative and special consents.
3. Identification process of the patient is initiated at the time of registration and continues throughout the perioperative process. The patient's identification bracelet is affixed. The identification of the patient is one element of the Universal Protocol.
4. Patient changes clothes.
5. **Vital signs** are taken.
6. Per physician request, patient may require preoperative hair removal and a preoperative antiseptic cleanse.
7. Surgical site is verified with patient and may be marked per health care facility policy.
8. Any necessary IVs are started.
9. Patient chart is reviewed by surgical team (including the preoperative RN, OR RN, surgeon, anesthesia provider).
10. Time is allowed with family and clergy as requested by the patient.
11. Preoperative medication is given if required.
12. Patient is transported to the OR.

Enemas

The enema is no longer a routine preoperative procedure, except in the case of certain gastrointestinal and gynecological procedures. Its purpose is the prevention of injury to the colon and to allow better visualization of the surgical area. Any time a patient has had barium studies performed immediately before surgery, enemas are indicated because the presence of barium in the bowel will predispose the patient to postoperative fecal impactions. If ordered, the enema should be administered 8–12 hours prior to the operation. When full bowel cleansing is not required, the patient may be given a mild laxative to provide for successful evacuation the evening before surgery.

Nail Polish

Prior to surgery, nail polish should be removed. The pulse oximeter, a device used intraoperatively to measure blood oxygen saturation, cannot function properly with nail polish present, as it relies on a light beam focused through the skin and nail of the finger. Colored nail polish also prevents proper assessment of nail bed color for capillary blanching and refill.

Sedation

Preoperative medications used to induce **sedation** are often administered by the anesthesia provider at the time of the preoperative visit. Other medications are given to decrease the secretion of saliva and gastric juices, prevent allergic reaction to anesthetic drugs, and decrease nausea. A preoperative antibiotic may be ordered by the surgeon to aid in preventing a postoperative surgical site infection. These medications are usually administered 1–2 hours prior to surgery. Any delay in the administration of these drugs should be reported to the anesthesia provider. All preoperative routines should be completed prior to the administration of preoperative medications, and the patient should be allowed to relax in a quiet place after receiving the medication. During this time, the side rails on the stretcher should be raised, and the patient should not be left alone. The patient must not be allowed to sign the surgical consent form after receiving this medication.

Preoperative Hygiene

The surgical patient should shower or bathe the night before or morning of the surgery and should be reminded to wash their hair, as it may be several days or longer before this can be done again. Surgeons may request that the patient shower with an antiseptic containing chlorhexidine or povidone-iodine in some cases where there is a particular risk of surgical site infection (SSI). Some studies have shown a decreased microbial count on the skin of surgical patients who have showered with an **antimicrobial** soap preoperatively. The patient should also be reminded to brush his or her teeth prior to surgery, as good oral hygiene is helpful in prevention of infection.

Preoperative Hair Removal

If ordered, hair removal may need to be performed prior to surgery. Patients may be provided with specific hair removal guidelines to follow at their home prior to their scheduled surgery. Preoperative hair removal that occurs in the health care setting can be performed by the preoperative RN, patient care assistant, or surgical technologist. Care should be taken to avoid cutting or nicking the skin, as breaks in the skin surface provide an easy opportunity for bacterial entry and wound infection. Some medical facilities will choose the use of a depilatory cream. After the cream has remained on the skin for the prescribed amount of time, it is wiped off and hair is removed. This method is beneficial in that it does not cut the skin. Often, patient hair removal is performed in the OR, although objections have been raised to this on the grounds that the operation is delayed and loose hair is released into the operative environment, where it may find its way onto the sterile field. Recent studies have shown that the preoperative use of clippers is the best method for hair removal if hair is to be removed at all, and the Centers for Disease Control and Prevention (CDC) recommends not removing hair preoperatively unless it interferes with the operation, as microbial counts have been shown to be increased in preshaved areas of the skin.

Diet

The day before surgery, a normal diet is usually indicated. In the case of bowel surgery, a low-residue diet may be necessary. No food or liquid is permitted by mouth for at least 6–8 hours prior to surgery. The presence of food or fluids in the stomach during surgery increases the danger of aspiration should the patient vomit while under anesthesia, which can lead to pneumonia and death. If it is discovered prior to surgery that the patient has consumed food or fluids despite having been ordered to take nothing by mouth (NPO), the surgeon should be notified immediately. The surgeon may then reschedule the procedure.

Makeup and Dress

The patient is instructed not to wear any makeup to the OR. While the danger of makeup shedding and entering the operative site is minimal, it does exist, and the use of makeup may prevent the anesthesia provider from monitoring skin tone and color properly. A psychological accommodation may be made, however, for the patient who is uncomfortable without the most basic makeup.

The patient is generally required to remove all personal clothing and wear a clean hospital gown. In the case of the weight-challenged patient, two gowns may be tied back to back to facilitate comfort and provide cover. In cases where the patient is allowed to keep some personal clothing items, such as the underwear under the gown, those items will need to be removed in the OR after induction of anesthesia and returned to the family or locked up for safekeeping with the rest of the patient's personal belongings. In cases where there is a high risk for postoperative thromboembolism, the patient may have antiembolic stockings or elastic bandages applied to their lower extremities. These use pressure to help prevent venous stasis, which can lead to thromboembolism and shock.

ATTIRE

The surgical technologist reports to the facility in street clothes at the designated time (or is "called in" to participate in an emergency procedure); signs in, if necessary; and enters the department. Authorized personnel in street clothes may pass through the nonrestricted area and proceed to the locker room to change into OR attire.

Three types of attire are required for personnel who enter the OR and perform various case management functions: OR attire, PPE, and sterile attire. Certain types of attire may be listed in more than one category. For example, the hair cover is a component of OR attire but is also considered protective attire.

OR Attire

OR attire is worn in the semirestricted and restricted areas of the OR to protect both the patient and the staff by keeping microbial counts to a minimum and limiting microbial spread (Figure 12-1). OR attire consists of a scrub suit and hair cover. A **mask** and shoe covers may also be required. The use of cosmetics (e.g., makeup, fragrance, nail polish, or artificial nails or tips) and wearing of jewelry of any type, including a wedding band, is restricted according to facility policy.

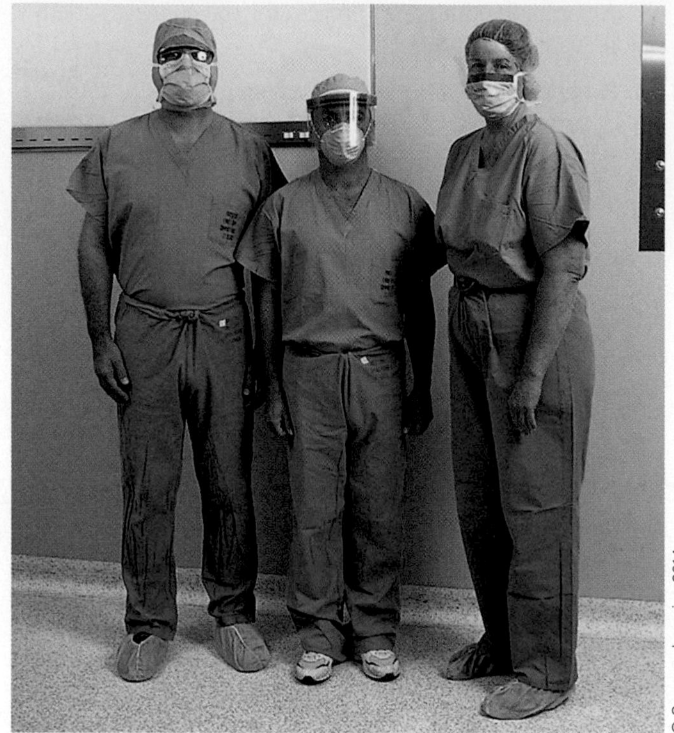

Figure 12-1 OR attire

TECHNIQUE

Operating Room Attire

1. Apply hair cover prior to donning scrub suit.
2. Don scrub suit.
3. Remove body adornments and excess cosmetics, as needed.
4. Apply identification badge and radiation monitoring device, if necessary.
5. Change into shoes appropriate to the OR; apply shoe covers, if necessary.
6. Apply mask and protective eyewear, as needed.

Scrub Suit

Each surgical team member must don a scrub suit ("scrubs") prior to entering any restricted or semirestricted area. Scrub suits come in a variety of sizes and styles.

The scrub suit has been shown to reduce particle shedding into the environment from the body, which helps maintain the clean operative environment. Scrub suits should therefore be close fitting and shirts and drawstrings should be tucked into the pants.

After each daily use they should be removed and placed in the appropriate receptacle to be laundered by the approved laundry facility. If scrubs become soiled or wet with blood, body fluids, sweat, or food, they should be changed immediately. This helps prevent cross-contamination and generally adds to the comfort of OR personnel. The surgical technologist will need to become familiar with the health care facilities policies on the wearing of the scrub suit, e.g., required or not required to wear a laboratory (lab) coat when leaving the department and laundry policies. However, scrubs worn outside the health care facility should not be worn in the OR; the individual should change into a clean scrub suit.

Hair Cover

While in the semirestricted and restricted areas of the surgery department, a cap or hood is worn to cover all hair of the head and face. Hair has been shown to be a major source of contamination; therefore, no hair should be left exposed while one is in the surgical environment. Hair covers are donned prior to the scrub suit to decrease the possibility of hair or dandruff being shed onto the scrub suit, prevent contamination of the wound, and decrease microbial dispersal. Head coverings include hats, caps, hoods, and even "space helmets" that completely enclose the head and provide their own ventilation system. Hoods that cover both the head and the sides of the face are provided for individuals with facial hair. "Space helmet" systems are usually used in high-infection-risk environments, such as open-joint orthopedic surgery. Skullcap-type hair covers should not be used unless the individual has very short hair that can be completely covered by this type of cap. Personnel with longer hair should wear bouffant-type caps or hoods. Most caps are disposable, single-use items, although some hospitals allow reusable head covers if they are laundered daily by a hospital-approved facility. If reusable head covers are used, they should be made of a densely woven, lint-free material. Disposable head covers are made of lint-free nonwoven material. After use, disposable hair covers should be immediately placed in a designated receptacle. Hair covers should be changed if they become wet or soiled.

Mask

A mask must be worn at all times in any restricted area where sterile supplies are open and while surgery is in progress (Figure 12-2). The mask should fit snugly over the mouth and nose. Most disposable masks have a metal or plastic noseband that can be contoured to fit over the bridge of the nose. To prevent fogging of protective eyewear, tape may be used to cover this portion of the mask, but care should be taken to use a nonirritating type of tape, because the skin under the eyes is very sensitive and prone to irritation.

The mask is secured to the head with either an elastic band or two pairs of strings. To ensure a snug, comfortable fit, the strings of the mask should not be crossed when tied. Some mask styles incorporate protective eyewear, for example, a mask with an attached eye protection shield. The CDC and the National Institute for Occupational Safety and Health (NIOSH) recommend the use of the N95 respirator when caring for patients with tuberculosis.

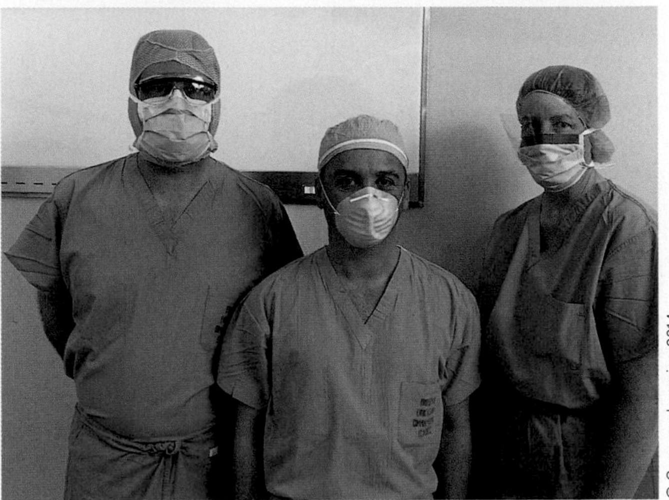

Figure 12-2 Examples of mask types

Masks are worn to contain and filter moisture droplets expelled from the mouth and nasopharynx during talking and normal breathing, as well as during sneezing and coughing. The mask also filters inhaled air and serves to protect the user from fluid splashes to the face.

Masks should be either on or off. *They should never be untied and allowed to hang down around the neck,* because they harbor many microorganisms that will further contaminate the scrub suit and the microbes can be dispersed into the environment. In addition, masks should be handled by the strings or elastic band and only handled minimally. If a mask is not in use, it should be removed and discarded in the proper container. *Masks should be changed between all cases.*

Shoe Covers

Protective shoe covers are worn in the semirestricted and restricted areas of the surgery department, primarily as PPE to shield the shoes and feet from gross fluid contamination. Shoe covers wear out quickly and should be changed as often as necessary. When a procedure will require large amounts of irrigation fluid or there is a possibility that large spills may occur, some individuals prefer to wear the larger impervious boot-style shoe covers (Figure 12-3).

Some health care facility policies allow individuals to provide their own shoes to be worn exclusively in the surgery department without shoe covers, as long as the shoes meet surgery department policies (e.g., no open toes). These shoes must not, however, be worn outside the surgical suite; this is necessary to prevent cross-contamination to and from the outside areas of the facility. Even if shoe covers are not required at a certain facility, their use may still be indicated for personal protection according to the situation. If shoe covers are used, they must be removed whenever they become soiled or wet and must always be removed when one leaves the surgical suite.

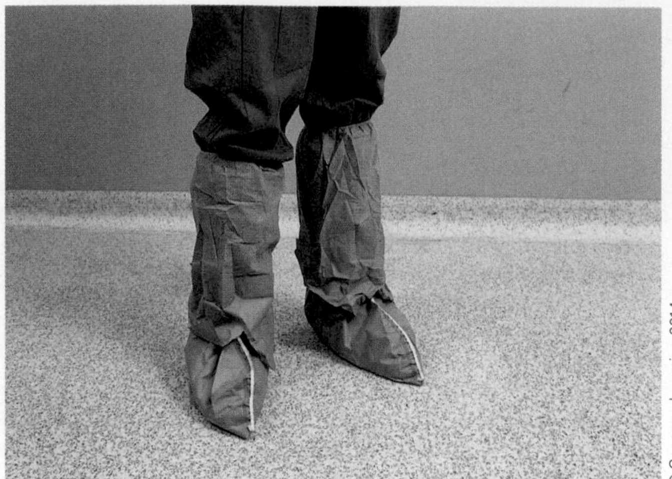

Figure 12-3 Impervious boots

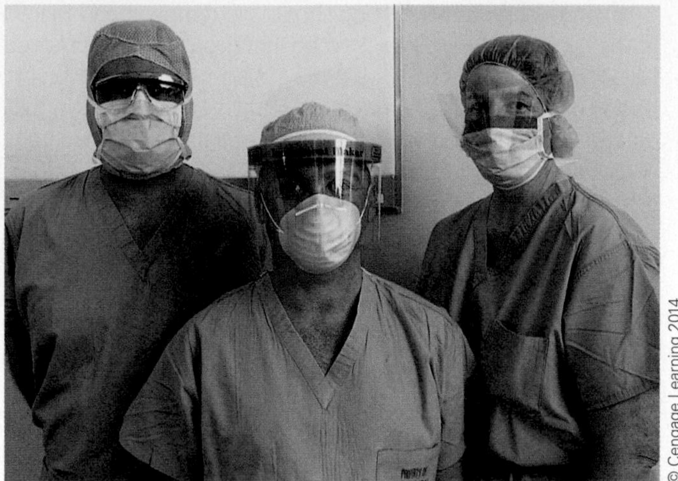

Figure 12-4 Examples of protective eyewear

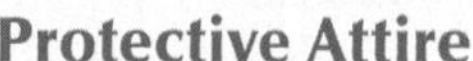

Protective Attire

Personal Protective Equipment (PPE) is worn to protect the health care provider and the patient not only from microbial contact, but also from environmental hazards (e.g., radiation, lasers). PPE includes nonsterile gloves, protective eyewear, and radiation protection.

Sterile team members must don some types of protective attire (e.g., protective eyewear and lead apron) prior to performing the surgical scrub. When a lead apron is required, the sterile attire is worn over the lead apron.

Nonsterile Gloves

As part of Standard Precautions, gloves must be worn any time contact with broken skin or body fluids is expected. When this contact is to occur outside the sterile field, nonsterile latex or vinyl gloves are available. Clean items should not be handled with soiled gloves, and gloves should be removed immediately after use and discarded in the appropriate receptacle. A **hand wash** should be performed immediately following glove removal.

Protective Eyewear

Protective eyewear should be worn any time an environmental hazard exists or exposure to blood or body fluids may occur (Figure 12-4). Eyewear or face shields that provide protection on all sides should be worn to reduce the risk of blood or body fluids splashing into the eyes.

Disposable plastic face shields that can be worn over the mask provide excellent protection for the eyes, nose, and mouth. Many have an attached foam brow band that offers protection from sweat or fluid falling into the eyes Mask-shield combinations without the upper foam band should be worn with caution, because they afford little protection from splashes from above. Regular eyeglasses with side and top shields applied or goggles are other options for eye protection. Prescription goggles are available. Experimentation with different types of face shields may be necessary to find one that offers protection, comfort, and maximum visibility. Specialized eyewear is also available to offer protection from radiation and laser injury. Use caution when selecting laser eyewear to ensure that the optical density of the lens is compatible for protection from the specific type of laser in use.

Radiation Protection

Radiation is routinely encountered in the OR in the form of x-rays; however, various other radioactive elements may also be used. Lead shielding devices are available to protect the staff and the patient from unnecessary exposure, including (see Chapter 5 for detailed information):

- Portable lead screen
- Lead apron
- Lead sternal/thyroid shield
- Leaded glasses
- Lead-impregnated gloves

Other Protective Attire

According to the situation, additional protective attire may also be required. A fluidproof apron may be worn by environmental services personnel and individuals working in the decontamination area of the sterile processing department.

Sterile Attire

Sterile attire is worn by the sterile surgical team members and is donned after performing the **surgical scrub**. Sterile attire is necessary for entry into the sterile field and consists of the sterile gown and gloves.

Sterile Gown

A sterile gown is worn by all sterile team members. Sterile gowns may be disposable or reusable and must be constructed of a lint-free woven or nonwoven fabric that offers a protective barrier. The front of the gown from the mid-chest level to the waist and the sleeves **circumferentially** to 2 inches proximal to the elbows is considered sterile. The cuffs of the gown are considered nonsterile and must always be covered by the cuff of the glove. Various types of gowns are available to provide protection from blood, body fluids, and irrigation solutions. *Fluid-resistant* gowns are cost effective but provide a low level of protection. *Impervious* gowns contain fluid-proof reinforcements in the front and in the sleeves. *Full-coverage systems,* sometimes referred to as space suits, are available for orthopedic and other high-risk procedures. The gown portion envelops the wearer's body to below the knees and has a hooded face shield or helmet that covers the head, neck, and shoulders. The full-coverage gown contains a ventilation system and many contain communication systems because the noise generated by the ventilation system and the wearing of the space helmet makes it extremely difficult to hear other surgical members.

Sterile Gloves

Sterile gloves are worn by all sterile team members. The sterile gloves are applied immediately after donning the sterile gown. Sterile gloves are available in a variety of styles and sizes and have been developed for specific surgical specialties (such as ophthalmology and orthopedics). Latex-free gloves are available for health care personnel who are allergic to latex. Latex-free gloves are also worn by members of the surgical team when caring for patients who may have a sensitivity or allergy to latex products. Extra protection from puncture or seepage of fluid through the gloves may be afforded by wearing glove liners (made of materials such as steel or Kevlar) or double gloving (Figure 12-5). Studies have shown that the incidence of disease contracted from puncture injuries decreases sharply when the injury occurs to a double-gloved hand. As a sharp item passes through the layers of the gloves, fluid and debris are removed and less bioburden is transmitted by the item if a skin puncture occurs.

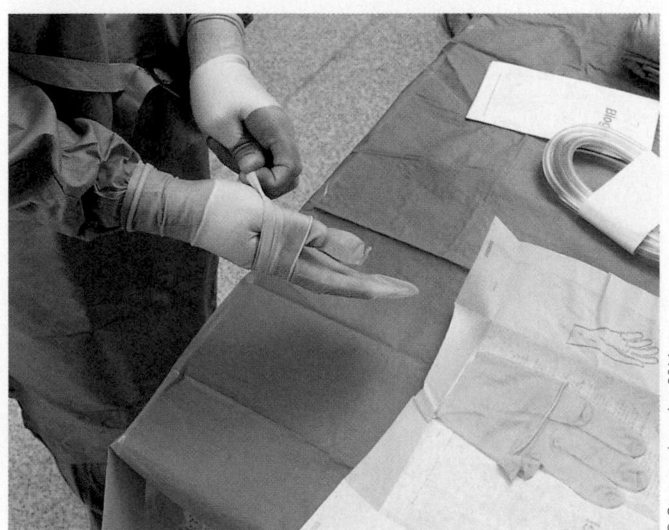

Figure 12-5 Double gloving

Additionally, double gloving is recommended for the following reasons:

- Fat is known to degrade latex.
- The barrier efficiency of latex decreases over time.
- The structure of latex is lattice-like, containing many spaces that fill with fluid during the surgical procedure. As the gloves become saturated with fluid, pathways may be created through the latex, allowing the passage of fluid to the wearer's skin.

Double gloving significantly reduces the amount of blood contamination of the hands.

When double gloving, extra comfort may be achieved by wearing an inner glove one-half to one full size larger than the wearer's normal glove size, and wearing an outer glove of normal size. While this method may seem backward, it often provides a greater level of comfort than two pairs of gloves of the same size. Experimentation with different glove types and sizes will allow the wearer to achieve the desired level of comfort and tactile awareness.

Note: Sterile gloves may be used without a sterile gown to allow a nonsterile team member to perform a sterile activity, such as urinary catheterization. However, in that situation they are not considered scrub attire.

PREPARING THE OPERATING ROOM

When properly attired, the surgical technologist reports to the main OR desk to obtain necessary information about that day's assignment. Preparation for the first surgical case of the day is slightly different from preparation for subsequent cases. Some of the activities need only be performed once each day or are included in the postoperative case management activities and do not have to be repeated. At many facilities, ancillary personnel may perform some of the tasks.

On entering the restricted area, a basic hand wash is performed. Depending on facility policy, application of the mask may be necessary at this time. All equipment and horizontal surfaces in the OR are wiped down with disinfectant solution and another hand wash should be performed after this activity.

OPERATING ROOM SETUP

Verify that all necessary furniture (e.g., IV stands, anesthesia provider's cart) and equipment (e.g., electrosurgical unit, microscope) is present in the OR and remove any unnecessary items. Furniture and equipment are arranged for ease of use, efficiency, and the best possible sterile technique. Whenever possible, the back table, Mayo stand, and ring stands should be positioned so that the sterile field is established in the area farthest from the door. When the OR doors open and close,

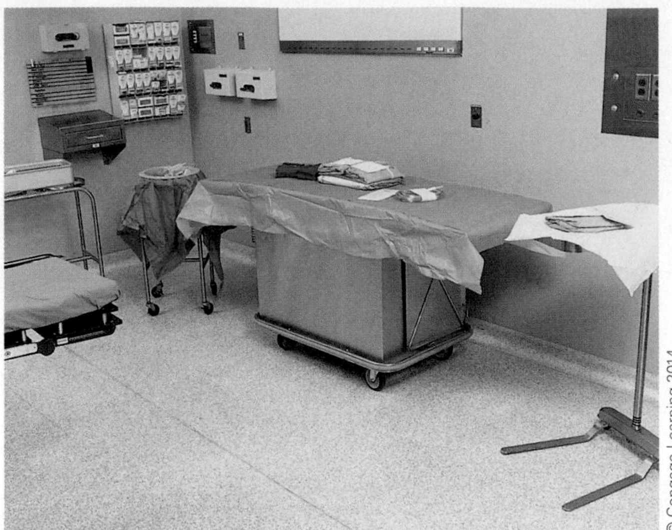

Figure 12-6 Furniture placement in the OR

air movement is at its highest; therefore, it is advantageous to establish the sterile field as far as possible from the doors and from human traffic into and out of the room. All tables that are to be set up as part of the sterile field should be placed at least 12 inches from the walls. All other furniture should be placed side by side and away from any major traffic paths (Figure 12-6).

The OR table is positioned under the operating lights in the orientation required for the procedure. The anesthesia machine is typically placed at the head of the table. The operating lights are checked at this time for functionality and positioned close to where they will be focused for the procedure. All other equipment (e.g., patient monitors, electrosurgical unit, tourniquet, suction system) is tested for functionality.

Bags for laundry, clean waste, and biohazardous waste should be in the hamper frames. These are positioned so that waste can be easily disposed of during initial setup, but at a safe distance from the sterile field. Kick buckets are lined with impervious **biohazard** liners. Suction canisters should have new suction liners. The suction tubing should be attached to the wall vacuum outlet. Confirm that a second suction apparatus is available and functional for management of the patient's airway.

GATHERING INSTRUMENTATION AND SUPPLIES

The surgeon's preference card is obtained and the necessary instrumentation and supplies are gathered for the surgical procedure and placed on a case cart. The preference card may be computer generated (Figure 12-7) or handwritten. Additional information concerning the procedure may be obtained from other sources such as the patient, the patient's chart, or other surgical team members. In some facilities the majority of instrumentation, supplies, and equipment is gathered by central sterile supply personnel; the surgical technologist must only locate the case cart and ensure everything is present. This case cart system is a good example of interdepartmental teamwork. The case cart is brought into the OR and the items are positioned for use. The back table pack is placed on the back table, the basin set is placed on the ring stand, and the instrument set is placed on a flat surface near the back table. If instruments or endoscopes must be sterilized, they are placed in the sterilizer (steam or peracetic acid) and processed at this time. Any items not needed immediately (e.g., dressing materials) are placed in a location where they will be convenient for the circulator to retrieve and open when needed.

CREATING AND MAINTAINING THE STERILE FIELD

The mask must be applied prior to creation of the sterile field and must be worn by all individuals in the OR. The door of the OR is closed prior to preparation of the sterile field and should remain closed as much as possible, as long as the sterile field needs to be maintained.

TECHNIQUE
Opening the Back Table Pack

Refer to Figure 12-8A–C.

1. Check the integrity of the outer packaging material.
2. Check the expiration dates (if present).
3. Remove the outer packaging material.
4. Check the integrity of the inner packaging material.
5. Orient the pack correctly on the back table.
6. Break or remove the seal.
7. Unfold the first flap away from you.
8. Unfold the second flap toward you.
9. Remove any accessory items, if included (some manufacturers place a sterile gown under the second flap for the surgical technologist to use).
10. Reposition yourself as necessary to open the third flap.
11. Insert your hands under the cuff, grasp, and extend the drape to cover the table.
12. Move to the opposite side of the table and open the fourth flap.

Preference Card

Surgeon:	**Dr. Mitchell**	
Procedure:	**Appendectomy - Adult (Traditional Approach)**	
Position:	**Supine**	
Glove Size/Style:	**8 white with 7½ ortho over**	Dominant Hand: **Right**
Equipment:	**Electrosurgical unit with dispersive electrode** **Standard setting: 40/40 Blend 1** **Suction Apparatus** **Headlamp (available)**	
Supplies:	**Basic pack (customized)** **Laparotomy sheet (vertical fenestration)** **Double basin set** **Gloves for all sterile team members** **Poole suction tip—disposable** **Electrosurgical pencil** **Aerobic and anaerobic culture tubes (available)**	
Instrumentation:	**Minor instrumentation set** **Medium Richardson retractor**	
Suture and Usage:	**Ties:**	**2-0 Vicryl Reel**
	Pursestring:	**3-0 Vicryl SH**
	Peritoneum:	**2-0 Vicryl CT-1**
	Fascia:	**2-0 Vicryl CT-1 x 3**
	Sub-Q:	**None or 3-0 Vicryl CT-1 (obese patient)**
	Skin:	**Staples or 3-0 Nylon (if ruptured)**
Dressings:	**Bacitracin ointment** **Telfa** **4x4 gauze** **2″ Paper tape**	
Skin Prep:	**Clip hair, if necessary** **Betadine—5 minute**	
Medications:	**Bupivacaine 0.5% (available for postoperative pain control)** **Control syringe (if needed)** **25-gauge 1½″ needle (if needed)**	

Figure 12-7 Sample surgeon preference card

Opening Sterile Supplies

Before opening any sterile item:

- Verify that the item has been exposed to a sterilization process by inspecting the chemical **indicator** for the appropriate color change.
- Examine the integrity of the packaging material to be sure that it is dry and does not have any tears, perforations, or watermarks.
- Ensure that the expiration date, if present, has not passed.

Any item that does not meet these criteria is not used. Because of its central location, it is recommended that the back table pack be opened first (Figure 12-8). This allows freedom of movement around the back table. As the outer wrap of the pack is opened it covers the back table, creating a sterile field and exposing the sterile supplies within. If an item is double wrapped, it will be necessary to open both wrappers at this time. If disposable packaging material is sealed with tape, the tape should be broken at the seal rather than removed because removal can damage the integrity of the packaging material. As additional items are opened, the

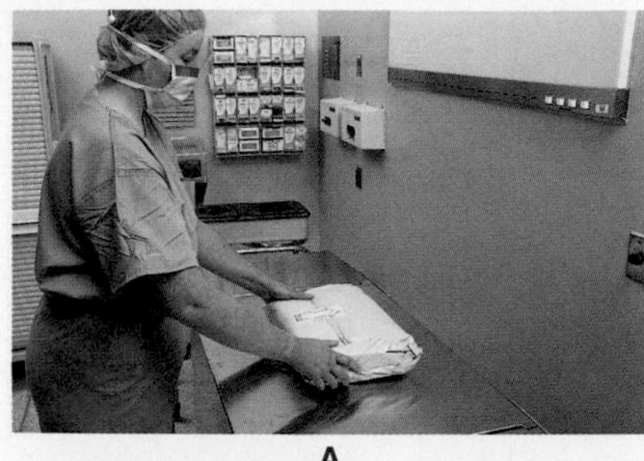
A

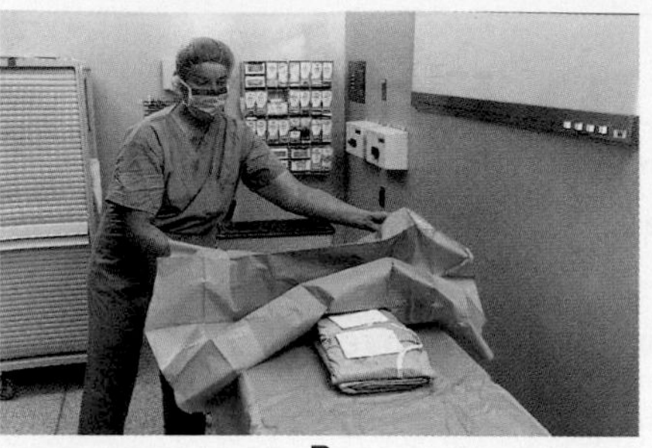
B

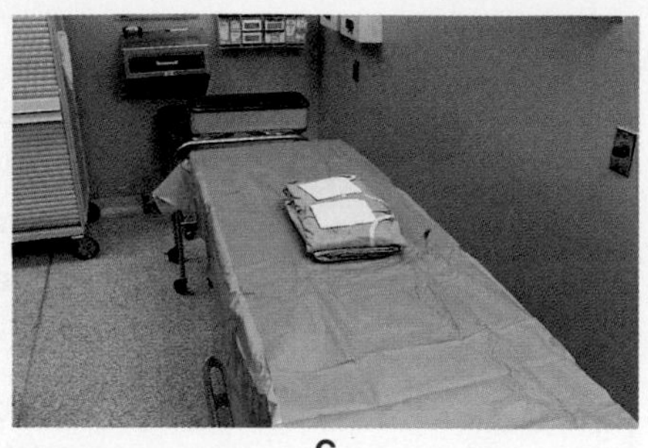
C

Figure 12-8 Opening the back table pack: (A) Position pack on back table, (B) place hands under the cuff and unfold, (C) pack opened

TECHNIQUE

Opening the Basin Set

Refer to Figure 12-9.

1. Check the integrity of the outer packaging material.
2. Remove the outer packaging material.
3. Check the integrity of the inner packaging material.
4. Orient the basin set on the appropriate-size ring stand.
5. Break or remove the seal.
6. Unfold the first flap away from you.
7. Grasp the tab and open the second and third flaps laterally.
8. Open the fourth flap toward you.
9. Place the ring stand in proximity to the back table.

TECHNIQUE

Opening a Small Wrapped Package (Such as Initial Gown) on a Clean Surface

1. Check the integrity of the packaging material.
2. Orient the gown package on the Mayo stand.
3. Break or remove the seal, if present.
4. Grasp the tab and open the first flap away from you.
5. Grasp the tab and open the second and third flaps laterally.
6. Grasp the tab and open the fourth flap toward you.
7. Open the appropriate-size gloves.

Figure 12-9 Opening the basin set

sterile field is expanded. Typically, the larger items such as the basin set and the instrument set are opened next and then smaller remaining wrapped and peel-packed items are placed onto the sterile field (Figures 12-9, 12-10, and 12-11). To reduce the risk of contamination of the sterile field, the surgical technologist's gown and gloves should be opened on a separate surface, such as the Mayo stand, rather than the back table.

Scrubbing and Donning Sterile Attire

Once the sterile field is established, the surgical technologist performs the surgical scrub and dons the sterile attire in preparation for entry to the sterile field. Be sure that all personal needs are taken care of and that all necessary PPE (e.g., protective eyewear, radiation shield) has been donned prior to initiating the surgical scrub.

TECHNIQUE

Opening a Small Wrapped Package onto the Sterile Field

Refer to Figure 12-10.

1. Check the integrity of the packaging material.
2. Orient the package in one hand so that the first flap will be opened away from you.
3. Break or remove the seal.
4. Grasp the tab and open the first fold away from you with your opposite hand.
5. Secure the flap in the hand that is holding the sterile package.
6. Open the second fold laterally and secure the flap without reaching over the exposed sterile item.
7. Open the third fold laterally and secure the flap.
8. Open the fourth fold toward you and secure the flap.
9. Transfer the item onto the sterile field by tossing it gently without crossing the boundary for the sterile field.
10. Retract your hands as soon as the item is airborne.
11. Discard the wrapper.

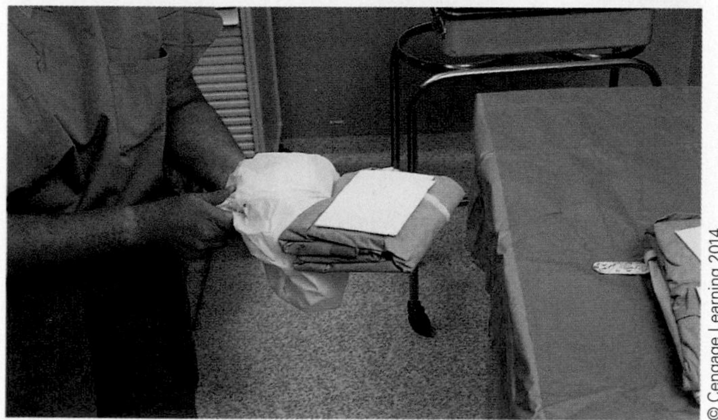

Figure 12-10 Opening a small wrapped package

The Surgical Scrub

Any individual who enters the sterile surgical field must scrub his or her hands and arms to 2 inches above the elbows with an antimicrobial scrub solution (refer to Chapter 7) prior to each surgical procedure. Some health care organizations also offer waterless/brushless surgical hand hygiene methods, for example, alcohol-based hand antiseptic. This surgical scrub is intended to remove as many microorganisms as possible from the hands and arms and to render the hands surgically clean prior to donning the sterile gown and gloves (Figure 12-12).

Two types of organisms live on and in the skin. **Transient organisms** are organisms that have been acquired by touching fomites contaminated with these organisms. These organisms are on the surface of the skin and are easily removed by hand washing or scrubbing. **Resident organisms** (flora) thrive deeper below the surface of the skin and are therefore more difficult to remove. The flora cannot be totally removed by scrubbing, although mechanical action does bring some of them to the

TECHNIQUE

Opening a Peel Pack

Refer to Figure 12-11.

1. Check the integrity of the packaging material.
2. Orient the package in both hands by grasping one edge of the peel pack in each hand.
3. Slowly separate the sides of the peel pack.
4. Balance the item within the package to prevent contamination.
5. Maintain a safe distance from the sterile field while continuing to open the package.
6. Transfer the item onto the sterile field by tossing gently without crossing the boundary for the sterile field.
7. Retract your hands as soon as the item is airborne.
8. Discard the wrapper.

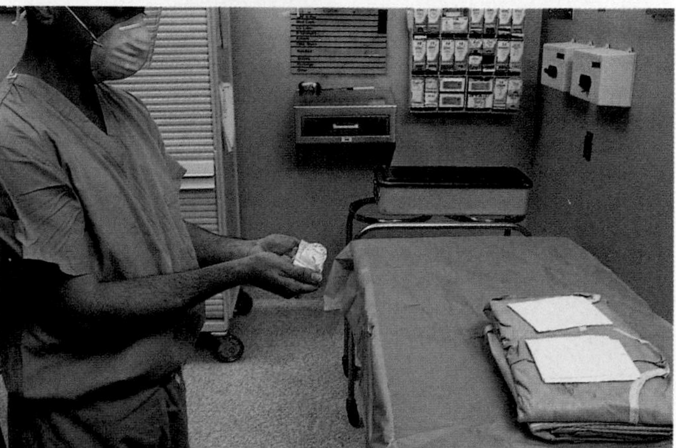

Figure 12-11 Opening a peel pack

surface. Over time, these microorganisms work their way to the surface of the skin, contaminating the skin. For this reason, it is preferable to use a surgical scrub solution that provides a film of protection lasting for several hours. This film will continue to kill any resident microbes that may reach the surface of the skin in the several hours following the surgical scrub.

Equipment and Methods for the Surgical Scrub

Each facility provides a variety of disposable scrub brushes impregnated with antiseptic solution. When a plain brush is used, containers of various antiseptic solutions (refer to Chapter 7)

TECHNIQUE

Opening the Instrument Set (Container System)

1. Place the instrument container on a suitable surface.
2. Verify the presence of filters and color change of external chemical indicator(s).
3. Break or remove the seals, ensuring that fragments of the seal do not become airborne.
4. Release the mechanism securing the lid.
5. Lift the lid vertically 12–18 inches above the container, then step back.
6. Invert the lid and inspect; verify that the inner surface of the lid is dry and that the filter is dry and intact.
7. Place the lid on the shelf of the back table or in the case cart.

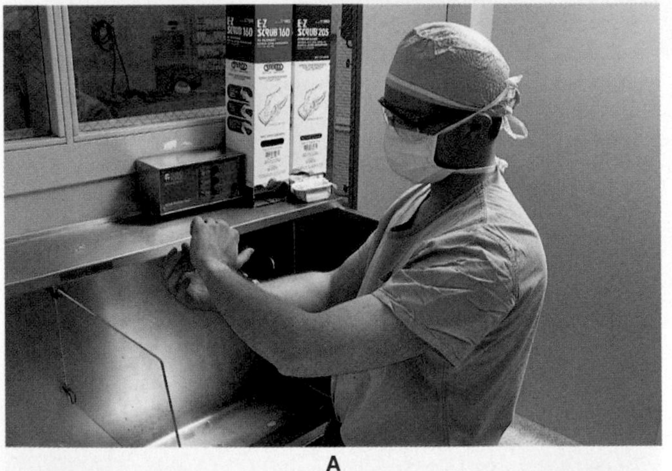
A

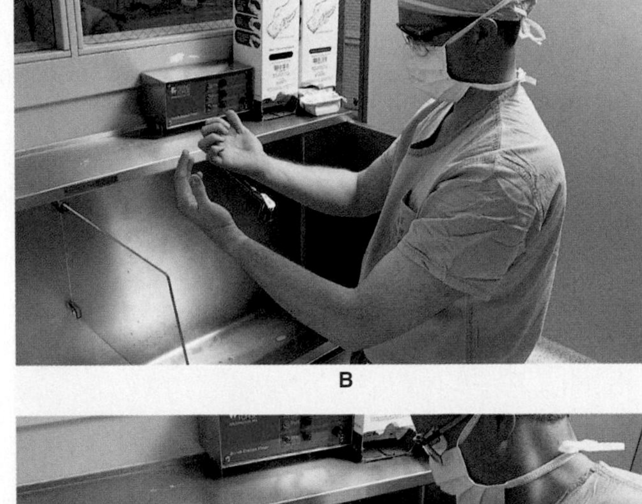
B

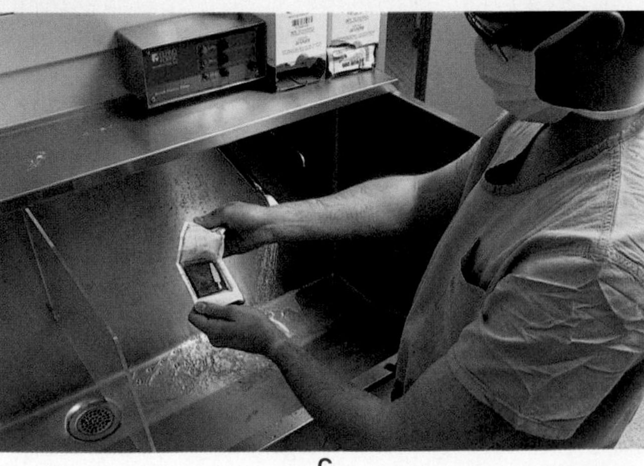
C

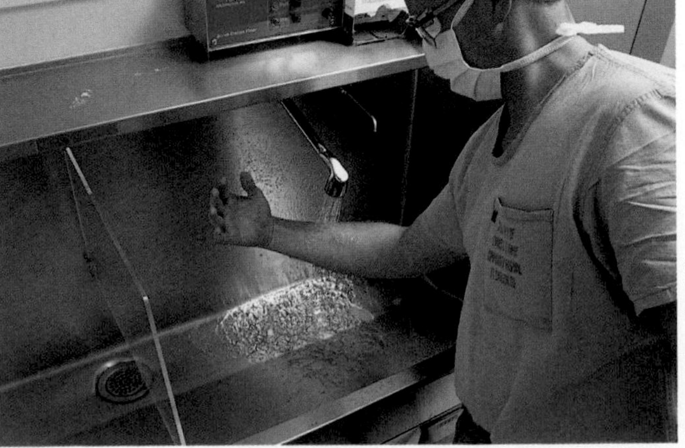
D

Figure 12-12 The surgical scrub: (A) Inspect hands and arms, (B) inspect nails and cuticles, (C) open brush package, (D) apply water

(continues)

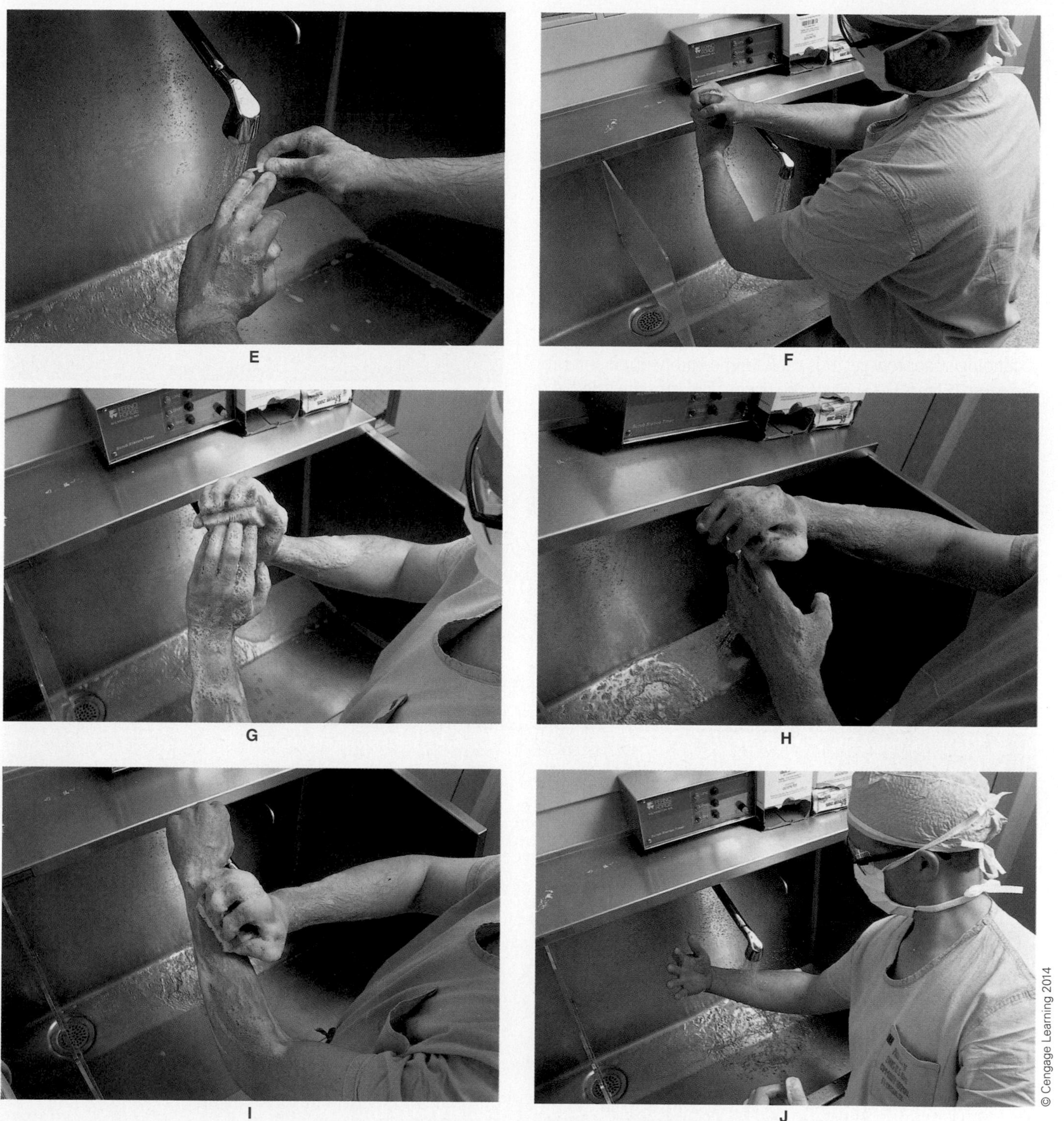

Figure 12-12 (*continued*) (E) clean under each nail, (F) apply antiseptic, (G) scrub nails, (H) scrub all planes of all fingers, (I) scrub hands and arms, (J) rinse thoroughly

are provided. These are operated with a foot pump so that the antiseptic can be dispensed without the use of the hands.

One of two methods for the surgical scrub may be used: the *timed method* or the *counted brush stroke method*. In the timed method, the hands and arms are scrubbed for a prescribed length of time. The counted brush stroke method requires a measured number of brush strokes for each anatomical area to be scrubbed. Health care facility policy will dictate the method of scrub to be performed. However, the student may encounter varying policies as related to the scrub. Studies have not definitively shown which method of scrubbing is best, or how long a scrub should last (5 minutes, 10 minutes, etc.). Additionally, some health care institutions now employ the use of alcohol-based antiseptic solutions, which are allowed to dry on the hands and forearms of the individual, negating the use of the drying towel prior to gowning and gloving.

Self-Drying and Gowning

As soon as the scrub is complete, the surgical technologist proceeds directly to the OR and enters by turning the back to the door, slightly bending forward, pushing it open, and rotating/stepping into the OR, keeping the hands between the waist and the mid-chest. He or she avoids touching anything with the hands or arms. The gown and gloves have already been opened by the surgical technologist onto a Mayo stand or other small table during the establishment of the sterile field. The surgical technologist approaches this table immediately upon entering the room (Figure 12-13). Once the hands and arms are dried, the surgical technologist is ready to don the gown.

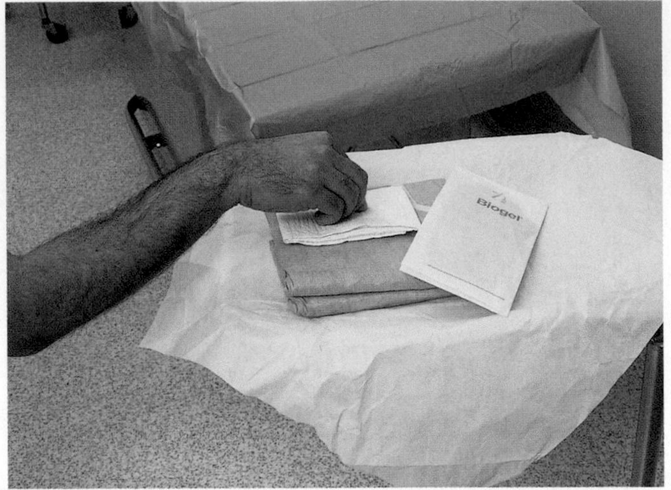

Figure 12-13 Drying the hands and arms

TECHNIQUE

The Surgical Scrub

Refer to Figure 12-12 A–J.

1. Don all PPE. Confirm scrub top is securely tucked into scrub pants and if necessary, sleeves of scrub top are slightly rolled up to allow access to 2 in. above the elbows.
2. Remove jewelry, watch, etc.
3. Inspect the integrity of the hands and arms to rule out the presence of wounds or infection.
4. Inspect nails and cuticles.
5. Open the brush package and place it in a convenient location.
6. Turn on the water and adjust the temperature.
7. Wet hands and arms, apply antiseptic, and lather to 2 inches above the elbows (basic hand wash).
8. Obtain the nail cleaner.
9. Clean each subungual space and around the cuticles (if necessary) under running water.
10. Discard the nail cleaner.
11. Rinse hands and arms starting at the fingers and moving arm forward in a sweeping motion without touching the sides of the scrub sink and faucet; do not go back over a clean area Always rinse fingers to 2 inches above elbows.
12. Keep the hands above the elbows and keep elbows bent to allow water to run off the elbows.
13. Obtain the scrub brush; wet and lather.
14. Begin scrubbing the first hand by placing the fingertips together and scrubbing all of the nails and cuticles.
15. Scrub each finger by dividing it into four planes.
16. Scrub each web space as a separate plane.
17. Add antiseptic, as needed.
18. Scrub the hand by dividing it into four planes; use circular motions.
19. Divide the arm into three sections and four planes; use circular motions.
20. Continue the scrub to 2 inches above the elbow.
21. Transfer the brush to the scrubbed hand and repeat the process on the opposite extremity.
22. Discard the brush.
23. Rinse one extremity from the fingertips to the elbows while keeping the elbows bent. Avoid touching the faucet, and sides and edges of the sink.
24. Repeat rinse on the opposite extremity.
25. Turn off the water.
26. Allow the excess water to drip into the sink.
27. Proceed to the OR with elbows bent and hands between the mid-chest and waist level. Do not touch anything.
28. Open the OR door by turning your back to the door, pushing it open, and rotating/stepping into the OR, and proceed to the table where the gown and gloves are open.

TECHNIQUE

Drying the Hands and Arms

Refer to Figure 12-13.

1. Approach the sterile field with caution, keeping the elbows bent.
2. Pinch and lift the towel from the sterile field without dripping on or touching the gown, gloves, or wrapper.
3. Step away from the sterile field with the arms extended.
4. Unfold the towel without allowing the edges to fall below the waist.
5. Bend slightly at the waist so that the towel does not come in contact with the scrubs.
6. Hold the towel in the palm of one hand while drying the opposite hand and arm using a circular motion.
7. Transfer the towel to the opposite hand without crossing the hands or passing the towel over the scrubbed hands.
8. Dry the opposite hand and arm.
9. Discard the towel.

Donning a surgical gown requires some movements (Figure 12-14) that should be minimized. The surgical technologist must have a heightened awareness of the total environment in order to avoid contamination.

After the gown has been donned, the fasteners at the shoulders and waist must be secured. The circulator will perform this task by pulling the gown all the way onto the shoulders and around the body. Care must be taken not to turn your back on the sterile field at any time.

Closed Gloving

The closed glove technique is used for donning the gloves after the sterile gown has been donned (Figure 12-15). The individual who is gloving should always work from a separate table, never the back table, to prevent contamination. Only the surgical technologist who scrubs first should use this technique. All other team members should be assisted by the surgical technologist.

Turning the Gown

The final step of gowning and gloving is called turning. The circulator assists in turning the **wraparound-style gown** (Figure 12-16). Because one sterile and one nonsterile team

TECHNIQUE

Self-Gowning

Refer to Figure 12-14A–F.

1. Approach the sterile field with caution.
2. Grasp the gown at the center near the neck without touching the gloves or the wrapper.
3. Lift the gown from the wrapper and step back with the gown still folded.
4. Hold the inside of the gown near the shoulders and allow the gown to unfold.
5. Begin donning the gown by slipping the hands and arms into the sleeves.
6. Slide the gown over the arms using a "swimming" motion.
7. Keep the hands within the cuff of the gown.
8. Flex the elbows to hold the gown in place.
9. Allow the circulator to assist with the final gown adjustments and secure the neck and back of the gown.

TECHNIQUE

Closed Gloving

Refer to Figure 12-15A–C.

1. Approach the sterile field with caution.
2. Secure the first glove, keeping the fingers within the cuff of the gown.
3. Align the glove on the palm of the hand that will be gloved first with the thumb side of the glove toward your palm and the fingertips toward the elbow.
4. Pull the cuff of the glove over the cuff of the gown.
5. Unfold the cuff of the glove to completely cover the cuff of the gown.
6. Grasp the glove and the gown at the wrist level.
7. Work the fingers into the glove as the glove is pulled into position.
8. Secure the second glove and apply using the same technique.
9. Double glove.

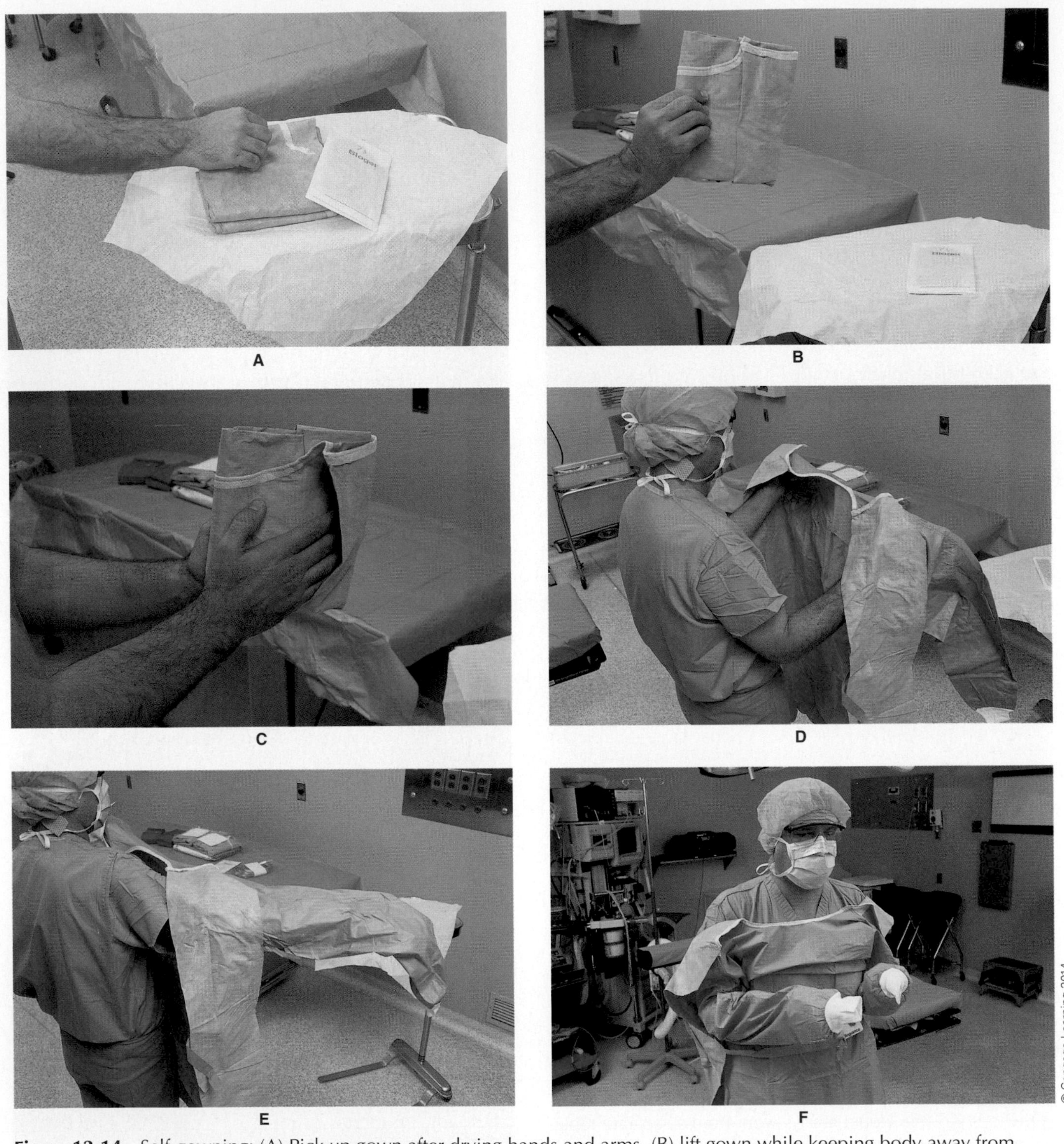

Figure 12-14 Self-gowning: (A) Pick up gown after drying hands and arms, (B) lift gown while keeping body away from Mayo stand, (C) identify collar and orient gown, (D) release lower portion and identify arm openings, (E) enter sleeves, (F) flex arms to hold gown in place

member and large movements are involved, extreme vigilance is required during this maneuver. The gowned individual maintains an appropriate distance from the other sterile areas until the gown has been completely secured, and should continue to face the sterile field at all times, never turning the back on a sterile area. Once the gown has been turned, the back of the wraparound-style gown is considered nonsterile since it cannot be seen by the surgical technologist. This technique is used not only for the surgical technologist but also for subsequent sterile team members.

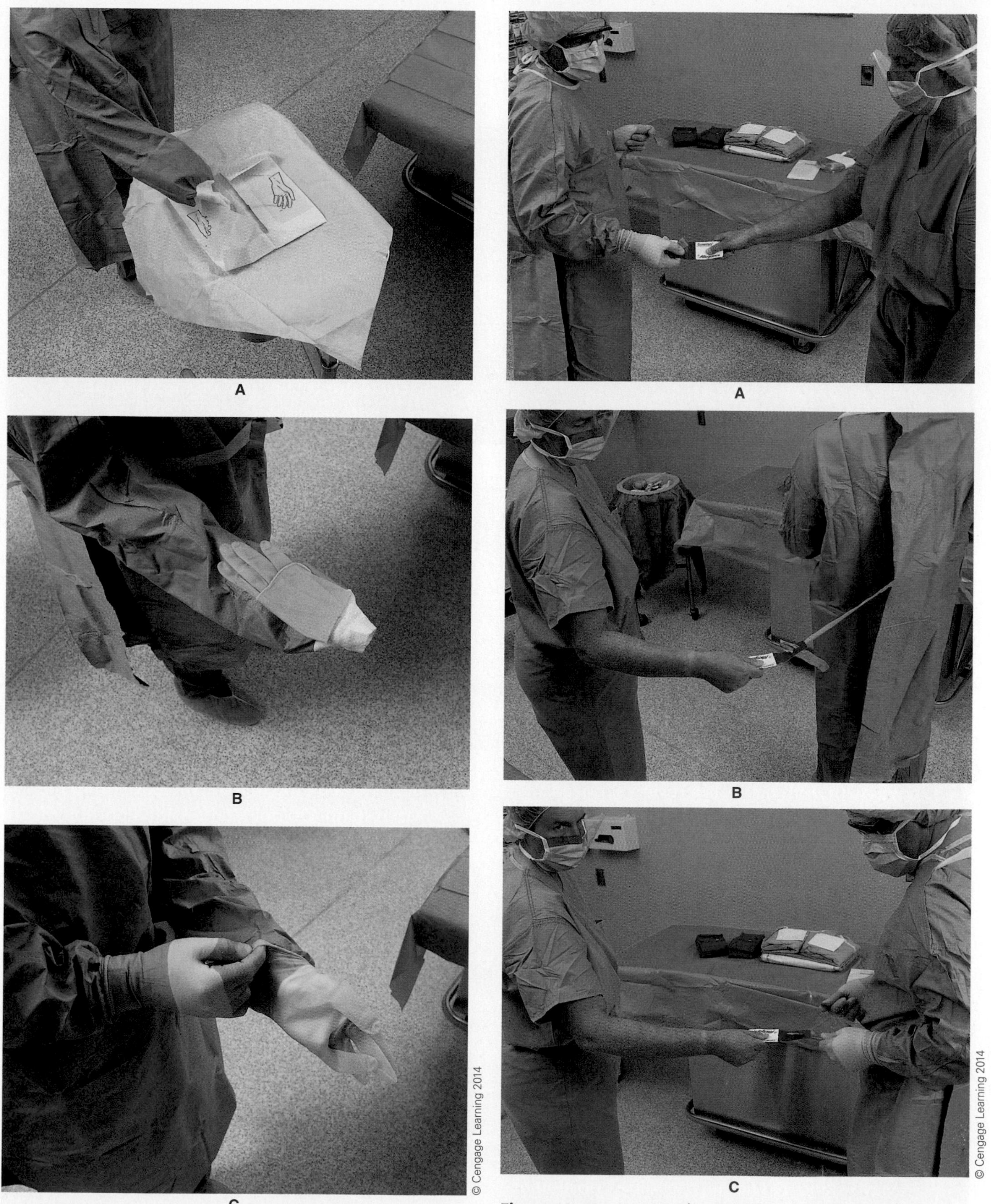

Figure 12-15 Closed gloving: (A) Keep hands in cuffs; remove glove from wrapper, (B) position first glove palm to palm, thumb to thumb, (C) pull on and adjust glove

Figure 12-16 Turning the gown: (A) Disengage the tag and hand it to the circulator, (B) circulator moves behind the surgical technologist, (C) surgical technologist rotates shoulders to receive the tie with the left hand

Preparation of the Sterile Field

Once the surgical technologist has entered the sterile field, a number of tasks must be performed quickly and efficiently prior to initiation of the surgical procedure. Keep in mind that practical realities conflict with the practice of strict sterile technique. For example, one of the concepts that relates to the second principle of asepsis states: "Sterile individuals must keep their hands in sight at all times,

TECHNIQUE

Turning the Gown

Refer to Figure 12-16A–C.

1. Remain facing the sterile field.
2. Secure the tag in the right hand and the gown tie in the left hand and separate.
3. Hold the tag in such a way that the circulator has space to grasp the tag.
4. Pass the tag to the circulator at the right side.
5. The circulator will move around to the left side.
6. Transfer the gown tie from the left to the right hand.
7. Receive the gown tie from the circulator at the left side.
8. The circulator retains and discards the tab.
9. Secure both gown ties.

TECHNIQUE

Draping the Mayo Stand

Refer to Figure 12-17A–C.

1. Partially open and orient the Mayo stand cover on the back table according to the manufacturer's instructions.
2. Insert hands into the cuff of the Mayo stand cover as directed.
3. Grasp all layers contained within the cuff of the cover with both hands to prevent slippage.
4. Open the pocket in the folded Mayo stand cover that will eventually present to the bare Mayo stand (*Tip:* Move hands from horizontal to vertical positions).
5. Approach the Mayo stand, ensuring that items that are to remain sterile do not touch the bare Mayo stand.
6. Secure the Mayo stand by placing one foot on the base of the stand.
7. Use the method that best suits your situation to apply the Mayo stand cover.

   Method A
   - Stand directly in front of the Mayo stand.
   - Begin to slide the Mayo stand cover onto the Mayo stand. Do not let the folded portion of the Mayo stand cover unfold and slip below the level of the Mayo stand.
   - Continue to slide the Mayo stand cover onto the Mayo stand until it is fully unfolded without reaching below the surface level of the Mayo stand.

   Method B
   - Stand slightly to the side of the Mayo stand.
   - Begin to slide the Mayo stand cover onto the Mayo stand. Do not let the folded portion of the Mayo stand cover unfold and slip below the level of the Mayo stand.
   - Keep one hand within the cuffed portion of the Mayo stand cover and begin to push the cover toward the back of the Mayo stand.
   - Extend the cover one fold at a time with your opposite hand.
   - Continue to slide the cover onto the Mayo stand until it is fully unfolded without reaching below the surface level of the Mayo stand.
8. Make any final adjustments.
9. Fold or tuck any excess material.
10. Place towels on the Mayo stand, if needed.
11. Continue with preoperative case management duties.

and within the sterile zone." This becomes impossible when the sterile individual is required to reach above his or her head to place sterile covers on the light handles. As long as direct contamination does not occur, the hand and arm of the individual applying the light handle covers are considered sterile.

A logical and efficient routine must be established and repeated during preparation for all types of surgical procedures. The following is a sample organizational routine for a laparotomy in which everything runs smoothly and according to plan. Be aware that variations (such as contamination, product differences, surgeon's preference, the patient's situation, and school or facility policy) can occur. Plan in advance the steps that will be taken when a variation does occur.

Draping the Mayo Stand

The sterile field is expanded to include the Mayo stand. The Mayo stand is draped by applying a sterile Mayo stand cover followed by placing a linen towel on top (Figure 12-17). The Mayo stand cover is a sterile **cylindrical** drape that is closed at one end and encircles the upper portion of the Mayo stand.

Organizing the Sterile Instruments and Supplies

The surgical technologist is now ready for the primary portion of preoperative case management, which is setting up the back table, Mayo stand, and basin set with the instruments, supplies, and equipment that will be used during the surgical procedure.

Organizing the Back Table

The back table provides a large sterile area for preparation and storage of sterile items. Instruments less likely to be used, redundant instruments, and instruments of specific and often one-time use are left on the back table. The back table is typically the first sterile area prepared by the surgical technologist.

Several principles of practice are applied while organizing the back table (Figure 12-18):

- Move about as little as possible.
- Keep the body centered in a "box" and move just the shoulders and hands.
- Work in sections at the table.
- Handle each item only once.
- Learn a logical and efficient pattern for back table organization and repeat it case after case.
- Be aware of the total environment, especially the movement of others.

Organization of the back table requires that drapes and supplies included in the back table pack itself be rearranged (Figure 12-19). This may be a relatively small number of items or quite complex. Small basins must be moved from the basin set and placed to receive sterile solutions. Instrument sets must be moved from a container system or wrapper to the back table. Sharps and medications must be arranged. Items must be organized in such a way as to allow for safe and efficient count procedures. Ultimately some items will be transferred to the Mayo stand.

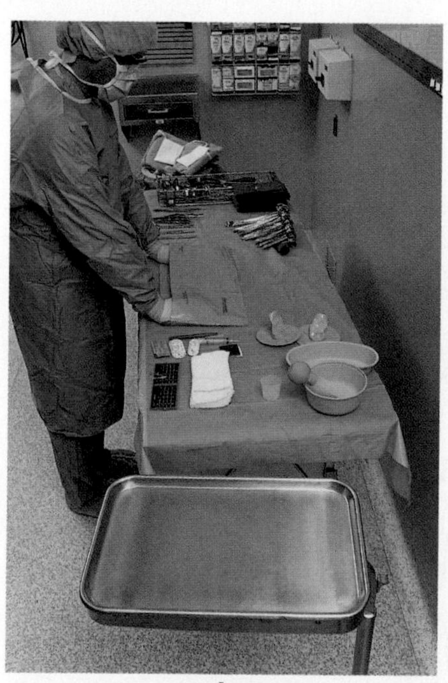
A

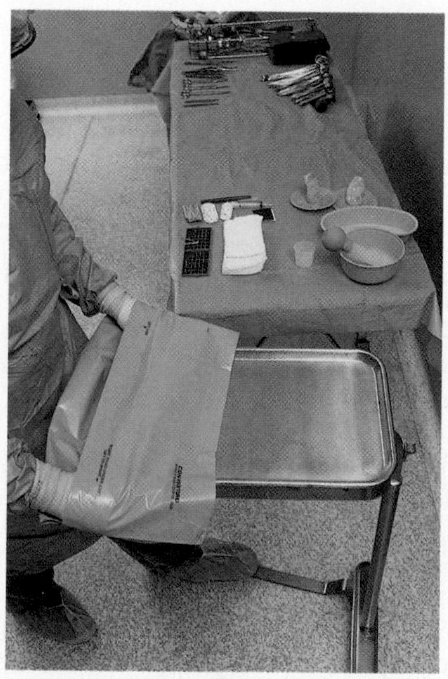
B

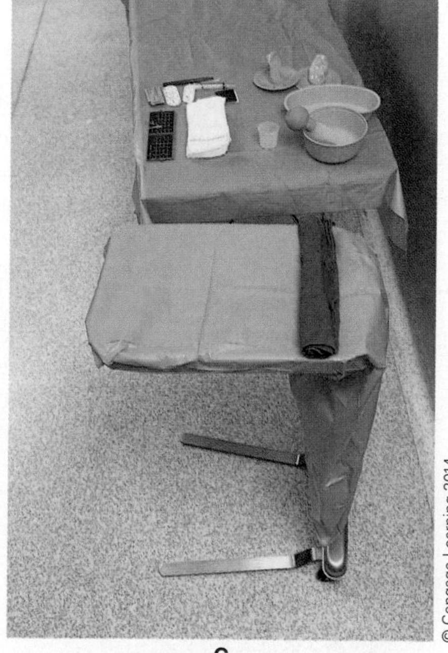
C

Figure 12-17 Draping the Mayo stand: (A) Orienting the Mayo stand cover on the back table, (B) initial placement of the Mayo stand cover, (C) Mayo stand draped

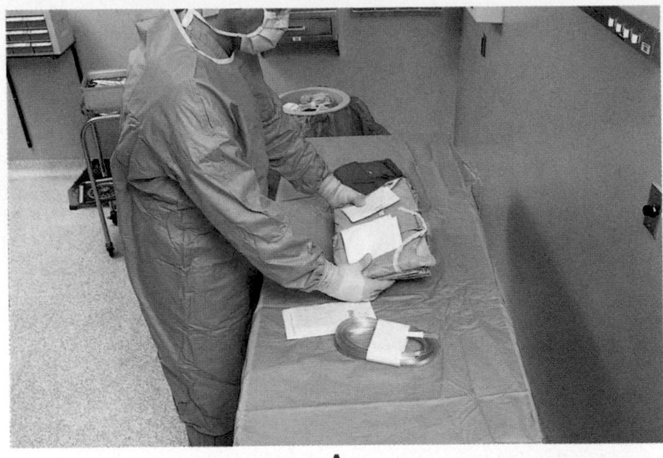

A

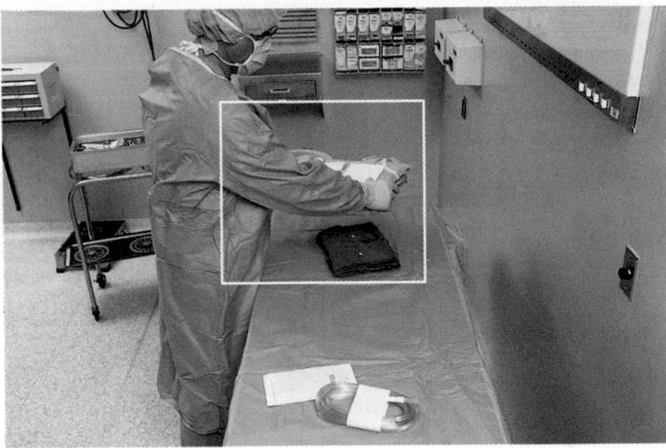

B

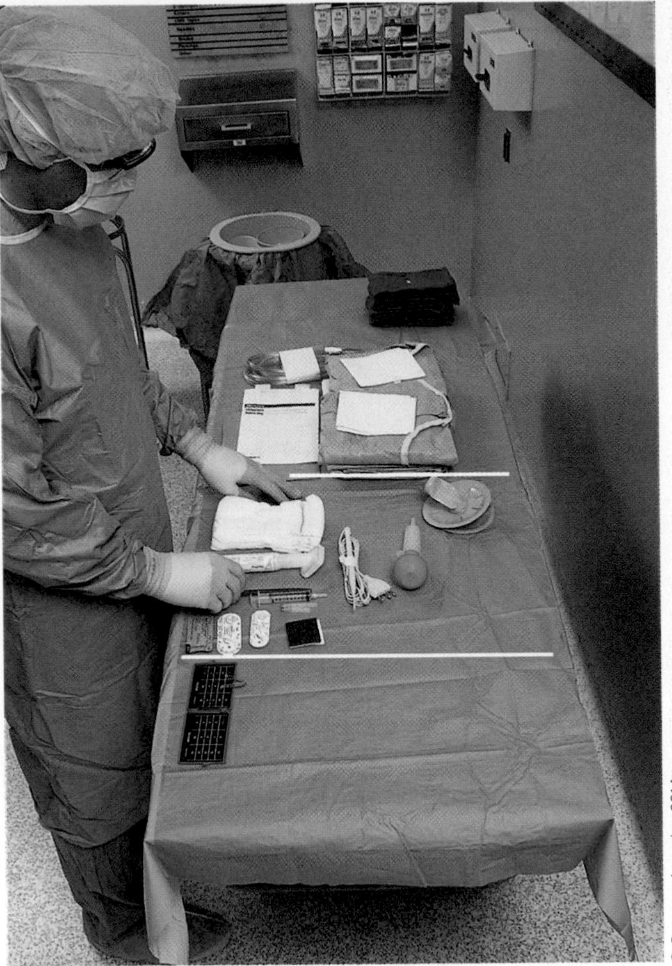

C

Figure 12-18 Principles of back table setup: (A) Move as little as possible, (B) keep body within an imaginary box, (C) work in sections at the back table

A good piece of advice is "Think fast but move carefully." The focus should be on moving at a good and efficient pace; but not so fast as to engage in wasted movements or to compromise safety. The surgical technologist should have a basic plan in mind before beginning back table organization. For the student, the time at the scrub sink is well spent mentally reviewing the first five or six steps that should be taken once the scrub attire is donned. As experience is gained, the time at the sink is better spent mentally reviewing the needs of the surgeon and the steps of the procedure. The surgical technologist with considerable experience will typically think of variations in anatomy and pathology and steps of the operative procedures and develop a mental game plan for responding to specific variations.

Preoperative Count

Instrument, sponge, and sharps counts are very important. They are important for both patient safety and legal reasons (Tables 12-1, 12-2, and 12-3). Counts should be performed according to health care facility policy and should be done with precision. Once items are counted the linen and trash bags should not be removed from the OR until the surgical procedure is completed and the patient is being transported out of the OR to the PACU or other designated area.

Sponges

Sponges are prepackaged by the manufacturer, typically in groups of 5 or 10. All sponges on the back table must be counted.

Dressing sponges should not be opened onto the back table until after the final closing count.

For all types of sponges, the count verifies the number of sponges and that each sponge has a radiologically detectable strip firmly attached.

The sponges are completely separated and counted one at a time. The surgical technologist and circulator should count the sponges simultaneously and in an audible fashion. The surgical technologist should set up the back table in such a

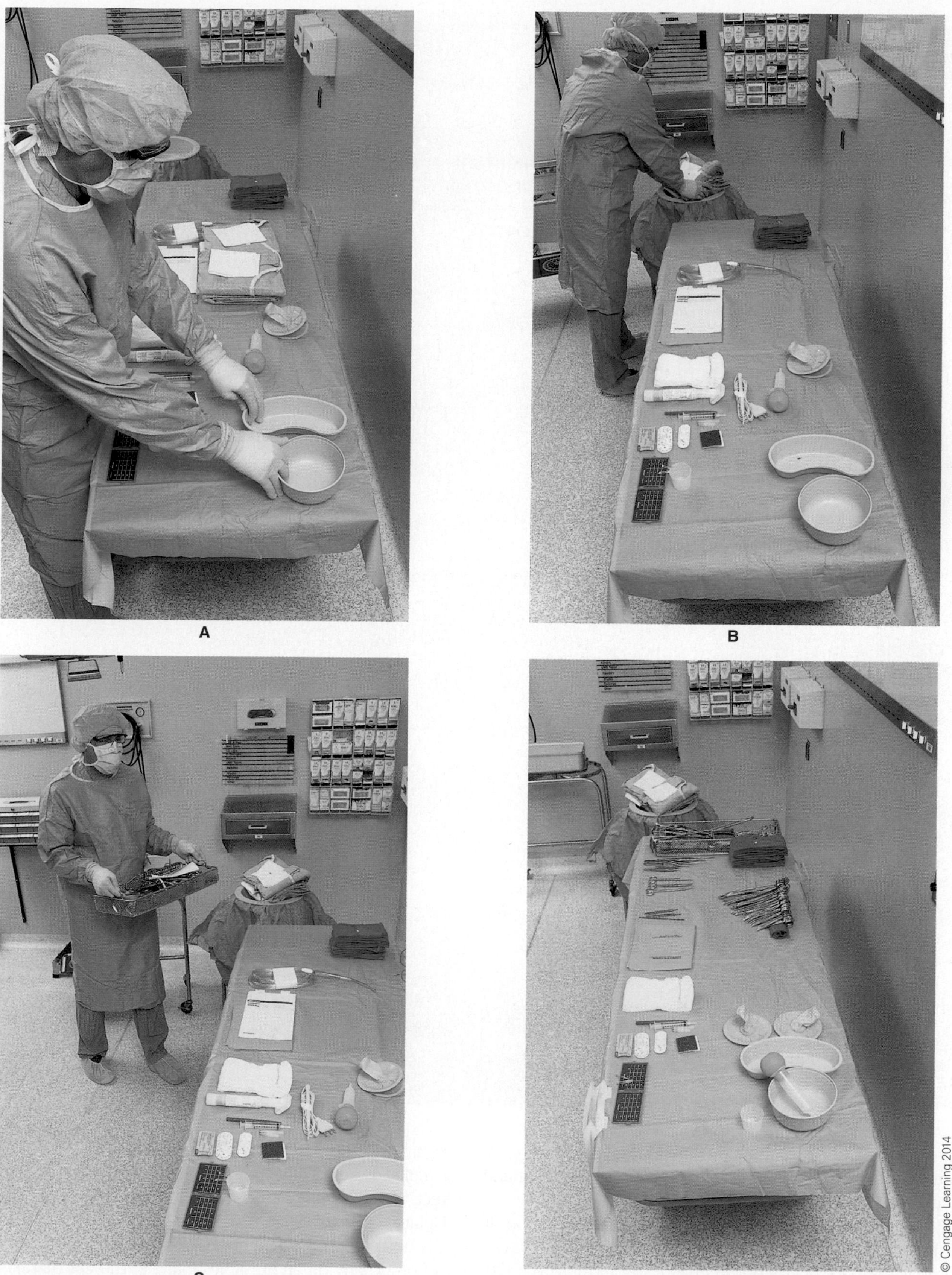

Figure 12-19 Organizing the back table: (A) Place the small basins near, but not over, the edge of the table, (B) move drapes, gowns, and gloves to the large basin area, (C) remove instrument tray from container; verify exposure to sterilization process, (D) back table setup complete

TECHNIQUE

Organizing the Back Table

Refer to Figure 12-19 A–D.

1. Arrange all items from the basin set and all items that were opened onto or contained within the back table pack by placing them in their final location on the back table. Handle each item only once.
   - Secure the sterile suture/trash bag in a convenient location.
   - Place small basins and medicine cups near the edge of the table to allow the circulator access for placement of solutions or medications (Refer to the Pouring Sterile Fluid technique. Medication handling techniques are presented in Chapter 9.)
   - Place all sharps in a common location.
   - Organize the suture material in the predicted order of need according to the surgeon's preference card.
2. Organize all drapes and accessory items related to the draping procedure and place on top of an empty basin in the order in which they will be needed. Complete each task prior to moving to the next item in the organizational routine.
   - Connect the Yankauer suction tip to the suction tubing and place it in the basin.
   - Prepare the electrosurgical pencil by removing and discarding any packaging material and placing the pencil in the basin.
   - Place the light handles or covers in the basin.
   - Place the laparotomy sheet over the items already in the basin. Be sure that it does not extend beyond the sterile field.
   - Prepare four drape towels and place them on top of the laparotomy sheet.
   - If a lower body sheet will be used, place it on top of the towels.
   - Place the surgeon's and assistant's gloves, gowns, and towels on the top of the stack.
3. Space is now available on the back table for the instrument set, which must be removed from its container (Refer to the Removal of the Instrument Set from the Container System technique.)
4. The instruments are organized by category. For example, all retracting instruments are placed in one area, all cutting instruments are placed in another, and so on. Instrument structure, classification, and usage information is found in Chapter 10.
5. The initial count is performed at a mutually convenient time by the circulator and the surgical technologist.
   - Items are counted in the same order for every procedure (e.g., sponges first, sharps second, and instruments last) according to facility policy.
   - The name of the item is stated prior to counting (e.g., "Lap sponges—1, 2, 3, 4, 5.").
   - Each item is separated by the surgical technologist and visualized by both team members.
   - Each item is verbally counted by both team members. This may be accomplished in unison or by repeating the count; follow facility policy.
   - The number of each item, or group of items, is recorded by the circulator.
   - Continue with preoperative case management duties.

manner as to keep each size and type of sponge separate and grouped together.

If a package of sponges contains an incorrect number it should be immediately handed off the sterile field to the circulator. If the patient has not been transported into the OR, the sponges may be removed from the room to prevent a miscount. If the patient has been transported into the OR, the circulator should bag the sponges, label the outside as incorrect, and place the bag somewhere in the OR that is relatively isolated, but the sponges should not be removed from the OR until the end of the case. The circulator will record the count, usually on an erasable board in the OR that easily allows recording the addition of sponges during the surgical procedure.

TECHNIQUE
Pouring Sterile Fluid

Note: This skill is typically performed by the circulator or other nonsterile individual once the surgical technologist has entered the sterile field.

1. Obtain sterile fluid (sterile water and saline are routinely used) according to the surgeon's preference card (first verification).
2. Verify that the " six rights" are met (refer to Chapter 9).
3. Verify the patient's allergy status.
4. Remove and discard the protective outer seal from the fluid container.
5. Remove the inner seal using sterile technique.
6. Approach the sterile field while maintaining a 12-inch minimum distance.
7. Ensure that the fluid does not spill, drip, or run down the outer surface of the container.
8. With the circulator, visually and verbally verify the name, strength, and expiration date of the fluid (second verification).
9. Hold the lip of the container approximately 12 inches above the basin and pour the solution without splashing or dripping. It may not be necessary to completely empty the solution container.
10. Once the fluid is poured, perform a third visual/verbal verification of the fluid label.
11. Either save the fluid container for future reference or discard it according to facility policy.
12. Do not recap the fluid container for later use of the remaining solution. However, it may be recapped for disposal.
13. The fluid is labeled by the surgical technologist according to facility policy.
14. Fluid is prepared for use (Refer to next technique, "Filling a Bulb Syringe").
15. Continue with preoperative case management duties.

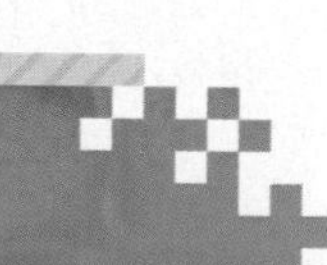

TECHNIQUE
Filling a Bulb Syringe

1. Assemble the components of the bulb syringe, if necessary.
2. Expel the air from the bulb.
3. Maintain pressure on the bulb.
4. Insert the tip of the syringe into the basin containing the sterile fluid.
5. Release the pressure on the bulb and allow the syringe to fill.
6. Hold the syringe upward allowing the sterile fluid to enter the bulb. If the syringe is not completely filled, repeat steps 2–5. Be sure that the sterile fluid within the syringe is not accidentally expelled while you are continuing to fill the syringe.
7. Label the bulb syringe (if necessary) according to facility policy.
8. Place the bulb syringe in a safe location until needed; usual placement is in the basin or emesis basin.
9. Continue with preoperative case management duties.
10. State the contents of the syringe when passing it to the surgeon or surgical assistant.
11. Keep track of the amount of fluid used and report usage to the anesthesia provider and/or circulator.

TECHNIQUE

Removal of the Instrument Set from the Container System

1. Request the circulator's assistance at a mutually convenient time.
2. Verify exposure to the sterilization process by observing the chemical indicator for the appropriate color change.
3. Approach the container cautiously, ensuring that the gown front and sleeves do not contact the exterior of the container.
4. Reach carefully into the container and grasp the handles of the tray/basket containing the instrumentation.
5. Lift the tray/basket vertically and step away from the container.
6. Hold the tray/basket (without allowing it to touch the sterile gown) while the circulator verifies that the container interior is dry and that the filter is intact.
7. Place the tray/basket gently in the prepared location on the back table.
8. Continue with preoperative case management duties.

TABLE 12-1 **Responsibility for Counts**

	Instruments	*Sponges*	*Sharps/Needles*
Prior to opening	Sterile processing	Manufacturer	Manufacturer
Opening/closing	Surgical technologist/circulator	Surgical technologist/circulator	Surgical technologist/circulator
Intraoperative additions	Surgical technologist/circulator	Surgical technologist/circulator	Surgical technologist/circulator
Circulator change	(Usually not possible)	Surgical technologist/incoming circulator	Surgical technologist/incoming circulator
STSR change	(Usually not possible)	Incoming surgical technologist/circulator	Incoming surgical technologist/circulator
Team change	Surgical technologist/circulator	Surgical technologist/circulator	Surgical technologist/circulator

TABLE 12-2 **When to Count**

Opening 1	All items open on back table prior to Mayo stand setup
Additional items	As added
Team changes	Before surgical technologist leaves room
Closing 1	As soon as closure of peritoneum or any first layer of a cavity is initiated (example: start closing count 1 while uterus is being closed on a cesarean section. Have an extra count on such procedures.)
Closing 2	As soon as closure of fascia or layer before subcutaneous is initiated
Final	As soon as skin closure is initiated

TABLE 12-3 **Problems with Counts**

Prior to Patient's Entry into OR	*Action*
Instruments	Change count sheet to match the actual count; initial change
Sponges	Count twice; if still incorrect, remove entire package from OR, document problem, open new package, and count again
Sharps/needles	Count twice; if still incorrect, remove entire package from OR, document problem, open new package and count again

Sharps

The initial count is accomplished by showing the circulator the needle picture on the suture packet. However, needle packets with multiple needles must be opened and the needles counted.

When opened, the circulator must be in a position to see each needle. If a suture packet indicates that there are five needles in the packet, five needles must be visualized and audibly counted by the surgical technologist and circulator and recorded. It is recommended that the surgical technologist open multiple needle packets and count the needles individually prior to the beginning of the procedure.

If a suture packet contains the wrong number of needles, the packet should be immediately handed off to the circulator. If the patient has not been transported into the OR, the needle packet may be removed from the room to prevent a miscount. If the patient has been transported into the OR, the circulator should bag the packet, label the bag as incorrect, and place the bag somewhere in the OR that is relatively isolated, but the needle packet is not removed from the OR until the end of the case.

The sharps count will include hypodermic needles, free needles, scalpel blades, and ESU tip(s).

Instruments

Instruments are counted in the sterile processing area and the initial instrument count sheet is signed by the individual preparing the instrument set. The count sheet is removed from the instrument set by the surgical technologist and handed to the circulator during the preoperative phase. The best time to complete the first count is when all items are on the back table but before preparation of the Mayo stand has begun.

Technique
Counting

1. State the name of the item to be counted (e.g., "4 × 4s").
2. Verify that the circulator can see the item.
3. Separate the items as they are counted.
4. State the numbers of items.
5. Circulator writes the number on count sheet or board.

Counts would not be performed if real problems did not exist. Most problems with counts result in the team correcting the problem immediately (Table 12-3). The failure to recognize or solve a problem can result in severe consequences for a patient later.

Counting requires that the surgical technologist and circulator visualize each individual instrument. Instruments should be audibly counted as listed on the count sheet. Any disagreement with the initial count from sterile processing should result in a recount. If the count remains at variance, the actual number should be written and initialed. If the facility has a policy and procedure for reporting this type of error, that procedure should be initiated. Extra instruments should be listed and counted.

For instruments that contain separate parts, such as a Balfour retractor, each part should be counted. No instruments should be removed from the OR during the procedure. Instruments dropped on the floor during setup that are not needed should be retrieved by the circulator and kept in a safe place to be included in the later counts.

There are times, although rare, when an initial count (and possibly the other counts) may be omitted. When an emergency procedure must be performed and the OR is given minimal notice of the arrival of the patient, the focus is placed on the patient and the emergent situation. There may be no time to perform the count when the priority is to save a life.

Two examples of emergency situations include a ruptured aortic abdominal aneurysm and an unplanned cesarean section. While the initial count may have been omitted, every attempt should be made to perform subsequent counts and to follow routine procedures. When a count is omitted, it must be documented on the patient's operative record. Count sheets must be retained for the purpose of conducting the closing counts. The surgeon may order a radiograph to be taken at the end of the procedure prior to the patient leaving the OR to confirm nothing was left inside the patient.

Electronic Methods of Tracking Surgical Counts

Technologies for performing counts include bar coding of sponges and instruments, which is a technology that is used to decrease the risk of retained items. Instruments and sponges that are uniquely identified are counted using a scanner at the beginning and end of each surgical procedure. This process is similar to bar code scanning methods at grocery stores. Bar coding technology produces a paper printout of the surgical counts.

Radiofrequency (RF) identification is another recent technology that uses RF identification tags to improve the detection of sponges intraoperatively. A handheld scanning wand is passed over the patient at key points of the surgical procedure in order to locate any retained sponges. The scanned information is displayed on a screen and an audible alarm will sound if a retained sponge is present. RF identification can be found in a variety of surgical sponges.

Organizing the Mayo Stand

The Mayo stand is prepared to receive the instruments and supplies that will be used most frequently during the surgical procedure. Items placed on the Mayo stand vary greatly. The instrumentation on the Mayo stand for a laparoscopic procedure varies greatly from a laparotomy setup, even if the intent is the same; for example, removal of the gallbladder. Instrumentation for orthopedic procedures is radically different from ophthalmic surgery. There is no way for a student to learn "the" setup because it does not exist. While facilities may require certain guidelines relative to basic setups, you, as an employee, may be able to initiate some minor adjustments that allow you to perform with greater efficacy. As with the back table, a logical and sequential routine for setting up the Mayo stand should be established and followed consistently. Some key principles of practice apply without regard to the particulars of instrument location:

- Place only those items (instruments and supplies such as sponges) most likely to be used on the Mayo stand.
- Instruments should be inspected for damage and functionality, then conveniently arranged on the Mayo stand.
- Instruments are placed on the Mayo stand in pairs (or in even numbers if more than two like items are required).
- Ratcheted instruments are closed to the first ratchet as they are moved from the back table to the Mayo stand.
- It is recommended that a rolled towel be used and that the ring handles not be placed over the edge of the Mayo stand, but placed over the rolled towel to facilitate order.
- Use caution when placing sharp items.

PATIENT TRANSPORT TO OR

While the surgical technologist is preparing the case, other activities concerning the patient are taking place, including notifying the same-day surgery department that the patient is going to be picked up for transport to the OR, positioning the patient, performing the patient's skin prep, and making other patient care preparations.

When the call comes that the OR is prepared, the patient should be notified. He or she should be instructed to void just prior to leaving for the OR; this allows better visualization of the abdominal organs and decreases the chances of injury to the bladder. If the procedure will require the bladder to be empty throughout the surgery, a Foley catheter may be inserted and attached to a closed drainage system. This is often done in the OR after anesthesia induction to ensure sterile conditions and for patient comfort. Prior to transportation to the OR, the patient's identification bracelet should be checked by the caregiver for accuracy and firmness of attachment. The patient identification bracelet is extremely important in that it helps ensure that the correct patient is brought to the OR and the correct procedure is performed by the correct physician. On admission to the hospital, the bracelet is typically affixed to the patient's wrist. It should not be removed unnecessarily until the patient has been discharged. When the transportation attendant or OR personnel arrive to transport the patient to the OR, nursing personnel should be notified. The individuals transporting the patient should introduce themselves and request that the patient state his or her name. The patient identification band should then be read and compared with the patient's chart and with the information on the surgical schedule. The information should also be confirmed with the patient's chart label. If any discrepancy is found it should be reported immediately to the nursing unit and OR personnel, and the patient should not be transported until patient identification can be absolutely verified.

A preoperative assessment including vital signs, consciousness and anxiety levels, skin condition, and personal information should be conducted and recorded prior to transport of the patient to the OR. This should also include personal data and any known allergies. This information provides the surgical team with a quick and concise view of the patient and his or her status prior to transport to the OR, so that any intraoperative or postoperative changes may be noted.

If possible, the patient should be allowed to visit with family or significant others prior to being transported to the OR. Some patients may request a visit by a member of the clergy at this time. This is psychologically important to the patient and aids in the relief of anxiety and mental preparation. Care should be taken that visitors do not cause the patient to become nervous or anxious at this time. Visitors should be informed at this time of the location of the waiting area and when and how to expect to receive information on the status of the patient.

Surgical patients are usually transported to the OR using a stretcher or the patient's bed. In some cases, the patient may be transported in a wheelchair or may even walk to the OR. Infants may be transported in an isolette and accompanied by a parent. Some hospitals provide a wagon, which may be more comfortable and familiar to a child. Whatever the mode of transportation, care must be taken to protect the patient as well as the individual providing transportation from injury. Proper body mechanics and lifting techniques should be observed by the transportation personnel to avoid personal injury. Side rails of the stretcher or bed should always be placed in the up and locked position to prevent falls. When using a wheelchair, the safety belt should be securely fastened, and the wheels should be locked before the patient sits and when the patient prepares to stand on arrival at the OR.

When a patient needs to have accessory equipment such as IV stands or traction apparatus moved along with the bed, extra personnel should be available to assist. Care must be taken not to catch such equipment on walls, doors, or ceilings, as patient injury or equipment damage could occur. The transporter should not attempt this alone, as use of improper body mechanics may result in injury to the individual moving the patient. Before the patient is moved, a check should be made to ensure that all drainage collection devices, IV tubing, and oxygen delivery devices are ready for transport. If the patient requires oxygen, a portable tank should be safely affixed to the stretcher and the oxygen should be connected to the delivery device from this site. Extra assistance in transport will also be necessary if the patient requires a ventilator. The respiratory therapy department of the hospital will provide personnel to assist with ventilator transport.

To avoid injury, the patient should be instructed to keep hands and feet inside the guardrails at all times. Care should be taken to protect the patient's dignity as well as his or her comfort. Blankets should be provided both for warmth and privacy. The patient's head should be raised or lowered into a position that is comfortable, unless physician orders or a patient condition will not permit this. The patient should be transported slowly, feet first, to maintain control of the stretcher at all times. When entering an elevator with a patient on a stretcher or in a wheelchair, the patient is taken in head first, so that when the elevator opens the patient is again being moved in the forward-facing position.

On arrival at the preoperative holding area, the surgical team is notified of the patient's arrival. The patient should not be left alone in the holding area. This is often the point of greatest anxiety for the patient, and feelings of abandonment may result if the patient is left alone. At the time of arrival at the holding area, the circulator will identify and interview the patient. The chart is reviewed to verify the presence of the surgical consent, history, physical assessment, radiology results, and laboratory reports.

Preoperative plans for positioning should be made before the patient enters the OR, to assure that all necessary positioning aids and accessory equipment for the OR table are available. In addition to the type of procedure and position to be used, any preoperative neuropathies, preexisting conditions, or diseases should be considered prior to positioning. Age, physical limitations, skin condition, and height and weight must also be considered to avoid injury to the patient. Muscles and nerves are easily injured from overstretching because muscle tone is lost during anesthesia. Pressure for any length of time on any part of the body may also easily injure the anesthetized patient. Very young, obese, elderly, or debilitated patients are at increased risk of compromise to the circulatory, respiratory, and integumentary systems. Prolonged procedures without position change can lead to a decrease in tissue perfusion, as can the use of positioning devices of inappropriate size.

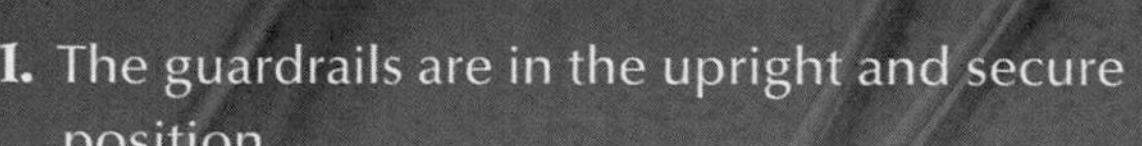

TECHNIQUE

Patient Transport

1. The guardrails are in the upright and secure position.
2. The safety belt is secured, if necessary.
3. The wheels are in the correct position (straight or swivel).
4. The patient is transported slowly, feet first.
5. The patient should enter an elevator head first and exit feet first.
6. Be certain that all parts of the patient's body are within the guardrails.
7. Use good body mechanics.
8. Never leave the patient unattended.

THERMOREGULATORY DEVICES

Control of patient body temperature is important in the OR environment, and several devices are available to assist with providing hypothermia, normothermia, or hyperthermia intraoperatively. During operative procedures, the body core temperature tends to drop due to heat loss in the cool, dry climate in the OR, the length of the operation, and the use of cold or room temperature irrigation fluids.

Most of a patient's heat loss occurs in the early stages of the procedure, when the patient is brought from a warm, humidified environment into a cold, dry one. In addition, the patient is no longer covered with clothing and bedding and is anesthetized, which further decreases the ability to control core temperature. Additionally, the patient is uncovered, and cold, wet skin prep solution is applied, which only adds to a rapid fall in body temperature.

The goal for every patient should be the maintenance of a normal core temperature, unless the procedure specifically calls for the use of hypothermia. The maintenance of a normal core temperature decreases the incidence of wound infection, may reduce blood loss, shortens the hospital stay, and helps decrease the incidence of fatal cardiac events.

Intraoperative heat loss occurs through the following mechanisms:

- *Radiation:* Loss of heat from the patient's body to the environment
- *Convection:* Loss of heat into the air currents (the "wind chill" effect)
- *Conduction:* Loss of heat from the patient's body into a cooler surface such as the operating table
- *Evaporation:* Loss of heat via perspiration or respiration

Radiation and convection are the major modes of patient heat loss.

Inadvertent hypothermia causes challenges intraoperatively and postoperatively in the surgical patient. These challenges include increased oxygen consumption due to shivering, cardiovascular and nervous system changes, and increased metabolism. Postoperative shivering is common and can cause serious cardiovascular and respiratory complications as well as discomfort, dental damage, and damage to the surgical repairs. Shivering also increases muscle metabolism, increasing oxygen consumption. Increased oxygen demand puts undue strain on the respiratory and cardiovascular systems. This undue stress may cause bradycardia and premature ventricular contractions. Hypothermia also causes vasoconstriction, leading to increased blood pressure, and tissue hypoxia, which increases the patient's susceptibility to wound infection. The central nervous system depression caused by hypothermia slows metabolism of medications, which in turn slows emergence from anesthesia.

Some of the safest methods of maintenance of normothermia are noninvasive, passive methods. These methods include keeping the OR at a warmer temperature until the skin is prepped and the patient is draped in order to maintain body temperature. An additional passive method of temperature control is the use of blankets, particularly on the extremities, including the hands and feet, and the head. Many hospitals have begun the use of thermal caps and blankets, especially in the preoperative waiting period, to reduce heat loss from the head and extremities.

The most effective, albeit most extreme and invasive, means of warming core temperature are direct treatments such as the use of warmed gastric lavage, peritoneal irrigation, and fluid warmers for blood and blood products and IV fluids. Special care must be taken to avoid burning the patient when using this technique.

Another type of temperature control is the use of active methods, which apply heat to the outside the body. These methods include the use of warmed blankets, warming blankets, and forced-air warmers. Infants are often placed on the operating table with warming lamps overhead. The use of active warming methods on the extremities causes vasodilation and a shift of cooler blood to the trunk, which reduces the core temperature. For certain procedures, such as cardiac procedures requiring cardiopulmonary bypass, hypothermia is desirable and necessary, in that it provides a lowered cellular metabolism and therefore a lower need for cellular perfusion. A warming device may then be used to return the patient to his or her normal body temperature. When these techniques are used, care should be taken that they are only applied to the patient's head, trunk, and groin. Special care must be taken to avoid burns.

If a blanket is to be used for warming, a sheet should be placed under the warming blanket to prevent direct contact that may overheat the skin. Blankets that circulate water or alcohol are placed on the table before the patient is positioned. Forced-air blankets are placed over unaffected parts of the patient's body prior to sterile draping. They pump warmed air through channels in the blanket to warm the patient. During the procedure, the circulator is able to adjust the temperature of the circulating-water or forced-air blanket for either warming or cooling to help achieve the desired patient body temperature.

TRANSFER AND POSITIONING

Usually, the patient is brought into the OR from the preoperative area on a stretcher and then transferred to the operating table. Patients who are not too heavily sedated and are ambulatory may move under their own effort onto the table. Typically, two individuals assist an awake patient who is capable of moving himself or herself from the stretcher onto the operating table. The stretcher is placed next to the operating table and the wheels are locked. One individual will stabilize the stretcher, while another stands on the opposite side of the operating table to receive the patient and assist in movement.

Many patients' first complaint about the OR relates to the low temperature, and the feet are often the first body part to feel uncomfortably cold. Booties and an additional blanket will provide warmth and comfort. A hair cover is placed on the patient's head. While the patient is moving or being moved from the stretcher to the operating table, care must be taken that IV tubing, O_2 tubings, and indwelling catheters do not become entangled or snagged in the bedding, on the patient, or on parts of the table, causing the tubings to be dislodged.

If the patient is too heavily sedated or is unable to move, he or she will need to be transferred onto the operating table by an appropriate number of personnel. Usually, four individuals are required for this process. If too few individuals attempt to move a patient, strained backs or other personnel injuries may occur. Always use the correct number of personnel when moving a patient to guarantee safe transfer of the patient and protection for the team members. The anesthesia provider supports the head, neck and shoulders, one lifts the feet and legs, and one stands on each side to lift and stabilize the patient's trunk. The movement is coordinated by the anesthesia provider and should be smooth to avoid injury to the patient. The use of a roller board, slider board, or draw sheet is recommended.

Once the patient has been moved onto the operating table, he or she must not be left alone for any reason. The safety strap should be securely placed 2 inches proximal to the knees. This strap should not be tight, but just snug enough to secure the patient. The patient should be assured that this strap is only placed for safety and is not being used for the purpose of restraint. The patient's arms are placed on the armboards; the armboards should not be abducted more than 90 degrees to avoid nerve damage, and safety straps are applied to prevent the arms from falling off of the table. Every effort should be made to make the patient comfortable on the operating table. A pillow may be placed under the head for comfort until the anesthesia provider needs it to be removed, pillow placed under the knees, and the heels padded. The patient's gown should be checked to make sure that it is not too tight and that free breathing is permitted. A warm cotton blanket may be placed over the patient for modesty and warmth. For the patient's psychological comfort, personnel around the table should introduce themselves and explain in as calm a manner as possible what the patient may expect. Noise in the OR should be kept to a minimum.

The patient is transferred to the operating table using one of the two methods described in the Patient Transfer technique.

TECHNIQUE

Patient Transfer

1. The mobile patient may be able to move to the operating table independently.
   - A minimum of two nonsterile team members should be available to assist with transfer of a mobile patient.
   - Position the stretcher next to the operating table.
   - Instruct the patient not to move until you give the command.
   - Be sure that the wheels of both the stretcher and the operating table are locked.
   - One individual should be positioned at the side of the stretcher and the other at the side of the operating table.
   - Brace your bodies against the stretcher and operating table to prevent any unexpected movement.
   - Instruct the patient to keep the blanket on and move to the operating table.
   - Assist the patient any way you can (e.g., move the pillow from the stretcher to the operating table or assist by lifting an extremity that is casted).
   - Apply the safety strap, then remove the stretcher.
2. The immobile patient will be unable to assist with the transfer and will have to be moved onto the operating table.
   - A minimum of four nonsterile team members should be available to assist with transfer of an immobile patient.
   - Position the stretcher next to the operating table.
   - If necessary, explain the transfer procedure to the patient.
   - One individual should be positioned at the side of the stretcher, another at the side of the operating table, anesthesia provider at the head, and an individual at the foot of the stretcher.
   - Brace your bodies against the stretcher and operating table to prevent any unexpected movement.
   - Keep the patient covered and transfer him or her to the operating table, using the draw sheet or roller board.
   - Apply the safety strap, then remove the stretcher.

VITAL SIGNS

Prior to placing the patient in the operative position the anesthesia provider will apply the monitoring equipment in order to monitor and record the patient's vital signs. Monitoring vital signs in the OR assists the surgeon and anesthesia provider in determining patient condition at any given time and can be an indicator of pathology. Baseline vital signs including height and weight are taken prior to the start of the procedure. These give a good basis on which to monitor changes. Taking vital signs involves the mechanical or automated electronic monitoring of such life functions as temperature, pulse, respiration (TPR), and blood pressure (BP). Intraoperatively, these functions are usually monitored electronically by the anesthesia provider.

Electronic monitoring equipment is able to monitor all of the vital functions simultaneously and to correlate the information into an easily readable format. Many of these devices are so small that they can be attached to an IV pole and transported along with the patient. These devices are now built into the anesthesia machine. When necessary, the health care provider should be able to manually monitor vital signs. This involves the use of some basic diagnostic equipment, including a stethoscope, sphygmomanometer, and thermometer. Regardless of whether they are monitored electronically or manually, preoperative, intraoperative, and postoperative vital signs must be recorded periodically to provide trends and timed information on the status of the patient. The recording of vital signs also protects the hospital and surgical team against potential liability.

Temperature

In the OR setting, body temperature can be affected by such outside factors as cold prep solutions, exposure, and anesthesia. Preoperatively, temperature is taken to establish a baseline for the patient and to help rule out preoperative infection (Table 12-4).

In the OR, temperature is closely monitored by automatic monitoring devices controlled by the anesthesia provider. It is important to monitor patient temperature carefully perioperatively to avoid undesirable hypothermia or hyperthermia. The methods for temperature monitoring are listed in Table 12-5.

TECHNIQUE

Temperature Assessment

1. Wash your hands.
2. Assemble equipment and supplies.
   - Thermometer of choice, including accessories
   - Gloves and lubricant, if necessary (*Note:* The patient's condition may require the use of gloves.)
   - Appropriate waste receptacle
3. Prepare equipment.
   - Apply gloves, if necessary.
   - Remove thermometer from package, as needed.
   - Place thermometer in ready mode, if electronic.
   - Apply lubricant, if necessary.
4. Introduce yourself, identify the patient, and explain the procedure, if necessary.
5. Position the patient, if necessary.
6. Place the thermometer according to site location.
7. Keep the thermometer in position for the prescribed length of time.
8. Support the thermometer, if necessary.
9. Carefully remove the thermometer according to protocol for site location.
10. Read the thermometer.
11. Wash your hands.
12. Record or report findings.
13. Care for the equipment as needed.

TABLE 12-4 **Normal Temperature Values**

Oral	98.6°F (37°C)
Rectal	99.6°F (37.6°C)
Axillary	97.6°F (36.4°C)

TABLE 12-5 **Temperature-Monitoring Methods**

Noninvasive	Touch Skin sticker Ear Axilla
Invasive	Oral Rectal Esophageal Bladder

TABLE 12-6 **Normal Pulse Values**

Birth	130–160 bpm*
Infants	110–130 bpm
Children (1–7 years)	80–120 bpm
Children (over 7)	80–90 bpm
Adults	60–80 bpm

*bpm = beats per minute.

Pulse

The pulse is measured when the health care provider palpates an artery, such as the radial artery (Table 12-6). If the pulse is being measured electronically, a pulse oximeter may be used.

The pulse may be felt in any point of the body that has near-surface arteries and bony understructures. These sites include the temporal, carotid, brachial, radial, femoral, popliteal, and dorsalis arteries. The pulse may also be monitored apically, or at the apex of the heart (referred to as the **apical pulse**), by using a stethoscope to listen at the level of the fifth and sixth ribs just to the left of the sternum and just below the nipple. The most commonly utilized pulse point is the radial artery, located about 1 inch proximal to the base of the thumb. Refer to Figure 12-20 for a diagram of the location of other pulse points in the body. To measure the pulse rate, the number of pulsations is counted for one minute. This number of beats is the pulse, or heart rate. The pulse may also be measured for 15 seconds, and the number is multiplied by 4 to obtain the heart rate. The rate will vary with age, level of activity, pain, medication, and emotional condition. Patients entering the OR will sometimes have an elevated pulse rate due to anxiety. In addition to the basic rate of pulse, or heart rate, several other pulse characteristics are monitored, including rhythm, volume, and strength. The rhythm of the pulse refers to the regularity of the beats.

Common pulse abnormalities include bradycardia (pulse rate less than 60) and tachycardia (pulse rate over 100) (Table 12-7). A dysrhythmia is an irregular pulse and may indicate heart disease. The most commonly felt dysrhythmia includes premature ventricular contraction (PVC), felt as a pulse beat earlier than expected. It can occasionally occur as a stress response or may be caused by caffeine, nicotine, alcohol, or sleep deprivation. The pulse strength is noted as full, strong, hard, soft, thready, or weak. Any pulse abnormalities should be noted and the surgeon or anesthesia provider should be alerted, as these can be serious and even fatal. An ECG may be needed prior to initiation of the surgical procedure (refer to Chapter 13).

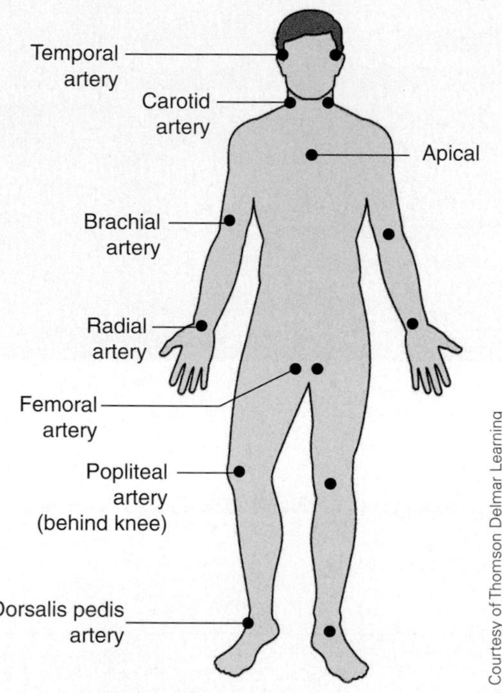

Figure 12-20 Pulse points in the body

Respiration

When monitoring respiration, rate, rhythm, and depth are noted. Rhythm of respiration is a measure of the pattern of breathing. This will vary with age, with adults having a regular

TECHNIQUE
Pulse Assessment

1. Wash your hands.
2. Assemble equipment and supplies.
   - Watch or clock with second hand
   - Stethoscope, if checking apical or fetal pulse
   - Gloves, if warranted by the patient's condition
3. Introduce yourself, identify the patient, and explain the procedure, if necessary.
4. Position the patient, if necessary.
5. Locate the site by gently palpating with the first two or three fingertips (don't use the thumb).
6. Gently compress the artery or listen with the stethoscope.
7. Note the time. *Note:* For accuracy, the pulse rate should be counted for one full minute.
8. Count the pulse rate and note the rhythm, volume, and condition of the arterial wall.
9. Wash your hands.
10. Record or report findings.
11. Care for equipment as needed.

TABLE 12-7 **Pulse Abnormalities**

Type	*Rate*	*Causes*
Normal	60–80 bpm	• Age, activity level, and gender variations (refer to Table 12-6)
Tachycardia	>100 bpm	• Stimulation of the sympathetic nervous system by stress or drugs • Exercise • Congestive heart failure, anemia
Bradycardia	<60 bpm	• Very fit athlete • Stimulation of the parasympathetic nervous system by certain drugs • Physical problems such as cerebral hemorrhage and heart blockage
Irregular	Uneven beat intervals	• Cardiac irritability or hypoxia • Chemical or drug issues such as potassium imbalance • If premature beats are frequent, this condition may indicate a serious dysrhythmia

pattern and infants having an irregular one. The depth of respiration is the amount of air taken in and exhaled with each respiration, an amount that is easily measured by anesthesia equipment in the OR. Manually, it is measured by watching the rise and fall of the chest. The rate is recorded, along with whether respirations are shallow or deep (Table 12-8).

Respiration rate abnormalities include apnea, bradypnea, Cheyne-Stokes, **dyspnea**, and tachypnea (Table 12-9). *Apnea* is the complete cessation of breathing. Apnea temporarily occurs upon induction of some types of anesthesia, hence the need for manual/mechanical ventilation during general anesthesia. Obstructive apnea occurs when there is a blockage in the airway. *Bradypnea* is the opposite of tachypnea; it is a decreased rate of respiration. *Cheyne-Stokes* respiration is a pattern of rhythmic waxing and waning of the depth of respiration. The patient breathes deeply for a short period of time and then breathes only very slightly or not at all for a period.

Table 12-8 Normal Respiration Rates

Infants	30–60 respirations per minute
Children (1–7 years)	18–30 per minute
Adults	12–20 per minute

Technique
Respiration Assessment

1. Wash your hands.
2. Assemble the equipment and supplies.
   - Watch or clock with second hand
   - Stethoscope, if necessary
   - Gloves, if warranted by the patient's condition
3. Introduce yourself, identify the patient, and explain the procedure, if necessary.
4. Position the patient, if necessary.
5. Note the time. *Note:* For accuracy, the respiratory rate should be counted for one full minute.
6. Obtain respiratory rate, depth, rhythm, and breath sounds.
7. Wash your hands.
8. Record or report findings.
9. Care for the equipment as needed.

Table 12-9 Breathing Patterns

Name	*Description*	*Cause*
Eupnea	Normal breathing	Normal
Apnea	No breathing	Obstructed airway Disruption or damage to lateral medulla oblongata (breathing center)
Bradypnea	Slow, even respirations	Normal during sleep Depression of respiratory center
Cheyne-Stokes	Fast, deep breaths for a period of time, followed by 20–60 seconds of apnea	Intracranial pressure increase Congestive heart failure Renal failure Cerebral anoxia
Dyspnea	Difficult, painful breaths	Respiratory pathologies Cardiovascular pathologies
Kussmaul's	Fast, deep, labored breaths over 20 per minute	Blood pressure systolic 140–160, diastolic 70–90
Tachypnea	Rapid breaths that rise with body temperature	Pneumonia Respiratory insufficiency Respiratory center lesions

Source: Data from Mednet (www.sermed.com).

This pattern repeats itself and can be caused by heart failure or brain damage. The term dyspnea refers to shortness of breath or difficulty breathing (e.g., during intense physical exercise or due to heart/lung disease). *Tachypnea* is very rapid respiration. This occurs in patients with a high fever when the body attempts to rid itself of excess body heat and also occurs when the patient is experiencing alkalosis and the body is attempting to rid itself of excess carbon dioxide.

Blood Pressure

Blood pressure is the pressure of the blood against the walls of the blood vessels. It is affected by several different factors. Pressure is affected and determined by the pumping of the heart, the resistance of the arterioles to the flow of blood, the elasticity of the arterial walls, the volume of blood in the body, and the blood thickness. The extracellular fluid volume also affects blood pressure. The pumping action of the heart is a measure of how hard the heart pumps, how much blood is pumped (cardiac output), and how efficiently the blood is pumped.

In the OR setting, BP may be measured manually for a baseline and then may be measured automatically via an electronically controlled recording sphygmomanometer (Table 12-10). To manually measure BP, an appropriately sized BP cuff is chosen. This device consists of a rubber cuff and a gauge. The rubber cuff is placed around the upper portion of the patient's arm and air is pumped into the cuff through an inflation device. As the cuff pressure increases, the arterial blood flow is momentarily stopped. A stethoscope is placed over the brachial artery at the antecubital portion of the elbow and the air in the cuff is slowly released. The health care practitioner auscultates, or listens, for Korotkoff's sounds, which will be heard as a tapping sound that gradually increases in intensity. These sounds take place in five distinct phases, which must be recognized for proper BP measurement:

Phase I: On hearing two initial tapping sounds, the gauge is read and the number is recorded as the systolic BP.

Phase II: Soft swishing sound as more blood passes through the vessels while the cuff is being deflated.

Phase III: Rhythmic tapping sound returns as more blood passes through the vessels while the pressure is slowly being released in the cuff. If phases I and II are missed, phase III may be improperly recorded as the systolic pressure.

Phase IV: Muffled, fading, tapping sounds heard as the cuff is deflated further.

Phase V: Sounds disappear altogether. The point at which these sounds disappear is recorded as the diastolic BP.

BP is recorded in a fraction format on the patient's chart; location of the measurement and the position of the patient (e.g., supine) are usually noted. For example: "120/80, left arm, supine." In children and patients where the BP sounds can still be heard at zero, the beginning of phase IV and zero should both be recorded. For example: "120/90/0".

TABLE 12-10 Normal Blood Pressure Values and Classifications of Abnormal Blood Pressure

	CHILDREN	
	Newborn	50–52 systolic/25–30 diastolic
	Child (under 6)	95/62
	Child (to 10 years)	100/65
	Adolescent	118/75
	ADULTS	
Category	*Systolic (mm Hg)*	*Diastolic (mm Hg)*
Normal†	Less than 120	Less than 80
Prehypertension	120–139	80–89
Hypertension‡		
Stage 1 (mild)	140–159	90–99
Stage 2 (moderate)	At or greater than 160	At or greater than 100

†Optimal BP with respect to cardiovascular risk is systolic less than 120 and diastolic less than 80. However, unusually low readings should be evaluated for clinical significance.

‡Based on the average of two or more readings taken at each of two or more visits following an initial screening. Thus, a reading in the OR of 140–159 would not necessarily classify a patient as clinically chronically hypertensive.

Source: National Heart, Lung, and Blood Institute; Nation Institutes of Health; U.S. Department of Health and Human Services

In some critically ill patients, and especially in the OR setting, BP will be monitored via a catheter inserted into an artery and attached to a catheter-monitor-transducer system called intra-arterial BP monitoring or "art-line" that provides constant, accurate BP data. The catheter is inserted by the anesthesia provider and the pressure displayed on a monitor at the head of the operating table.

TECHNIQUE

Blood Pressure Assessment

1. Wash your hands.
2. Assemble the equipment and supplies.
   - Sphygmomanometer
   - Stethoscope, if necessary
   - Gloves, if warranted by the patient's condition
3. Introduce yourself, identify the patient, and explain the procedure, if necessary.
4. Position the patient and expose the site, if necessary. *Note:* Left upper extremity is preferred.
5. Apply the appropriate-size blood pressure cuff.
6. Place the stethoscope.
   - Stethoscope is placed over the brachial artery.
   - Stethoscope is secured with fingers only (not the thumb).
7. Inflate the blood pressure cuff to the desired pressure.
8. Deflate the blood pressure cuff slowly, while listening for Korotkoff's sounds.
   - Listen for Korotkoff phase I; note systolic blood pressure.
   - Continue to listen for sequential Korotkoff phases.
   - Note diastolic blood pressure; listen for Korotkoff phase V.
9. Continue deflation of blood pressure cuff and note auscultatory gap, if present.
10. Continue deflation of blood pressure cuff and remove it.
11. Wash your hands.
12. Record or report findings.
13. Care for the equipment as needed.

URETHRAL CATHETERIZATION

When preparing the patient for a surgical procedure, several sterile tasks are performed by the nonsterile team members. Two of the more common, Foley catheter insertion and the surgical skin prep, are presented here. However, first we will discuss the gloving procedure required before these sterile tasks can be performed.

Open Gloving

Prior to the nonsterile individual performing a sterile task, sterile gloves must be applied using the open-gloving technique (Figure 12-21). The open-gloving technique is not recommended when wearing a sterile gown.

Hands should always be washed and dried before gloves are donned and as soon as feasible following removal. Soiled gloves are removed and discarded as described in the technique that follows Open Gloving, entitled Removal of Soiled Gloves.

Indications for Urethral Catheterization

The most commonly used method of draining the bladder is urethral catheterization. **Catheterization** involves the introduction of a flexible tube via the urethra into the bladder for the purpose of drainage and/or irrigation. Foley catheterization is considered an invasive procedure (Figure 12-22). A physician's order is required for catheterization. The health care provider must use strict sterile technique to prevent infection.

Foley catheter insertion may be indicated for one or more reasons. Some of the indications for urethral catheterization are as follows:

- Decompression of the bladder
  - To prevent bladder trauma during pelvic procedures
  - To provide better surgical site visualization during pelvic procedures
  - To facilitate healing of urinary tract structures following genitourinary procedures
- Preoperative monitoring of urine output to aid in assessing kidney function and fluid balance. Output is documented in the patient's chart.
- Drainage of urine
  - To prevent overfilling of the bladder during lengthy surgical procedures
  - To measure urinary output
  - To obtain a sterile urine specimen
  - To relieve urinary retention
  - To treat incontinence
- Irrigation of the bladder
- Control of bleeding
  - A balloon may be used to place pressure on the bladder neck, such as after a transurethral resection of the prostate.

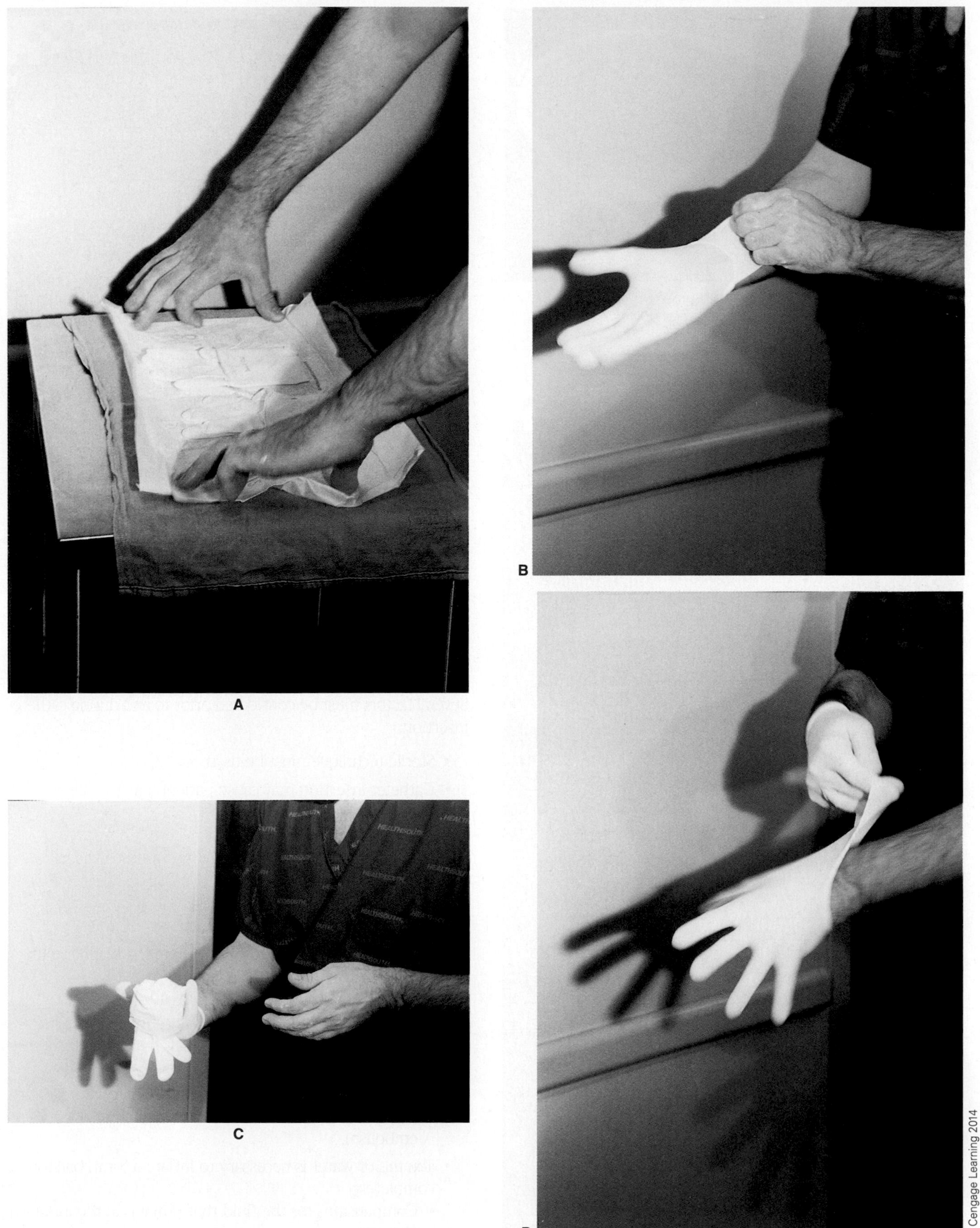

Figure 12-21 Open gloving: (A) Open inner glove wrapper, (B) don first glove, (C) secure and lift second glove, (D) second glove is donned

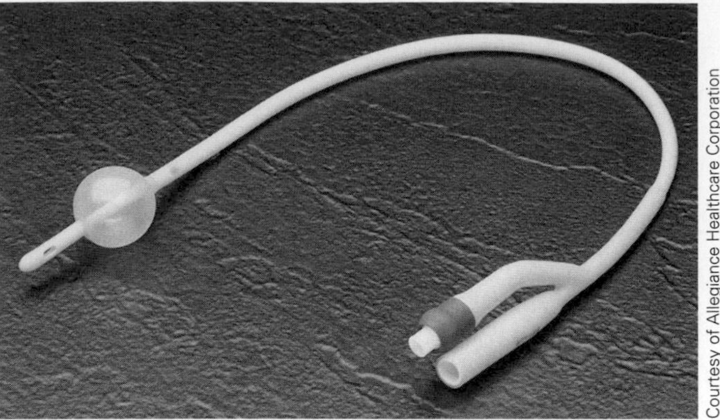

Figure 12-22 Two-way Foley catheter

TECHNIQUE

Open Gloving

1. Remove the wrapper containing the gloves from the outer package.
2. Place the glove wrapper on a suitable surface.
3. Open the wrapper to create a small sterile field by touching only the outer edges of the inside of the wrapper (up to 2 inches of the perimeter are considered nonsterile).
4. Secure the first glove from the wrapper by pinching the cuffed edge and lifting the glove up and away from the wrapper.
5. Orient the fingertips of the glove downward.
6. Apply the glove to the opposite hand by inserting the fingers and pulling the glove over the palm without touching the glove exterior.
7. Unfold the cuff of the glove without touching the exterior.
8. Release the second glove from the wrapper by inserting the fingertips of the already gloved (sterile) hand under the cuffed edge of the glove.
9. Keep the gloved thumb tucked under the cuff or well out of the way.
10. Lift the glove up and away from the wrapper.
11. Apply the glove in the manner previously described and make any minor adjustments.
12. The gloved hands are now considered sterile and the planned task (e.g., skin prep, Foley catheter insertion) is performed.

TECHNIQUE

Removal of Soiled Gloves

1. Grasp the palm of the glove to be removed first with your opposite hand.
2. Remove the glove by inverting it as you remove it; be sure that you do not touch your skin with your gloved hand.
3. Use slow movements to prevent snapping of the glove and splattering of debris.
4. Keep the removed glove in the hand that remains gloved.
5. Begin to remove your second glove by sliding your degloved hand between the skin of your wrist and the glove. Touch only your skin and the inner aspect of the glove.
6. Invert the glove as you remove it to contain both gloves.
7. Dispose of the gloves.
8. Wash your hands.

Considerations for Urethral Catheterization

Several factors must be considered prior to and during catheter insertion:

- Sterile technique must be used.
- Catheter insertion may cause patient injury or illness.
  - Urethral injury
  - Urinary tract infection
  - Be aware of the patient's allergy status; use a latex alternative if necessary.
- Catheters are available in a variety of styles, materials, and sizes.
  - Use the smallest size that will drain the bladder without leakage.
  - The surgeon will order the style catheter desired.
  - The Foley catheter is the most common style.
- The balloon is inflated with water, rather than air or saline.
  - Saline may break down the catheter material.
  - Air may escape from the balloon and cause an embolism.
- Ten mL of water is necessary to inflate a 5-mL balloon completely.
  - Compensates for the fluid that remains in the inflation channel

- Drainage of urine occurs by gravity.
  - Be sure the tubing is not kinked or compressed.
  - The urinary collection bag must be placed lower than the level of the bladder.
  - Do not raise the collection unit above the level of the bladder to prevent retrograde urine flow.
- Secure the catheter tubing to the patient's thigh.
  - Prevents unnecessary tension on the urethra
  - Prevents accidental catheter removal

Urethral Catheterization Supplies

The surgical technologist may be responsible for inserting the catheter preoperatively, intraoperatively, or postoperatively. Knowledge of the perineal anatomy is essential to proper technique in catheter insertion. Sterile technique is essential; urinary tract and/or kidney infections, blood infections, septicemia, or urethral injury can result from improper catheter insertion and care.

Catheters come in a large variety of sizes, from 8 French (pediatric) up to the largest size, 30 French. They are available in various materials, including latex, silicone, and Teflon, and types, including Foley, straight (Robinson), and coude tip. The smallest-gauge catheter that will drain the bladder is recommended. Commonly, a size 14 French or size 16 French catheter is used for adults. Although larger catheters are more likely to cause urethral damage, some people will require larger catheters to control leakage of urine around the catheter. Some people have developed allergies or sensitivity to latex; these people should be catheterized using silicone or Teflon catheters. Catheterization is usually performed after the induction of anesthesia to prevent undue patient pain and discomfort. For the male patient, the supine position is used. For the female patient, the legs should be spread, or "frog-legged." The following supplies should be gathered prior to catheterization and are often available as a kit:

1. Sterile drapes, one fenestrated
2. Sterile gloves
3. Lubricant (KY)
4. Antiseptic cleansing solution (iodine solution or chlorhexidine solution)
5. Gauze squares
6. Forceps
7. Syringe prefilled with sterile water (amount determined by balloon size of catheter)
8. Catheter of correct size and type
9. Sterile drainage tubing and collection bag
10. Sterile basin (bottom of sterile catheterization tray or basin containing prep solution may be used)

Prior to catheterization the items are set up on a Mayo stand or prep stand or the catheter prep kit is opened. Sterile catheter trays contain all of the above. With these premade setups, one need only open the tray using sterile technique and pour the antiseptic solution into the tray as well as open the packet of KY lubricant.

POSITIONING THE SURGICAL PATIENT

Positioning for surgery usually takes place after the administration of anesthesia. The goal of proper positioning is to provide the best possible access and visualization of the surgical site while causing the least possible compromise in physiological function and stress to joints, skin, and other body parts, and preserving patient safety. Positioning should also provide access to the patient for the administration of IV fluids and anesthetic agents.

When a patient is awake, physical indicators such as pain and pressure that warn when the limits of stretching and twisting are being reached maintain the range of motion (ROM) of the body. Muscle tone also helps prevent strain and stress to muscle groups. Under anesthesia, these protective devices are no longer active. After anesthetic agents have been administered, the patient is completely relaxed and paralyzed and has no ability to react to movements that could potentially damage joints or stress muscle groups. This is especially important to note with the arthritic patient, who may have joint changes that will prevent even slight movement beyond the normal ROM. Patients with demineralizing bone diseases such as osteoporosis are also at increased risk for injury. Patients are at higher risk in long surgical procedures and during vascular surgery, where blood perfusion may be low or even interrupted. The pooling of blood in dependent areas is a major problem and causes sudden shifting of blood when the patient is returned to the supine position following surgery. This places a strain on the cardiovascular system and may cause a rapid rise or drop in blood pressure. The patient should always be returned slowly from the operative position back to the supine position. This gives the cardiovascular system time to adjust. Patients with cardiovascular conditions and the elderly are at particular risk and should be closely monitored. Several factors must be considered prior to positioning the patient for a procedure:

- Basic anatomy and related physiology must be understood.
- Factors specific to each patient must be considered.
  - Planned surgical procedure
  - Primary condition
  - Co-morbid conditions
  - Allergy status
  - Age
  - Size
  - Nutritional status
  - Planned anesthetic

TECHNIQUE

Urethral Catheterization

Note: If a sterile kit with plastic tray is used, this may be placed between the patient's thighs; otherwise, work from a sterile Mayo setup specifically designed for catheterization.

1. Don sterile gloves using the open-glove technique.
2. Drape the patient.
   - For female patient, place sterile bottom drape just under patient's buttocks using sterile technique and taking care not to touch contaminated surfaces. Apply fenestrated drape over perineum, leaving labia exposed.
   - For male patient, place fenestrated drape over thighs below the penis and unfold up over the penis with penis exposed through the fenestration, using sterile technique.
3. Prepare supplies in order of use. Test balloon.
4. Cleanse urethral meatus.
   - For female patient, use nondominant hand to retract the labia and expose the urethral meatus. This hand should remain in place for the entire procedure and should not return to the sterile setup. Using the dominant hand and forceps, pick up gauze pad soaked in antiseptic solution and use it to cleanse perineal area. This should be done with a wiping motion anterior to posterior from the clitoris toward the anus. A new gauze or cotton ball should be used for each wiping motion, cleansing along each labial fold and then along the meatus.
   - For male patient, if present retract foreskin (be sure to replace at end of procedure) with nondominant hand. The penis should be grasped at the shaft below the glans, and the urethral meatus retracted between the thumb and forefinger. The nondominant hand should remain in this position for the duration of the procedure and should not return to the sterile setup. Using the dominant hand and forceps, pick up gauze pad or cotton ball and cleanse the penis, wiping once around the penis. Begin at the meatus and work toward the base.
5. Pick up catheter with the dominant hand and lubricate the tip. Catheter should be grasped about 5 cm (2 inches) from the tip and held with the end of the catheter coiled loosely in the palm of the hand. The distal end of the catheter should be placed in the prep tray receptacle unless it is already attached to the drainage bag.
6. Insert catheter.
   - For a female patient, slowly insert catheter through meatus. If no urine appears, it is likely that the catheter has been inserted in the vagina. If this occurs, another sterile catheter should be obtained and inserted, leaving the first one in the vagina until the second catheter insertion is complete, to prevent contamination.
   - Insert catheter approximately 5 cm (2 inches) in adult female patient, 2.5 cm (1 inch) in female child, or until urine is seen flowing out the end of the catheter.
   - Labial retraction may now be released and catheter held with the nondominant hand.
   - For a male patient, insert catheter approximately 17.5–22.5 cm (7–9 inches) in an adult or 5–7.5 cm (2–3 inches) in a child, or until urine is seen flowing out the end of the catheter. Catheter should not be forced against resistance. If resistance is felt, catheter should be withdrawn slightly. The catheter should be advanced another 5 cm (2 inches) after urine appears for retention catheters.
   - The penis should now be released and catheter should be held securely with the nondominant hand.
7. Inflate balloon.
   - Holding the catheter with the thumb and little finger of the dominant hand at the meatus,

(continues)

TECHNIQUE

Urethral Catheterization (*continued*)

place the end of the catheter between the first two fingers of the nondominant hand.

- With the dominant hand, attach the syringe (if not already attached) to the injection port.
- Inject solution slowly. If resistance is felt, the solution should be aspirated back and the catheter inserted farther. Do not push against resistance, as this may cause urethral damage.
- After the balloon is fully inflated, release the catheter and pull gently to feel resistance, and move the catheter back into the bladder. Disconnect the syringe.

8. Connect the end of the catheter to the drainage system, unless already connected. The drainage tube should be placed under the patient's leg and the bag should be hung on the operating table so that it cannot be pulled off. The catheter may be taped to the patient's leg using hypoallergenic tape.

- Knowledge of positioning equipment and supplies is imperative.
- Proper body mechanics must be implemented.
- Injury to the patient and surgical staff must be avoided.
  - Chemical
  - Electrical
  - Mechanical (gravity, friction, shearing)
  - Thermal
- Surgeon and anesthesia provider preferences must be considered.

For the safety and comfort of the patient—as well as personnel safety—many basic safety measures must be followed each time the patient is transferred or positioned.

- Patient identification and assessment (including allergy status and surgical site confirmation) occurs prior to transportation to the OR, and preparations to meet special needs are made in advance.
- A minimum of two individuals should be available to assist the mobile patient.
- A minimum of four individuals should be available to assist the immobile patient.
- All patient care devices (e.g., oxygen and IV administration equipment, Foley catheter, and drainage collection devices) must be protected during transfer or positioning.
- The patient must be adequately covered to provide warmth and privacy.
- Provide comfort devices (such as a pillow) and adjust the head of the transport device or operating table to a comfortable level, as the patient's condition allows.
- The wheels of the transportation device and operating table must be locked and the mattress stabilized.
- The patient is lifted, rather than slid, to prevent friction and shearing injuries. The use of transfer devices is recommended.
- The patient is moved slowly to maintain control of the body and allow for circulatory changes.
- Pressure points and bony prominences should be padded to prevent gravity-related injuries.
- The patient's skin should not come in direct contact with any metallic operating table parts, accessories, or unpadded surfaces that may cause electrical and gravity-related injuries.
- No part of the patient may extend beyond the operating table surface.
- Safety belt or straps are to be used whenever indicated.
- The anesthetized patient is not moved without permission from the anesthesia provider. The anesthesia provider directs movement of the patient.
- The anesthesia provider is responsible for maintaining the patient's airway and may not be able to help lift the patient.
- The armboards must not extend beyond a 90-degree angle.
- The patient's legs should not be crossed.
- The patient must be protected from injury during movement of the operating table.
- Patient care supplies, furniture, and personnel may not rest on the patient.
- The patient's eyes must be protected from drying and abrasion.
- Excessive torsion, flexion, and/or extension of any part of the patient's body must be avoided.

There are three basic surgical positions—supine, **prone**, and lateral—and each may be varied to accommodate specific patient needs. Body region(s) that may be accessed when the patient is in each position, the potential hazards to the patient, and the precautions that must be taken to prevent injury to the patient are discussed next. Keep in mind that variations may occur due to the specific patient's situation, surgeon and anesthesia provider preferences, product differences, and facility policy.

Supine Position

The **supine** position is the most natural position for the body at rest (Figure 12-23). The patient lies flat on the back with the arms extended on armboards with the palms facing upward. The armboards should not be positioned at more than a 90-degree angle to the operating table to prevent hyperextension nerve damage. Some surgical procedures require the arms to be positioned along the side of the patient's body, but this presents additional safety precautions. The arms should be slightly bent at the elbows and the palms facing inward. The draw sheet is placed over the arms extending 2 inches above the elbows and the sheet is tucked under the mattress. The draw sheet should be secure, but not too tight to avoid circulatory compromise. A small pad or donut should be used to stabilize the head, as extreme rotation of the head intraoperatively can lead to occlusion of the vertebral artery. Small pillows may be placed under the head, lumbar curvature, and knees.

The legs are straight and parallel, in line with the head and spine, placing the cervical, thoracic, and lumbar vertebrae in a straight line with the hips. The feet must not be in prolonged plantar flexion, which may cause stretch injury. A pillow or padded footboard may support the soles of the feet. Care should be taken that the ankles are not crossed to prevent pressure injury. The feet must not extend beyond the end of the operating table to prevent damage to the peroneal nerve, which can cause "foot drop." A table extension can be added to the end of the table. A safety belt is placed across the thighs 2 inches proximal to the knees.

Areas of the body that are in direct contact with the table will be under pressure during the procedure and are therefore at risk of tissue injury. These may include the occiput, scapula, olecranon, sacrum, ischial tuberosity, and calcaneus. The use of egg-crate padding and gel pads helps to minimize the pressure.

Typically, the patient is placed in the supine position prior to the administration of anesthesia. The patient may remain in the supine position for the procedure or be repositioned as needed once anesthetized. Any additional procedures such as application of antiembolic stockings, insertion of a Foley catheter, or application/insertion of additional monitoring devices are performed prior to repositioning. Once the patient is anesthetized, permission must be sought from the anesthesia provider to reposition the patient. Body regions that may be accessed with the patient in the supine position include:

- Head and neck
- Anterior upper extremity

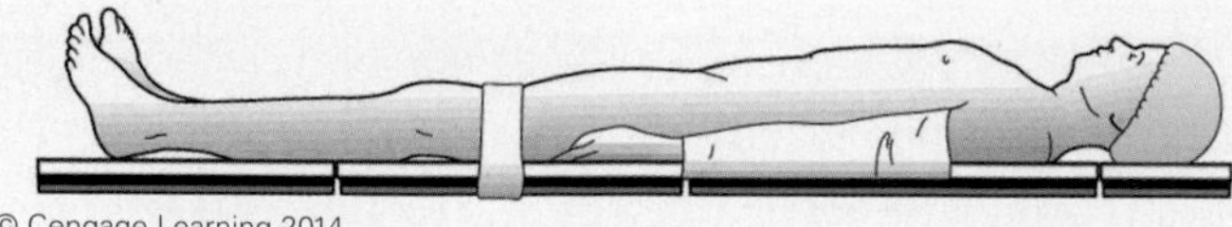

Figure 12-23 Supine position

- Chest/breast
- Abdomen
- Pelvis
- Anterior lower extremity

Potential hazards and necessary precautions that apply to the patient in the supine position are presented in Table 12-11.

Trendelenburg Position

The Trendelenburg position is a modification of the supine position (Figure 12-24; note head down positioning). It is used to displace the abdominopelvic organs cephalad to provide better visualization of the surgical site. Another benefit of the Trendelenburg position is that blood flow to the lower body is reduced and venous drainage is promoted. Conversely, the position may be used to increase blood flow to the upper body, as in the treatment of shock or for distention of blood vessels to be cannulated. Body regions that may be accessed with the patient in the Trendelenburg position include the pelvis and the lower abdomen. Potential hazards and necessary precautions that apply to the patient in the Trendelenburg position (in addition to those previously listed for the supine position) are presented in Table 12-12.

Reverse Trendelenburg Position

The reverse Trendelenburg position is a modification of the supine position (Figure 12-25; note head up position). It is used to displace the abdominal organs caudad to provide better visualization of the surgical site. Other benefits of the reverse Trendelenburg position are that blood flow to the upper body is reduced, venous drainage is promoted, and respiration is facilitated. Body regions that may be accessed with the patient in the reverse Trendelenburg position include the upper abdomen and the head and neck.

Potential hazards and necessary precautions that apply to the patient in the reverse Trendelenburg position (in addition to those previously listed for the supine position) are presented in Table 12-13.

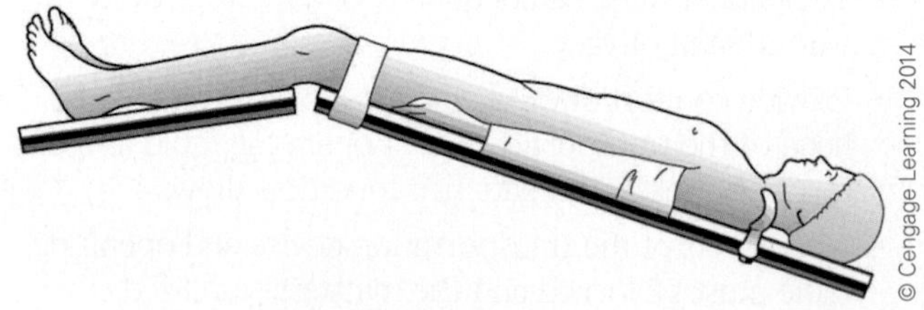

Figure 12-24 Trendelenburg position

TABLE 12-11 Patient Safety—Supine Position

Potential Hazard	*Precautionary Action(s)*
Brachial plexus injury	• Position armboard at less than a 90-degree angle.
Ulnar nerve injury	• Pad elbows. • Place arms on armboards with palms facing upward. • Place arms next to patient's body with palms facing inward.
Pressure injury to skin, blood vessels, and nerves	• Pad all bony prominences. • Uncross ankles. • Be sure restraining devices are not restrictive. • Use egg-crate padding or gel pads on the operating table. • Do not let any part of the patient's body extend beyond the padded operating table. • Avoid excessive torsion, flexion, or extension of any part of the patient's body.
Back and neck pain	• Ensure legs are parallel and the spine is in alignment. • Provide lumbar support pillow. • Stabilize head on a pillow or foam headrest.
Hypo-hyperthermia	• Adjust OR temperature. • Provide or remove blankets. • Implement use of hypo/hyperthermia unit. • Ensure solutions (IV and irrigation) are at correct temperature. • Provide warm humidified inhalation agents.
Corneal drying and abrasion	• Lubricate eyes. • Secure eyes in the closed position. • Prevent pressure on the eyelids.
Foot drop	• Use padded footboard.
Electrical injury	• Do not let any part of the patient's body contact any metal object.

Fowler's Position and Sitting Position

The Fowler's position is a modification of the supine position (Figure 12-26). The Fowler's position reduces blood flow to the upper body, promotes venous drainage, and facilitates respiration. Air embolism is a potential concern when the patient is in the Fowler's position. Body regions that may be accessed with the patient in the Fowler's position include the breast, head and neck, and shoulder.

Potential hazards and necessary precautions that apply to the patient in the Fowler's position (in addition to those previously listed for the supine position) are presented in Table 12-14.

The sitting position is a modification of Fowler's position (Figure 12-27). The torso is in an upright position. The flexed arms rest either on a lap pillow or on an adjustable padded table in front of the patient. A body strap should

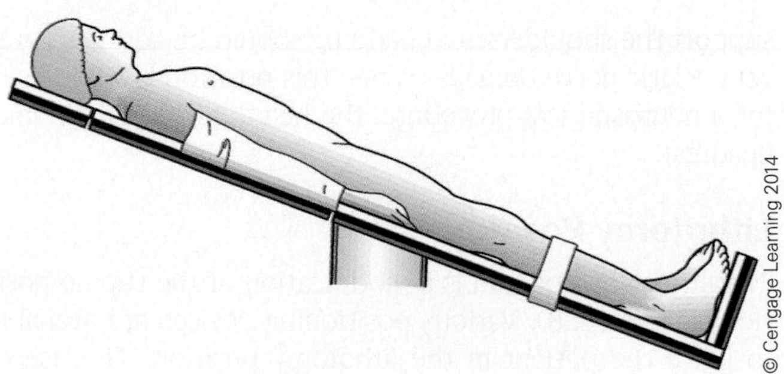

Figure 12-25 Reverse Trendelenburg position

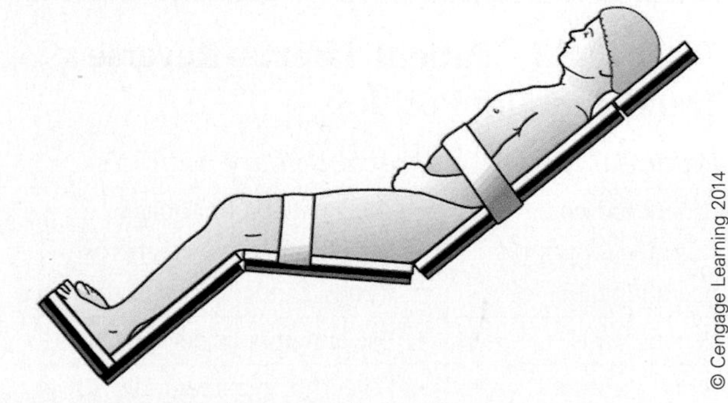

Figure 12-26 Fowler's position

Table 12-12 Patient Safety—Trendelenburg Position

Potential Hazard	*Precautionary Action(s)*
Cardiovascular and respiratory compromise	• Decrease angle of operating table. • Return patient to supine position as soon as possible.
Pressure injury to skin, blood vessels, and nerves *Note:* Special attention is given to the peroneal nerves.	• Pad areas as indicated for supine position.
Patient movement toward the head of the table	• Use padded shoulder braces.
Venous stasis	• Use antiembolic devices.
Blood pressure changes	• Level the operating table slowly.

TECHNIQUE

Supine Position

1. Transfer the patient onto the operating table.
2. Instruct the awake patient to keep the arms crossed over the abdomen temporarily (the arms of the unconscious patient must be held by a team member).
3. Apply the safety strap snugly across the thighs approximately 2 inches proximal to the knees. Allow approximately two finger breadths of space beneath the strap.
4. Be sure the patient is comfortable (offer pillow and warm blanket).
5. Be sure the patient's spine and lower extremities are in alignment.
6. Be sure the legs are parallel and the heels are resting on the table. Heel pads may be applied. The ankles may not be crossed.
7. There are two options for positioning the arms. Arm position will be determined by patient situation, surgeon, and anesthesia provider preference.
   - The arms may be placed on armboards, palms up, at no greater than a 90-degree angle. The elbows may be padded. A safety strap is snugly applied approximately 2 inches proximal to the wrist. Allow approximately one finger breadth of space beneath the strap. Be sure the strap does not interfere with IV infusion. A blanket may be placed across the arms.
   - The arms may be placed, palms facing the body, along the patient's sides. The elbows are slightly flexed and may be padded. The arms are secured with the draw sheet; the draw sheet is placed 2 inches above the elbows and tucked under the mattress. The sheet should not be too tight to prevent circulatory compromise.

Table 12-13 Patient Safety—Reverse Trendelenburg Position

Potential Hazard	*Precautionary Action(s)*
Patient movement toward the foot of the operating table	• Use a padded footboard. • Safety strap is placed approximately 2 inches distal to the knees.
Venous stasis	• Use antiembolic devices.
Blood pressure changes	• Level the operating table slowly.

support the shoulders, and padding should be added to prevent sciatic nerve damage. When this position is to be used for a neurosurgical procedure, the head will be in a cranial headrest.

Lithotomy Position

The lithotomy position is a modification of the supine position (Figure 12-28). Various positioning devices are available to place the patient in the lithotomy position. The use of candy-cane-style stirrups is presented here. Body regions

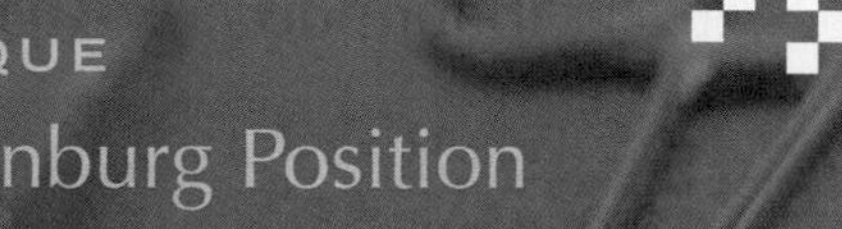

TECHNIQUE

Trendelenburg Position

1. Place the patient in the supine position.
2. Apply the safety strap snugly across the thighs approximately 2 inches proximal to the knees.
3. Padded shoulder braces may be applied to both sides of the operating table.
4. Secure permission to move the patient.
5. Tilt the operating table head downward to approximately 45 degrees or to the desired angle.

TECHNIQUE

Reverse Trendelenburg Position

1. Place the patient in the supine position as previously described.
2. Apply the safety strap snugly approximately 2 inches distal to the knees.
3. A padded footboard may be applied to the operating table.
4. Secure permission to move the patient.
5. Tilt the operating table foot downward to approximately 45 degrees or to the desired angle.

that may be accessed with the patient in the lithotomy position include:

- Vagina
- Urethra
- Perineum
- Anus and rectum

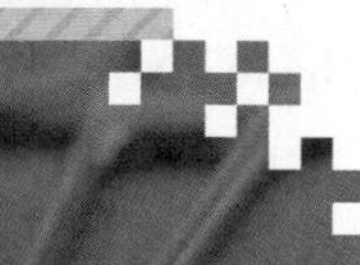

TECHNIQUE

Fowler's Position

1. Place the patient in the supine position as previously described.
2. The patient's arms may be secured on armboards or across the abdomen; a pillow may be placed on the patient's lap to place the arms.
3. Be sure the patient's hips are positioned at the table flex.
4. A padded footboard may be applied to the operating table.
5. Lower the leg section of the table to the desired angle.
6. Raise the body section of the table to 45 degrees or to the desired angle.
7. The entire operating table may be tilted head downward to achieve the desired level.

TABLE 12-14 **Patient Safety—Fowler's Position**

Potential Hazard	*Precautionary Action(s)*
Blood pressure changes *Note:* Postural hypotension is of special concern.	• Make adjustments to the operating table slowly. *Note:* A pneumatic compression device may be useful in combating postural hypotension.
Respiratory compromise	• If arms are not placed on an armboard, place and restrain them on a pillow resting across the abdomen, not on the chest.
Venous stasis	• Use antiembolic devices.
Patient movement on the operating table	• Padded footrest may be used. • Upper body may be restrained. • Neurosurgical headrest may be used.
Pressure injury to skin, blood vessels, and nerves *Note:* Special attention is given to the sciatic nerves.	• Pad pressure points. *Note:* Give special attention to the ischial tuberosities.

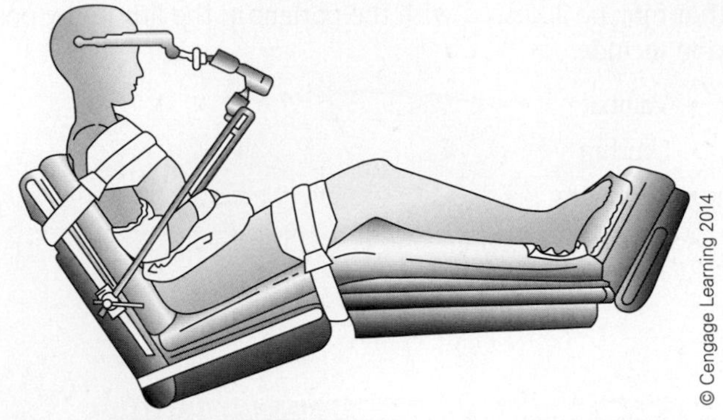

Figure 12-27 Sitting position

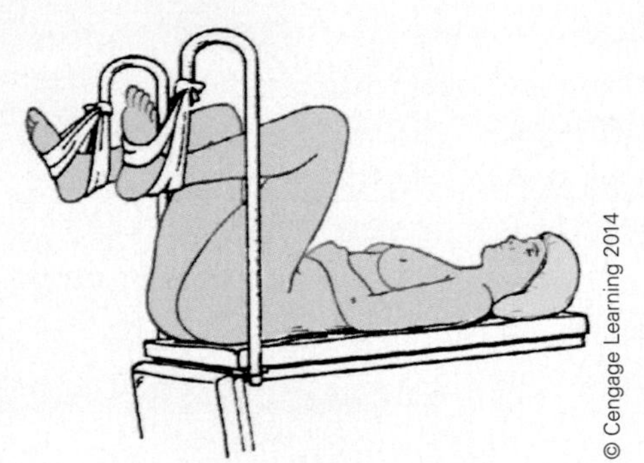

Figure 12-28 Lithotomy position

Potential hazards and necessary precautions that apply to the patient in the lithotomy position (in addition to those previously listed for the supine position) are presented in Table 12-15.

Prone Position

Prior to placement in the prone position, the patient is anesthetized on the stretcher (Figure 12-29). All preoperative procedures, such as Foley catheter insertion, must be performed prior to placement of the patient in the prone position. Body regions that may be accessed with the patient in the prone position include:

- Posterior cranium
- Dorsal body surface
- Spine
- Posterior lower extremity

Potential hazards and necessary precautions that apply to the patient in the prone position (in addition to those previously listed for the supine position) are presented in Table 12-16.

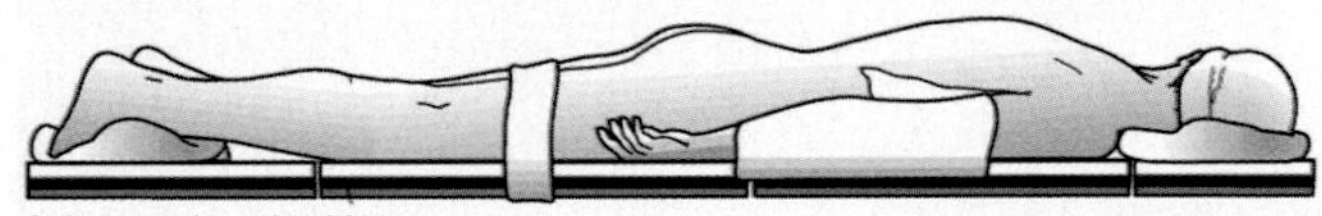

Figure 12-29 Prone position

TABLE 12-15 Patient Safety—Lithotomy Position

Potential Hazard	*Precautionary Action(s)*
Crushing or shearing injury to the hand	• Place arms on armboards. • If arms are positioned at the patient's sides, the hands must be observed during movement of the operating table.
Pressure injury to skin, blood vessels, and nerves	• Pad feet and ankles. • Be sure restraining devices are not restrictive. • Avoid excessive torsion, flexion, or extension of any part of the patient's body. • The legs may *not* come in direct contact with the stirrups. • Adjust stirrups to an equal height and length. • Raise and lower legs slowly and simultaneously by two individuals. *Note:* Give special attention to the peroneal nerves.
Back, knee, and hip pain	• Buttocks rest completely on the operating table. • Adjust stirrups to an equal height and length. • Raise and lower legs slowly and simultaneously by two individuals.
Blood pressure changes	• Raise and lower legs slowly and simultaneously by two individuals.
Venous stasis	• Use antiembolic devices.
Cardiovascular and respiratory compromise	• Restrict accompanying use of Trendelenburg's position. • Decrease leg height and hip flexion. • Return patient to the supine position as soon as possible.

TECHNIQUE

Lithotomy Position

The operating table is prepared in the following manner prior to patient placement:

1. Remove the head section of the operating table and place at the foot; secure.
2. Position the indentation in the mattress to allow access to the operative site.
3. Apply the sheet and draw sheet to the table.
4. An absorbent pad may be placed.

The procedure for placing the patient in the lithotomy position is as follows:

1. Place the patient in the supine position as previously described, with the arms on armboards, if possible.
2. Be sure the patient's hips are positioned at the table break.
3. Pad the patient's lower extremities as needed.
4. Apply the sockets and stirrups of choice to the operating table bilaterally.
5. Adjust the height and length of stirrups as needed.
6. Secure permission to move the patient.
7. Remove the safety strap.
8. Two nonsterile team members raise the patient's legs slowly and simultaneously by grasping the sole of the foot in one hand and supporting the calf with the other. The hips are rotated externally.
9. Place and secure the extremities in the stirrups.
10. Make any final height and length adjustments to the stirrups.
11. Release and remove the head section from the foot of the table and place it in a convenient location.
12. Remove the mattress and Bakelite portion from the leg section of the table and place them in a convenient location.
13. Lower the leg section of the table as far as possible.
14. If the patient's arms will be tucked at the sides, always check the location of the hands and fingers before lowering or raising the leg section of the table to prevent crushing them.

TABLE 12-16 Patient Safety—Prone Position

Potential Hazard	*Precautionary Action(s)*
Pressure on abdominal contents and thoracic compression *Note:* The vena cava and abdominal aorta are of particular concern.	• Use chest rolls. • Use axillary rolls. • Use antiembolic devices. • Move breasts laterally.
Pressure injury to skin, blood vessels, and nerves	• Place arms on armboards, rather than at the patient's sides. • Be sure all pressure on the male genitalia is removed. • Place pillows under the knees and ankles. • Flex arms on armboards with the palms facing downward or along the sides of the body with the palms facing inward.
Venous stasis	• Use antiembolic devices. • Elevate the lower portion of the legs.
Shoulder injury	• Lower and rotate arms for placement on armboards.

TECHNIQUE

Prone Position

1. Place necessary accessories within reach.
2. Apply pads to the ankles, knees, and elbows as needed.
3. A minimum of four nonsterile team members is required to place the patient in the prone position.
4. Align the stretcher alongside the operating table and be certain that both are in the locked position.
5. Chest rolls may be positioned on the operating table at this time.
6. Secure permission from anesthesia provider to move the patient.
7. Be sure that any patient care equipment is not disrupted when moving the patient.
8. Position the patient's arms alongside the body.
9. Roll the patient onto the operating table.
10. Be sure to secure the patient's arms.
11. Remove the stretcher.
12. Verify the position of the chest rolls if they are already in position; if not, they may be placed at this time.
13. Position breasts and external genitalia to alleviate any pressure.
14. The head may be turned to the side and placed on a pillow or foam headrest or be placed face down on a foam headrest designed for this purpose.
15. The arms may be secured alongside the body with the palms facing upward or toward the body, or the arms may be placed palms facing downward on angled armboards. This is accomplished by slowly lowering the arms toward the floor, then rotating them upward. The armboard is placed after the arm is positioned. Secure the arm on the armboard.
16. Place a pillow under the ankles.
17. Apply the safety strap 2 inches proximal to the knees.

TECHNIQUE

Kraske Position

1. Place the patient in the prone position as previously described.
2. Be sure the patient's hips are positioned at the table break.
3. Flex the operating table to the desired angle.
4. Tilt the operating table head downward to elevate the hips.
5. Apply the safety strap proximal to the knees.
6. Tape may be used to expose the anal area.

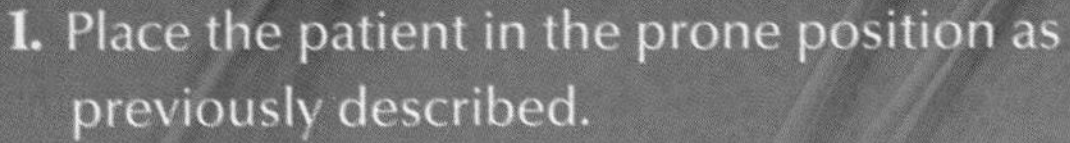

TABLE 12-17 **Patient Safety—Kraske Position**

Potential Hazard	*Precautionary Action(s)*
Blood pressure changes	Return the patient to the horizontal position slowly.

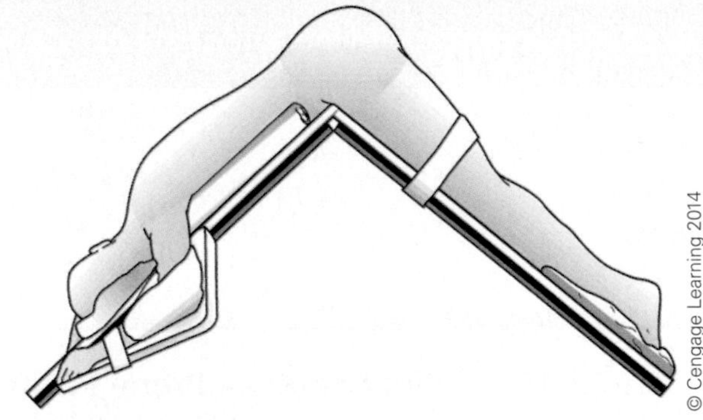

Figure 12-30 Kraske position

Kraske (Jackknife) Position

The Kraske (jackknife) position is a modification of the prone position (Figure 12-30). Body regions that may be accessed with the patient in the prone position include the anus and the pilonidal area.

Potential hazards and necessary precautions that apply to the patient in the Kraske position (in addition to those previously listed for the supine and prone positions) are presented in Table 12-17.

Lateral Position

The lateral position is also referred to as the lateral recumbent or lateral decubitus position (Figure 12-31). The patient in the

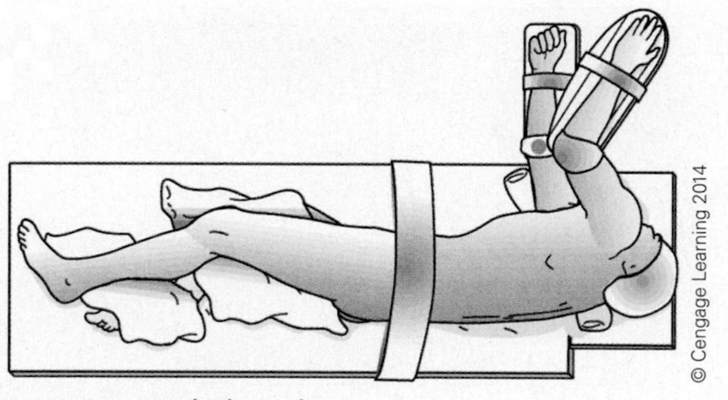

Figure 12-31 Right lateral position

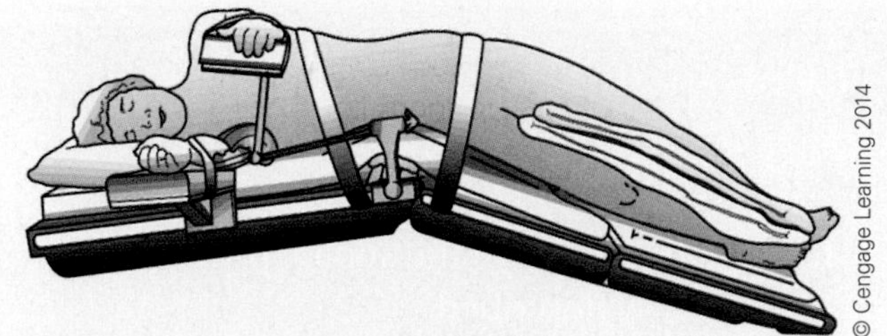

Figure 12-32 Right kidney position

right lateral position is placed on the operating table with the right side downward, exposing the left side of the body. The patient in the left lateral position is placed on the operating table with the left side downward, exposing the right side of the body. All preoperative procedures, such as Foley catheter insertion, must be performed prior to placement in the lateral position. Body regions that may be accessed with the patient in the lateral position include the retroperitoneal space, hip, and hemithorax.

Potential hazards and necessary precautions that apply to the patient in the lateral position (in addition to those previously listed for the supine position) are presented in Table 12-18.

Kidney Position

The kidney position is a modification of the lateral position (Figure 12-32). Body regions that may be accessed with the patient in the kidney position include the retroperitoneal space.

Potential hazards and necessary precautions that apply to the patient in the kidney position (in addition to those listed for the supine and lateral positions) are presented in Table 12-19.

Sims' Position

Sims' position is a modification of the left lateral position. This is the preferred position for endoscopy performed via the anus. Typically, the patient remains on the stretcher (rather than being transferred to the operating table) and is awake and able to assist with positioning.

The potential hazards and necessary precautions that apply to the patient in the supine and lateral positions also apply to the Sims' position.

TABLE 12-18 **Patient Safety—Lateral Position**

Potential Hazard	*Precautionary Action(s)*
Respiratory compromise *Note:* Due to gravitational forces the lower lung is better perfused, but contains less residual air due to diaphragmatic and mediastinal compression.	• Implement positive pressure ventilation. • Maintain cervical alignment. • Place an axillary roll.
Circulatory compromise *Note:* Arterial circulation to the lower body is restricted, as is venous return.	• Use antiembolic devices. • Avoid excessive compression of the abdomen. • Measure blood pressure from the lower arm.
Movement on the operating table	• Flex the lower leg. • Apply a safety strap over the hip, if possible. Tape may be used instead of a safety strap. • An upper body restraint may be necessary.
Pressure injury to skin, blood vessels, and nerves *Note:* The peroneal nerve, brachial plexus, and the vascular structures of the axilla are of special concern.	• Place pillows between the knees and ankles. • Place an axillary roll. • Place arms on a double-padded armboard. The palm of the lower hand faces upward and the palm of the upper hand faces downward. • The head is in alignment with the spine.
Foot drop	• Support foot and ankle of upper leg.

TECHNIQUE

Right Lateral Position

1. Place the patient in the supine position as previously described.
2. Apply pads to the ankles, knees, and elbows as needed.
3. Place necessary accessories within reach.
4. A minimum of four nonsterile team members is required to place the patient in the lateral position.
5. Secure permission from anesthesia provider to move the patient.
6. Remove the safety strap.
7. Be sure that any patient care equipment is not disrupted when moving the patient.
8. Use the draw sheet to slide the patient as far as possible to the left side of the operating table.
9. Roll the patient onto his or her right side.
10. Stabilize the patient's torso.
11. Place an axillary roll.
12. A pillow or foam headrest may be used to stabilize the patient's head.
13. Flex the lower leg.
14. Place two pillows between the legs.
15. The upper leg remains straight.
16. Apply the safety strap over the hip; tape may be used instead of the safety strap.
17. Ensure that shoulders and spine are aligned.
18. The arms are placed on a double armboard. The palm of the lower arm faces upward and the palm of the upper arm faces downward. The elbows may be slightly flexed.
19. The upper torso may be secured if necessary. *Note:* An alternate method for stabilizing the patient in the lateral position is to use a beanbag.

TABLE 12-19 **Patient Safety—Kidney Position**

Potential Hazard	*Precautionary Action(s)*
Abdominal compression	• The large kidney rest is attached anteriorly. • Both kidney rests must be well padded. • Be sure patient is positioned correctly over the kidney lift. • Lower kidney lift as soon as possible.
Circulatory compromise	• Reduce table flexion as soon as possible. • Be sure patient is positioned correctly over the kidney lift. • Lower kidney lift as soon as possible. *Note:* Reducing table flexion will also facilitate tissue approximation.
Venous stasis *Note:* The dependent arm and leg are at greatest risk.	• Use antiembolic devices.
Shoulder pain	• Place a chest roll.
Muscle strain to the torso	• Use the least possible amount of table flexion. • Reduce table flexion as soon as possible. • Be sure patient is positioned correctly over the kidney lift. • Lower kidney lift as soon as possible.
Blood pressure changes	• Ensure fluid management.

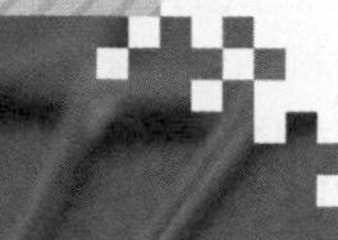

TECHNIQUE

Right Kidney Position

1. The patient should be rolled onto the right side as previously described.
2. Be sure the patient's flank is located over the kidney lift of the operating table.
3. The small kidney rest is attached to the kidney lift behind the patient.
4. The large kidney rest is attached to the kidney lift in front of the patient.
5. The operating table is flexed to the desired angle.
6. The kidney lift is raised to the desired height.
7. The safety strap is applied over the hip; tape may be used instead of the safety strap.
8. Shoulders and spine are aligned.
9. The arms are placed on a double armboard. The palm of the lower arm faces upward and the palm of the upper arm faces downward. The elbows may be slightly flexed.
10. The upper torso may be secured if necessary.
11. The table is tilted head downward until the flank area is horizontal.

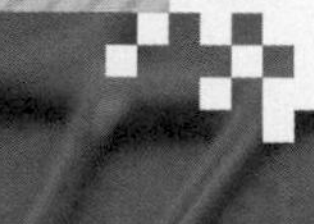

TECHNIQUE

Sims' Position

1. Apply padding to the knees, ankles, and elbows, if needed.
2. Ask the patient to roll onto the left side using the side rail for support as necessary.
3. A pillow or foam headrest may be used.
4. Request that the left leg be kept straight.
5. Have the patient slide the left hip back and flex the right leg.
6. The arms are either flexed or placed on the stretcher (a pillow may be placed between the arms) or the left arm may be placed behind the patient along the back and the right arm flexed and placed on the stretcher.
7. A safety strap is not generally used; the side rail is lowered and the area exposed just prior to the start of the procedure.

PATIENT SKIN PREPARATION

The surgical skin prep is performed on the surgical patient for the same reasons that the sterile surgical team members perform the surgical scrub prior to entry into the sterile field:

- To remove transient organisms from the patient's skin
- To reduce the number of resident organisms on the patient's skin

Living human tissue cannot be sterilized. Therefore, the goal related to the principles of asepsis is the basis for performance of the surgical skin prep: to keep the microbial count within the sterile field to an irreducible minimum.

Several factors must be considered prior to and during the surgical skin prep. Probably the most controversial of these is hair removal from the surgical site. Hair that may interfere with electrode placement, the surgical site, wound closure, and dressing application may be removed according to surgeon preference, facility policy, age and gender of the patient, and the planned operative site. Hair removal should occur as close as possible to the time of the planned surgical procedure to reduce the risk of microbial growth in any breaks in the skin surface caused by the hair removal. Be sure that the privacy of the awake patient is ensured to avoid embarrassment during the hair removal procedure.

Other factors related to the skin prep are as follows:

- All necessary procedures must be carried out prior to performing the surgical skin prep.
  - Anesthesia administration
  - Foley catheterization
  - Positioning
  - Exposure of the surgical site
  - Hair removal
  - Skin marking
- Gross soil and skin oils must be removed from the planned operative site.
  - May require use of a fat solvent or degreaser
  - May require use of a scrub brush and/or nail cleaner
- Prep fluids may not be allowed to accumulate adjacent to or under the patient.
  - May cause chemical irritation or burn the skin
  - Increases the risk of electrosurgical or laser burn
- Consider the patient's allergy status prior to application of any chemical; an alternate antiseptic may be needed, in particular if the patient is allergic to iodine.
  - Certain areas are considered contaminated and may require special attention. The general rule in prepping these areas is to prep the surrounding areas first and the contaminated area last and to use a separate sponge for each area. These areas are:
  - Mucous membranes
  - Stomas
  - Nonintact skin

  - Sinus tracts
  - Umbilicus
- Two separate skin preps may be necessary in certain situations (e.g., skin graft—donor and recipient sites).
- The prep is initiated at the planned incision site and carried toward the periphery, using a widening circular motion.
- An assistant may be necessary to elevate an extremity that must be circumferentially prepped.
- The recommendations of the antiseptic manufacturer must be followed (e.g., exposure time).
- Preoperative skin markings are not removed during the surgical skin prep.

Note: Some of the preparatory steps (e.g., hair removal and skin degreasing) may also apply to the skin sites selected for placement of the dispersive electrode for the electrosurgical unit and the ECG electrodes.

Types of skin prep solutions used in the OR are:

- *Alcohol*—Provides a rapid and significant reduction in skin microbial counts.
- *Iodophors*—Less likely to cause skin irritation and do not need to be removed.
- *Chlorhexidine*—Does not provide as rapid a reduction in skin microbial counts as alcohol, but provides a longer residual effect (5–6 hours).

TECHNIQUE

Preoperative Skin Preparation—Abdominal

If a commercial skin prep tray is not available, a sterile tray will need to be set up with the following items using sterile technique:

1. Two small basins for solution filled with the scrub solution and "paint" of choice.
2. Disposable, nonradiopaque sponges: 4 × 4 or foam sponges. The sponges used must not be counted radiopaque sponges but must be disposable.
3. Cotton-tipped applicators for cases where the umbilicus will need to be prepped. This is used to clean any detritus out of the umbilicus prior to applying the prep solutions.
4. Sterile towels to be used to soak up solutions along the sides of the patient in order to prevent pooling.
5. Forceps

Steps

1. Don sterile gloves using the open-glove technique.
2. Place sterile towels along the sides of the patient to absorb solutions.
3. Soak sponge in antiseptic scrub solution and apply the agent. The gloved hand must not be allowed to touch the skin, so that the hand may remain sterile.
4. Sponges used in scrubbing must be discarded as each one is used, and a fresh one is used to replace it. A soiled sponge must never be brought back over a scrubbed or "clean" surface.
5. Scrub skin starting at the incision site in a circular motion working in widening circles toward the outer edges of the area to be prepped. Effective cleansing requires both mechanical and chemical action, so enough friction must be applied to cleanse the skin and the pores.
6. After the periphery is reached with the first sponge, discard it, and use a second sponge to start at the incision site and work outward again.
7. Again, when prepping contaminated areas, prep those areas last. If a stoma is in the area to be prepped, cover it with 4 × 4-inch gauze soaked in the antiseptic scrub solution. At the end of the prep, discard this sponge.
8. Repeat this process for at least 5 minutes, or in some cases, until the counted number of prepared sponges has been used.
9. After scrubbing sterile towels are placed over the prep site to absorb excess scrub solution. The towels are removed and, the antiseptic agent is applied using more sterile sponges placed on a sponge stick or preferably foam sponges, and utilizing the same incision-site-outward technique until the entire area is covered with a film of the antiseptic agent, or "paint."
10. After the completion of the prep, cover any stomas or intestinal fistulas with a plastic transparent adhesive drape.

Several products are available for use in skin preparation, including scrub soaps, scrub solutions, and single-use prep applicators. The agent should be a broad-spectrum antimicrobial that provides residual protection. The choice of agent should be based on the patient's skin sensitivity and the surgical site.

The items necessary for skin preparation should be arranged on a separate sterile Mayo stand or prep stand. Sterile commercial prep trays are available, containing all the necessary equipment except for the antiseptic scrub solution and "paint" solution.

Single Use

Single-use applicators are available for the skin prep. These contain an alcohol-based antiseptic solution that leaves an antimicrobial film. They are self-contained units, and after activation as per manufacturer's instructions, the solution flows into the applicator sponge. These are used in the same manner as sponges for prepping the skin incision site by performing an outward circular motion and are discarded after use. To prevent ignition of the alcohol fumes, the solution should be allowed to dry. These have shown to have a long-lasting antimicrobial effect and leave an antimicrobial film on the skin.

Abdominal and Thoracoabdominal Preparations

Abdominal and thoracoabdominal preps are the most common preoperative skin prep performed in most ORs. The area covered for an abdominal prep is indicated in Figure 12-33.

Chest and Breast

For procedures in the area of the chest and breast, the arm on the affected side is elevated by an assistant during the prep (Figure 12-34). The areas to be prepped include the shoulder, upper arm extending down to the elbow, axilla, and chest to the table line and to the shoulder opposite from the affected side.

Eyes, Ears, Face, and Nose

For preparation of these areas, a piece of sterile plastic sheeting may be used to protect the eyes. The area to be prepped will vary, but as much of the area surrounding the incision site should be prepped and the prep should always extend to the hairline. Extreme care must be taken to prevent the prep solutions from entering the eyes, nares and mouth. The solutions can burn the delicate tissues of the eyes as well as the mucosa of the nares and inside of mouth and back of throat.

Extremities

When an extremity is to be prepped, an assistant should don sterile gloves and elevate the extremity so that it may be prepped around its entire circumference. For prep of the leg or legs, the assistant holds the extremity at the foot, and the leg is prepped around the entire circumference (Figure 12-35). A moisture-proof pad should be placed under the extremity to collect any excess solution that may drip. The pad is removed after the prep is completed and before draping. A sterile plastic adhesive drape is used to cover the tourniquet. The adhesive edge of the plastic drape is placed along the lower edge of the tourniquet and is opened toward the head of the patient to cover the tourniquet.

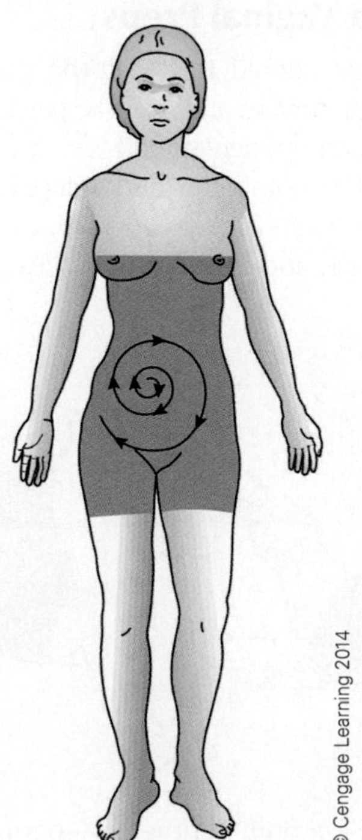

Figure 12-33 Skin prep perimeters—abdominal

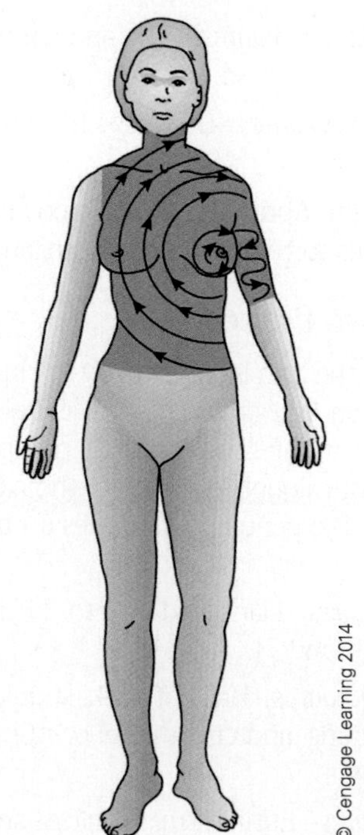

Figure 12-34 Skin prep perimeters—left chest/breast

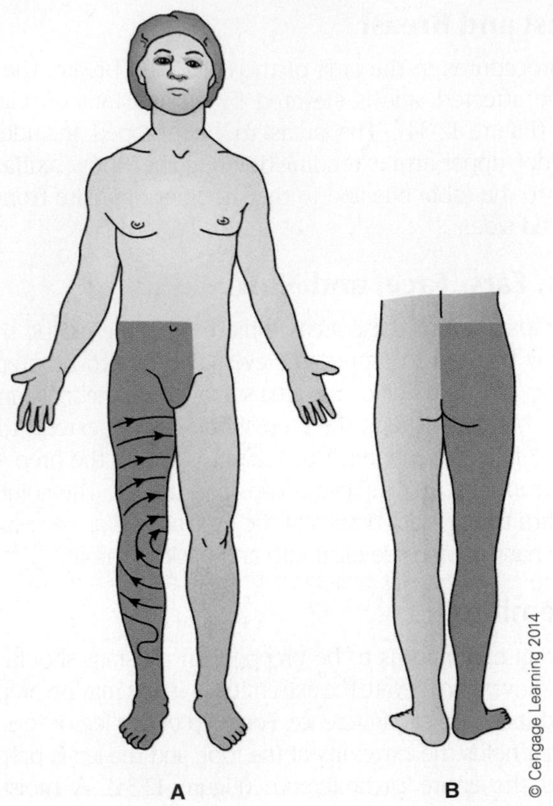

Figure 12-35 Skin prep perimeters (circumferential)—right lower extremity: (A) Anterior view, (B) posterior view

Leg and Hip Procedures

The general boundaries for leg and hip preps are:

- *Foot and ankle procedures*—Foot and leg from ankle to knee
- *Bilateral leg procedures*—Both legs from toes to waist level
- *Hip procedures*—Abdomen on affected side, entire leg and foot, buttocks to the table line, groin, and pubis

Hand and Arm Procedures

To prep the arm, the arm is elevated by the individual performing the prep or an assistant. The arm is held by the hand so that the entire circumference may be prepped (Figure 12-36). If a pneumatic tourniquet is not used, the axillary area should also be prepped. The general boundaries for hand and shoulder preps are:

- *Hand procedures*—Hand and arm to 7.5 cm (3 inches) above the elbow
- *Shoulder procedures*—Base of neck, shoulder, scapula, chest to midline, and circumference of upper arm down to the elbow
- *Arm procedures*—Entire arm, shoulder, and axilla, including hand

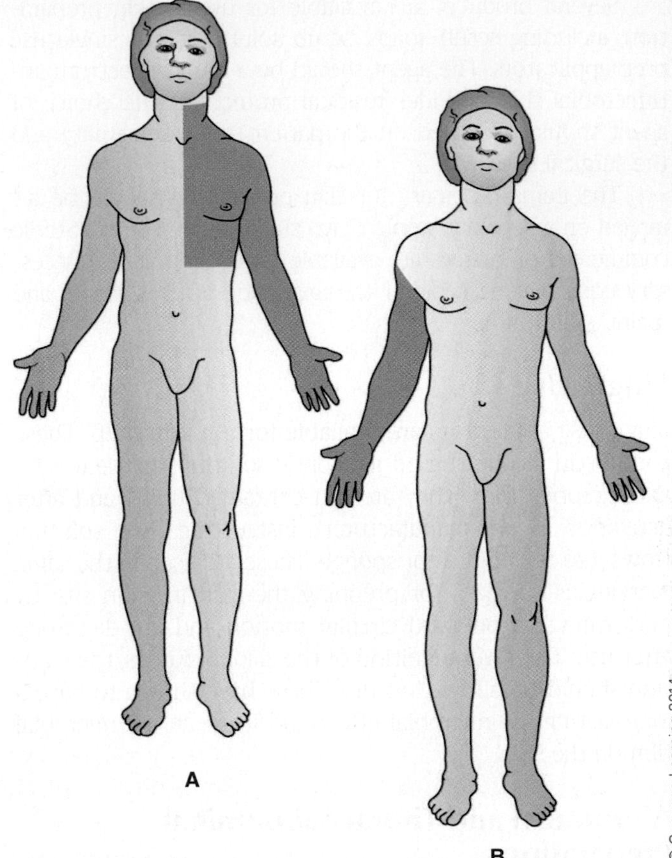

Figure 12-36 Skin prep perimeters (circumferential)—upper extremity: (A) Left proximal portion, (B) right distal portion

Perineal and Vaginal Preps

The perineal prep should begin at the pubic area, using a downward motion toward and over the genitalia and perineum (Figure 12-37). Each sponge should be discarded after going over the anus. For combined abdominoperineal operations, two separate prep sets should be used, one for the perineal area and one for the abdominal area. Gloves should be changed between areas.

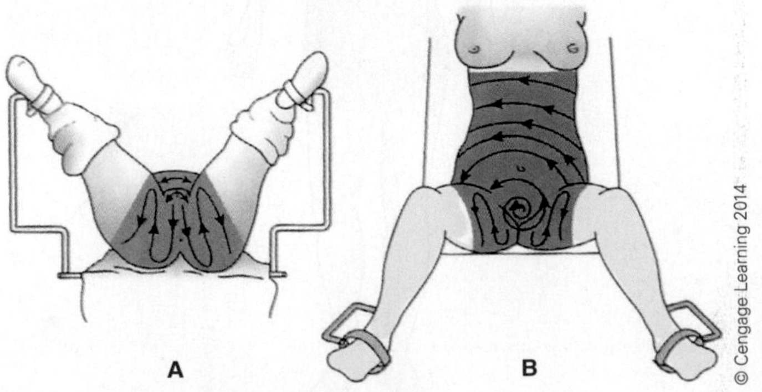

Figure 12-37 Skin prep perimeters—perineum: (A) Perineal view, (B) anterior view

For the vaginal prep, forceps will be necessary for the internal portion of the prep. Some surgeons will require no vaginal prep, as this is considered a contaminated area. Disposable prepackaged vaginal prep trays are available. A leakproof pad should be placed under the buttocks to capture excess fluids. The pubis, vulva, labia, perineum, and anus are prepped, including the upper thighs. To prep the vaginal area, begin over the pubic area and move downward over the vulva and perineum. Each sponge must be discarded after going over the anus. Sponges on sponge forceps are used to cleanse the vagina. After scrubbing the vagina, a dry sponge may be used for internal drying.

ASSISTING A TEAM MEMBER

The surgical technologist (or another team member) who has already scrubbed and donned sterile attire assists other team members who have performed their surgical scrub and are ready to enter the sterile field (Figure 12-38). Typically, the surgeon and surgical assistant begin their surgical scrub when the circulator begins the patient's skin prep and enter the OR just about the time the prep is finished.

DRAPING THE SURGICAL PATIENT

Drapes are applied to expose the surgical site, create a sterile barrier, and maintain a sterile field. Drape styles are introduced in Chapter 10.

Draping is another variable procedure. Draping for most abdominal procedures is common to several specialty areas; however, many specialty areas require specific kinds of drapes and draping techniques. In this section, several key principles that apply to all draping activities and four types of draping procedures—abdomen, perineum, extremity, and craniotomy—are presented in detail.

The surgical technologist may pass drapes in order to the surgeon, who drapes with the surgical assistant, or the surgical technologist may drape with the surgeon or with the surgical assistant. The surgical technologist must know the draping procedures, details about the drapes themselves, folding patterns, and potential difficulties associated with specific drape types. Because some drapes are large and because the possibility of contamination is increased during

A

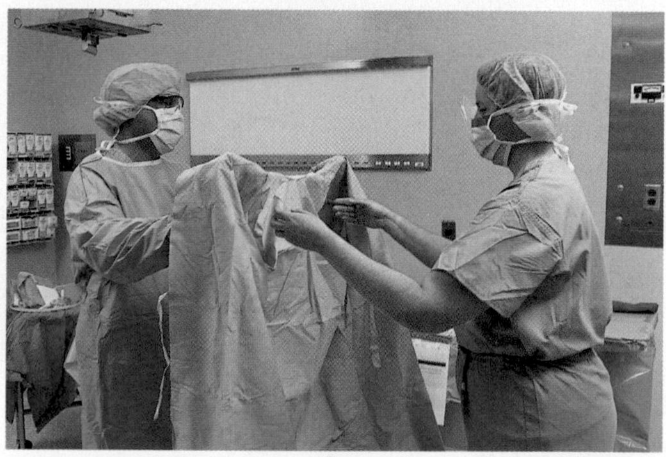
B

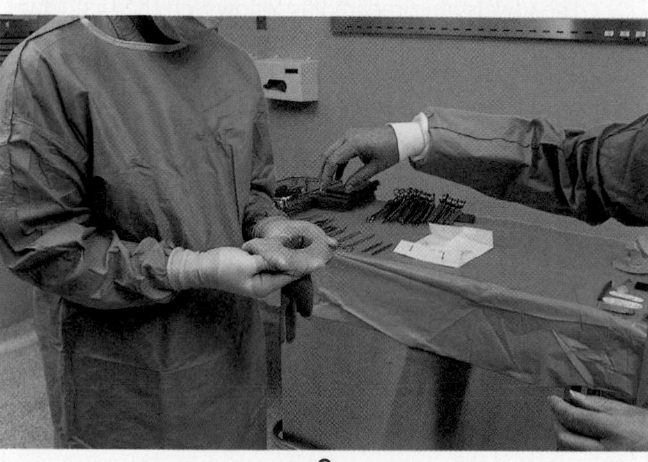
C

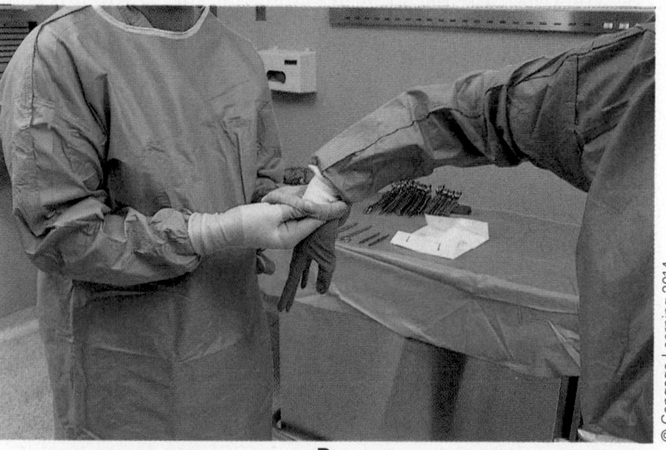
D

Figure 12-38 Assisting a team member with drying, gowning, and gloving: (A) Handing the towel, (B) presenting the gown, (C) glove position, (D) applying the glove

TECHNIQUE

Assisting a Team Member: Drying, Gowning, and Gloving

Refer to Figure 12-38A–D.

1. Lift the towel from the sterile field and step away from the field without turning your back on the sterile field.
2. Unfold the towel without allowing the ends of the towel to fall below waist level.
3. Protect your gloved hands by rolling the towel over the gloved fingers.
4. Present the towel to the team member by holding it taut and placing the edge of the towel on the team member's extended palm without making contact.
5. Lift the folded gown from the sterile field while the team member is drying his or her hands and arms.
6. Step away from the sterile field without turning your back on the sterile field and unfold the gown so that the outside of the sterile gown is toward you.
7. Place your hands near the shoulder area of the gown, allowing the neck/shoulder area of the gown to fold back over your hands, protecting them from contact with the individual you are assisting.
8. Present the gown to the team member by extending your arms.
9. Remain still while your team member places his or her arms into the gown sleeves.
10. Drop the gown onto the team member's upper arms.
11. Expose the team member's hands by pulling upward on the forearm section of each sleeve.
12. Secure the right glove from the wrapper.
13. Step back from the sterile field and prepare the glove by unfolding and orienting it with the thumb of the glove facing the team member.
14. Roll the glove cuff over your fingertips and slightly stretch to create a circular opening.
15. Extend the glove toward the team member and hold securely while he or she inserts his or her right hand.
16. Ensure that the cuff of the glove completely covers the cuff of the gown.
17. Repeat the procedure for the left glove; the team member will use a gloved hand to assist with slightly stretching the glove outward.
18. The circulator will assist with the final gown adjustments, secure the neck and back of the gown, and assist with turning the back of a wraparound-style gown.

draping, the circulator should participate as a careful observer of the procedure.

The core principles that relate to draping, without regard to the type of surgical procedure or the type of draping, are discussed below.

1. Typically, the following is accomplished prior to drape application:
   - The patient is anesthetized.
   - A Foley catheter is inserted, if necessary.
   - The patient is positioned.
   - The patient is prepped.
   - The dispersive electrode for the ESU is applied, if necessary.
2. Drapes are applied to expose the surgical site.
3. Organize the drapes in advance of need.
   - Drapes are stacked in order of intended use (Refer to the earlier technique, Organizing the Back Table).
   - Towels are prepared with a 2-inch cuffed edge. Four towels are used to initially square off the incision. The towels are prepared as follows: on the first towel the cuffed edge faces away from the surgical technologist, and on the next three towels the edge faces toward the surgical technologist.
4. Drapes and towels are not passed over nonsterile areas. It may be necessary to carry the drape to the opposite side of the operating table.
5. Towel placement follows a specific protocol.
   - All four towels and the four nonperforating towel clips, if needed, are carried together to the individual applying the drapes.
   - Towels are presented one at a time to the individual applying the drapes.
   - Towels are placed with the folded edge down and the gloved hands protected from contamination.
   - The first towel is placed on the side of the patient nearest the individual applying the drapes.

- The second and third towels are placed superiorly and inferiorly.
- The fourth towel is placed opposite the first towel.

9. Drapes are passed in the folded position.
10. Maintain a safe distance from the operating table until the drapes have been applied.
11. The protective covering is removed from a self-adherent drape prior to use.
12. Place the folded drape on the patient and unfold it, using sterile technique.
13. A folded towel may be useful in applying and smoothing the self-adherent impervious drape.
14. The sterile gown and gloves may not contact nonsterile personnel or items.
15. Drapes are not repositioned after initial placement. Misplaced drapes may be covered with another drape, if necessary.
16. Sterile gloved hands are covered by a cuff of the drape when extending the drape to the periphery of the sterile field.
17. A contaminated drape is removed by the circulator and discarded; it may be necessary to re-prep the area.
18. Any portion of the drape that falls below waist or table level is considered contaminated.
19. Sterile gloved hands are not allowed below waist or table level at any time during draping.
20. Nonperforating towel clips are used to secure cords and tubing to the drapes.

Problem Solving

- Any contamination offers two possible responses: discard and replace or cover.
- Holes discovered or made after draping must be covered immediately or the drape must be replaced. Covering small holes with an impermeable towel that has an **adhesive** edge works well in many cases.
- Perforating towel clips, if unfastened after initial placement, should be removed from the sterile field and the area should be covered with a sterile half- or three-quarters-drape or towel. Do not touch the tips of the towel clip while handing off the clip to the circulator, because the tips are contaminated.
- Small foreign bodies (e.g., hair) are grasped with a hemostat and handed to the gloved hand of the circulator and the area covered. The hemostat should be placed in a convenient place off the sterile field for inclusion in closing counts.

Draping the Abdomen

The technique for draping the abdomen is illustrative of the most basic type of draping (Figure 12-39). This technique is also used when draping the back, side, or any relatively flat surface that does not require manipulation of an extremity. Slight variations will occur due to patient position, surgical site, size of the area to be draped, and surgeon's preference.

Draping the Perineum

One-piece lithotomy drapes that will cover the legs while in stirrups and provide access to the perineum are available. However, a series of special drapes, including an under-the-buttocks sheet, special drapes for each leg and stirrup (leggings), and a fenestrated sheet, are more typically used (Figure 12-40). The technique described presumes an isolated vaginal procedure and not a laparoscopic combination. This type of draping runs an unusually high risk of glove contamination; therefore, double gloving is recommended and the outer gloves should be removed after the draping procedure is completed.

Draping an Extremity

Draping an extremity provides four unique challenges not faced in the first two draping scenarios:

- The body part to be draped for surgery is cylindrical in shape.

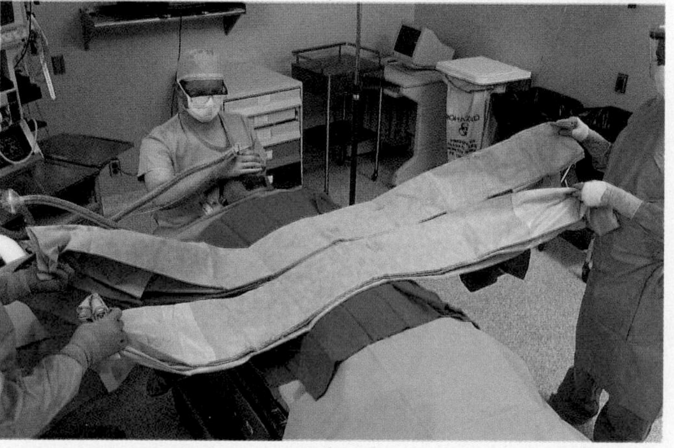

A

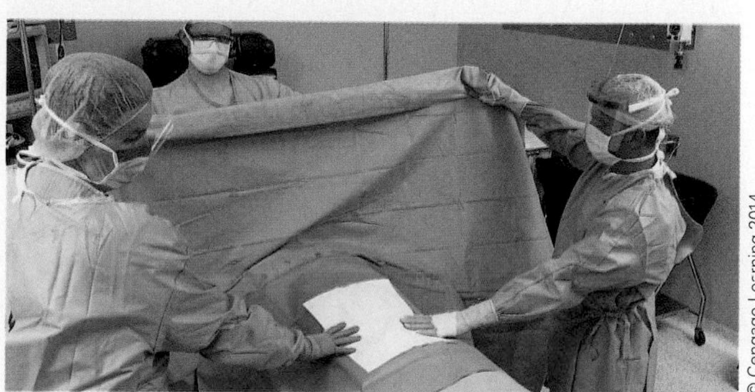

B

Figure 12-39 Draping the abdomen: (A) Unfold laparotomy sheet, (B) protect hands as laparotomy sheet is unfolded

TECHNIQUE

Draping the Abdomen

Refer to Figure 12-39A–B.

1. A half or three-quarters nonfenestrated drape may be used to cover the patient's lower body.
   - Present the edge of the sheet to the individual assisting with application of the sheet.
   - Unfold the sheet as both individuals approach the patient.
   - Protect the gloved hands by cuffing the sheet.
   - Do not reach below the surface of the operating table.
2. Four towels are used to outline the intended surgical site.
3. Provide nonperforating towel clips.
4. If desired, a self-adherent impervious drape may be placed; provide a folded towel to be used to smooth the surface of the drape.
5. Standing on the opposite side of the OR table across from the surgeon, remove the protective covering from the adhesive-backed portion of the drape and orient the fenestration of the laparotomy sheet over the surgical site and place on the patient.
6. Hand off one end of the drape to the surgeon and unfold the sheet toward the patient's feet.
   - Protect the gloved hands from contamination by cuffing the sheet.
   - Do not reach below the surface of the operating table.
7. Extend the head end of the sheet.
   - Be sure the arm boards are adequately covered.
   - Protect the gloved hands from contamination by cuffing the sheet.
   - Hold the sheet until a nonsterile team member (usually the anesthesia provider) is able to take it from you and secure it to the IV poles situated on each side.
8. Proceed with other preoperative activities, such as placement of the electrosurgical cord, suction tubing, and light handles.

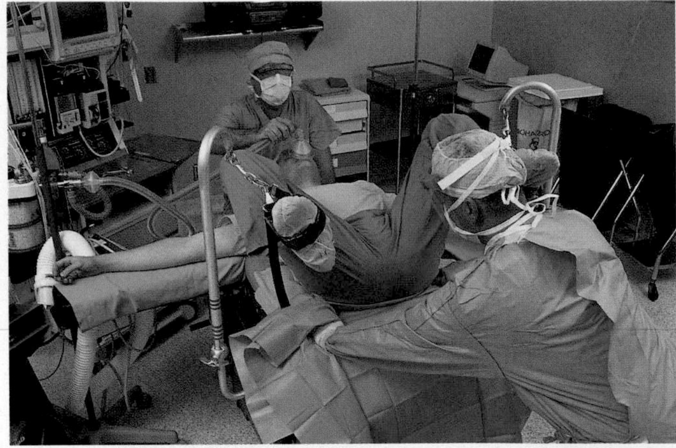

A

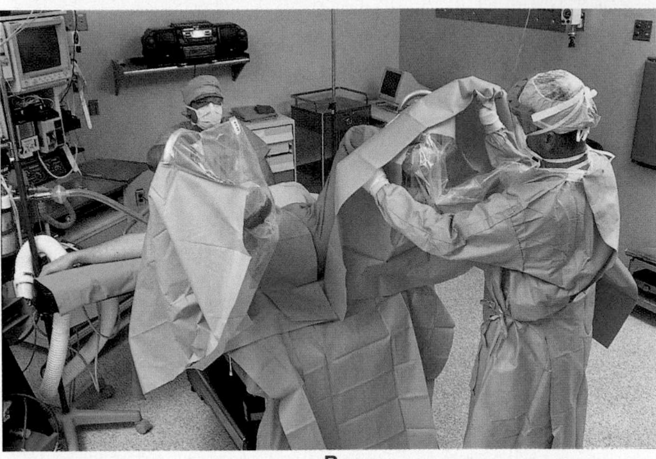

B

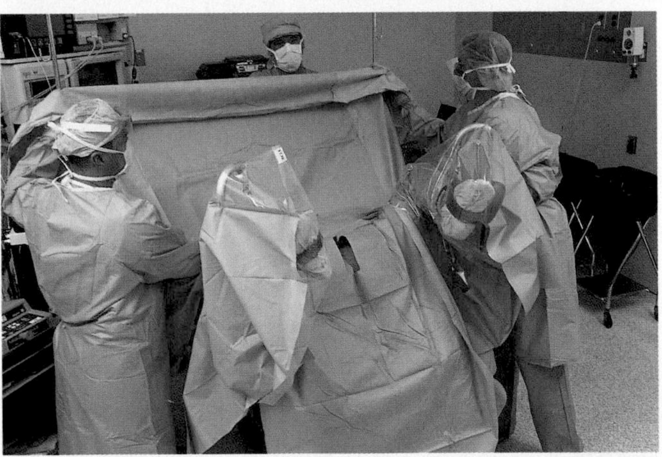

C

Figure 12-40 Draping the perineum: (A) Place the under-the-buttocks sheet, (B) place the leggings, (C) place the fenestrated sheet

- Because the cylindrical shape requires a nonsterile team member to hold the extremity while the skin is being prepped, the extremity must be received from the nonsterile team member. Typically, the nonsterile team member wearing sterile gloves will be holding the extremity

TECHNIQUE

Draping the Perineum

Refer to Figure 12-40A–C.

1. Present the under-the-buttocks drape to the team member applying the drapes so that the hands may be inserted into the cuff of the drape.
2. Let the drape unfold toward the floor.
3. Tuck the drape under the patient's buttocks with the hands protected within the cuff of the drape and an awareness of environmental hazards (e.g., the patient's legs).
4. Two or three towels may be applied to outline the intended surgical site.
   - Present the first two towels that have been folded diagonally, one at a time, to the team member applying the drapes.
   - If necessary, place a third towel horizontally to isolate the anal area.
   - Provide nonperforating towel clips, if necessary.
5. Present the first legging to the team member applying the drapes so that the hands may be inserted into the cuff of the drape.
6. The legging is unfolded while it is being applied to the leg suspended in the stirrup.
7. Present the second legging to the team member applying the drapes so that the hands may be inserted into the cuff of the drape.
8. The legging is unfolded as it is applied to the leg suspended in the stirrup.
9. The fenestrated sheet is applied to expose the perineum. Alternatively, a drape sheet or towel may be applied across the abdomen.
10. Proceed with other preoperative activities, such as placement of the electrosurgical cord, suction tubing, and light handles and positioning of the sitting stool for the surgeon, back table, and basin set.
11. A common variation to this draping technique is to apply the leggings prior to placement of the under-the-buttocks drape.

in an elevated position at approximately a 45-degree angle (Figure 12-41). If the patient's condition allows, the extremity may also be abducted.

- The body part will most likely be manipulated through some range of motion during the procedure.

Note: Studies have shown that for orthopedic procedures, contamination occurs most often during the draping procedure of an extremity. Double gloving and removal and replacement of the outer glove at the end of the draping procedure is recommended.

Draping for Craniotomy

Draping for a **craniotomy** illustrates another type of draping with unique specifications. It also presents two unique challenges:

- The patient and the operating table may be in a variety of positions (e.g., sitting, lateral, or supine).
- A relatively small access area is required but it is on a rounded surface.

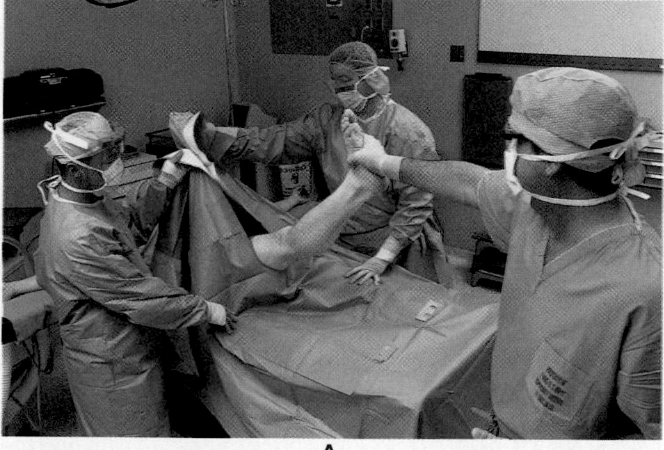

A

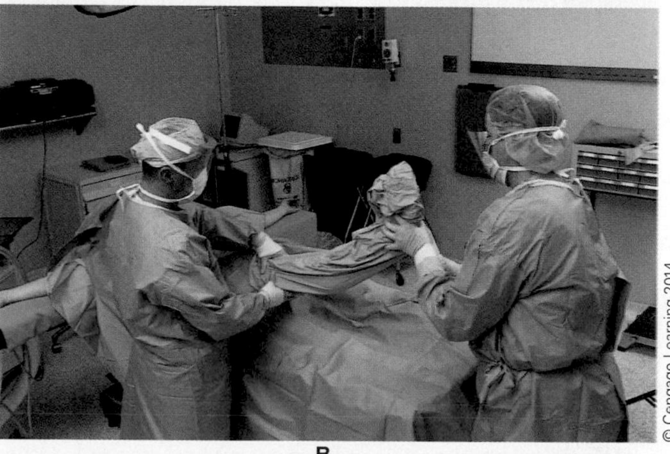

B

Figure 12-41 Draping an extremity: (A) Place the split sheet under the extremity, (B) place the cylindrical covering (stockinette)

TECHNIQUE

Draping the Extremity

Refer to Figure 12-41, A and B.

1. The circulator maintains elevation of the extremity following the prep.
2. A sheet or towels may be placed superiorly.
3. A sheet is placed under the extremity.
   - Present the edge of the sheet to the individual assisting with application of the sheet.
   - Unfold the sheet as both individuals approach the patient.
   - Be aware of the position of the circulator to avoid contamination.
   - Protect the gloved hands by cuffing the sheet.
   - Do not reach below the surface of the operating table.
   - When placing the sheet under the operative leg, the other portion of the sheet covers the nonoperative leg.
4. Adherent split ("U") sheets may be placed superiorly and/or inferiorly.
5. Present the prepared stockinette to the team member assisting with draping.
   - As the stockinette is applied, the responsibility for elevating the extremity is transferred from the circulator to the sterile team member as the extremity is accepted into the sterile field.
   - The surgical technologist may be required to hold the extremity while the stockinette is unrolled to the proper level.
   - If necessary, the stockinette is secured by wrapping it with an elastic or adherent bandage.
6. Standing on the opposite side of the OR table across from the surgeon, prepare the fenestration of the extremity drape for insertion of the extremity.
7. Unfold the sheet bilaterally and place over the extremity and slide upwards to the level of the planned procedure.
8. Extend the foot end of the sheet as far as possible.
   - Protect the gloved hands from contamination by cuffing the sheet.
   - Do not reach below the surface of the operating table.
9. Extend the head end of the sheet.
   - Protect the gloved hands from contamination by cuffing the sheet.
   - Do not reach below the surface of the operating table.
10. Place the extremity on the sterile surface. Alternatively, the surgeon may prefer that the extremity remain elevated while the tourniquet is inflated.
11. Cut the stockinette with bandage scissors to expose the surgical site.
12. Proceed with other preoperative activities, such as placement of the electrosurgical cord, suction tubing, and light handles and positioning of the Mayo stand, back table, and basin set.

There is little room for error in craniotomy draping. Since the critical steps of the surgical intervention take place inside the skull, the opening must be in precisely the correct place or access to the corresponding brain area will be difficult or denied. Many times, the preoperative skin prep routine will include the surgeon marking the skin incision with a scalpel or sterile marking pen prior to draping.

The craniotomy drape is normally a large fenestrated sheet with a round opening that can be adjusted in circumference (Figure 12-42). Some surgical units use Mayfield tables for neurosurgical instrumentation and some use Mayo stands. In either case the instrument stand is positioned over the patient's body. The craniotomy drape may be placed over the Mayo stand or over the Mayfield table. This prevents gravity from pulling the drapes toward the floor. If using a Mayo stand, the surgical technologist can use a sterile Mayo stand tray to place the instruments while setting up. Once the drape is in place the surgical technologist will place the tray on the Mayo stand.

POSITIONING OF THE STERILE TEAM MEMBERS AND THE FURNITURE

Following drape application, the sterile team members take their places around the operating table and the furniture is moved into position. Positioning of the sterile team members

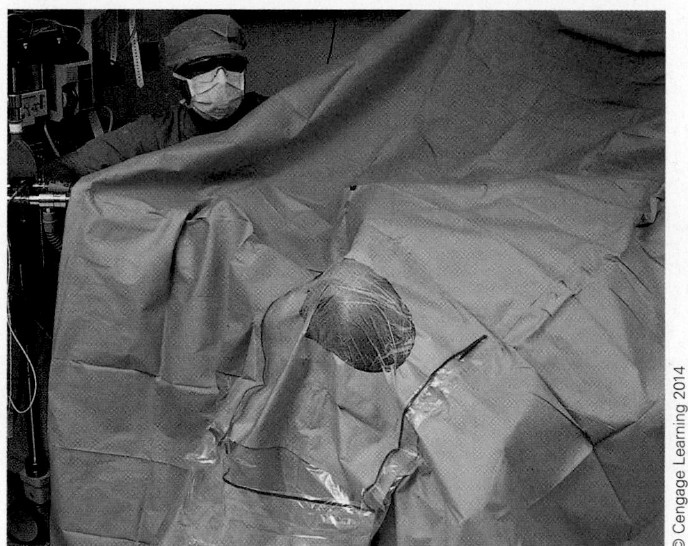

Figure 12-42 Patient draped for a craniotomy

and the furniture is affected by a number of factors. Variations are often necessary to accommodate a specific situation. Factors affecting positioning of sterile individuals and items include:

- Planned surgical procedure and incision site
- Planned patient position
- Size of the patient
- Preference of the sterile team members (e.g., a right-handed surgeon may prefer the surgical technologist to consistently be to his or her right)
- Heights of the sterile team members
- Dominant hands of the sterile team members
- Configuration of the OR
- Placement of nonsterile personnel or items (e.g., anesthesia provider or X-ray machine)

Following drape application the surgeon and surgical assistant may be provided with the light handles or covers, suction apparatus, and electrosurgical pencil for placement on the sterile field while the surgical technologist moves the furniture into position.

The Mayo stand is typically the first sterile item that is moved into position. To move the Mayo stand, the surgical technologist lifts the front of the Mayo stand slightly, without disturbing the items that have been placed thereon, and carefully rolls it into position. The Mayo stand is constructed to allow the tray portion to be placed over the draped patient. This allows the surgical technologist to stand behind the Mayo stand (with access to the foot pedal, should height adjustment be necessary) facing the instruments and supplies on the Mayo stand while observing the procedure, and allows efficient passing of instruments and supplies to other sterile surgical team members.

The ring stand containing the basin(s) may be positioned next, followed by the back table or vice versa, according to the situation. The surgical technologist maneuvers the sterile item into position by placing the hands on the surface of the back table or ring stand and rolling it into position. The circulator may independently move or assist the surgical technologist with movement of the ring stand or back table by grasping the item below the level of the sterile drape, and maneuvering the item into position, being careful that the bouffant hair cover does not touch any sterile item or surface.

The back table should be positioned to allow the surgical technologist to retrieve items without turning his or her back to the remainder of the sterile field. Since this may be a practical impossibility, the back table must be distant enough from

TECHNIQUE

Draping for a Craniotomy

Refer to Figure 12-42.

1. The intended surgical site is outlined with three or four sterile towels.
   - If cloth towels are used, they may be sutured in position or secured with nonperforating towel clips.
2. The craniotomy drape is applied.
   - If necessary, remove the protective covering from the adhesive portion of the drape.
   - Hand one end of the craniotomy drape to the surgeon.
   - Unfold the drape bilaterally.
   - Position the fenestration to expose the surgical site.
   - The superior end of the drape with fluid collection pouch is allowed to fall toward the floor.
   - The inferior end of the drape is extended over the patient.
   - The drape may be allowed to rest on the patient's body or may be placed on the Mayo stand or Mayfield table and secured by the weight of the instruments and supplies or with adhesive or clamps.
3. Additional sheets may be used as necessary.
4. Proceed with other preoperative activities, such as placement of the electrosurgical cord, suction tubing, and light handles and positioning of the back table and basin set.

the surgical technologist to allow safe movement between the sterile areas.

While the circulator connects and activates the electrosurgical unit, suction apparatus, and any other necessary items, the surgical technologist places two surgical sponges on each side of the operative site for use by the surgeon and surgical assistant. The surgical technologist also ensures that everything is ready, and prepares to pass the scalpel to the surgeon. The preoperative case management phase ends just prior to initiation of the incision.

MARKING THE SKIN INCISION

Sterile skin markers are available for the surgeon's use for marking incision lines on the skin preoperatively. In some instances, the surgeon may prefer to use a cotton applicator dipped in methylene blue or gentian violet. These markers may also be used intraoperatively, although the original skin marker should be discarded and a fresh sterile marker should be used.

PART II: Intraoperative Case Management

The intraoperative phase of case management begins when the incision is made. The intraoperative responsibilities of the surgical technologist extend far beyond passing the instrumentation and supplies to the surgeon and other sterile team members. An awareness of the total surgical environment is necessary to allow the surgical technologist to anticipate the needs of the patient, the surgeon, and other surgical team members.

GENERAL PRINCIPLES

The information in this section is not intended to serve as a memorization aid for the steps related to particular surgical procedures. Rather, it is meant to help the surgical technologist focus on organization of thoughts and activities to enable application of the information to management of virtually any surgical procedure. (Specific technical considerations are presented in Chapters 14 through 24.)

It is the intraoperative activity of the surgical technologist that is most illustrative of the classic role of the surgical technologist. Throughout this period, the surgical technologist should constantly compare the anatomy and pathology being seen to what should be expected and the progress and success of the procedure to the norm. The specific variations observed should lead to predictions about procedural sequence and needs of the surgeon. The efficient and effective surgical technologist always:

- Observes the details of anatomy, pathology, and procedure
- Handles the specific skills of instrument care and passing proficiently; additionally, keeps the instruments clean and maintains an orderly work area
- Anticipates actions and needs two to three steps in advance
- Pays attention to the entire OR environment: physical and mental
- Communicates effectively with all members of the surgical team, particularly the surgeon and the circulator
- Understands the nature of the pathology causing the intervention and its variations, and is prepared for unknown or unpredictable pathology
- Is prepared for differences in surgeons' approaches to the procedure
- Anticipates problems with equipment, instruments, and technology, and can problem-solve equipment break-downs

The surgical technologist should be familiar with the basic normal anatomy of all bodily systems and well versed in those specialty areas in which he or she works frequently. The first question is always something like this: Does the basic gross anatomy appear normal? Normal variations are found frequently and include:

- The arterial branches to the liver and gallbladder, which have several well-documented patterns
- The course of the recurrent laryngeal nerve, which has several well-documented patterns
- Female pelvic structure, which has several defined types

Each of these is a variation of the norm. However, each may affect the decisions made in patient intervention. It is important to ligate and cut the cystic artery and not the hepatic artery or any of its branches during a cholecystectomy. The course of the recurrent laryngeal nerve must be identified and preserved during a thyroidectomy to avoid postoperative speech complications. Pelvic structure is a significant contributor to the decision to perform a cesarean section. In each case, the anatomy determines changes from the routine. The surgical technologist must prepare for these changes in advance. In the first two examples, the changes may be subtle. The surgical technologist may verify that there are enough ligating clips remaining or recognize that the pattern of dissection will follow a different sequence. In the third instance, the variation may cause a change in procedure from normal delivery to cesarean section or may affect visibility during a hysterectomy, resulting in the use of different retractors. Sometimes the surgical technologist cannot actually see the variation but can identify it from the surgeon's comments. In every instance, the surgical technologist should use the information to predict the sequence of events to follow.

Pathological variations in anatomy also affect the procedure. At times the abnormality may be the reason the procedure is being done (e.g., aortic aneurysm, bowel obstruction, or congenital anomaly). At other times, the abnormality may be discovered as part of the procedure (e.g., adhesions, bicornuate uterus, or retrocecal appendix). Each condition affects the procedural sequence and presents unique technical problems. The surgical technologist should immediately ask himself or herself: What are the possible solutions to this problem and how will it affect the procedure?

Several examples of pathological conditions and some of the problems presented by each condition are described briefly below.

- Meningiomas usually have a rich vascular supply from their meningeal origin. Excessive bleeding may begin with the perforation of the bone and may be problematic throughout the procedure.
- A severely infected and friable gallbladder may need decompression prior to any attempt to remove it.
- A bowel obstruction resulting in leakage of intestinal contents may lead to the use of retention sutures.
- Abnormal placental position may cause a change from a low cervical to a classical incision into the uterus during a cesarean section.

Each problem of pathology usually has several different solutions. Some of the responses are determined more by the anatomical and pathological variables combined than by any other factor. Some are more affected by the training and preference of the surgeon. Some are affected by current research studies. All responses are ultimately affected by a combination of these variables. The effective surgical technologist must be conscious of the variables and use them to predict the future path of the procedure.

Probable changes or special needs should be communicated as early as possible to the circulator. For instance, if there is a bowel obstruction with spillage and the surgical technologist knows that the specific surgeon always uses retention sutures in this circumstance, this information should be communicated as early as possible. This allows for efficient and effective case management in the circulator's role. For instance, one might state, "There is spillage of bowel contents. We may anticipate copious irrigation and the use of retention sutures. Dr. Doe usually uses No. 1 nylon, double armed." This allows the circulator to plan an efficient course of action. The circulator will be thinking: When will these be needed? Are there other items (such as bolsters) that will be needed? When is it best for me to leave the room in order to obtain the supplies?

As knowledge and experience grow, the surgical technologist becomes more adept at seeing subtle changes and predicting the effects of the changes on the procedure.

Safety

Standard Precautions must be followed at all times. Additionally, a number of intraoperative safety measures must be employed to protect the patient and the surgical team members. Some examples include

- Placement of the electrosurgical pencil in the holster when not in use
- Cautious handling of sharps (e.g., use of the **neutral zone**, use of sharps container/counter)
- Double gloving and other PPE
- Appropriate protection from environmental hazards (e.g., lasers, X-rays)

INTRAOPERATIVE COMMUNICATION

Along with the ability of the surgical technologist to anticipate the needs of the patient and surgical team members, verbal and nonverbal methods of communication are also used to facilitate the surgical procedure.

Verbal Communication

Verbal communication occurs between all members of the surgical team. However, the majority of the intraoperative verbal communication takes place within the sterile field. The surgeon or surgical assistant typically calls out the name of the desired item and the surgical technologist responds by providing it directly to the individual requesting the item. For example, if the surgeon asks for a scalpel, the surgical technologist responds by placing the scalpel in the preestablished "neutral zone." If the requested item is readily available, a verbal response from the surgical technologist may not be necessary. However, if a requested item is not readily available, the surgical technologist should acknowledge the request and inform the team member(s) when the item is expected. For example, if the surgeon calls for culture tubes that were not opened onto the sterile field, the surgical technologist may respond with, "I'm getting them now" and provides them to the surgeon as soon as the circulator provides the item(s). It is important to remember to be courteous and professional with all team members.

Nonverbal Communication

Hand signals are often used to keep talking, and its resultant microbial contamination, to a minimum (Figure 12-43). Additionally, hand signals often replace verbal requests if the patient is not under general anesthesia. The surgical technologist must be vigilant of the activities at the surgical site to receive and accurately respond to nonverbal requests.

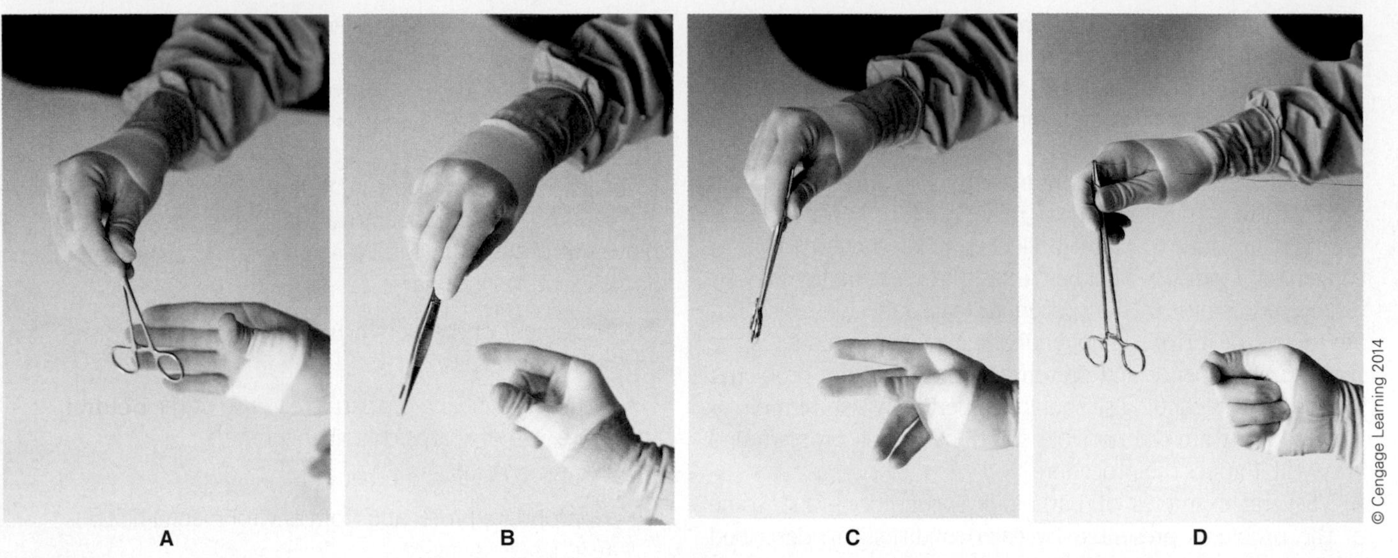

Figure 12-43 Hand signals: (A) Request for a hemostat, (B) request for a tissue forceps, (C) request for a scissors, (D) request for a suture

PASSING THE INSTRUMENTS (AND OTHER SUPPLIES)

Specific techniques are used for handling each of the types of instruments used in surgery. This section considers general techniques for passing instruments and the specific problem of handling sharps. The reader is also referred to the sections on the neutral zone and sharps safety in Chapter 5. The basic principle of instrument passing is simple: Pass the instrument so that it is received in a position ready for use.

The discussion on instrument passing presumes a laparotomy procedure. The Mayo stand is placed in the area of the patient's lower thighs. Surgeon and assistant are positioned on each side of the patient at the level of the abdomen. The surgical technologist should be directly behind the Mayo stand. The surgeon may be positioned on the same or opposite side of the operating table as the surgical technologist. Generally, the surgical technologist standing opposite of the surgeon promotes greater efficiency in the passing of instruments. The surgical technologist must be aware of the visual field of the surgeon. The surgeon's field of vision should not be obstructed when passing instruments to the assistant. Passing techniques are described in Table 12-20.

TABLE 12-20 Techniques for Passing Instruments: Which Hand to Use

Receiver's Position	*Surgical Technologist's Passing Hand*	*Special Technique*
Surgeon on same side of table as surgical technologist and to surgical technologist's left		
Pass to surgeon's right hand	Surgical technologist uses right hand	
Pass to surgeon's left hand	Surgical technologist uses right hand	Arm must be bent to avoid surgeon's right hand
• These passes must be made without hitting Mayo stand with side or back		
• May use left hand if the pass does not interfere with surgeon's right hand		
Surgeon on same side of table as surgical technologist and to surgical technologist's right		
Pass to surgeon's left hand	Surgical technologist uses left hand	
Pass to surgeon's right hand	Surgical technologist uses left hand	Arm must be bent to avoid surgeon's right hand
• These passes must be made without hitting Mayo stand with side or back		
• May use right hand if the pass does not interfere with surgeon's right hand		
Surgeon across table from STSR		

The scalpel is one of the more dangerous instruments used. Several practices have been defined and practiced, including:

- Handing the scalpel to the surgeon and receiving the scalpel back from the surgeon
- Handing the scalpel to the surgeon but having the surgeon place it in a designated safe area on the Mayo stand where it is retrieved by the surgical technologist (Chapter 5)
- No-hand technique where the scalpel is placed in the neutral zone by the surgical technologist, retrieved and used by the surgeon, returned to the neutral zone by the surgeon, and retrieved by the surgical technologist
- No-hand technique using a basin as the safe area (beware of reaching into basin with sharps; refer to Chapter 5)

It is not clear if any of the above techniques are any safer than the others in the long run. Practical experience suggests that the most dangerous component is the return exchange from surgeon to surgical technologist. The surgeon is solely focused on the procedure and there is no clear, safe technique for this pass. However, OSHA guidelines recommend the use of the third or fourth options for purposes of safety. The surgical technologist may then secure the scalpel and return it to its designated location on the Mayo stand. It is probably best to remove both the skin and deep "knives" to a secure sharps area on the back table as soon as they are no longer needed. If handed, the scalpel is placed into the surgeon's hand "pencil" style. The surgical technologist should use the fingers of the passing hand to protect the others from the blade. This is accomplished by holding the scalpel handle with the index and middle finger near the blade. With the palm of the passing hand facing the OR table and the scalpel blade edge also facing toward the OR table away from the palm, the blade rests in the open area formed by the cupped hand. The knife handle is placed firmly in the surgeon's hand. When the surgeon has securely grasped the knife, the surgical technologist moves the passing hand up and away from the blade (Figure 12-44).

Ringed instruments are passed by holding the box lock of the instrument and placing the rings in the palm of the surgeon's open receiving hand. The instrument should be placed firmly into the surgeon's hand. Remember that the surgeon's eyes and thoughts are on the next step of the procedure. A quick snap of the wrist will place the rings into the surgeon's palm with a slight "snap." This is the proper pressure (The student should note that microsurgical instruments are not passed with the same speed or pressure at which general laparotomy instruments are passed.) The surgeon will know the instrument is there and close the receiving hand around the rings. Curved instruments should be placed in the hand with the point curving in the same direction as the surgeon's fingers. Ringed instruments are passed closed. During the procedure, all instruments are returned to a designated area by the surgeon where they are retrieved, cleaned, and replaced on the Mayo stand by the surgical technologist.

Needle holders are ringed instruments with the added complexity of having a sharp needle held at the end (Figure 12-45). As mentioned above, the instrument should be passed from the surgical technologist to the surgeon but placed in the safe area by the surgeon after use to be retrieved

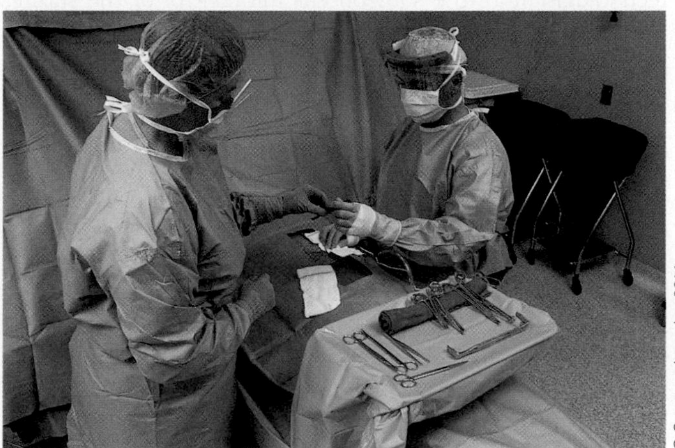

Figure 12-44 Passing the scalpel to the surgeon

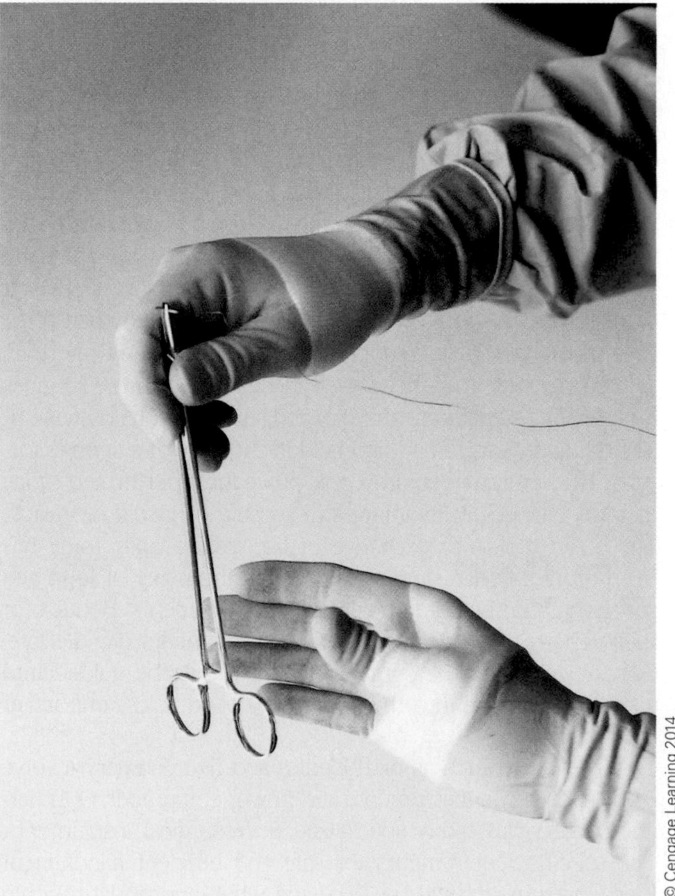

Figure 12-45 Passing the suture to the surgeon

by the surgical technologist. Typically, needles are placed near the tip of the needle holder and set at a 90-degree angle to the long line of the needle holder. Other needle positions are used for specific purposes, but the surgeon will ask for these variations when needed. Suture should be draped over the back of the hand so the surgical technologist's delivering hand prohibits the suture from entering the surgeon's hand with the instrument. Long sutures should be controlled by the surgical technologist until the surgeon has full control of the suture. The use of a neutral zone is recommended to minimize the incidence of sharps injury; other passing methods should only be employed when the neutral zone cannot be safely utilized.

Retractors come in a variety of shapes, weights, and types. They should be passed carefully. The handles of handheld retractors are placed in the palm of the surgeon's or surgical assistant's hand with gentle pressure. Self-retaining retractors are presented according to the type of retractor. Those with rings are held along the box lock with the rings presented. Some retractors (e.g., Gelpi) must be handled according to sharps rules. Some retractors are large and require the addition of multiple pieces. These must be passed with extra care because of their weight.

Lap sponges are passed unfolded. The sponges may be used moistened or dry. If moistened, they are soaked in body-temperature saline and squeezed out before use. The solution in which sponges are soaked should not be used as irrigation; fiber particles may contribute to the formation of adhesions. Laparotomy sponges are sometimes "packed" into the abdominal cavity to hold some portion of the contents away from the operative site. The best practice is to count the sponges as they are packed into the abdomen, report the count to the circulator, and record it on a count board. Keep an ongoing count of these sponges. If you are preparing to close and you notice that four sponges were packed into the abdomen but only three are marked as removed, you should notify the surgeon. It is easier to retrieve the sponge before closure has started than after. Four-in. × 4-in. raytec sponges are usually opened one fold, converting them to 4 inches × 8 inches. Use of these sponges is generally restricted to the skin and subcutaneous tissues unless the sponge is folded and held in the jaws of a sponge forceps. The volume of laparoscopic procedures performed today dictates changes in handling and passing of instrumentation. The often rapid-fire exchange of the classic laparotomy has been replaced with slow and methodical passing of long and somewhat cumbersome laparoscopic instruments. Because of their length and thin shafts, these instruments are delicate. Once received by the surgeon, the tips must be guided into a port for passage into the abdomen. Speed is less important than precision.

Specialties such as orthopedics and neurosurgery involve many specialized instruments and power equipment. Ophthalmic surgery has many specialized microsurgical instruments. The specific requirements for safe and efficient handling of these instruments will be discussed when appropriate within the procedural chapters.

MAINTAINING ORDER WITHIN THE STERILE FIELD

The surgical technologist must not only keep up with the needs of the sterile team members, but must also maintain the sterile field in a safe and orderly fashion to facilitate the surgical procedure and counting.

All instruments and supplies are arranged on the Mayo stand so that each one is picked up and passed using one smooth movement, ensuring a safe transfer and conserving time and movement within the sterile field.

Each time the electrosurgical pencil is used, the tip should be checked for cleanliness and cleaned if necessary; the cord may need to be untangled; and the pencil must be returned to the holster for safe storage.

Clean sponges are added to the field as needed and the used ones are removed and placed in the kick bucket.

With the exception of the scalpel, most instruments are placed on the drapes when no longer needed by the surgeon or surgical assistant. Loose instruments are picked up as soon as feasible, cleaned if necessary, and returned to their location on the Mayo stand or back table.

Blades, suture needles, and other sharps not in use are typically placed on the back table in the sharps container and organized in an orderly fashion to facilitate counting. Excess suture material is removed from the needle and discarded to prevent entanglement.

Additional instruments and supplies may be added to the field during the procedure and must be placed in position and accounted for.

ADDITIONAL SUPPLIES

Often, it is necessary to add instruments and supplies to the sterile field. The surgical technologist typically verbally requests the additional item(s); however, the circulator may anticipate a specific need and provide the item(s) without being asked. The circulator obtains the item, inspects and opens the package, and places the item in a convenient location on the sterile back table or allows the surgical technologist to retrieve the item from the packaging material. Any additional packaging material is removed and discarded by the surgical technologist and the item is either used immediately or left on the back table or Mayo stand for future use. Countable items (e.g., sponges) are immediately counted and added to the count by the circulator. Addition of items to the sterile field should not disrupt the progression of the surgical procedure.

INTRAOPERATIVE COUNTS

The following general guidelines pertain to counts performed during the procedure and keeping track of the soiled sponges and sharps.

Sponges

The surgical technologist should discard soiled sponges into the kick bucket. The circulator retrieves the sponges, keeping the same type together; counts the sponges with the surgical technologist according to their packaging (e.g., 4 × 4 sponges come in packs of 10 and lap sponges in packs of 5); places them in an impermeable plastic bag; closes the bag; and labels it with the type and number of sponges inside. The bag is set aside.

When closure of a wound or cavity is begun, the surgical technologist and circulator complete the second count. The surgical technologist is responsible for knowing where all the sponges are on the sterile field, and verifying that all lap sponges have been removed from the cavity and accounted for. Remember that all counts are performed in a verbal fashion.

The surgical technologist should establish a routine for counting; most often the count is begun with the smallest sponges and progresses to the largest. Additionally, it is recommended the surgical technologist follow this sequence for counting of sponges, sharps, and instruments: sterile operative field (remember the needle the surgeon may be using); Mayo stand; back table; basin; off the sterile field.

Third count is performed when closure of the subq and skin is begun. The surgeon is notified if the counts are correct. Refer to Table 12-21 for actions to be taken when counts are incorrect.

Sharps Management

Just as with sponges, the surgical technologist is responsible for keeping track of and knowing where the sharps are located on the sterile field. Sharps that are added during the procedure are recorded by the circulator on the erasable board.

The surgical technologist should place used needles in the magnetic or foam type needle pad that is positioned on the back table. Additionally, if a scalpel blade is removed from a knife handle, it should be placed in the needle pad.

Needle pads that become full can be handed off to the circulator. The surgical technologist and circulator count the needles and any other sharps in the needle pad; the surgical technologist hands it off; and the circulator places it in an impermeable bag, labeling it with the number of needles inside and the initials of the surgical technologist and himself or herself as the individuals who did the count. Remember, all pieces of a broken sharp must be accounted for. Closing counts are performed the same as for sponges.

Instruments

Instruments added during the procedure are recorded on the instrument count sheet. The pieces of instruments that can be disassembled must be counted. The pieces of broken instruments must be accounted for. Closing counts are performed the same as for sponges.

MEDICATION HANDLING

No amount of vigilance can prevent some patients from reacting negatively to a medication, but vigilance can reduce medication errors to an absolute minimum. The surgical technologist should be familiar with anesthetic agents, medications, and solutions used during surgical intervention. Procedures and practices concerned with the safe handling of medications are covered in Chapter 9.

SPECIMEN CARE

According to the situation, specimen care may occur during the intraoperative or postoperative phases of case management. For example, a specimen obtained for frozen section (e.g., breast biopsy) is generally removed from the sterile field intraoperatively, prepared and identified according to facility policy, and sent to pathology as soon as possible. However, a specimen obtained for permanent section (e.g., an appendix) may remain on the sterile field until the procedure is completed and will be cared for postoperatively. A general discussion of

Table 12-21 Incorrect Closing Counts

Closing Count	*Action*
Instruments	Inform surgeon immediately; recount; if still incorrect, inform surgeon again; check cavity; document all actions and findings
Sponges	Inform surgeon immediately; recount; if still incorrect, inform surgeon again; check cavity; document all actions and findings
Sharps/needles	Inform surgeon immediately; recount; if still incorrect, inform surgeon again; check cavity; document all actions and findings

Note: Diagnostic imaging may be used to demonstrate the presence or absence of the item in a body cavity or wound. However, every effort should be made to find the missing items.

specimen care is found in Chapter 13, and details that are more specific to each surgical specialty are available in each of the procedural chapters as needed.

REPLACEMENT OF CONTAMINATED GLOVE OR GOWN

During the course of the surgical procedure the glove(s) and/or gown of the surgical technologist or one of the other sterile team members can become contaminated. The technique for removal of the gown and gloves during the procedure if contamination occurs varies from the technique for removing the gown and gloves at the end of the procedure, which is discussed later in this chapter in the postoperative case management section.

DRESSING APPLICATION

There are too many types of postoperative wound dressings to list the technique for application of each. However, it is important to recognize that the last skin suture or staple does not end the team's responsibility for wound care. Given our presumed laparotomy, it is to be expected that the area around the incision is both bloody and covered with prep solution. It is also true that for comfort reasons the best time to clean the patient is immediately following the completion of the procedure.

For our hypothetical laparotomy, the following are four examples of dressings that could be used:

Example 1

- Wound and surrounding area is cleaned and dried using a wet lap sponge soaked in saline and a dry sponge.
- The 4 × 4 sponges are unfolded into 4 × 8s, stacked, and placed on the wound. If the incision is long, several dressing

TECHNIQUE

Gown and Glove Removal for Replacement During a Procedure

The following methods for replacement of a contaminated glove reflect best practice as well as routine practice; method one is optimal, down to method four, which is least optimal. The following information is from the AST *Recommended Standards of Practice for Gowning and Gloving* (2008).

1. Step away from the sterile field and inform the circulator that you have a contaminated glove.
2. Method 1: Assisted Gloving
   - Surgical technologist extends arm and hand with contaminated glove, palm upward.
   - Circulator, wearing nonsterile gloves, grasps the palm of the glove and removes without touching the gown. The circulator should not include the cuff of the gown by pulling it over the team member's hand since the cuff is not considered sterile.
   - A member of the sterile team re-gloves the surgical technologist.
3. Method 2: Re-gown and Re-glove
   - If a member of the sterile team cannot perform assisted gloving, the surgical technologist should remove the gown and gloves, and re-gown and re-glove.
   - Remain still with your back toward the circulator so that the gown can be unfastened.
   - Face the circulator once the gown is unfastened.
   - Remain still and maintain an appropriate distance from the circulator while he or she removes the gown.
   - Extend both arms with palms upward to allow the circulator to grasp the palms of the gloves and remove.
   - Rescrub if necessary.
   - Don the new gown and gloves, and return to the sterile field.
4. Method 3: Open Gloving—See Open Gloving Technique
5. Method 4: Open Gloving over Contaminated Glove
   - Don sterile glove over contaminated glove using open-gloving technique.
   - When time permits, utilize one of the methods above to remove both gloves and don new gloves.

Note: Information courtesy of the Association of Surgical Technologists, *Recommended Standards of Practice.*

sponges may be needed in order to completely cover the area.
- Tape is applied to keep the sponges in place.

Example 2

- Gauze strips impregnated with antibiotic ointment (Adaptic and Xeroform are two trade names) are placed on the incision.

Example 3

- The 4 × 4 sponges are unfolded into 4 × 8s, stacked, and placed on the wound.
- One to two ABD pads are then placed on top of the sponges and the dressing is taped into place.

Example 4

- The same procedure can be performed and with a Montgomery strap placed in order to hold the bulky dressings in place and allow for wound inspection and frequent dressing changes.

The intraoperative phase of case management ends with application of the sterile dressing.

TECHNIQUE

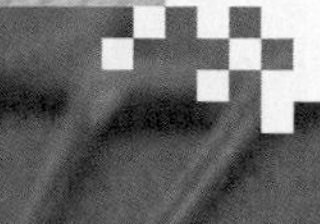

Dressing Application

1. All necessary items are prepared in advance.
   - Moist and dry sponges are prepared.
   - Dressing materials are obtained (following wound closure and completion of the final count) and arranged in the order in which they will be applied.
2. The area around the wound is cleaned and dried, using caution not to disrupt the wound edges.
3. The dressing is applied. Use of a temporary dressing is not recommended because the risk of contamination of the wound is increased when replacing it with the permanent dressing.

PROGRESSION OF THE SURGICAL PROCEDURE

Although each patient and procedure differs in detail, most open procedures follow the same sequence of events. During each event within the sequence, the surgical technologist must anticipate the needs of the patient and the surgical team members. The surgeon should not have to ask for each item; the surgical technologist must be able to predict and anticipate the sequence of the needed items. A sample sequence of events for an open operative procedure and the technical considerations for the surgical technologist are found in Table 12-22.

PART III: Postoperative Case Management

The postoperative phase of case management begins after the sterile dressing is applied. The OR furniture and equipment must be returned to their original placement, instruments transported to the decontamination room, patient transported to PACU, and OR cleaned.

PRESERVATION OF THE STERILE FIELD

Following dressing application, the surgical technologist ensures that all sharps and nondisposable items are removed from the drapes. The sterile back table, Mayo stand, and basin set are moved away from the operating table and kept sterile until the patient is out of the OR, being transported to the PACU. Maintaining the sterility of those three items until the patient is transported out of the OR is considered "best practice." The surgical technologist should keep a minimum number of sterile instruments on the Mayo stand, including two to four hemostats and a knife handle with attached knife blade. When a patient is waking up from general anesthesia and the intraoperative drugs are wearing off, a number of complications can occur, including respiratory distress. The surgical team should be prepared to treat the emergency situation in the OR, such as by performing an emergency tracheotomy.

Drape Removal

As soon as the items that must remain sterile are moved away from the operating table, the surgical technologist removes his or her outer pair of gloves (if double gloved) and returns to the operating table to assist with drape removal. In some situations, the surgical technologist may be required to remain sterile while other surgical team members remove the drapes.

TABLE 12-22 Sample Sequence of Events for an Open Procedure

Steps of the Operative Procedure	*Technical Considerations for the Surgical Technologist*
1. An incision is made.	• Pass the scalpel or "skin knife" to the surgeon's dominant hand (or use a safe transfer method). • Prepare the electrosurgical pencil and suction for use. • Expect the surgeon to return the scalpel to the Mayo stand (or neutral zone) and keep hands out of the way.
2. Hemostasis is achieved.	• Place the electrosurgical pencil in the surgeon's dominant hand. • The surgical assistant may use the suction apparatus to remove excess blood and electrosurgical plume, as needed—the surgical assistant will likely be able to retrieve the suction apparatus without the assistance of the surgical technologist due to its location on the sterile field. • Anticipate the use of hemostats if the electrosurgical pencil is not effective in achieving hemostasis. • Retrieve the skin knife and place it in its storage location on the back table—reuse of the skin knife is not anticipated. • Clean surgical sponges are added to the field as needed, and then the used ones are removed and placed in the kick bucket—it may be necessary to switch from small sponges to larger ones as the wound size/depth increases.
3. Dissection continues through the necessary tissue layers.	• Sharp dissection may be carried out with the "deep knife" or with scissors. • Blunt dissection may be carried out with the use of a dissecting sponge (e.g., peanut) or with the surgeon's fingers. • Retrieve the electrosurgical pencil, clean the tip if necessary, and place the pencil in the holster—reuse of the electrosurgical pencil is anticipated. • If hemostats are used to control bleeding, anticipate the use of the electrosurgical pencil or suture material and the suture scissors. • As the wound deepens, anticipate the need for longer instruments. • Any instrument not in use is secured, cleaned as needed, and replaced on the Mayo stand; contaminated items are isolated as needed (e.g., bowel technique).
4. The wound edges are retracted to provide exposure.	• Expect the surgical assistant to retract the wound edges and provide the appropriate-size retractor or pair of retractors when needed—as the incision deepens, larger/deeper retractors will be used. • Exposure and isolation of structures may also be achieved with the use of surgical sponges (e.g., moistened laparotomy sponges).
5. The procedure is performed.	• Provide specialty instrumentation and suture material for the specific procedure. • Anticipate the continuing need for hemostasis. • Retrieve and care for sharps and other items as needed. • Care for the specimen as needed.
6. Hemostasis is maintained.	• Prior to closure, a final wound inspection is made to ensure that there is no active bleeding. • If necessary, hemostasis may be achieved mechanically (e.g., ligating clips), thermally (e.g., electrosurgery) , or pharmaceutically (e.g., topical thrombin)—provide necessary items.
7. Wound is irrigated.	• Prior to wound closure, the surgeon may irrigate the wound with body-temperature normal saline (or antibiotic solution according to the situation). • Pass the container (e.g., bulb syringe or pitcher) containing the irrigation fluid and be sure to state the name of the contents (e.g., normal saline). • Provide the Poole suction tip if necessary with wet lap sponge wrapped around the suction tip. • A small basin (e.g., kidney basin) placed near the dependent wound edge may be useful for collection of excess irrigation fluid. • Make a mental note of the amount of irrigation fluid used. • Retrieve and refill the fluid container if necessary. • Remove and replace the Poole suction tip with Yankauer tip as needed.

(continues)

TABLE 12-22 (continued)

Steps of the Operative Procedure	*Technical Considerations for the Surgical Technologist*
8. Wound is closed.	• Provide appropriate retractors to the surgical assistant. • Hemostats may be needed to secure the wound edges prior to closure. • Provide necessary wound closure material to the surgeon's dominant hand and a tissue forceps to the nondominant hand. • Provide the suture scissors to the surgical assistant. • Perform necessary counts as needed and report the results. • Provide additional wound closure material as needed. • Retrieve and care for sharps and other items as needed. • As closure of the wound progresses, smaller/shallower retractors will be used.
9. Dressing is applied.	• Dressing materials are provided after the skin is closed and the final count is performed. • The dressing materials are organized in the order in which they will be applied. • The skin around the wound is cleaned and dried, using caution not to disrupt the wound edges. • The dressing is applied.

Gown and Glove Removal

Following removal of the drapes, the surgical technologist removes his or her soiled gown and gloves, disposes of them in the appropriate receptacle(s), and dons a pair of nonsterile gloves in order to assist with the immediate postoperative care of the patient.

Gown Removal

Careful removal of the gown is necessary to prevent cross-contamination. The soiled gown should never be thrown any distance to the waste container. The gown is removed prior to glove removal. Following the case, the gown removal is typically accomplished by the individual. If necessary, another individual may assist you with unfastening the back of the gown. Do not touch an area with your soiled gloves that you cannot visualize. The fasteners on a disposable gown may simply be torn to allow removal. Grasp the unfastened gown at the shoulders and pull down. As you remove the gown from your arms, roll it so that the exterior of the gown is contained within itself. The gloves will remain on the hands as the gown is totally removed and disposed of. Be sure to touch only the gown with your soiled gloves to prevent cross-contamination.

TECHNIQUE

Drape Removal

1. The surgical technologist gently holds the dressing in place while the anesthesia provider releases the suspended portion of the drape.
2. The drape is rolled as it is removed, containing any biohazardous material or disposable items.
3. It will be necessary for the surgical technologist to switch hands to hold the dressing as the drape is rolled over that area to facilitate removal of the remainder of the drape.
4. The drape is placed in the linen or waste receptacle as needed.
5. The towels and towel clips are removed.
6. The towels are placed in the linen or waste receptacle and the towel clips are set on the back table.

Note: The following steps are not part of the drape removal process, but are carried out immediately following drape removal.

7. If necessary, the patient's skin adjacent to the dressing is cleaned and dried.
8. The dressing is secured with tape by the circulator.

Glove Removal

Careful removal of the gloves is necessary to prevent splash injuries to either the wearer or others in the room. Gloves should never be thrown any distance to the waste container, as splash contamination may occur. After the gown has been removed and disposed of in the waste container, the gloves are removed one layer at a time. This allows the wearer to identify if one or both pairs of gloves were breached by a tear or puncture. A common method of glove removal is to grasp the outer cuff of the glove with the thumb and middle finger of the opposite hand and then pull the hand outward, removing the glove. This is repeated to remove all the gloves. This prevents the wearer from having to touch contaminated areas of the gloves with bare hands, and at the same time turns the gloves inside out so that further contamination does not occur. Gloves should be disposed of immediately, and the hands should be washed and dried after glove removal at the end of each case.

TECHNIQUE

Gown and Glove Removal at End of Procedure

1. If necessary, the circulator unfastens the back of a reusable gown. The back of a disposable gown may be torn by the surgical technologist.
2. Touch the gown only with the gloved hands. Grasp the gown near the shoulders and roll the gown away from you; roll the gown up to contain biohazardous material and place in the proper receptacle.
3. Grasp the palm of the glove to be removed first with your opposite hand without touching your bare skin.
4. Remove the glove by inverting it.
5. Retain the removed glove in the hand that remains gloved.
6. Initiate removal of the remaining glove by sliding the degloved hand between the skin of the wrist and the glove.
7. Invert the second glove as it is removed to contain both gloves.
8. Dispose of the gloves in the proper receptacle.
9. Wash your hands as soon as feasible.

Immediate Postoperative Patient Care

Several tasks must be performed before the patient is ready to be transferred onto the stretcher and transported to the PACU. Some of these tasks include:

- Any excess prep solution is removed from the patient's skin.
- If used, the dispersive electrode is removed and the condition of the patient's skin is noted.
- The patient may be extubated.
- Monitoring devices are removed.
- A warm blanket may be provided if necessary.

Patient Transfer and Transportation

In preparation for transfer to the stretcher, the stretcher is brought into the OR and positioned adjacent to the operating table, and the wheel locks are applied. A transfer device, such as a roller, is obtained and positioned for use. The IV bag is moved onto the IV pole that is attached to the stretcher and the tubing is freed.

Typically, four individuals are needed to transfer an anesthetized patient from the operating table to the stretcher. The anesthesia provider remains at the patient's head and coordinates the transfer. Additional team members position themselves at the patient's sides and feet. When the anesthesia provider gives the signal, the patient's head and feet are supported and the patient is rolled away from the stretcher using the draw sheet. The transfer device is placed under the patient's torso and the patient is gently rolled back onto the transfer device. Be sure that the individuals at the patient's sides brace their bodies against the operating table and the stretcher to prevent slippage and verify that no tension will be placed on the IV tubing (or any other tubing such as a Foley catheter or chest tube) during the transfer. The anesthesia provider will again signal when he or she is ready to complete the transfer. The patient's head and feet are supported while the patient is gently moved onto the stretcher. Following transfer, the transfer device is removed, the side rails are raised, and the wheel locks are released.

When the anesthesia provider determines that the patient is ready, he or she is transported to the PACU. Typically, the anesthesia provider and the circulator transport the patient; however, in certain situations (e.g., if additional equipment must be moved with the patient), the STSR may be required to assist with the transport.

BREAKDOWN OF THE SETUP

Once the patient leaves the OR, the surgical technologist may begin breakdown of the setup. If needed, additional PPE (e.g., nonsterile gloves) is donned. A sample routine for breakdown of the setup follows.

- The specimen is cared for as needed.
- All sharps are placed in the sharps container on the back table.

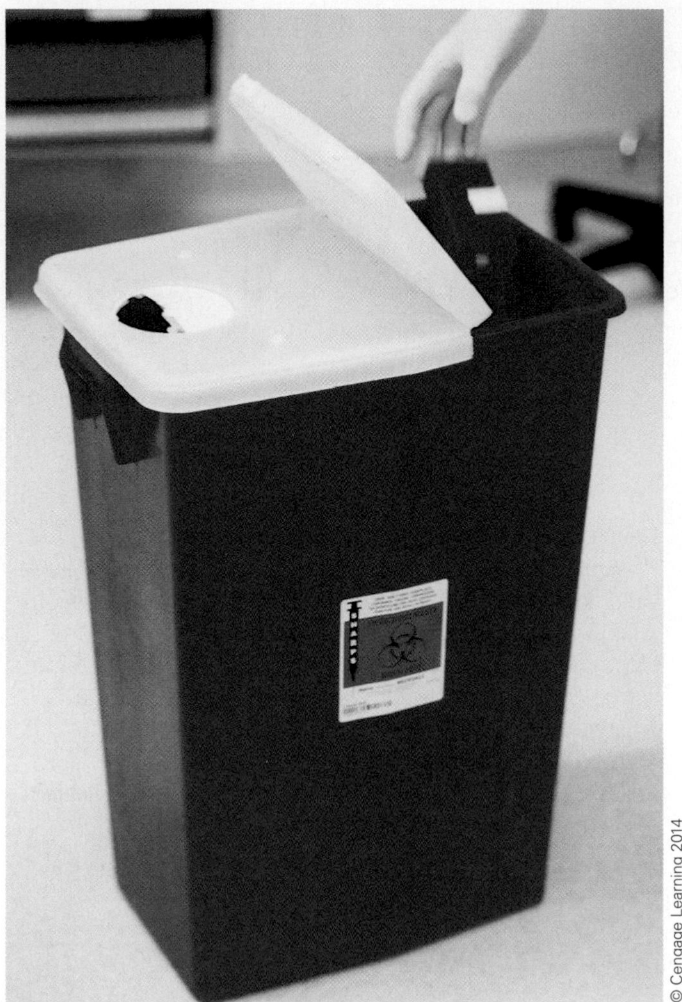

Figure 12-46 Disposal of the sharps container

- The sharps container is closed and placed in a large puncture-proof biohazardous sharps container (Figure 12-46).
- Instruments are removed from the Mayo stand, opened or disassembled as needed, and placed in a basin of containing a mixture of water and enzymatic detergent.
- The basin containing the soiled instruments is placed in or on the case cart.
- Instruments on the back table that were not used for the procedure may be placed into the instrument tray.
- The instrument tray is placed in or on the case cart.
- All linen items are placed in the hamper.
- All disposable items are placed in the waste receptacle.
- Suction canisters and tubing are discarded.
- The OR furniture is positioned.
- The case cart is taken to the decontamination area.
- Environmental decontamination of the OR is performed.
- PPE is removed and discarded.
- A hand wash is performed.
- The OR is set up for the next patient and the preoperative case management phase begins again.

Case Study During the repair of a midline episiotomy, the family practice resident closing the episiotomy said, "Something's wrong but I can't identify it." The surgical technologist said, "I'm worried too. Do you think this patient may have DIC (disseminated intravascular coagulopathy)?" "Why do you ask?" the resident asked. "I've seen this before and the blood doesn't look right. I placed some of the patient's blood in a plain test tube. It's been 7 minutes, and there is no clot forming." The resident asked the circulator to call the obstetric faculty to the room and alerted the anesthesia provider. The patient's blood pressure dropped for a while, but the quick response of the team held off any severe complications and the patient was dismissed several days later without further complications.

1. What observation did the surgical technologist make that helped the patient?
2. Was the surgical technologist's response appropriate? Discuss your opinion.

Questions for Further Study

1. Why is it important to anticipate the needs of the patient and surgical team members?
2. What are the procedures for correct counting of instruments and sponges?
3. What steps must be taken if any part of the count is incorrect?
4. Describe the OR cycle and explain how the surgical technologist participates in the OR cycle.
5. What corrective options are available to the surgical team members when a breach in sterile technique occurs?

BIBLIOGRAPHY

Association of Surgical Technologists. (2008). *Recommended standards of practice for gowning and gloving.* Retrieved from http://www.ast.org/pdf/Standards_of_Practice/RSOP_Gowning_Gloving.pdf

Association of Surgical Technologists. (2011). *Core curriculum for surgical technology* (6th ed.). Littleton, CO: Association of Surgical Technologists.

Ball, K. A. (2004). *Lasers: The perioperative challenge* (3rd ed.). Parker, CO: Association of periOperative Registered Nurses.

Deitch, E. A. (1997). *Tools of the trade and rules of the road: A surgical guide.* Philadelphia: Lippincott Williams & Wilkins.

Goldman, M. A. (2007). *Pocket guide to the operating room* (3rd ed.). Philadelphia: F.A. Davis.

Harrington, L., & Kennerly, D. (2011). Safety issues related to the electronic medical record (emr): Synthesis of the literature from the last decade, 2000–2009. *Journal of Healthcare Management, 56*(1), 31–43.

Phillips, N. F. (2007). *Berry & Kohn's operating room technique* (11th ed.). St. Louis: Mosby.

Section 3

Surgical Procedures

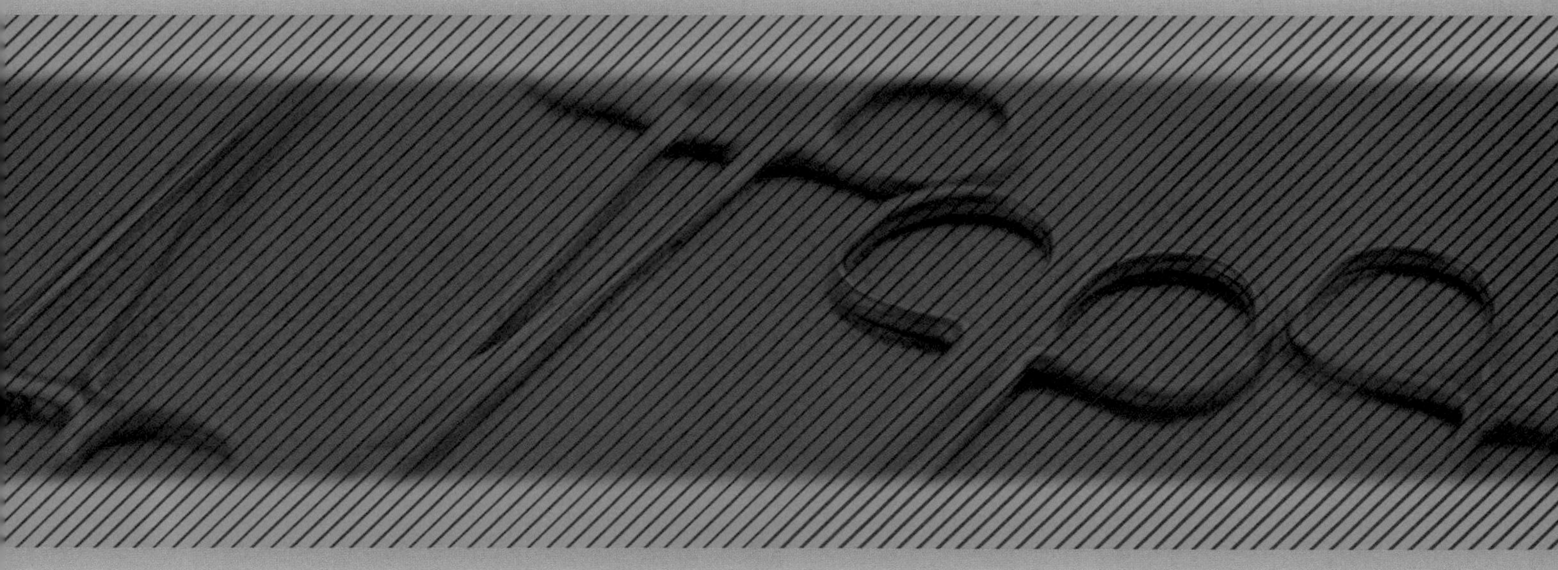

CHAPTER

13

Diagnostic Procedures

CASE STUDY Dathan, an 8-year-old male, was brought to the emergency department by his parent. He complained of generalized periumbilical pain that has now localized to the right lower quadrant. His mother states that his appetite has been poor and that he is now experiencing nausea, vomiting, and a fever.

1. What structures might be involved in the right lower quadrant?
2. What diagnostic studies might be performed?
3. What diagnostic study will indicate the presence of infection?

OBJECTIVES

After studying this chapter, the reader should be able to:

A 1. Apply knowledge of anatomy and physiology to determine which diagnostic examinations will be useful.

P 2. Indicate the sources of patient data.

3. Compare and contrast techniques used to establish the diagnosis.

O 4. Determine which diagnostic procedures will require surgical intervention.

S 5. Recognize the major indications for surgical intervention.

Select Key Terms

angina	CSF	-graph	roentgenography
auscultation	cystoscopy	indwelling	sign
biopsy	EEG	isotope scanning	symptom
capnography	electrocardiogram (ECG)	obstruction	ultrasonography
C-arm	frozen section	palpation	urinalysis (UA)
cholangiography	-gram	prosthesis	
contrast medium	Gram stain		

SOURCES OF PATIENT DATA

Information about a patient's condition can be obtained in several ways from many sources, including

- History and physical examination
- Diagnostic imaging
- Laboratory findings
- Electrodiagnostic studies
- Endoscopic studies
- Pulmonary diagnosis
- Plethysmography and phleborheography

History and Physical Examination

The first step in determining the etiology of a patient's condition is gathering medical, social (including any ethnic and/or religious information that may impact the course of treatment), and psychological information about the patient and, if applicable, the patient's family. This is generally achieved in a personal interview with the patient or some other responsible party (parent, spouse, paramedic) if the patient is unable to respond as a result of age or condition. The examination may be routine, or the individual may have one or more **symptoms** that have caused the patient to seek medical attention.

A physical examination should be performed. The physician performing the examination will verify the symptoms that the patient is experiencing and may discover other **signs** that will indicate the presence of a pathological condition. The physical exam should not focus on just the area of complaint, but should be inclusive of all body systems. The patient's height, weight, temperature, pulse, respiration, and blood pressure (BP) information should be recorded.

Several tools and methods are available to the physician to facilitate the physical exam, including:

- Direct visualization
- Enhanced visualization (otoscope/ophthalmoscope)
- Indirect visualization (pharyngeal mirror)
- **Palpation:** external (abdominal or thyroid) and/or internal (pelvic exam or digital rectal exam)
- **Auscultation** (stethoscope)

In addition to the physical exam, the physician may request that the patient undergo one or more imaging or laboratory tests. Once the results of the physical examination and the ordered tests have been assimilated, treatment may begin or more advanced diagnostic procedures may be advised.

The same tools used for preliminary diagnosis continue to be available during treatment (surgical or otherwise) for reevaluation of the patient's condition; they may also have therapeutic applications.

Diagnostic Imaging

Diagnostic imaging is a term that refers to the various techniques now available for producing images of the human body. Historically, the radio**graph** or X-ray was the predominant, if not the only, imaging technique available. *Radiography,* or **roentgenography**, remains a viable source of diagnostic information. Large surgical departments may have diagnostic imaging personnel assigned solely to the OR.

Radiography (Roentgenography)

X-rays used to view internal structures for diagnostic purposes are high-energy electromagnetic radiation. The X-rays are produced by the collision of a beam of electrons with a metal target within an X-ray tube. Penetrability of the X-ray beam is related to the unit of energy called a joule measured in rads (radiation absorbed dosage), the standard unit of an absorbed dose of ionizing radiation.

Preoperative plain radiographic films of the chest are frequently ordered by the anesthesia provider for identification of lung abnormalities that may interfere with the exchange of gases during anesthesia.

Thoracic surgeons can discover a good deal about the status of the ribs, sternum, and internal thoracic organs from a plain chest film. Fractures of the bones of the thorax may be revealed, as well as primary or metastatic tumors. Examination of the lung fields may reveal lung disease patterns or a collapsed lung, and examination of the pleural space may reveal effusion (escape of fluid) or a tumor. Examination of the vessels in the lung field can reveal pulmonary arterial or venous hypertension. Interstitial edema appears as a diffuse haziness, and alveolar edema will produce a lung opacification (nontransparency). Structures within the mediastinum may also be examined for lesions.

In the OR, plain radiographic films from a fixed X-ray tube (may be included in **cystoscopy** rooms for retrograde urography or cystography) or portable X-ray machines are used for these purposes:

- Identify the location of abnormalities and foreign bodies (such as bullets, ingested items, or calculi).
- Locate retained sponges, sharps, or instruments.
- Discover fluid or air within body cavities.
- Verify the correct location for an operative procedure (such as the level of a cervical disk to be removed).
- Aid in bone realignment and **prosthesis** placement.
- Verify placement of **indwelling** catheters, tubes, and drains.

A portable X-ray machine must be moved into the OR in order to make radiographs (Figure 13-1). The making of a radiograph requires that a cassette, containing unexposed X-ray film, be positioned opposite the tube. Anteroposterior (AP) radiographic views require that the film be placed underneath the patient; lateral views demand placement next to the body. In the radiology department, film placement is not difficult; in the OR, however, specially developed assistive devices may be required. The primary goal of the surgical technologist during intraoperative radiography is to protect the sterile field from contamination. The surgical technologist may accomplish the dual goals of keeping the field sterile and allowing for the radiographic study using several methods. The X-ray cassette can be covered by the surgical technologist with a sterile cassette cover to allow the cassette to be placed within the sterile field. If the X-ray tube is to be positioned over the operative field, the tube itself may be covered with a sterile drape or the wound may be protected with a sterile towel. Lateral films require the use of a portable cassette holder that can be positioned opposite the tube. This portable holder should be covered with a sterile drape before it is positioned near the OR table.

Once the film has been exposed to the radiation, it must be processed prior to viewing. The film is removed from the cassette in a darkroom and passed through a developing machine. Many ORs are equipped for this procedure; otherwise the film must be taken to the radiology department for processing, which can be time consuming. Often, the surgeon will

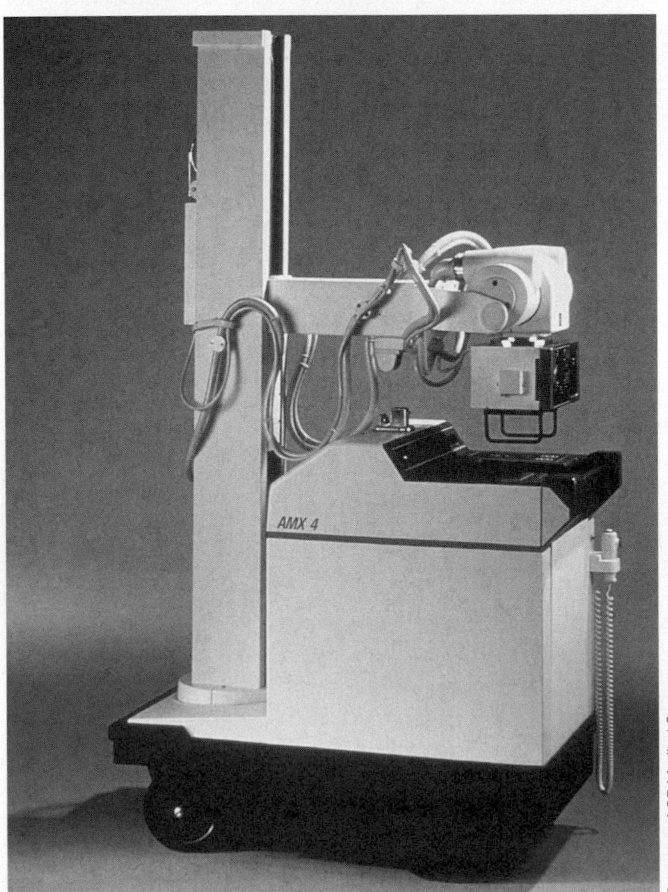

Figure 13-1 Portable X-ray machine

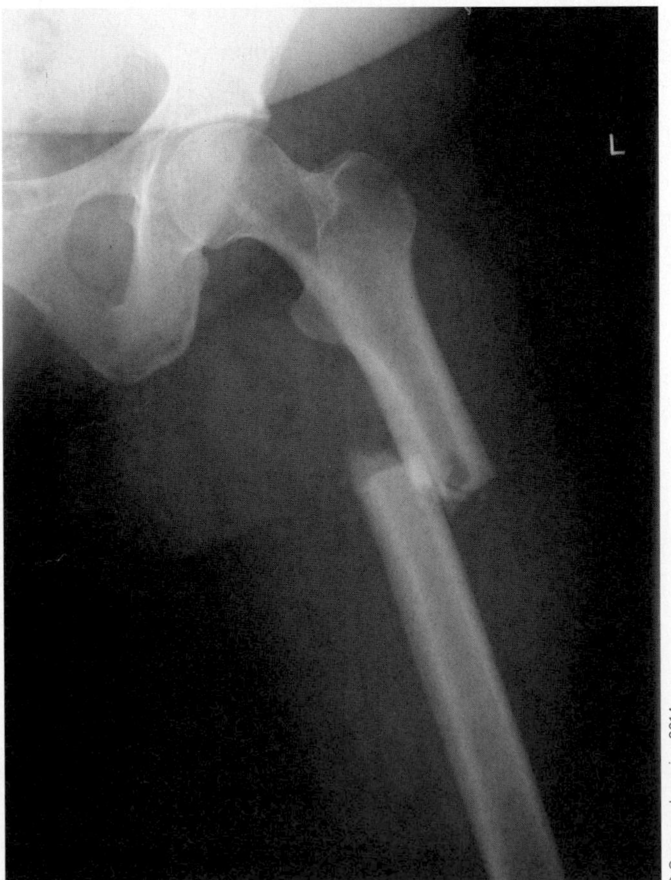

Figure 13-2 X-ray depicting a femur fracture

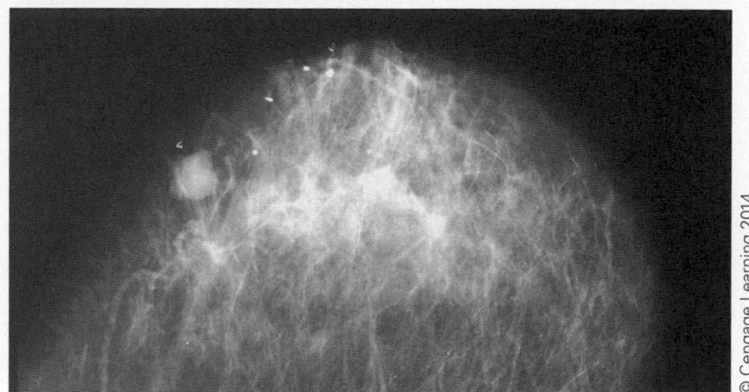

Figure 13-3 Mammogram depicting a sarcoma

"read" the film intraoperatively; in some situations, the expertise of the radiologist may be requested (Figure 13-2).

Mammography

Mammography utilizes X-rays to locate tumors of the breast in their early stages (Figure 13-3). The breast is tightly held in a device intended to decrease the density of the tissue for better visualization. Mammography should not be painful, but the positioning of the breast can be uncomfortable for the patient.

Mammography can be performed in conjunction with a needle aspiration biopsy during which a very fine, long needle may be used to **biopsy** a tumor after it is localized on the X-ray film.

A mammo**gram** may be sent with the patient to the OR for breast biopsy and local excision of breast masses.

Myelography

Myelography is used to evaluate the spine for patients with neck, back, or leg pain. Magnetic resonance imaging (MRI) has largely replaced this technique, but it may still be used in some cases. MRI is useful in imaging the spinal cord, nerve roots, and disks, but myelography has the added benefit of clearly outlining bone tissue. Myelography is also useful for patients who are unable to undergo MRI because of metallic implants.

For myelographic studies, **contrast medium** is injected into the cerebrospinal fluid at the lower lumbar level. This contrast medium outlines the spinal cord and nerve roots on X-ray film studies. Computed axial tomography (CAT) studies may also be performed along with plain radiography to identify osteophytes (bony spurs) or disk extrusions.

Fluoroscopy

A fluoroscope utilizes X-rays to project images of body structures onto a monitor. Amplification is achieved with the use of an image intensifier. The images may be viewed during movement and projected in "real time," allowing the action of joints and organs to be viewed directly. Fluoroscopic images taken during angiography can be digitalized with background images subtracted for enhanced visualization of the structures.

The portable image intensifier is referred to as the **C-arm** because of its configuration (Figure 13-4). It is designed so that

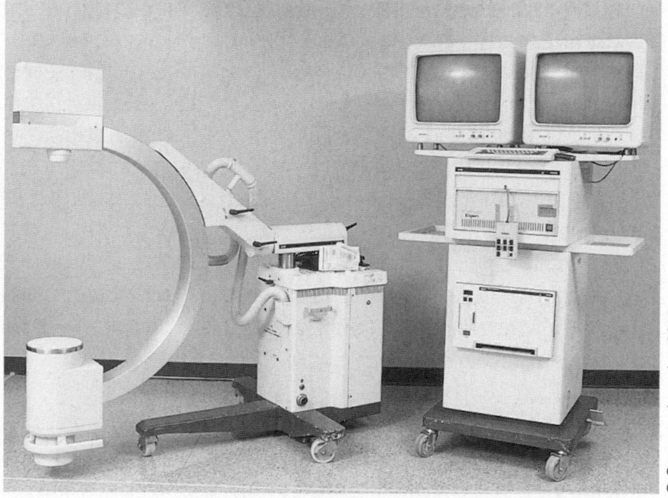

Figure 13-4 C-arm with monitor

the image intensifier and tube are always in opposition. The C-arm is frequently used in conjunction with a special radiographic table that allows X-rays to pass through the tabletop, which is referred to as being radiolucent.

Fluoroscopy has many intraoperative applications:

- Angiography (including cardiac catheterization)
- **Cholangiography**
- Retrograde urography
- Aid in bone realignment and prosthesis placement
- Verification of catheter placement (epidural/central venous pressure) and lead (pacemaker) introduction
- To direct instrumentation (neurosurgery/orthopedics)

Angiography

Angiography remains the reference standard for assessing the cause and severity of peripheral vascular disease. It is the preliminary diagnostic technique necessary for planning of many therapeutic procedures, including endarterectomy, angioplasty, bypass grafting, and embolectomy. Angiography is an invasive procedure that must be accomplished under sterile conditions.

The technique, using videotape and subtraction of background (digital subtraction angiography), allows the visualization of most veins and arteries of the body following the intravenous or intra-arterial injection of a contrast medium. Most angiographic studies are carried out in specially equipped rooms, such as the cardiac catheterization laboratory, or the special studies room of the radiology department, although intraoperative arteriograms are frequently performed in the OR (usually without the benefit of digital subtraction).

Essential equipment for angiography includes an X-ray unit that is capable of making both fluoroscopic (recorded on videotape) and still pictures, film changers for still shots, pressure injectors, contrast media, catheters, guidewires, and needle/cannula assemblies.

The film changer allows tracking of the course of the injected contrast medium as it travels through the portion of the arterial or venous system being studied. It exchanges film rapidly after each exposure so that the area under study is completely outlined. Rapid serial film changers capable of at least two films per second are essential for areas of high-velocity blood flow (e.g., thoracic and abdominal aorta or cerebral vessels).

Single-plane units (using only one film) are sufficient for angiographic studies done in the OR during the surgical procedure, but generally biplane studies are necessary to truly evaluate the anatomy of a vessel, particularly the posterior wall.

A pressure injector is useful for areas of nonselective angiography where large amounts of contrast solution must be injected quickly. It is universally used for angiography of the aorta and left ventricle.

Contrast, as defined in radiology, is the difference in optical density in a radiograph that results from a difference in radiolucency or penetrability of an object. Contrast materials are solutions that are injected into the arteries or veins during angiography that are not penetrable by X-rays (that is, they are radiopaque) and therefore stand out in contrast to the surrounding tissues during angiographic study.

The modern contrast materials are water-soluble organic molecules with bound iodine. There are many brand names, such as Hypaque, Cystografin, or Renografin, each with varying iodine concentration. It is the iodine content that determines the radiodensity of the material. The exact concentration of iodine is listed on the label. Often the brand name reflects the area of intended use (e.g., the brand name Renografin implies that the intended target area is the kidney).

The trade names and numbers of the various agents can be confusing to the surgical technologist. For example, the iodine contents of Renografin 60 (meglumine diatrizoate) and Hypaque 50 (sodium diatrizoate) are almost identical. Most contrast media are hypertonic, viscid solutions, some with high sodium as well as iodine content. In proper dosage, they are quite safe, but they are toxic in overdosage and when allowed to remain in tissues for extended periods of time due to low cardiac output or dehydration. Additionally, a patient may be allergic to a contrast medium; the patient should be tested for allergy to a contrast medium prior to injection.

The site of the injection of the contrast medium may vary with each patient as well as the amount of the contrast medium that is injected. Nonselective aortography may require 30–50 mL of the more concentrated solutions at a rate of 10–25 mL/sec. Selective arterial injections—for example, carotid studies—require 10–12 mL at 7–8 mL/sec. Less-concentrated solution is recommended for the selective studies. The volume and the flow rate of the contrast material into the vessel are the determining factors in the quality of the angiogram. In the demonstration of peripheral arteriosclerosis, relatively slow rates and large volumes of contrast solution make the best combination for successful study.

Catheters (needle/cannula combinations that may include a stylet or guidewire) are tubular, flexible instruments for intra-arterial or intravenous injection of contrast solutions. New catheter materials are continually appearing on the market. Selective catheterization of vessels often requires specially designed, preformed catheters. The smaller the radius of the catheter, the safer is the procedure. Thin-wall catheters of sizes 5–7 French (Fr) are sufficient for most applications. Catheters with multiple side holes are necessary for nonselective aortograms. All catheters should be frequently irrigated (flushed) with a normal saline/heparin mixture (1,000–2,000 u/500 mL) to prevent clots from forming within the catheter.

Many different needle/cannula assemblies are available for angiography. Most consist of an innermost obturator within a sharp, pointed needle and an external cannula with a blunt, tapered end. The most common size is 18 Fr. The Potts-Cournand arterial needle/cannula assembly is frequently used for angiography.

Flexible, atraumatic guidewires protect the intima of the vessel from the catheter tip and "guide" the catheter to the proper location within the cardiovascular system. The guidewires come in various diameters, lengths, and tip styles. The guidewire length and diameter must correspond with the internal diameter and length of the catheter being used. The typical guidewire is called a *J-wire* because the flexible tip at the end is shaped like the letter J. The floppy curve at the end of the guidewire is useful for negotiation of tortuous, sclerotic vessels.

The percutaneous intra-arterial catheter placement described by Seldinger and called the *Seldinger technique* allows easy entrance into most vessels of the body. The femoral route is the method of choice for study of the entire aorta and its branches, including the cerebral vessels and those of the lower limbs.

With the Seldinger technique, the skin and subcutaneous tissues in the femoral region are injected with xylocaine 1%, and a small incision is made with a #11 knife blade. The subcutaneous tissues are spread with a hemostat for free passage of the catheter and guidewire. The needle/cannula is then inserted into the femoral artery at an angle of 45–60 degrees, and the stylet is gently and slowly withdrawn until blood spurts forcefully from the proximal end of the cannula. The guidewire is then inserted through the cannula and into the artery. The cannula is removed over the guidewire and, while pressure is applied to the puncture site, the catheter is threaded over the guidewire and into the artery. With the tip of the guidewire protruding from the distal end, the catheter is positioned at the proper level under fluoroscopy, and the guidewire is removed. The catheter is then flushed with heparinized saline. Contrast material is injected and X-rays are taken.

Cardiac Catheterization

Cardiac catheterization permits the evaluation of heart function, visualization of coronary arteries and cardiac chambers (especially the left ventricle), and the measurement of pressures within the cardiac chambers. It is used to diagnose coronary artery, valvular, pulmonary, and congenital heart disease (Figure 13-5).

Studies may be made of the left and right sides of the heart with catheters introduced into the femoral artery and

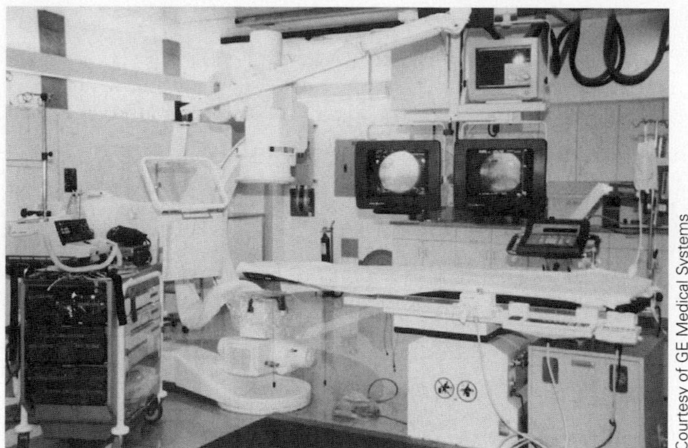

Figure 13-5 Cardiac catheterization laboratory

femoral vein, or the brachial artery and brachial vein, right subclavian, or internal jugular vein. Because the introduction of a catheter into the brachial artery involves an incision and "cut-down" of the vessel (the term "cut-down" refers to making an incision and dissecting through the tissue layers to expose the vessel and making an incision into the vessel for the introduction of the catheter), the percutaneous femoral route is by far the most popular.

Left heart studies include left ventriculogram, coronary artery arteriogram, and measurement of left ventricular pressures. The term *ejection fraction* refers to the percentage of blood that is pumped out of a filled ventricle with each heartbeat. This is a good indicator of the heart's health and may also be an indicator of a cardiac condition such as cardiomyopathy. Since the left ventricle is responsible for pumping out the blood into the aorta, the ejection fraction is usually only measured in the left ventricle. A normal ejection fraction is 55% to 75%. The gold standard for determining the ejection fraction is the use of ventriculography.

Using the Seldinger technique described previously for peripheral vessel angiography, a catheter is introduced into the femoral artery and positioned into the ostia of the left coronary system under fluoroscopy. Contrast medium is injected, and, with the aid of computerized digital subtraction, cinefluorograms are taken. Any lesions of the left coronary system are clearly outlined. Catheters are exchanged, and the technique is repeated for the right coronary system.

After coronary angiograms are completed, coronary catheters are exchanged for a multihole pigtail catheter that is positioned across the aortic valve and into the left ventricle. Chamber pressures are measured and recorded, and the catheter is hooked up to a pressure injector capable of injecting a large volume of contrast material into the left ventricle. A ventriculogram is made outlining the left ventricular wall. Wall movement is examined for any deficiencies related to myocardial infarction, and the ejection fraction is calculated from the ventriculogram.

Right heart studies are accomplished with the aid of a balloon-tipped, Swan-Ganz pulmonary artery catheter attached to a transducer and monitor. Pressures are taken in the right atrium to rule out right or left ventricular failure, hypovolemia, or embolism. Pressures are also taken in the right ventricle to rule out mitral valve insufficiency, left ventricular failure, or congestive heart failure and in the pulmonary artery to rule out changes in pulmonary vascular resistance that may occur in hypoxemia, respiratory insufficiency, pulmonary edema, or pulmonary embolism.

The catheter is inserted into the femoral vein (or, occasionally, the subclavian or internal jugular vein), advanced through the inferior or superior vena cava, and positioned into the right atrium for chamber pressure measurements. When a right atrial waveform appears on the oscilloscope, the balloon is inflated with air to facilitate catheter advancement with blood flow across the tricuspid valve and into the right ventricle, where a typical right ventricular waveform appears on the oscilloscope. After recording, the catheter is advanced across the pulmonary semilunar valve and into the pulmonary artery, where a pulmonary artery waveform is noted and recorded. The flow of blood through the pulmonary artery carries the catheter balloon into one of the smaller pulmonary artery branches, where it wedges and occludes the vessel. This wedge has a distinct waveform and is referred to as the pulmonary capillary wedge pressure (PCWP). PCWP reflects end-diastolic pressures and is an important determinant in the functioning of the left side of the heart. After recording of the PCWP, the balloon is deflated and the catheter slips back into the pulmonary artery, where a pulmonary artery pressure is measured and recorded.

Cholangiography

As a diagnostic tool preoperatively, and intraoperatively during cholecystectomy or common bile duct exploration, a catheter can be inserted and contrast medium injected into the biliary system to outline calculi or other **obstructions** under fluoroscopy. Accomplished either with plain films or fluoroscopy, cholangiography may be done during open or laparoscopic cholecystectomy (Figure 13-6).

Computed Axial Tomography (CAT Scan)

Computed axial tomography (CT or CAT scan) is the use of a specialized X-ray machine that produces pictures of a body part in "slices" for evaluation by a radiologist (Figure 13-7). The CT scanner is adjustable to make the slices as thick or thin as desired. Most slices are 2–10 mm thick. The CT scan uses electromagnetic radiation to create an image from approximately 4,000 different tissue densities that are sorted into 16 different groups. Each group is assigned a shade of gray. The detailed cross sections of the CT scan are useful for detection and examination of masses within the body. The CT image can sometimes be enhanced with the use of an iodine-based contrast medium, which is given to the patient intravenously. The contrast medium cannot be used in individuals who are allergic to iodine.

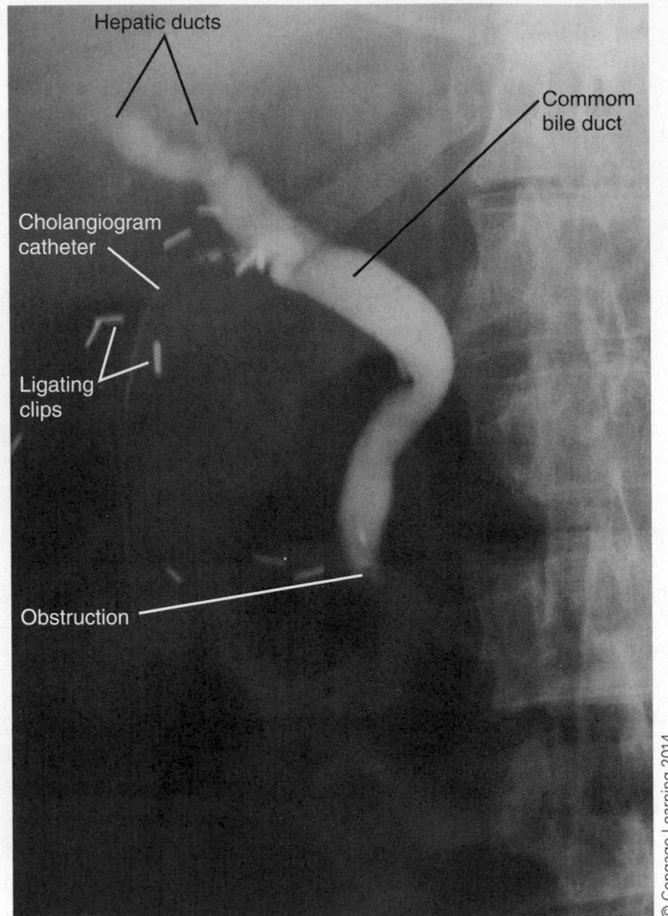

Figure 13-6 Intraoperative cholangiogram depicting gallstones

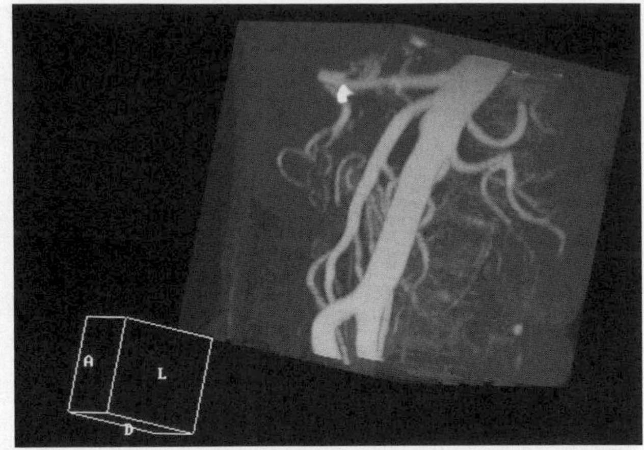

A

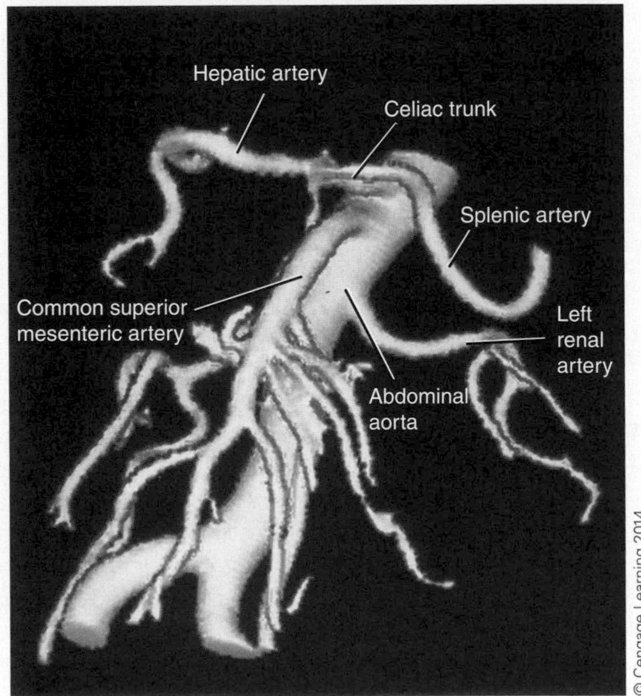

B

Figure 13-7 Computed tomography angiography: (A) Demonstration of the abdominal aorta with its main branches, (B) 3D reconstruction

As a neurological diagnostic tool, CT scanning is better than MRI for emergencies related to the brain because it is faster and better able to detect fresh bleeding. The CT scan is also useful for the detection of cerebral infarction and can be used with contrast for the detection of tumors and infection. This iodinated solution tends to leak into brain tissues that have suffered damage from tumor or infection, causing them to be seen as bright spots on the CT scan.

To undergo a CT scan, the patient must enter the scanning device, which is tubular in shape. The exam can be lengthy and the patient is expected to remain still for the duration of the scan. This is difficult for young children who may become frightened, or for an adult patient who may experience a feeling of claustrophobia. Either of these situations may require the patient to be sedated or placed under general anesthesia.

Positron Emission Tomography

Positron emission tomography (PET scanning) combines CT and radioisotope brain scanning. PET scanning helps to identify how different areas of the brain function by highlighting chemical or metabolic activity.

Magnetic Resonance Imaging

Magnetic resonance imaging (MRI) uses two different forms of energy to create an image. A spinning hydrogen atom is placed into a magnetic field, forcing the atoms to line up and "spin" at a particular frequency. Applied radio waves force the hydrogen atoms to cycle in phase. As the radio waves shut down, the atoms release a radio wave of the characteristic frequency that is measured and transformed into an image. MRI uses these radio waves in a strong magnetic field to form pictures of parts of the body in slices, much like a CT scan. However, MRI slices may be taken from any direction, a feature that CT scanners are unable to provide. (CT scanners generate images taken around

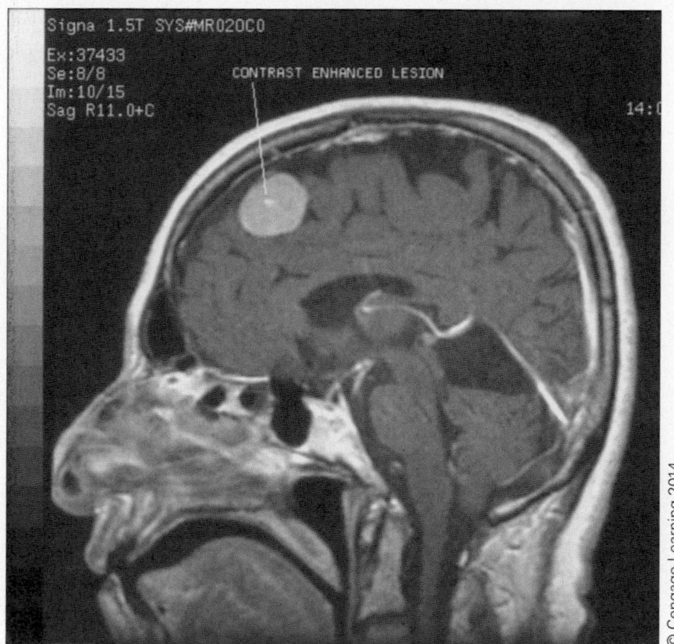

Figure 13-8 MRI depicting a brain tumor

a single axis of rotation in the axial or transverse plane of the body.) In addition, MRI uses no X-ray radiation.

MRI is especially good for imaging soft tissue, so it is often used for the evaluation of brain disorders and for providing images of a herniated disc and its relationship to the spinal cord (Figure 13-8).

As with CT scanning, contrast media may be injected intravenously to help spotlight tumors and infections. For detection of brain or spine tumors and infections, MR images are taken before and after injection of contrast. The contrast medium used for MRI is not iodine based, so that patients with iodine allergy are not adversely affected.

Like the CT scan, the MRI exam is lengthy and the unit is tubular in shape, potentially causing fear and anxiety in the patient. In addition, the MRI device makes repeated loud noises that can complicate the patient's ability to remain calm and still. Again, sedation or general anesthesia may be used.

Ultrasonography

During an ultrasound examination, high-frequency sound waves are directed into the body and reflected from the tissues to a recording device for diagnostic purposes. Frequencies of 1–10 million Hz are necessary for diagnostic studies. The lower the frequency, the greater is the depth of sound wave penetration into the body.

Ultrasonic waves are produced when a crystal (transducer) is stimulated electrically. The beam that is produced is directed into the body and variances in tissue density are reflected back to the transducer as echoes. These echoes are then converted into electrical impulses that can be viewed as images.

Ultrasound is a useful diagnostic tool for examination of the heart and abdominopelvic cavity. It is also useful

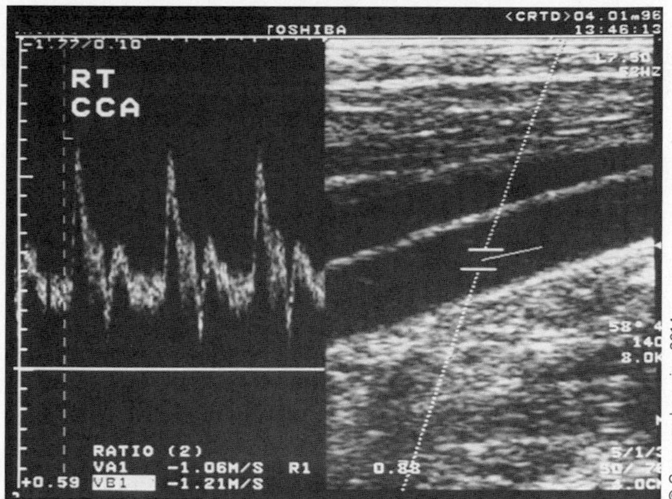

Figure 13-9 Doppler ultrasound, venous system

for identifying carotid artery stenosis. Because ultrasound waves cannot pass through structures that contain air, **ultrasonography** is not used to examine the lungs. Ultrasonography is ideal for examination of the fetus because it does not use ionizing radiation.

Echocardiography

Echocardiography is a noninvasive study that provides a two-dimensional image of the heart by directing beams of ultrasonic waves from a sonar-like device through the chest wall. These sound waves echo from the heart and surrounding structures to provide information about cardiac structural abnormalities. Color Doppler techniques of echocardiography are useful for mapping blood flow through the heart.

Transesophageal echocardiography (TEE), a slightly more invasive procedure, involves the introduction of a transducer attached to the end of a gastroscope into the esophagus, bringing the probe into closer approximation with the heart. It is useful for the assessment of valvular function and intraventricular blood volume during cardiac surgery and for the detection of cardiac chamber enlargement and septal defects.

Doppler Ultrasonography

A measurement can be taken of the shift in frequency of a continuous ultrasonic wave proportional to the velocity of blood flow in vessels (Figure 13-9). The Doppler monitor measures blood flow that transmits the sound of moving red blood cells to the transducer. The difference in pitch between the transmitted and reflected sounds produces a tone that can be amplified by the machine. *Doppler ultrasonography* is used in the OR to determine the patency of arterial anastomosis. The Doppler probe is covered with a sterile drape for use within the sterile field.

The measurement of segmental limb pressures is easily achieved with the Doppler probe. Pressure in the thigh can be determined by applying a tourniquet and determining the

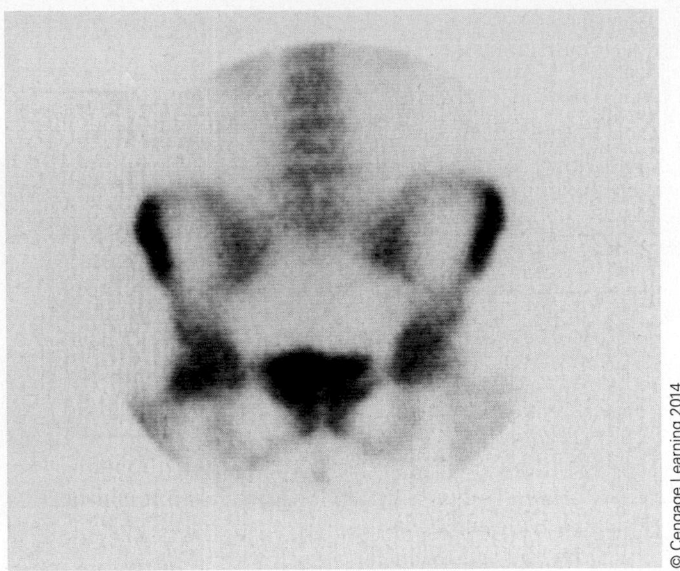

Figure 13-10 Radionuclide scan, lumbar

pressure at which flow is extinguished in the popliteal or tibial artery using the Doppler probe. By placing the cuff around the calf, pressure measurements of the calf can be obtained as the examiner determines which pressure is associated with the loss of pedal flow. Calf and thigh pressures are compared with each other and with the brachial artery pressure to provide an objective assessment of the degree of arterial disease.

Isotope Scanning

Isotope scanning, sometimes referred to as a nuclear medicine study or radionuclide imaging, involves the intravenous injection of a radioactive isotope into the patient prior to the imaging study (Figure 13-10). Various isotopes are available that are taken up metabolically by specific types of tissue. The metaiodobenzylguanidine (MIBG) scan will be specifically discussed in Chapter 20 as it relates to the adrenal gland. Collections of isotopes in a certain area are referred to as a "hot spot" and may indicate the presence of a pathological condition. A bone scan is an example of an isotope scan.

Radiation Therapy

Radiation kills cells by interfering with their metabolic activity. *Radiation therapy* is used in predetermined doses to treat specific types of neoplasms that are susceptible to radiation by exposure to the radiation source. Radiation can be administered to the patient with a beam that passes through the tissue or by direct tissue contact with an implantable radiation source.

Laboratory Reports

The laboratory or pathology department is responsible for countless types of examinations on every type of body fluid and tissue that exists. Findings from these studies are extremely valuable in sorting out what may be normal for one patient and abnormal for another. Every type of exam cannot possibly be listed here simply because they are too numerous; only the basics will be covered in this text. A blood test, for example, may be run to provide the practitioner with some broad general information, or may be ordered to obtain one specific value. Only normal values are listed here. Abnormalities as they pertain to a patient's pathological condition will be discussed in the procedural chapters.

The surgical technologist plays an important role in specimen care and handling. This is more thoroughly discussed in the procedural chapters. As always, whenever handling any body substances, Standard Precautions are used.

Hematological Studies

Venous or arterial blood is drawn from the patient for visual or computerized examination in the laboratory setting. Normal laboratory findings are illustrated in Table 13-1, and normal blood gas findings are listed in Table 13-2.

Urinalysis

Urine collection methods vary according to the type of test to be performed. A simple voided specimen is collected as the patient urinates into a clean container. A clean-catch sample involves cleaning the urinary meatus prior to voiding and "catching" the sample midstream into a sterile collection device. Catheterized specimens are obtained under sterile conditions and placed in a sterile specimen container. Normal **urinalysis (UA)** and chemistry values are shown in Table 20-5.

Urine may be collected over a 24-hour period and the entire sample tested for electrolytes and nitrogenous wastes.

Tissue Specimens

The excision of tissue or aspiration of fluid to determine the nature of the disease or for treatment of a condition is called a **biopsy** and the tissue or fluid is referred to as a specimen. The specimen is sent to the pathology department where the pathologist performs histologic examination (study of tissue) or cytologic examination (study of cells) to determine a diagnosis that is communicated to the surgeon (Figure 13-11). With very few exceptions, all tissue and objects removed from a patient are considered specimens and sent to the pathology department. The following is general information pertaining to the care and handling of specimens; this is followed by information pertaining to specific types of biopsies and handling of specific types of specimens.

- *Loss of specimen*—The loss of a specimen can have devastating effects for the patient. It could necessitate a second procedure to be performed to obtain another specimen and delay postoperative treatment, such as chemotherapy or antibiotic therapy.
- *Correct labeling*—Specimens must be correctly labeled. The STSR should confirm the identity of the specimen (name) and origin (left arm) with surgeon, and when handing off the specimen to the circulator should confirm this information with him or her. Additionally, the orientation of the specimen becomes important when

TABLE 13-1 Hematology Values

Red blood cell (RBC) count	
Male:	4.3–5.9 × 10^6/mm^3, 4.3–5.9 × 10^{12}/L (SI units)
Female:	3.5–5 × 10^6/mm^3, 3.5–5.0 × 10^{12}/L (SI units)
RBC indices	
Mean corpuscular hemoglobin (MCH):	27–33 pg (standard and SI)
Mean corpuscular hemoglobin concentration (MCHC):	33–37 g/dL, 330–370 g/L (SI units)
Mean corpuscular volume (MCV):	76–100 μm^3, 76–100 fL
Hemoglobin	
Male:	13.5–18 g/dL, 135–180 g/L (SI units)
Female:	11.5–15.5 g/dL, 115–155 g/L (SI units)
Glycosylated (HbA1-C):	<7.5%, 5–6% (desired)
Hematocrit	
Male:	40–52% (0.40–0.52)
Female:	35–46% (0.35–0.46)
Platelets	130–400 × 10^3/mm^3
White blood cells (leukocytes)	5,000–10,000/mm^3
Neutrophils	50–70%
Segments	50–65%
Bands	0–5%
Basophils	0.25–0.5%
Eosinophils	1–3%
Monocytes	2–6%
Lymphocytes	25–40%
T-lymphocytes	60–80% of lymphocytes
B-lymphocytes	10–20% of lymphocytes
Bleeding time	1–3 min (Duke)
	1–5 min (Ivy)
Coagulation time (Lee White)	5–15 min
Prothrombin time	10–15 sec (same as control)
Partial thromboplastin time (PTT)	60–70 sec
Thrombin time	Within 5 sec of control
INR recommended range	
Standard therapy	2.0–3.0
High-dose therapy	2.5–3.5
Activated partial thromboplastin time (APTT)	30–45 sec

TABLE 13-2 Blood Gas Values

Whole blood oxygen, capacity	17–24 vol%
Arterial	
Saturation	96–100% of capacity
pCO_2	35–45 mm Hg
pO_2	75–100 mm Hg
pH	7.38–7.44
Bicarbonate, normal range	24–28 mEq/L
Base excess (BE)	+2 to −2 (±2 mEq/L)
Venous	
Saturation	60–85% capacity
pCO_2	40–54 mm Hg
pO_2	20–50 mm Hg
pH	7.36–7.41
Bicarbonate, normal range	22–28 mEq/L

the margins of the wound must be proven to be free of tumor. The surgeon may mark the edges with suture and the STSR should accurately communicate the information to the circulator, e.g., "left breast biopsy, suture marker on superior quadrant of biopsy."

- *Incorrect labeling*—Again, this can have devastating effects for the patient. For example, imagine that a biopsy is taken from the right breast, but is labeled left breast and, the diagnosis comes back as invasive breast cancer. If the mistake is not caught the patient could mistakenly undergo a mastectomy of the left breast, which is healthy, while the cancer remains in the right breast.

Foreign bodies must be cared for according to health care facility policy. Foreign bodies could have legal value and are often turned over to the police as evidence. It is recommended that the circulator or person who turns over the foreign body to the law enforcement officials receive a written receipt or record of who received the specimen.

Containers should be large enough to contain the specimen and, if warranted, tissue preservative. The STSR must pass off the specimen in a sterile manner to the circulator. Small

SPECIMEN COLLECTION SHEET
(DO NOT USE FOR FROZEN SECTIONS)

SOURCE OF SPECIMEN: ______________________________

O.R. ROOM# __________ LOC/GEN ______________________

SURGEON: __________ PLEASE CALL OR # __________ WITH RESULTS

CALL FRONT DESK WITH ORDERS
ORDERS MUST ACCOMPANY THIS FORM

PATHOLOGY #5139

______ 1. FOR A FAXIGRAM
(SEND PATH CARD & X-RAYS)

______ 2. FOR MD TO LOOK AT
(SEND PATH CARD)

______ 3. ROUTINE
(WRITE MD COMMENTS ON BACK OF CARD)

______ 4. RETURN SPECIMEN TO O.R.

DO NOT MARK LOOK AT AND ROUTINE TOGETHER!

*****MUST BE FILLED IN*****

I CERTIFY THE CORRECT PATIENT LABEL IS ON TISSUE CONTAINER FOR PATHOLOGY.

SIGN: ______________ LABELER

SIGN: ______________ WITNESS

PLACE PATIENT LABEL HERE

______ BONE-BANK-CULTURE FEMORAL HEAD

MICROBIOLOGY #5137

- TISSUE (ANY TISSUE)
3057-CULTURE TISSUE & GRAM STAIN
INCLUDES AEROBES & ANAEROBES
3065-AFB CULTURE & SMEAR
3005-FUNGAL CULTURE & KOH
- BODY FLUIDS IN CUP OR SYRINGE
DO NOT USE FOR URINE OR CSF!!!!!
3054-CULTURE BODY FLUID & GRAM STAIN
3065-AFB CULTURE & SMEAR
3005-FUNGAL CULTURE & KOH
3021-ANAEROBIC CULTURE & GRAM STAIN
4510-CRYSTAL ID
5122-CYTOLOGY FLUID
- SWAB SPECIMEN (KNEE & HIP)
3047-CULTURE MISCELLANEOUS & GRAM STAIN
3021-ANAEROBIC CULTURE & GRAM STAIN
- CSF IN A CUP OR SYRINGE
3056-CULTURE CSF & GRAM STAIN
1019-GLUCOSE CSF
1074-PROTEIN CSF
5110-CYTOLOGY CSF
- URINE (CATH-VOIDED-KIDNEY-URETER)
3046-CULTURE URINE
3008-GRAM STAIN ONLY
4524-URINALYSIS
5110-CYTOLOGY URINE
- BRONCH WASH-SPUTUM
3053-SPUTUM CULTURE & GRAM STAIN
3006-AFB CULTURE & SMEAR
3005-FUNGAL CULTURE & KOH
5119-CYTOLOGY SPUTUM
- OTHER CULTURES
3048-STOOL CULTURE
3058-GENITAL CULTURE (CERVIX-VAGINAL)
2093-GC & CHLAMYDIA DNA PROBE
5107-PAP SMEAR
3047-PELVIC WASHING
3017-KOH ONLY
1383-VIRUS ISOLATION CULTURE

Figure 13-11 Specimen documentation

tissue specimens can be passed off on a Telfa pad. Large specimens can be placed in a basin and passed off to the circulator. A counted sponge must never be used for passing off and transporting a specimen. The circulator should wear gloves when receiving the specimen, if necessary transfer it to the appropriate container, place a lid or seal the container, wipe the outside of the container with a disinfectant solution and label the container.

If the STSR cannot immediately pass off the specimen to the circulator, he or she should place it in a sterile container, such as a basin, and submerge it in sterile water to keep the tissue from drying out.

The most common type of tissue preservative used is formalin. However, occasionally sterile water may be used.

General recommendations for the handling of specific types of specimens are as follows:

Smear and Brush Biopsy

Fluid with cells can be smeared and fixed on a microscopic slide. This is often done during endoscopic procedures. The specimen is fixed on the slide by spraying it with a fixative. The pathologist will then stain the slide and examine the cells under the microscope to obtain a diagnosis. One type of smear is a brush biopsy. During an endoscopic procedure such as a bronchoscopy, the surgeon may insert a long flexible wire with a small brush on the tip through a port in the scope. The surgeon will rub the brush against the targeted tissue, remove the instrument, and hand it to the STSR. The STSR is responsible for wiping the brush on a slide using aseptic technique to create a smear and then cutting off the tip of the brush to be placed in formalin. The slide and brush are examined by the pathologist.

Aspiration Biopsy

Aspiration biopsy is the removal of fluid through a needle attached to a syringe. Examples of aspiration biopsies include fluid taken from a cyst, a joint such as the knee joint, a body cavity such as the peritoneal cavity, or a solid lesion in the breast, thyroid or lymph nodes. Cells are present in the fluid in the syringe for the pathologist to examine.

Incisional Biopsy

Incisional biopsy entails the removal of a portion of the tissue mass or lesion for pathological study. The types of incisional biopsies that will be discussed are **frozen sections** (FS) and permanent sections. The surgeon may want to have an immediate diagnosis for two reasons: (1) to determine if it is necessary to excise more tissue, or (2) to be able to begin postoperative therapy as soon as possible. Use of FS allows for an immediate diagnosis; however, the method is not 100% accurate and the final diagnosis is determined by the "permanent section" that is performed by the pathologist. (See below for a description of a permanent section.) The tissue that is targeted to undergo FS must be kept dry; it is placed in a specimen container of the right size with no tissue preservative of any type added. Formalin or normal saline will alter the freezing process. The pathologist freezes the tissue sample, slices it into thin sections, stains the sections, and views the tissue under the microscope. When complete, the pathologist will report the results directly to the surgeon in the OR. When reporting results, sensitivity is required if the patient is under local anesthesia and awake. This is one reason that computers in the OR are useful: for presenting information for the surgeon to read.

Permanent sections are placed in a preservative such as formalin. The specimen is then placed in a machine that removes the fluid and water from the tissue, replacing it with paraffin. The specimen is sliced into thin sections which are placed on slides and stained or dyed for viewing under the microscope.

The following information pertains to the correct handling of other specific types of specimens.

- *Calculi (gallstones, kidney stones)*—Calculi must be sent to pathology dry. If a preservative is added it will dissolve the stones or permanently alter them.
- *Amputated limbs*—Amputated limbs are sent to the pathology department dry. They are carefully bagged and wrapped for transfer. It must be confirmed with the family if they want the limb; some cultures or religions believe that when the person dies the amputated limb must be buried with the person.

- *Bullets*—Bullets must be handled carefully. Do not use forceps or clamps to handle the bullet because the instrument could scratch the bullet. The barrels of all guns are unique and leave markings on the bullet; forensics matches the bullet to the gun by analyzing these markings. If there are additional scratches this could prevent the law enforcement officials from making a correct match between bullet and gun. Therefore, handle the bullet with gloved hands at all times.
- *Removed prostheses (orthopedic implants)*—Prostheses should be kept dry and sent to pathology.

Bacteriological Tests

Tissue or fluid that is suspected of being infected may be cultured so that the pathogen can be identified and treated. This is called *culture and sensitivity*. The culture is performed to determine the exact organism; once the organism is identified, a determination is made as to which form of treatment it will be sensitive to. Sterile cotton-tipped swabs are exposed to the tissue or fluid to be cultured, and then placed into the transport container. Aerobic and anaerobic studies may be ordered, each requiring its own specialized transport container. Anaerobic bacteria die quickly if exposed to air; therefore the swab should be placed quickly into the growth medium or vacuum transport tube for incubation in the laboratory.

Gram Stain

The **Gram stain**, developed in 1844, remains a valuable tool in identifying bacteria. Bacteria to be cultured are collected in the sterile transport tube and taken to the laboratory for analysis. There the bacterium is exposed to stains of crystal violet and iodine, then exposed to alcohol and stained again. Bacteria that retain the blue dye are called *gram positive* and those that fade to pink are *gram negative*. This quick method of identification helps the physician determine an initial course of treatment, which may be altered when the culture and sensitivity results are available.

Many other staining techniques for specific organisms have been developed following Gram's principles.

Spinal Tap

Cerebrospinal fluid (**CSF**) is withdrawn ("tapped") from the lumbar area of the spinal column for analysis. The fluid is normally clear. The physician can make a preliminary diagnosis by observing if the fluid is bloody or cloudy, allowing initial treatment to begin. Final diagnosis is reserved until the CSF has undergone laboratory analysis (Table 13-3).

Thoracentesis

Thoracentesis involves the placement of a needle into a posterior portion of the pleural space for the analysis of pleural effusion. The procedure is generally performed as an aid in the diagnosis of inflammatory or neoplastic diseases of the pleura or the lung. Therapeutic applications for thoracentesis include the removal of fluid accumulations from within the thoracic cavity. CT scan or ultrasonography may accompany thoracentesis to ensure accurate needle placement.

Table 13-3 Cerebrospinal Fluid Values

Cell count	0–8/mm^3
Chloride	118–132 mEq/L
Culture	No organisms
Glucose	40–80 mg/dL
Pressure	75–175 cm water
Protein	15–45 mg/dL
Sodium	145–150 mg/dL

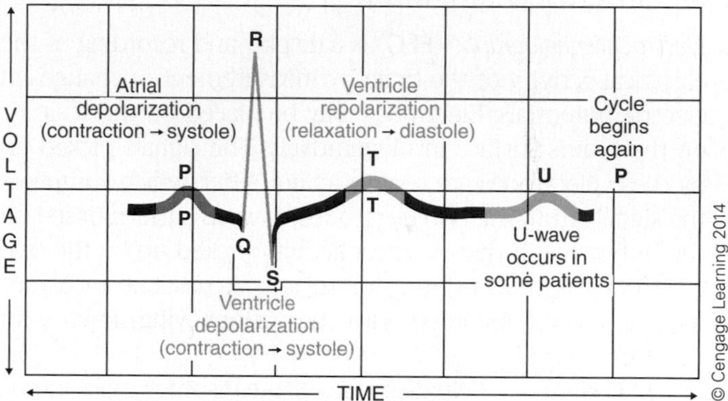

Figure 13-12 ECG and cardiac cycle

Electrodiagnostic Studies

The body consists of cells that contain polarized molecules. The communication systems of the body are bioelectrical or biochemical. Microelectrical impulses can be measured and provide useful diagnostic information.

Electrocardiography

The **electrocardiogram (ECG)** is a valuable tool for the detection and evaluation of all forms of heart disease, especially myocardial infarction (Figure 13-12). However, the ECG should not be the only diagnostic tool used because, in certain instances, it may appear normal in patients with cardiac conditions. It may also appear abnormal in patients in good cardiac health; therefore, the ECG is best utilized in the detection and evaluation of cardiac dysrhythmias and conduction disturbances. Cardiac dysrhythmias are discussed in Chapter 22.

Electrocardiography is performed by placing a number of electrodes in predetermined locations on the skin of the arms, legs, and torso to record the electrical activity of the heart. The number of electrodes (also referred to as *leads*) varies according to the patient situation and the type of information desired. Typically, a five-lead configuration is utilized in the operating room.

The Holter monitor allows 24-hour monitoring for asymptomatic and symptomatic dysrhythmias. The system is composed of a portable tape recorder, one or two electrocardiographic leads, and a computer system capable of quantifying rhythm disturbances. The patient wears the monitor while attending to daily activities.

ECG is also useful for graded exercise testing, often referred to as a stress test. The patient walks on a treadmill at an increasing rate while heart rate, blood pressure, and ECG are closely monitored for significant changes. Exercise testing evaluates the delivery of oxygen via coronary circulation in response to increased demands. It also indicates the presence of myocardial ischemia for patients with **angina**.

Electroencephalography

Electroencephalography (**EEG**) is a display and recording of the electrical activity of the brain by measurement of changes in electric potentials. Electrodes may be placed on the scalp or on the brain's surface intraoperatively. The signals picked up by these electrodes are sent to an amplifier, which compares the signals from the two electrodes. A wave pattern based on the difference in the electrical activity picked up by the two electrodes is then printed for review. A baseline measurement is usually recorded with the patient lying down with the eyes closed.

EEG is used to help diagnose seizure disorder, brain tumor, epilepsy, and other diseases and injury to the brain. In addition, EEG is used intraoperatively during certain cranial, spinal, and vascular procedures for monitoring of neurological function.

When used in the diagnosis of seizures, EEG measurements are taken during a seizure and during a period of normal brain activity. This helps to localize the origin of the seizure within the brain and to confirm seizure activity. EEG patterns are also analyzed to help determine the area of the brain affected by a tumor or other abnormality.

EEG brain topography uses computers to simultaneously record a large number of digitized EEG channels. This information is analyzed and plotted on a screen or printer using different colors to depict EEG activity. This method gives a more accurate view of the location of alterations in brain wave activity in relation to the surface of the skull.

Electromyography

Electromyography (EMG) is the study and recording of the electrical activity of skeletal muscle. Electric stimulation is applied to the muscle via a probe that is inserted through the skin into the muscle. Information about muscle contractility and innervation can be assembled.

Pulmonary Diagnosis

Respiratory status and the severity of several pulmonary conditions are evaluated in several ways. One of them, blood gas analysis, has already been mentioned.

Pulse Oximetry

Arterial saturation of hemoglobin with oxygen is measured by passing a light through the tissues to determine the optical density of the blood. The lighted noninvasive device is most often placed on the finger, toe, or earlobe. The pulse oximeter measures the oxygen saturation in percentages. The normal value is 95%–97%. Oxygen administration should increase the percentage.

Capnography

Capnography was designed to estimate arterial levels of carbon dioxide noninvasively for surgical patients requiring mechanical ventilation. Measurement of the amount of carbon dioxide that is exhaled makes the estimation. This is referred to as the *end-tidal* CO_2. The sensor is located within the anesthesia circuit or ventilation tubing and sends the information to a monitor, which displays the information in graph (wave) form. This is helpful in detecting dislocated endotracheal tubes and acidosis.

Spirometry

Spirometry is another noninvasive technique used for evaluating the patient's respiratory status. Information about the lung capacity, resistance, and ventilatory pressure is obtained and displayed in numerical and graph form on a monitor. This technique is useful in detecting leaks in the ventilatory system and patient conditions such as chronic obstructive pulmonary disease (COPD) and adult respiratory distress syndrome (ARDS).

Endoscopy

Endoscopes can be used preoperatively or intraoperatively to directly visualize internal structures for diagnostic purposes. Chapter 10 provides a detailed description of the various types of endoscopes and their uses for diagnosis and therapy. Refer to individual procedural chapters for specific endoscopic procedures.

Plethysmography and Phleborheography

Plethysmography is useful in patients with diffuse small vessel arterial disease, especially diabetics. A plethysmograph is an instrument for determining and registering variations in the volume of an extremity and in the amount of blood present in the extremity or passing through it. Common plethysmographic techniques include a mercury strain gauge and air plethysmography (pulse volume recorder). With the use of a mercury strain gauge, changes in leg volume that accompany arterial pulsation are sensed by the strain gauge and translated as a waveform on a strip chart recorder. A pulse volume recorder detects changes in the volume of an inflated air bladder that is expressed on a strip chart recorder. In each case, changes in the volume of the examined part are measured, rather than changes in blood velocity of a particular artery, as in Doppler studies. Thus, while their waveforms are similar, plethysmography and Doppler ultrasonography are measuring two related but separate parameters and provide different information. Although plethysmography measures blood flow quite well, it does not measure the flow of a particular artery in the way that Doppler studies can.

Diagnosis of deep-vein thrombosis can be made by *phleborheography*, a plethysmographic technique in which rhythmic changes in venous volume in the legs associated with respiration are recorded.

Case Study Fredrick is scheduled as the surgical technologist on a laparoscopic cholecystectomy for a patient diagnosed with cholecystitis and cholelithiasis. He is assembling supplies and preparing the operating room for the case.

1. **What laboratory studies do you expect to find on the patient's chart?**
2. **Are diagnostic image studies likely to be part of the patient's preoperative workup? If so, what kind? How will they be viewed in the OR?**
3. **Is it likely that any studies will be performed during the procedure? What kind? How might this affect the room preparation?**

Questions for Further Study

1. Would a CT scan or X-ray best demonstrate a soft tissue tumor? Why?
2. What is the first priority of the STSR when an intraoperative X-ray is being taken?
3. What is a cholangiogram?
4. Contrast media and isotopes are both used to enhance diagnostic imaging studies. How do they differ?

BIBLIOGRAPHY

Association of Surgical Technologists. (2011). *Core curriculum for surgical technology* (6th ed.). Littleton, CO: Association of Surgical Technologists.

Delmar Cengage Learning. (1999). *Delmar's radiographic positioning and procedures: Image library* [CD-ROM]. Clifton Park, NY: Author.

Estes, M. E. Z. (2010). *Health assessment and physical examination* (4th ed.). Clifton Park, NY: Delmar Cengage Learning.

O'Toole, M. (Ed.). (2005). *Miller-Keane encyclopedia & dictionary of medicine, nursing, and allied health* (7th ed.). Philadelphia: W. B. Saunders.

Phillips, N. F. (2007). *Berry & Kohn's operating room technique* (11th ed.). St. Louis: Mosby.

Spratto, G. R., & Woods, A. L. (2011). *Delmar's nurse's drug handbook 2011: Special 20 year anniversary*. Clifton Park, NY: Delmar Cengage Learning.

Townsend, C. M., Beauchamp, R. D., Evers, B. M., & Mattox, K. (Eds.). (2007). *Sabiston textbook of surgery: The biological basis of modern surgical practice* (18th ed.). Philadelphia: W. B. Saunders.

Chapter 14

General Surgery

Case Study Laura is a 45-year-old woman who is somewhat overweight, eats a typical American diet, and is generally healthy. She has been developing severe colicky pain in her right upper quadrant about 2 hours after meals. After a history and physical, she was diagnosed with cholelithiasis.

1. What does cholelithiasis mean?
2. What causes the condition?
3. Name three possible treatments for cholelithiasis.

Objectives

After studying this chapter, the reader should be able to:

A 1. Indicate the pathology and related terminology of each system or organ that prompts surgical intervention.

P 2. Indicate special preoperative preparation procedures related to general surgery procedures.

3. Recall the names and uses of general surgery instruments, supplies, and specialty equipment.
4. Propose the intraoperative preparations of the patient specific to the illustrative procedures.

O 5. Summarize the surgical steps of the illustrative general surgery procedures in this chapter.

6. Identify the purpose and expected outcomes of the illustrative procedures.
7. Determine the immediate postoperative care of the patient and possible complications of the illustrative procedures.

S 8. Determine any specific variations related to the preoperative, intraoperative, and postoperative care of the general surgery patient.

Select Key Terms

absorption	-ectomy	–oma	portal venous system
anastomosis	excision	–ostomy	–stasis
ascites	incision	–otomy	stenosis
bile	lysis	parietal	ulcer
chole-	necrosis	peritoneum	viscera
-docho-			

PART I: General Information

INTRODUCTION

General surgery involves many organ systems but most commonly involves the abdominal cavity and the organs contained within the cavity. However, there are surgical procedures that may be considered in the realm of another surgical specialty, but the general surgeon often performs the procedures; for example, vein ligation and stripping is a vascular procedure for treating varicose veins or a muscle and nerve biopsy. Additionally, the general surgeon performs procedures on tissues and organs outside of the abdominal cavity, including breast and thyroid procedures. This chapter will address the general surgery procedures that provide a basis for the student to carry the knowledge into surgical rotation.

INSTRUMENTATION, ROUTINE EQUIPMENT, AND SUPPLIES

Instrumentation, equipment, and supplies vary widely with geographic region, hospital availability, and the surgeon's preference. The following sections provide information on a broad basis to provide students with a starting point from which to further their learning in the classroom, mock operating room (OR), and surgical rotation.

Instrumentation

Many factors influence the selection of instrumentation for both the facility and the surgeon. For this reason, the instrumentation lists that follow are basic and relatively standard.

Major Set

The foundation set for many surgical procedures is the major *lapar**otomy*** set (Table 14-1).

Many types and sizes of retractors are used in general surgery. An illustrative sample is shown in Figure 14-1. Additionally, there are many types and sizes of forceps, clamps or hemostats, and miscellaneous instrumentation used in general surgery. When a surgical procedure calls for performing in a deep cavity such as the abdominal cavity or bariatric surgery is scheduled, instruments called "long and deep" instruments will be needed. Long and deep instruments refer to those that are longer than normal and used in deep cavities. For example, routinely used Metzenbaum scissors are usually 7″ in length; long Metzenbaum scissors are available up to 14″ in length.

Table 14-1 Major Laparotomy Set

Yankauer suction tip	1 ea.	Mayo scissors straight	1 ea.
Poole suction tip	1 ea.	Mayo scissors curved	1 ea.
8″, 10″, and 12″ DeBakey forceps	2 ea.	7″ and 9″ Metzenbaum scissors	1 ea.
#3, #4, and #7 knife handles	1 ea.	Ferris-Smith forceps	2 ea.

Table 14-1 (continued)

Adson tissue forceps with teeth (Figure 14-2A)	2 ea.	U.S. Army retractor (Figure 14-1H)	2 ea.
Brown-Adson tissue forceps (Figure 14-2B)	2 ea.	Ribbon retractor ¾″	1 ea.
Russian tissue forceps	2 ea.	Ribbon retractor 1¼″	1 ea.
Cushing thumb tissue forceps (Figure 14-2C)	2 ea.	Deaver retractor 1″ (Figure 14-1F)	1 ea.
Halsted mosquito forceps curved (Figure 14-2D)	6 ea.	Deaver retractor 2″	1 ea.
Crile hemostats 5½″ straight (Figure 14-2E)	6 ea.	Richardson retractor, small	2 ea.
Crile hemostats 5½″ curved (Figure 14-1L)	12 ea.	Richardson retractor, large	1 ea.
Rochester-Pean forceps 8″ (Figure 14-2F)	6 ea.	Kelly retractor, 2½″ (Figure 14-1A–D)	1 ea.
Kocher clamp 6¼″ (Figure 14-2G)	4 ea.	Gelpi retractor (Figure 14-1N)	1 ea.
Mixter forceps 7¼″ curved	1 ea.	Beckman-Weitlaner (Figure 14-1O)	1 ea.
Mixter forceps 9″	1 ea.	Balfour retractor and blades (Figure 14-1E)	1 ea.
Baby Mixter forceps 5¼″ curved	1 ea.	Harrington retractor (Figure 14-1G)	3 ea.
Backhaus towel clamp (Figure 14-2L)	8 ea.	Lahey gall duct forceps 7½″	2 ea.
Foerster sponge forceps (Figure 14-2K)	2 ea.	Allis tissue forceps 6″ (Figure 14-2I)	2 ea.
Mayo-Hegar needle holder 6″	2 ea.	Allis tissue forceps 10″	2 ea.
Mayo-Hegar needle holder 7″	2 ea.	Babcock tissue forceps 6¼″ (Figure 14-2H)	2 ea.
Mayo-Hegar needle holder 8″	2 ea.	Babcock tissue forceps 9¼″	2 ea.
Mayo-Hegar needle holder 10½″	2 ea.	Pennington clamp (Figure 14-2J)	2 ea.
Green retractor (Figure 14-1J)	2 ea.	Stainless steel ruler	1 ea.
Goelet retractor (Figure 14-1I)	2 ea.	Schnidt tonsil forceps 7½″	2 ea.

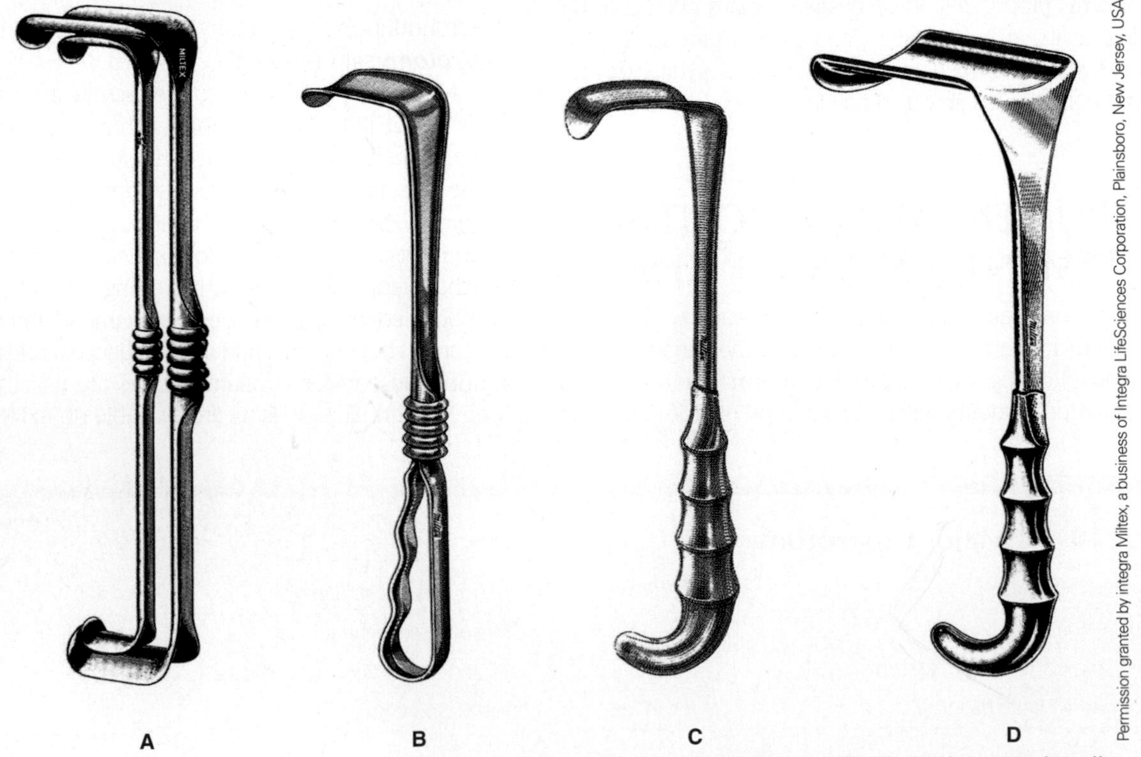

Figure 14-1 Retractors: (A) Richardson-Eastman (double end), (B) Kelly (loop handle), (C) Kelly (hollow grip handle), (D) Kelly (3½-in blade)

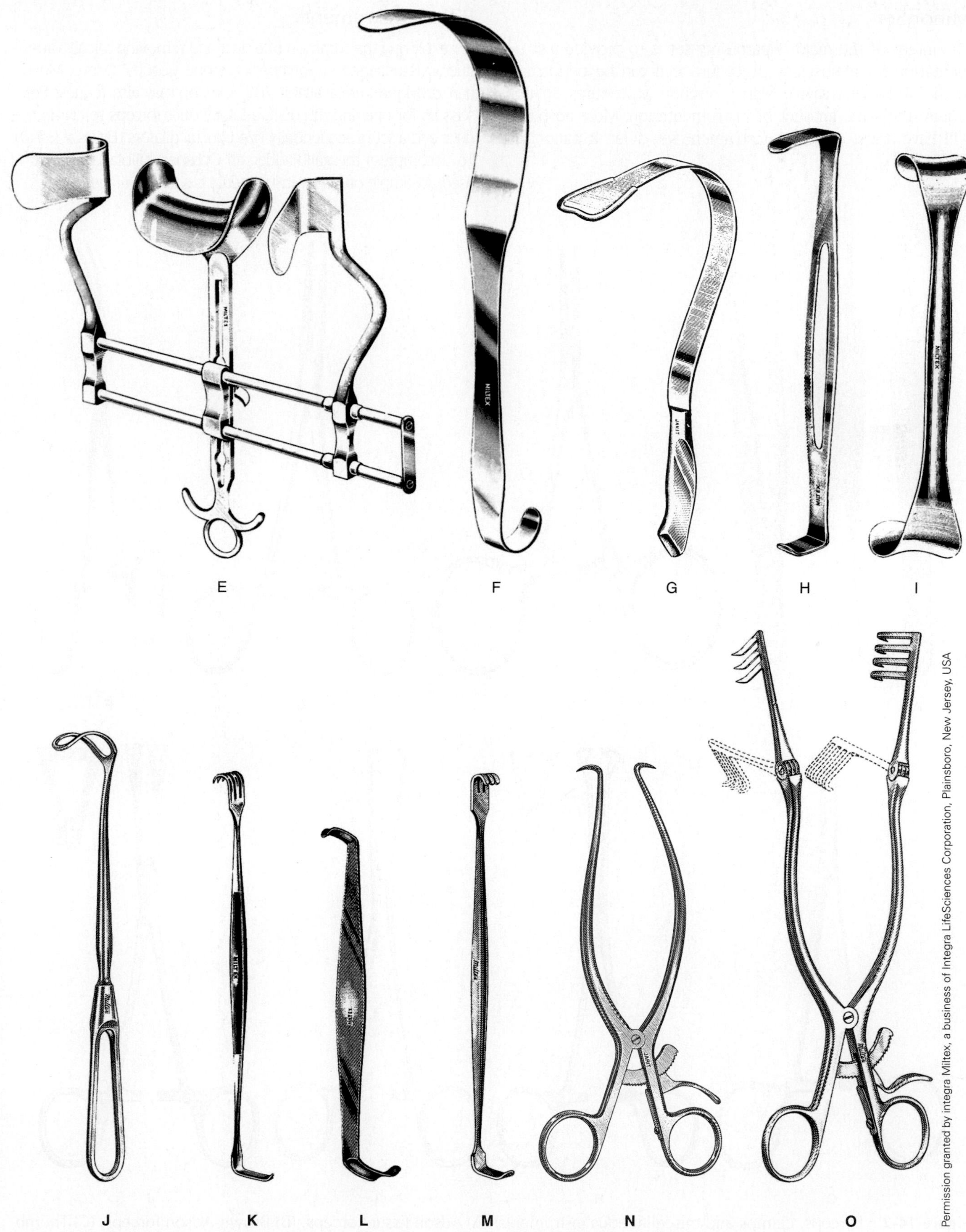

Figure 14-1 Retractors: (E) Balfour (solid side blades), (F) Deaver, (G) Harrington retractor, (H) U.S. Army, (I) Goelet, (J) Green, (K) Senn, (L) Crile, (M) Mathieu, (N) Gelpi, (O) Beckman-Weitlaner

Minor Set

The intent of the major laparotomy set is to provide instrumentation for almost any procedure that can be performed in the abdominal cavity. Many common procedures do not require the same amount of instrumentation. Most hospitals will have a less extensive instrument set called a minor set (Table 14-2).

Biliary Instruments

For exploring the common **bile** duct and removing calculi, various ductal (Randall stone) forceps and stone "scoops" (Mayo, Moynihan, or Moore) are available. The surgeon may also request Potts scissors for opening the duct, a Lahey duct forceps to clamp the duct, and a set of sequentially sized ductal dilators (Bakes #3–#10). To decompress the gallbladder, an Ochsner gallbladder trocar is used. A sample of biliary instruments is shown in Figure 14-3.

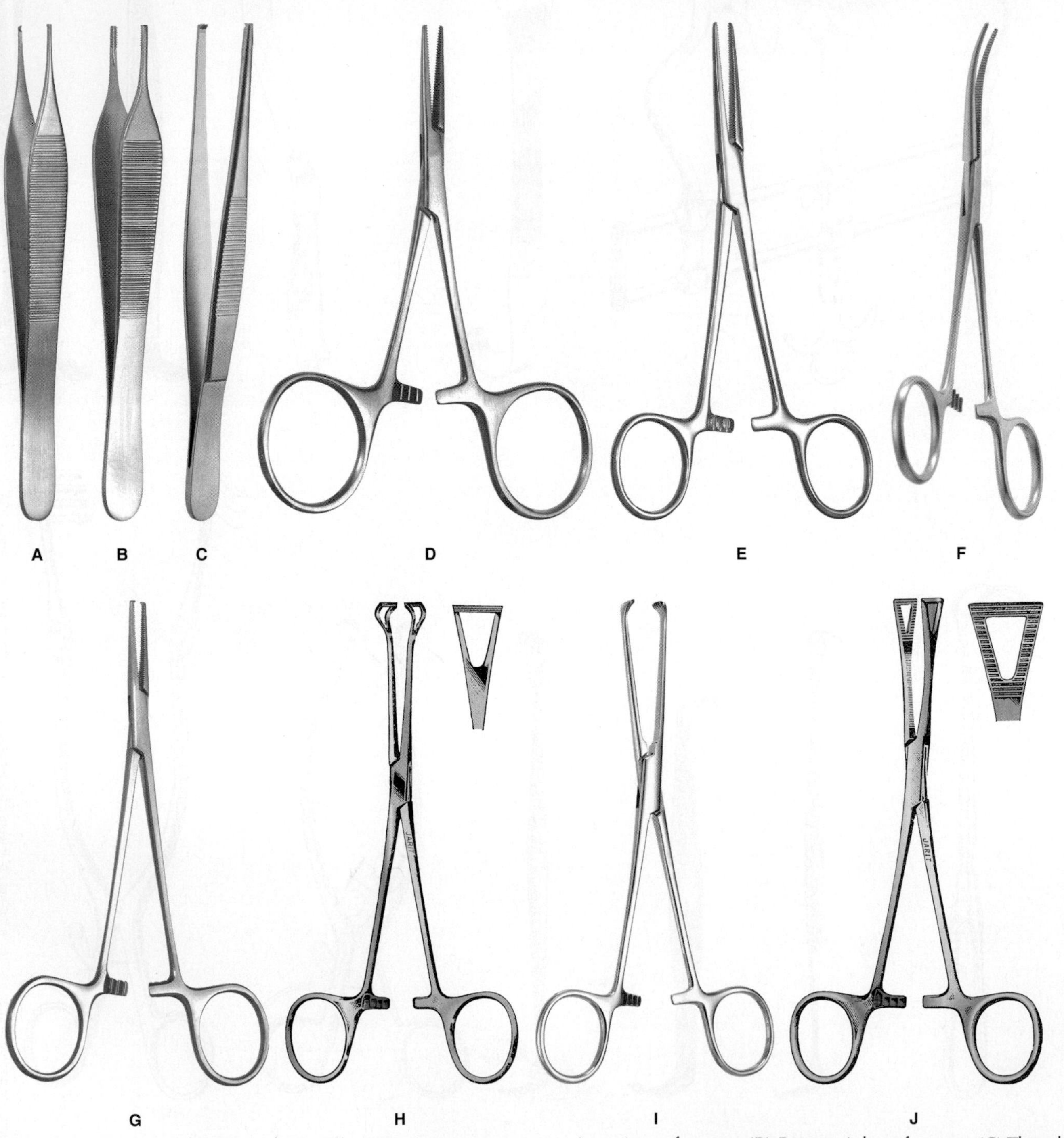

Figure 14-2 Forceps, clamps and miscellaneous instruments: (A) Adson tissue forceps, (B) Brown-Adson forceps, (C) Thumb tissue forceps, (D) Mosquito forceps, (E) Crile hemostats, (F) Rochester-Pean clamp, (G) Kocher clamp, (H) Babcock tissue clamp, (I) Allis clamp, (J) Pennington clamp

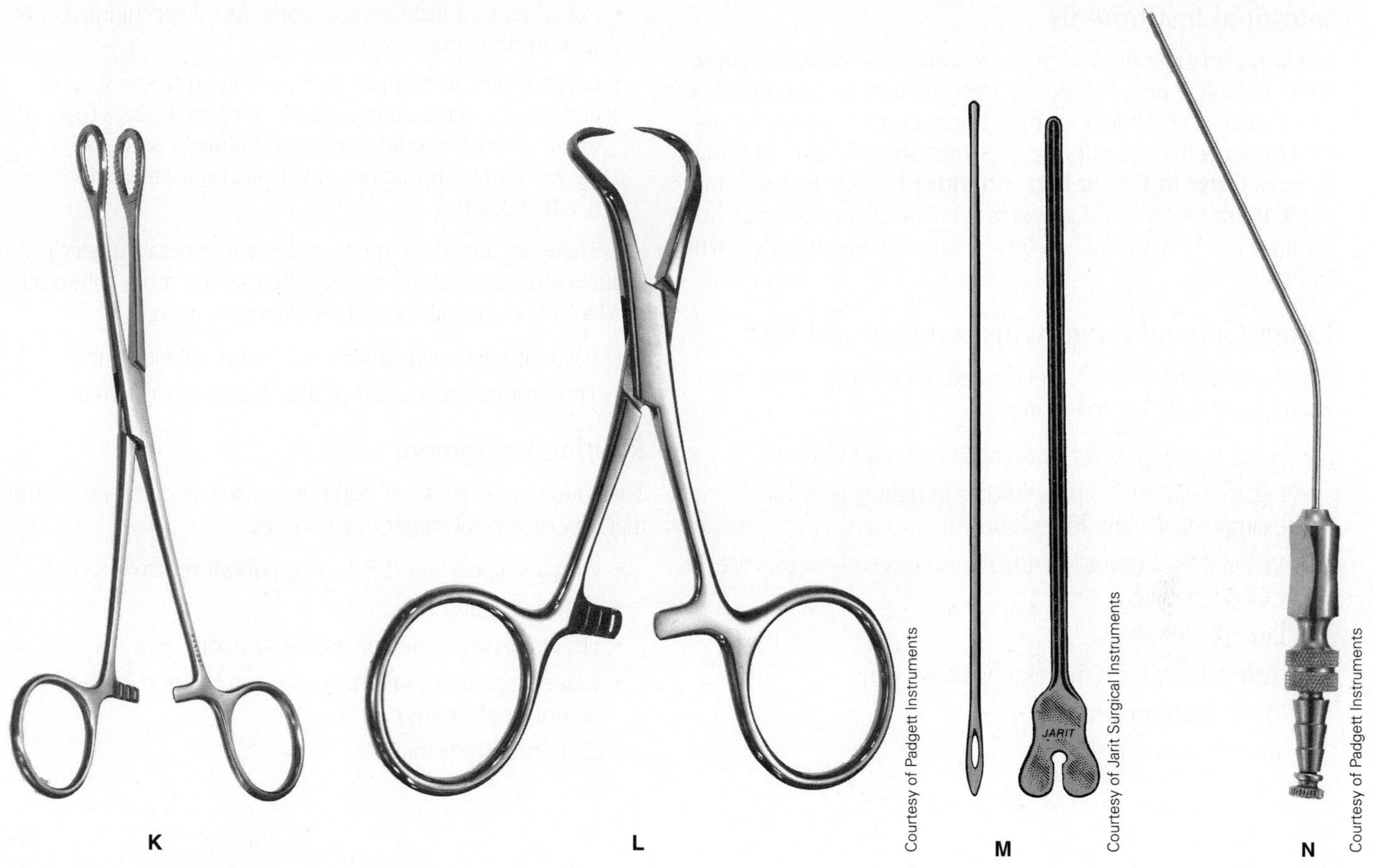

Figure 14-2 Forceps, clamps, and miscellaneous instruments: (K) Foerster sponge- holding forcep, (L) Backhaus towel clamp, (M) Probe and grooved director, (N) Frazier suction tip

TABLE 14-2 **General Surgery—Minor Set**

Yankauer suction tip	1 ea.	U.S. Army retractor	2 ea.
#3 knife handles	2 ea.	Allis tissue forceps 6″	2 ea.
Mayo scissors straight	1 ea.	Babcock tissue forceps 6¼″	2 ea.
Mayo scissors curved	1 ea.	Probe with eye 5½″ (Figure 14-2M)	1 ea.
7″ Metzenbaum scissors	1 ea.	Grooved director with probe tip 5½″ (Figure 14-2M)	1 ea.
Adson tissue forceps with teeth	2 ea.	Senn retractor, double ended, sharp (Figure 14-1K)	2 ea.
Halsted mosquito forceps curved	6 ea.	Mathieu retractor (Figure 14-1M)	2 ea.
Crile forceps 5½″ curved	6 ea.	Volkman retractor, three prong	2 ea.
Backhaus towel clamp	6 ea.	Frazier Ferguson suction tip (Figure 14-2N)	1 ea.
Foerster sponge forceps	2 ea.	Schnidt hemostatic forceps	2 ea.
Mayo-Hegar needle holder 6″	2 ea.		
Mayo-Hegar needle holder 7″	2 ea.		

Intestinal Instruments

Intestinal instruments include a variety of bowel clamps, such as Payr, Allen, Doyen, or Best, as well as stapling devices such as the linear stapler, linear cutter, and the circular stapler with accompanying sizers and circular suturing devices (refer to Chapter 11). An intestinal set may also include extra forceps and an extra Poole suction tip for intraluminal work. A sample of intestinal instruments is shown in Figure 14-4.

Other General Surgery Instruments and Sets

Some procedures require specific and unique instrumentation. Examples include the following:

- Adair tenaculums for grasping large breast masses
- Ligature carriers to pass sutures in tight spaces, for example low sigmoid resection
- Maloney esophageal dilators; these types of dilators are called a bougie
- Liver retractors
- Vein stripper for removal of varicose veins
- Thyroid**ectomy** set
- Tracheotomy set
- Rectal set that includes anoscope, rectal speculum, rectal dilators, Buie pile forceps
- Laparoscopic instrumentation, including trocar sheaths and trocars, and laparoscopes of varying degrees (e.g., 0°, 30°), Verres needle, curved and straight scissors, curved clamps, retractors of various types and sizes, needle holders

There are instances in which specific general surgery procedures require instruments and sets that are more commonly used in other surgical specialties; examples include:

- Vascular set (repair of liver laceration; splenectomy)
- Thoracotomy set (repair of liver laceration; trauma)

Routine Equipment

The following is a list of equipment that is common to the majority of general surgery procedures:

- Electrosurgical unit (ESU) with patient return electrode
- Suction apparatus
- Headlamp (available for use by surgeon)
- Laser (procedures in which laser can be used, such as hemorrhoidectomy)
- Cell-Saver (available)

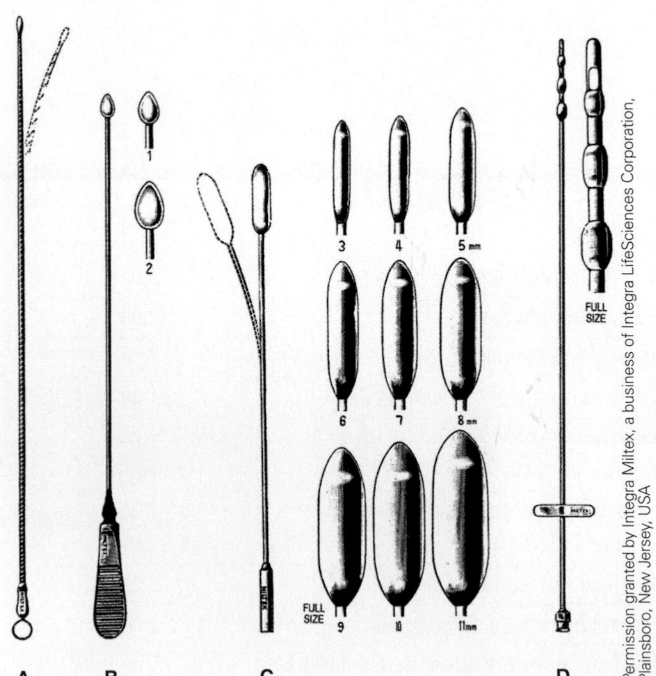

Permission granted by Integra Miltex, a business of Integra LifeSciences Corporation, Plainsboro, New Jersey, USA

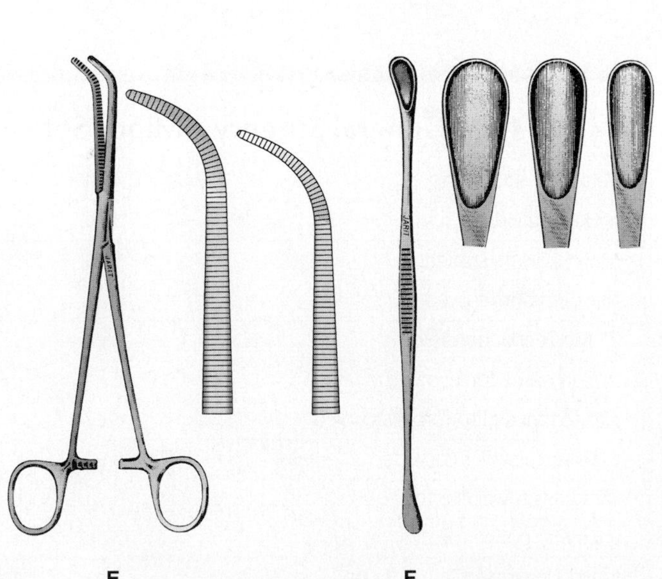

Courtesy of Jarit Surgical Instruments

Figure 14-3 Gallbladder instruments: (A) Ochsner (Fenger) gall duct probe, (B) Mayo common duct probe, (C) Bakes common duct dilator set, (D) Mixter irrigating dilaprobe, (E) Desjardin gallstone forceps, (F) Ferguson gallstone scoops

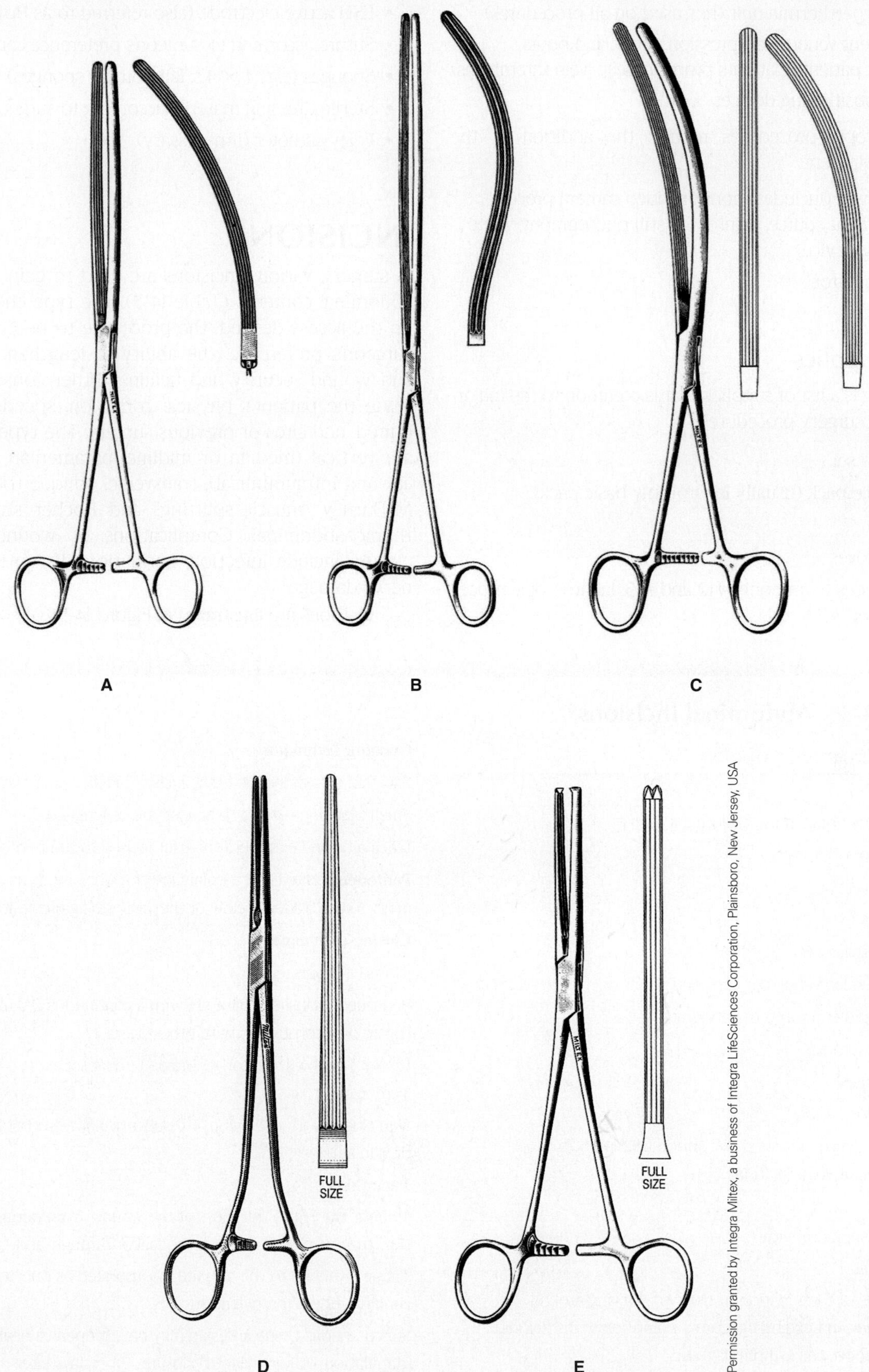

Figure 14-4 Intestinal instruments: (A) Doyen forceps, (B) Kocher forceps, (C) Mayo-Robson forceps, (D) Dennis clamp, (E) Allen clamp

- Hypo-/hyperthermia unit (not used on all procedures)
- Intermittent venous compression device and boots (bariatric patients; patients prone to deep-vein thrombosis)
- Patient positioning devices

Laparoscopic procedures require the addition of the following equipment:

- Video tower (includes monitor, video camera processing unit, light source, printer for still photography, video recording device)
- "Slave" monitor
- Insufflator

Routine Supplies

The following is a list of supplies that is common to the majority of general surgery procedures:

- Skin prep set
- Back table pack (usually laparotomy basic pack)
- Basin set
- Sterile gloves
- Knife blades (commonly #10 and #15; laparoscopic procedures need #11)
- ESU active electrode (also referred to as Bovie pencil)
- Suture according to surgeon's preference card
- Sponges (e.g., 4 × 4's; laparotomy sponges)
- Sterile dressing material according to surgeon's preference
- Foley catheter (if necessary)

INCISIONS

In surgery, various incisions are used to gain access to the abdominal contents (Table 14-3). The type chosen depends on the access desired, the procedure to be performed, the surgeon's preference, the ability to lengthen the **incision**, and wound security and healing. Other considerations include the patient's physical condition, speed of entry required, and sites of previous surgery. The types of incisions are vertical (median or midline, paramedian, supraumbilical, and infraumbilical), transverse, oblique (oblique lateral, McBurney "muscle-splitting," and Kocher subcostal), and thoracoabdominal. Complications of wounds and their closure include infection, herniation, disruption, pain, and nerve damage.

Incisions are illustrated in Figure 14-5.

Table 14-3 Abdominal Incisions

Vertical Incision—Median

Use
Access to any organ in the abdominal cavity
Ventral herniorrhaphy
Trauma
Advantages
Provides good access
Can be extended caudad or cephalad
Provides rapid entry into the abdomen
Least hemorrhagic
Disadvantages
Wide scar formation
Highest incidence of wound disruption (dehiscence) and postoperative herniation
Types
Epigastric (supraumbilical)
Subumbilical
Full midline—a combination of the two, curving around the umbilicus and extending from a point below the xiphoid to a point above the symphysis pubis
Opening Technique
Skin and subcutaneous tissue incised in a line over the linea alba
Small bleeding vessels, "bleeders," are coagulated
Linea alba and extraperitoneal fat incised to the peritoneum
Peritoneum entered at a point closest to the umbilicus to avoid injury to the bladder below or the falciform ligament above
Closing Technique
Closed in layers
Peritoneum closed separately with a continuous 2-0 absorbable suture or incorporated with other layers
Fascia closed with #0 or #1 braided nonabsorbable sutures placed 1 cm apart
Skin closed with 4-0 nylon, 4-0 subcuticular absorbable sutures, or skin staples
Variations
Trauma: the entire thickness of the wound, from peritoneum to skin, may be closed in one layer, called "through-and-through"
Tissue layers up to the skin are incorporated as one layer, using running #2 polypropylene sutures
Subcutaneous tissue and skin may be left open to heal by granulation, or for "delayed" closure 3 to 5 days later

Table 14-3 (continued)

Vertical Incision—Paramedian

Use
Same as median except for trauma
Lower left excellent for sigmoid surgery
Advantages
Better wound strength than median
Better cosmesis
Lower incidence of incisional herniation
Disadvantages
Increased intraoperative bleeding
Increased infection rates
Greater postoperative pain
Nerve damage
Atrophy of the rectus abdominus muscle
Types
Upper (may require an oblique extension toward the xiphoid)
Lower
Lateral (junction of the middle and outer thirds of the rectus sheath)
Opening Technique
Skin and subcutaneous tissue incised to the anterior rectus sheath
Anterior rectus dissected away from the muscle
Rectus muscle retracted laterally
Posterior rectus sheath and peritoneum are incised in the same plane as the anterior sheath
Closing Technique
Peritoneum and posterior rectus sheath are closed as one layer, 2-0 or 0 absorbable suture
Anterior sheath closed, 0 absorbable or nonabsorbable
Subcutaneous tissue may be approximated with interrupted 3-0 catgut or similar suture
Skin closed as in median incision

Oblique Incision—General Features

Use
Access to specific structures, especially those located laterally in the abdominal cavity
Advantages
Access to specific organ(s)
Strong closure
Disadvantages
Hemorrhagic
Muscle splitting
May endanger nerves
Types
Subcostal (Kocher)
McBurney's
Lateral

Oblique Incision—McBurney's

Use
Access to the appendix and extraperitoneal drainage of an abscess
Opening Technique
Obliquely downward and inward over "McBurney's point," the junction of the middle and outer third of the line that joins the umbilicus and the anterior superior iliac spine
External oblique muscle is divided in the direction of its fibers
Small incision is made in the underlying internal oblique adjacent to the rectus sheath
The opening is then spread with the tips of scissors until it is big enough to allow two fingers to be placed within
Small retractors (e.g., U.S. Army or small Richardson) are then placed to retract the muscle and expose the peritoneum
Peritoneum is grasped with forceps, incised, and the resultant hole is spread with the index finger, creating a circular opening
Note: A variation of this incision is the Rocky-Davis incision, which encounters the same abdominal structures, but runs more transversely.
Note: If further surgery (e.g., colon resection) is needed, the entire incision can be extended in either a medial or lateral direction.
Closing Technique
Begins with a "pursestring" closure of the peritoneum, or by incorporating the peritoneum with the transversalis fascia in a running closure with 2-0 absorbable suture
Transverse abdominis and internal oblique may be approximated with two or three interrupted 2-0 absorbable sutures
External oblique approximated with 2-0 absorbable or polypropylene sutures
Subcutaneous tissues may be closed with interrupted 3-0 or 4-0 absorbable sutures
Skin is closed with a subcuticular 4-0 suture or skin staples

(continues)

Table 14-3 (continued)

Oblique Incision—Kocher Subcostal

Use

Biliary tract (right) and spleen (left)

Opening Technique

Incision begins at the midline 2.5–5 cm below the xiphoid and extends obliquely lateral about 12 cm, staying 2.5 cm below the costal margin

Rectus sheath and muscle are divided electrosurgically

Underlying lateral musculature is incised in an outward direction for a short distance and retracted to expose the peritoneum

The small eighth dorsal nerve may be divided; however, the ninth dorsal nerve must be preserved to prevent subsequent weakening of the abdominal musculature

Peritoneum is incised the length of the incision

Closing Technique

Peritoneum and fascia closed with 0 synthetic absorbable or nonabsorbable suture

Subcutaneous tissue may be approximated with 2-0 absorbable suture

Skin is closed with interrupted 4-0 nylon subcuticularly, or with staples

Transverse Incision

Use

Curved transverse upper abdominal incision is used for access to the pancreas and abdominal exploration in cases of blunt trauma

Lower transverse incision used for access to pelvic **viscera**

Advantages

Access to specific organ(s)

Strong closure

Disadvantages

Hemorrhagic

Muscle splitting

May endanger nerves

Types

Upper transverse (a bilateral subcostal incision that is joined through the midline)

Lower transverse (Pfannenstiel, Maylard, and Cherney; see Chapter 15)

Opening Technique

Upper transverse: incised bilaterally as described in the subcostal incision, and joined at the midline

Lower transverse: see Chapter 15

Closing Technique

Peritoneum and fascia closed with 0 absorbable or nonabsorbable suture

Subcutaneous tissue may be approximated with a 2-0 absorbable suture

Skin closed with interrupted or running 4-0 nylon suture, subcuticularly or with staples

Thoracoabdominal

Use

Converts the pleural and peritoneal spaces into one cavity, and is used when particular access is required for extensive esophagogastric surgery (left) or emergency hepatic resection (right)

Advantages

Access to specific organ(s)

Access to both pleural and peritoneal spaces

Disadvantages

Difficult patient positioning

Hemorrhagic

Same as median

Same as thoracic (requires chest tube)

Difficult for patient postoperatively

Opening Technique

Incision begins as a standard midline or left upper paramedian incision

Extended obliquely over the thorax along the eighth costal interspace

Diaphragm is divided radially toward the esophageal hiatus for as far as necessary

Closing Technique

Begins with repair of the diaphragm with #1 silk

A chest tube is placed through a stab wound in the ninth intercostal space along the posterior axillary line

Standard closure of the chest

Standard median or paramedian closure

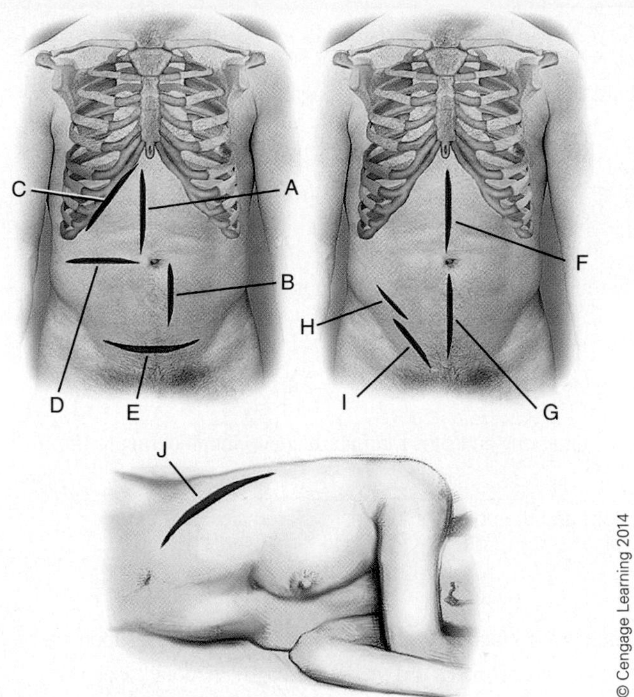

Figure 14-5 Abdominal incision options: (A) Right upper paramedian, (B) left lower paramedian, (C) right subcostal, (D) right midline transverse, (E) Pfannenstiel, (F) upper longitudinal midline, (G) lower longitudinal midline, (H) McBurney's, (I) right inguinal oblique, (J) right thoracoabdominal

HERNIAS

A hernia (Latin for "rupture") is defined as a protrusion of a viscus through an opening in the wall of the cavity in which it is contained. The hernial orifice is the defect in the abdominal wall and the hernia sac is the outpouching of the peritoneum. A hernia is termed external if it protrudes through the abdominal wall, interparietal if the sac is contained within the abdominal wall, and internal if the hernia is within the visceral cavity. A hernia may be congenital, acquired, or a combination thereof.

The anatomical features of the abdomen and the various types of pathology result in several different but recognizable types of hernia. These are summarized in Table 14-4.

Indirect, direct, and femoral distinctions are illustrated in Figure 14-6.

Hernia Repair

All hernia repairs have some common goals, and the procedures have some common features, also. These are listed in Table 14-5.

The classic procedures that remain in current use are:

Bassini or Bassini-Shouldice repair—A new inguinal canal is made by uniting the edge of the internal oblique muscle to the inguinal ligament.

McVay (Cooper ligament) repair—The transversus abdominis muscle and its associated fasciae (transversus layer) are sutured to Cooper's ligament (see Cooper's ligament repair).

Endoscopic approaches are increasingly common today. These approaches typically place a synthetic mesh over the defect. The mesh may or may not be sutured or stapled in place. Figure 14-7 illustrates this technique with a mesh repair of the defect. The following lists the surgical steps for a laparoscopic herniorraphy using the totally extraperitoneal patch (TEP) repair.

Table 14-4 Hernia Types

Category	*Features: Anatomical Location*
Groin	Hernias of the inguinal and femoral areas
	Inguinal: above the abdominocrural crease (>95% male)—direct or indirect
	Femoral: below the abdominocrural crease (97% female)
Ventral	Present on the anterior abdominal wall at any point other than the groin
	May present along the linea alba (epigastric, umbilical, and hypogastric) or at the semilunar lines (Spigelian hernia)
Incisional	Hernias at sites of previous surgery and at stomal sites
Diaphragmatic	Hernias in the diaphragm, usually at the esophageal hiatus
Type	*Features: Condition*
Reducible	Manual manipulation can return the hernia contents to the abdominal cavity
Irreducible or incarcerated	Manual manipulation cannot return the hernia contents to the abdominal cavity
Strangulated	Hernia with luminal viscera entrapment that compromises the vascularity of the viscera

Table 14-4 (continued)

Richter's	Incarcerated or strangulated bowel spontaneously reduces and the subsequent gangrenous portion of bowel may be overlooked during hernia repair
Sliding	The abdominal viscera forms part of the hernia sac
Direct	Inguinal hernia
	Acquired type
	Presents within Hesselbach's triangle (bounded by the inguinal ligament, the inferior epigastric vessels, and the lateral border of the rectus abdominis)
Indirect	Inguinal hernia
	Congenital type
	Follows congenital defects that dilate the internal inguinal ring and pass through the deep inguinal ring to the scrotum
	Hernia sac is generally confined to the spermatic cord and the posterior inguinal wall remains intact
Pantaloon	Both direct and indirect hernias are present
Femoral	More common in females than males
	The fossa ovalis is the passageway of the iliopsoas muscle and blood vessels, nerves, and lymphatics that supply the lower extremity. The femoral sheath is divided into three compartments and the smallest is the femoral canal. The iliopubic tract, connected to the transversalis fascia, is the medial border of the canal; Cooper's ligament and the femoral vein form the other borders. The hernia sac originates from the femoral canal through a defect in the medial femoral sheath and emerges through the fossa ovalis of the pelvis into the subcutaneous tissues of the thigh, inferior to the inguinal ligament. The lymph nodes in this area are commonly caught in the hernia sac, forming a palpable mass
	Prone to incarceration and strangulation
Epigastric	Midline hernias above the umbilicus
Hypogastric	Midline hernias below the umbilicus
Umbilical	In children: usually congenital; often spontaneously close
	In adults: usually acquired
	Hernia consists of a peritoneal sac (or sacs) and omentum or abdominal viscera contents protruding through the umbilical ring

Procedure 14-1 Laparotomy

A surgical opening through the skin layer and abdominal wall into the peritoneal cavity is called a laparotomy. Many surgical procedures, such as bowel procedures, begin with a laparotomy, or if the surgeon is not completely sure of a diagnosis the procedure can be listed on the surgery schedule as an exploratory laparotomy. As an aid in understanding other open procedures of the peritoneal cavity and to prevent having to repeat the steps of a laparotomy, the following is an outline of the procedural steps for laparotomy opening and closure.

Anatomy and Pathology

Layers of the abdominal wall:

- Subcutaneous fat
- Scarpa's fascia
- External oblique muscle
- Internal oblique muscle
- Transversus abdominus muscle
- Transversalis fascia
- Peritoneum

Pathology according to procedure to be performed

Equipment and Instrument Sets Unique to Procedure

- Major laparotomy set

PROCEDURE 14-1 (continued)

Supplies Unique to Procedure	• Laparotomy back table pack
Preoperative Preparation	• Supine position • General anesthesia • Skin prep: mid-chest to symphysis pubis and laterally as far as possible; may be extended to mid-thigh for extensive procedures • Foley catheter (if necessary) • Abdominal draping procedure
Practical Considerations	• Have Yankauer and Poole suction tips available. When using the Poole suction tip within the abdominal cavity, the surgeon may want to wrap a wet lap sponge around the tip to prevent tissue attaching to the tip and being damaged. • Depending on the procedure, the surgeon may irrigate the abdominal cavity with an antibiotic solution that is mixed by the surgical technologist at the back table in a graduated pitcher. • A variety of retractors will be needed (e.g., handheld and self-retaining).

Opening

1. Midline skin incision is made and extended around the umbilicus.

   Procedural Consideration: Place two lap sponges on each side of the incision. Skin knife used. Have ESU pencil and forceps ready.

2. The incision is deepened.

   Procedural Consideration: Deep knife used. As the surgeon goes deeper into the abdominal cavity, the larger, deeper retractors will be used.

3. Bleeding vessels are clamped with small hemostats and either ligated with nonabsorbable ties or cauterized.

   Procedural Consideration: Keep ESU cautery blade clean using scratch pad or if using Teflon cautery tip wipe clean with a sponge.

4. Using curved Mayo scissors, electrosurgery, or scalpel, the external oblique muscle is opened the length of the skin incision. This is referred to as a muscle splitting incision because the incision is in the direction of the muscle fibers. Bleeding vessels are controlled through methods listed in #3.

   Procedural Consideration: Keep clean lap sponges on the field.

5. Medium retractors are placed to retract the external oblique muscle.

   Procedural Consideration: Richardson retractors are often used.

Opening

6. The internal oblique muscle, transverse muscle, and transversalis fascia are split in the direction of the muscles fibers up to the rectus sheath using a scalpel or curved Mayo scissors. The medium retractors are replaced with large Richardson retractors that have longer blades in order to retract the internal oblique and transverse muscle.

7. The peritoneum is now exposed. A small incision is made in the peritoneum using the smooth forceps to grasp the peritoneum to elevate to prevent the underlying bowel from being injured, and the scalpel.

   Procedural Consideration: Surgeon may prefer using a small hemostat to elevate the peritoneum.

8. If abnormal fluid is encountered, sponges and suction are used as needed. Cultures will also be taken at this time if necessary.

   Procedural Consideration: Instruments and suctions tips that come into contact with the infectious fluid are considered contaminated and should not be used when the wound is being closed.

9. The edges of the peritoneum and transversalis fascia are grasped with a Kocher on each lateral edge and slight traction is placed on the Kochers laterally.

10. Using Metzenbaum scissors, curved Mayo scissors, or scalpel, the peritoneal incision is lengthened. The surgeon may insert the index and middle finger beneath

(continues)

Procedure 14-1 (continued)

Opening

the peritoneum to aid in elevating it and carefully cut the tissue between the two fingers in the direction of the pelvis.

11. Be prepared to encounter one or two blood vessels in the fatty layer between the fascia and peritoneum in the region of the umbilicus. These vessel(s) will need to be quickly clamped and ligated.

    Procedural Consideration: Surgeon may use ties or cautery.

12. The Richardson retractors are repositioned to allow the surgeon to conduct an initial exploration of the abdominal cavity.

13. Once the affected and nonaffected organs have been identified, and anatomical landmarks are also identified, the Richardson retractors will be replaced with a large self-retaining retractor such as the Balfour or Bookwalter.

Closure

1. The peritoneum may be closed separately or as a single unit with the internal oblique fascia.

   Procedural Consideration: Sponge, sharp, and instrument counts must be completed before the abdominal cavity is closed.

   a. Peritoneum closed separately: Edges of transversalis fascia grasped with toothed forceps to expose the peritoneum. The edges of the peritoneum are grasped with clamps and the clamps are crossed to bring the edges together. The peritoneum may be closed with synthetic absorbable suture in continuous fashion or interrupted nonabsorbable sutures. A medium-width malleable (ribbon) retractor may be placed under the peritoneal layer to keep the underlying organs pushed away from the suture line to avoid being sutured to the peritoneum. The internal oblique fascia is then closed with absorbable or nonabsorbable sutures in continuous or interrupted fashion.

   b. Single-unit closure: The peritoneum and internal oblique fascia are closed together as a single unit. A heavy looped synthetic absorbable or nonabsorbable suture is used, #0 or #1 size; it is usually placed in continuous fashion.

2. The muscle tissue may or may not be sutured. Because the incision is in the direction of the muscle fibers, the edges approximate in a natural fashion.

3. The external oblique fascia and Scarpa's fascia are separately closed with a few interrupted 3-0 absorbable sutures. Some surgeons may not close Scarpa's fascia and proceed directly to the skin. However, other surgeons are of the opinion that closure of Scarpa's fascia lessens the incidence of dead space in the subcuticular layer.

   Procedural Consideration: Use of retractors is easy to remember because it is opposite of the order used when opening the abdomen. As the surgeon closes a layer, the wound cavity becomes shallower; therefore, deeper retractors are replaced with smaller retractors.

4. A few 3-0 or 4-0 absorbable sutures are placed in interrupted fashion to close the subcuticular layer.

5. The skin is closed in one of the following three most frequently employed methods:

   Procedural Consideration: Last count must be completed before the skin closure is completed.

   a. Skin edges are grasped on both sides with toothed forceps, preferably Adsons. The skin edges are brought together and approximated with interrupted 3-0 or 4-0 silk or nylon on a cutting needle.

   b. Subcuticular closure is achieved using interrupted or continuous 3-0, 4-0, or 5-0 synthetic absorbable or nonabsorbable sutures.

   c. Skin staples are often used to approximate the skin edges. The skin edges are grasped and everted using the toothed Adsons. The skin staples are then placed.

Postoperative Considerations

According to the procedure that was performed.

Procedure 14-2 McVay (Cooper Ligament) Inguinal Herniorraphy

Surgical Anatomy and Pathology	In order of descent:
	• Skin and subcutaneous tissues
	• Scarpa's fascia: membranous sheet attached to iliac crest, linea alba, pubis
	• Innominate fascia: separates aponeurosis of external oblique muscle from overlying tissues and contains the intercrural fibers
	• External oblique muscle
	• Inguinal (Poupart) ligament
	• Interparietal fascia: located between external and internal oblique muscles, and between internal and transverse abdominis muscles; zone for interparietal herniation
	• Internal oblique muscle
	• Transverse abdominis muscle
	• Transversalis fascia: separates abdominal musculature from preperitoneal fat; continuation of fascia containing the abdominal cavity
	• Cooper's ligament: periosteum of the pubis
	• Rectus abdominis muscle
	• Peritoneum
	• Other associated anatomical structures
	  • Inguinal canal: Consists of internal and deep inguinal rings. Internal inguinal ring is located superolateral to the pubic tubercle, and deep inguinal ring is located halfway between symphysis pubis and iliac spine along the abdominocrural crease. The canal is located in oblique fashion medial from the internal ring to the external ring and contains the spermatic cord and vessels.
	  • Epigastric vessels
	  • Iliofemoral vessels
	  • Spermatic cord
	  • Iliohypogastric and ilioinguinal nerves
	  • Cremaster muscle
	• The transversalis fascia is main focus of inguinal herniation; it is inherently weak and the hernia occurs through a tear in the fascia

Preoperative Diagnostic Tests and Procedures	• History and physical exam
	  • Obvious inguinal hernia observed as bulge in inguinal region
	  • Scrotal digital exam to feel for hernia pathway; may have patient cough while standing to increase abdominal pressure

Equipment and Instrument Sets Unique to Procedure	• Bowel clamps (available) • GI stapling devices (available)
Supplies Unique to Procedure	• ½″ or 1″ Penrose drain • Synthetic mesh (available) • Suture or staples for mesh (available) • Aerobic and anaerobic cultures
Preoperative Preparation	• Supine position • General, spinal, epidural, or local anesthesia • Skin prep: Lower right or left quadrant; umbilicus down to the symphysis pubis and laterally as far as possible • Draping: Square off with four towels using skin prep anatomical points of reference; laparotomy drape
Practical Considerations	• Anticipate use of mesh requiring additional sutures. • Anticipate strangulated inguinal hernia that requires cultures and bowel resection.

(continues)

Procedure 14-2 (continued)

Surgical Procedure

1. An oblique or transverse incision is made using the #10 knife blade. The incision is carried deeper through the superficial fascia and Scarpa's fascia using the knife, Metzenbaum scissors, and electrosurgery. Hemostats are placed on the edges of the fascia for retraction purposes.

   Procedural Consideration: The surgical technologist may place tension on the skin to facilitate the skin incision.

2. The external oblique aponeurosis is opened by making a small incision with the knife over the inguinal canal. The iliohypogastric and ilioinguinal nerves are identified and preserved.

   Procedural Consideration: The surgical technologist should have a number of curved hemstats available for placement on the edges of the fascia.

3. The cremaster muscle is incised or separated in the direction of its fibers to expose the spermatic cord.

4. The cord is bluntly and sharply dissected free from surrounding tissues in a circumferential manner. A saline-moistened Penrose drain is placed around the cord and a clamp placed on the ends; the drain is used to gently retract the cord. The area next to the cord is then examined to confirm the presence of an indirect hernia.

   Procedural Consideration: A Penrose drain should be placed in a small basin with saline. When the spermatic cord is dissected free, it should be handed to the surgeon with a curved hemostat attached to one end to facilitate placing the drain aroud the cord. The surgeon may request the surgical technologist to attach the clamp to the drapes to facilitate puttig gentle retraction on the drain.

5. The indirect hernia sac is dissected away from the cord using blunt and sharp dissection down to the neck of the hernia sac. The sac is opened and the surgeon pushes the contents of the sac back into the abdominal cavity with his or her finger(s) or a 4 × 4 sponge stick; the sponge should be moistened with saline if used.

6. A pursestring suture technique is used to place the suture around the neck of the sac and the sac is excised. As the suture is tightened, the sponge stick will be removed.

   Procedural Consideration: Once the hernia sac is excised and the repair begins, the surgical technologist should have 4–5 suture packets on the sterile field for use; depending on the size of the repair the surgical technologist may need to request the circulator to open additional sutures.

7. Repair of the transversalis fascia now begins; the transversalis fascia is either sutured to Cooper's ligament, or if the defect is large, mesh is sutured in place. The surgeon begins suturing at the pubic tubercle in an interrupted fashion and continues in a lateral direction suturing the transversalis fascia to Cooper's ligament up to the femoral sheath and the repair is then continued laterally, suturing the fascia to the inguinal ligament.

8. Once the transversalis fascia is sutured to Cooper's ligament, a relaxing incision is made in the rectus sheath, using a #15 knife blade to relieve excess tissue tension.

   Procedural Consideration: The surgical technologist should have the #15 knife blade loaded ahead of time for the surgeon to use for the relaxing incision.

9. If mesh is used, it is sutured in place. The surgeon will size the mesh according to the size of the inguinal floor canal. The mesh will be sutured or stapled into place. One edge of the mesh is sutured to the inguinal ligament, the other edge is sutured to the conjoined tendon, and the lateral edge is cut into tails to be placed around the spermatic cord and sutured into place.

Procedure 14-2 (continued)

Procedural Consideration: If the mesh is going to be used, the surgical technologist requests that the circulator open the package containing the mesh. In some instances, the package may come with suture. The surgical technologist provides the mesh to the surgeon for sizing. Since mesh cannot be resterilized and is expensive, it should not be opened unless the surgeon requests the use of the mesh.

10. The surgeon examines the repair; if the patient is awake the surgeon may request that he or she cough 2–3 times as a test of the repair. The cremaster muscle is now sutured around the spermatic cord. The wound is closed in layers: external oblique aponeurosis, Scarpa, fascia and skin.

Postoperative Considerations	**Immediate Postoperative Care**	**Prognosis**	**Wound Classification**
	• Transport to PACU. • Instruct patient not to strain (increases intraabdominal pressure).	• No complications: return to normal activities in 6–8 weeks. • Complications: hernia recurrence; nerve injury; postoperative SSI.	• Class I: Clean, or • Class III: Contaminated (strangulated bowel)

Procedure 14-3 TEP Hernia Repair

Surgical Anatomy and Pathology; Preoperative Diagnostic Tests and Procedures	• Same as for open prodedure		
Equipment and Instrument Sets	• See previous list of laparoscopic equipment and instrumentation	• 30° laparoscope • Laparoscopic stapling device	
Supplies Unique to Procedure	• Dissecting balloon	• Polypropylene mesh and suture	• Loop ligature
Preoperative Preparation	• Position and anesthesia same as for open procedure • Skin Prep: Wide abdominal prep; anatomical points of	reference: mid-chest to symphysis pubis and laterally as far as possible • Draping: Square off with four towels using skin prep anatomical	points of reference; abdominal laparoscopy drape (some health care facilities may have a specialty laparoscopic hernia drape available)

(continues)

PROCEDURE 14-3 (continued)

Practical Considerations

- Surgical technologist must know how to set up all of the laparoscopic equipment and instruments, e.g., trocars and trocar sheaths, Verres needle, connecting insufflation tubing, connecting cautery to laparoscopic instruments, connecting camera to laparoscope, connecting light source cord to laparoscope, loading laparoscopic staplers and needle holders.
- Surgcial technologist may be responsible for "running" the camera and holding instruments in place; therefore he or she must learn how to "triangulate"—looking at the video monitor while moving the camera and holding instruments.
- Surgical technologist may also be responsible for assisting the surgeon by inserting laparoscopic instruments into the trocar sheath.

Surgical Procedure

(Procedural Considerations are the same as the Practical Considerations)

1. Infraumbilical incision is made using a #15 knife blade.
2. Anterior rectus sheath is incised and ipsilateral rectus abdominis muscle retracted laterally.
3. Blunt dissection is used to create a space beneath the rectus abdominis muscle.
4. Dissection balloon is inserted and placed on the anterior surface of the posterior rectus sheath. The balloon dissector is moved forward creating a tunnel to the pubic symphysis in the preperitoneal space where the balloon is inflated creating a cavity. The balloon is removed and a blunt-tip trocar is inserted to take the place of the balloon.

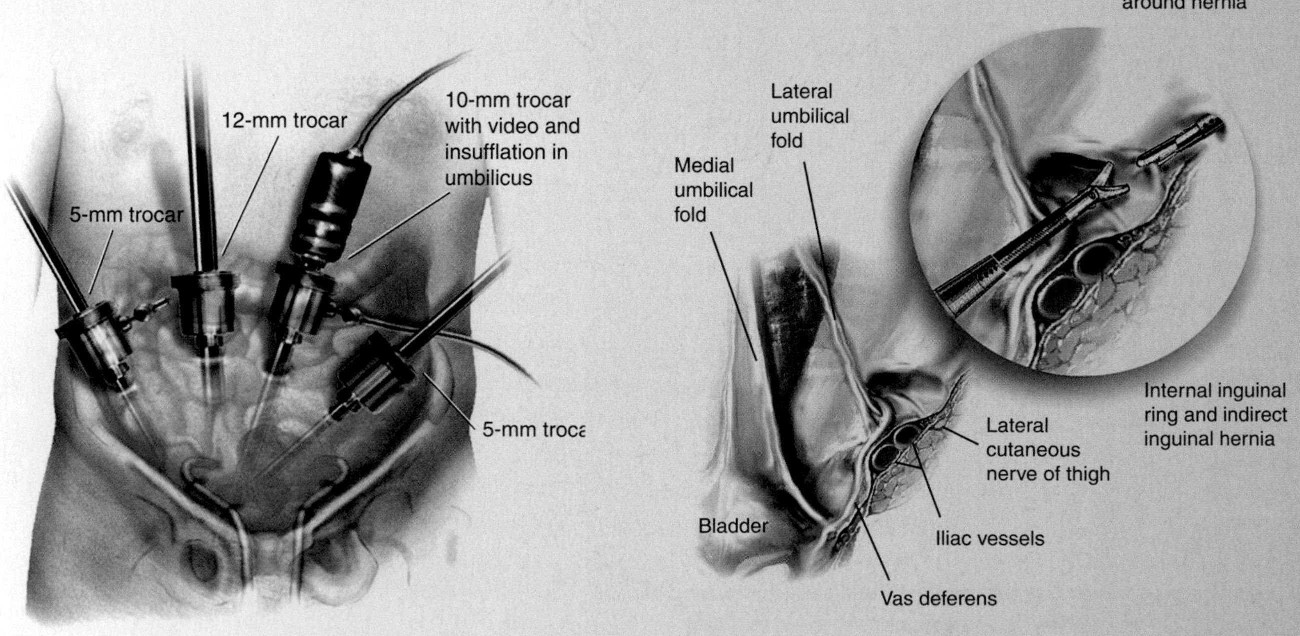

Figure 14-7 Endoscopic herniorrhaphy: (A) Trocar positions, (B) peritoneal incision at internal ring

PROCEDURE 14-3 (continued)

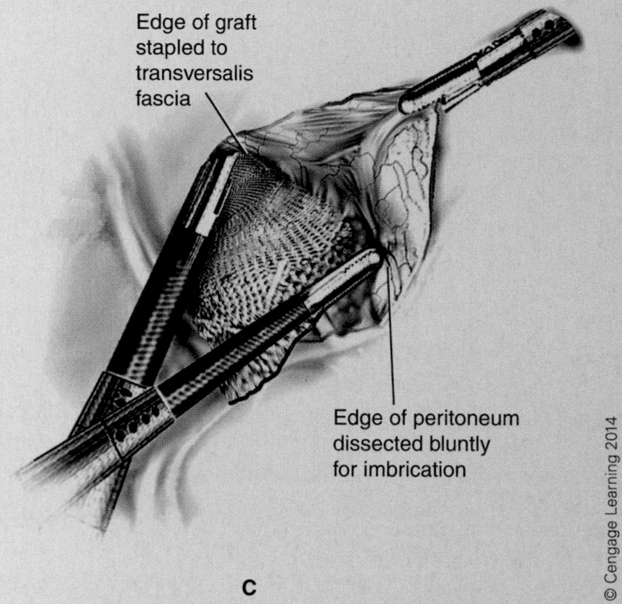

Figure 14-7 Endoscopic herniorrhaphy: (C) application of polypropylene mesh

5. The preperitoneal space is insufflated and additional trocars inserted. A 30° laparoscope is used to perform the surgical procedure (Figure 14-7A).
6. The inferior epigastric vessels are identified and retracted anteriorly.
7. Cooper's ligament is identified and dissected free from the pubic symphysis medially to the level of the external iliac vein.
8. The iliopubic tract is identified as well as the genitofemoral and lateral femoral cutaneous nerves in order to avoid injuring the nerves.
9. Lateral dissection is completed to the anterior iliac spine and the spermatic cord is dissected free (Figure 14-7B).
10. A direct hernia sac will be reduced by traction. A small indirect hernia sac is freed from the spermatic cord and reduced into the peritoneal cavity. Large indirect hernia sacs are divided with cautery near the internal inguinal ring. The proximal peritoneal sac is closed with a loop ligature.
11. Upon reduction of the hernia, a polypropylene mesh is inserted through the trocar and unfolded to cover the direct, indirect, and femoral spaces as well as the spermatic cord. The mesh is secured in place with a tacking stapler (Figure 14-7C).
12. The balloon, laparoscope, and trocars are removed; skin incisions may be closed with suture and/or skin closure strips.

Postoperative Considerations

Immediate Postoperative Care

- Transport to PACU.
- Instruct patient not to strain.

Prognosis

- No complications: Discharged same day of surgery; return to normal activities in 2–4 weeks.
- Complications: hernia recurrence; nerve injury; fluid build-up at site of mesh; postoperative SSI.

Wound Classification

- Class 1: Clean

Procedure 14-4 Ventral (Incisional) Herniorrhaphy

Surgical Anatomy and Pathology	• Anatomy depends on location of the ventral hernia. Postoperative ventral hernias, referred to as incisional hernias, usually occur when a vertical midline incision has been used; refer to the Laparotomy procedure for the abdominal anatomy • Ventral hernia is a weakened area that occurs near or directly aloing a primary abdominal incision, allowing the internal abdominal organs to protrude through the hernial defect, identified by a bulge in the abdomen
Preoperative Diagnostic Tests and Procedures	• Diagnosis primarily obtained by history and physical
Equipment, Instruments and Supplies Unique to Procedure	• Laparoscopic equipment, instruments, and supplies same as for laparoscopic inguinal herniorraphy • Need #10 knife blade and Allis clamps for removal of old scar incision
Preoperative Preparation	• Same as for laparoscopic inguinal herniorraphy
Practical Considerations	• Same as for laparoscopic inguinal herniorraphy
Surgical Procedure	1. The old abdominal scar incision is removed with a #10 knife blade. **Procedural Consideration:** An Allis clamp will be placed on the end of the scar tissue; the surgical technologist should place gentle traction and hold up the tissue while following the surgeon as he or she removes the tissue. This is a surgical specimen.
	2. The Verres needle is placed and the abdomen insufflated.
	3. The three trocars are placed lateral to the incision; the middle trocar is for the laparoscope and other two are for instrumentation.
	4. An atraumatic laparoscopic curved clamp is used to pull the internal abdominal contents such as the omentum from the hernia site and back into normal anatomical position.
	5. With the use of cautery or Harmonic scalpel, adhesions are lysed.
	6. A spinal is placed through the skin and visualized with the laparoscope to aid in measure the size of the defect, and therefore, the size of mesh that is required. The mesh is cut to size so that it is several centimeters larger than the defect. The surgeon uses a marking pen to mark the correct side of the mesh as well as placing non-absorbable monofilament sutures in the corners of the mesh to serve as markers for the correct placement of the mesh over the defect. **Procedural Consideration:** The surgical technologist must confirm prior to the procedure that a large size of mesh is available for the procedure.

Procedure 14-4 (continued)

7. The mesh is placed into the abdomen through the trocar and positioned over the defect.

   Procedural Considerations: The surgical technologist should hand the mesh to the surgeon or place into the trocar rolled up.

8. A suture passer/retriever is inserted and used to grasp the corner sutures; they are brought out and tied at the skin level. The mesh is secured to the anterior abdominal wall with the use of mattress sutures that were placed through separate incision sites. The number of sutures depends on the size of the hernia defect; the sutures are placed at the corners and middle of the sides of the mesh.

9. Tacking staples are placed in-between the sutures to further secure the mesh and prevent abdominal tissue from protruding underneath.

Postoperative Considerations

Immediate Postoperative Care

- Transport to PACU.
- Instruct patient not to strain.

Prognosis

- No complications: Discharged same day of surgery; return to normal activities in 2–4 weeks.
- Complications: hernia recurrence; nerve injury; fluid build-up at site of mesh; postoperative SSI.

Wound Classification

- Class 1: Clean

Procedures 14-5 Umbilical Herniorraphy

Surgical Anatomy and Pathology	• Umbilicus is formed by the umbilical ring of the linea alba. • Ligamentum teres (round ligament) and paraumbilical veins join superiorly at the umbilicus and the obliterated urachus (umbilical ligament) enters the umbilicus inferiorly.	• Umbilical hernias in infants are congenital and usually close spontaneously. If the hernia is present after the age of 5 it is often surgically treated.
Preoperative Diagnostic Tests and Procedures	• History and physical confirms the presence of the hernia.	
Equipment and Instrument Sets Unique to Procedure	• Minor instrument set.	• Radiant overhead heater for patients 2 years and younger.
Supplies Unique to Procedure	• Synthetic mesh (available).	• Suture for mesh (available).

(continues)

Procedures 14-5 (continued)

Preoperative Preparation

- Supine position
- General anesthesia
- Skin prep: mid-chest to symphysis pubis and laterally as far as possible
- Draping: Square off with four towels around infraumbilical incision site; pediatric laparotomy drape

Practical Considerations

- Umbilical herniorraphy is often a same-day surgery procedure.
- Several surgical approaches are used; the infraumbilical incision is the most common.

Surgical Procedure

1. Infraumbilical incision is made with a #15 knife blade.
2. Senn retractors (or small retractors of surgeon's preference) are used to retract the skin and subcutaneous tissue to visualize the rectus fascia and hernia defect.
3. The hernia sac is located between the rectus muscle sheaths at the midline and is bluntly dissected free.
4. Once dissected free, the hernia sac may be ligated or excised.

   Procedural Consideration: If excised, the hernia sac is a specimen.

   If ligated, a peanut sponge placed on the end of a mosquito clamp may be placed within the sac to gently push down the hernia sac contents while the surgeon places the suture. A Brown or Crile-Wood needle holder should be loaded with the suture.
5. The peritoneum is closed with a continuous suture technique.

   Procedural Consideration: The surgical technologist should always remember to follow the surgeon when the continuous technique is used in order to keep slight tension on the suture and keep it out of the way.
6. The rectus fascia is closed using interrupted suture technique using 3-0 or 4-0 nonabsorbable suture.
7. Continuous suture technique with a small-gauge absorbable suture is used to close the subcutaneous layer.
8. A small pressure dressing is placed.

Postoperative Considerations

Immediate Postoperative Care

- Transport to PACU.
- Patient carefully monitored while recovering from anesthesia, including ensuring dressing is not removed.
- Once the first set of vitals has been recorded indicating the patient is stable, the parent(s) are often allowed to come into the PACU.

Prognosis

- No complications: Discharged same day of surgery; return to normal activities in 2–4 weeks. Parent(s) will have received postoperative education, in particular to be alert for signs and symptoms of an SSI.
- Complications: hernia recurrence; hemorrhage; postoperative SSI.

Wound Classification

- Class 1: Clean

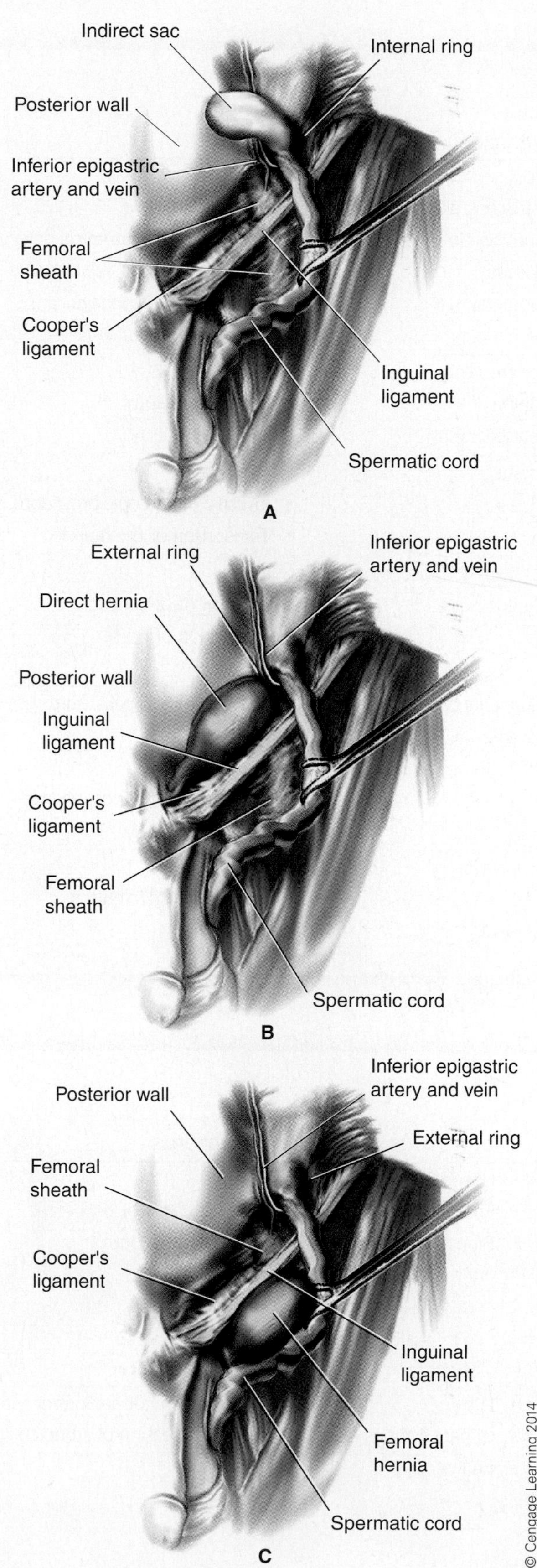

Figure 14-6 Hernia types: (A) Indirect inguinal, (B) direct inguinal, (C) femoral

SURGERY OF THE ALIMENTARY CANAL

Surgery on the digestive system constitutes the major portion of surgery performed by the general surgeon. Many of the procedures are variations on a common theme because of the tubular anatomical structure of the digestive tract. This section will look at surgery of the alimentary canal moving from cephalad to caudad.

ESOPHAGEAL PATHOLOGY

Pathological conditions of the esophagus fall into four major categories: hiatal hernia and reflux esophagitis, esophageal motility disorders, neoplasms, and trauma (Table 14-5).

LAPAROSCOPIC NISSEN FUNDOPLICATION

Laparoscopic Nissen fundoplication is a surgical procedure that is performed to correct a hiatal hernia. The laparoscopic approach has become the preferred operative procedure.

Pathological Conditions of the Stomach

The stomach is a common area for a number of pathologic conditions that eventually lead to surgery (Table 14-6).

GASTROSTOMY

A gastr**ostomy** is the surgical creation of an opening (fistula tract) from the gastric mucosa to the skin and is performed to provide nutrition "feeding" to the patient or to decompress and drain the stomach. A gastrostomy may be lined with mucosa for long-term or permanent usage, or serosa for temporary measures, depending on technique. Often tumors of the larynx, pharynx, esophagus, and proximal stomach, as well as esophageal stricture, dictate this need. Gastrostomy may be performed in conjuction with a gastrectomy. There are a variety of ways in which this fistula tract can be created, including

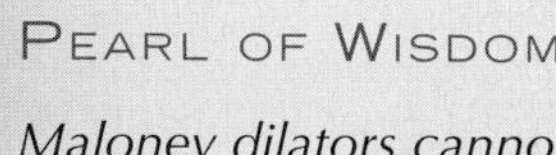

PEARL OF WISDOM

Maloney dilators cannot be inserted from the sterile field. They are passed down the esophagus by the anesthesia provider. Be sure everyone knows where the Maloney dilators are and remind team members when you are nearing the time of use.

TABLE 14-5 Pathology of the Esophagus

Condition	Symptoms/Signs	Diagnostics	Treatments
Hiatal hernia	• Acid reflux • Mucosal erosion, ulceration, scarring • Stricture • Burning, nonradiating pain • Pain is positional	• History • Fluoroscopy during barium swallow • Endoscopy • Manometry	Medical treatment Surgical • Correction of anatomical defect • Reconstruction of valve mechanism in lower esophagus
Motility disorders	• Dysphagia • Regurgitation of undigested food	• X-ray with contrast medium • Cineradiography	Medical • Usually unhelpful
Achalasia	• Weight loss • Pain is uncommon • Aspiration pneumonia	• Manometry	Surgical • Invasive endoscopic procedure • Transection of the muscle
Diverticula	• Regurgitation of recently swallowed material • Choking • Foul breath odor	• X-ray with contrast medium	Surgical • **Excision** of diverticula • Correction of cause
Neoplasm (benign tumors are rare)	• Asymptomatic early • Dysphagia • Weight loss • Pain	• Barium contrast studies • CT scan	May be limited to palliation • Radiotherapy • Tracheostomy • Extirpation of the esophagus • Reconstruction
Trauma	• Perforation (usually the result of instrumentation) • Ingestion of caustic substances	• Varies with type	Surgical • Immediate intervention

TABLE 14-6 Pathologic Conditions of the Stomach

Condition	Symptoms/Signs	Diagnostics	Treatments
Gastric ulcer disease	• Epigastric pain radiating to the back • Pain on ingestion of food • Weight loss	• Upper GI series • Endoscopy • Biopsy to rule out malignancy	Medical • Dietary control • Medication control • Antacids Surgical • Vagotomy • Excision of **ulcer**
Gastritis	• Diffuse erythema • Mucosal disruption • Nausea • Vomiting • Bleeding	• History • Upper GI series • Endoscopy	• Withdrawal of noxious agents • Decompression of stomach • Antacids • H_2 blockers

TABLE 14-6 (continued)

Condition	Symptoms/Signs	Diagnostics	Treatments
Gastric polyp (rare)	• Typically asymptomatic	• Endoscopy	• Biopsy • Conservative treatment related to histological findings
Bezoar (mass of indigestible vegetable fiber)	• Pain • Indigestion	• History • Endoscopy	• Endoscopic removal • Surgical removal
Carcinoma	• Asymptomatic early • Weight loss • Epigastric pain • Dysphagia • Hematemesis • Melena	• Laboratory studies • Upper GI • Endoscopy • Biopsy	• Surgical resection
Lymphoma, leiomyoma, leiomyosarcoma	• Same as above	• Same as above	• Same as above • Benign have good results • Malignant, very poor results

placement of synthetic tubes (Stamm or Witzel procedures), rolling the gastric tissues into a tube (Spivak-Watsuji gastrostomy), raising a flap of gastric tissue (Janeway gastrostomy), and utilizing a transected portion of the jejunum. A gastrostomy can be created by open, percutaneous, endoscopic, and laparoscopic means. The Stamm procedure is described. It is a temporary measure that can often be performed under local anesthesia (if not performed with a gastrectomy). It is quick, has the widest application, and is technically easy to perform, providing sufficient venting of the stomach.

PROCEDURE 14-6 Laparoscopic Nissen Fundoplication

Surgical Anatomy and Pathology (lower esophagus)	• Abdominal esophagus extends from the esophageal hiatus to the opening of the cardia of the stomach. • Abdominal esophagus lies in the esophageal groove on the posterior surface of the left lobe of the liver. • At the point where it joins the stomach is a layer of circular muscle fibers called the lower esophageal sphincter (LES), which contracts to close the opening to the stomach and prevent food and gastric juices from reentering the esophagus. • Hiatal hernia occurs when the esophageal hiatus is weak, which allows the abdominal esophagus and superior portion of the stomach to protrude into the thoracic cavity.
Preoperative Diagnostic Tests and Procedures	• See Table 14-6.
Equipment and Instruments Unique to Procedure	• Harmonic scalpel • Laparoscopic equipment • Insufflator • Laparoscopy instrumentation: • 0° and 30° laparoscopes • Liver retractor (fan retractor) • Coagulation hook • Grasping forceps • Laparoscopic ligating clip applier with various sizes of clips • Trocars: 10 mm × 3; 5 mm × 2 • Minor instrument set • Laparotomy instrument set (available for conversion from laparoscopic to open procedure)

(continues)

PROCEDURE 14-6 (continued)

Supplies Unique to Procedure	• Abdominal laparoscopic drape	• Maloney dilators • #11 and #15 knife blades	
Preoperative Preparation	• Supine position with thighs slightly abducted and flexed; surgeon may prefer legs placed in low stirrup position • 20° reverse Trendelenburg • General anesthesia	• Skin prep: Nipple line to mid-thighs and laterally as far as possible • Draping: Apply leggings if stirrups are used; square off with four towels–edge of upper towel placed	mid-chest; lateral towels placed using anterior superior iliac spines as guide; edge of lower towel placed just above line of symypsis pubis; abdominal laparoscopic drape
Practical Considerations	• X-rays and barium studies in OR • Check all equipment prior to patient's arrival in the OR	• Surgeon usually stands between the patient's legs, surgical assistant on the patient's left, and the surgical technologist on patient's right	• Be prepared for conversion from laparoscopic to open procedure if complications arise

Surgical Procedure

1. Five trocars are typically used in the following locations
   - Above umbilicus in midline
   - Right subcostal
   - Left subcostal
   - Between the umbilical and left subcostal
   - Under the xiphoid process

   A 30° angled laparoscope is used in the periumbilical port

   Procedural Consideration: Probable order of trocar use is 10 mm, 5 mm, 5 mm, 10 mm, 10 mm.

2. Surgical assistant retracts left lobe of liver, exposing esophageal hiatus.

   Procedural Consideration: Have liver retractor ready.

3. The lesser omentum is opened. Extragastric vagal branches may be sacrificed. The right pillar of the hiatus is identified.

   Procedural Consideration: Have ready laparoscopic scissors, coagulation hook, and ligating clips.

4. An incision is made into the peritoneum covering the phrenoesophageal ligament and the phrenogastric ligament is severed.

   Procedural Consideration: Have grasper and dissector of surgeon's choice ready.

5. The right pillar of the crus is dissected until lower left pillar is reached.

   Procedural Consideration: Prepare grasping forceps of surgeon's choice.

6. Grasping forceps are placed on the stomach and the stomach is retracted caudally and laterally.

   Procedural Consideration: Grasping forceps are placed through the uppermost trocar.

7. The left pillar is localized and the posterior vagus nerve identified. The retroesophageal areas are dissected.

PROCEDURE 14-6 (continued)

Procedural Consideration: Have ready laparoscopic scissors, coagulation hook, ligating clips.

8. The left pillar is dissected cephalad.

   Procedural Consideration: Prepare needle holder with 2-0 silk and have ready a second grasping forceps, coagulation hook, and ligating clips.

9. Grasping forceps are applied to stomach and counter traction is applied to expose gastrosplenic ligament. Vessels are isolated with coagulation hook and clipped.

   Procedural Consideration: Check with anesthesia provider to verify that Maloney dilators are ready.

10. The fundus is grasped and passed behind the esophagus and regrasped from other side. Maloney dilator introduced to prevent torsion or stricture.

11. Interrupted 2-0 silk sutures are placed through stomach and the anterior wall of the esophagus, creating the gastric "wrap." Maloney dilator is removed and replaced with nasogastric tube (Figure 14-8).

    Procedural Consideration: Anticipate use of 4–6 sutures.

    Perform counts.

12. Hemostasis is achieved; instruments are removed; and the incisions are closed in normal laparoscopic manner.

    Procedural Consideration: Have dressing supplies ready.

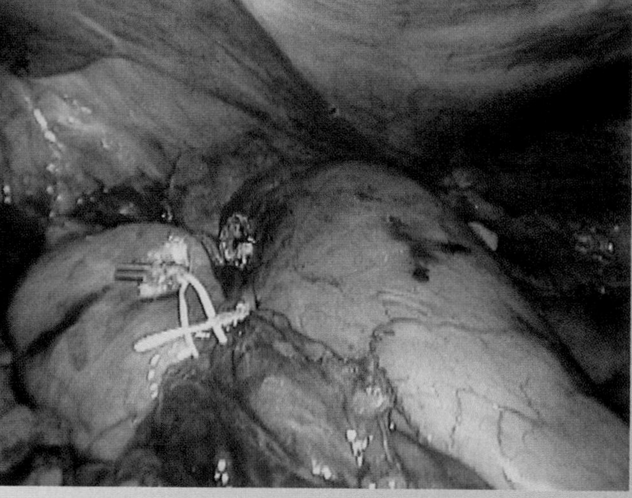

Figure 14-8 Laparoscopic Nissen fundoplication—wrap is completed

Postoperative Considerations

Immediate Postoperative Care

- Transport to PACU.

Prognosis

- No complications: Return to normal activities within 2–4 weeks.
- Complications: esophageal or gastric perforation; pleural perforation; conversion to laparotomy; dysphagia; **necrosis** of wrap; pulmonary infection; incisional hernia; SSI; hemorrhage; failure to gain relief from preoperative complaint.

Wound Classification

- Class 1: Clean

PROCEDURE 14-7 Gastrostomy

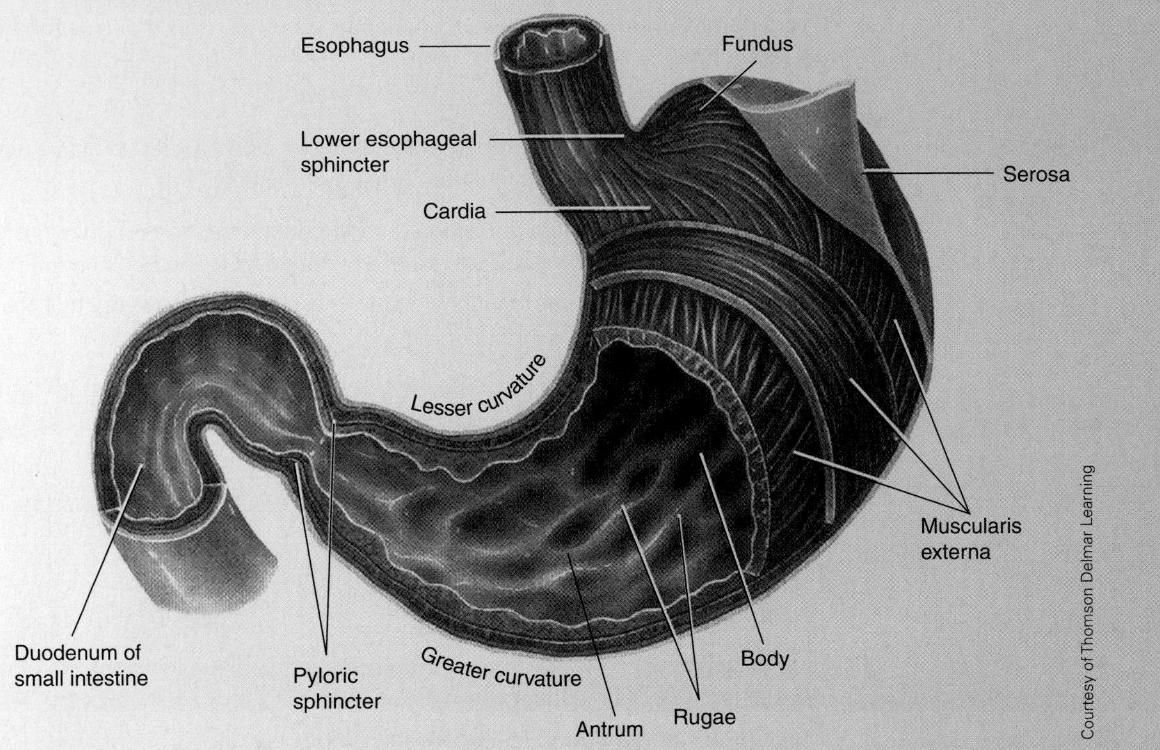

Figure 14-9 Stomach anatomy

Surgical Anatomy and Pathology	• Muscularis coat of the stomach is composed of three layers of smooth muscle: inner oblique that is continuous with the circular layer of the	esophagus; middle circular; outer longitudinal that is continuous with the longitudinal fibers of the esophageal muscle (Figure 14-9).	• Procedure performed due to tumors of the larynx, pharynx, esophagus, and proximal stomach as well as esophageal strictures.
Preoperative Diagnostic Tests and Procedures	• See Table 14-6.		
Equipment and Instruments Unique to Procedure	• Headlamp • Minor instrument set	• Hemoclip appliers and clips	
Supplies Unique to Procedure	• #10 and #15 knife blades	• Gastrostomy tube of surgeon's choice (e.g., Foley or Pezzer)	• Sterile catheter plug • Gastrostomy drainage bag of surgeon's choice
Preoperative Preparation	• Supine position • General anesthesia (preferred); MAC or local • Skin prep: mid-chest to mid-thighs and laterally as far as possible	• Draping: square off with four towels–edge of upper towel placed mid-chest; lateral towels placed using anterior superior iliac	spines as guide; edge of lower towel placed just above line of sympysis pubis; laparotomy drape

PROCEDURE 14-7 (continued)

Practical Considerations	• Have a variety of gastrostomy tubes available in the OR; do not open until surgeon indicates choice.
Surgical Procedure	1. An upper midline incision is made. **Procedural Consideration:** Verify gastrostomy tube type prior to incision if possible.
	2. The stomach is identified, and a site on the middle anterior wall of the stomach is selected for tube placement. **Procedural Consideration:** Have ready small abdominal wall retractors (U.S. Army or small Richardsons).
	3. The gastric site is grasped with a Babcock and elevated, and a small puncture wound is made through the layers of the gastric wall. **Procedural Consideration:** Have ready Babcock clamps and deep knife (do not re-use), verify size of catheter desired, and prepare the pursestring suture. Also have suction ready to prevent any spillage of stomach contents into the abdominal cavity.
	4. #20 to #26 French Foley, Malecot, or Pezzer catheter is inserted 3 to 5 cm into the stomach and secured with two concentrically placed pursestring sutures in the gastric wall. **Procedural Consideration:** Hand first pursestring and prepare second.
	5. The exit site at the skin level in the left hypochondriac region is identified and a stab wound is made in the abdominal wall and the catheter is passed through the opening to the skin. **Procedural Consideration:** Be sure to use the skin knife. A hemostat is usually passed through the incision to receive the catheter.
	6. The stomach is secured to the anterior abdominal wall with several heavy sutures placed through the gastric serosa and **parietal** peritoneum. **Procedural Considerations:** Prepare sutures. Closure happens quickly, so be prepared to perform counts.
	7. The tube is then secured to the skin and the midline incision is closed. **Procedural Consideration:** Place a sterile plug in the catheter or connect to drainage bag. Prepare dressings.
Postoperative Considerations	**Immediate Postoperative Care** • Transport to PACU. **Prognosis** • No complications: Response to treatment is usually optimal; return to normal activity in 1–2 weeks. • Complications: hemorrhage; SSI; erosion of the skin; leakage. **Wound Classification** • Class II: Clean-contaminated

Endoscopic developments allow for another variation on the traditional gastrostomy, the percutaneous endoscopic gastrostomy (PEG). The procedure uses an industry-prepared kit and the procedural steps are as follows:

1. Skin site exit point is one-third of the way between the midclavicular line at the rib margin and the umbilicus.
2. Placement site for gastrostomy incision is midstomach.
3. Pediatric gastroscope is introduced and the stomach is insufflated with air.
4. A finger is pressed into the abdominal wall and indention of the stomach is observed through the endoscope.

5. Local anesthesia is injected at the incision site and a trocar needle is passed into the stomach.
6. Placement of the needle is confirmed visually and the trocar is removed.
7. A wire or nylon loop is passed through the needle and snared by a loop from the gastroscope.

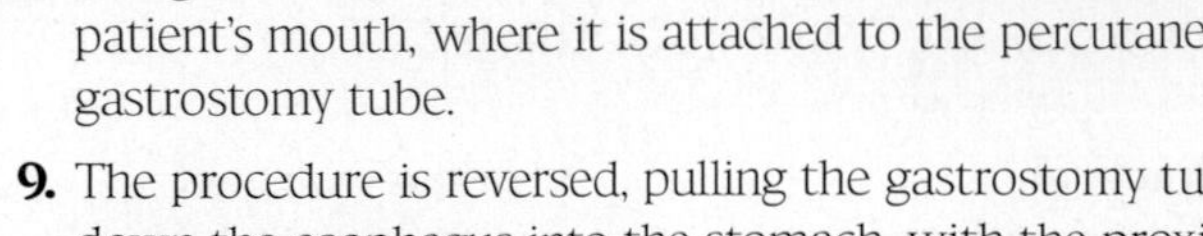

8. The gastroscope is removed, pulling the snare out of the patient's mouth, where it is attached to the percutaneous gastrostomy tube.
9. The procedure is reversed, pulling the gastrostomy tube down the esophagus into the stomach, with the proximal end being drawn through the stab incision and secured.

> **Pearl of Wisdom**
>
> *The stomach may have considerable gastric material inside. Have the suction ready for use as soon as the incision is made into the stomach.*

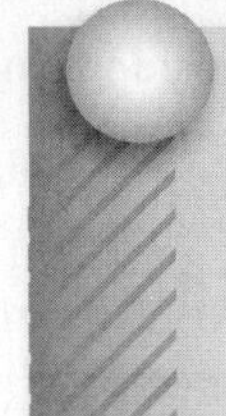

> **Pearl of Wisdom**
>
> *Patients routinely have nasogastric tubes in place. Be sure the position of the nasogastric tube is identified before the linear cutter is placed and activated.*

TOTAL GASTRECTOMY

Total gastrectomy involves removal of the stomach and reconstitution of the alimentary tract. A subtotal gastrectomy is referred to as a Billroth I or II procedure. The Billroth I procedure involves removal of the pylorus of the stomach and an end-to-end anastomosis of the remaining stomach and duodenum. Billroth II is the same except the cut ends of the duodenum are closed and the jejunum is anastomosed to the stomach (a procedure called a gastrojejunostomy). The most common reasons for total gastrectomy are malignancy and bleeding that is uncontrollable by conservative means.

Table 14-7 Procedures Related to Ulcers and Neoplasm

Procedure	*Definition/Purpose*	*Notes*
Gastroduodenostomy Billroth I	Antrectomy removes the distal portion of the stomach and the pylorus Reanastomosis is to the duodenum	Preferred approach
Gastrojejunostomy Billroth II	Antrectomy removes the distal portion of the stomach and the pylorus Reanastomosis is to the jejunum	Preferred when the duodenum is scarred End of duodenum must be closed
Gastrectomy	Removal of the stomach Partial or total gastrectomy may be performed for other conditions	More difficult technically Requires a Roux-en-Y antecolic esophagojejunostomy or end-to-side antecolic esophagojejunostomy

Procedure 14-8 Total Gastrectomy

Surgical Anatomy and Pathology

- The lesser omentum is connected to the lesser curvature of the stomach and extends to the posterior surface of the liver to hold the stomach in place.
- The gastrophrenic ligament extends from the diaphragm to the cardia of the stomach to also help keep the stomach in normal anatomic position.
- The inferior border of stomach is the greater curvature.
- Arterial blood supply: Left gastric artery; branches of the celiac artery; branches of the splenic artery; branches of the left gastroepiploic; one branch of the left gastric artery; gastroduodenal artery (Figure 14-10).
- Gastrectomy performed due to cancer or perforating bleeding ulcer that is unresponsive to conservative treatment.

PROCEDURE 14-8 (continued)

Preoperative Diagnostic Tests and Procedures	• See Table 14-6.		
Equipment and Instruments Unique to Procedure	• Upper arm or Bookwalter self-retaining abdominal retractor • Headlamp	• Laparotomy instrument set • Long instruments • Gastric or bowel resection instrument set	• Hemoclip appliers with ligating clips (open several of each) • Staplers of surgeon's choice
Supplies Unique to Procedure	• #10 knife blades × 5 • Chest tubes and drainage unit if	thoracoabdominal approach	
Preoperative Preparation	• Supine position • General anesthesia • Skin prep: mid-chest to mid-thigh and laterally as far as possible	• Draping: square off with four towels–edge of upper towel placed mid-chest; lateral towels placed using anterior superior iliac	spines as guide; edge of lower towel placed just above line of sympysis pubis; laparotomy drape
Practical Considerations	• Have X-rays in OR. • Confirm blood has been ordered from the blood bank. • Blood loss should be carefully monitored; keep close track of the amount of irrigation used.	• Thoracoabdominal approach may be used. • Notify pathology department if frozen sections will need to be performed prior to patient entering OR.	• Use bowel technique • Headlamp available • Staplers of choice • Chest tubes and drainage unit if thoracoabdominal approach
Draping	• Anticipated surgical area is outlined with towels secured with	adhesive or towel clips. • Laparotomy sheet.	• Be prepared to use clean closure technique.

Surgical Procedure

1. An upper midline incision, bilateral subcostal incision (chevron), or thoracoabdominal incision is made.

   Procedural Consideration: Be prepared for incision of surgeon's choice and have self-retaining retractor of surgeon's choice assembled and ready for use.

2. The lesser sac is entered and the greater and lesser curvatures mobilized. Any adhesions or peritoneal attachments to the pancreas and posterior peritoneum are divided to mobilize the entire stomach.

   Procedural Consideration: Have ready for use on the Mayo stand regular and long Metzenbaum scissors; regular and long hemostatic clamps; hemoclip appliers loaded.

3. The vessels of the greater curvature of the gastroepiploic and inferior short gastrics are ligated and divided. The right and left gastric vessels are ligated and divided. The dissection moves toward the duodenum and extends to include at least one centimeter of the duodenum.

   Procedural Consideration: Prepare stapler of surgeon's choice.

(continues)

Procedure 14-8 (continued)

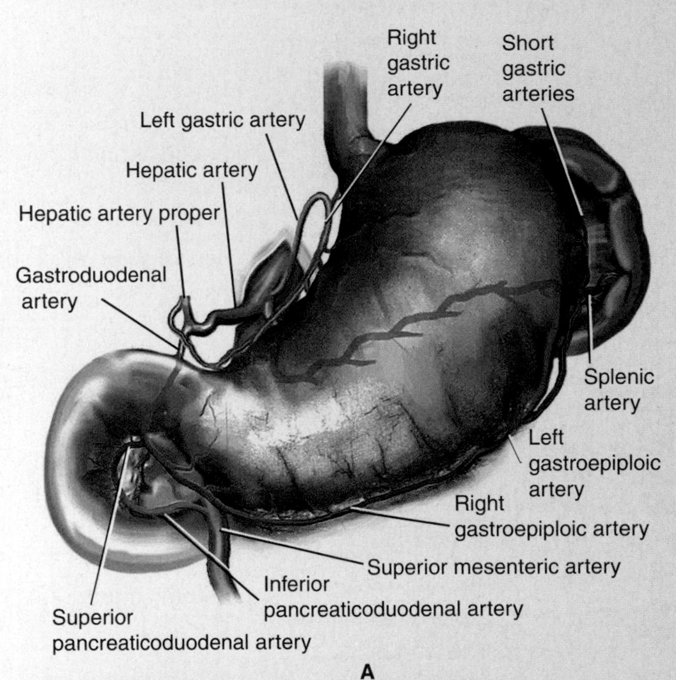

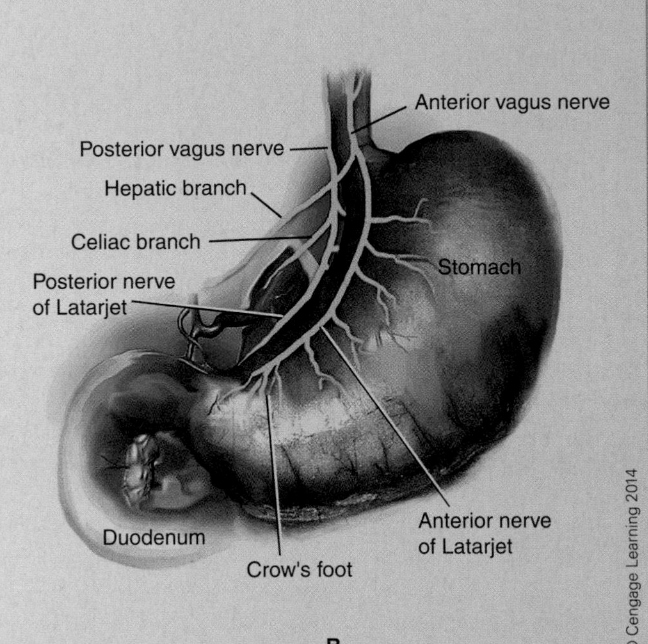

Figure 14-10 Stomach: (A) Arterial supply, (B) neural supply

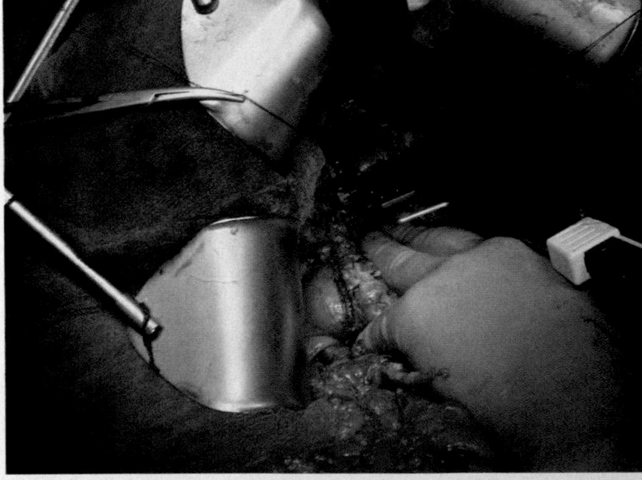

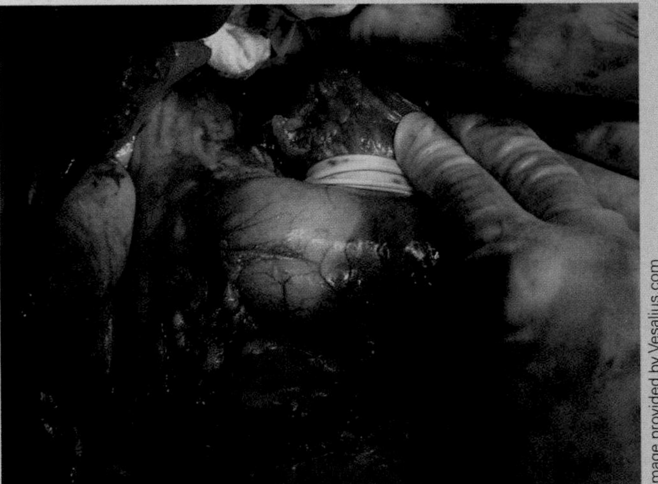

Figure 14-11 Gastrectomy: (A) Esophagus stapled, (B) pylorus mobilized

4. The duodenum is divided with a linear cutter. Devascularization of the stomach is completed. The duodenum and stomach are left attached while the posterior row of anastomosis sutures is placed.

   Procedural Consideration: Prepare for "bowel" technique procedures.

5. The dissection is completed and the esophagus is transected.

   Procedural Consideration: Prepare stapler for reuse.

PROCEDURE 14-8 (continued)

6. The reconstruction of choice is a Roux-en-Y esophagojejunostomy. Eighteen inches of jejunum is needed for a tension-free loop that prevents reflux. Transection is made as far proximal as possible with a linear cutter. Anastomosis can be antecolic or retrocolic as needed. Reconstruction requires two anastomoses: esophagojejunal and an end-to-end jejunojejunal anastomoses.

   Procedural Consideration: Sutures commonly used are 3-0 absorbable and nonabsorbable on GI needle.

7. Abdomen is closed in the usual manner.

Postoperative Considerations

Immediate Postoperative Care

- Transport to PACU, ICU, or CCU.

Prognosis

- No complications: Return to majority of normal activities in 4–6 weeks; however, lifestyle will be somewhat restricted, with diet being the most important adjustment.
- Complications: hemorrhage; SSI; failure of anastomosis.

Wound Classification

- Class II: Clean-contaminated

BOWEL PATHOLOGY

The pathological conditions that affect the bowel are summarized in Table 14-8.

Principles of Bowel Resection and Anastomosis

There are numerous variations in pathology and anatomy that result in variations in procedures of the bowel; however, most procedures are more alike than different. Surgically the overriding characteristic of the bowel is that it is a flexible tube that must allow for the movement of contents. No matter what area is resected or anastomosed, some common principles apply. These are summarized as follows:

- The affected bowel must be mobilized.
- Pathological tissue is removed with a margin of healthy tissue. The site of injury or pathology is identified and the margins of resection are selected.
- An adequate blood supply to the remaining bowel must exist. The mesentery is inspected to ensure good blood flow to the remaining segments of bowel.

TABLE 14-8 **Pathological Conditions of the Bowel**

Condition	*Symptoms/Signs*	*Diagnostics*	*Treatments*
Small Bowel Pathology			
Meckel's diverticulum	• Peptic ulceration • Inflammation of the ileal mucosa • Congenital umbilical fistula, iron deficiency anemia • Malabsorption • Neoplastic formation • Impacted foreign body • Fistula • Incarcerated hernia • Sudden profuse and painless hemorrhage in a child	• History • Radionuclide scans • GI series	Simple diverticulum • Diverticulectomy • Bowel resection

(continues)

Table 14-8 **(continued)**

Condition	*Symptoms/Signs*	*Diagnostics*	*Treatments*
Benign neoplasm	• Obstruction • Volvulus • Bleeding • Pain	• GI series • CT scan	• Resection
Malignant neoplasms	• Obstruction • Bleeding • Pain	• GI series • CT scan	• Wide resection
Obstruction	• Various complaints • Fluid and electrolyte imbalance • CT scan • Sepsis • Colic • Distension • Nausea and vomiting • Constipation	• GI series • Barium studies • CT scan	• Treat the cause (e.g., **lysis** of adhesions) • Resection
Crohn's disease	• Decreased body weight • Chronic illness • Hypoproteinemia • Edema • Muscle weakness • Increased basal metabolic rate • Vitamin deficiencies	• GI series • Barium studies	Medical • Treat symptoms • Manage complications Surgical • Treat obstruction, perforation, abscess formation, bleeding fistulas • Resection if necessary
Colon Pathology			
Diverticular disease (diverticulosis, diverticulitis)	• Subacute onset of left lower quadrant pain • Alteration in bowel habits • Palpable mass • Fever	• History • Physical examination • Abdominal X-rays • Barium studies • Fiberoptic endoscopy	Medical • Treat complications Surgical • Colectomy
Neoplasm (polyps and carcinoma)	• Determined by anatomical location	• History • Physical examination • Abdominal X-rays • CT or ultrasound • Barium enema studies • Colonoscopy	Surgical • Adequate local incision • Hemicolectomy or colectomy
Ulcerative colitis and Crohn's disease	• See small bowel pathology • Watery diarrhea • Cramping • Abdominal pain	• History • Physical examination • Abdominal X-rays • Barium studies • Fiberoptic endoscopy	Medical • Treat symptoms Surgical • Colectomy with ileostomy • Continent ileostomy
Obstruction, volvulus, intussusception, impaction	• Abdominal distension • Cramping abdominal pain • Nausea • Vomiting	• Histoy • Physical examination • Abdominal X-rays • Barium studies • Fiberoptic endoscopy	Surgical • Relieve condition • Resection if necessary

TABLE 14-9 **Bowel Anastomosis Options**

Type	*Feature*	*Notes*
End-to-end	Attachment of two ends of approximately the same sized structures	• Best accomplished by a two-layer closure technique • Continuous 3-0 absorbable for mucosa-to-mucosa anastomosis • 3-0 silk interrupted sutures for seromuscular closure • Entire staple line from transection is excised electrosurgically on the distal and proximal ends prior to anastomosis • Open ends of bowel may be suctioned to remove any residual fecal material prior to anastomosis
End-to-side	Attachment of the end of one section of bowel into the side of another section (T-like)	• Best accomplished by a two-layer closure technique • Continuous 3-0 absorbable for mucosa-to-mucosa anastomosis • 3-0 silk interrupted sutures for seromuscular closure • Staple line from transection is removed electrosurgically on the "end" section prior to anastomosis • Open ends of bowel may be suctioned to remove any residual fecal material prior to anastomosis • End-to-side positioning has one oriented at right angle to other to maintain opening
Side-to-side	Creation of parallel opening in two sections of bowel with anastomosis	• Especially good technique between lumens of unequal dimensions • Best realized with staplers • Technique requires opening the bowel minimally to allow passage of the "halves" of the linear cutter into each lumen, followed by activation of the device to divide the bowel, thereby creating a terminal tube pouch twice the diameter of the bowel • End of the "tube" is closed with a linear stapler
Roux-en-Y	Roux-en-Y is a specific technique of anastomosis that allows for a variety of applications in gastric, intestinal, biliary, and pancreatic surgery. Roux-en-Y is used in partial or total gastrectomy, with pancreatic resection, and in surgery of the bile duct, and is an integral part of the Whipple pancreaticoduodenectomy	Using the small intestine as an example, the proximal end of the divided intestine is anastomosed end-to-side to the distal loop and a section of the distal loop is anastomosed to another organ of the digestive system such as the stomach, which forms the shape of the letter Y

- Relatively equal-diameter segments of bowel should be sewn together.
- The **anastomosis** must be tension-free and leak-proof.
- The mesenteric defect is closed.
- Functional and anatomical continuity is maintained.

There are several options for the type of anastomosis to be used that accomplish the above-stated principles; see Table 14-9.

Appendectomy

Appendectomy is performed for acute appendicitis or incidentally during other surgery as a prophylactic measure. Acute appendicitis is usually caused by obstruction of the appendiceal lumen, which manifests as inflammation that can affect other nearby organs. Perforation of the appendix or gangrene can result. Pylephlebitis, septic thrombosis of the **portal venous system**, can also occur. Symptoms of acute appendicitis include pain, which can be diffuse, central, or localized in the right lower quadrant; nausea and vomiting; and constipation or diarrhea. An elevated white blood cell count and fever are also common. Physical examination reveals tenderness especially on rebound or a palpable abdominal mass in the area of the appendix. The laparoscopic and open procedure is described. The anatomy, pathology, and preoperative diagnostic tests and procedures are the same for both procedures and are provided in the open procedure.

Procedure 14-9 Laparoscopic Appendectomy

Equipment and Instruments Unique to Procedure

- Laparoscopic equipment (see listing at beginning of chapter)
- Insufflator
- Veress needle
- 10/12-mm trocar × 2
- 5-mm trocar
- Hasson trocar
- Laproscopic instruments to include Babcock, curved grasping forceps, curved scissors, endoscopic linear stapler, ligating loop instrument, needle holder, suction irrigator

Supplies Unique to Procedure

- Specimen pouch
- Local anesthetic of the surgeon's choice

Preoperative Preparation

- Supine position with slight Trendelenburg and right side of OR table slightly elevated
- General anesthesia
- Skin prep: mid-chest to symphysis pubis and laterally as far as possible
- Draping: square off with four towels–edge of upper towel placed mid-chest; lateral towels placed using anterior superior iliac spines as guide; edge of lower towel placed just above line of sympysis pubis; laparotomy drape

Practical Considerations

- Same as for other laparoscopic procedures

Surgical Procedure

1. Patient is placed in supine position. Pneumoperitoneum of the abdominal cavity can be established using one of two methods depending on surgeon's preference.
   a. *Veress needle method:* Using their hands, the surgeon and surgical technologist elevate the skin and subcutaneous fat on each side of the umbilicus to allow the underlying viscera to fall away and avoid its being punctured by the needle. Entry with the Veress needle is made in the periumbilical region and inserted into the abdominal cavity. The insufflation tube is attached to the needle and the abdominal cavity is insufflated with 3–4 liters of CO_2 to reach an intra-abdominal pressure of 12 to 15 mm Hg. The needle is removed and replaced with 10–12-mm umbilical port trocar and the insufflation tube is attached to the port.

   Procedural Consideration: Due to the skin prep solution the skin may be slippery and difficult to hold; using a 4 × 4 raytec sponge aids in being able to elevate the skin.

   b. *Hasson technique:* Using a #15 knife blade, a periumbilical incision is made down to the fascia. The Hasson trocar is introduced through the incision into the abdominal cavity and secured with stay sutures. The insufflation tube is attached to the sheath of the trocar.
2. The 0° 5-mm or 10-mm rigid laparoscope with video camera is inserted through the port and the cord to the light source attached to the side of the laparoscope. The surgeon completes a brief visualization of the abdominal cavity and confirms position of the appendix and that it is inflamed.
3. The light of the laparoscope is used to transilluminate the abdomen at the proposed site for the placement of the next trocar; the trocar is placed in the right upper quadrant (RUQ). The surgeon may infiltrate the site with local anesthetic. A small skin incision is made using the #15 knife blade. The subcutaneous tissue is slightly separated down to the fascia using a mosquito hemostat. Another 10/12-mm trocar with sheath is inserted under visualization with the use of the laparoscope. This serves as the working port through which instruments are placed.

PROCEDURE 14-9 (continued)

4. The same process is repeated for placement of a 5-mm trocar in the midline suprapubic site to avoid the bladder. This serves as the traction port.
5. The patient may be placed in slight Trendelenburg position and right side of the OR table slightly elevated to facilitate the small bowel falling away from the right lower quadrant.
6. A laparoscopic Babcock instrument is inserted through the RUQ trocar to grasp the cecum and retract it cephalad.
7. A grasping forceps is inserted through the suprapubic trocar to grasp the tip of the appendix and hold it in an upward position. This forceps is kept in place for the entire procedure.

   Procedural Consideration: The surgical technologist will be responsible for holding the grasping forceps throughout the procedure.
8. The cecum is released and the Babcock removed. A dissecting instrument is inserted through the RUQ trocar and used to create an opening/window in the mesoappendix at the base of the appendix.
9. According to surgeon's preference, the mesappendix may be divided one or more times using an endoscopic linear stapler. The lower jaw of the stapler is placed through the mesenteric window and closed to lay down the line of staples. Some surgeons may not perform this step and staple the mesoappendix and appendix together for removal.

   Procedural Consideration: Confirm extra staple packets are in the OR; however, do not open unless needed.
10. According to the surgeon's preference, the appendix can be transected in one of three methods: (a) endoscopic linear stapler, (b) ligating loop instrument, (c) suturing instrument.
11. Use of the linear stapler:
    a. If the surgeon is removing the mesoappendix and appendix together, the lower jaw of the stapler is placed through the mesenteric window and the stapler is fired.
    b. If the surgeon already transected the mesoappendix, the jaws of the stapler are placed on both sides of the base of the appendix.
12. The grasping forceps are used to rotate the appendix 180° in order to visualize the entire length of the appendix and place the stapler to the base of the appendix.

    Procedural Consideration: Gently rotate the appendix to prevent perforation and spillage of contents.
13. The stapler is closed and fired and withdrawn. The staple line is inspected.
14. If the appendix is minimally inflamed it can be removed through the RUQ port. If the appendix is highly inflamed the laparoscope is inserted through the RUQ port and using the grasping forceps a specimen pouch is inserted through the umbilical port. The appendix is placed inside the pouch and brought out through the port. Care is taken not to perforate the appendix and spill the contents.
15. The appendiceal stump and line of staples is inspected one last time. Using the suction irrigator, the area is irrigated. The ports are removed and the abdomen allowed to deflate.
16. Routinely only the 10/12-mm sites require fascial closure with 2-0 absorbable suture. The subcutaneous layer is not sutured. The skin of each trocar site is approximated with 3-0 or 4-0 nonabsorbable sutures. Adhesive skin strips and band-aids are applied to each site.

(continues)

Procedure 14-9 (continued)

Postoperative Considerations	**Immediate Postoperative Care** • Transport to PACU.	**Prognosis** • No complications: Discharged same day of surgery; return to normal activities in 4–6 weeks.	• Complications: same as for open procedure. **Wound Classification** • Class 2: Clean-contaminated

Procedure 14-10 Appendectomy

Surgical Anatomy and Pathology	• Attached to cecum by the mesoappendix, which contains the appendiceal artery.	• Frequently located upward and inward, behind the cecum called retrocecal.	• Inflamed, infected appendix called appendicitis; often due to impacted feces.
Preoperative Diagnostic Tests and Procedures	• Physical: pain and tenderness in the right lower quadrant upon palpation	• White blood cell count	
Equipment and Instruments Unique to Procedure	• Minor instrument set		
Supplies Unique to Procedure	• Aerobic and anaerobic culture tubes (do not open until requested by surgeon)	• ¼″ and ½″ Penrose drain (do not open until requested by surgeon)	• Antibiotic irrigation solution
Preoperative Preparation	• Supine position • General anesthesia	• Skin prep: umbilicus to symphysis pubis and bilaterally as far as possible	• Draping: square off RLQ with four towels; laparotomy drape
Practical Considerations	• Have major instrument set available.	• For female patient, a laparoscopy may be first performed to rule	out ovarian cyst or ectopic pregnancy.

Surgical Procedure

1. The McBurney's incision is typically used.

   Procedural Consideration: Small retractors (e.g., U.S. Army) are placed and may be redirected several times as the incision proceeds through the muscle layers.

2. The appendix is identified by following the cecal taenia to the appendiceal base. This may require the gentle mobilization of the cecum into the wound (see Figure 14-12A and B). The appendix is identified, brought out of the wound, and grasped with a Babcock.

   Procedural Consideration: Be prepared to culture fluid, if present, as soon as the peritoneum is entered and have suction ready.

Procedure 14-10 (continued)

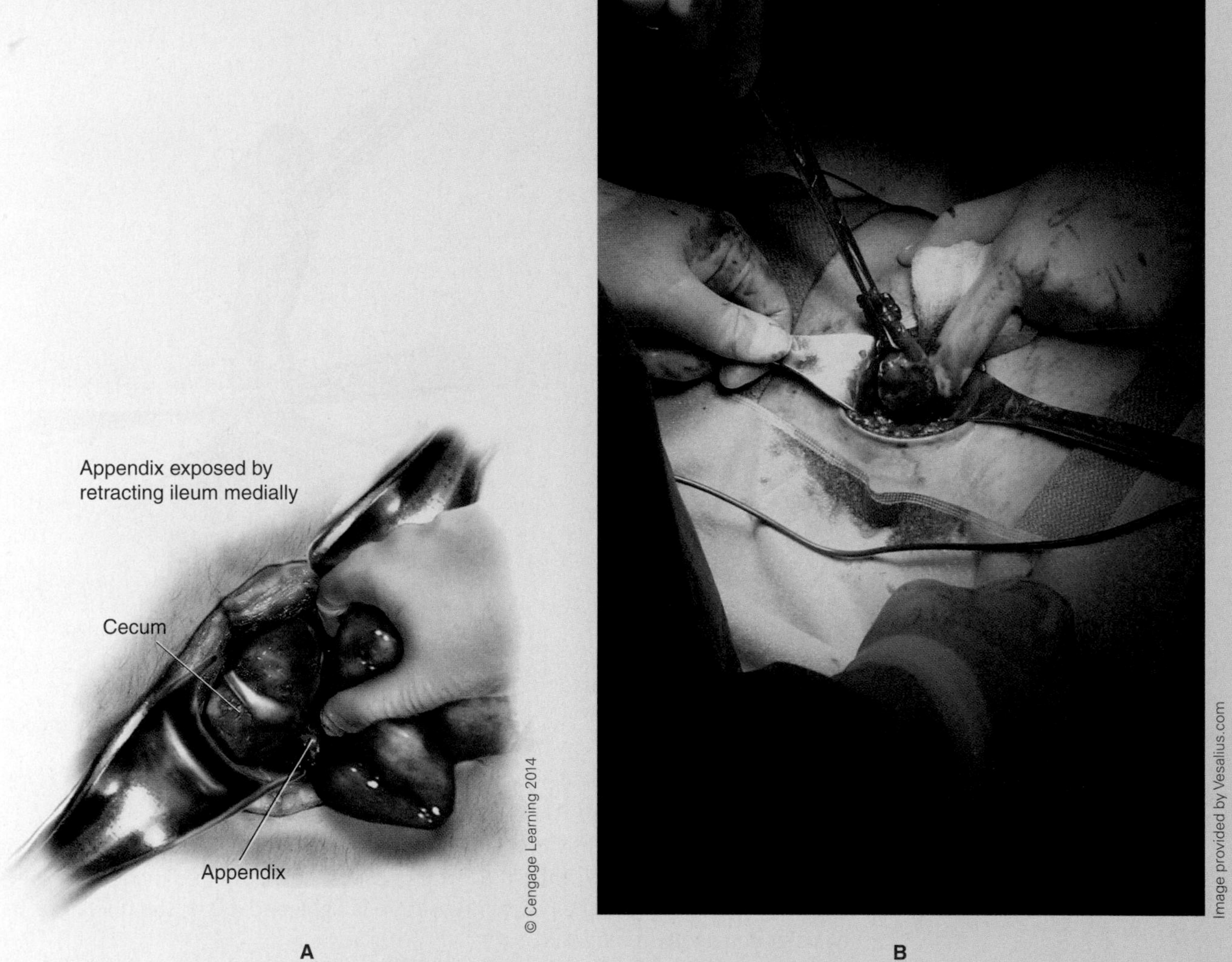

Figure 14-12 Appendectomy: (A) Cecum and appendix identified, (B) mobilization of appendix

3. The mesoappendix is transected from the free end tip of the appendix toward the base, by a series of double clamping, cutting, and ligation with 3-0 absorbable ties (Figure 14-12C).

   Procedural Consideration: This step of the procedure may be reversed if the appendix is severely adhered or retrocecal.

4. A clamp is placed across the appendix near the base, crushing the appendix, and is then removed and reapplied slightly distally.

   Procedural Consideration: Prepare pursestring suture if surgeon uses that technique. Replace Babcock with Crile hemostat to grasp the tip of the appendix.

5. A 3-0 absorbable suture on a small taper needle may be passed through the cecum, around the base of the appendix, in a pursestring manner (see Figure 14-12D).

   Procedural Consideration: Suture and needle are contaminated and must be isolated after use; try to avoid touching them or change glove(s) if necessary.

(*continues*)

PROCEDURE 14-10 (continued)

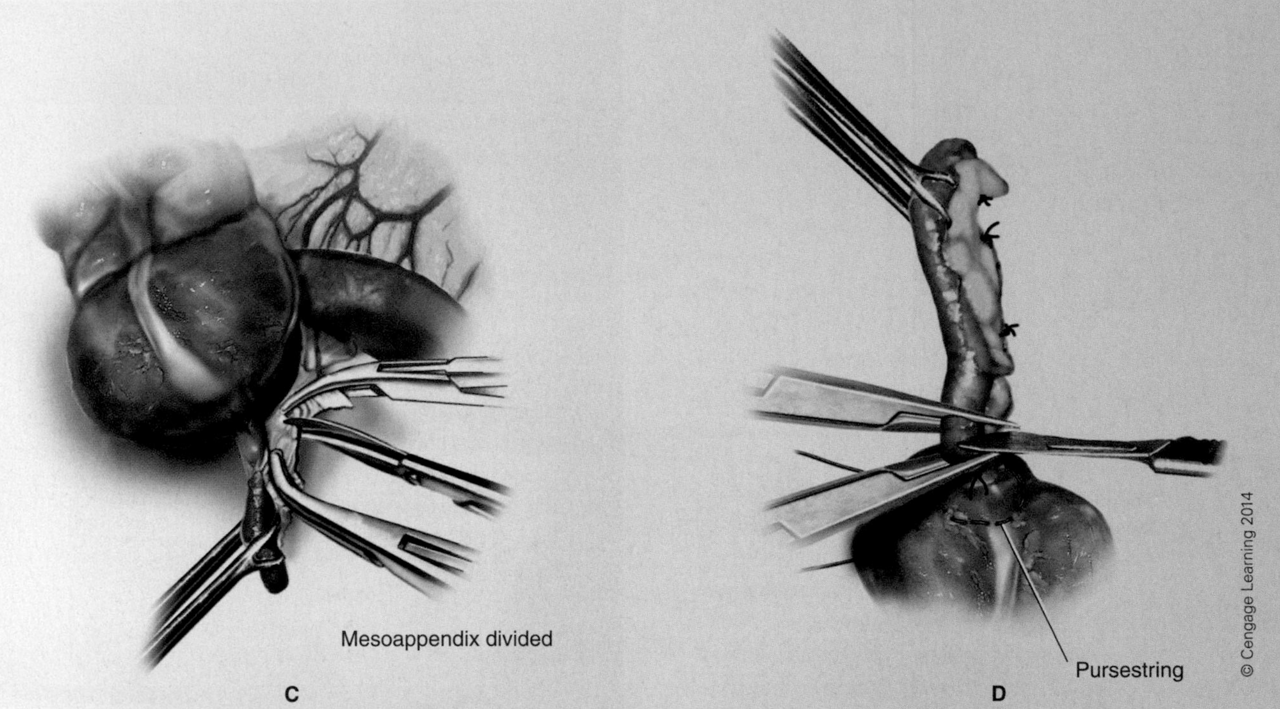

Figure 14-12 Appendectomy: (C) appendiceal artery ligated, (D) excision of appendix

6. The crushed base is then ligated with an 0 absorbable tie and the appendix is amputated electrosurgically or with scissors or a scalpel.

   The appendiceal stump is inverted within the lumen of the cecum and the pursestring suture is tightened and tied. The STSR gently pushes the stump into the lumen with the Crile hemostat and as the pursestring suture is tightened, he or she unclamps the hemostat and gently removes it.

   Procedural Consideration: Have a kidney basin on the sterile field for placement of the appendix and contaminated instruments and pass off to the circulator. A Penrose drain may be placed in particular if the appendix was perforated; size according to surgeon's choice. Antibiotic irrigation solution may be used, especially in presence of wound contamination; have a small basin ready on the back table for the circulator to pour the saline and antiobiotic in order to mix.

7. The incision is closed in layers.

   Procedural Consideration: The incision is small; be prepared to perform the counts quickly.

Postoperative Considerations

Immediate Postoperative Care

- Transport to PACU.

Prognosis

- No complications: Return to normal activities in 4–6 weeks.
- Complications: hemorrhage; SSI; intestinal obstruction due to postoperative adhesions forming; appendicial stump rupture; sepsis.

Wound Classification

- Class II: Clean contaminated
- Class III: Contaminated; ruptured appendix

Table 14-10 Pathological Conditions of the Colon

Condition	Symptoms/Signs	Diagnostics	Treatments
Diverticular disease (diverticulosis, diverticulitis)	• Subacute onset of left lower quadrant pain • Alteration in bowel habits • Palpable mass • Fever	• History • Physical examnination • Abdominal X-rays	Medical • Treat complications Surgical • Colectomy
Neoplasm (polyps and carcinoma)	• Determined by anatomical location	• History • Physical examination • Abdominal X-rays • Barium studies • Fiberoptic endoscopy	Surgical • Adequate local excision • Hemicolectomy or colectomy
Ulcerative colitis and Crohn's disease	• See small bowel pathology • Watery diarrhea • Cramping • Abdominal pain	• History • Physical examination • Abdominal X-rays • Barium studies • Fiberoptic endoscopy	Medical • Treat symptoms Surgical • Colectomy with ileostomy
Obstruction, volvulus, intussusception, impaction	• Abdominal distension • Cramping abdominal pain • Nausea • Vomiting	• Histoy • Physical examination • Abdominal X-rays • Barium studies • Fiberoptic endoscopy	Surgical • Relieve condition • Resection if necessary

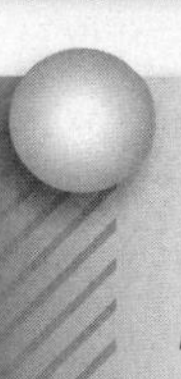

Pearl of Wisdom

The appendix and all instruments and needles associated with its removal are contaminated. They are placed in a basin and removed from the immediate field. The basin is placed in a predefined area on the back table and left there until the case is completed. Instruments and needles are counted by pointing, not by touching.

Procedure 14-11 Colon Resection

Surgical Anatomy and Pathology

- Colon divided into seven sections: cecum, ascending colon, transverse colon, descending colon, sigmoid colon, rectum and anal canal.
  - Cecum held in position by peritoneum.
  - Ascending colon begins at ileocecal valve and ends at hepatic flexure; held in place by peritoneum and hepato-renal ligament at the hepatic flexure.
  - Transverse colon begins at hepatic flexure, travels across top of abdominal cavity, and ends at splenic flexure; most mobile section of the colon attached to the posterior surface of the diaphragm by the phrenocolic ligament.
  - Descending colon begins as splenic flexure and is supported by peritoneum and attachment to the posterior abdominal wall.

(continues)

PROCEDURE 14-11 (continued)

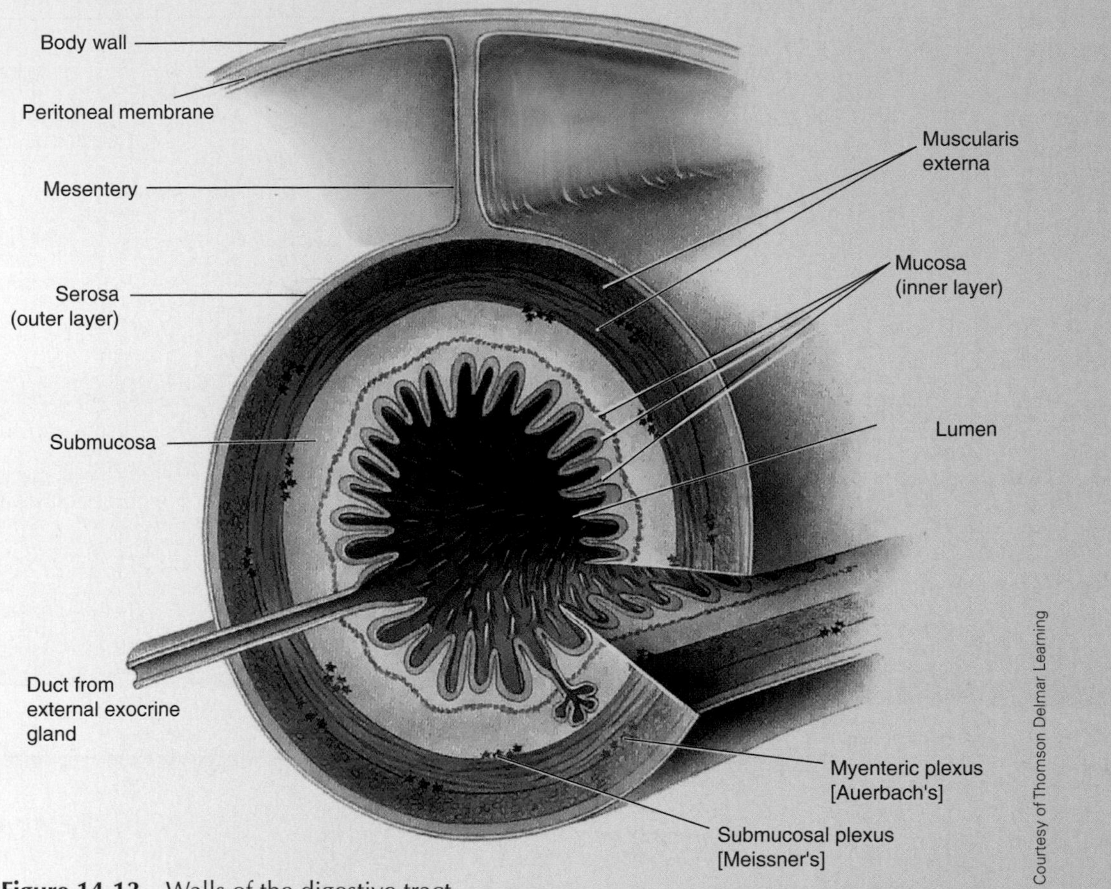

Figure 14-13 Walls of the digestive tract

	• The sigmoid colon is held in place by fold of peritoneum called the iliac mesocolon and it ends at the rectum; it is the most frequent site of colon cancer and volvulus. • Colon has four layers: serosa, muscular, submucosa, mucosa (Figure 14-13). • Arterial vessels encountered during a colon resection can include the right, middle, and left colic arteries; inferior and superior mesenteric arteries; intercolic and sigmoid arteries; superior rectal artery (Figure 14-14). • See Table 14-10 for pathologies. • See Figure 14-15 for colon resection options.
Preoperative Diagnostic Tests and Procedures	• See Table 14-10.
Equipment and Instruments Unique to Procedure	• Major instrument set; include extra Crile hemostats and large hemostats such as curved Kelly and Pean due to large vessels • Long and deep instrument set • GI instrument set with bowel clamps • GI staplers (type of staplers needed according to resection and anastomosis to be performed) • Large self-retaining retractor (e.g., Balfour)

PROCEDURE 14-11 (continued)

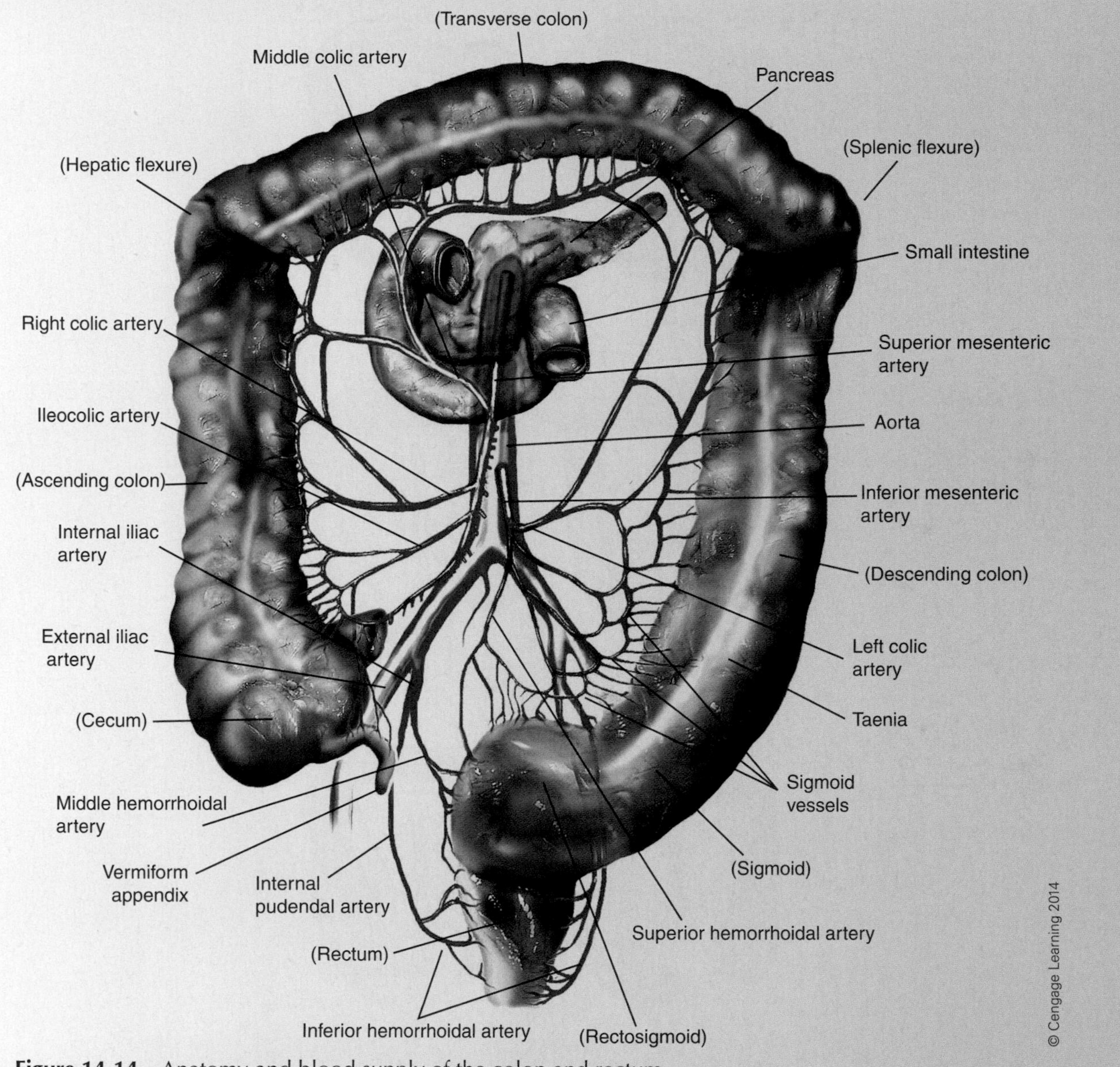

Figure 14-14 Anatomy and blood supply of the colon and rectum

Supplies Unique to Procedure	• Large-diameter ties due to size of vessels that will be encountered; will need a large	number of ties opened and ready to use • Foley catheter	• Active drain (e.g., Hemovac or Jackson-Pratt)
Preoperative Preparation	• Colon has the largest population of intestinal flora; therefore the chances of a postoperative SSI are higher than normal. • Bowel prep performed on the ward to cleanse	the colon of fecal matter and bacteria. • Prophylactic antibiotics given by anesthesia preoperatively, possibly intraoperatively and postoperatively by IV.	• Supine position • General anesthesia with nasogastric tube inserted

(continues)

Procedure 14-11 (continued)

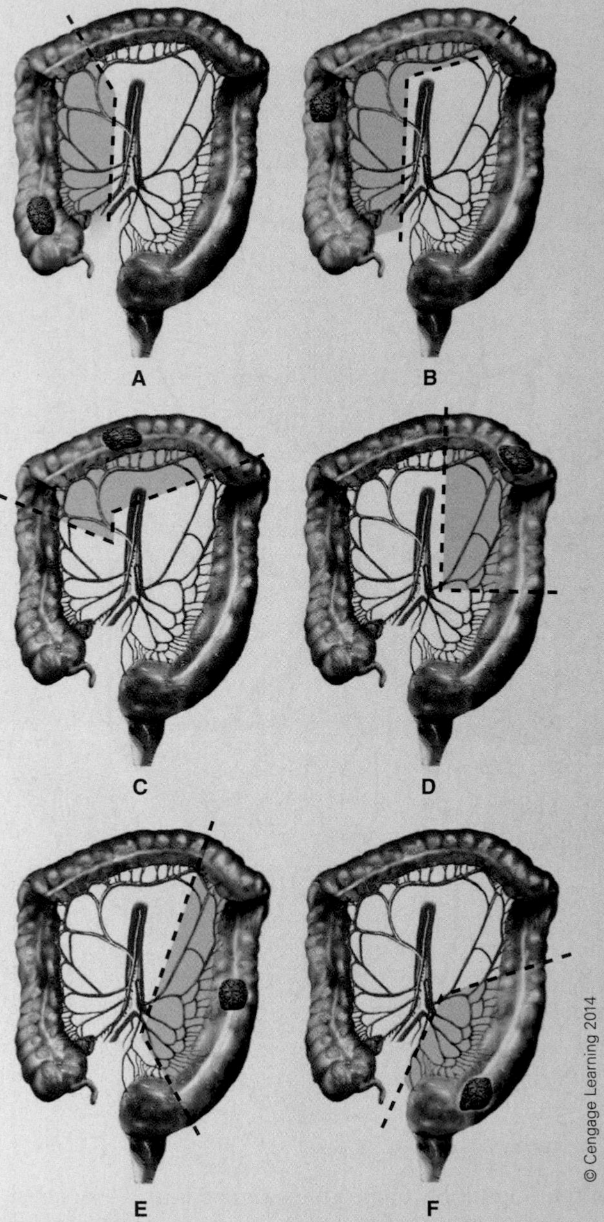

Figure 14-15 Colon resection options: (A) Right colectomy, (B) right hemicolectomy, (C) transverse colectomy, (D) left colectomy, (E) left hemicolectomy, (F) abdominoperineal resection

- Skin prep: mid-chest to symphysis pubis and laterally as far as possible. Care must be taken to avoid removing the markings made by the surgeon for the site of a colostomy.
- Draping: square off with four towels–edge of upper towel placed mid-chest; lateral towels placed using anterior superior iliac spines as guide; edge of lower towel placed just above line of sympysis pubis; laparotomy drape. Surgeon may want to place an incise drape that is impregnated with an antimicrobial iodine agent; the incise drape is placed prior to the placement of the laparotomy drape.

Procedure 14-11 (continued)

Practical Considerations

- The surgical technologist along with the other members of the sterile team must use "bowel technique" once the bowel is opened.
  - Instruments, sponges, and gloved hands that come into contact with the open bowel are considered contaminated.
- It is recommended the surgical technologist create two Mayo stand set ups, one for surgical wound and colon resection, and the other for wound closure. The instruments and supplies set aside for closure should not be handled until the colon is closed and the sterile team members have changed gown and gloves.
  - A stoma may be created as part of the surgical procedure. See information below about stomas.

Surgical Procedure

1. A midline incision is made and laparotomy opening performed. The surgeon "runs" the colon to inspect it and determine the section to be removed. If the procedure is being performed due to cancer, a wide margin of colon on each end will be removed to ensure that all of the affected tissue is removed.

   Procedural Consideration: Resection of cancerous colon requires a distal margin of at least 5 cm from the pathology and proximal margin is determined by the colonic blood supply.

2. The colon is freed from mesenteric, colic ligaments and posterior peritoneal attachments. A window is created in the mesentery and division begins; the surgeon will double clamp, divide, and ligate the mesentery several times until it is dissected free from the colon. The surgical technologist should have quite a few Pean or other large clamps available for use, as well as silk ties of the surgeon's preference, in sizes that may include 1-0, 2-0, and 3-0. The section of colon to be removed is fully mobilized (Plates 14-1 to 14-4).

3. Once the colon is freed, the surgeon may cover the surgical wound with towels or sponges soaked in saline to isolate the section of colon to be removed and protect the peritoneal cavity from possible spillage when the colon is opened.

   Procedural Consideration: Towels should not be placed within the surgical wound/abdominal cavity because they do not have an X-ray-detectable strip.

4. Four intestinal clamps are placed; each end of the segment to be excised is double clamped (Plate 14-5). Using a #10 knife blade or cautery, the surgeon divides the colon between each set of intestinal clamps and passes off the specimen by placing it into a basin that the surgical technologist should have available at the sterile field; the surgical technologist then passes off the basin to the circulator. An intestinal clamp may still be attached to each end of the specimen; the surgical technologist must remember this when performing the counts.

   Procedural Consideration: The surgeon may use a linear cutter that transects and staples the colon.

5. The surgeon is now ready to perform the anastomosis. If a linear cutter was used, a #10 knife blade is used to cut a small section of each bowel ends to remove the staples and create openings. The assistant, using the two intestinal clamps, brings the two bowel ends together. The surgeon places the first layer of interrupted sutures using silk or Vicryl (Plate 14-6). The first and last sutures should be cut long, leaving tails for the purpose of traction.

   a. Colon resection can require anastomosis between lumens of unequal diameter, such as anastomosis to the ileum. To overcome this challenge, the smaller lumen is cut using the #10 knife blade at a slant to provide a wider aperture for anastomosis or a side-to-side technique is used.

(*continues*)

Procedure 14-11 (continued)

b. Rather than using suture to perform the anastomosis, the surgeon may use a linear stapler; the surgical technologist should have multiple packets of staples available in order to reload the stapling device.

c. At this point a colostomy may be performed rather than the anastomosis. A Kocher clamp is used to grasp the skin at the center of the colostomy site and elevated. Using a #10 knife blade, the surgeon makes the skin incision and removes a circular section of subcutaneous tissue; electrocautery is used to dissect down to the anterior fascia. The muscle fibers are separated by blunt and sharp dissection, and dissection continues down to the peritoneum, which is opened with scissors or electrocautery. Then 2–3 cm of colon is delivered through the opening using a Babcock clamp, which also serves to keep the end of the colon closed somewhat to prevent spillage. Inside the abdominal cavity the colon is tacked to the peritoneum. Externally, four sutures are placed at each quadrant of the colon through the cut end of the colon and dermis to keep the colon in position. Additional sutures are needed to "mature" the stoma, which refers to everting the mucosa of the colon to create an opening for the feces to pass into the drainage bag.

6. The second layer of suture is placed; an absorbable suture is often used. The sutures are placed until the anastomosis is complete.

7. A third layer of interrupted suture (silk or Vicryl) is placed (Plate 14-6).

8. At this point bowel technique ends (Plate 14-7). Health care facility policies will vary, but optimally the sterile surgical team removes the lap sponges, suction tubing with tip, Bovie pencil, and contaminated instruments from the field. The circulator assists the team members in removing gown and gloves, and gives the surgical technologist a new sterile gown and gloves. Once the surgical technologist dons the gown and gloves, he or she will gown and glove the surgeon and assistant. A sterile laparotomy drape may be placed over the contaminated drape, or the surgeon may square off the operative site with towels, placing them on the contaminated drape. New suction tubing with tip and Bovie pencil are positioned, clean lap sponges are placed on the field, and the clean closure instruments are brought up to the field by the surgical technologist.

9. Laparotomy closure is performed.

Postoperative Considerations

Immediate Postoperative Care

- Transport to PACU.
- Instruct patient not to strain and bolster wound with a pillow if he or she must cough or sneeze.

Prognosis

- No complications: Return to most normal activities in 6–8 weeks. Depending on location of resection, bowel habits may be altered. Lifestyle and diet will be somewhat altered if colostomy is performed.
- Complications: hemorrhage; SSI; intestinal obstruction due to formation of postoperative adhesions; stump rupture if colostomy performed; sepsis; ureteral injury; thromboembolism; stoma complications (see section on stomas).

Wound Classification

- Class II: Clean contaminated
- Class III: Contaminated (if spillage from the GI tract occurred)

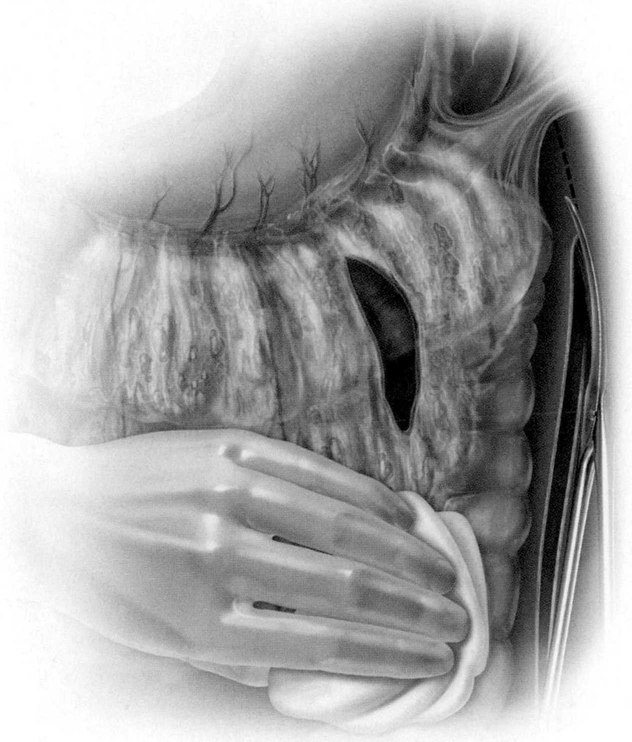

Plate 14-1 Colon is freed from mesenteric and peritoneal attachments

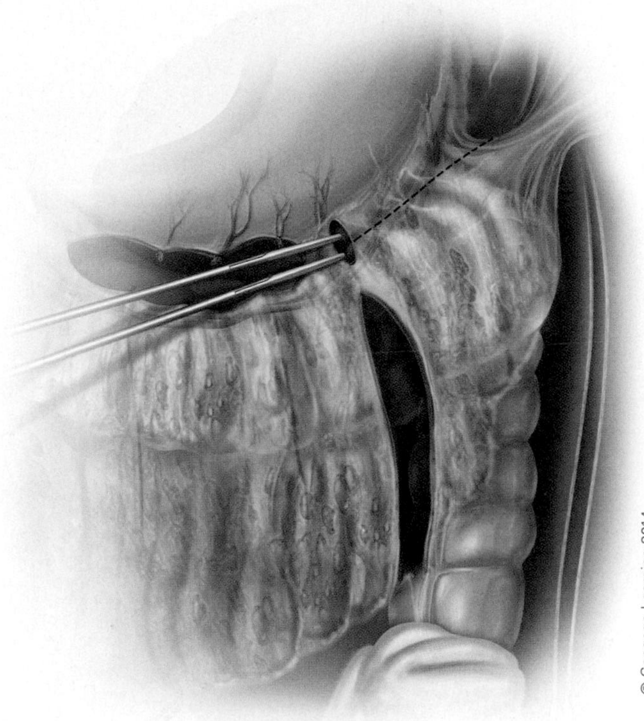

Plate 14-2 Dissection continues

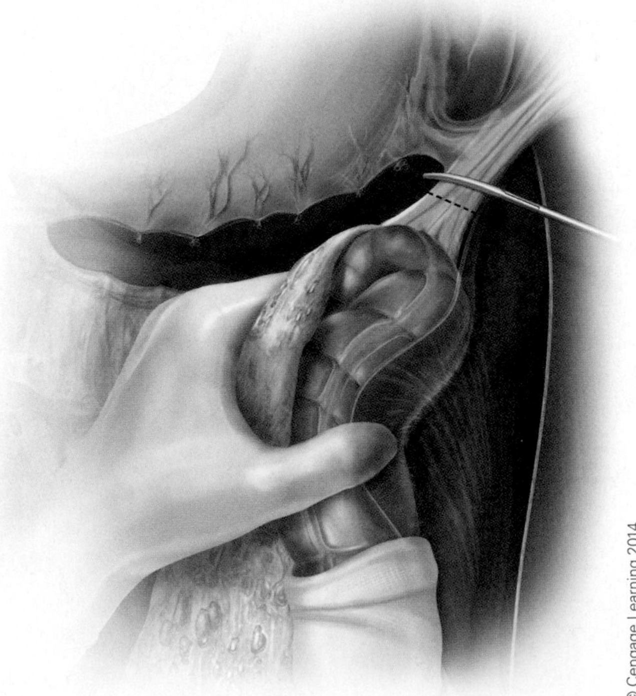

Plate 14-3 Dissection continues further

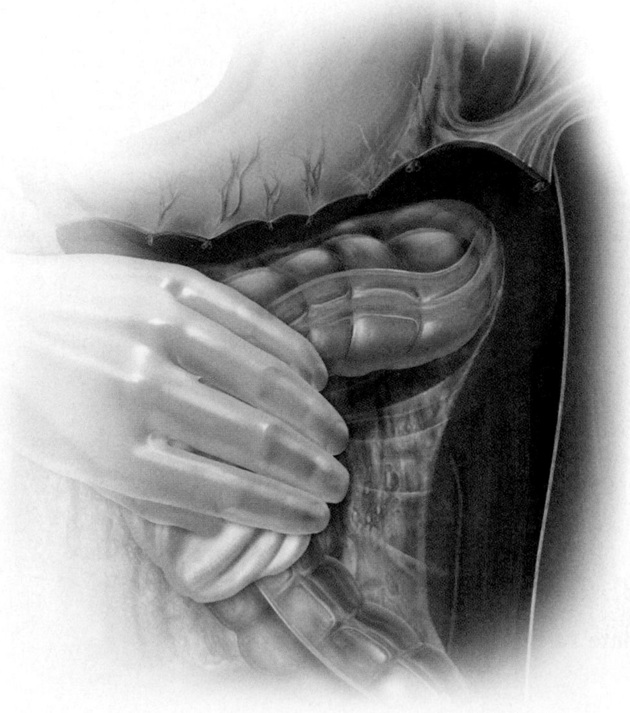

Plate 14-4 Colon is freed from attachments

(*continues*)

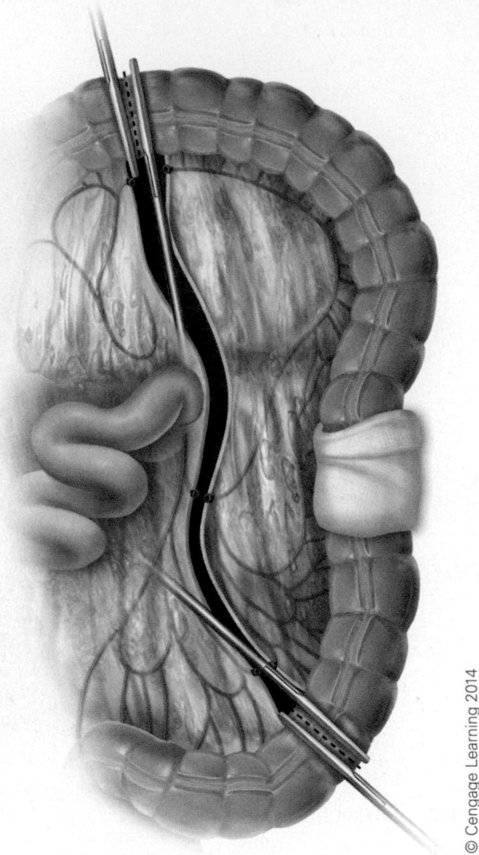

Plate 14-5 Intestinal clamps are placed

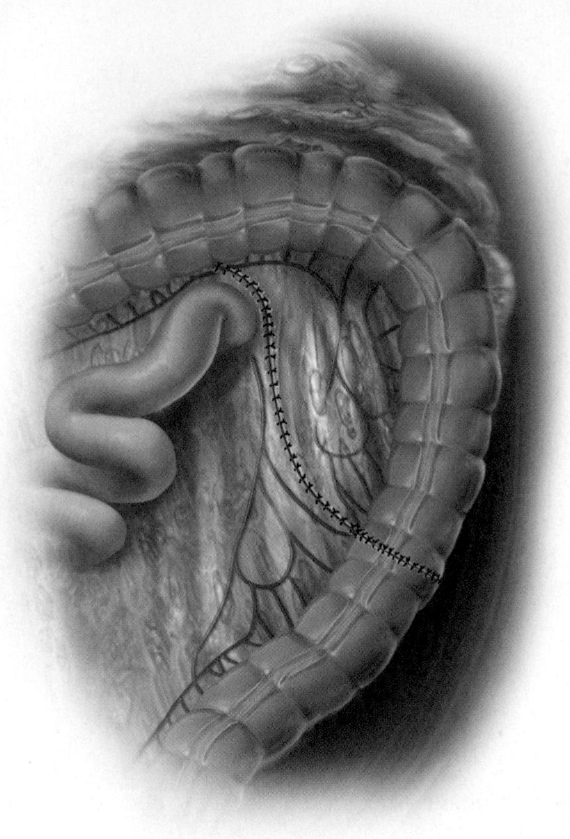

Plate 14-7 Completed anastomosis

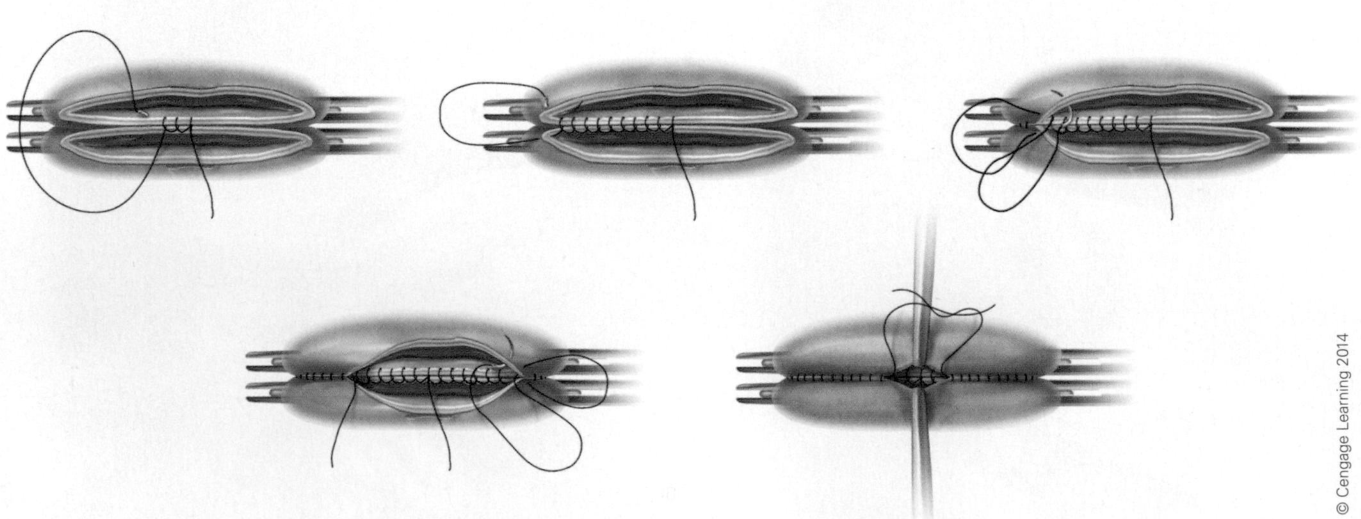

Plate 14-6 End-to-end anastomosis

STOMAS

A stoma ("ostomy") is a communication of a section of bowel with the outside of the abdominal cavity that is created to divert the fecal stream. This diversion is done temporarily to protect a recent intestinal anastomosis, to avoid potential abdominal spillage postoperatively, or as an end (permanent) result of bowel resection. In this section of the chapter, a stoma is in reference to an ileostomy or colostomy.

Stomas are created from either an end section or loop of the ileum (ileostomy) or colon (colostomy). The sigmoid colon is also used as an "end" colostomy following abdominoperineal (A/P) resection. Stomas created as end stomas have a single aperture at the skin surface, and those created from loops generally have two apertures in the same wound. Loop-type stomas have an afferent functioning aperture and an efferent nonfunctioning aperture, and may be created with the bowel in continuity or separated.

There are numerous potential complications common to all stomas. They include ischemia, **stenosis**, stomal prolapse, stomal retraction, parastomal hernia, fistula formation, bleeding from varices around the stoma, leakage from the appliance, offensive odors, contact dermatitis, laceration, urinary tract calculi, gallstones, infection, hyperplasia, and bowel obstruction secondary to stomal creation.

In stoma creation, a site is selected at a point below the costal margin, above the belt line, and usually at the appropriate lateral edge of the rectus abdominis muscle. Site selection is preferably accomplished prior to surgery, with the site marked on the patient after review of the area in both the standing and sitting positions. This provides maximum comfort for the patient. In some cases, of course, stoma creation is a result of intraoperative decision making, and therefore pre operative site selection is a moot point. However, selection of the site will still follow the basic guidelines just described. Stoma types are listed in Table 14-11.

ANORECTAL PATHOLOGY

Pathological conditions of the anorectal area are summarized in Table 14-12.

Anorectal pathology presents with a variety of signs and symptoms (Table 14-13). For most conditions, a conservative approach to treatment is followed before surgical options are exercised.

SELECT PATHOLOGY OF THE LIVER AND BILIARY TRACT

Liver pathology and surgical conditions are diagnosed via patient history, physical examination, changes in laboratory data, sonography, liver scan, CT scan, and biopsy. Arteriograms may be required to diagnose suspected vascular lesions. The biliary tract is subject to the same diagnostic examinations (Table 14-14). Some biliary stones will appear on routine X-ray.

TABLE 14-11 **Stoma Types**

Stoma Type	*Description*
End ileostomy	• Constructed from a terminal portion of ileum • Temporary or permanent
Loop ileostomy	• Primarily a temporary stoma for fecal diversion
End-loop ileostomy	• A modification of the loop method in which the loop is divided with a linear cutter and both ends are brought out through the skin incision
End colostomy	• Created from the descending colon and sigmoid
Loop colostomy	• Utilizes the transverse colon • Not generally used as a permanent colostomy because it discharges a semiliquid stool • The most frequently used method of stoma creation for temporary fecal diversion
End-loop colostomy	• A modification of the loop method in which the loop is divided with a linear cutter and both ends are brought out through the skin incision
Sigmoid colostomy	• Most common type of permanent colostomy • Created at the time of A/P resection • Created as an end colostomy in the lower left quadrant

Table 14-12 Anorectal Pathology

Condition	Definition/Types
Fistula-in-ano	A chronic form of perianal abscess that fails to heal after draining and becomes an inflammatory tract characterized by primary internal and secondary external openings. Categorized into four groups based upon their relation to the sphincter muscles: • Intersphincteric • Transsphincteric • Suprasphincteric • Extrasphincteric Causes: infectious diseases, malignancy, and trauma; associated with active pulmonary tuberculosis and Crohn's disease
Anal fissure	• Tears in the epidermis of the anal canal extending from the dentate line to the margin of the anus • Primary fissures: trauma, childbirth, or the passage of hard stools • Secondary fissures: associated with other systemic conditions, such as Crohn's disease, leukemia, aplastic anemia, superinfection in HIV patients, and agranulocytosis
Pilonidal disease	• An acute abscess in the sacrococcygeal area, exclusively in the midline, that ruptures spontaneously, resulting in an unhealed sinus tract with chronic drainage • Sinus tract is generally 2 to 5 cm and can be mistaken for a fistula-in-ano • Lesions are often secondarily invaded by hair
Hemorrhoids	• Congestion and dilatation of the submucosal and subcutaneous venous plexuses that line the anal canal; caused by persistent or repeated intra-abdominal pressure, heavy physical exertion, constipation, heredity, age, and diet • Most common anal lesions • Classified as external or internal and by location

Table 14-13 Anorectal Pathology—Diagnosis and Treatment

Condition	Symptoms/Signs	Diagnostics/Treatment
Fistula-in-ano	• Purulent or serosanguinous drainage • Palpable fistula tract may be evident • External opening at skin level • Internal opening	Diagnosis • Anoscopy • Hydrogen peroxide injection study • Fistulography • Examination under anesthesia • Probing of the fistula tract • MRI (complex fistulas) • Ultrasonography (complex fistulas) Treatment • Fistulotomy • Fistulectomy • Placement of a seton
Anal fissure	• Pain in the anus during and after defecation • Bleeding (over 70% of patients) • Swelling that can form a "sentinel pile" • Fibrosis, which may lead to skin tag formation • Constipation • Spasm • Pain may be severe and incapacitating	Diagnosis • Visualization • Anoscopy under anesthesia • Digital examination Treatment • Acute fissures usually heal spontaneously in 6 weeks • Chronic fissures generally require surgical intervention • Conservative treatment: application of topical anesthetics or hydrocortisone ointments; warm baths; addition of bulk-forming agents, such as bran or psylliumseed, to the diet to relieve constipation; anal hygiene • Surgical treatment: lateral internal sphincterotomy

Table 14-13 (continued)

Condition	*Symptoms/Signs*	*Diagnostics/Treatment*
Pilonidal disease	• More frequent in obese males in their 20s or 30s • Acute abscess; pain can be severe • Chronic sinus formation; pain is minimal, but a seropurulent drainage is present • A pit is evident in the midline approximately 5 cm above the anus	Diagnosis • Visual examination Treatment • Incision and drainage: wound may be left open and allowed to heal by second intention (granulation). • Various techniques used for the sinus path
Hemorrhoids	• Generally asymptomatic • Painful protrusions that bleed and itch • Mucoid discharge • Inspection of the anal orifice reveals thickening of the columns of Morgagni that appear as bluish lumps beneath the skin or as distinct, prolapsed purplish bodies	Diagnosis • Anoscopy Treatment • Nonoperative treatments: sitz baths, dietary supplements, topical medications, and injections • Hemorrhoidectomy for severe prolapse or other complications • Rubber-band ligation is a conservative intervention that is usually done in the office setting

Table 14-14 Select Pathology and Treatment of Liver Disorders

Pathology	*Symptoms/Signs*	*Treatment*
Primary malignancy	• Abdominal pain and weight loss • Palpable mass, arterial bruit, friction rub, **ascites**	• Partial hepatectomy • Arterial ligation • Chemotherapy
Secondary malignancy (metastasis)	• Same as primary	• Chemotherapy for the primary neoplasm
Hepatic adenoma	• Right upper quadrant pain in females taking birth control pills • Right upper quadrant mass • Massive intra-abdominal hemorrhage	• Discontinue birth control pills and observe • Enucleation • Partial hepatectomy when symptomatic
Nodular hyperplasia	• Usually asymptomatic • Right upper quadrant discomfort not associated with birth control pills	• Surgical removal only if symptomatic
Hemangioma	• Occasional pain or discomfort • Palpable mass • May rupture	• Excision if symptomatic • Radiotherapy • Arterial ligation
Hepatic cysts	• Occasional right upper quadrant discomfort • Occasional mass	• Usually none • Percutaneous or open drainage if symptomatic
Hepatic abscess	• High fever • Right upper quadrant pain • Jaundice • Enlarged and tender liver	• Percutaneous or open drainage • Antibiotics
Trauma/laceration	• Intra-abdominal bleeding • Hypovolemic shock	• Surgical repair of laceration • Partial resection • Arterial ligation

PROCEDURE 14-12 Hemorrhoidectomy

Surgical Anatomy and Pathology

- Rectum descends in an anteroposterior curve called the sacral flexure traveling through the pelvic cavity and joins the anal canal. A layer of muscle surrounds the rectum.
- Last portion of the colon is the anal canal that opens to the outside of the body through the anus.
  - Two sphincter muscles are located around the anus: internal sphincter composed of involuntary smooth muscle supported by the levator ani muscles; external sphincter composed of voluntary skeletal muscle.
- Mucous membrane of the anal canal consists of longitudinal folds called anal columns that contain arteries and veins.
- Anal valves are located just above the anus and just above the valves are the anal sinuses.
- A hemorrhoid is an abnormal enlarment of a vein or veins, referred to as a *varicosity* or *varicose vein,* in the lower rectum or anus. Hemorrhoids can be internal or external. Internal hemorrhoids occur above the internal sphincter of the anus. External hemorrhoids appear outside the anal sphincter.

Preoperative Diagnostic Tests and Procedures

- History and physical
- Hemorrhoidectomy indicated in cases of third- and fourth-degree hemorrhoids

Equipment and Instruments Unique to Procedure

- CO_2 laser may be used for vaporization and coagulation of hemorrhoid tissue
- Headlamp available
- Rectal set that includes:
  - Anscope (Figure 14-16)
  - Rectal speculum
  - Rectal dilators
  - Buie pile forceps
  - Crypt hook

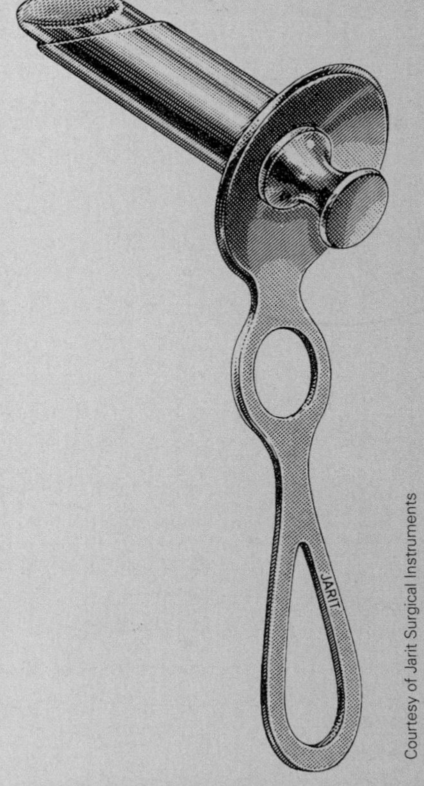

Courtesy of Jarit Surgical Instruments

Figure 14-16 Hirschmann anoscope

Procedure 14-12 (continued)

Supplies Unique to Procedure

- #10 knife blades × 2
- Surgical or Gelfoam
- Local anesthesia of surgeon's choice; often 0.5% lidocaine with epinephrine
- K-Y jelly lubricant
- Benzoin spray
- Tape

Preoperative Preparation

- Kraske, lithotomy, or lateral position
- General, spinal, or local anesthesia
- Skin prep: Enema 1–2 hours preoperatively; shaving of hair may be required, especially for the male patient; formal prep not required; benzoin sprayed onto skin and tape applied to retract buttocks.

Practical Considerations

- Do not overuse benzoin; used to protect skin from tape and aids in securing tape in place.
- If spinal or local anesthesia is used, be aware that the patient may be embarrassed and uncomfortable when placed in the surgical position and words of comfort will be helpful.

Surgical Procedure

1. A Fansler speculum is inserted to expose the anal canal past the anorectal ring dentate line.

   Procedural Consideration: Lubricate rectal speculum for ease of insertion.

2. Hemostats are placed on the protruding components.

   Procedural Considerations: The largest, most redundant group is approached first.

3. The area around the hemorrhoid group is incised in an elliptical manner with care taken not to cross the dentate line.

   Procedural Consideration: Pass scalpel.

4. External hemorrhoids are dissected from the external and internal sphincters.

   Procedural Consideration: Have hemorrhoidal clamp ready.

5. A hemorrhoid clamp is then applied to the internal hemorrhoids, and all tissue above the clamp is removed.

   Procedural Consideration: Specimens are labeled and sent to pathology for examination. Have suture ready.

6. The resultant pedicle is suture ligated with 3-0 chromic, released, and oversewn.

   Procedural Consideration: Assist with suture as needed.

7. The mucosa is then approximated with interrupted 3-0 chromic.

   Procedural Consideration: Prepare to repeat process.

8. The excision procedure is repeated on the other group(s) of hemorrhoids.

   Procedural Consideration: Have suture ready. Perform counts.

9. Gelfoam or Surgicel sheet may be flattened, rolled, and inserted into the anal canal to provide hemostasis, and a dry dressing is applied over it.

Postoperative Considerations

Immediate Postoperative Care

- Transport to PACU.

Prognosis

- No complications: May be discharged same day of surgery; return to normal activities 48–72 hours. Patient education includes how to protect area during healing, cleaning area after bowel movements. Stool softener should be used for short period of time.
- Complications: pain; hemorrhage; SSI; recurrence of hemorrhoids; constipation.

Wound Classification

- Class II: Clean contaminated

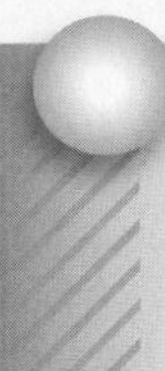

PEARL OF WISDOM

If the width of the hemorrhoidal elliptical excision surpasses 1.5 cm, the wound may be left open to heal by second intention and the packing will need to be changed while healing is occurring.

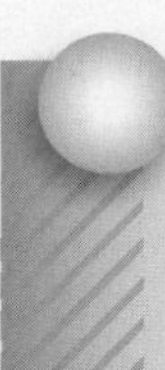

PEARL OF WISDOM

Prioritize! This is the key concept in preparing for trauma surgery. What must be ready first in order to save a life? What must be ready to correct the condition? Then, what must be ready to create a better outcome? Organize your mind and instruments accordingly.

LIVER RESECTION

Liver resection is most commonly performed to excise hepatocellular tumor. It may also be performed as part of the course of treatment for carcinoma of the gallbladder, to resolve uncontrollable bleeding or parenchymal maceration following abdominal trauma, or for transplant. Liver cancer is one of the most common solid organ cancers; the liver is a common site for metastatic disease from other organs as well. Although resection is an effective intervention, many patients are not good candidates. Factors such as associated liver disease, extrahepatic metastases, large tumor size, or major hepatic vascular involvement may make resection untenable. The ideal setting for liver resection is a small (2- to 5-cm) tumor in a noncirrhotic liver, but this is uncommon. Cirrhosis of the liver is associated with hepatocellular carcinoma as a result of viral hepatitis or alcohol abuse.

PROCEDURE 14-13 Liver Resection

Surgical Anatomy and Pathology	• Liver is located inferior to the diaphragm in the right abdominal quadrant. • It is covered by a fibrous and serous coat called Glisson's capsule. • Divided into two lobes: right and left lobes, which are divided by the falciform ligament that also attaches the organ to the diaphragm and abdominal wall anteriorly.	• Two additional smaller lobes located in the right lobe: quadrate lobe located next to the gallbladder; caudate lobe located next to the vena cava. • Porta hepatic: surgical anatomical landmark; region where the right and left lobes join; also region where the hepatic artery and portal vein enter the liver, and the common heptic duct exits the liver.	• On the superior side of the liver the coronary ligament anchors the liver to the diaphragm. • Liver is highly vascular organ in which the vessels subdivide many times. The primary vessels are the hepatic artery, portal vein, and hepatic vein. • See section "Liver Resection" for information pertaining to pathology.
Preoperative Diagnostic Tests and Procedures	• History and physical • Laboratory tests: blood tests • Liver scan	• CT scan • Liver biopsy (only procedure that provides a definitive diagnosis)	
Equipment and Instruments Unique to Procedure	• Hypo-/hyperthermia unit • Cell-saver available • Cavitron or plasma knife available • Suction apparatus × 2 • Headlamp available	• Major instrument set • Long and deep instruments • Peripheral vascular instrument set • Gallbladder instruments	• Thoracotomy instrument set available • Hemoclip appliers with ligating clips–will need several appliers and clips

PROCEDURE 14-13 (continued)

Supplies Unique to Procedure	• Several #10 knife blades • Gelfoam or Surgical– according to surgeon's preference	• Vessel loops • Suction tips and tubing × 2	• Long Bovie tip
Preoperative Preparation	• Supine or modified lateral position • General anesthesia • Skin prep: shoulders bilaterally (use the clavicle as anatomical landmark) to mid-thighs and bilaterally as far as possible	• Fole catheter inserted • Draping: square off with four towels–edge of upper towel placed mid-chest; lateral towels placed using anterior superior iliac spines as guide; edge of lower towel placed just above line of	sympysis pubis; laparotomy drape. Surgeon may want to place an incise drape that is impregnated with an antimicrobial iodine agent; the incise drape is placed prior to the placement of the laparotomy drape.
Practical Considerations	• Confirm availability of blood with the blood bank. • X-rays and CT scans in OR. • Blood loss must be carefully monitored; keep track of irrigation that is used in order to assist with determing blood loss in suction container.	• Be prepared to set up and use the cell-saver. • Liver is highly vascular; have several types of hemostatic clamps as well as a large number of ties. Electrocautery will be often used; keep the tip clean. Have other methods to control bleeding immediately available, such as Gelfoam or Surgicel.	• Sutures of choice are absorbable with a short **absorption** rate as the liver tissue tends to heal quicky. In the absence of hemorrhage, small-size sutures will most likely be used. The surgeon may prefer to use suture attached to a blunt tip needle to aid in preventing bleeding.

Surgical Procedure

1. Incision choice varies but most common is an ipsilateral subcostal (Kocher) incision.
2. After entering the abdomen, the liver is appropriately mobilized and inspected for extent and possibility of resection.

   Procedural Consideration: Handheld retractors may be used for initial evaluation. Long instruments may be needed. Procedure may be terminated at this point.
3. Prior to beginning liver resection, the Pringle maneuver is often performed to control blood flow (allows up to 60 minutes before tissue damage occurs). The Pringle maneuver involves clamping a large hemostat across the lesser omentum to temporarily interrupt the flow of blood through the hepatic artery and the portal vein to help control bleeding from the liver. Control of blood supply may also be performed by balloon occlusion or clamping of the infrahepatic and suprahepatic inferior vena cava.

   Procedural Consideration: Have vascular clamp available for Pringle maneuver or other methods such as Gelfoam to control hemorrhage. Be prepared to use cell-saver until a tumor is present.

(*continues*)

PROCEDURE 14-13 (continued)

4. Division of the parenchyma is undertaken in a "segmental" or "lobular" fashion, utilizing a scalpel and/or electrosurgery, and ligation of the artery/vein/duct triad is performed, addressing each structure individually, as it is encountered.

   Procedural Consideration: May need to replace regular-length Bovie tip with long tip. Make sure to have several hemoclip appliers loaded and ready to use. Right-angle clamps will be used for separation of liver tissue. Have suture loaded on long needle holders to use for the control of bleeding.

5. Resection continues until the desired amount of liver is excised, preserving as much of the functional liver parenchyma as possible.

6. After resection, occlusive devices (refer to Step 3) are released, and hemostasis is achieved. Hemostatic agents may be applied to the parenchyma, and the abdomen is closed.

   Procedural Considerations: Hemostatic agents should be ready for use. The surgeon may use a large amount of warm saline for irrigation.

Postoperative Considerations

Immediate Postoperative Care

- Transport to PACU or ICU.

Prognosis

- No complications: Return to normal activities in 6–8 weeks; however, depending on health condition of patient and follow-up treatment for cancer such as chemotherapy, lifestyle may be altered.
- Complications: hemorrhage; SSI; bile leak; liver failure; tumor recurrence; liver resection has a 5% mortality rate.

Wound Classification

- Class I: Clean
- Class II: Clean contaminated (if gallbladder included in procedure)

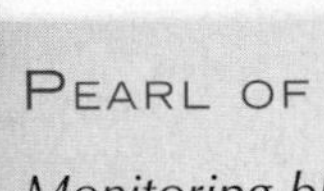

PEARL OF WISDOM

Monitoring blood loss is always important. In procedures such as liver trauma and resection it is essential. Keep a sterile marker and a sterile piece of paper to write notes on. Log how much irrigation has been used. Place a scale in the room so the circulator can weigh sponges. Listen for the anesthesia provider to ask questions about blood loss. Be prepared to communicate how many sponges and how much irrigation have been used.

As important as the liver is to life, loss of significant portions of the liver can be survived. The liver is divided into eight segments, each with its own arterial supply, venous drainage, and ductal system (Figure 14-17). For this reason liver resection of up to 80–90% of the organ can be safely performed. Compensatory hypertrophy and hyperplasia, occurring within 3 to 6 weeks after resection (partial hepatectomy), can result in regeneration of the liver to almost normal size.

Surgical Treatment of Gallbladder Disease

Gallbladder disease is seen daily in the OR. In this section, a logical sequence will be presented so the student can appreciate the pathology, conservative interventions, and a progressively complicated series of surgical interventions. The sequence is as follows:

- Conservative, noninvasive treatment
- Open **chole**cystectomy with cholangiogram
- Laparoscopic cholecystectomy

Cholelithiasis represents a significant health problem in the United States. Gallstones (calculi) are classified as being either cholesterol or pigmented. Cholesterol gallstones are a by-product of liver bile that is supersaturated with cholesterol, which then precipitates from the bile to form crystals that grow to macroscopic stones. Pigmented gallstones are composed of calcium bilirubinate, bilirubin polymers, bile acids, iron, and phosphorus, and may be black, dark brown, yellow, or green.

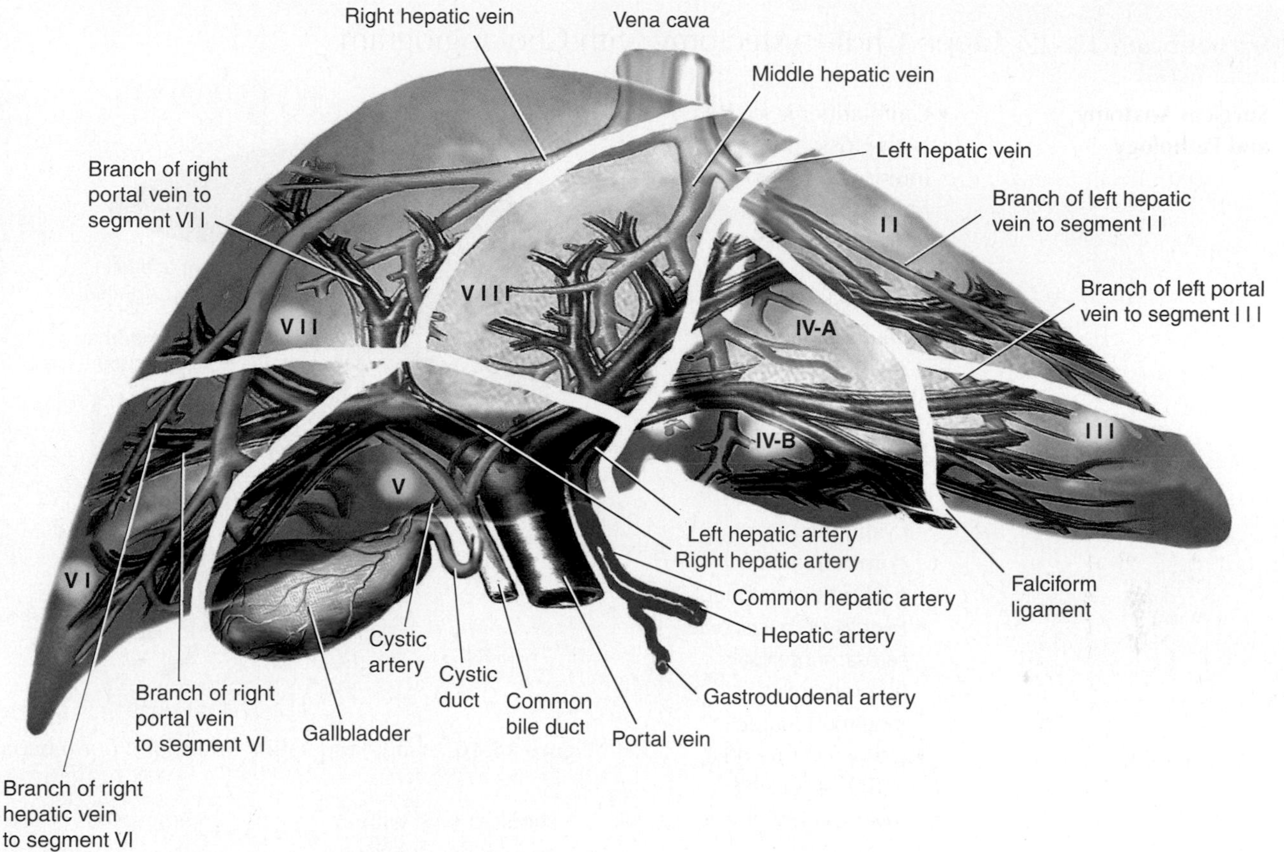

Figure 14-17 Segmental blood supply and ductal system of the liver

Conservative Treatment for Cholelithiasis

Cholelithiasis can be treated with medications designed to dissolve them or by extracorporeal shock-wave lithotripsy (ESWL). The electro-generated shock waves pass through soft tissue without harm, but the solid gallstones absorb them and become fragmented. ESWL fragments the gallstones into pieces that are small enough to pass down the cystic duct and common bile duct (CBD) into the alimentary system, where they can be expelled with fecal material. Ultrasound is used to compute the exact location of the target gallstones. The ideal patient for ESWL will have a solitary gallstone less than 2 cm in diameter.

Medications for treatment of cholelithiasis include ursodiol, which reduces cholesterol saturation, and oral bile acids. These medications attack only calcium free gallstones; about 15% of patients with gallstones are candidates for pharmaceutic treatment. This form of therapy may follow ESWL to dissolve the fragments created by that procedure. Although dissolution is usually achieved (50% success rate) within 2 years, half of all patients will develop more gallstones within 5 years of treatment. Methyl tert-butyl ether (MTBE) may also be used to dissolve gallstones by direct injection into the gallbladder through a 7 Fr catheter introduced via the percutaneous transhepatic method. Liver hemorrhage may occur; packing the tract with Gelfoam lowers this risk.

CHOLECYSTECTOMY AND CHOLANGIOGRAPHY

Cholecystectomy is excision of the gallbladder. This procedure is primarily performed for acute cholecystitis.

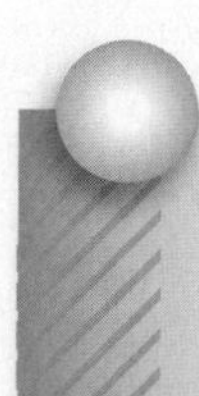

Pearl of Wisdom

Ensure that all air has been expelled from the cholangiography system—air bubbles can resemble stones on an X-ray. Hold the syringe with the plunger up so microscopic bubbles do not get injected.

Procedure 14-14 Open Cholecystectomy with Cholangiogram

Surgical Anatomy and Pathology

- Gallbladder is located in the fossa on the inferior surface of the right lobe of the liver above the transverse colon and next to the duodenal cap.
  - Divided into four regions: fundus, body, infundibulum, neck
  - Hartman's pouch located at the junction with the cystic duct; a common area for gallstones to collect
  - Four tissue layers: outer serosa; subserosal; fibromuscular; innermost mucosa
  - Common bile duct (CBD) is formed from joining of the cystic duct and hepatic duct.
  - Triangle of Calot: anatomic triangle formed by cystic duct, common hepatic duct, and inferior boder of liver; used to locate the cystic artery, which is usually within the triangle
  - Arterial blood supply: cystic artery, right hepatic artery, posterior superior pancreaticoduodenal artery (Figure 14-18)
  - Sympathetic nerve innervation: splanchnic nerve and hepatic plexus that have motor and sensory function and communicate with fibers of the right phrenic nerve, which explains the "referred" shoulder pain with gallbladder disease

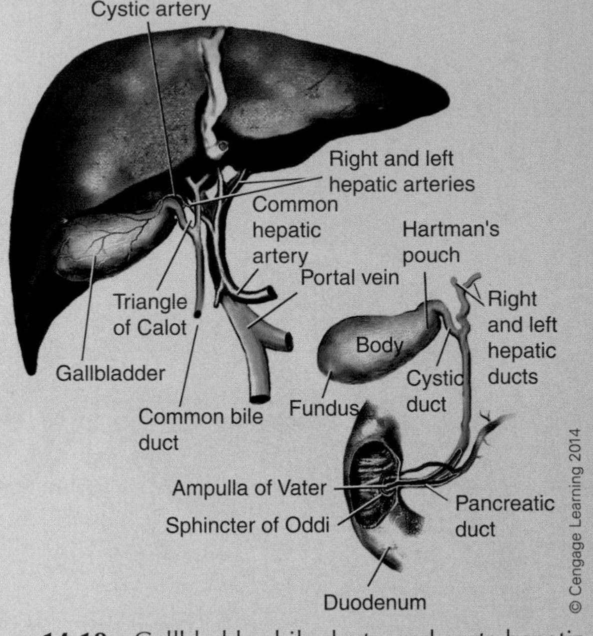

Figure 14-18 Gallbladder, bile ducts, and porta hepatic

- Cholecystitis commonly results from obstruction of the cystic duct by gallstones trapped in Hartman's pouch.
  - Other indications include chronic cholecystitis, calcified gallbladder, tumor of the gallbladder, presence of asymptomatic gallstones larger than 2 cm, biliary peritonitis, traumatic rupture of the gallbladder.
  - Acute cholecystitis produces severe pain in the RUQ, fever, nausea, vomiting, jaundice, and tenderness along the right costal margin; the pain may be referred to the shoulder. Acute cholecystitis is also associated with bacterial inflammation; *E. coli*, salmonella, streptococci, and clostridia have all been implicated. Left untreated, acute cholecystitis can lead to empyema, perforation of the gallbladder, abscess formation, cholecystenteric fistula, ischemia, impairment of venous return, and necrosis.
  - Cholecystitis is most common in females who are over 40 years of age, premenopausal, and obese.
- Contraindications for performing gallbladder surgery include liver cirrhosis, advanced age, presence of small asymptomatic gallstones

PROCEDURE 14-14 (continued)

Preoperative Diagnostic Tests and Procedures	• History and physical • Abdominal X-rays	• Laboratory blood tests (usually reveal an increased white cell	count and elevated serum bilirubin)
Equipment and Instruments Unique to Procedure	• OR table that is compatible with using X-ray cassettes or C-arm • Major instrument set	• Long and deep instruments • Gallbladder instrument set that includes CBD exploration instruments	• Upper Hand or Thompson retractor • Hemoclip appliers with ligating clips • C-arm
Supplies Unique to Procedure	• Knife blades: #10 × 2; #11 or #15 • Long Bovie tip • Cholangiogram supplies: Cholangiogram catheter; syringe × 2 (one for saline; other	for contrast medium); contrast medium • Magnetic instrument pad • Aerobic and anaerobic cultures • C-arm drape (available; do not open unless needed)	• Have ties of various sizes available; usually 1-0, 2-0, and 3-0 silk ties • Active drainage system (Hemovac; Jackson-Pratt)
Preoperative Preparation	• Supine position with slight reverse Trendelenburg • General anesthesia • Skin prep: mid-chest to symphysis pubis and	bilaterally as far as possible • Draping: square off with four towels–edge of upper towel placed mid-chest; lateral	towels placed using anterior superior iliac spines as guide; edge of lower towel placed at umbilical level; laparotomy drape
Practical Considerations	• Have X-rays in the OR. • Anticipate intraoperative cholangiogram and know how to set up the cholangiogram catheter. • Wear an X-ray apron under sterile gown for protection unless existing OR into	sub-sterile room while X-ray is taken during cholangiogram. • Have smooth, fine forceps for the surgeon to use for the insertion of the cholangiogram as well as a grooved director to help guide the catheter into the CBD.	• Place magnetic instrument pad on the sterile field to facilitate the surgeon quickly grabbing instruments that are frequently used and not having to wait for them to be passed.

Surgical Procedure

1. Several incisional options exist; right subcostal (Kocher) is preferred.

   Procedural Considerations: Prior to the incision being made, provide the crossbar/horizontal bar of the Upper Hand or Thompson retractor to be placed into the rail clamps that were slid into position on the OR table before the patient was brought into the OR. Next, provide the joints that slide onto the crossbar that hold the retracting blades in place. Provide two green towels that will be wrapped around the arms of the crossbar at the level of the drape to prevent contamination because the arms are inserted through the drape in order to attach to the rail clamps. Prepare for routine laparotomy; normal incision and exposure procedures will be followed. Kocher incision is a muscle-splitting incision. Electrocautery will be heavily used and a suction will be necessary to evacuate the plume. As the surgeon dissects down to the gallbladder, provide retractors such as Richardsons for deep retraction.

(continues)

Procedure 14-14 (continued)

2. The gallbladder is explored and any apparent adhesions are first released by blunt or sharp dissection. Packs are placed to protect adjacent visceral structures and to further isolate the gallbladder, and retractors are placed.

   Procedural Consideration: Prepare warm, moist lap sponges for packing; loosely roll up each sponge to facilitate the surgeon placing in the abdomen. Provide the Upper Hand or Thompson retractor blades of surgeon's choice. Peanut sponges loaded on a Pean may be used for blunt dissection.

3. The lesser omentum is opened and the associated ducts and vasculature are identified.

   Procedural Consideration: Long curved Metzenbaum scissors, tissue forceps such as the DeBakey, and right-angle clamps will be used. Have hemoclip appliers loaded and ready for use.

4. Once the gallbladder is exposed, a Kelly clamp is placed near the ampulla and traction is applied inferiorly and medially to place the peritoneum overlying the cystic duct and artery under tension.

   Procedural Consideration: Electrosurgery may used to free the gallbladder from the liver bed; replace the regular Bovie tip with longer tip if necessary. Keep the Bovie tip clean using the scratch pad because it will be often used.

5. The peritoneum is incised with Metzenbaum scissors. Using a right angle and blunt dissection, the cystic artery is identified and followed toward the gallbladder until it is certain that the structure is not the right hepatic artery.

   Procedural Consideration: Long scissors, tissue forceps, right-angle clamp, and electrosurgery will be used repeatedly. Keep available for immediate reuse; some surgeons prefer the instruments be kept on the sterile field to be easily retrieved from the magnetic instrument pad.

6. The cystic artery is then double ligated with 2-0 silk or ligating clips are placed across it near the gallbladder, and the artery is transected between the ties or clips.

   Procedural Consideration: Ties will likely be used on passers; load the ties onto tonsil or Pean clamp and have them loaded in advance.

7. The cystic duct, which lies inferior and lateral to the cystic artery, is then isolated by blunt dissection, and its junction with the CBD is identified.

   Procedural Consideration: Anticipate the same procedure for securing and transecting the cystic duct as was carried out on the cystic artery.

8. If necessary, an intraoperative cholangiogram is performed at this point. A stab incision is made in the cystic duct, about 2 cm from the CBD, and 4-0 chromic stay sutures are placed on either side of the wound.

   Procedural Consideration: Prepare the cholangiogram catheter when setting up the back table and Mayo stand. When it is close to the time to perform the cholangiogram, the circulator will contact the X-ray department to have a technician come to the OR If a C-arm is being used, the surgical technologist will need to place a C-arm drape. Request the circulator to pour the contrast solution into a small basin on the back table. When drawing up the saline and contrast solution, make sure no bubbles are present in the syringes before handing the cholangiocath with syringes attached to the surgeon; tap the syringes gently to make the bubbles rise to the top and gently remove by pushing on the plunger. Tie a silk tie around the syringe with saline as a marker; saline and contrast medium are both clear in color and the surgeon needs to know the

Procedure 14-14 (continued)

difference between the two syringes. A #11 or #15 knife blade followed by 45° angled Potts scissors will be used for chole**docho**tomy. Two stay sutures, 4-0 of surgeon's choice, and hemostats to tag the sutures will be needed.

9. The duct is gently probed for patency and usually bile will ooze out. A cholangiogram catheter is introduced into the duct and secured with a ligating clip across the duct.

   Procedural Consideration: Surgeon may request culture of bile; request circulator to open aerobic and anaerobic cultures. Suction will be needed to remove bile. A probe with grooved director should be available for the surgeon to probe the CBD. Provide fine-tipped forceps for the surgeon to grasp the end of the catheter and insert into the CBD.

10. The duct is aspirated until bile is drawn into the saline syringe and the duct is flushed with the saline. The dilute contrast medium is then instilled into the duct and an X-ray is taken.

    Procedural Consideration: Be sure to remind the surgeon the syringe with the silk tie contains saline. Be sure all team members are protected from the radiation before the X-ray is taken.

11. The X-ray should reveal the structure of the CBD and hepatic duct, as well as demonstrate spillage into the duodenum without any sign of ductal gallstones. (Percutaneous cholangiography requires the same basic steps.)

    Procedural Consideration: Anticipate instruments needed for a CBD exploration if gallstones are visible on X-ray.

12. Traction is then reapplied to the gallbladder in changing directions as needed. With blunt and sharp dissection, the gallbladder is excised from the liver bed. Small bleeders in this area are controlled electrosurgically.

    Procedural Considerations: Electrosurgery will be heavily used to dissect the gallbladder from the liver bed. Place a scratch pad near the surgeon, who will need to clean the tip frequently.

13. Excision of the gallbladder is usually performed from the cystic duct to the fundus. However, if these structures are difficult to discern, dissection may begin at the fundus and proceed to the duct.

    Procedural Consideration: Have a kidney basin available for the surgeon to place the gallbladder. Do not immediately pass off the kidney basin to the circulator; the surgeon may want to open the gallbladder to examine the contents and take additional cultures of the fluid. Give the surgeon the skin knife to open the gallbladder. Once the surgeon is finished with the specimen the circulator can prepare it for transport to pathology.

14. The specimen is removed from the wound, the area is irrigated and checked for hemostasis, and the abdomen is closed.

    Procedural Consideration: The active drain may be placed at this time. The deep knife with #10 knife blade will be needed to make the stab incision for the drain tube. A copious amount of warm irrigation will be used to irrigate the liver bed and abdomen, which will also help to identify any small bleeders in the liver bed to be cauterized.

(*continues*)

Procedure 14-14 (continued)

Postoperative Considerations	**Immediate Postoperative Care** • Transport to PACU. **Prognosis** • No complications: Return to normal activities in 8–10 weeks.	• Complications: hemorrhage; SSI; atelectasis; ileus; hepatic artery injury; hepatic bile duct injury; injury to the porta hepatic structures; persistent bile drainage; retention of duct stones; spillage from ducts or gallbladder contaminates abdomen.	**Wound Classification** • Class II: Clean contaminated • Class III: Contaminated (if gross spillage occurred)

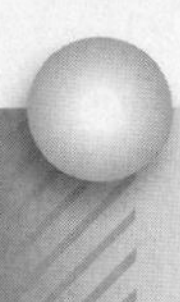

Pearl of Wisdom

Cholecystectomy with cholangiogram is one of those procedures that illustrates a routine problem: significant movement by nonsterile team members around the sterile field. Observe carefully the movement of the radiology technologist and protect the sterile field from potential contamination.

Cholecystectomy is performed through laparoscopic means in up to 90% of all cases, and this route is successful 95% of the time. However, conversion to the open procedure does occur and some patients are best treated in this manner. The open cholecystectomy and laparoscopic procedures are presented; the anatomy and pathology, preoperative diagnostic tests and procedures, and preoperative preparation are the same for both procedures.

Procedure 14-15 Laparoscopic Cholecystectomy

Intraoperative cholangiogram will not be repeated; refer to the open procedure.

Equipment and Instruments Unique to Procedure (Plate 14-8)	• 30° laparoscope • Two 5-mm trocars • Two 10- or 11-mm trocars (surgeon's preference; for purposes of continuity the surgical procedure will refer to 10-mm trocars)	• Endoscopic instrumentation, including Babcock, curved clamps, spatula, electrocautery hook, endoscopic hemoclip appliers, endoscopic suction/irrigator, and curved Metzenbaum scissors	• Laparoscopic tower with additional "slave" monitor for assistant • Insufflator with tubing • Have laparotomy instruments and supplies available in the event the procedure converts to an open procedure
Supplies Unique to Procedure	• #11 knife blade (have #10 and #15 knife blades unopened but available in case laparoscopic procedure is converted to an open procedure) • Long endoscopic Bovie tip		• 10-cc syringe • Endobag • T-tube
Preoperative Preparation	• Only variation from open procedure is draping; the bottom towel will be placed at the symphysis pubis		

PROCEDURE 14-15 (continued)

Practical Considerations	• The surgical technologist will often be responsible for manipulating the camera during the procedure and holding the grasping forceps
Surgical Procedure	1. Using a #11 knife blade, a small incision is made in the umbilicus. The pneumoperitoneum is established by inserting the Verres needle through the incision and the CO_2 is introduced into the peritoneal cavity (Plate 14-9). Some surgeons may use the saline drop test to confirm the position of the Veress needle. A 10-cc syringe with saline is attached to the Verres needle and the saline is injected. Absence of resistance to injecting confirms the Verres needle is positioned in the peritoneal cavity. **Procedural Consideration:** The surgeon and surgical technologist will elevate the skin on each side of the umbilicus to facilitate abdominal contents falling away and prevent injury when the Verres needle is inserted.
	2. The Verres needle is removed and replaced with a 10-mm trocar and sheath; the trocar is removed and the laparoscope with camera is inserted (Plate 14-10). The patient is now placed in slight Trendelenburg position. **Procedural Consideration:** The laparoscope will be inserted and the surgical technologist may be responsible for attaching the camera and light cord.
	3. The three other trocars are placed as follows: 10-mm placed subxiphoid; two 5-mm trocars placed in the right upper quadrant, subcostally at the midclavicular and anterior axillary lines (Plate 14-11).
	4. Grasping forceps are placed through a 5-mm port and the gallbladder is grasped cephalad. The gallbladder is gently retracted to elevate the edge of the liver, thus exposing the entire gallbladder, cystic duct, and cystic artery. Another grasper is inserted through the other 5-mm port to grasp the gallbladder infundibulum. Gentle traction is placed on the gallbladder and the triangle of Calot can now be viewed (Figure 14-19; Plate 14-12). **Procedural Consideration:** As mentioned, the gallbladder must be gently retracted to prevent perforation as well as damage to the delicate liver tissue.
	5. If the gallbladder is highly distended by bile fluid, it may be suctioned using an endoscopic needle aspirator to decrease the size of the organ.
	6. The cystic duct and artery are identified. Using scissors, grasper, and electrocautery hook, the duct and artery are dissected free from surrounding tissue (Plates 14-13 to 14-15). Next, the cystic duct is divided. Some types of ESU hooks have a port through which suction can be applied in order to suction the smoke plume during the dissection. Two to three hemoclips are placed on the duct and it is divided (Plates 14-16 and 14-17). Prior to dividing the cystic duct, a cholangiogram may be performed. **Procedural Consideration:** if the ESU hook does not have a port for suction, an endoscopic suction/irrigator may need to be placed down a trocar in order to remove the plume from the use of the electrocautery hook in order to make sure the surgeon can visualize the surgical site.
	7. Two to three hemoclips are placed on the cystic artery and it is divided (Plate 14-18).

(*continues*)

PROCEDURE 14-15 (continued)

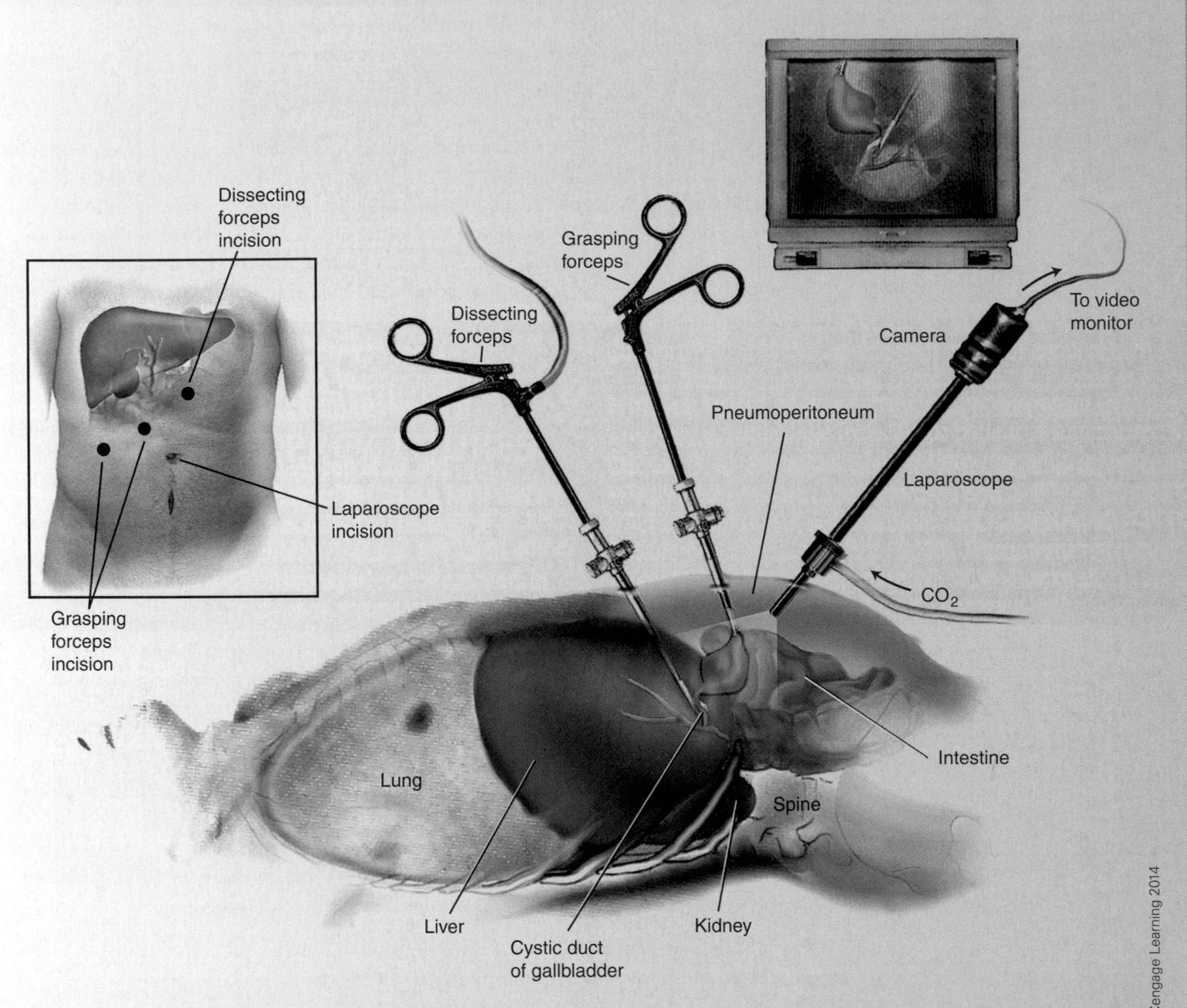

Figure 14-19 Laparoscopic cholecystectomy: (A) Lateral view

8. The gallbladder can now be dissected from the underside of the liver. Continuous upward traction is maintained on the gallbladder with the use of the graspers to facilitate dissection of the tissue. The surgeon will use scissors and, frequently, the ESU hook to dissect the tissue and free up the gallbladder (Plates 14-19 to 14-21).

9. Once free, the gallbladder is removed through the umbilical port with the aid of a grasper (Plate 14-22). Prior to removal the gallbladder may be placed in an endobag to contain the specimen and prevent spillage of bile into the peritoneal cavity. If the gallbladder is distended, the neck may be brought out through the umbilical incision, hemostats applied to the edges, and the bile suctioned out to decompress it; the gallbladder can then be removed in its entirety (Plates 14-23 and 14-24).

PROCEDURE 14-15 (continued)

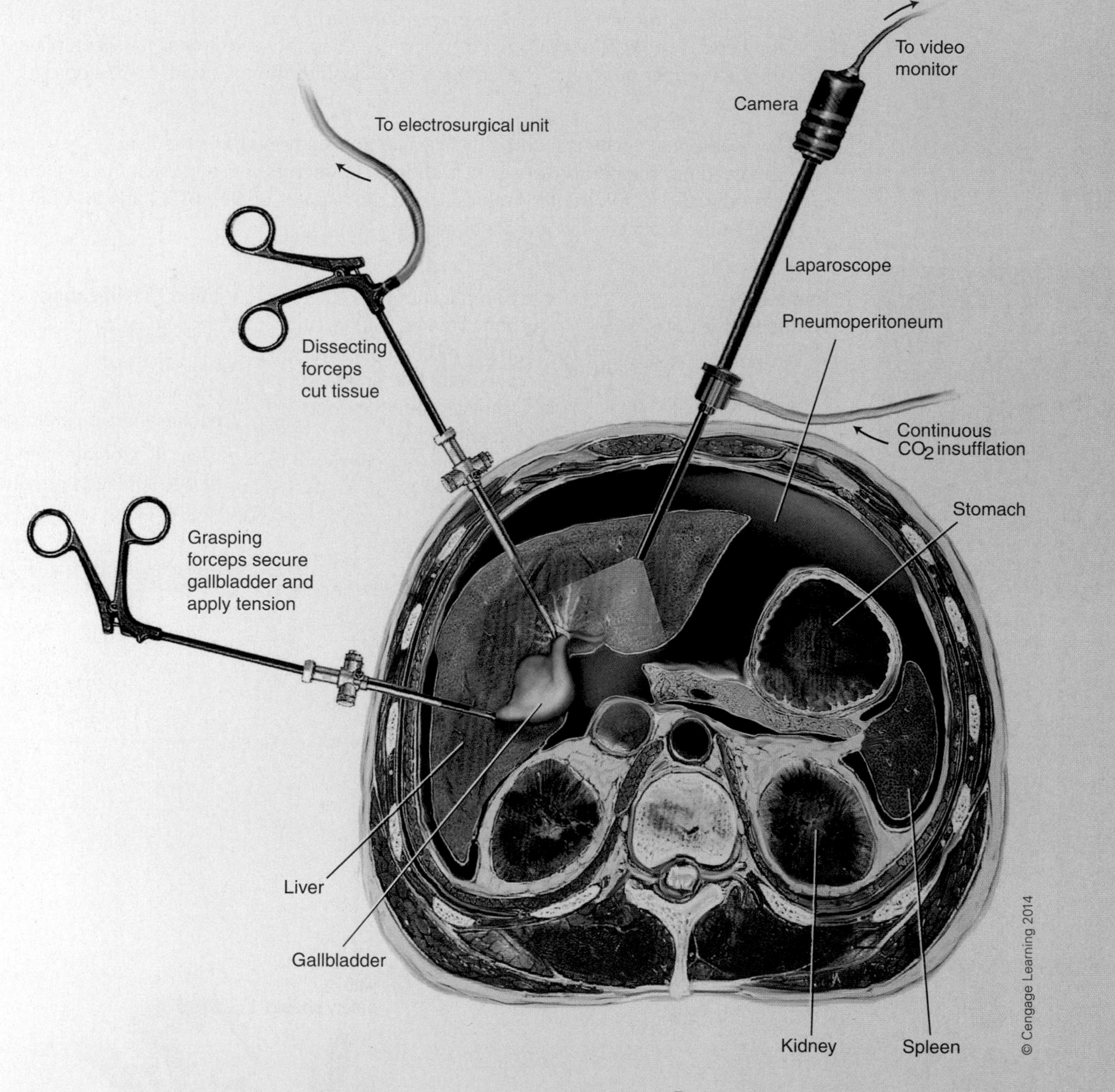

Figure 14-19 Laparoscopic cholecystectomy: (B) Cross-section view

Procedural Consideration: The umbilical incision may need to be slightly widened with the #15 knife blade.

10. The surgical technologist receives the specimen by having it placed into a kidney basin and passes it off to the circulator. Occasionally the surgeon may request that a culture of the gallbladder be completed prior to passing it off to the circulator.

11. If necessary, a T-tube is placed to provide postoperative drainage of bile. The limbs of the T-tube are cut to size by the surgeon and the tube is inserted through the

(continues)

Procedure 14-15 (continued)

subxyphoid trocar. The limbs are placed superiorly and inferiorly in the CBD and the long end is brought out through the incision where a 5-mm trocar has been placed in the right upper quadrant. The CBD is closed around the tube with endoscopic sutures.

12. The peritoneal cavity is thoroughly irrigated and suctioned and the liver bed checked for bleeding. The peritoneal cavity is allowed to decompress and each trocar site is closed with 1–2 interrupted sutures and/or skin staples (Plates 14-25 and 14-26). The T-tube is attached to the drainage bag.

Postoperative Considerations

Immediate Postoperative Care

- Transport to PACU.

Prognosis

- No complications: Hospital stay is usually less than 24 hours; return to normal activities in 1–2 weeks.
- Complications: hemorrhage; SSI; hepatic artery or bile duct injury; persistent bile drainage; spillage from bile ducts or gallbladder contaminating the peritoneal cavity.

Wound Classification

- Class I: Clean
- Class II: Clean contaminated (if cholangiogram performed)
- Class III: Contaminated (if bile spillage from duct or gallbladder occurs)

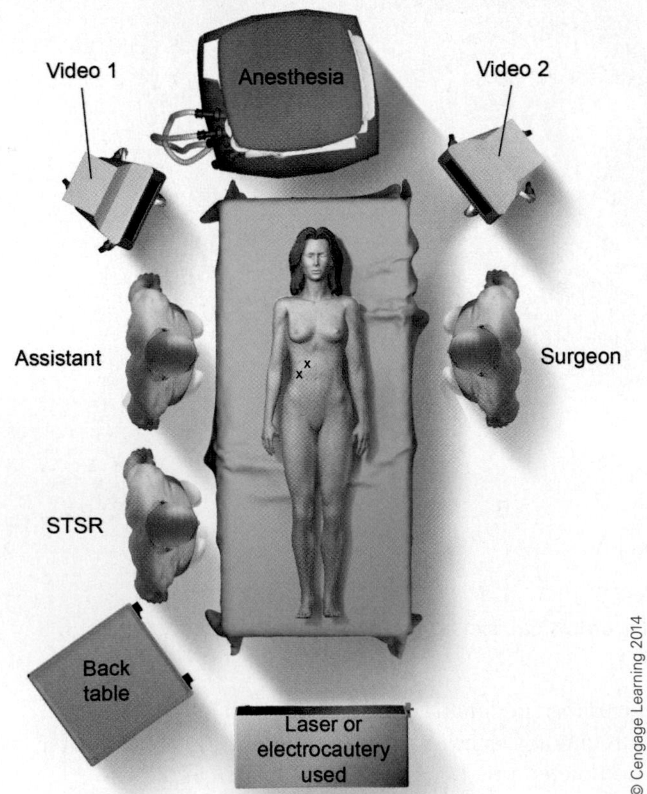

Plate 14-8 Room setup and patient position

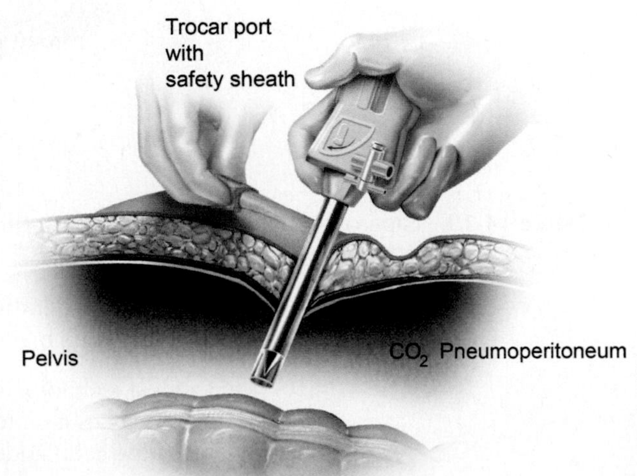

Plate 14-10 Trocar with sheath is inserted

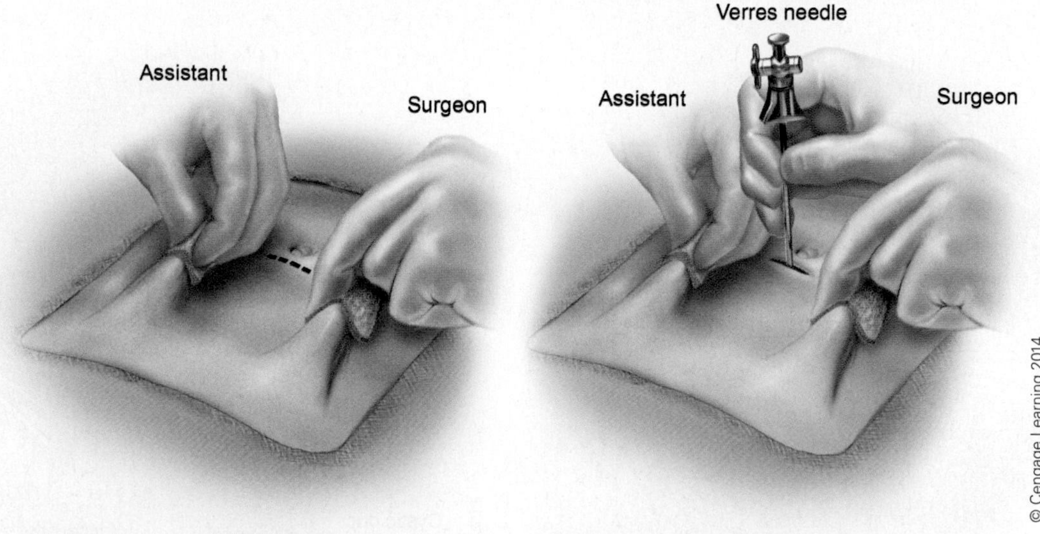

Plate 14-9 Umbilical incision and insertion of Verres needle

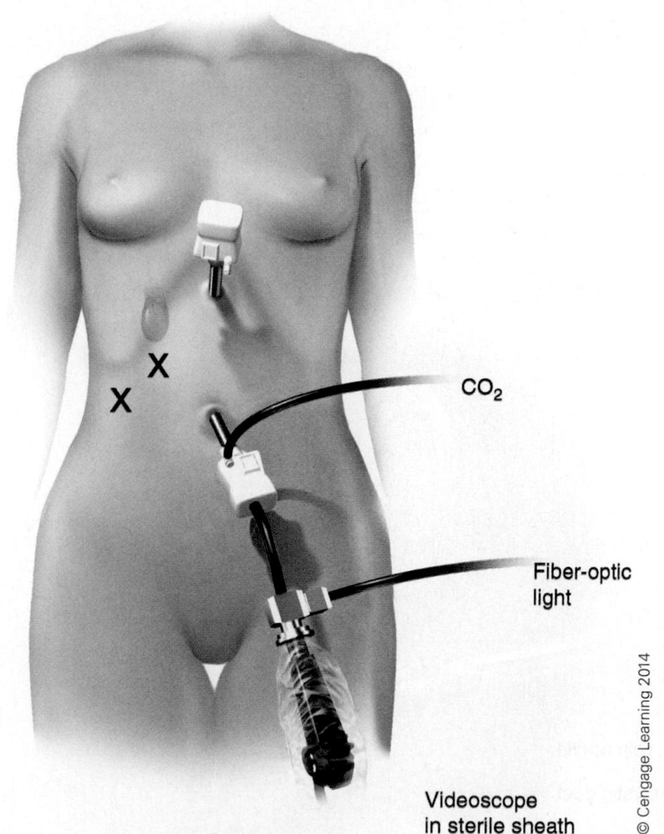

Plate 14-11 Camera and additional trocars are placed

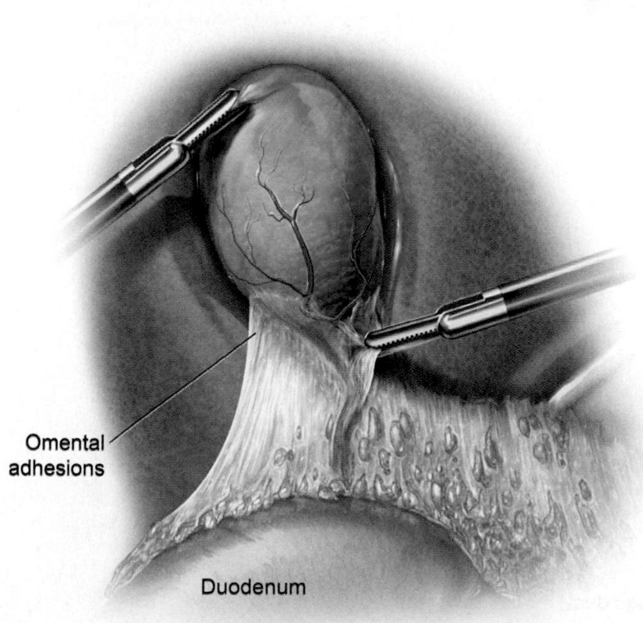

Plate 14-12 Retraction of gallbladder and exposure of triangle of Calot

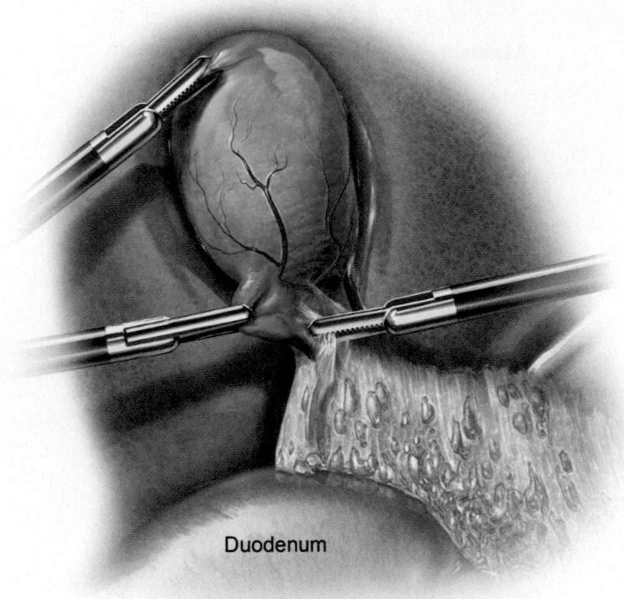

Plate 14-13 Cystic duct and artery are dissected free

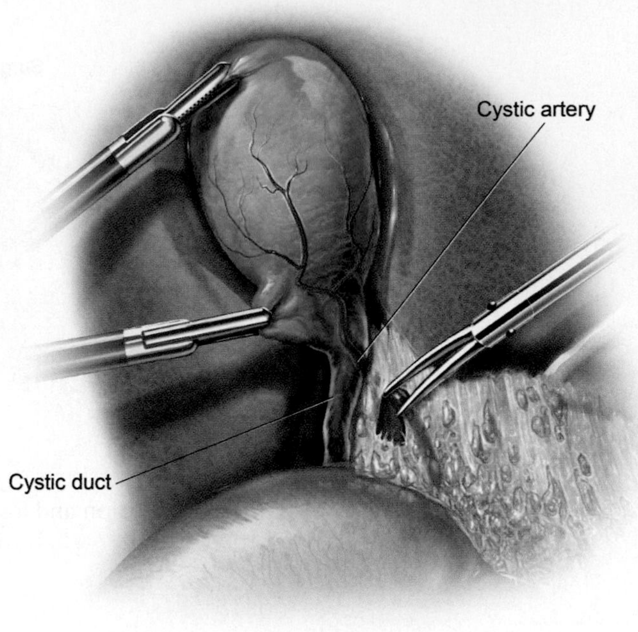

Plate 14-14 Dissection continues

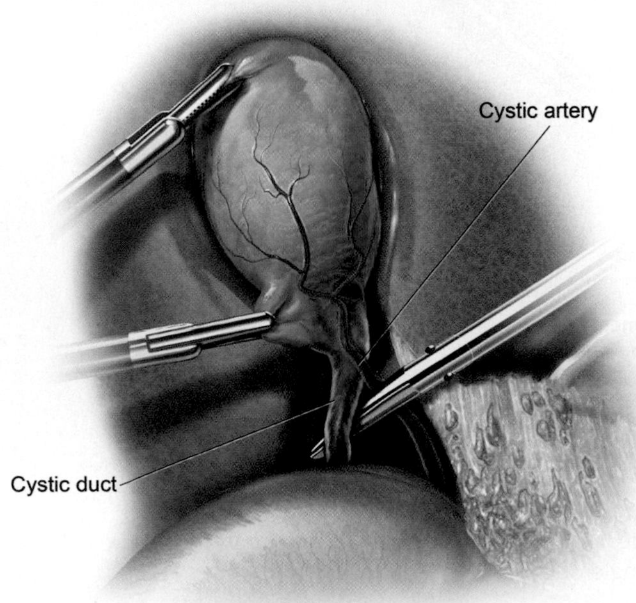

Plate 14-15 Cystic duct and artery are freed from tissue

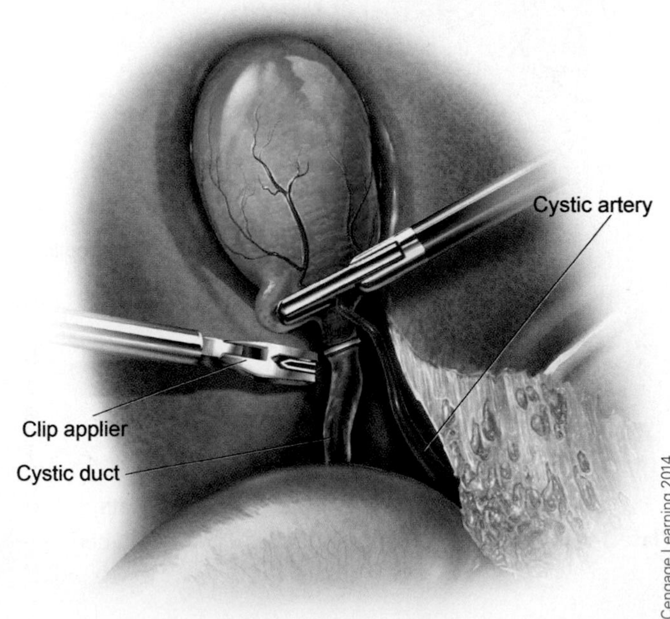

Plate 14-16 Hemoclips are applied to cystic duct

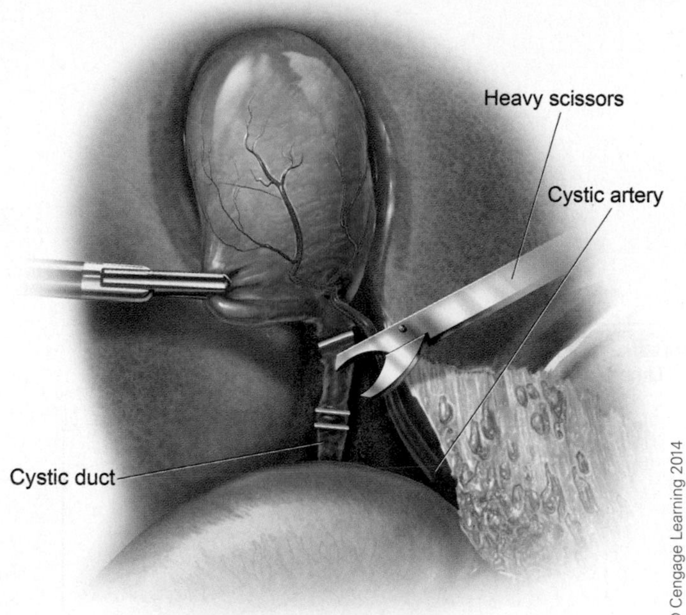

Plate 14-17 Division of cystic duct

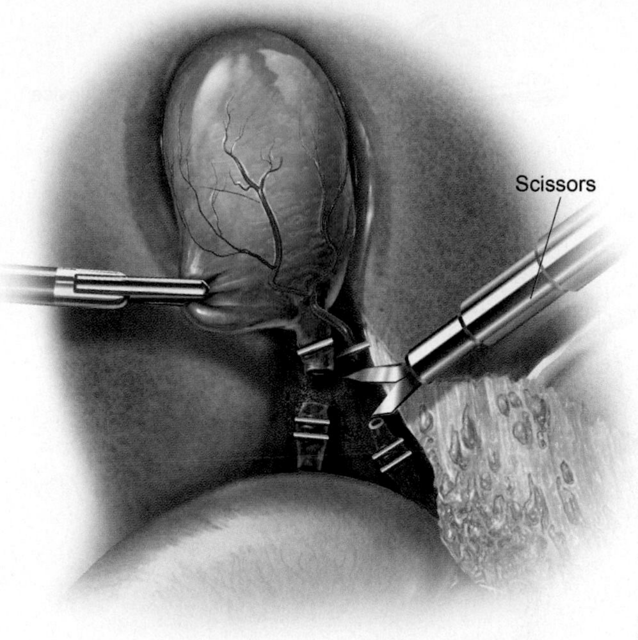

Plate 14-18 Hemoclips are placed and cystic artery is divided

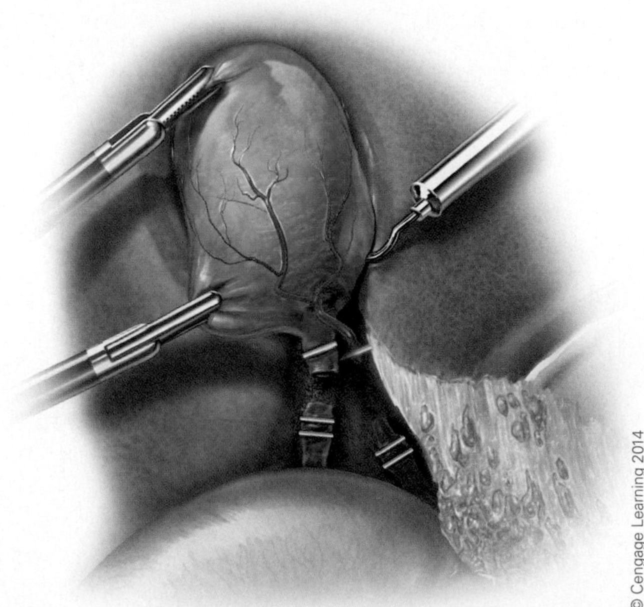

Plate 14-19 Dissection of gallbladder from liver bed begins

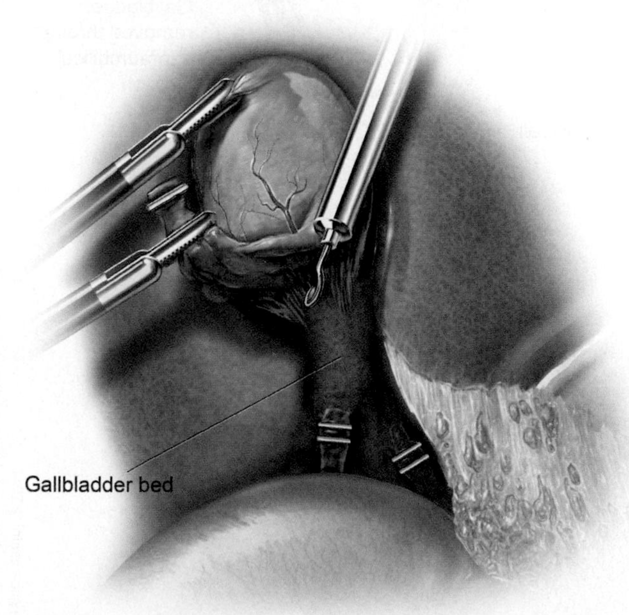

Plate 14-20 Dissection of gallbladder from liver bed continues

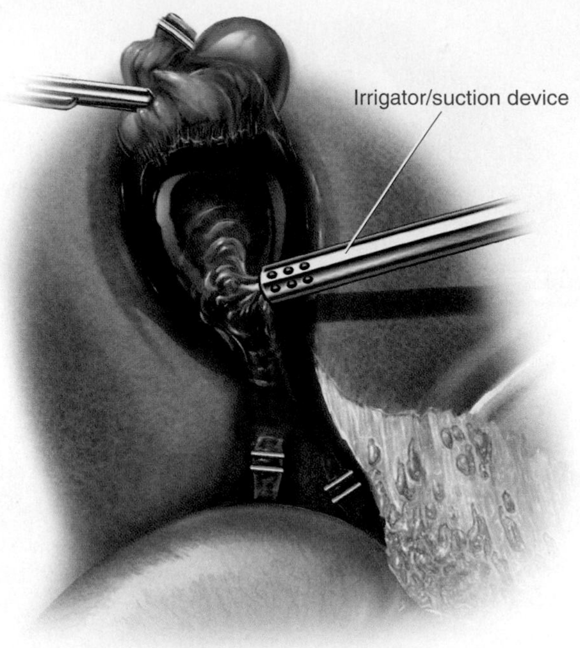

Plate 14-21 Irrigating liver bed and checking for bleeding

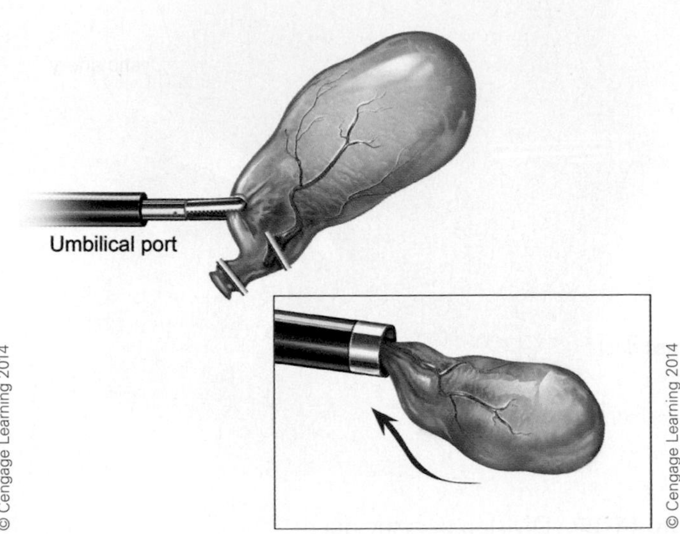

Plate 14-22 Removal of gallbladder through umbilical port

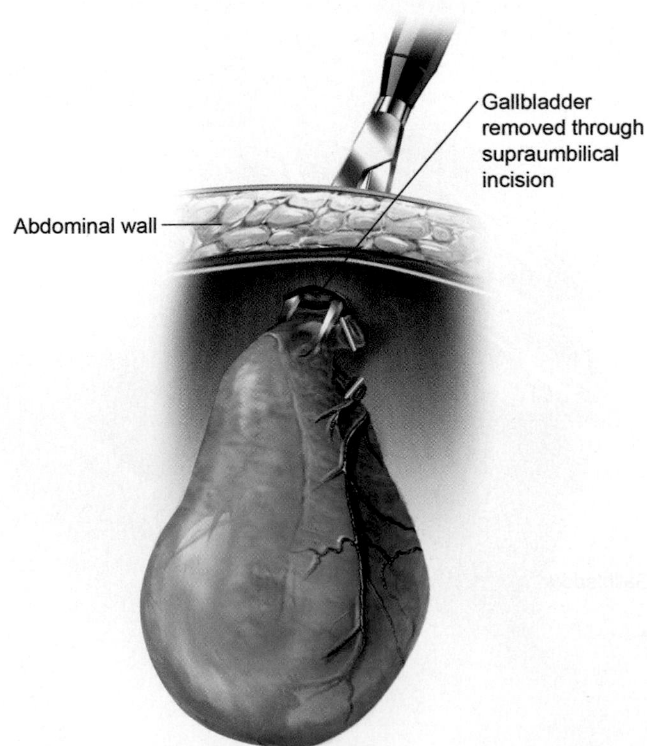

Plate 14-23 Distended gallbladder is removed through supraumbilical incision

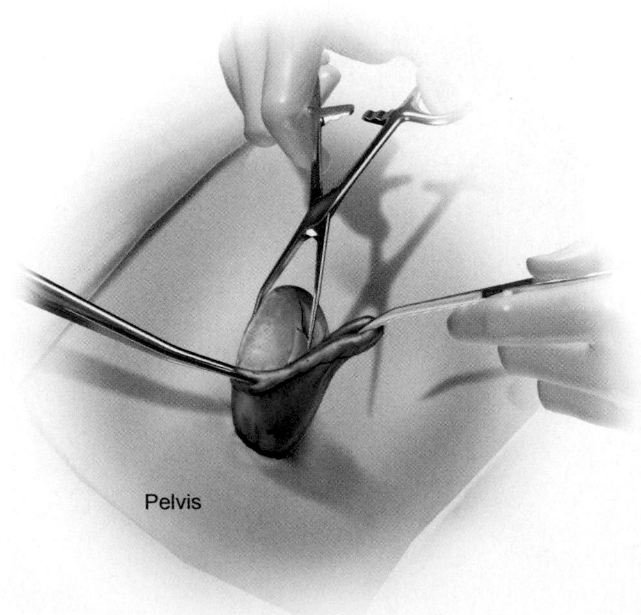

Plate 14-24 Removal of distended gallbladder

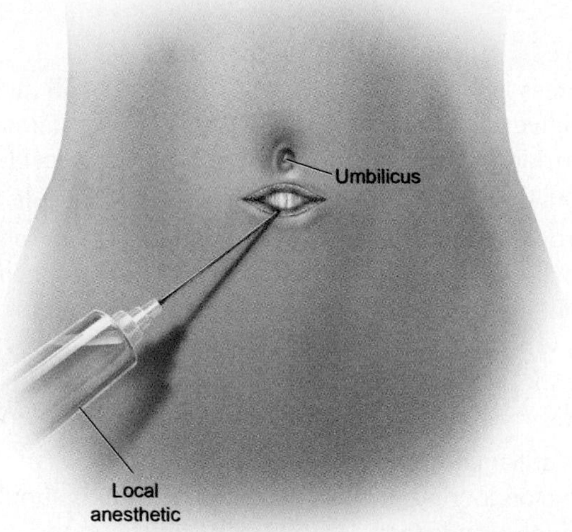

Plate 14-25 Local anesthetic is injected at umbilical trocar site

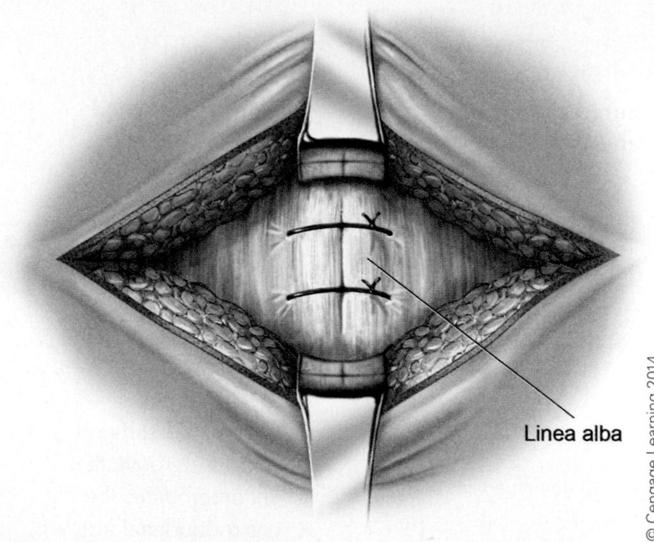

Plate 14-26 Placement of sutures at umbilical trocar site

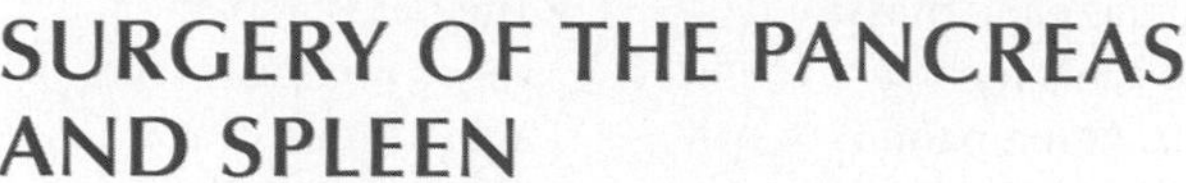

SURGERY OF THE PANCREAS AND SPLEEN

Throughout much of history the pancreas was essentially unapproachable. Modern surgical methods and a better understanding have made pancreatic surgery possible and effective. The spleen is commonly traumatized and removed during emergency surgery.

Cancer of the Pancreas

Symptoms and diagnosis of pancreatic cancer are listed in Table 14-15.

PANCREATECTOMY

Pancreatectomy is the surgical removal of the pancreas. It is most often performed as part of a combination procedure, the pancreaticoduodenectomy (Whipple procedure).

Pancreaticoduodenectomy

The Whipple procedure is performed for managing tumors of the head of the pancreas, the most common site of pancreatic cancer. The head of the pancreas and the duodenum share the same arterial supply. Both organs are removed because removal of only the head of the pancreas would disrupt the blood supply to the duodenum.

TABLE 14-15 Pancreatic Cancer, Symptoms and Diagnosis

Cancer	*Symptoms and Diagnostics*
• Pancreatitis is associated with both primary pancreatic tumors and metastases, primarily from gastric cancer. • Although the inflammatory process of chronic pancreatitis can involve the whole organ, in 20% to 30% of cases it is limited to the pancreatic head. • Carcinoma of the pancreas is the fourth most common malignancy in the United States. • The incidence of pancreatic cancer is the highest in the pancreatic head and ampulla of Vater, and lesions in these areas tend to grow to a large size and metastasize prior to the onset of symptoms. • The majority of patients (over 80%) with pancreatic cancer never undergo curative surgical intervention, whereas the remainder will be treated by the Whipple pancreatoduodenectomy.	• The most common symptom (95% of patients) is intractable upper abdominal (epigastric) pain that is constant and dull. • Other signs and symptoms include malabsorption of nutrients leading to diarrhea and weight loss, nausea, vomiting, low-grade fever, respiratory problems, absence of normal bowel sounds, jaundice secondary to CBD compression, and diabetes. • Diagnosis is commonly made through physical examination that reveals a large palpable mass, low serum bilirubin levels, abnormal radiographs of the abdomen, needle biopsy, CT scan, ERCP, and ultrasonography. • Laparoscopy may also be performed prior to submitting the patient to a laparotomy.

Procedure 14-16 Pancreatectomy

Surgical Anatomy and Pathology

- Pancreas is divided into three regions: head, body and tail.
  - Head lies within the duodenal curve and can be embedded into the wall of the second portion of the duodenum.
  - The boundary between the head and neck is a groove that accommodates the gastroduodenal artery.
  - Neck of the pancreas adjoins the pylorus and merges into the body of the pancreas. It extends obliquely upward and to the left to the tail.
  - Tail is narrow and usually reaches the gastric surface of the spleen. It is contained between two layers of the splenorenal ligament along with the splenic vessels.
- Pancreas lacks a definitive capsule and is surrounded by connective tissue.
- Approximately 80% of the parenchyma is divided into lobules consisting of acini, the exocrine secreting glands.
- Islets of Langerhans are the endocrine-secreting glands that number about 1,000,000 and account for only 1% of the pancreatic mass.
  - The islets receive 25% of the pancreatic blood supply.
  - The islets are composed of glucagon-secreting alpha cells, insulin-secreting beta cells, somatostatin-secreting delta cells, and pancreatic-peptide-secreting cells. The primary function of all these cells are to maintain blood sugar levels.
- The arterial supply of the pancreas is from branches of the celiac artery and superior mesenteric artieres and great pancreatic branch of the splenic artery (Figure 14-20).
- Innervation is supplied by the vagus and splanchnic nerves by way of the hepatic and celiac plexuses.
  - The parasympathetic vagus innervates the acini, ducts, and islets and mediates visceral pain.
  - The sympathetic nerves influence the pancreatic blood vessels.
- Refer to Table 14-15 for pancreatic cancer symptoms.

Preoperative Diagnostic Tests and Procedures

- See Table 14-15.

Equipment and Instruments Unique to Procedure

- Headlamp available
- Suction apparatus × 2
- Major instrument set
- Peripheral vascular instrument set
- Gallbladder instruments
- Long and deep instruments
- GI resection instruments
- Deep retractors (e.g., Harrington retractors)
- GI linear stapling devices
- Yankauer and Poole suction tips
- Hemoclip appliers and ligating clips (several clip appliers and clips)
- Self-retaining abdominal retractor (Balfour or Bookwalter)

Supplies Unique to Procedure

- Knife blades: several #10; #11 and/or #15
- Hemostatic agents (e.g., Gelfoam or Surgicel)
- Active drain available (Hemovac or Jackson-Pratt)

PROCEDURE 14-16 (continued)

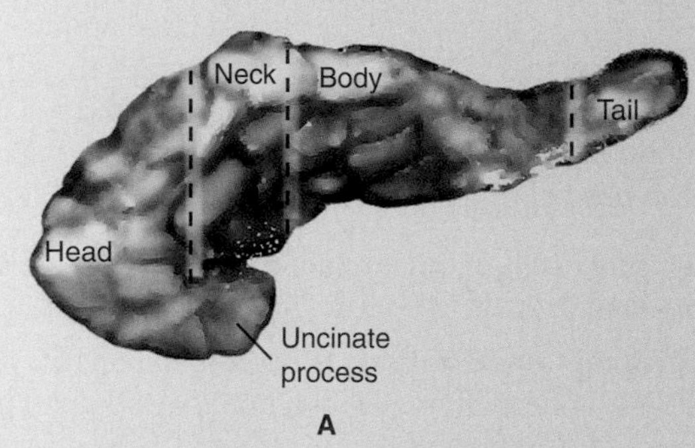

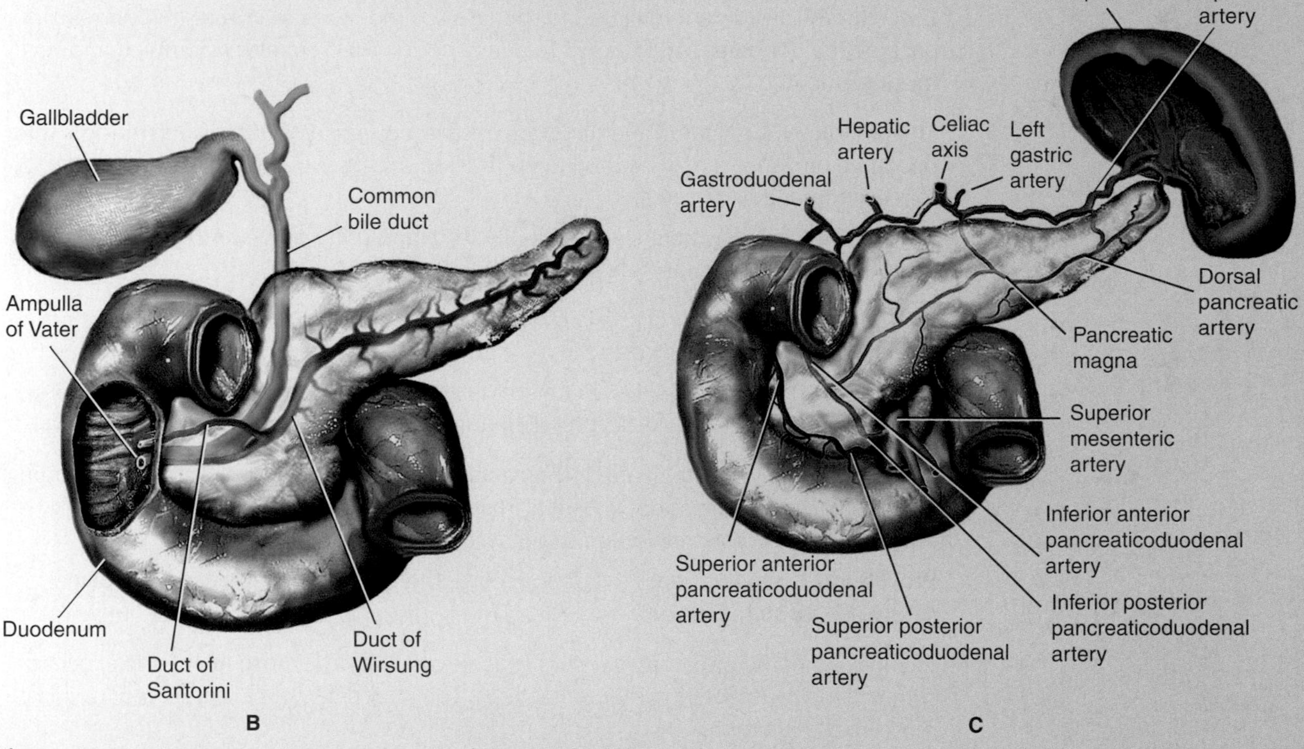

Figure 14-20 Pancreas: (A) Segments, (B) ducts, (C) blood supply

Preoperative Preparation

- Supine position
- General anesthesia
- Foley catheter inserted if ordered by surgeon
- Skin prep: mid-chest to mid-thighs and bilaterally as far as possible
- Draping: square off with four towels–edge of upper towel placed mid-chest; lateral towels placed using anterior superior iliac spines as guide; edge of lower towel placed at symphysis pubis; laparotomy drape

(*continues*)

Procedure 14-16 (continued)

Practical Considerations

- Confirm blood is available with blood bank.
- Monitor blood loss carefully; keep track of the amount of irrigation used in order to estimate blood loss in suction container.
- Have a large number of lap sponges available for the procedure.
- Prepare several hemoclip appliers while setting up back table and Mayo stand.
- Have a large supply of 1-0, 2-0, and 3-0 ties.

Surgical Procedure

1. A left subcostal or upper midline incision is made and retractors are placed for exposure.

   Procedural Considerations: All considerations for a cholecystectomy, choledochojejunostomy, and small bowel resection may apply to pancreatectomy.

2. The entire anterior surface of the pancreas is exposed by opening the lesser sac of the omentum and mobilizing the hepatic flexure of the colon.

   Procedural Consideration: Have lap sponges soaked in warm saline solution ready for packing the abdomen, and the self-retaining abdominal retractor assembled and ready for placement.

3. The pathology is palpated and the extent of the required resection is determined. Intraoperative ultrasound may be used to outline the structure of the pancreatic duct prior to resection and anastomosis.

   Procedural Consideration: Have available throughout the procedure: suture ligatures, ties-on-a-pass, and ligating clips loaded.

4. A Satinsky-type vascular clamp is placed across the pancreas distal to the point of resection. The pancreatic parenchyma is divided sharply with a scalpel.

   Procedural Consideration: Long curved Metzenbaum scissors, long fine-tipped tissue forceps such as the DeBakeys, long right angles and tonsil hemostats available.

5. The posterior vessels are divided. The pancreas is dissected from the spleen, including division of the splenic artery and vein. The tail and body of the pancreas are removed and any retained pancreatic stump is closed.

   Procedural Consideration: Prepare to receive the pancreas specimen. Anticipate suture use for stump closure.

6. Hemostasis of the proximal pancreas is achieved with fine mosquito clamps, electrosurgery, and 3-0 silk ties or suture ligatures. The pancreatic duct is prepared for anastomosis to the jejunum.

   Procedural Consideration: GI clamps and suture or GI linear staplers for bowel closure should be available. Prepare for and maintain bowel technique per facility policy.

7. Reconstruction (pancreaticojejunostomy) is carried out by use of a jejunal loop that is defunctionalized by a Roux-en-Y anastomosis.

   Procedural Consideration: Plan for the surgeon to use a copious amount of warm saline to irrigate; the surgeon may want to use a Poole suction tip. Wrap a wet sponge around the Poole tip. Prepare for placement of the active drain.

8. The pancreatic duct is anastomosed end-to-side to the jejunal loop with a mucosa-to-mucosa closure. The parenchyma of the pancreas is then secured to the jejunal serosa.

PROCEDURE 14-16 (continued)

Postoperative Considerations	**Immediate Postoperative Care** • Transport to PACU or ICU. **Prognosis** • No complications: Return to normal activies in 8–10 weeks; however, lifestyle may be altered by health condition of patient and additional treatments such as chemotherapy. • Complications: hemorrhage; SSI; fistula formation; recurrence of tumor; leakage of anastomosis; nutritional/digestive complications; ileus. **Wound Classification** • Class II: Clean contaminated.

The Whipple procedure requires both resection and reconstruction. Resection is an en bloc excision of the head of the pancreas, the distal one-third (antrum and pylorus) of the stomach, all of the duodenum, the proximal 10 cm of the jejunum, the gallbladder, the cystic and common bile ducts, and the peripancreatic and hepatoduodenal lymph nodes. Resection is performed in eight steps (Figure 14-22A), and reconstruction in three steps (Figure 14-22B), with variable methods employed for each.

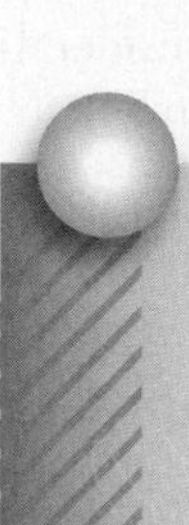

PEARL OF WISDOM

Listen carefully to the conversation between the surgeon and surgical assistant. It will help you determine which options and procedures will be required. These are very complex procedures but they are made up of a series of smaller procedures. Organize for one basic procedure at a time.

PROCEDURE 14-17 Pancreaticoduodenectomy (Whipple Procedure)

Anatomy and Pathology	• See previous surgical procedures on the gallbladder and biliary tract, bowel, pancreas and liver for surgical anatomy. • See previous information for pathology.
Preoperative Diagnostic Tests and Procedures; Equipment and Instruments; Supplies; Preoperative Preparation	• Same as for pancreatectomy
Practical Considerations	• Whipple procedure can take 5–6 hours and the transfusion of many units of blood and/or blood products. • Due to the length of the procedure, hypothermia is a concern; a forced-air warming device should be used. • Upon opening and exploration of the abdomen, if the surgeon discovers that the tumor has invaded the base of the mesocolon, aorta, vena cava, portal vein, or superior mesenteric vessels, the Whipple procedure will not be performed and a bypass of the biliary tract and possibly the stomach will most likely be performed.

(continues)

Procedure 14-17 (continued)

Surgical Procedure

1. A upper transverse, paramedian incision or bilateral subcostal skin incision is made and laparotomy performed.
2. The abdomen is explored and the extent and resectability of the tumor is assessed. As mentioned in Practice Considerations, if the tumor has spread and invaded key anatomical structures, it is considered unresectable and the Whipple procedure will not be performed.
3. Laparotomy sponges are placed in the surgical wound to pack off and protect abdominal structures not involved in the procedure as well as to aid in visualization. The self-retaining abdominal retractor is placed.

   Procedural Consideration: The lap sponges should be soaked in warm saline before being placed in the abdominal cavity. The self-retaining abdominal retractor should be assembled when setting up the back table and Mayo stand.
4. The entire duodenum and head of the pancreas are dissected free with Metzenbaum scissors, electrosurgery, and blunt dissection; silk ties on passers as well as suture ligatures will be needed to control bleeding.

   Procedural Consideration: At this point long and deep instruments may be needed for the rest of the resection portion of the procedure. Silk ties on passers such as tonsil hemostat or Pean should be loaded ahead of time.
5. The gastrohepatic omentum and ligament are double clamped, divided with scissors or electrosurgery, and ligated.
6. The right gastric and gastroduodenal arteries are double clamped, divided with scissors, and ligated. The surgeon may use hemoclips and the arteries are divided between the ligating clips.
7. The distal section of the stomach is mobilized using scissors and electrosurgery.

   Procedural Consideration: Hemoclips may be frequently used due to the number of vessels that supply the stomach.
8. The surgeon may want towels placed on the operative field to protect and isolate the area in preparation for the anastomoses.
9. Two long Payr or Allen clamps are placed across the stomach and the stomach is resected; the surgeon may use a linear stapler for the resection.

   Procedural Consideration: The various stapling devices will be used multiple times during the procedure; the surgical technologist must be able to quickly and skillfully reload the staplers. Several packets of clips should be available in the OR.
10. The duodenum is retracted downward; the CBD is identified and resected distally.
11. The proximal end of the jejunum is clamped with two Allen clamps and divided with scissors.
12. The area between the head of the pancreas and body is clamped with two Allen clamps (or GI clamps of surgeon's choice) and divided; the surgeon may use a GI linear stapler.
13. The duodenum may require further mobilization and the gastroduodenal artery is identified, double clamped, divided, and ligated in order to be able to remove the specimen en bloc (Figure 14-21A).

PROCEDURE 14-17 (continued)

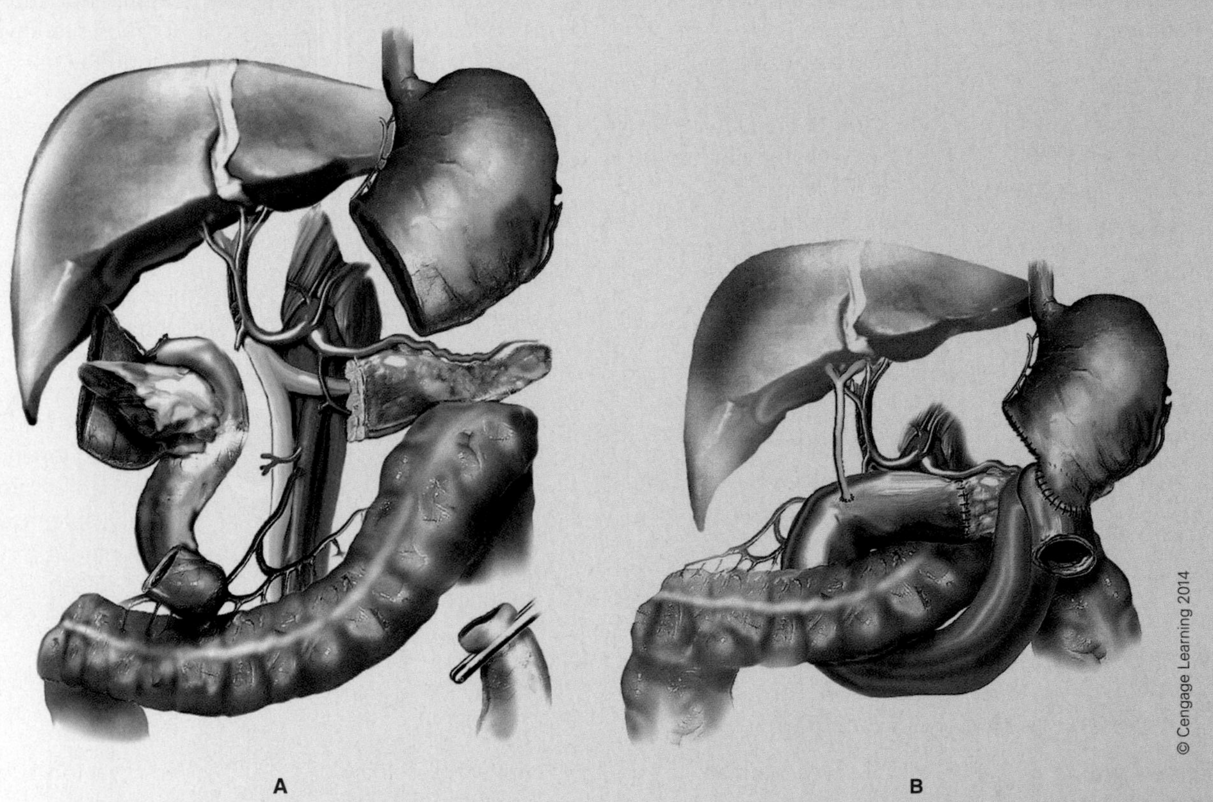

Figure 14-21 Whipple procedure: (A) Resection, (B) reconstruction

14. The anastomoses are usually performed in the following order:
    a. Proximal end of jejunum is anastomosed to the pancreatic body.
    b. CBD is anastomosed to the jejunum in end-to-side technique.
    c. Distal stomach is anastomosed to the jejunum end-to-side (Figure 14-21B).
15. The abdominal cavity is thoroughly irrigated with warm saline solution; lap sponges are removed; self-retaining retractor is removed; one or two active drains (Hemovac) are placed behind the pancreatic and biliary anastomoses.
16. Abdomen is closed in usual fashion.

Postoperative Considerations

Immediate Postoperative Care

- Transport to PACU or ICU.

Prognosis

- No complications (rare): Return to activities, but lifestyle will be altered due to change in diet and bowel habits, and follow-up treatments such as chemotherapy.
- Complications: Some degree of complications will be experienced by 20–40% of patients. Complications include abdominal sepsis, pancreatic fistula formation, diabetes, hemorrhage, possibility of reoperation, peptic ulcer formation, disrupted nutrient absorption, delayed gastric emptying, and death. Postoperative hospital mortality has been reduced to under 5%.

Wound Classification

- Class II: Clean contaminated
- Class III: Contaminated (if spillage from bowel or biliary tract occurs)

PROCEDURE 14-18 Splenectomy

Surgical Anatomy and Pathology	• Spleen is the single largest mass of lymphatic tissue in the body. • It lies in the LUQ, between the fundus of the stomach and the diaphragm. • It is kept in anatomical position by the gastrosplenic, splenorenal, splenophrenic, and pancreaticosplenic ligaments. • The spleen is made up of "red pulp," which is predominantly vascular (75% of its volume), and "white pulp," which is primarily lymph tissue. • Arterial blood supply is via the splenic artery from the celiac trunk of the aorta, but in about 15% of patients the splenic artery is a direct aortic branch. The splenic artery divides into two branches that in turn divide into 3 to 40 branches. • The splenic vein arises from the hilum of the spleen and is eventually joined by the superior and inferior mesenteric veins to form the portal vein. • Pathologies • Primary indicator for a splenectomy is trauma with intraperitoneal hemorrhage. • Other disorders that may require a splenectomy: intraoperative injury; thrombocytopenia; neutropenia; splenomegaly; splenic abscess; parasitic cysts of the spleen.
Preoperative Diagnostic Tests and Procedures	• History and physical • CT scan • Laboratory blood tests
Equipment and Instruments Unique to Procedure	• Cell-saver available • Suction apparatus × 2 • Headlamp available • Major instrument set • Gastrointestinal instrument set • Peripheral vascular instrument set (includes large Sarot clamps) • Long and deep instruments, including deep retractors such as the Harrington • Hemoclip appliers with ligating clips (several)
Supplies Unique to Procedure	• Knife blades: #10 × 2; #15 • Large number of silk ties, 0, 1-0 and 2-0 • Kitners or Peanuts • Yankauer suction tips and tubing × 2 • Hemostatic agents (e.g., Thrombostat, Avitene, Gelfoam) • Active drains (Hemovac or Jackson-Pratt)
Preoperative Preparation	• Supine position • General anesthesia • Skin prep: mid-chest to symphysis pubis; bilaterally as far as possible • Draping: square off with four towels–edge of upper towel placed mid-chest; lateral towels placed using anterior superior iliac spines as guide; edge of lower towel placed at symphysis pubis; laparotomy drape • Foley catheter inserted (if ordered by surgeon)

Procedure 14-18 (continued)

Practical Considerations

- Contact blood bank to confirm availability of blood, especially in instances of trauma. Many units of blood may be needed if the splenectomy is being performed due to trauma.
- Monitor blood loss carefully; keep track of the amount of irrigation that is used in order to estimate the blood loss in the suction canister.
- The OR team may not have much notification of a trauma patient being transported from the emergency department to the surgery department. The team will need to move quickly, but coordinate actions in order to prepare the OR. The surgical technologist may not have time to put all needed instruments on the Mayo stand and concentrate on getting a knife handle loaded, ties situated, and needle holder loaded; he or she may have to grab instruments off the back table as the procedure progresses.

Surgical Procedure

1. An upper midline or left subcostal incision is used. Appropriate retractors are placed.

   Procedural Consideration: Prioritize if patient is hemorrhaging; for example, dry laps may need to be initially used.

2. Left upper quadrant is explored. Suspensory splenic ligaments are identified and ligaments are then divided by blunt dissection or scissors as required (Figure 14-22).

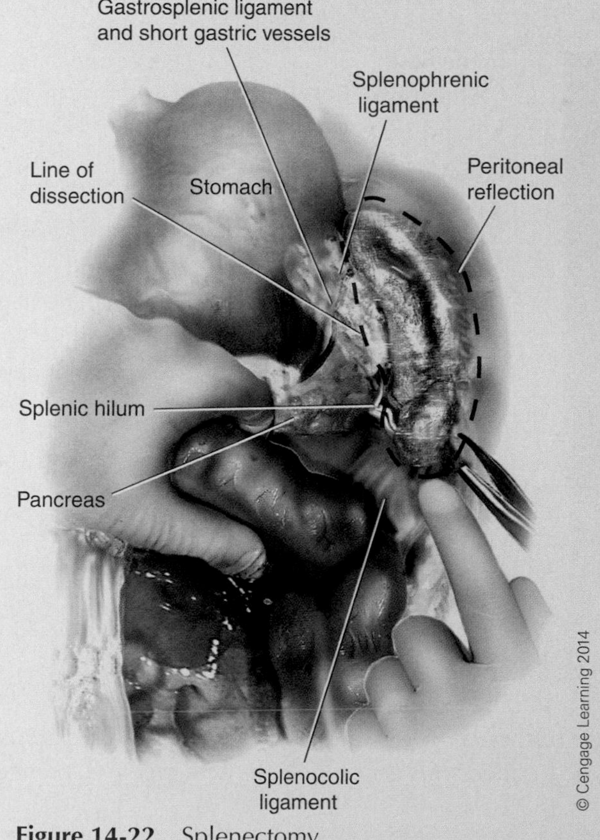

Figure 14-22 Splenectomy

(continues)

PROCEDURE 14-18 (continued)

Procedural Consideration: When hemostasis is somewhat under control, remove used sponges and replace with clean sponges soaked in warm saline.

3. The short gastric veins that run to the stomach are identified, ligated, and cut. The spleen is "mobilized" into the wound.

   Procedural Consideration: Load 0 silk ties on right-angle passer and have suture ligatures loaded on needle holder. Also have several hemoclip appliers loaded and available.

4. Dissection is carried out at the splenic hilum to identify splenic vessels. The splenic artery is double ligated, suture ligated, and divided. The splenic vein is double ligated and divided.

   Procedural Consideration: Throughtout procedure, two suction tips may be needed to maintain visualization of the wound for the surgeon.

5. The spleen can now be removed and hemostasis is achieved.

   Procedural Consideration: In trauma procedures, the entire abdomen will be explored once the hemorrhage is controlled and the spleen removed. Injury to the pancreas, stomach, and bowel is common.

6. A drain may be placed and the wound is closed.

   Procedural Consideration: Assemble the drain and have available.

Postoperative Considerations

Immediate Postoperative Care

- Transport to ICU.

Prognosis

- No complications: Return to normal activities in 8–10 weeks; however, other trauma injuries may affect lifestyle.
- Complications: Immunologic response may be impaired; hemorrhage; SSI; dehiscence.

Wound Classification

- Class II: Clean-contaminated
- Class III: Clean-contaminated (fresh traumatic wound from clean source; spillage from GI tract).
- Class IV: Dirty-infected (traumatic wound from dirty source or due to delayed treatment)

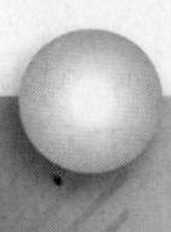

PEARL OF WISDOM

Splenectomy for trauma usually involves a large amount of bleeding. The procedure is relatively straightforward but visualization may be a problem. Large clamps such as Sarot clamps and many lap sponges may be needed (this is not the case with elective splenectomy).

Procedure 14-19 Laparoscopic Splenectomy

Surgical anatomy and pathology, preoperative diagnostic tests and procedures, and preoperative preparations the same as for the open procedure.

Equipment and Instruments Unique to Procedure

- See list of laparoscopic equipment earlier in chapter.
- 30° laparoscope
- Verres needle
- Hasson trocar
- 12-mm trocars × 4 (surgeon's preference–surgeon may want two 12-mm trocars and two 5-mm or 3-mm trocars)
- Curved endoscissors
- Curved endograspers
- EndoBabcock
- Fan retractor
- Endoclip applier with ligating clips
- GIA linear endostapler
- Endosuction/irrigator
- Endocautery

Supplies Unique to Procedure

- Endobag

Practical Considerations

- Surgical technologist may be responsible for manipulating the camera during the procedure as well as holding graspers.

Surgical Procedure

1. Verres needle is inserted and the pneumoperitoneum established.

   Procedural Consideration: The surgeon and surgical technologist will elevate the skin to allow the abdominal contents to fall away and facilitate the insertion of the Verres needle without injuring the internal organs.

2. A 12-mm trocar is inserted at the midline 2–3 cm above the umbilicus; the laparoscope is inserted through this trocar. The other three trocars are inserted.

   Procedural Consideration: The surgical technologist should connect the camera and light cord to the laparoscope.

3. A endograsper, endoBabcock, or fan retractor is used to retract the stomach medially to expose the spleen; the instrument is placed through the most lateral trocar on the right. The abdomen is thoroughly explored for any accessory spleen, which is first excised.

4. The dissection to free up the spleen begins with use of the endoscissors and endocautery to dissect the splenic flexure from the colon.

5. The splenocolic ligament is divided using the endoscissors to free up the inferior section of the spleen. An endoBabcock is used to carefully retract the spleen cephalad.

   Procedural Consideration: If the surgical technologist is responsible for holding any of the graspers during the procedure, just enough tension and traction should be placed in order to avoid injury to the stomach and rupturing the splenic capsule.

6. The peritoneal attachment on the lateral side of the spleen is divided with endoscissors.

7. A window is created in the lesser sac adjacent to the greater curvature of the stomach and along the medial border of the spleen. The laparoscope is placed within the lesser sac.

8. The gastric vessels are divided with endoclips or endovascular stapler. The splenic pedicle is identified and dissected free with the endoscissors.

(*continues*)

PROCEDURE 14-19 (continued)

9. The laparoscope is removed from the lesser sac. The tail of the pancreas is identified in order to avoid injury. The splenic artery is carefully dissected free and endoclips are placed, but not yet divided. The splenic vein is also dissected free and endoclipls are placed. The vessels are now divided, starting with the artery, using the endovascular stapler.

   Procedural Consideration: Several other vessels may be encountered that must be ligated and divided. The surgical technologist will need to be able to quickly re-load the endostaplers.

10. The spleen is now completely freed up and is placed inside an endobag. The end of the bag is brought upward through the supraumbilical or epigastric port site. The drawstring on the bag is opened and the spleen is morcellated inside the bag and removed in small pieces. The bag is fully removed.

    Procedural Consideration: All pieces of the spleen are specimens and can be sent to pathology together.

11. The laparoscope is re-inserted and the splenic bed is visualized to confirm hemostasis has been achieved. The suction/irrigator may be used.

12. The trocars are removed and the trocar sites are closed.

Postoperative Consideration

Immediate Postoperative Care

- Transport to PACU.

Prognosis:

- No complications: Discharged from hospital within 24 hours; return to normal activities in 4–6 weeks.
- Complications: Same as for open procedure.

Wound Classification

- Class I: Clean
- Class II: Clean contaminated (spillage occurs due to intraoperative injury to stomach or bowel)

BREAST SURGERY

Although the vast majority of breast cancer cases are female, breast cancer is not limited to the female breast. Today, treatment of breast cancer is multidisciplinary and has received emphasis in finding a cure for this devastating diseasee.

Breast and Axilla: Pathology and Diagnosis

Like most conditions involving malignancy, breast cancer has been staged. One system is presented in Table 14-16.

Diagnosis of breast cancer clinical Stages I to IV or ductal carcinoma *in situ* usually begins with initial detection through breast examination or mammography. Follow-up endeavors include chest X-ray and bone scanning.

Some general facts about breast cancer that affect surgical intervention are:

Tumor size is directly related to the presence of regional metastases and progressive deterioration after treatment

Breast-conserving surgery is possible in 90% of cases

Men suffer from breast disorders such as breast enlargement (gynecomastia) and less commonly cancer.

The trend in breast surgery is an evolution from the total removal of all breast tissue to the conservation of as much breast tissue as possible while excising the entire tumor (Figure 14-23). This approach is often combined with dissection of lymph nodes for cancer staging, and postoperative chemotherapy and/or irradiation therapy. (Staging refers to the classification of breast cancer by anatomical extent.)

Biopsy

Breast biopsy may be accomplished with a needle or by surgical removal (excisional biopsy). Biopsy is used for diagnostic purposes; its aids the surgeon is determining the stage and course of treatment if the biopsy is considered malignant.

Table 14-16 Breast Cancer Staging

Cancer in Situ	
Stage I	• Tumor 2 cm or less in greatest diameter • No evidence of regional or distal spread
Stage II	• Tumor greater than 2 cm but not more than 5 cm in greatest diameter • With or without movable axillary nodes • Without distal spread
Stage IIIa	• Tumor up to 5 cm in diameter • May or may not be fixed • Homolateral clinically suspicious regional spread or • Tumor greater than 5 cm diameter • May or may not be fixed • With or without clinically suspicious homolateral regional spread • No evidence of distant metastases
Stage IIIb	• Tumor of any dimension • Unequivocal homolateral metastatic supraclavicular or interclavicular nodes or • Edema of the arm, but without distant metastases
Stage IV	• Tumor of any size • With or without regional spread • Evidence of distant metastases

Adapted from *Essentials of Obstetrics and Gynecology,* 3rd ed., by N. F. Hacker and J. G. Moore. Copyright 1998 by W. B. Saunders.

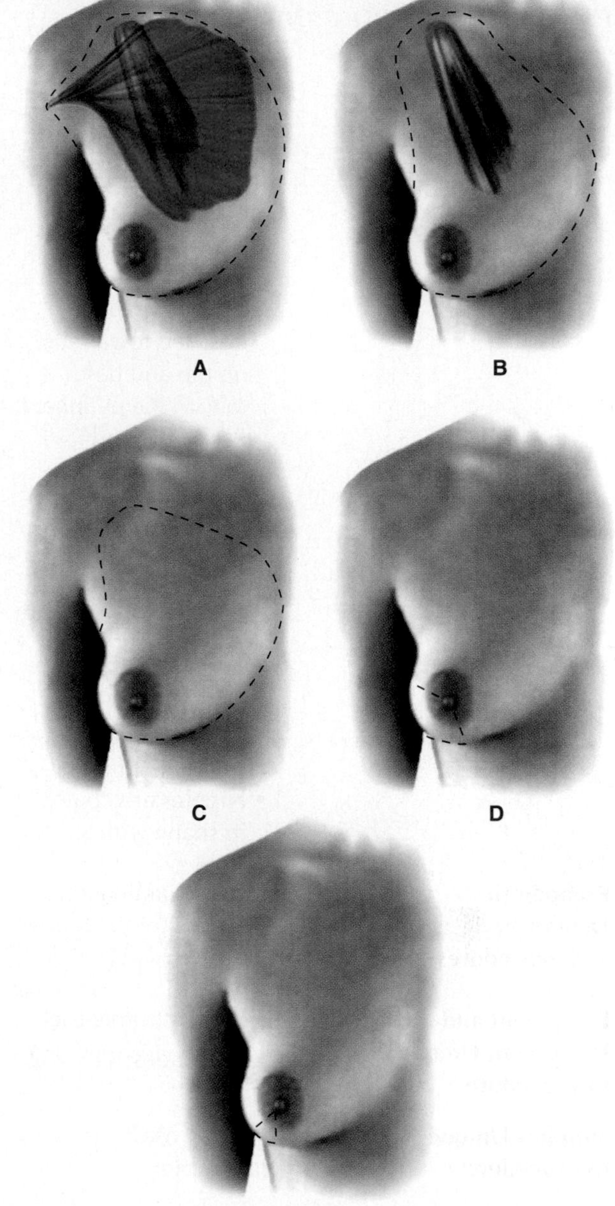

Figure 14-23 Breast surgery options: (A) Radical mastectomy, (B) modified radical mastectomy, (C) simple mastectomy, (D) segmental resection, (E) lumpectomy

Procedure 14-20 Breast Biopsy

Surgical anatomy and pathology	• Mammary glands are located anterior to the pectoralis major muscle between the second and sixth ribs (refer to Plate 12A in Appendix A), lateral to the sternum and extend to the axilla. • Mammmary glands consists of glandular tissue.

(*continues*)

PROCEDURE 14-20 (continued)

	• The tissue is thicker underneath the nipple and thinner at the periphery. • The tissue contains 15–20 lobes that are pyramidal in shape with their apexes oriented toward the nipple and bases toward the periphery. Each lobe and lobules are surrounded by loose connective tissue and the entire gland is surrounded by connective tissue. • Each lobe contains a lactiferous duct. • The nipples lies at the level of the fifth rib. • Nipples are conical in shape with a rounded and fissured tip. • The nipples receive the openings of the lactiferous ducts. • The pigmented skin around the nipple that covers smooth muscle is the areola.	• Arterial supply to the breast is via the internal thoracic, lateral mammary, and intercostals, which are branches for the subcutaneous vessels of the anterior thorax. • The vessels enter the breasts at their superomedial and superolateral borders. • Venous drainage follows the same course at the arteries.	• Lymphatic drainage is of particular importance because tumor cells often follow the lymphatic network. • The anteriolateral thoracic wall contains a cutaneous lymphatic network that is continuous with the neck and abdomen. The mammary cutaneous lymphatics are part of this lymphatic network. • Pathology can be cystic disease or malignant tumor (see Table 14-16).
Preoperative Diagnostic Tests and Procedures	• Breast examination: Palpation of the breasts • Mammography	• Breast biopsy is a diagnostic procedure	
Equipment and Instrument Unique to Procedure	• Minor instrument set • Knife blades: #15 × 2		
Supplies Unique to Procedure	• ¼″ Penrose drain (available)		
Preoperative Preparation	• Supine position • Local anesthesia with IV conscious sedation (MAC) • Skin prep: ONLY paint solution is gently applied starting at the site of the lesion extending to the level of the clavicle to the sternum downward, including a wide margin of the abdomen and laterally as far as possible to include the axilla. The scrub is NOT performed in order to avoid spreading cancer cells. The surgeon may order the paint to be applied by spraying the prep area.		• Draping: Four towels to square off breast–the towels are NOT placed in a manner to just square off the incision site; they are placed in a manner that squares off the entire breast. Laparotomy drape is positioned.

PROCEDURE 14-20 (continued)

Practical Considerations

- The surgical team must be sensitive to the fact that the patient is under local anesthesia and may be alert enough to hear the conversations that are taking place. Additionally, if a frozen section is to be performed by pathology, the report should be communicated to the surgeon in the OR in a confidential manner and not through a speaker phone.
- The surgical technologist and circulator should confirm before the patient is brought into the OR if a frozen section has been ordered by the surgeon and the pathology department has been notified.
- Tissue being sent to pathology for frozen section must NOT be placed in formalin.
- If the patient has undergone a needle localization procedure in the radiology department just prior to the breast biopsy, the circulator must be extremely careful not to dislodge the needle when applying the paint solution. Additionally, when assisting with the draping procedure, the surgical technologist must make sure not to dislodge the needle.

Surgical Procedure

1. A curvilinear incision is made in order to follow the skin lines directly over the tumor mass or along the border of the areola (circumareolar incision) if it is a centrally located mass.
   a. If a needle localization procedure has been performed in the radiology department, the incision is placed as directly over the location of the tumor mass as possible using the needle as a guide. The needle should NOT be removed.

   Procedural Consideration: The surgeon may have the surgical technologist place gentle traction on the skin to facilitate the skin incision.

2. The incision is carried down to the tumor mass with the knife and Metzenbaum scissors. Electrocautery will be used to control bleeding.
   a. Needle localization: The surgeon will follow the needle down to the tumor mass.

   Procedural Consideration: If the mass is deep within the breast tissue the surgeon may need to inject additional local anesthesia.

3. The surgeon will grasp the tumor mass with DeBakey forceps, Babcock, or Allis clamp. A small margin of tissue will be excised along with the tumor mass as the surgeon works in a circular fashion using the Metzenbaum scissors to free up the mass.

   Procedural Consideration: The surgical technologist may be responsible for holding the Babcock or Allis and will follow the surgeon by gently moving the mass to provide visualization.

4. The tissue specimen is removed en bloc.
   a. Needle localization: The tissue with wire is sent to pathology for frozen section. Closure of the surgical wound is not performed until the pathologist communicates confirmation that the tumor mass has been excised. During the wait the surgeon will gently irrigate the wound and control small bleeders with the electrocautery.
   b. Non-needle localization: The surgeon will use a sterile marking pen or silk suture ligature to mark the breast tissue as to its anatomical position to the breast; the superior and inferior poles will most likely be marked. The surgical technologist should cut the suture in such a manner that it has long tags.

(continues)

Procedure 14-20 (continued)

c. The surgical technologist should NOT pass off the tissue specimen on a counted 4 × 4 raytec sponge. If the specimen does not have a needle, the surgical technologist should use a DeBakey forcep to place the specimen inside a specimen cup the circulator will be holding. If a needle is present, the surgical technologist can place the specimen on a sterile Telfa pad and pass off to the circulator.

5. When the pathology report has been received, hemostasis will be checked one last time. The surgical wound is closed with interrupted absorbable suture. The skin will be closed with a running subcuticular closure and skin closure tapes.

Postoperative Considerations

Immediate Postoperative Care

- Transport to PACU.

Prognosis

- No complications: Discharged same day of surgery; return to normal activities in 1–2 weeks.
- Complications: hemorrhage; SSI.

Wound Classification

- Class I: Clean

Procedure 14-21 Sentinel Node Biopsy with Isosulfan Blue Dye

- Anatomy and pathology, preoperative diagnostic tests and procdures, and preoperative considerations are the same as for breast biopsy.

Equipment and Instruments Unique to Procedure

- Minor instrument set

Supplies Unique to Procedure

- 5-mL syringe
- 25-gauge needle
- Alcohol wipes
- Isosulfan blue dye
- Multiple specimen containers with several pathology request forms
- Crash cart immediately available (allergic reactions to dye)

Practical Considerations

- The sentinel lymph nodes are the first nodes along the lymphatic channel from the tumor site; removal and examination aids in making patient care decisions and forming a treatment plan. Confirmation of positive nodes indicates that at a minimum an axillary dissection procedure will be performed and the patient will most likely undergo chemotherapy.
- An alternative to the use of isosulfan blue dye is technetium 99, a radioactive sulfur colloid that is injected into the patient in the nuclear medicine department just prior to surgery. The rest of the surgery procedure is the same as when using isosulfan blue dye.
- Patients can be allergic to isosulfan blue dye.

1. Steps 1 and 2 of the breast biopsy procedure are performed.
2. The surgeon will inject isosulfan blue dye directly into the tumor mass. This is usually completed before the patient skin prep if the patient is under general anesthesia or early in the procedure to allow the dye to travel through the lymphatic system.
   a. The "Rule of 5s" is followed: 5-mL of dye is injected at 5 sites spanning a 5-cm diameter and the site massaged for 5 minutes
   b. The patient must be carefully observed for an allergic reaction to the dye.

Procedure 14-21 (continued)

3. Axillary dissection is carried out.
   a. The stained sentinel nodes are identified and excised. The surgeon may want each node placed in a separate specimen container and numbered each with its own pathology request form.
   b. The specimens are sent to the pathology deparment.
4. The surgeon will continue with either the planned surgical procedure or possibly a less invasive procedure based on the pathology results.

Postoperative Considerations

Immediate Postoperative Care

- Transport to PACU.

Prognosis

- Based on extent of surgical procedure that was performed.
- Complications from sentinel node biopsy include allergic reaction to dye; sensory or motor nerve damage (rare); pneumothorax that occurs with internal mammary node biopsy.

Wound Clasification

- Class I: Clean

Modified Radical Mastectomy

Modified radical mastectomy is the removal of the entire breast including axillary lymph nodes. This approach is used in Stage I and II breast cancer or in conjunction with chemotherapy and radiation treatments for Stage III and IV breast cancer.

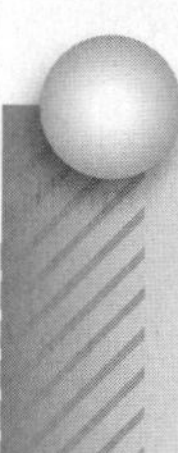

Pearl of Wisdom

Two setups may be required if reconstruction is being done immediately following the mastectomy to prevent seeding (spread of cancer cells).

Procedure 14-22 Modified Radical Mastectomy

Surgical anatomy and pathology, and preoperative tests and procedures are the same as for breast biopsy (procedure 14-19).

Equipment and Instruments Unique to Procedure

- Major instrument set
  - Additional Crile hemostats
  - Additional Allis-Adair clamps
  - Additional rake retractors of various sizes
- Hemoclip appliers with ligating clips

Supplies Unique to Procedure

- Knife blades #10 × 5 (or more)
- Magnetic instrument pad
- Impervious stockinette
- Marking pen
- Active wound drain 3 2 (usually Jackson-Pratt; may have drainage tube that bifurcates to allow the insertion of the two ends in the surgical wound and one tube that connects to the drain)

(continues)

Procedure 14-22 (continued)

Preoperative Preparation	• Supine position.
	  • Arm on affected side should be on an armrest.
	• General anesthesia
	• Skin prep: Starting at the site of the lesion, extend upward to include the neck, medial to the sternum, downward to mid-abdomen, as far as possible laterally including axilla and arm on affected side up to the wrist.
	  • A towel or sheet should be placed on the armboard while the arm is being prepped.
	• Draping: Four towels to square off breast. Nonsterile towel or sheet removed from the armboard by a nonsterile team member; a sterile 3/4 sheet placed on the armboard. Stockinette placed on arm. Laparotomy sheet placed.

Practical Considerations	• Mammograms in the OR. • If the mastectomy is following a biopsy, the patient should be reprepped and redraped, the surgical team should regown and reglove, and the mastectomy instrumentation should be brought up to the OR table. • The surgical technologist will have to change out the #10 knife blade multiple times due to the toughness of the fibrous tissue; communicate to the surgeon each time a knife blade is new. • The electrocautery will be used multiple times; keep the Bovie tip clean using the scratch pad. • At the end of the procedure, make sure there is warm water for irrigation.
Surgical Procedure	1. The extent of the skin flaps is marked and an elliptical transverse incision is made along these markings allowing for a 4-cm margin around any lesion. The elliptical incision extends laterally into the axilla through the subcutaneous layer. Bleeding is controlled with electrocautery. **Procedural Consideration:** Have marking pen available. Place laparotomy sponges on the field.
	2. Tapering skin flaps are developed with the #10 knife blade and held upward with the use of rake retractors Dissection continues down to the chest muscles and laterally to the border of the pectoralis minor muscle. Breast tissue and underlying pectoralis fascia are resected from the pectoralis major muscle. The axillary area including the tail of Spence is dissected (see Figure 14-24). The intercostal arteries and veins are identified,

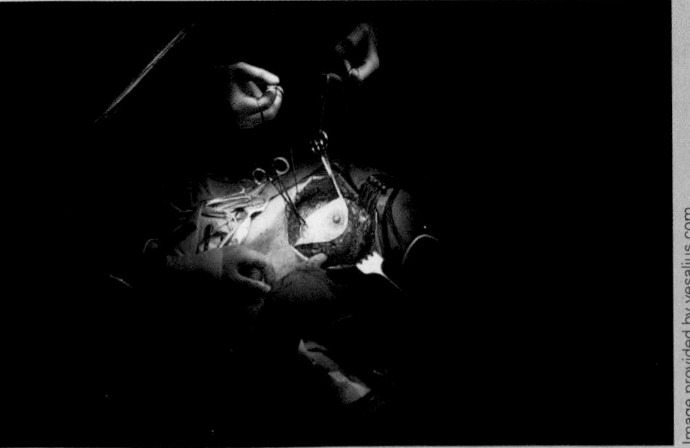

Figure 14-24 Mastectomy—Skin flaps developed

PROCEDURE 14-22 (continued)

double clamped and ligated. The axillary vein and medial and lateral nerves that supply the pectoralis major muscle should be identified and preserved during dissection.

Procedural Consideration: The majority of the procedure is soft tissue dissection; have the scalpel, scissors, electrocautery, and hemostats available at all times. Large vessels will be ligated.

3. Dissection of the fascia from the lateral edge of the pectoralis major muscle and serratus anterior muscle is completed.

   Procedural Consideration: The long thoracic and thoracodorsal nerves are identified and preserved; the surgeon may want vessel loops to gently retract the nerves.

4. Dissection is completed by resecting the breast and axillary fascia from the latissimus dorsi muscle and suspensory ligaments. The entire specimen is passed off the sterile field to the circulator.

   Procedural Consideration: The surgical technologist may have to provide a large round basin for the specimen to be placed and pass it off to the circulator.

5. Bleeding is controlled with electrocautery. The wound is irrigated with warm water.

   Procedural Consideration: Warm water is used for irrigating, NOT saline. The warm water is absorbed by cells, including cancerous cells that may be present and due to osmosis, the cells burst.

6. Two wound drains are usually placed, one in the anterior chest and the other in the axilla. Excess skin is excised and the wound is closed.

   Procedural Consideration: The drain tubes are brought out through stab incisions and secured to the skin using a 2-0 or 3-0 silk suture on a cutting needle. The surgeon may place some interrupted absorbable sutures in the subcutaneous layer to aid in approximating the skin edges. The incision is usually closed with skin staples. The dressing is usually a bulky dressing using Kerlix (Kerlix is opened and "fluffed" by the surgical technologist prior to placement).

Postoperative Considerations

Immediate Postoperative Care

- Transport to PACU.

Prognosis

- No complications: Return to normal activities in 6–8 weeks; however, follow-up treatment may alter lifestyle for a period of time.
- Complications: hemorrhage; SSI; numbness of the skin and anterior chest wall–temporary or permanent; impaired arm and shoulder range of motion ("frozen shoulder"); skin flap necrosis; seromas; lymphedema; phantom breast syndrome; cellulitis; hematoma formation.

Wound Classification

- Class I: Clean

SURGERY OF THE THYROID AND PARATHYROID

The thyroid gland may fall within the realm of other specialties in some locales; however, the general surgeon commonly operates on the thyroid and parathyroid glands.

Pathological conditions affecting the thyroid and parathyroid glands are summarized in Tables 14-17 and 14-18.

Thyroidectomy

Thyroidectomy is the surgical removal of the thyroid gland. The parathyroid glands, intimately related to the thyroid glands, must be spared. A life-threatening condition associated with the parathyroid glands is tetany. When surgery is performed on the thyroid gland, as many of the parathyroids should be identified as possible and at least one parathyroid gland left in place to guarantee the secretion of calcium into the circulation. If all four glands are removed, the patient will experience hypoparathyroidism, which causes hypocalcemia that leads to the neuromuscular symptoms of tetany.

Table 14-17 Pathological Conditions of the Thyroid

Condition	Symptoms/Signs	Diagnostics	Treatments
Hyperthyroidism or thyrotoxicosis	• Nervousness • Restlessness • Emotional lability • Fast speech • Tachycardia • Palpitations • Arrhythmias • Dyspnea • Heat intolerance • Sweating • Fatigue • Weakness • Tremor • Hair loss • Nail separating from nail bed • One complication of thyrotoxicosis is "thyroid storm"	• History • Physical examination • Serum levels of TSH	• Medical blocking of the hormone and its effects • Radioiodide ablation of active thyroid tissue • Surgical resection
Thyroid carcinoma	• May be asymptomatic • May show signs of hyper- or hypothyroidism according to tumor type • Hoarseness • Signs of tracheal or esophageal compression	• History • Physical examination • Serum levels of TSH • Ultrasound • Laryngosocopy • Scans • Biopsy	• Surgical resection for localized carcinoma (unless anaplastic carcinoma or lymphoma)

Table 14-18 Pathological Conditions of the Parathyroid

Condition	Symptoms/Signs	Diagnostics	Treatments
Hyperparathyroidism	• Asymptomatic early on • Skeletal damage	• Laboratory studies • Ultrasound • Biopsy • CT/MRI scan	• Varies with cause • Surgical resection of affected gland
Hypoparathyroidism	• Anxiety, depression, irritability • Brittle nails • Very dry skin • Thin hair • Tetany, which can be caused by an abnormal low level of calcium or *Clostridium tetani* that invades a surgical wound, is a severe complication	• Laboratory studies • Serum levels of PTH	• Calcium • Vitamin D • Controlled diet • Antibiotic therapy in case of wound infection

PROCEDURE 14-23 Thyroidectomy

Surgical Anatomy and Pathology	• Thyroid gland consists of two lobes that are anterior to the larynx.
	  • The lobes are connected by the thyroid isthmus at the level of the second tracheal ring.
	  • A pyramidal lobe may extend cephalad from the isthmus or its junction with one of the lobes.
	  • A fibrous capsule invests the thyroid.
	  • The infrahyoid muscles and their fascia overlie the thyroid.
	  • The thyroid crosses the trachea and esophagus.
	  • The superior portions of the lateral lobes connect to the cricoid and thyroid cartilages.
	  • The parathyroid glands lie on the dorsal side of the thyroid gland.
	• The gland consists of two groups of cells that produce hormones (refer to Plate 5 in Appendix A).
	  • Follicular cells produce, store, and release thyroxine and triiodothyronine.
	  • Parafollicular cells secrete calcitonin.
	• Arterial blood supply is from the superior and inferior thyroid arteries.
	  • The superior thyroid artery is the first branch of the external carotid artery; it courses downward and toward the apex of the lateral lobe.
	  • The inferior thyroid artery is the largest branch of the thyrocervical trunk of the subclavian artery; it ascends along the medial margin of the anterior scalene muscle and lies behind the lateral lobe of the thyroid, and continues downward to the inferior pole.
	• Veinous drainage is via the superior thyroid, middle thyroid, and inferior thyroid veins.
	• Nerve supply is via the cardiac, superior laryngeal, and inferior laryngeal nerves.
	• Thyroid pathology (refer to Table 14-17)

Preoperative Diagnostic Tests and Procedures	• Refer to Table 14-17.
Equipment and Instruments Unique to Procedure	• Harmonic scalpel • Thyroidectomy instrument set that includes several sizes of rake retractors, Green loop retractors, self-retaining retractor such as a Weitlaner, straight mosquito and Crile hemostats, right-angle clamps and Lahey thyroid clamps • Bipolar forceps electrocautery • Hemoclip appliers with ligating clips • Headlamp
Supplies Unique to Procedure	• Knife blades: #10 × 2; #15 × 2 • Bulb syringe • ¼″ Penrose drain
Preoperative Preparation	• Supine position with roll towel or padded sandbag placed between the scapulae to extend the neck. • Surgeon may want patient placed in reverse Trendelenburg; therefore, a padded footboard will need to be placed on the OR table. • General anesthesia. • Skin prep: Point of chin to mid-chest and bilaterally as far as possible following the jaw line to include the entire neck and shoulders. • Draping: Square off incision site with four towels: Upper towel placed along chin to follow jaw line; lower towel placed at level of clavicles; lateral towels placed along sides of neck using sternal end of clavicles as a landmark. Transverse drape or thyroid drape with a transverse opening placed.

(*continues*)

Procedure 14-23 (continued)

Practical Considerations

- A Queen Anne's dressing or thyroid collar may be used at the end of the procedure (refer to Chapter 10 for description of dressing).
- Surgeon may use a silk tie to mark the line of incision on the neck.
- Often straight mosquito and Crile hemostats are used rather than curved.
- The surgical technologist should keep the back table and Mayo stand sterile until the patient has been transported from the OR in case an emergency tracheotomy needs to be performed.
- A tracheotomy tray should be transported with the patient to PACU and the ward.

Surgical Procedure

1. A symmetrical, transverse incision following the Langer lines is made over the thyroid. Size varies to provide optimal access, but is typically two fingerbreadths above the clavicular head. The incision is through the skin and cervical fascia and the platysma muscle is divided (Figure 14-25A).

   Procedural Consideration: Electrocautery or bipolar electrocautery, hemoclips, and ties will be used to control bleeding.

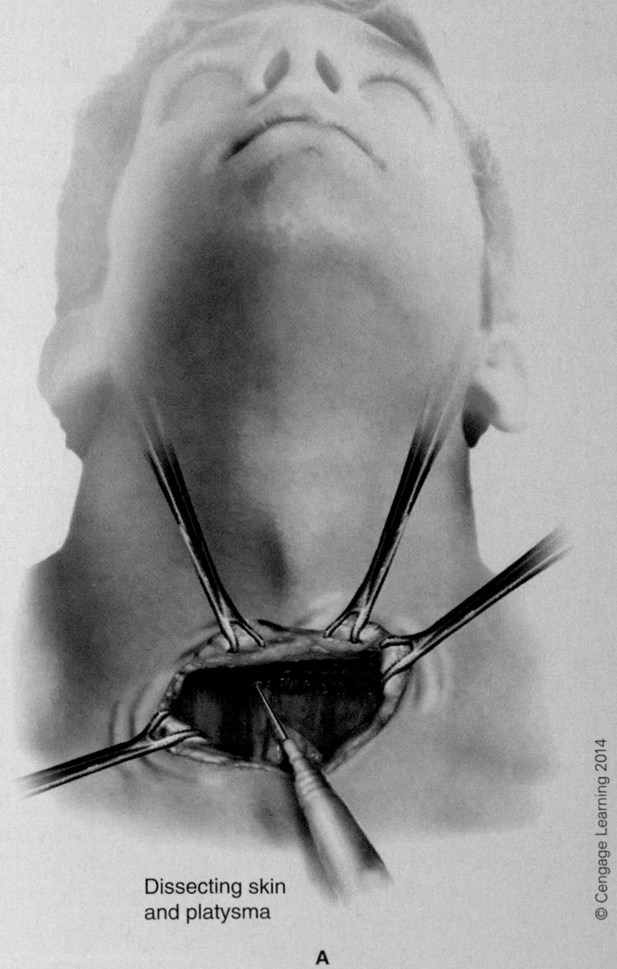

Figure 14-25 Thyroidectomy: (A) Incision

PROCEDURE 14-23 (continued)

2. Superior and inferior flaps are mobilized and retractors placed. The upper skin flap is created to the level of the thyroid notch; two double skin hooks are placed to retract the flap superiorly. The lower skin flap is created down to the sternoclavicular joint. Bleeding continues to be controlled primarily with clamps and ties.

   Procedural Consideration: A self-retaining retractor such as a Weitlaner may be placed.

3. The fascia between the strap muscles is incised and the muscles are separated and the thyroid lobe is exposed. The sternocleidomastoid muscle is retracted with a Green loop retractor. The middle and inferior thyroid veins are identified, clamped, divided, and ligated.

   Procedural Consideration: Thyroidectomy procedures will move carefully and methodically. Keep clean dry sponges on the field. Procedural steps are often repeated when careful dissection is being performed; the surgeon will use a right-angle clamp to spread a small piece of tissue, cut the tissue with Metzenbaum scissors, and ligate with ties.

4. The superior poles are retracted caudally with Lahey thyroid clamps and the tissue between the trachea and superior poles is dissected with the Metzenbaum scissors. The recurrent and superior laryngeal nerves must be identified at this point and must be preserved. The superior thyroid artery is doubly clamped, divided, and ligated (Figure 14-25B).

5. The parathyroid glands and inferior thyroid artery are identified. The parathyroid glands are mobilized and the vascular supply is preserved (Figure 14-25C).

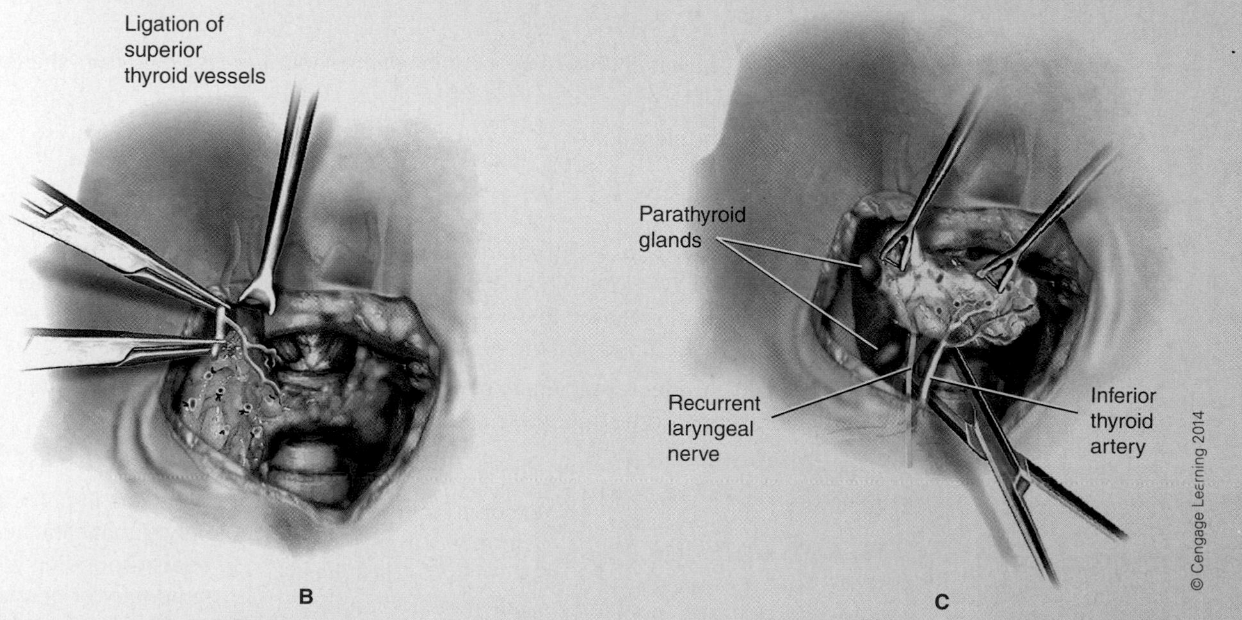

Figure 14-25 Thyroidectomy: (B) ligation of superior thyroid vessels, (C) identification of parathyroid glands and recurrent laryngeal nerve

(continues)

PROCEDURE 14-23 (continued)

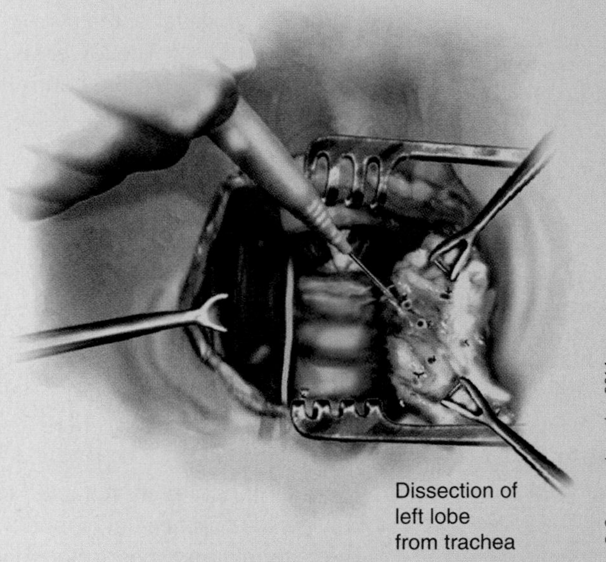

Figure 14-25 Thyroidectomy: (D) dissection from trachea

6. Branches of the inferior thyroid artery that do not supply the parathyroid glands are clamped, divided, and ligated. The superior connective tissue is divided. Hemostasis is achieved with electrosurgical unit (ESU). *Note:* Recurrent nerve must be preserved.

   Procedural Consideration: May alternate between sharp and blunt dissection, and electrocautery.

7. The thyroid is elevated with Allis or Lahey clamps and it is dissected from the trachea (Figure 14-25D).

   Procedural Consideration: If only one lobe is taken, the isthmus is divided so that it is removed with the resected lobe.

8. Hemostasis is achieved after lobe or lobes removed. If the strap muscles were incised, they are reapproximated with suture of the surgeon's choice. A Penrose drain may be placed and exteriorized at the midline. The platysma muscle is reapproximated and a subcuticular closure is used to bring the skin edges together. Skin closure tapes may be applied to the wound and the dressing of the surgeon's choice applied.

   Procedural Consideration: Sequence is irrigation, placement of wound drain, closure, and application of dressings while counts are completed.

Postoperative Considerations

Immediate Postoperative Care

- Check voice as soon as possible.
- Transport to PACU with tracheotomy tray.

Prognosis

- No complications: Return to normal activities in 2-4 weeks; medications usually required for life.
- Complications: hemorrhage; SSI; tetany; damage to nearby structures in particular nerves that can cause hoarse-sounding voice–temporary or permanent.

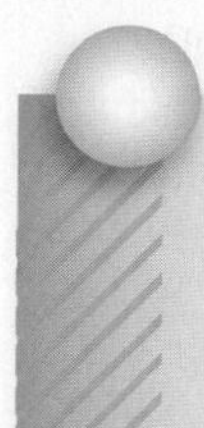

PEARL OF WISDOM

Maintain the integrity of the sterile field until the patient is extubated, breathing freely, and has been transported to the PACU. Emergency tracheotomy is a possibility.

CASE STUDY Jesse is a surgical technology student assigned to a Whipple procedure with his preceptor. The preceptor told Jesse that he should be an expert at several procedures before the case was finished.

1. What did the preceptor mean?
2. What individual procedures comprise the Whipple procedure?
3. What instrument sets will be used?

QUESTIONS FOR FURTHER STUDY

1. Why is everyone concerned about a patient's voice following a thyroidectomy?
2. Name and describe all of the variations for large bowel anastomosis.
3. Imagine a gunshot wound that entered a patient's left chest and exited above the right iliac crest. How many structures can you name that the bullet could have passed through?
4. Describe the patient position that is necessary when a thoracoabdominal approach is planned.

BIBLIOGRAPHY

Adams, R. D. (2009). Electrophysiologic testing and laboratory aids in the diagnosis of neuromuscular disease. In R. D. Adams et al. (Eds.), *Principles of neurology* (9th ed. New York: McGraw-Hill.

Asensio, J. A., & Buckman, R. F., Jr. (2007). Duodenal injuries. In G. D. Zuidema (Ed.), *Shackelford's surgery of the alimentary tract* (6th ed.). St. Louis: Elsevier.

Association of Surgical Technologists. (2011). *Core curriculum for surgical technology* (6th ed.). Littleton, CO: Association of Surgical Technologists.

August, D. A., & Sondak, V. K. (2005). Breast. In M. W. Mulholland, K. D. Lillemore, G. M. Doherty, R. V. Maier, & G. R. Upchurch (Eds.), *Greenfield's surgery: Scientific principles and practice* (4th ed.). Philadelphia: Lippincott Williams & Wilkins.

Banks, P. A. (2006). Acute and chronic pancreatitis. In M. Feldman, M. H. Sleisenger, & B. F. Scharschmidt (Eds.), *Sleisenger and Fordtran's gastrointestinal and liver disease* (8th ed.). Philadelphia: W. B. Saunders.

Bannister, L. H. (1995). Alimentary tract. In P. L. Williams et al. (Eds.), *Gray's anatomy: The anatomical basis of medicine and surgery* (38th ed.). New York: Churchill Livingstone.

Bannister, L. H. (1995). Haemolymphoid system. In P. L. Williams et al. (Eds.), *Gray's anatomy: The anatomical basis of medicine and surgery* (38th ed.). New York: Churchill Livingstone.

Bannister, L. H. (1995). Integumental system. In P. L. Williams et al. (Eds.), *Gray's anatomy: The anatomical basis of medicine and surgery* (38th ed.). New York: Churchill Livingstone.

Barnett, J. L., & Raper, S. E. (2008). Anorectal disease. In T. Yamada, D. H. Alpers, L. Laine, N. Kaplowitz, & C. Owyang (Eds.), *Textbook of gastroenterology* (5th ed.). Hoboken, NJ: Wiley-Blackwell.

Beger, H. G., & Buchlet, M. W. (1995). Surgical management of chronic pancreatitis. In W. S. Haubrich, F. Schaffner, & J. E. Berk (Eds.), *Bockus' gastroenterology* (5th ed.). Philadelphia: W. B. Saunders.

Behar, J. (1995). Anatomy and anomalies of the biliary tract. In W. S. Haubrich, F. Schaffner, & J. E. Berk (Eds.), *Bockus' gastroenterology* (5th ed.). Philadelphia: W. B. Saunders.

Bell, R. H. (2005). Neoplasms of the exocrine pancreas. In M. W. Mulholland et al. (Eds.), *Greenfield's surgery: Scientific principles and practice* (4th ed.). Philadelphia: Lippincott Williams & Wilkins.

Bennion, R. S., Williams R. A., & Wilson, S. E. (2003). Principles of vascular access surgery. In F. J. Veith et al. (Eds.), *Vascular surgery* (3rd ed.). New York: Informal Healthcare.

Bennion, R. S., & Wilson, S. E. (2001). Hemodialysis and vascular access. In W. S. Moore (Ed.), *Vascular surgery: A comprehensive review* (6th ed.). Philadelphia: W. B. Saunders.

Bergan, J. J. (2001). Varicose veins: Chronic venous insufficiency. In W. S. Moore (Ed.), *Vascular surgery: A comprehensive review* (6th ed.). Philadelphia: W. B. Saunders.

Berne, T. V., & Ortega, A. (2006). Appendicitis and appendiceal abscess. In J. E. Fischer, K. I. Bland, M. P. Callery, G. P. Clagett, & D. B. Jones (Eds.), *Mastery of surgery* (5th ed.). Philadelphia: Lippincott Williams & Wilkins.

Biancani, P., & Behar, J. (2008). Esophageal motor function. In T. Yamada et al. (Eds.), *Textbook of gastroenterology* (5th ed). Hoboken, NJ: Wiley-Blackwell.

Bland, K. I., & Vezeridis, M. P. (2006). Anatomy of the breast. In J. E. Fischer et al. (Eds.), *Mastery of surgery* (5th ed.). Philadelphia: Lippincott Williams & Wilkins.

Bockus, M. S. (1995). Anatomy of the small intestine. In W. S. Haubrich, F. Schaffner, & J. E. Berk (Eds.), *Bockus' gastroenterology* (5th ed.). Philadelphia: W. B. Saunders.

Britt, L. D., & Berger, J. (2006). Splenic repair and partial splenectomy. In J. E. Fischer et al. (Eds.), *Mastery of surgery* (5th ed.). Philadelphia: Lippincott Williams & Wilkins.

Brophy, M. T., Fiore, L. D., & Deykin, D. (2006). Hemostasis. In D. Zakim & T. D. Boyer (Eds.), *Hepatology: A textbook of liver disease* (5th ed.). Philadelphia: W. B. Saunders.

Brown, S. D., van Sonnenberg, E., & Mueller, P. R. (2006). Interventional radiology in the liver, biliary tract, and gallbladder. In *Schiff's diseases of the liver* (10th ed). Philadelphia: Lippincott Williams & Wilkins.

Bubrick, M. P., & Rolstad, B. S. (2007). Intestinal stomas. In P. H. Gordon & S. Nivatvongs (Eds.), *Principles and practices of surgery for the colon, rectum, and anus* (3rd ed). Boca Raton, NM: Informa Healthcare.

Camilleri, M., & Prather, C. M. (2006). Gastric motor physiology and motor disorders. In M. Feldman, M. H. Sleisenger, & B. F. Scharschmidt (Eds.), *Sleisenger and Fordtran's gastrointestinal and liver disease* (8th ed.). Phildelphia: W. B. Saunders.

Carey, L. C., & Ellison, E. S. (2006). Cholecystostomy, cholecystectomy, and intraoperative evaluation of the biliary tree. In J. E. Fischer et al. (Eds.), *Mastery of surgery* (5th ed.). Philadelphia: Lippincott Williams & Wilkins.

Carter, D. C. (1998). Pain-relieving procedures in chronic pancreatitis. In M. Trede, Sir D. C. Carter, & W. P. Longmire, Jr. (Eds.), *Surgery of the pancreas* (2nd ed.). New York: Churchill Livingstone.

Cello, J. P. (2006). Pancreatic cancer. In M. Feldman, M. H. Sleisenger, & B. F. Scharschmidt (Eds.), *Sleisenger and Fordtran's gastrointestinal and liver diseasei* (8th ed.). Philadelphia: W. B. Saunders.

Chang, A. E., & Sondak, V. K. (2007). Clinical evaluation and treatment of soft tissue tumors. In F. M. Enzinger & S. W. Weiss (Eds.), *Soft tissue tumors* (5th ed.). St. Louis: Mosby-Yearbook.

Chapman, W.C., & Newman, M. (2008). Disorders of the spleen. In G. R. Lee et al. (Eds.), *Wintrobe's clinical hematology* (12th ed.). Baltimore: Williams & Wilkins.

Condon, R. E. (2006). Iliopubic tract repair of inguinal hernia: The anterior inguinal canal approach. In J. E. Fischer et al. (Eds.), *Mastery of surgery* (5th ed.). Philadelphia: Lippincott Williams & Wilkins.

Condon, R. E. (2001). The anatomy of the inguinal region and its relation to groin hernia. In L. M. Nyhus & R. E. Condon (Eds.), *Hernia* (5th ed.). Philadelphia: J. B. Lippincott.

Cotton, P. B., & Williams, C. B. (2008). *Practical gastrointestinal endoscopy* (6th ed.). Hoboken, NJ: Wiley-Blackwell.

Crist, D. W., & Gadacz, T. R. (2006). Anatomy, embryology, congenital anomalies, and physiology of the gallbladder and extrahepatic biliary ducts. In G. D. Zuidema (Ed.), *Shackelford's surgery of the alimentary tract* (6th ed.). Philadelphia: W. B. Saunders.

Daly, J. M. (2009). Abdominal wall, omentum, mesentery, and retroperitoneum. In F. C. Brunicardi, D. K. Andersen, T. R. Billiar, D. L. Dunn, J. G. Hunter, & R. E. Pollock (Eds.), *Schwartz's principles of surgery* (9th ed.). New York: McGraw-Hill Professional.

Dempsey, D. T., & Ritchie, W. P., Jr. (2006). Anatomy and physiology of the duodenum. In G. D. Zuidema (Ed.), *Shackelford's surgery of the alimentary tract* (6th ed.). Philadelphia: W. B. Saunders.

Dempsey, D. T., & Ritchie, W. P., Jr. (2006). Anatomy and physiology of the stomach. In G. D. Zuidema (Ed.), *Shackelford's surgery of the alimentary tract* (6th ed.). Philadelphia: W. B. Saunders.

Deveney, K. E. (2005). Hernias and other lesions of the abdominal wall. In G. M. Doherty (Ed.), *Current surgical diagnosis and treatment* (12th ed.). New York: McGraw-Hill Medical.

Donegan, W. L. (2002). Staging and primary treatment. In W. L. Donegan & J. S. Spratt (Eds.), *Cancer of the breast* (5th ed.). Philadelphia: W. B. Saunders.

Dong-Weng Eu, & Oakley, F. R. (1997). Stoma construction. In R. N. Allan et al. (Eds.), *Inflammatory bowel diseases* (3rd ed.). New York: Churchill Livingstone.

Eastwood, G. L. (2008). Stomach: Anatomy and structural anomalies. In T. Yamada et al. (Eds.), *Textbook of gastroenterology* (5th ed.). Hoboken, NJ: Wiley-Blackwell.

Eisenbert, M. M., Fondacaro, P. F., & Dunn, D. H. (1995). Applied anatomy and anomalies of the stomach. In W. S. Haubrich, F. Schaffner, & J. E. Berk (Eds.), *Bockus' gastroenterology* (5th ed.). Philadelphia: W. B. Saunders.

Ellis, H. (2006). Cholecystostomy and cholecystectomy. In M. J. Zinner & S. W. Ashley (Eds.), *Maingot's abdominal operations* (11 th ed.). New York: McGraw-Hill Professional.

Ellis, H. (2006). Incisions and closures. In M. J. Zinner et al. (Eds.), *Maingot's abdominal operations* (11 th ed.). New York: McGraw-Hill Professional.

Ellis, H. (2006). Incisions, closures, and wound management. In M. J. Zinner et al. (Eds.), *Maingot's abdominal operations* (11 th ed.). New York: McGraw-Hill Professional.

Ellis, H., & Nathanson, L. K. (2006). Appendix and appendectomy. In M. J. Zinner et al. (Eds.), *Maingot's abdominal operations* (11 th ed.). New York: McGraw-Hill Professional.

Fazio, V. W., & Erwin-Toth, P. (1995). Stomal and pouch function and care. In W. S. Haubrich, F. Schaffner, & J. E. Berk (Eds.), *Bockus' gastroenterology* (5th ed.). Philadelphia: W. B. Saunders.

Fazio, V. W., & Tjandra, J. J. (2007). The management of perianal disease. In J. L. Cameron et al. (Eds.), *Surgery* (9th ed.). St. Louis: Mosby Yearbook.

Feliciano, D. V. (2006). Trauma and the liver. In D. Zakim & T. D. Boyer (Eds.), *Hepatology: A textbook of liver disease* (5th ed.). Philadelphia: W. B. Saunders.

Fernandez-del Castillo, C., Rivera, J. A., & Warshaw, A. L. (1999). Cystic tumors. In M. Trede, Sir D. C. Carter, & W. P. Longmire, Jr. (Eds.), *Surgery of the pancreas* (2nd ed.). New York: Churchill Livingstone.

Flesch, L. (2006). Care of stomas. In J. E. Fischer et al. (Eds.), *Mastery of surgery* (5th ed.). Philadelphia: Lippincott Williams & Wilkins.

Fong, Y., & Blumgart, L. H. (2006). Surgical therapy of liver cancer. In D. Zakim & T. D. Boyer (Eds.), *Hepatology: A textbook of liver disease* (5th ed.). Philadelphia: W. B. Saunders.

Frey, C. F., Wardell, J. W., & McMurtry, A. L. (1998). Injuries to the pancreas. In M. Trede, Sir D. C. Carter, & W. P. Longmire, Jr. (Eds.), *Surgery of the pancreas* (2nd ed.). New York: Churchill Livingstone.

Gabella, G. (1995). Cardiovascular system. In L. H. Bannister (Ed.), *Gray's anatomy: The anatomical basis of medicine and surgery* (38th ed.). New York: Churchill Livingstone.

George, J. N., & El-Harake, M. (2008). Thrombocytopenia due to enhanced platelet destruction by nonimmuno-logic mechanisms. In Beutler, E. Lichtman, B. S. Coller, & T. J. Kipps (Eds.), *Williams hematology* (6th ed.). New York: McGraw-Hill.

Goldstone, J. (2005). Veins and lymphatics. In G. M. Doherty (Ed.), *Current surgical diagnosis and treatment* (12th ed.). New York: McGraw-Hill Medical.

Gordon, P. H. (2007). Anorectal abscesses and fistula-in-ano. In P. H. Gordon & S. Nivatvongs (Eds.), *Principles and practices of surgery for the colon, rectum, and anus* (3rd ed.). Boca Raton, FL: Informa Healthcare.

Gorelick, F. S. (2008). Acute pancreatitis. In T. Yamada et al. (Eds.), *Textbook of gastroenterology* (5th ed.). Hoboken, NJ: Lippincott-Blackwell.

Green, R. M., & Ouriel, K. (2009). Venous and lymphatic disease. In F. C. Brunicardi et al. (Eds.), *Schwartz's principles of surgery* (9th ed.). New York: McGraw-Hill Professional.

Grendell, J. H. (1995). Embryology, anatomy, and anomalies of the pancreas. In W. S. Haubrich, F. Schaffner, & J. E. Berk (Eds.), *Bockus' gastroenterology* (5th ed.). Philadelphia: W. B. Saunders.

Grendell, J. H., & Ermack, T. H. (2006). Anatomy, histology, embryology, and developmental anomalies of the pancreas. In M. Feldman, M. H. Sleisenger, & B. F. Scharschmidt (Eds.), *Sleisenger and Fordtran's gastrointestinal and liver disease* (8th ed.). Philadelphia: W. B. Saunders.

Guice, K. S. (2005). Acute pancreatitis. In M. W. Mulholland et al. (Eds.), *Greenfield's surgery: Scientific principles and practice* (4th ed.). Philadelphia: Lippincott Williams & Wilkins.

Hacker, N. F. (2009). Breast disease: A gynecologic perspective. In N. F. Hacker & J. G. Moore (Eds.), *Essentials of obstetrics and gynecology* (5th ed.). Philadelphia: W. B. Saunders.

Hays, A. P., & Younger, D. S. (1994). Muscle and nerve biopsy. In L. P. Rowland (Ed.), *Merritt's textbook of neurology* (9th ed.). Baltimore: Williams & Wilkins.

Hoover, H. C., Jr. (2006). Pancreatic and periampullary carcinoma nonendocrine. In G. D. Zuidema (Ed.), *Shackelford's surgery of the alimentary tract* (6th ed.). Philadelphia: W. B. Saunders.

Huibregtse, K., & Kimmey, M. B. (2008). Endoscopic retrograde cholangiopancreatography, endoscopic sphincterotomy and stone removal, and endoscopic biliary and pancreatic drainage. In T. Yamada et al. (Eds.), *Textbook of gastroenterology* (5th ed.). Hoboken, NJ: Wiley-Blackwell.

Jesseph, J. M. (2006). Open gastrostomy. In J. E. Fischer et al. (Eds.), *Mastery of surgery* (5th ed.). Philadelphia: Lippincott Williams & Wilkins.

Joehl, R. J. (2006). Gastrostomy and gastroenterostomy. In G. D. Zuidema (Ed.), *Shackelford's surgery of the alimentary tract* (6th ed.). Philadelphia: W. B. Saunders.

Jones, A. L., & Aggeler, J. (1995). Structure of the liver. In W. S. Haubrich, F. Schaffner, & J. E. Berk (Eds.), *Bockus' gastroenterology* (5th ed.). Philadelphia: W. B. Saunders.

Kafie, F. E., & Wilson, S. E. (1998). Complications of vascular access surgery. In J. S. T. Yao & W. H. Pearce (Eds.), *Techniques in vascular and endovascular surgery.* Stamford, CT: Appleton & Lange.

Karan, J. A., & Roslynn, J. J. (2006). Cholelithiasis and cholecystectomy. In M. J. Zinner et al. (Eds.), *Maingot's abdominal operations* (11 th ed.). New York: McGraw-Hill Professional.

Kaunitz, J. D., Barrett, K. E., & McRoberts, J. A. (2008). Electrolyte secretion and absorption: Small intestine and colon. In T. Yamada et al. (Eds.), *Textbook of gastroenterology* (5th ed.). Hoboken, NJ: Wiley-Blackwell.

Keljio, D. J., & Squires, R. H., Jr. (2006). Anatomy and anomalies of the small and large intestines. In M. Feldman, M. H. Sleisenger, & B. F. Scharschmidt (Eds.), *Sleisenger and Fordtran's gastrointestinal and liver disease* (8th ed.). Philadelphia: W. B. Saunders.

Kirsner, J. B., & Shorter, R. G. (1999). *Inflammatory bowel disease* (5th ed.). St. Louis: Elsevier.

Kodner, I. J. (2007). Colon, rectum, and anus. In G. D. Zuidema (Ed.), *Principles of Shackelford's surgery of the alimentary tract* (6th ed.). St. Louis: Elsevier.

Kuster, G. G. R. (1995). The appendix. In W. S. Haubrich, F. Schaffner, & J. E. Berk (Eds.), *Bockus' gastroenterology* (5th ed.). Philadelphia: W. B. Saunders.

Lance, P. (2008). Tumors and other neoplastic disease of the small bowel. In T. Yamada et al. (Eds.), *Textbook of gastroenterology* (5th ed.). Hoboken, NJ: Wiley-Blackwell.

Langnas, A. N., & Shaw, B. W., Jr. (2006). Surgical therapy for hepatocellular carcinoma. In E. R. Schiff, M. F. Sorrell, & W. C. Maddrey (Eds.), *Schiff's diseases of the liver* (10th ed.). New York: Lippincott Williams & Wilkins.

Lavery, I. C. (2006). Technique of colostomy construction and closure. In J. E. Fischer et al. (Eds.), *Mastery of surgery* (5th ed.). Philadelphia: Lippincott Williams & Wilkins.

Lefkowitch, J. H. (2006). Pathologic diagnosis of liver disease. In D. Zakim & T. D. Boyer (Eds.), *Hepatology: A textbook of liver disease* (5th ed.). Philadelphia: W. B. Saunders.

Lin, E., Lowry, S. F., & Calvano, S. E. (2006). The systemic response to injury. In M. Feldman, M. H. Sleisenger, & B. F. Scharschmidt (Eds.), *Sleisenger and Fordtran's gastrointestinal and liver disease* (8th ed.). Phildelphia: W. B. Saunders.

Low, P. A. (2004). Diseases of the peripheral nerves. In R. J. Joynt & R. C. Griggs (Eds.), *Clinical neurology.* Philadelphia: Lippincott Williams & Wilkins.

Lucas, C. E., & Ledgerwood, A. M. (2006). Treatment of the injured liver. In J. E. Fischer et al. (Eds.), *Mastery of surgery* (5th ed.). Philadelphia: Lippincott Williams & Wilkins.

Martindale, R. G., & Gadacz, T. R. (2007). Open cholecystectomy and cholecystostomy. In G. D. Zuidema (Ed.), *Shackelford's surgery of the alimentary tract* (6th ed.). St. Louis: Elsevier.

Martindale, R. G., & Gadacz, T. R. (2007). Treatment of common duct stones. In G. D. Zuidema (Ed.), *Shackelford's surgery of the alimentary tract* (6th ed.). St. Louis: Elsevier.

McArthur, K. E. (2006). Hernias and volvulus of the gastrointestinal tract. In M. Feldman, M. H. Sleisenger, & B. F. Scharschmidt (Eds.), *Sleisenger and Fordtran's gastrointestinal and liver disease* (8th ed.). Philadelphia: W. B. Saunders.

Minei, J. P., & Shires, G. T., III. (1999). Trauma of the liver. *Schiff's diseases of the liver.* New York: Lippincott-Raven.

Morrow, M. (2006). Segmental mastectomy and axillary dissection. In J. E. Fischer et al. (Eds.), *Mastery of surgery* (5th ed.). Philadelphia: Lippincott Williams & Wilkins.

Mulholland, M. W. (2006). Chronic pancreatitis. In M. W. Mulholland et al. (Eds.), *Greenfield's surgery: Scientific principles and practice* (4th ed.). Philadelphia: Lippincott Williams & Wilkins.

Mulholland, M. W., Moossa, A. R., & Liddle, R. A. (2008). Pancreas: Anatomy and structural anomalies. In T. Yamada et al. (Eds.), *Textbook of gastroenterology* (5th ed.). Hoboken, NJ: Wiley-Blackwell.

Nance, F. C. (1995). Diseases of the peritoneum, retroperitoneum, mesentery, and omentum. In W. S. Haubrich, F. Schaffner, & J. E. Berk (Eds.), *Bockus' gastroenterology* (5th ed.). Philadelphia: W. B. Saunders.

Neglen, P. (1997). Cosmetic excision and stripping of varices. In S. Raju & J. L. Villavicencio (Eds.), *Surgical management of venous disease.* Baltimore: Williams & Wilkins.

Nivatvongs, S. (2006). Anorectal disorders. In M. W. Mulholland et al. (Eds.), *Greenfield's surgery: Scientific principles and practice* (4th ed.). Philadelphia: Lippincott Williams & Wilkins.

Nivatvongs, S. (2007). Pilonidal disease. In P. H. Gordon & S. Nivatvongs (Eds.), *Principles and practices of surgery for the colon, rectum, and anus* (3rd ed.). Boca Raton, FL: Informa Healthcare.

Nivatvongs, S. (2009). Hemorrhoids. In P. H. Gordon & S. Nivatvongs (Eds.), *Principles and practices of surgery for the colon, rectum, and anus* (3rd ed.). Boca Raton, FL: Informa Healthcare.

Nordestgaard, A. G., & Williams, R. A. (1994). Varicose veins. In F. J. Veith et al. (Eds.), *Vascular surgery* (2nd ed.). New York: McGraw-Hill.

Nyhus, L. M. (2006). Iliopubic tract repair of inguinal and femoral hernia: The posterior preperitoneal approach. In J. E. Fischer et al. (Eds.), *Mastery of surgery* (5th ed.). Philadelphia: Lippincott Williams & Wilkins.

Osborne, M. P. (1998). Breast development and anatomy. In J. R. Harris et al. (Eds.), *Diseases of the breast.* New York: Lippincott-Raven.

Owhyang, C., & Levitt, M. D. (2008). Chronic pancreatitis. In T. Yamada et al. (Eds.), *Textbook of gastroenterology* (5th ed.). Hoboken, NJ: Wiley-Blackwell.

Pachter, H. M., & Hofstetter, S. (2007). The spleen: Splenic salvage procedures. In J. L. Cameron (Ed.), *Current surgical therapy* (9th ed.). St. Louis: Mosby.

Palovan, D. (2004). Intestinal problems in gynecologic surgery. In J. J. Sciarra (Ed.), *Gynecology and obstetrics.* New York: Lippincott Williams & Wilkins.

Patino, J. E. (2004). A history of the treatment of hernia. In L. M. Nyhus & R. E. Condon (Eds.), *Hernia* (4th ed.). Philadelphia: Williams & Wilkins.

Patten, R. M., & Moss, A. A. (1995). Computed tomography. In W. S. Haubrich, F. Schaffner, & J. E. Berk (Eds.), *Bockus' gastroenterology* (5th ed.). Philadelphia: W. B. Saunders.

Pearl, R. K. (1995). Indications for and techniques of ileostomy. In C. Wastell, L. M. Nyhus, & P. E. Donahue (Eds.), *Surgery of the esophagus, stomach, and small intestine.* Philadelphia: Williams & Wilkins.

Pellegrini, C. A., & Quan-Yang Duh. (2008). Gallbladder and biliary tree: Anatomy and structural anomalies. In T. Yamada et al. (Eds.), *Textbook of gastroenterology* (5th ed.). Hoboken, NJ: Wiley-Blackwell.

Pollak, R. (2006). Miscellaneous surgical techniques for the small intestine. In J. E. Fischer et al. (Eds.), *Mastery of surgery* (5th ed.). Philadelphia: Lippincott Williams & Wilkins.

Pratt, J. S., & Donegan, W. L. (2002). Surgical management. In W. L. Donegan & J. S. Spratt (Eds.), *Cancer of the breast* (5th ed.). Philadelphia: W. B. Saunders.

Ratych, R. E. (1995). Anorectal disease. In W. S. Haubrich, F. Schaffner, & J. E. Berk (Eds.), *Bockus' gastroenterology* (5th ed.). Philadelphia: W. B. Saunders.

Ratych, R. E., & Smith, G. W. (2007). Anatomy and physiology of the liver. In G. D. Zuidema (Ed.), *Shackelford's surgery of the alimentary tract* (6th ed.). St. Louis: Elsevier.

Read, R. C. (2006). Anatomy of abdominal herniation: The parietoperitoneal spaces. In J. E. Fischer et al. (Eds.), *Mastery of surgery* (5th ed.). Philadelphia: Lippincott Williams & Wilkins.

Read, R. C. (2007). Basic features of abdominal wall herniation and its repair. In G. D. Zuidema (Ed.), *Shackelford's surgery of the alimentary tract* (6th ed.). St. Louis: Elsevier.

Read, R. C. (2007). Femoral hernia. In G. D. Zuidema (Ed.), *Shackelford's surgery of the alimentary tract* (6th ed.). St. Louis: Elsevier.

Read, R. C. (2009). Ventral herniation in the adult. In G. D. Zuidema (Ed.), *Shackelford's surgery of the alimentary tract* (6th ed.). St. Louis: Elsevier.

Redel, C. A., & Zwiener, R. J. (2006). Anatomy and anomalies of the stomach and duodenum. In M. Feldman, M. H. Sleisenger, & B. F. Scharschmidt (Eds.), *Sleisenger and Fordtran's gastrointestinal and liver disease* (8th ed.). Philadelphia: W. B. Saunders.

Rees, W. D. W., & Brown, C. M. (1995). Physiology of the stomach and duodenum. In W. S. Haubrich, F. Schaffner, & J. E. Berk (Eds.), *Bockus' gastroenterology* (5th ed.). Philadelphia: W. B. Saunders.

Romolo, J. L. (2007). Embryology and anatomy of the colon. In G. D. Zuidema (Ed.), *Shackelford's surgery of the alimentary tract* (6th ed.). St. Louis: Elsevier.

Rosch, T. (1997). Endoscopic ultrasonography. In M. Trede, Sir D. C. Carter, & W. P. Longmire, Jr. (Eds.), *Surgery of the pancreas* (2nd ed.). New York: Churchill Livingstone.

Roubenoff, R. (1995). The musculoskeletal system. In W. S. Haubrich, F. Schaffner, & J. E. Berk (Eds.), *Bockus' gastroenterology* (5th ed.). Philadelphia: W. B. Saunders.

Rout, W. R. (2007). Abdominal incisions. In G. D. Zuidema (Ed.), *Shackelford's surgery of the alimentary tract* (6th ed.). St. Louis: Elsevier.

Rout, W. R. (2007). Exposure of the thoracic alimentary tract. In G. D. Zuidema (Ed.), *Shackelford's surgery of the alimentary tract* (6th ed.). St. Louis: Elsevier.

Rubin, D. C. (2008). Small intestine: Anatomy and structural anomalies. In T. Yamada et al. (Eds.), *Textbook of gastroenterology* (5th ed.). Hoboken, NJ: Wiley-Blackwell.

Runyon, B. A., & Hillebrand, D. J. (2006). Surgical peritonitis and other diseases of the peritoneum, mesentery, omentum, and diaphragm. In M. Feldman, M. H. Sleisenger, & B. F. Scharschmidt (Eds.), *Sleisenger and Fordtran's gastrointestinal and liver disease* (8th ed.). Philadelphia: W. B. Saunders.

Sabiston, D. C., Jr. (1994). Hernias. In D. C. Sabiston, Jr. & H. K. Lyerly (Eds.), *Sabiston essentials of surgery* (2nd ed.). Philadelphia: W. B. Saunders.

Salmons, S. (1995). Muscles. In L. H. Bannister (Ed.), *Gray's anatomy: The anatomical basis of medicine and surgery* (38th ed.). New York: Churchill Livingstone.

Salvati, E. P., & Eisenstat, F. E. (2007). Hemorrhoidal disease. In G. D. Zuidema (Ed.), *Shackelford's surgery of the alimentary tract* (6th ed.). St. Louis: Elsevier.

Schaffner, F., & Thung, S. N. (1995). Liver biopsy. In W. S. Haubrich, F. Schaffner, & J. E. Berk (Eds.), *Bockus' gastroenterology* (5th ed.). Philadelphia: W. B. Saunders.

Schrock, T. R. (2005). Large intestine. In G. M. Doherty (Ed.), *Current surgical diagnosis and treatment* (12th ed.). New York: McGraw-Hill Medical.

Schrock, T. R. (2007). Colon and rectum: Diagnostic techniques. In G. D. Zuidema (Ed.), *Shackelford's surgery of the alimentary tract* (6th ed.). St. Louis: Elsevier.

Schrock, T. R. (2006). Appendicitis. In M. Feldman, M. H. Sleisenger, & B. F. Scharschmidt (Eds.), *Sleisenger and Fordtran's gastrointestinal and liver disease* (8th ed.). Philadelphia: W. B. Saunders.

Schrock, T. R. (2006). Examination and diseases of the anorectum. In M. Feldman, M. H. Sleisenger, & B. F. Scharschmidt (Eds.), *Sleisenger and Fordtran's gastrointestinal and liver disease* (8th ed.). Philadelphia: W. B. Saunders.

Schwartz, S. I. (2006). The spleen: Anatomy and splenectomy. In J. E. Fischer et al. (Eds.), *Master of surgery* (5th ed.). Philadelphia: Lippincott Williams & Wilkins.

Schwartz, S. I. (2007). The spleen: Splenectomy for hematologic disorders. In J. L. Cameron (Ed.), *Current surgical therapy* (9th ed.). St. Louis: Mosby.

Schwartz, S. I. (2009). Gallbladder and extrahepatic biliary system. In F. C. Brunicardi et al. (Eds.), *Schwartz's principles of surgery* (9th ed.). New York: McGraw-Hill Professional.

Selub, S. E. (1995). Digestion and absorption: Water, electrolyte, and vitamin transport. In W. S. Haubrich, F. Schaffner, & J. E. Berk (Eds.), *Bockus' gastroenterology* (5th ed.). Philadelphia: W. B. Saunders.

Sherlock, S., & Dooley, J. (Eds.). (2002). Anatomy and function. *Diseases of the liver and biliary system* (11th ed.). Hoboken, NJ: Wiley-Blackwell.

Sherlock, S., & Dooley, J. (Eds.). (2002). Gallstones and inflammatory disease. *Diseases of the liver and biliary system* (11th ed.). Hoboken, NJ: Wiley-Blackwell.

Sherry, R. M., & Gadacz, T. R. (2007). Cholelithiasis and cholecystitis. In G. D. Zuidema (Ed.), *Shackelford's surgery of the alimentary tract* (6th ed.). St. Louis: Elsevier.

Shires, G. T. (2007). Trauma. In G. D. Zuidema (Ed.), *Principles of Shackelford's surgery of the alimentary tract* (6th ed.). St. Louis: Elsevier.

Smith, D. L., & Meyer, A. A. (2007). Anatomy, immunology, and physiology of the spleen. In G. D. Zuidema (Ed.), *Shackelford's surgery of the alimentary tract* (6th ed.). St. Louis: Elsevier.

Solomon, T. E. (1995). Physiology of the exocrine pancreas. In W. S. Haubrich, F. Schaffner, & J. E. Berk (Eds.), *Bockus' gastroenterology* (5th ed.). Philadelphia: W. B. Saunders.

Stirling, M. C., & Orringer, M. B. (2007). Esophageal varices. In G. D. Zuidema (Ed.), *Shackelford's surgery of the alimentary tract* (6th ed.). St. Louis: Elsevier.

Stolz, A. (2006). Liver physiology and metabolic function. In M. Feldman, M. H. Sleisenger, & B. F. Scharschmidt (Eds.), *Sleisenger and Fordtran's gastrointestinal and liver disease* (8th ed.). Phildelphia: W. B. Saunders.

Suchy, F. J. (2006). Anatomy, anomalies, and pediatric disorders of the biliary tract. In M. Feldman, M. H. Sleisenger, & B. F. Scharschmidt (Eds.), *Sleisenger and Fordtran's gastrointestinal and liver disease* (8th ed.). Phildelphia: W. B. Saunders.

Telford, G. L., & Condon, R. E. (2007). Appendix. In G. D. Zuidema (Ed.), *Shackelford's surgery of the alimentary tract* (6th ed.). St. Louis: Elsevier.

Tominaga, G. T., & Jakowatz, J. G. (2002). Placement of indwelling venous access systems. *Vascular access: Principles and practice* (4th ed.). St. Louis: Elsevier.

Trede, M. (1997). Approaches to the pancreas and abdominal exploration. In M. Trede, Sir D. C. Carter, & W. P. Longmire, Jr. (Eds.), *Surgery of the pancreas* (2nd ed.). New York: Churchill Livingstone.

Trede, M. (1998). Approaches to the pancreas and abdominal exploration. In M. Trede, Sir D. C. Carter, & W. P. Longmire, Jr. (Eds.), *Surgery of the pancreas* (2nd ed.). New York: Churchill Livingstone.

Trede, M. (1998). Embryology and surgical anatomy of the pancreas. In M. Trede, Sir D. C. Carter, & W. P. Longmire, Jr. (Eds.), *Surgery of the pancreas* (2nd ed.). New York: Churchill Livingstone.

Trede, M. (1998). Technique of Whipple pancreatoduodenectomy. In M. Trede, Sir D. C. Carter, & W. P. Longmire, Jr. (Eds.), *Surgery of the pancreas* (2nd ed.). New York: Churchill Livingstone.

Trede, M., & Carter, C. (1998). The complications of pancreatoduodenectomy and their management. In M. Trede, Sir D. C. Carter, & W. P. Longmire, Jr. (Eds.), *Surgery of the pancreas* (2nd ed.). New York: Churchill Livingstone.

Veith, F. J. (1994). Vascular surgical techniques. In F. J. Veith et al. (Eds.), *Vascular surgery* (2nd ed.). New York: McGraw-Hill.

Wanless, I. R. (2006). Anatomy and developmental anomalies of the liver. In M. Feldman, M. H. Sleisenger, & B. F. Scharschmidt (Eds.), *Sleisenger and Fordtran's gastrointestinal and liver disease* (8th ed). Phildelphia: W. B. Saunders.

Wantz, G. E. (2009). Abdominal wall hernias. In F. C. Brunicardi et al. (Eds.), *Schwartz's principles of surgery* (9th ed.). New York: McGraw-Hill Professional.

Way, L. W. (2005). Biliary tract. In G. M. Doherty (Ed.), *Current surgical diagnosis and treatment* (12th ed.). New York: McGraw-Hill Medical.

Weiss, L. (2005). The structure of the spleen. In Beutler, M. A. Lichtman, B. S. Coller, & T. J. Kipps (Eds.), *Williams hematology* (7th ed.). New York: McGraw-Hill.

Werner, J., & Warshaw, A. L. (1998). Pseudocysts, post-inflammatory cystic fluid collections, and other nonneoplastic cysts. In M. Trede, Sir D. C. Carter, & W. P. Longmire, Jr. (Eds.), *Surgery of the pancreas* (2nd ed.). New York: Churchill Livingstone.

White, R. A., & Fogarty, T. J. (1999). Devices and techniques for vascular access: Utility and limitations of current methods. In R. A. White & T. J. Fogarty (Eds.), *Peripheral endovascular interventions.* New York: Springer.

Wile, A. (2002). Indications and devices for chronic venous access. *Vascular access: Principles and practice* (4th ed.). St. Louis: Elsevier.

Wilson, S. E. (2002). Complications of vascular access procedures: Thrombosis, venous hypertension, arterial steal, and neuropathy. *Vascular access: Principles and practice* (4th ed.). St. Louis: Elsevier.

Wood, D. K. (2006). Liver biopsy techniques. In J. E. Fischer et al. (Eds.), *Mastery of surgery* (5th ed.). Philadelphia: Lippincott Williams & Wilkins.

Wright, P. E., II. (2007). Hand infections. In S. T. Canale (Ed.), *Campbell's operative orthopaedics* (11 th ed.). St. Louis: Mosby.

Zucker, S. D., & Gollan, J. L. (1995). Physiology of the liver. In W. S. Haubrich, F. Schaffner, & J. E. Berk (Eds.), *Bockus' gastroenterology* (5th ed.). Philadelphia: W. B. Saunders.

CHAPTER

15

Obstetric and Gynecologic Surgery

CASE STUDY Meredith is in labor for the first time. She had a normal pregnancy and good prenatal care. Labor proceeded normally until she was dilated to 4 centimeters. Since that point, no progress has taken place. It has been 12 hours; Meredith is tired and frustrated. The fetus demonstrates no stress as of yet. Meredith is scheduled for a cesarean section.

1. What is the term used to describe this condition?
2. Is the condition a common reason for cesarean section?
3. What are the procedural steps for a cesarean section?

OBJECTIVES

After studying this chapter, the reader should be able to:

A 1. Recognize the relevant anatomy and physiology of the female reproductive system.

P 2. Summarize the pathology of the female reproductive system that prompts surgical intervention and the related terminology.

3. Determine any special preoperative obstetric and gynecologic diagnostic procedures/tests.

O 4. Determine any special preoperative preparation procedures related to obstetric/gynecologic procedures.

5. Indicate the names and uses of obstetric and gynecologic instruments, supplies, and drugs.

6. Indicate the names and uses of special equipment related to obstetric/gynecologic surgery.

7. Determine the intraoperative preparations of the patient undergoing an obstetric or gynecologic procedure.

8. Summarize the surgical steps of obstetric/gynecologic procedures.

9. Interpret the purpose and expected outcomes of the obstetric/gynecologic procedure.

10. Recognize the immediate postoperative care and possible complications of the obstetric/gynecologic procedure.

S 11. Assess any specific variations related to the preoperative, intraoperative, and postoperative care of the obstetric/gynecologic patient.

SELECT KEY TERMS

adnexa	episiotomy	labium (sing.)	parity
breech	exenteration	LEEP	perineum
cesarean section	fimbria	ligament	Pfannenstiel
curettage	fistula	marsupialization	vestibule
DUB	gravida	myoma	
dystocia	labia (pl.)	occiput anterior	

INTRODUCTION TO OBSTETRIC AND GYNECOLOGIC SURGERY

Obstetric and gynecologic surgery is a specialty in the field of medicine. This specialty area focuses its attention on females after the beginning of menstruation. The obstetrician's attention is given to the pregnant patient and issues concerned with fertility. Gynecologists focus on the female reproductive system and related problems outside pregnancy. Traditionally and typically, a practicing physician in this specialty field sees patients for both obstetric and gynecologic reasons. However, physicians may narrow their focus to either an obstetric or gynecologic practice. Some subspecialties exist. For instance, some physicians may specialize in infertility and its related treatment modes. Some surgeons specialize in the treatment of gynecologic cancer. In some locales, nonreconstructive types of breast surgery are considered the domain of the gynecologist.

INSTRUMENTATION, EQUIPMENT, AND SUPPLIES IN OBSTETRIC AND GYNECOLOGIC SURGERY

Instrumentation

The basic instrumentation for obstetric surgery and **cesarean section** is similar to general surgery (see Chapter 14); however, there are specialty instruments as shown in Figures 15-1 through 15-5. Major abdominal sets are used for gynecologic laparotomy. Obstetrics requires unique instruments because of the purpose and the anatomical relationship between mother and fetus. Laparoscopic instrumentation is discussed in some detail in this chapter because of its historical roots in gynecologic surgery.

The instrumentation lists that follow are provided to give the student some insight into the equipment and instrumentation related to obstetric and gynecologic surgery. Some basic instrument sets are listed in Table 15-1 and illustrative examples are shown in the illustrations that follow (Figures 15-1, 15-2, 15-3, 15-4, and 15-5).

Equipment

In obstetric surgery, special beds are usually available in the delivery room. These beds function as normal facility beds but have foot ends that separate or drop down for the delivery. These beds will accept one or more varieties of stirrups and other devices developed to accommodate the patient in various delivery positions. They may be electrically or manually operated.

The delivery room will also contain a fetal monitor and a warming bed for the fetus.

Gynecologic surgery requires the same equipment as the abdominal procedures of general surgery. Since many of the procedures are performed with the patient in the lithotomy position, various types of stirrups and leg holders will be used. Likewise, the high percentage of laparoscopic procedures will require the surgical technologist to be familiar with the video equipment and insufflators used in this type of surgery, which are later illustrated, including their use. Additionally, lasers are used relatively frequently in obstetric and gynecologic surgery (see Chapter 10).

Supplies

Most of the supplies used in obstetric and gynecologic surgery are the same as those used in general surgery (refer to Chapter 14).

PATIENT POSITIONING, DRAPING, AND/OR SETUP

Positioning for abdominal cases is supine. Vaginal and combination procedures require the lithotomy position (Figure 15-6). For obstetric and gynecologic procedures, a standard operating table, with both Trendelenburg and foot-drop capability, is used. The table must accommodate sockets for leg holders such as "candy cane" or Allen stirrups. Because the patient's horizontal

TABLE 15-1 Examples of Basic Instrument Sets in Obstetric and Gynecologic Surgery

Vaginal Prep Set	(Commonly a disposable set)
	Graves vaginal speculum
	16 Fr urethral catheter
	Dressing forceps
	Sponge forceps
	Solution cups
Vaginal Delivery	Kelly hemostats
	Medium needle holder
	Tissue forceps with teeth
	Russian tissue forceps
	Straight Mayo scissors
	Curved Mayo scissors
	Placenta basin
	Cord clamps
	Cord blood tube
D&C	Knife handles, #3 and #4 long
	Dressing forceps, 8 in.
	Russian tissue forceps
	Towel clamp(s)
	Sponge forceps, 9.5 in.
	Bozeman dressing forceps, 10.5 in.
	Heaney needle holder
	Graves vaginal speculum
	Auvard weighted speculum
	Jackson vaginal retractor
	Hegar uterine dilator set
	Sims uterine sound
	Tenaculum forceps
	Sims uterine curette set
Basic Vaginal Set	Knife handles, #3 and #4
	Mayo scissors, several lengths
	Metzenbaum scissors, 7 in.
	Dressing forceps
	Tissue forceps, different lengths
	Kelly hemostats
	Rochester-Pean clamps
	Heaney clamps
	Kocher clamps
	Towel clamps
	Sponge forceps
	Vaginal retractors
	Deaver retractors
	Allis tissue forceps
	Auvard weighted speculum
	Tenaculum forceps
Gynecologic Abdominal	Basic laparotomy set plus:
	Mayo scissors, different lengths
	Jorgensen scissors
	Long and short tissue forceps with and without teeth
	Long and short Russian tissue forceps
	Rochester-Ochsner clamps
	Heaney needle holders
	O'Sullivan-O'Connor retractor
	Tenaculum, triple toothed
	Heaney hysterectomy clamps
	Heaney-Ballantine hysterectomy clamps
Cesarean Section	Knife handles, #3
	Needle holders
	Tissue forceps, short and long Russian, with teeth, and Adson's
	Kelly hemostats, short and medium
	Rochester-Pean clamps
	Rochester-Ochsner clamps
	Mayo scissors
	Metzenbaum scissors
	Bandage scissors
	De Lee universal retractor or bladder blade from Balfour
	Richardson retractors
	Goelet retractors
	Cord clamps
	Cord blood tubes
	Bulb syringe
Laparoscopic	Basic laparotomy set (in room)
	"Minor" set open
	Modified Graves vaginal speculum

TABLE 15-1 (continued)

Auvard weighted speculum	Hook scissors
Sims uterine sound	Grasping forceps
Cervical dilators	Needle holder
Tenaculum forceps	Atraumatic grasping forceps
Camera and adapters	Knife electrode
Appropriate set of telescopes	Veress needle
Trocar set or individual trocars	Kleppinger
Appropriate laparoscopic instruments:	Tubing for insufflator
Peritoneal scissors	Cords and connectors for fiber-optics and electrosurgical unit (ESU)

orientation may be changed frequently in some procedures, the surgical technologist must be familiar with the operation of the operating table. Furthermore, the frequently used lithotomy position requires careful handling of both equipment and the patient's extremities. All equipment should be tested before the patient is placed on the operating table. See Chapter 12 for draping procedure.

The anesthesia provider is invariably positioned at the head of the table. The OR should be arranged with this in mind. A Mayo stand is frequently used for abdominal approaches but may not be used for vaginal approaches. A back table of adequate size to accommodate the required instrumentation without clutter is necessary for all procedures and may be used alone for vaginal approaches. Suction devices, an ESU with the appropriate sterile hand piece(s), kick buckets, and sitting stools (if required) are basic components of any operation.

SURGICAL PROCEDURES: OBSTETRICS

Obstetric and gynecologic surgery are part of the same specialty area of medicine, but they are significantly different to warrant special consideration for each. This chapter will present obstetric and fertility-related procedures and gynecologic procedures in separate sections.

The obstetric patient presents an unusual situation in medicine. The "patient" exhibits a normal condition, pregnancy. The patient seeks medical support and help because the condition, while normal, may result in danger to the mother and/or fetus. Care, monitoring, and diagnosis of the pregnant patient begin at the physician's office. An outline of the routine obstetric visit is presented in Table 15-2.

The obstetrician performs surgery to facilitate or inhibit the natural state of pregnancy. Pregnancy is a physiologic condition that may place both mother and fetus in jeopardy. Pregnancy brings changes to the female body and presents a condition that can lead directly to surgery or contribute to other conditions that lead to surgery. Obstetrics has a language of its own related to the specific events of pregnancy and childbirth (Table 15-3).

Labor

The progress of the labor process is defined by four stages. Stage one begins with the onset of true labor and is considered complete when the cervix is fully dilated. Stage two begins with complete dilatation of the cervix and terminates with the birth of the infant. The third stage is initiated with the birth of the infant and ends when the placenta is delivered. The fourth stage begins at that point and is considered completed when the mother's condition has stabilized. The length of each stage is highly variable under normal conditions. Many factors contribute to the length of labor (Table 15-4).

The obstetrician and labor and delivery nurse routinely evaluate the progress of the patient during labor. Their findings are documented in the patient's chart. Many labor and delivery units maintain a monitoring board so the team, including the surgical technologist, may be alert to changing conditions, developing problems, deliveries, and cesarean sections. A typical monitoring board contains the information illustrated in Table 15-5. Because the board may be open to public viewing, patients' names are often excluded.

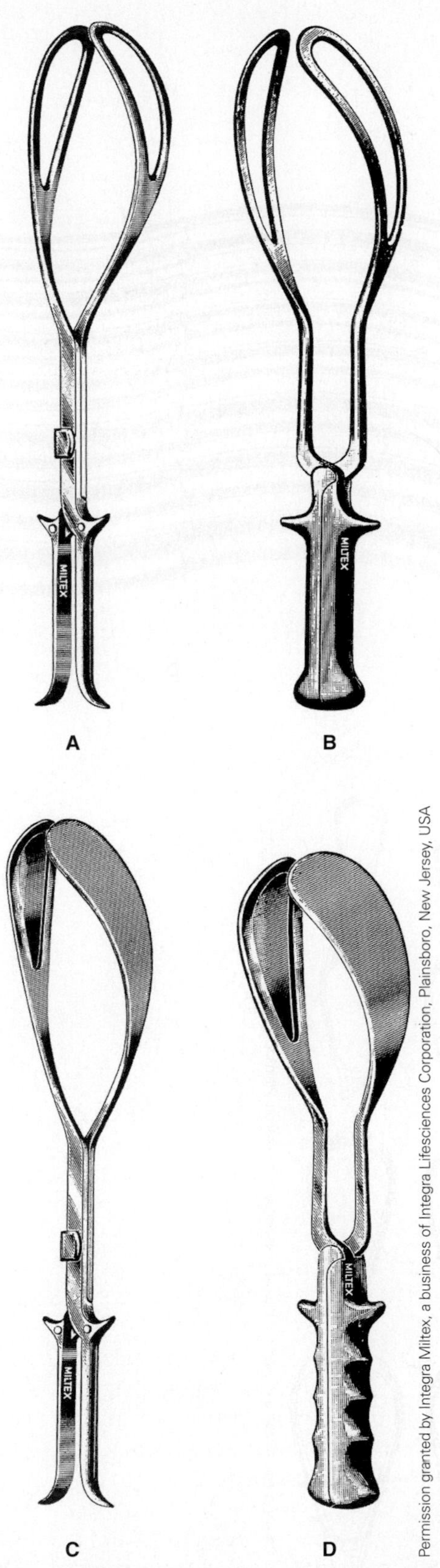

Figure 15-1 Delivery forceps: (A) Kielland, (B) De Lee, (C) Luikart, (D) Simpson-Luikart

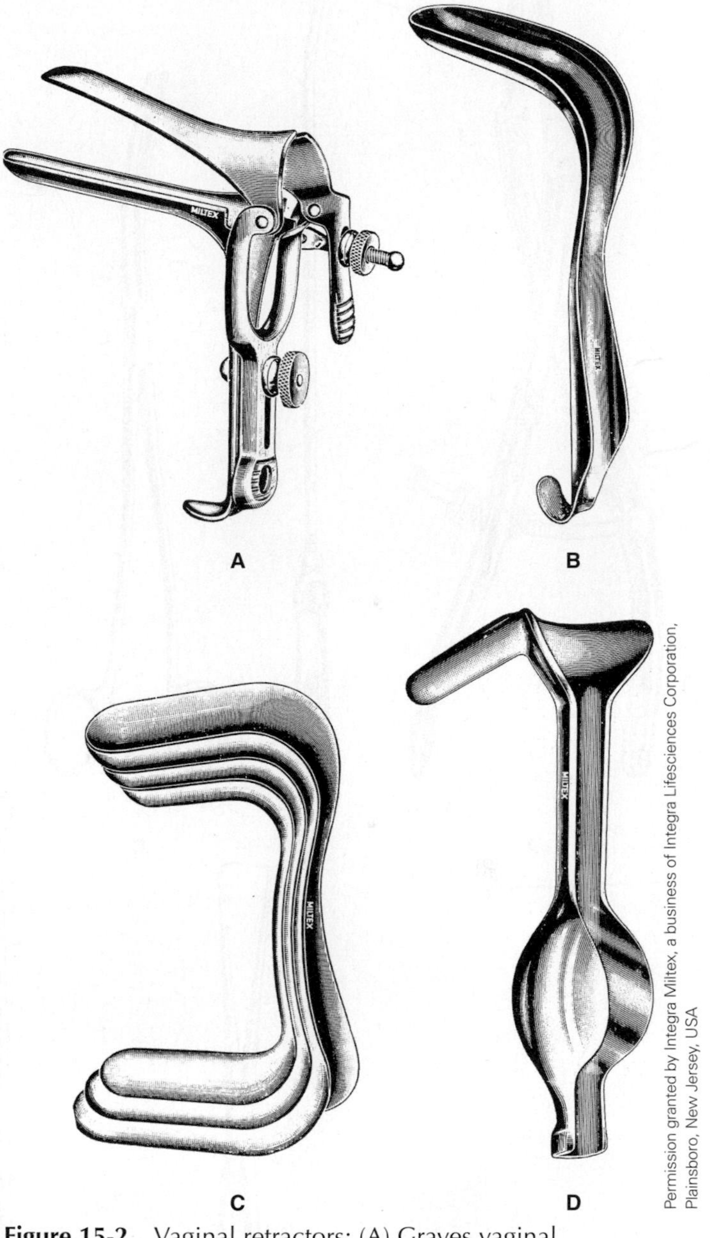

Figure 15-2 Vaginal retractors: (A) Graves vaginal speculum, (B) Sims vaginal speculum (single end), (C) Sims vaginal speculum (double end), (D) Auvard weighted vaginal speculum

Normal Role of Surgical Technologist in Delivery

Most deliveries occur in a natural and normative pattern. The surgical technologist is there as part of the team to assist the obstetrician, support the mother, and prepare for any developing problems. It is common to help with clamping and cutting

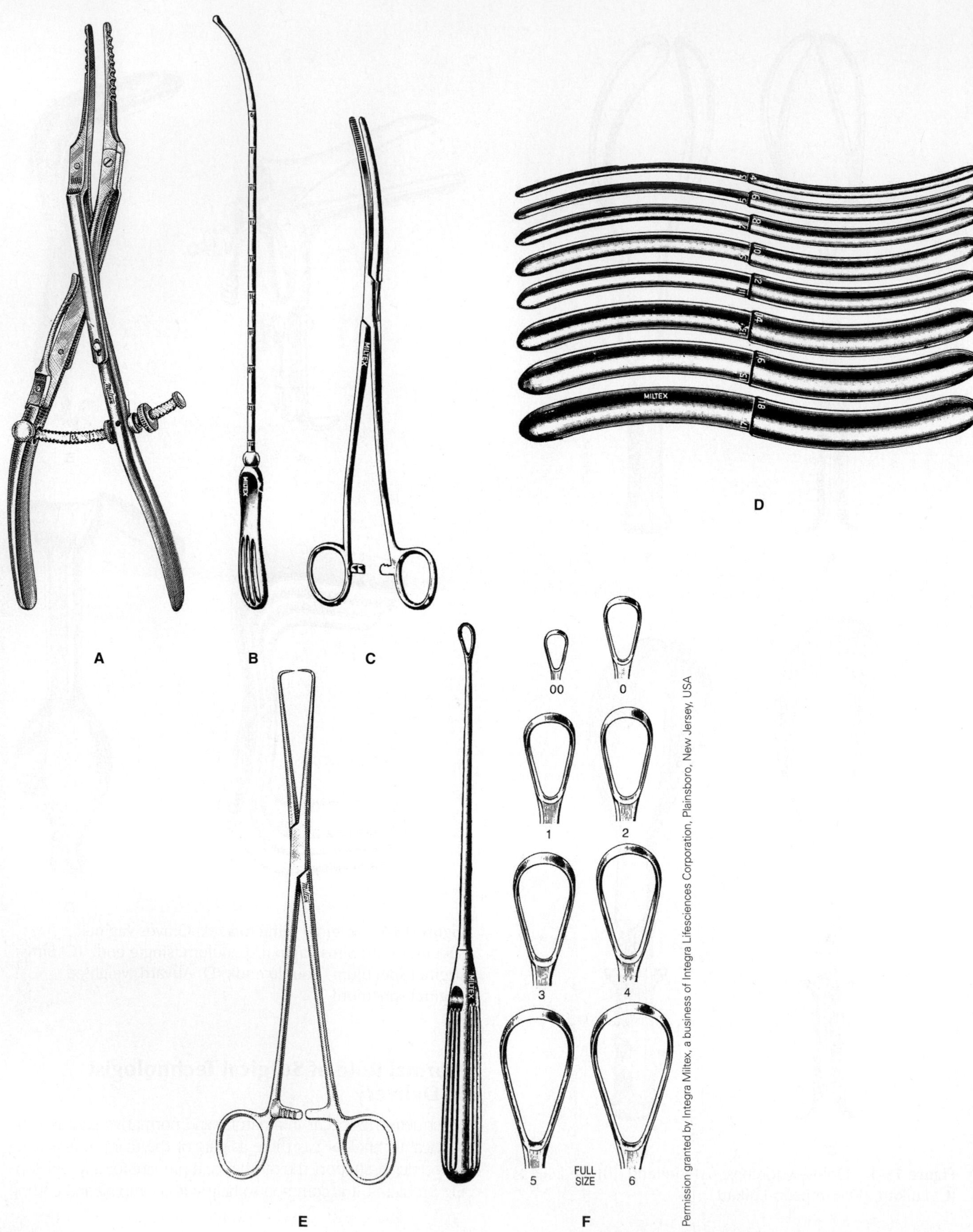

Figure 15-3 Cervical and intrauterine instruments: (A) Goodell uterine dilator, (B) Sims uterine sound, (C) Bozeman uterine dressing forceps, (D) Hegar uterine dilators, (E) Schroeder-Braun uterine tenaculum, (F) Sims uterine curettes (sharp blades)

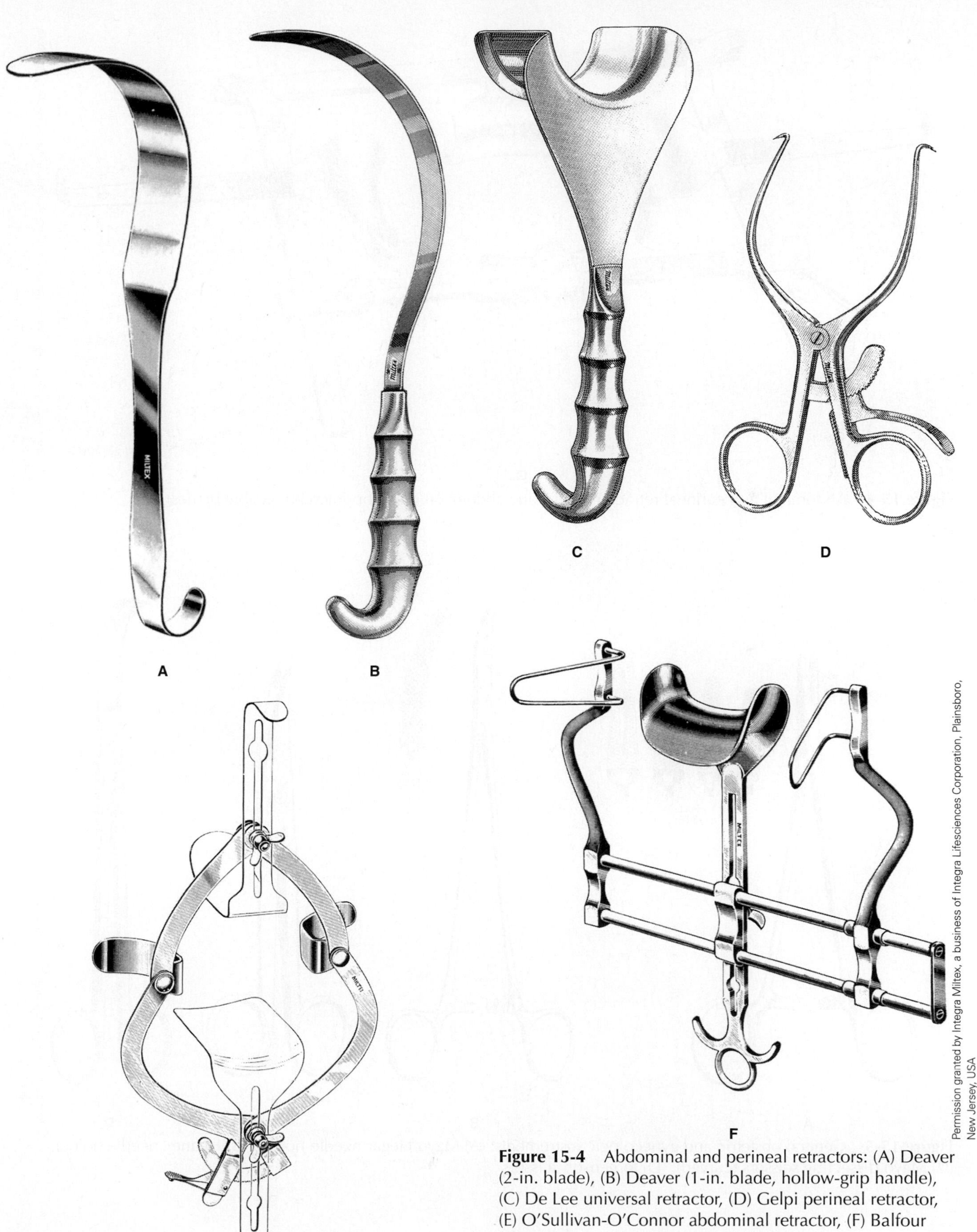

Figure 15-4 Abdominal and perineal retractors: (A) Deaver (2-in. blade), (B) Deaver (1-in. blade, hollow-grip handle), (C) De Lee universal retractor, (D) Gelpi perineal retractor, (E) O'Sullivan-O'Connor abdominal retractor, (F) Balfour abdominal retractor (fenestrated blades)

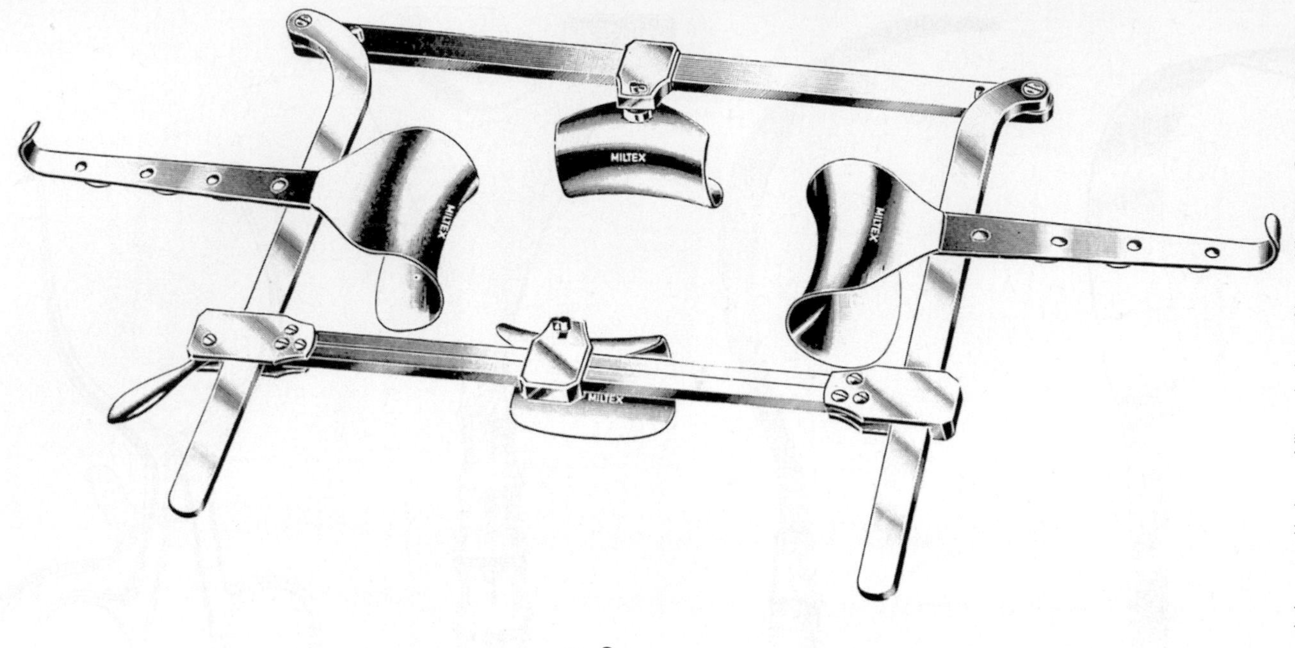

Figure 15-4 Abdominal and perineal retractors: (G) Franz abdominal retractor (interchangeable blades)

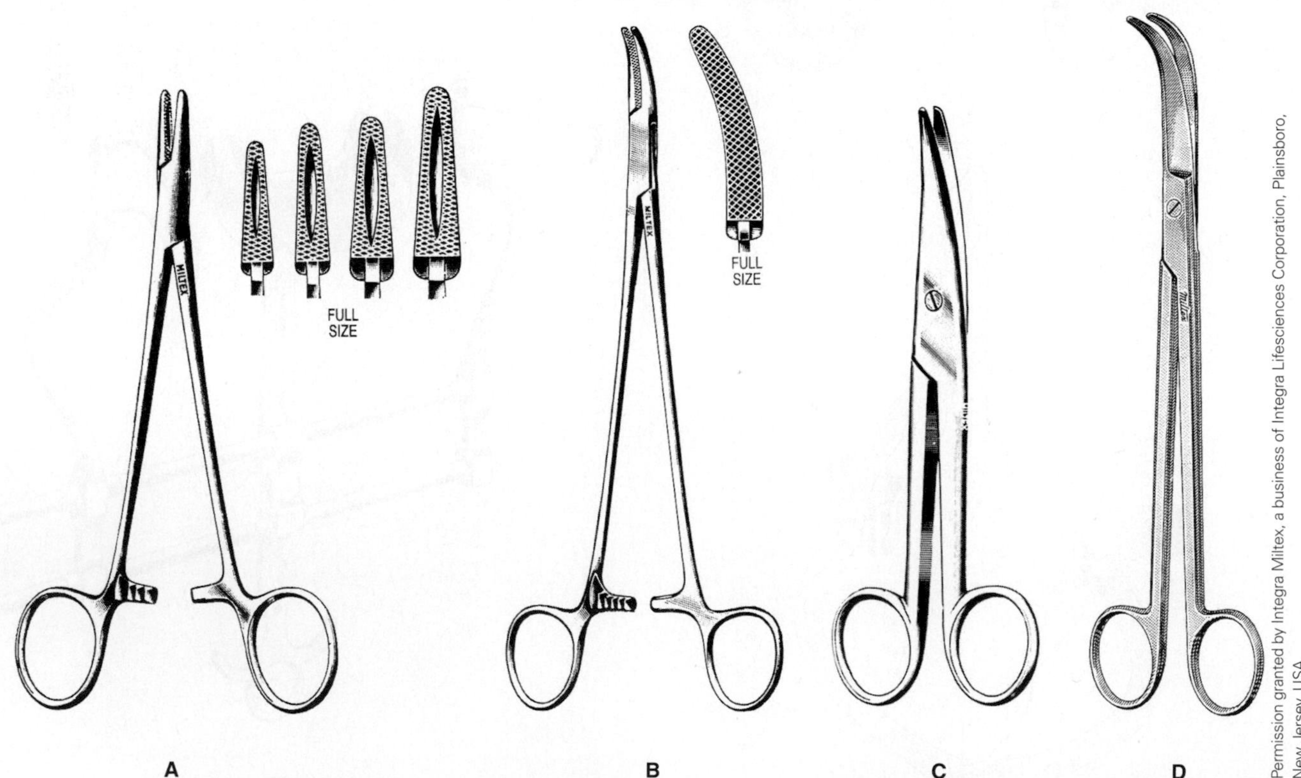

Figure 15-5 General obstetric and gynecologic instruments: (A) Mayo-Hegar needle holder, (B) Heaney needle holder, (C) Mayo dissecting scissors (curved), (D) Jorgenson scissors

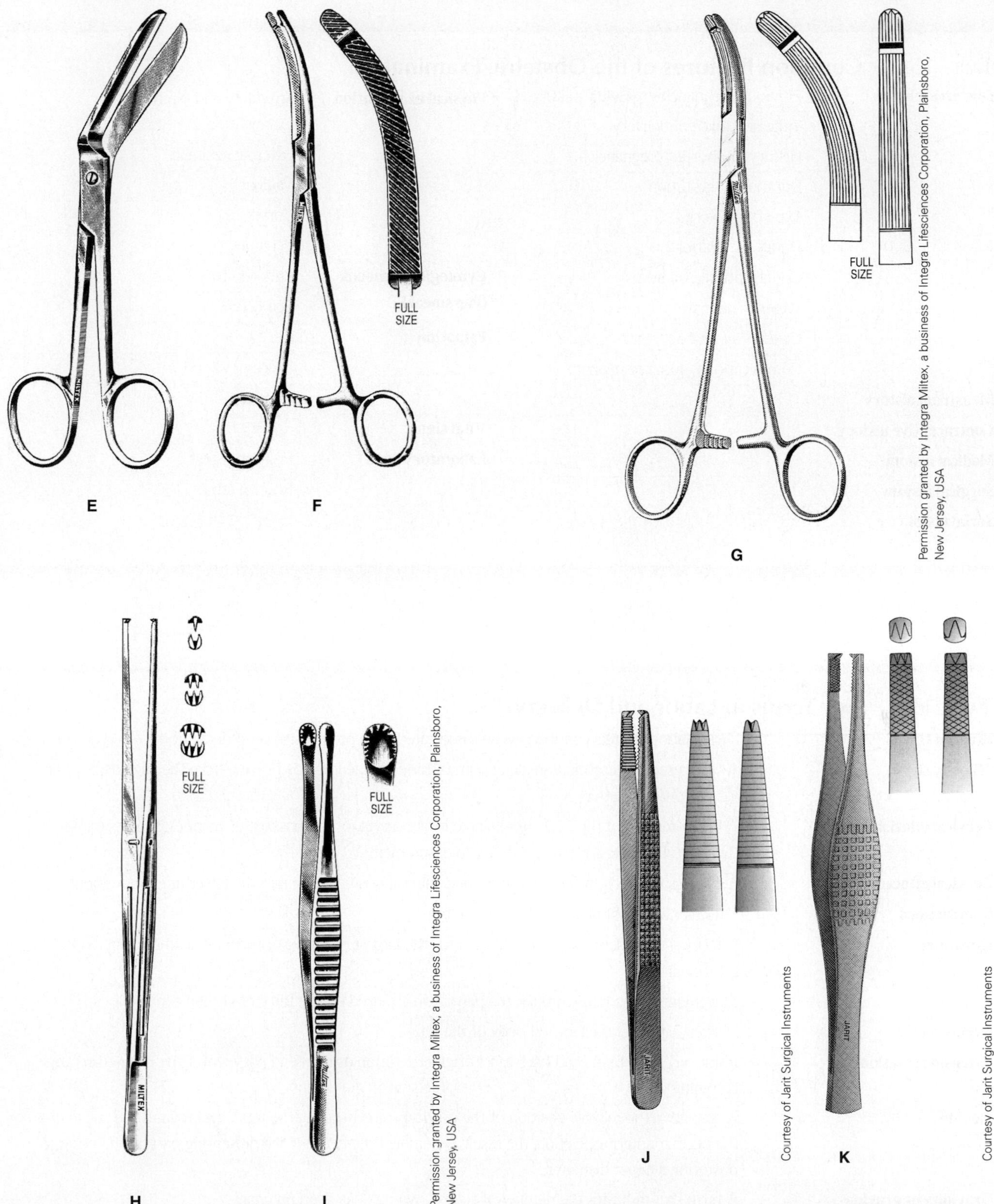

Figure 15-5 General obstetric and gynecologic instruments: (E) Braun episiotomy scissors, (F) Heaney hysterectomy clamp, (G) Heaney-Ballantine hysterectomy clamp, (H) Kelley tissue forceps, (I) Russian tissue forceps, (J) Bonney tissue forceps, (K) Ferris-Smith tissue forceps

Table 15-2 Common Features of the Obstetric Examination

Obstetric history	Previous pregnancies (**gravida**, para)	**Physical examination**	Speculum and bimanual examination
	Time and place of delivery		External genitalia
	History of aborted pregnancies		Vagina
	Duration of gestation		Cervix
	Type of delivery		Pelvimetry
	Duration of labor	**Cytologic specimens (Pap smear)**	Endocervix
	Complications—maternal		Ectocervix
	Weight—neonate	**Palpation**	Cervix
	Gender—neonate		Uterus
	Complications—fetus or neonate		**Adnexa**
Menstrual history		**Vital signs**	
Contraceptive history		**Laboratory tests**	Pregnancy test
Medical history			Routine labs
Surgical history			
Social history			

Table 15-3 Key Terms in Labor and Delivery

Braxton Hicks	"False" labor; normal contractions not associated with progressive cervical dilation
"Bloody show"	A term used to describe a small amount of blood-tinged mucus flowing from the vagina; may herald the onset of labor
Cervical dilation	A measurement of the opening available in the cervix for the passage of uterine contents (closed, 0 cm to fully dilated, 10 cm in obstetric measurements)
Cervical effacement	A process in which the cervix softens and thins and is taken up into the lower uterine segment
Contractions	Muscular action of uterus to expel the fetus
Crowning	A term used to describe the event in which the largest diameter of the fetal head is encircled by the vulvar ring
Descent	Movement of the fetus through the pelvic canal caused by the force of uterine contractions
Expulsion	Delivery of the shoulders and body of the fetus
Extension rotation	Rotation of the fetal head back to its original position as the head passes over the **perineum** (after crowning)
Flexion	A change in the relative position of the cervical spine bringing the fetal head toward the chest; in the occipitoanterior position, the result is a smaller diameter of the presenting part; in the occipitoposterior, a larger diameter
Gravidity or gravida	A term that indicates the number of times a woman has been pregnant
Internal rotation	Rotation of the fetal head as it meets the musculature of the pelvic floor; precise movements depend on initial position of the fetus relative to the pelvis
Lie	Relationship that exists between the long axis of the fetus and the long axis of the mother
Lightening	A term used to describe the settling of the fetal head into the brim of the pelvis

Table 15-3 (continued)

Para or parity	A term that indicates the number of times a woman has given birth; a multiple-birth experience is considered one birth
Position	Relationship between the presenting fetal part and the maternal body pelvis (most common is **occiput anterior** [OA])
Presentation	A term referring to the fetal part overlying the pelvic inlet (normally the fetal head but may be **breech** [buttocks] or compound [more than one part])
Station	In obstetrics, 'station' is the level of the fetal head relative to the level of the ischial spine of the mother's pelvis.

Table 15-4 Normal Labor—Characteristics

Event or Characteristic	*Primapara*	*Multipara*
Stage one—duration	6–18 hr	2–10 hr
Stage two—duration	0.5–3 hr	5–30 min
Stage three—duration	0–30 min	0–30 min
Stage four—duration	6 hr average	6 hr average
Cervical dilatation	1 cm/hr	1.2 cm/hr

Source: Adapted from *Essentials of Obstetrics and Gynecology*, 3rd ed., by N. F. Hacker and J. G. Moore, 1998, Philadelphia: W. B. Saunders.

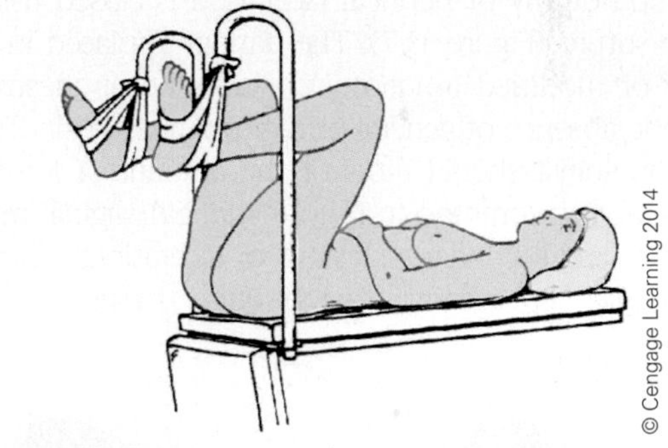

Figure 15-6 Lithotomy position

the umbilical cord, collecting blood for cord gases, and assisting as needed. The surgical technologist working in the labor and delivery unit should be familiar with basic fetal monitoring equipment, infant resuscitation procedures, and signs of a developing crisis with either the mother or the fetus. An understanding of delivery techniques, including vacuum and forceps extraction, is mandatory. The most common surgical interventions in vaginal birth are the **episiotomy** and the repair of perineal lacerations.

Episiotomy and Perineal Lacerations

Episiotomy is an intentional midline surgical incision in the perineum to ease the birth process or to protect the mother from uncontrolled perineal lacerations. Both surgical episiotomy and perineal laceration are classified according to the depth of the wound. The commonly used definitions are found in Table 15-6.

Table 15-5 Sample Labor and Delivery Monitoring Board

Room	*Doctor*	*Gravida/Parity*	*Dilation*	*Effacement*	*Station*	*Care Notes*
1	Johnson	3/2	8 cm	90%	0	Diabetes

Table 15-6 Definitions: Perineal Lacerations and Incisions

First degree	Involves the vaginal mucosa or perineal skin
Second degree	Extends into the vaginal submucosa or perineum with or without the perineal body musculature being involved
Third degree	Involves the anal sphincter
Fourth degree	Involves the rectal mucosa

An episiotomy or perineal laceration is closed using absorbable suture (Figure 15-7). The patient is placed in the lithotomy or modified lithotomy position. Local anesthesia is used in the absence of general or regional anesthesia. The surgical technologist should monitor the amount of local anesthetic used. It is common to use a handheld vaginal retractor for primary and secondary incisions or lacerations. Third- and fourth- degree episiotomies may require the use of a Gelpi perineal retractor. Improperly closed wounds can lead to postpartum hemorrhage, sepsis, **fistulas**, and coital pain.

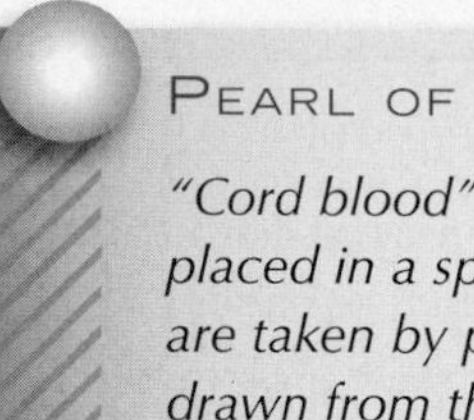

Pearl of Wisdom

"Cord blood" is routinely collected and placed in a special tube. "Cord gases" are taken by physician's order. Blood is drawn from the cord artery in a prepared, heparinized syringe and sent immediately to the laboratory.

Incompetent Cervix

A woman with an incompetent cervix is at a high risk for delivering prematurely. An incompetent cervix is prone to dilating and effacing prematurely in particular during the second trimester. The fetus places pressure on the cervix that can lead to miscarriage or premature delivery. Risk factors for incompetent cervix include previous premature delivery, previous trauma to the cervix, congenital weakness of the cervix and abnormalities of the uterus or cervix. To address the situation a cervical cerclage (Shirodkar's Procedure) is performed (Procedure 15-1).

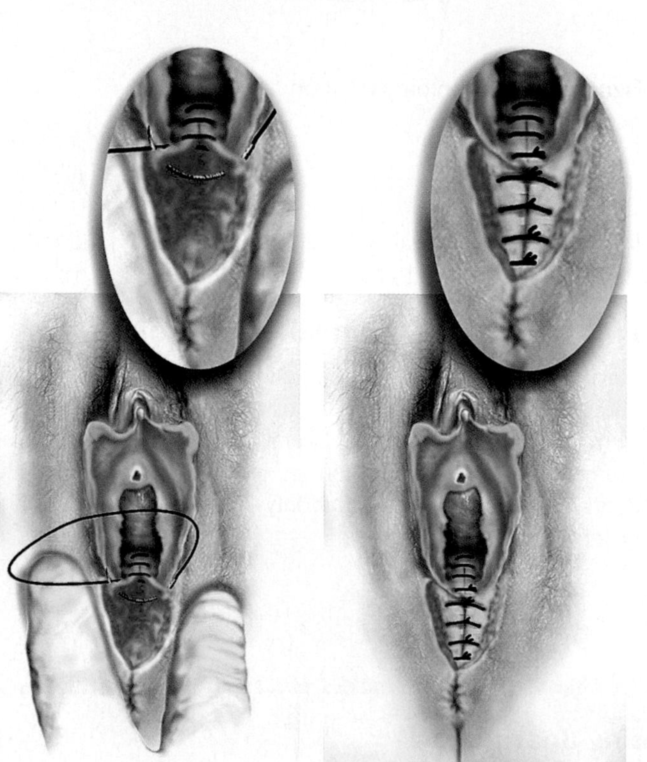

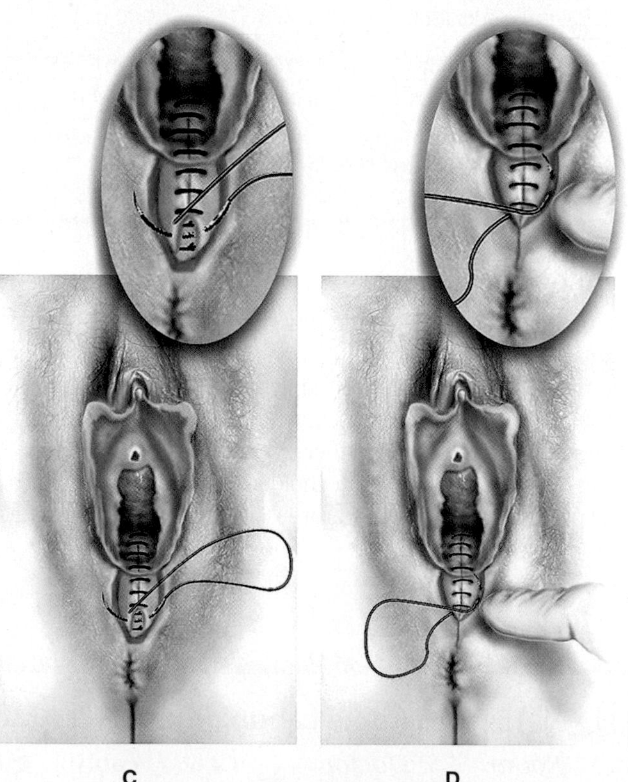

Figure 15-7 Episiotomy repair: (A) Closure of vaginal epithelium from apex to hymenal ring, (B) interrupted sutures to close perineal fascia and levator ani muscles, (C) continuous closure of superficial fascia to the anal edge, (D) continuous closure of subcutaneous layer

PROCEDURE 15-1 Cervical Cerclage (Shirodkar's Procedure)

Surgical Anatomy and Pathology

- Uterus is a hollow, thick-walled, pear-shaped organ situated between the bladder and rectum (Figure 15-8). The middle portion is the body and the superior portion called the fundus.
- The body narrows to a lower portion called the cervix. At the junction of the body and cervix is an aperture called the internal os; the cervix opens into the vagina at the external os.
- The uterus is lined with endometrium and at the internal os the lining becomes the mucous-secreting tissue of the cervix.
- Several layers of muscle of the myometrium lie beneath the endometrium. The outermost layer is longitudinal muscle; the innermost layer consists of longitudinal and oblique muscles. Between the muscle layers is a vascular layer of smooth muscle and many blood vessels. This structure allows the uterus to aid in hemostasis by mechanical contraction of the muscle fibers that surround the blood vessels.
- The visceral peritoneum lies over the pelvic surface of the uterus.
- Paired **ligaments** that extend to the pelvic walls to suspend the uterus are the broad, cardinal, round, and uterosacral. The broad ligament contains the round and ovarian ligaments.
- The uterine arterial supply is the uterine branch of the internal iliac arteries.
- Cervical cerclage is performed in late second trimester or early third trimester to prevent spontaneous abortion due to an incompetent cervix. Incompetency is often related to laceration, previous conization, or a congenital weakness of the cervix.

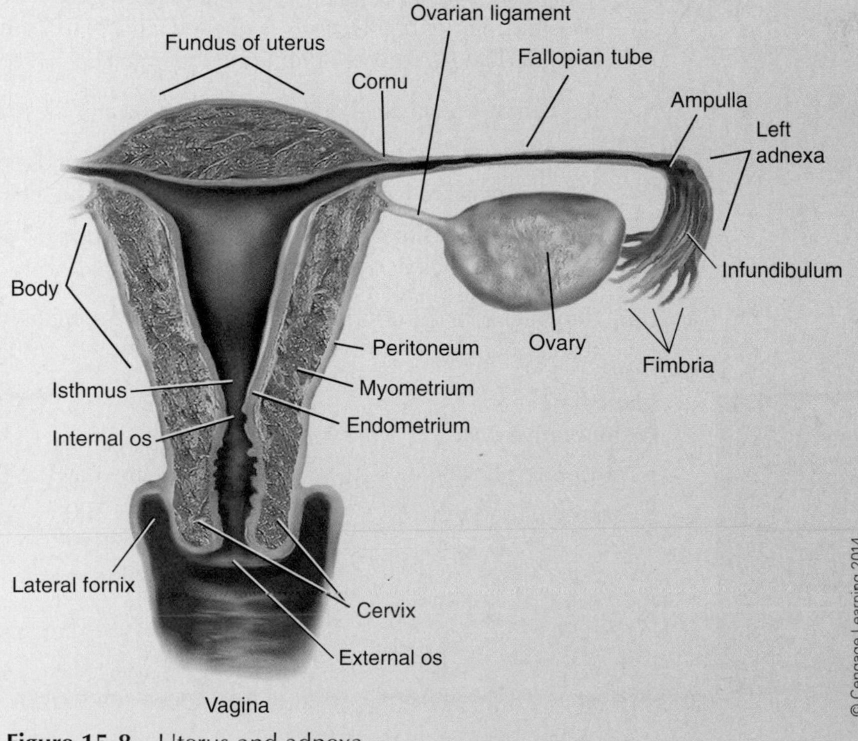

Figure 15-8 Uterus and adnexa

(*continues*)

PROCEDURE 15-1 (continued)

Preoperative Diagnostic Tests and Procedures	• Ultrasound (reveals abnormal short length and funneling of cervix)		
Equipment, Instruments, and Supplies Unique to Procedure	• D&C or basic vaginal instrument set	• Cervical cones of various sizes • Deschamps ligature carriers	• 5 mm Dacron or Mersilene tape
Preoperative Preparation	• Position: Lithotomy • Anesthesia: Spinal, epidural or general anesthesia	• Patient skin prep: Gentle vaginal preparation including inner thighs	• Draping: Perineal
Practical Considerations	• Procedure is performed before the cervix is dilated.	• The vaginal preparation must be carefully performed so as to disturb the cervix as little as possible.	

Surgical Procedure

1. The Auvard weighted speculum is placed posteriorly into the vagina and a Deaver retractor is placed anteriorly.

   Procedural Consideration: The surgical technologist will be responsible for holding the Deaver retractor in place. The surgeon and surgical technologist will be working off the back table; therefore, the table should be positioned to allow the surgeon easy access to the instruments and supplies.

2. The cervix is grasped with sponge-holding forceps and pulled downward inside the vaginal vault.
3. Using long smooth tissue forceps and long curved Metzenbaum scissors, the mucosa over the anterior of the cervix is opened. This permits the bladder to be pushed back and out of the way to avoid injuring the organ.
4. The cervix is lifted anteriorly with the forceps and the posterior vaginal mucosa is incised.
5. Using the smooth forceps, the tape is placed around the cervix and both ends exit at the anterior incision. The tape is drawn tightly to close the cervix and tied.

   Procedural Consideration: The surgeon will use the Deschamps ligature carrier to facilitate placement of the tape.

6. The anterior and posterior muscosal incisions are closed with continuous 1-0 or 2-0 absorbable suture.

Postoperative Considerations	**Immediate Postoperative Care** • Transport to PACU. • Short-term bed rest.	**Prognosis** • No complications: Discharged same day or next day of surgery; return to activities with some restrictions in 3–5 days.	• Complications: Postoperative SSI; cervix dilates due to poor placement of tape; hemorrhage. **Wound Classification** • Class II: Clean-Contaminated

Procedure 15-2 Cesarean Section

Surgical Anatomy and Pathology	• See Procedure 15-1 for uterine anatomy.	• See Table 15-7 for pathology.	
Preoperative Diagnostic Tests and Procedures	• History and physical, including measurement of pelvis	• Fetal and maternal monitoring during labor	
Equipment, Instruments, and Supplies Unique to Procedure	• Cesarean section back table pack • Bulb syringe (one per infant if multiple birth) • Cord clamps (two per infant)	• De Lee suction device available • Cord blood container • Blood gas containers available • Cesarean section instrument set that	includes delivery forceps and bladder retractor • Fetal monitor • Overhead radiant heater (infant warming bed) • Two suction tubes and Yankauer suction tips
Preoperative Preparation	• Position: Supine with roll placed under right hip to reduce the uterine pressure on the vena cava	• Spinal and Epidural preferred; General anesthesia for emergency	• Patient skin prep: Abdominal • Draping: Laparotomy
Practical Considerations	• Emergency cesarean sections will move very fast. There may not be time to do an initial count or perform routine abdominal skin prep; the circulator may only have time to spray scrub solution onto the abdomen.	• The surgical technologist should learn how to apply fundal pressure to assist in the delivery of the infant from the uterus. • There may only be time for the surgeon and surgical technologist to	perform the cesarean section. The surgical technologist should learn how to apply the two clamps to the umbilical cord and once it is cut take cord blood samples.

Surgical Procedure

1. Skin incision may be midline or low transverse (Pfannenstiel). The most common incision is the low transverse. Using a #10 knife blade, the incision is carried to the level of the fascia.

   Procedural Consideration: Initial steps vary with type of anesthesia. With an epidural or spinal anesthetic, the patient should be tested for sensitivity to skin pain prior to initiation of the incision. In the case of general anesthesia, all preoperative preparation should be completed prior to the induction. Once the patient is intubated, the procedure should progress rapidly.

2. The fascia is incised at the midline with a #10 blade and the incision is carried laterally using Mayo scissors. This is repeated on both sides.

   Procedural Consideration: Goulet or U.S. Army retractor is commonly used.

3. A longitudinal plane is developed in the midline by bluntly dissecting the posterior fascia from the rectus abdominus muscle and cutting the aponeurosis superiorly to near the umbilicus and inferiorly to the symphysis pubis.

   Procedural Consideration: Two Kocher clamps are typically placed on the fascia near the midline during this phase. Mayo scissors are used in the horizontal plane for the sharp dissection.

(*continues*)

Procedure 15-2 Cesarean Section

Table 15-7 Cesarean Section—Indications

Category	Indication
Maternal	Diseases
	Eclampsia or severe preeclampsia
	Cardiac disease
	Diabetes mellitus
	Cervical cancer
	STD such as Herpes or AIDS
	Prior surgery of the uterus
	Cesarean section (especially classical type)
	Previous rupture of the uterus
	Full-thickness myomectomy
	Obstruction to birth canal
	Fibroids
	Ovarian tumors
	Other
	Uterine rupture
	Failure to progress (etiology unknown)
	Maternal demise
Fetal	Fetal distress (sustained low heart rate)
	Prolapse of the umbilical cord
	Malpresentation
	Breech
	Transverse
	Brow
	Multiples (depends on number and presentation)
	Fetal demise
Maternal/Fetal	**Dystocia**
	Cephalopelvic disproportion (Figure 15-9)
	Failed induction of labor
	Abnormal uterine action
Placental	Placenta previa
	Placental abruption

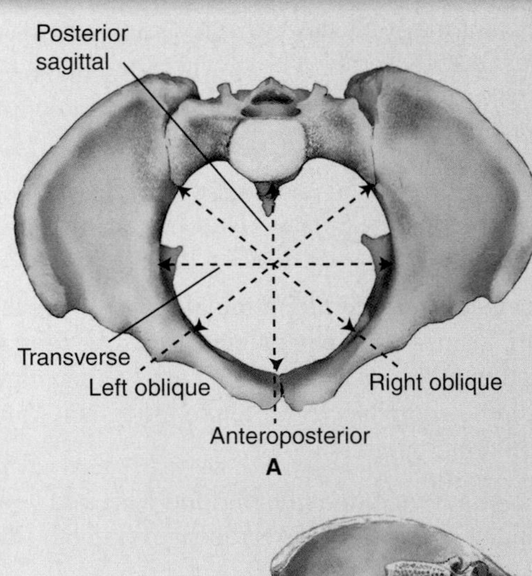

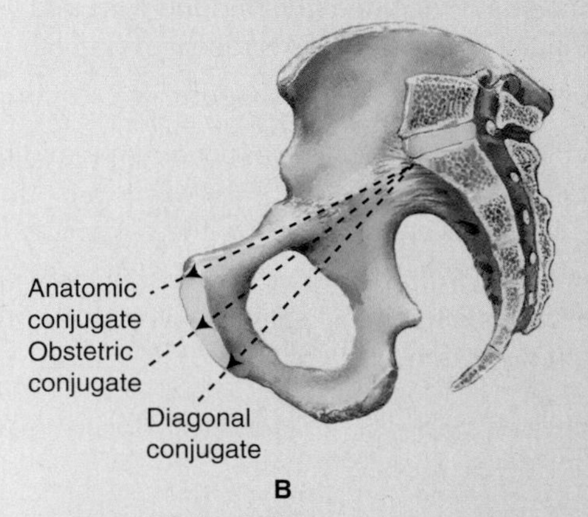

Figure 15-9 Pelvic girdle and diameters

PROCEDURE 15-2 (continued)

4. A longitudinal peritoneal incision is made and extended the length of the facial opening.

   Procedural Consideration: Metzenbaum scissors are commonly used on the peritoneum.

5. The uterus is palpated to determine fetal placement and position.

   Procedural Consideration: Some fetal positions may require the use of delivery forceps.

6. To perform the uterine incision, the line representing the bladder peritoneal reflection on the uterus is identified. The bladder is freed from the uterus and retracted inferiorly (Figure 15-10A).

   Procedural Consideration: The surgical technologist should be prepared to assist with exposure using a bladder retractor of the surgeon's preference. (The bladder retractor is removed before the infant's head is elevated out of the uterus.)

7. A small transverse incision is made in the lower uterine segment and carried bilaterally with blunt or sharp dissection (Figure 15-10B).

   Procedural Consideration: The surgical technologist should perform a visual double check at this time to be sure all supplies related to the infant are available and ready for use.

8. The amniotic sac may or may not need incising.

   Procedural Consideration: The surgical technologist should note the nature of the amniotic fluid. Meconium-stained fluid may require suction with a De Lee suction catheter. The surgical technologist should be prepared to keep the field clean of amniotic fluid if necessary.

9. The obstetrician places a hand inside the uterus and manipulates the fetus to draw it from the uterus. To further aid in delivering the fetus from the uterus the surgical technologist will gently push downward on the upper region of the abdomen. The nares and mouth of the fetus are suctioned immediately.

   Procedural Consideration: Once the head (typically) is controlled, all sharp and metal objects are removed from the field prior to elevating the infant's head.

10. The umbilical cord is clamped and cut with curved Mayo scissors or Lister bandage scissors (Figure 15-10C). A cord blood sample is collected (Figure 15-10D).

    Procedural Consideration: Cord blood gases may or may not be drawn. In the case of multiple births, each cord is marked for individual identification. This can be accomplished by using a different type of clamp on each cord (e.g., straight clamp—neonate A). Cord Blood Unit for donation may or may not be collected.

11. The neonate is passed to the pediatrician or neonatal nurse.

    Procedural Consideration: Be especially aware of the movements of the pediatrician and other nonsterile team members. Protect the sterile field and Mayo stand.

12. The placenta is delivered, inspected, and removed to the back table (Figure 15-10E).

    Procedural Consideration: The surgical technologist will bring a large basin onto the sterile field in which the placenta is placed. The basin is passed off to the circulator; the placenta may or may not routinely be sent to pathology.

(continues)

PROCEDURE 15-2 (continued)

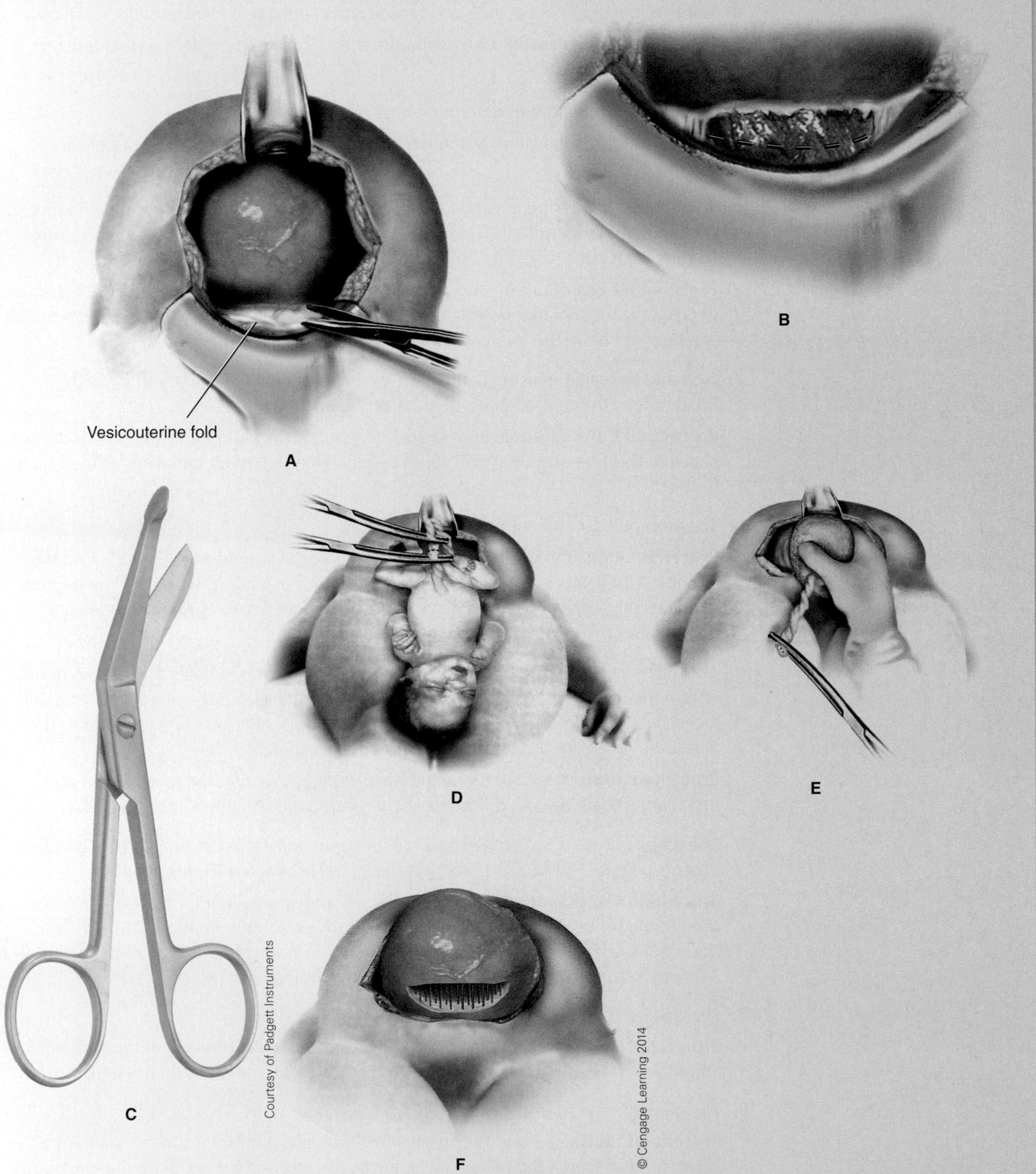

Figure 15-10 Cesarean section: (A) Creation of bladder flap at vesicouterine fold, (B) bladder flap retracted and transverse incision made in lower uterine segment, (C) Lister bandage scissors, (D) delivery of infant with umbilical cord clamped, (E) dissection of the placenta from the uterine wall, (F) uterine incision closed in two layers

PROCEDURE 15-2 (continued)

13. The uterine interior may be cleaned with a laparotomy sponge, and oxytocin may be injected into the uterus to help with hemostasis secondary to contraction.

    Procedural Consideration: Sponge should be moist. Oxytocin is drawn up in advance.

14. The uterus is usually closed in two layers using 2-0 or 0 absorbable suture (Figure 15-10F).

    Procedural Consideration: The surgical technologist may need to help with exposure during this phase. The surgical technologist should request a "uterine count" as soon as the first suture is handed to the surgeon.

15. The bladder flap may be approximated or not. If approximated, a 3-0 nonabsorbable suture is commonly used.

    Procedural Consideration: There will be four counts on cesarean sections: (A) prior to skin incision; (B) prior to closure of the uterus, (C) prior to closure of the abdominal cavity, and (D) prior to closure of the skin.

16. The abdominal cavity should be examined for uncontrolled bleeding, sponges, and other potential problems. The abdominal cavity may be irrigated.

    Procedural Consideration: Prepare closing sutures during this time. Prepare for second count.

17. Closure of the abdominal wall and skin follow the usual procedure for low transverse incisions.

    Procedural Consideration: A subcuticular stitch or staples are commonly used for skin closure.

18. Blood clots are expressed from the uterus. The wound and vaginal area are cleaned and dressing and perineal pad applied.

Postoperative Considerations

Immediate Postoperative Care

- Transport to PACU.
- Support abdominal incision if patient coughs.

Prognosis

- No complications: Discharged from hospital next day or within 2 days after surgery; return to normal activities in 6–8 weeks; neonate–prognosis depends on nonsurgical factors.
- Complications: Postoperative SSI; hemorrhage; injury to surrounding structures such as the bladder; morbidity of mother or fetus due to anesthetic complications; cesarean sections can result in a weakened uterus and may need to be performed for future pregnancies.

Wound Classification

- Class I: Clean (Membranes Intact)

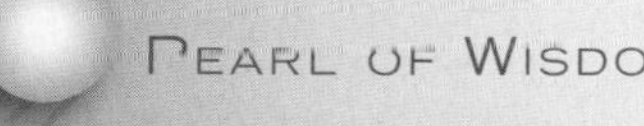

PEARL OF WISDOM

Bulb syringes are normally used to suction the nares and mouth of neonates; however, a De Lee suction may be preferred in the presence of meconium. Be sure to know the surgeon's preference before the procedure begins.

PROCEDURE 15-3 Tubal Sterilization

Surgical Anatomy and Pathology

- Each tube is located in the mesosalpinx of the broad ligament. The tubes are attached to and open into the uterus at the uterine os in the area called the cornu; each open end is near an ovary located in the infundibulum.
- The fallopian tubes are divided into four sections: **fimbria** (also called infundibulum), ampula, isthmus, and intramural (Figure 15-18).
  - The fimbria are finger-like projections at the terminal end of the tube that guide oocytes released by the ovaries into the tube's lumen.
  - The ampula is the largest and longest portion of the tube.
  - The isthmus is heavily muscled, acting as a "sphincter"; this effect is important in preventing endometriosis.
  - The isthmus opens to the intramural portion of the tube, which is located within the wall of the uterus. The intramural communicates with the uterus at the cornu.
- The muscularis of the tubes consists of external longitudinal and internal circular layers of smooth muscle.
- The outer serosal layer of the tubes is continuous with the broad ligament.
- The tubes are lined with simple ciliated and secretory epithelium.
  - The lining provides motility and lubrication for the captured oocytes as they travel down to the uterus.
- The blood supply to the tubes is the ovarian and uterine arteries and veins.
- No pathology—an elective procedure.

Preoperative Diagnostic Tests and Procedures

- History and physical

Equipment, Instruments, and Supplies Unique to Procedure

- Basic or minor laparotomy instrument set and/or Gyn. Laparoscopy instrument set
- Depending on surgeon's preference: Hemoclip appliers with hemoclips of various sizes; ligature; Silastic bands or clips

Preoperative Preparation

- Position: Open procedure – supine; laparoscopic – lithotomy
- Anesthesia: Local or general
- Patient skin prep: Abdominal
- Draping: Open procedure – laparotomy drape; laparoscopic – laparoscopy drape with leggings

Practical Considerations

- Tubal sterilization is performed as an outpatient or inpatient procedure.
- Careful patient counseling is necessary to make sure the patient definitely wants and is psychologically prepared for a tubal sterilization.
- Several techniques are used by the surgeon for performing the tubal portion of the procedure, including Irving, Pomeroy, Parkland, Madlener, and Kroener fimbriectomy (Figure 15-11). The Pomeroy technique is most often used since it provides the best potential for tuboplasty in case the patient changes her mind as to wanting more children.
  - Interruption of the tube's lumen can be done by sharp division, ligature placement, electrosurgery, or application of Silastic bands or clips.
  - Laparoscopy is commonly performed when the procedure does not follow childbirth.
- The right and left sections of tube that are excised must be kept as separate specimens. The separate specimen containers must be labeled right and left fallopian tube.

PROCEDURE 15-3 (continued)

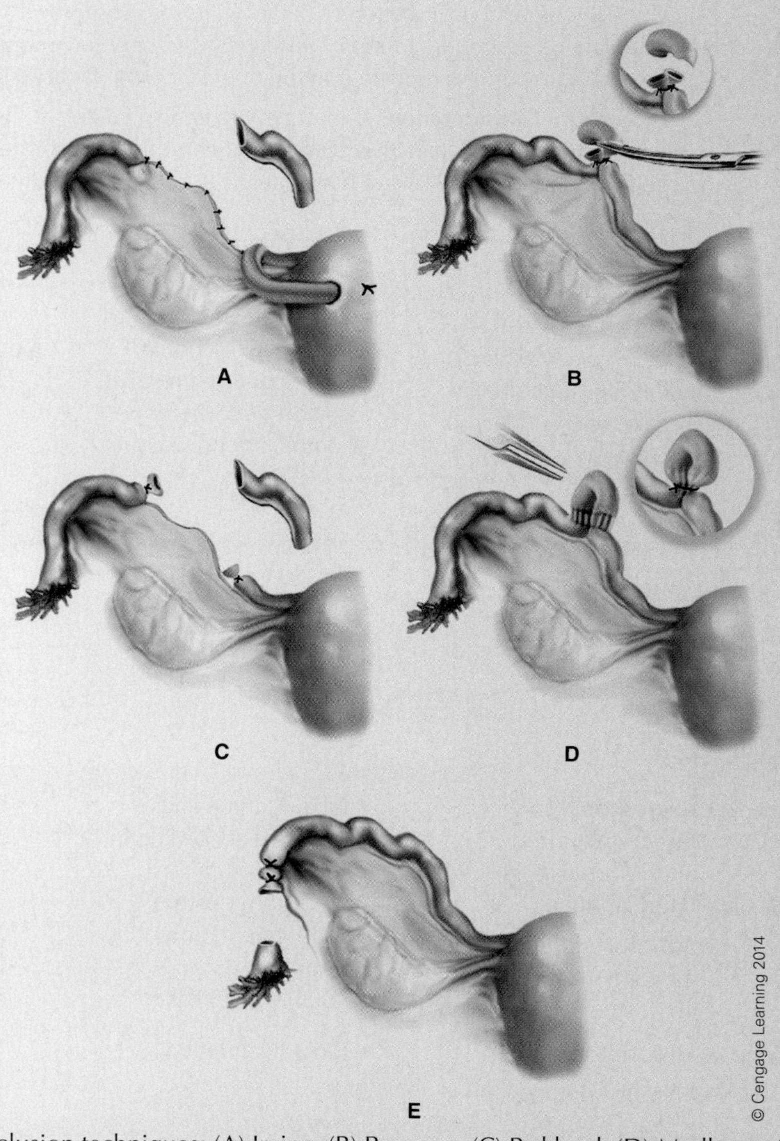

Figure 15-11 Tubal occlusion techniques: (A) Irving, (B) Pomeroy, (C) Parkland, (D) Madlener, (E) Kroener fimbriectomy

Surgical Procedure

1. The supraumbilical incision is performed and a small opening into the peritoneal cavity is made.
2. The surgeon identifies the right and left fallopian tubes and their condition.

   Procedural Consideration: The surgical technologist may be holding small retractors in place, but should have placed the Babcock forceps on the sterile field for easy access by the surgeon or easily available to retrieve from the Mayo stand.

(continues)

Procedure 15-3 (continued)

3. The first tube is grasped with the Babcock and brought upward through the incision.
4. The surgeon excises a section of the tube (Irving, Pomeroy, Parkland techniques), places a Silastic band around a loop of the tube (Madlener technique), or performs the Kroener fimbriectomy. This is repeated on the opposite tube (Figure 15-11).

   Procedural Consideration: The surgeon may also cauterize the end of each side of the tube if the Irving, Pomeroy, or Parkland technique is performed. Depending on surgeon's preference, he or she may want to use the electrosurgery needle tip.
5. The small peritoneal incision is closed in layers.

Postoperative Considerations	• Transport to PACU. • No complications: Release from health care facility on same day of surgery; return to normal activities in 2–4 weeks.	• Complications: Postoperative SSI; intra-abdominal bleeding; pelvic pain that resolves in short period of time. Complications are rare due to limited intervention. **Wound Classification** • Class II: Clean-contaminated if manipulator utilized.

Procedure 15-4 Tuboplasty

Surgical Anatomy and Pathology	• Microscopic surgical resection and anastomosis of the fallopian tube. • See Procedure 15-3 for anatomy (Figure 15-8).	• Tubal reanastomosis is classified according to anatomic location, e.g., isthmic-isthmic, midsegment, ampullary-ampullary, isthmic-ampullary.	• Pathology is tubal obstruction due to tubal sterilization or constriction of the tubes by adhesions from previous abdominal surgery.
Preoperative Diagnostic Tests and Procedures	• History and physical • Hysterosalpingogram	• Tubal insufflation	
Equipment, Instruments, and Supplies Unique to Procedure	• Major laparotomy instrument set • Microsurgical instruments (Figure 15-12) • Bipolar coagulating forceps • Electrosurgery needle tip • Lacrimal duct probes • Operating microscope or loupes	• Microscope drape • Microsurgical sutures of surgeon's preference • 2-0 monofilament sutures or stents to place in fallopian tubes • Tongue blade • Low-molecular-weight dextran • Indigo carmine dye	• Variety of syringes, needles, and injection catheters • Laparoscopy equipment, instrumentation and supplies for laparoscopic approach • Vaginal instrumentation for Endocervical balloon tuboplasty

PROCEDURE 15-4 (continued)

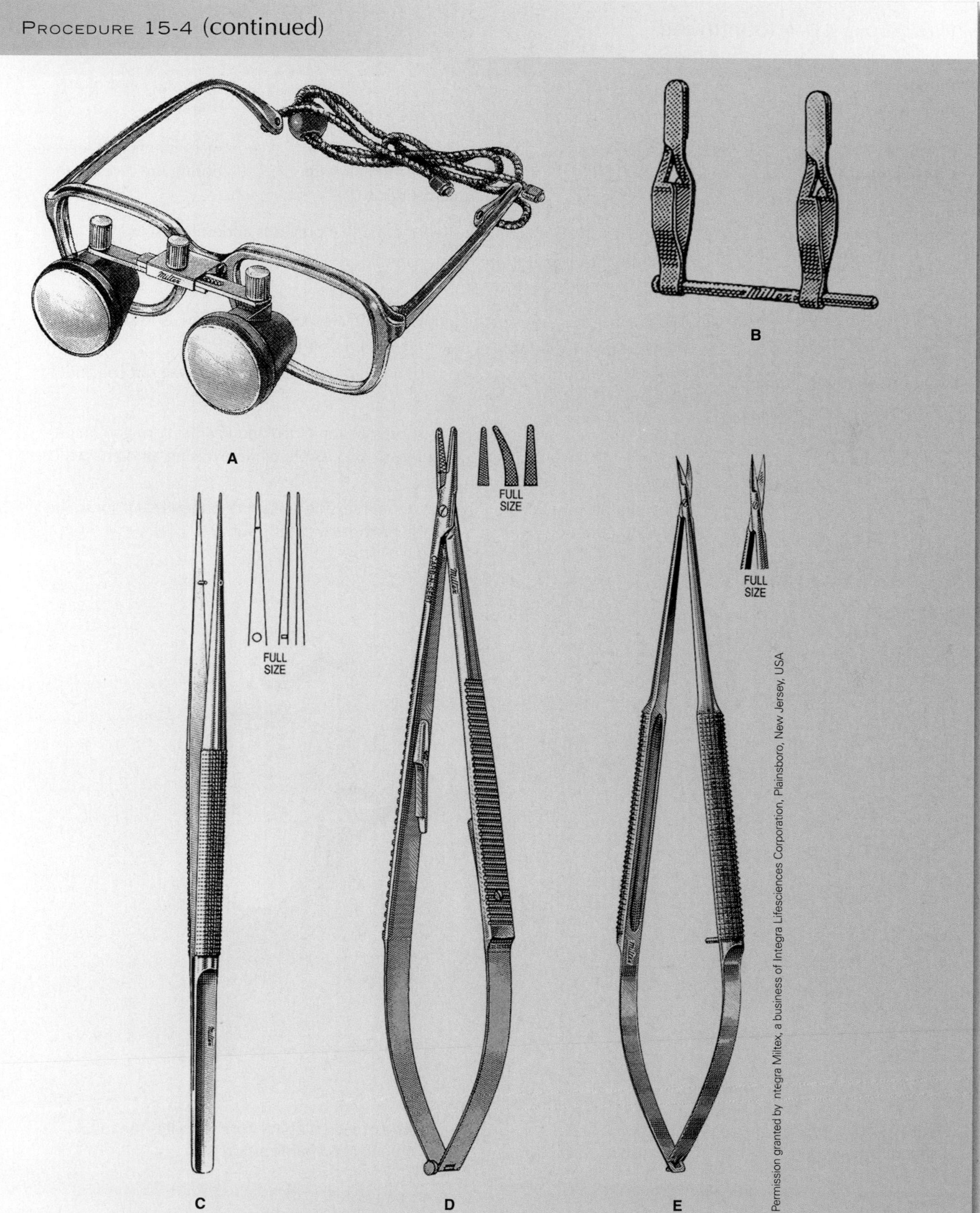

Figure 15-12 Microsurgical instruments: (A) Binocular magnifying loupe, (B) micro approximation clips, (C) Rhoton micro forceps, (D) Jacobson microvascular needle holder, (E) microsurgical scissors

(continues)

PROCEDURE 15-4 (continued)

Preoperative Preparation	• Position: Supine • Anesthesia: General	• Patient skin prep: Abdominal	• Draping: Laparotomy drape
Practical Considerations	• Have diagnostic studies in OR	• Surgical technologist must be familiar with microsurgical	instruments that are used during the procedure

Surgical Procedure

1. Abdominal incision: Pfannenstiel or through a previous abdominal scar.

   Procedural Consideration: Be prepared for routine opening of the abdomen. Drape the microscope early.

2. The damaged portions of the fallopian tube are isolated. The tube is freed from its attachments to the mesosalpinx with careful dissection.

   Procedural Consideration: Dissection will require atraumatic tissue forceps and dissecting scissors.

3. Fallopian tube is transected with iris scissors or #11 blade against a tongue blade at a point that maintains as much length as possible while excising all damaged portions (Figure 15-13).

   Procedural Consideration: Be sure to identify the surgeon's preference prior to the procedure. If used, the tongue blade provides a cutting surface.

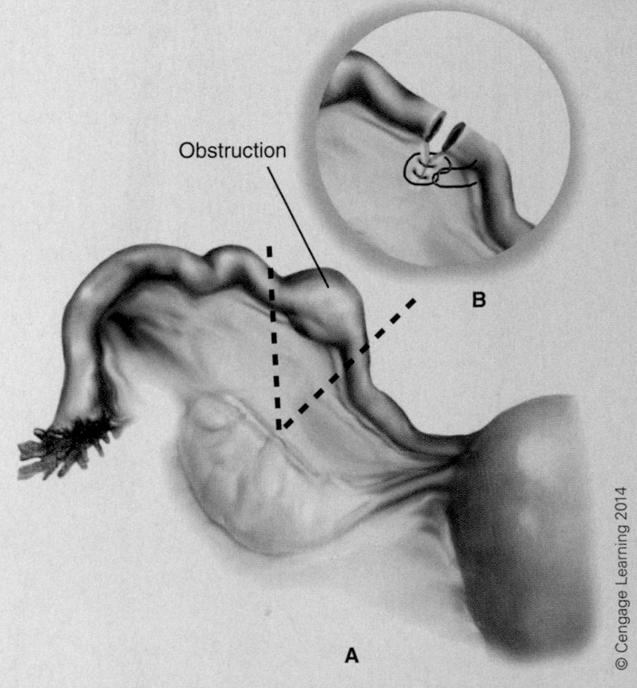

Figure 15-13 Tuboplasty: (A) Obstruction must be removed, (B) closure of mesosalpinx approximates the tubal segments; anastomosis is then accomplished with 7-0, 8-0, or 9-0 synthetic absorbable suture.

Procedure 15-4 (continued)

4. Proximal luminal patency is demonstrated by gentle probing with a lacrimal duct probe and injection of dye solution into the uterus.

   Procedural Consideration: Have indigo carmine dye ready in a syringe with the desired needle or catheter attached.

5. Distal tubal patency is also tested by probing, followed by cannulation with a pediatric catheter, or 18-gauge angiocatheter, and similar dye study that displays spillage through the fimbrial end.

   Procedural Consideration: Observe fimbria for evidence of dye.

6. The mesosalpinx is approximated to reduce tension on the tubal ends and an approximation clamp may be used to bring the tubal ends into close proximity.

   Procedural Consideration: Needle holders and needles will be very fine for the procedure. Handle them with extreme care. The surgeon may ask to have the needles loaded at a specific angle other than 90°.

7. A 2-0 monofilament suture (stent) may be threaded through the lumen to assist with approximation and protection of the lumen.

   Procedural Consideration: This suture is usually passed with a fine-eyed probe.

8. The sections of tube are sutured together at the 3-, 6-, and 9-o'clock positions with interrupted 8-0 synthetic absorbable suture. Sutures are placed in the muscularis only. No suture material should pass though the mucosa of the tube.

   Procedural Consideration: Remember that the surgeon and surgical assistant are looking through a microscope. Place instruments into their hands carefully and precisely. Do not pass instruments under the microscope lens.

9. The 2-0 monofilament stent is removed and a similar suture is passed at the 12-o'clock position.

   Procedural Consideration: Hemostasis is critical in these procedures. Microscopic bipolar coagulation will usually be the method of choice.

10. A second layer of sutures is placed circumferentially in the serosa and outer muscle layer with 8-0 or 9-0 absorbable sutures.

    Procedural Consideration: Suture is loaded in advance if possible.

11. The area is then irrigated, dextran is poured into the abdominal cavity, and the abdomen is closed.

    Procedural Consideration: Prepare for closure. Count is performed.

Postoperative Considerations

Immediate Postoperative Care

- Transport to PACU.

Prognosis

- No complications: Discharged same day of surgery or next day; return to normal activities in 4–6 weeks; successful potential to become pregnant.
- Complications: Postoperative SSI; hemorrhage; ectopic pregnancy; continued infertility; abdominal adhesions.

Wound Classification

- Class I: Clean

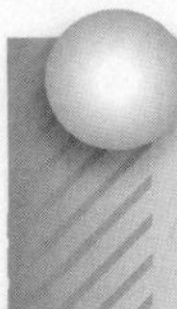

Pearl of Wisdom

Low-molecular-weight dextran may be poured into the pelvic area like irrigation fluid but is left in place. The solution helps keep tissues separated for several days, thus reducing adhesions and scar tissue formation.

Table 15-8 Risk Factors for Ectopic Pregnancy

- A history of pelvic inflammatory disease
- Previous ectopic pregnancy
- Pregnancy following sterilization procedure
- Prior tubal reconstructive surgery
- IUD usage
- Prolonged infertility
- Exposure to diethylstilbestrol

Procedure 15-5 Laparoscopic Resection of Unruptured Tubal Pregnancy

Surgical Anatomy and Pathology	• See Procedure 15-3 for anatomy. • Ectopic pregnancy is pregnancy that occurs outside the uterine cavity.	• It can occur in the fallopian tubes, ovaries, cervix, or peritoneal cavity. • Most common causes are physiological	interruption of the normal mechanism for the transport of the oocyte and anatomical changes to the fallopian tubes (Table 15-8).
Preoperative Diagnostic Tests and Procedures	• History and physical • Laparoscopy	• Pelviscopy • Ultrasound	• Pregnancy test • Culdocentesis
Equipment, Instruments, and Supplies Unique to Procedure	• Laparoscopic equipment • Laparoscopic instrumentation	• Major laparotomy instrument set in OR • Vaginal hysterectomy instrument set in OR	• D&C instrument set in OR
Preoperative Preparation	• Position: Lithotomy with Trendelenburg at 15° • Anesthesia: General	• Patient skin prep: Abdominal including vaginal prep	• Draping: Combined laparoscopic and lithotomy drape
Practical Considerations	• Pelviscopy with salpingostomy may be performed if ectopic pregnancy is unruptured and implantation is in the ampulla of the fallopian tube. • Other possible procedures include salpingotomy, resection of affected tubal segment, and salpingectomy.	• Unruptured tubal pregnancy can be laparoscopically treated. • Ruptured ectopic pregnancy is an emergency situation and a laparotomy is performed. • The surgical technologist should anticipate a large volume of blood in the abdominal cavity due	to hemorrhaging; two suction setups will be needed and a large number of laparotomy sponges. • The surgical team will need to move quickly to open the patient, control the hemorrhage, and perform a tubal resection.

PROCEDURE 15-5 (continued)

Surgical Procedure

1. Normal laparoscopy technique is employed (see Procedure 15-6 Laparoscopy, pp. 543–548).
2. The site of the tubal pregnancy is visually identified (Figure 15-14A).

   Procedural Consideration: Visual confirmation is diagnostic. One critical goal is preservation of the tube.
3. A longitudinal incision is made in the tube electrosurgically (Figure 15-14B).

   Procedural Consideration: Pass the electrosurgical instrument through access port.
4. Grasping forceps are placed in the tube and the trophoblastic tissue is removed (Figure 15-14C).

   Procedural Consideration: A laparoscopic Babcock is often used. Check patency of the tips before the procedure begins.
5. Hemorrhage is controlled electrosurgically (Figure 15-14D).

   Procedural Consideration: Smoke evacuator/suction may be needed.
6. The tubal incision is left open.

   Procedural Consideration: Prepare for closure while hemostasis is being achieved.
7. The laparoscopic procedure is terminated in the normal manner.

   Procedural Consideration: Closure suture passed. Count is performed.

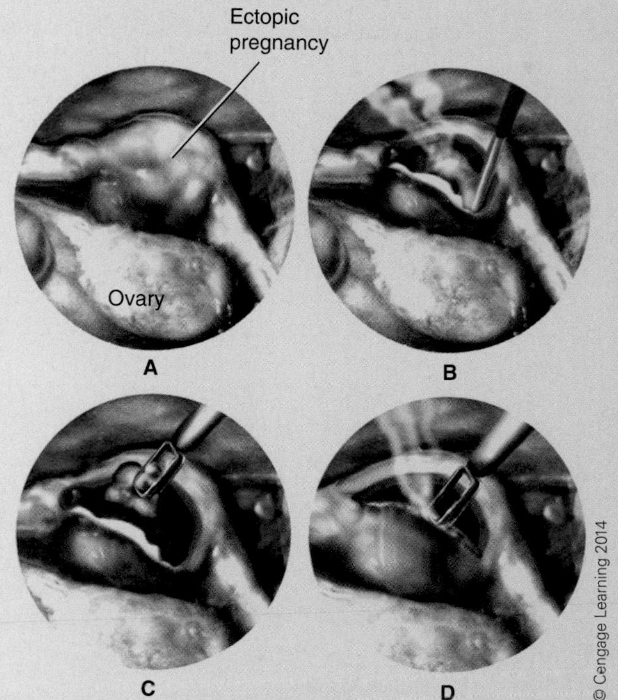

Figure 15-14 Laparoscopic resection of unruptured tubal pregnancy: (A) Site of implantation identified, (B) longitudinal incision into fallopian tube, (C) removal of tissue, (D) hemostasis achieved

(continues)

PROCEDURE 15-5 (continued)

Postoperative Considerations	**Immediate Postoperative Care** • Transport to PACU. • PACU team must be aware of the psychological grief associated with the loss of the fetus, which can increase the physiological vital signs, e.g., BP, heart rate, respiration rate. **Prognosis** • No complications: Discharged 1–2 days from health care facility; return to normal activities in 4–6 weeks. • Complications: Postoperative SSI; hemorrhage; increased risk for future ectopic pregnancy. **Wound Classification** • Class II: Clean-contaminated if manipulator used

SURGICAL PROCEDURES: GYNECOLOGIC PROCEDURES

Gynecologic surgery is surgery on the female reproductive system. The gynecologic patient typically seeks medical help on the basis of a complaint. The patient has identified some symptom or set of symptoms that cause concern. The routine examination of the gynecologic patient is summarized in Table 15-9. The categories of conditions treated in gynecologic practice are found in Table 15-10, along with some diagnostic considerations. Table 15-11 summarizes surgical interventions by anatomic area.

TABLE 15-9 Common Features of the Gynecologic Examination

Gynecologic history	Present complaint	Abnormal vaginal bleeding
		Abdominal pain
		Amenorrhea
		Amenorrhea
Contraceptive history		
Obstetric history		
Marital history		
Medical history		
Review of systems	Head and neck	
	Breasts	
	Heart and lungs	
	Abdomen	
	Back	
	Extremities	
Physical examination	Vital signs	
	Pelvic examination	
	Rectal examination	
Laboratory test	Urinalysis	
	Complete blood count	
	Erythrocyte sedimentation rate	
	Blood chemistry	
	Other	

TABLE 15-10 **Select Gynecologic Conditions, Symptoms, and Diagnostic Tests**

Condition or Disease	*Symptoms/Signs*	*Typical Diagnostic Tests*
Genital anomalies	Symptoms	Physical examination, including pelvic examination
	Primary amenorrhea	Sonography
	Dyspareunia	Intravenous pyelogram
	Dysmenorrhea	Hysterosalpingogram
	Cyclic pelvic pain	Hysteroscopy
	Inability to achieve penile penetration	Magnetic resonance imaging
	Infertility	Examination under anesthesia
	Habitual abortion	Laparoscopic visualization
	Spontaneous second-trimester abortion	
	Premature labor	
	Postpartum hemorrhage	
	Leakage with tampon in place	
	Signs	
	Vaginal mass	
	Abdominal mass	
	Absence of normal structures	
	Ambiguous genitalia	
	Fetal malpresentation	
	Retained placenta	
Benign lesions of the vagina		
Inclusion cysts	Usually asymptomatic	Visual examination
Endometriosis	Steel-gray or black cysts that bleed at time of menses	Visual examination Biopsy
Gartner's duct cysts	Usually asymptomatic	Visual examination
Urethral diverticula	Recurrent urethral infection	Visual examination
	Dribbling of urine	Urethroscopy
	Dyspareunia (pain during intercourse)	
	Dysuria	
Benign lesions of the cervix		
Chronic cervicitis	Persistent infections	Visual examination
	Leukorrhea	Papanicolaou smear
	Lower abdominal discomfort	Colposcopy to rule out dysplasia or cancer
	Dyspareunia	
Cervical polyp	Pedunculated lesion	Removal and pathologic examination to rule out cancer
Benign lesions of the vulva	Types	Physical examination
	Inflammatory vulvar dermatosis	Biopsy of gross lesions
	Vulvar dystrophies	
	Benign cysts and tumors	

(*continues*)

TABLE 15-10 **(continued)**

Condition or Disease	*Symptoms/Signs*	*Typical Diagnostic Tests*
	Dermatosis not unique to vulvar infections	
	Infectious disease	
Benign lesions of the uterus		
Leiomyomas	Majority are asymptomatic	Bimanual examination
	Symptoms	Ultrasonography
	Lower abdominal pain	MRI
	Pelvic pressure or congestion	Computed tomographic scan
	Menorrhagia	Hysterosalpingography
	Secondary dysmenorrhea	X-ray
	Increased infertility	Laparoscopic visualization
	Signs	
	Abdominal mass	
Endometrial hyperplasia	Postmenopausal bleeding	Endometrial biopsy
	Prolonged or irregular bleeding	D&C to rule out carcinoma
	Anemia	
Benign lesions of the ovaries and fallopian tubes		
Functional ovarian tumor	Usually asymptomatic	Bimanual examination
	Pelvic pain	Regression of cyst after menstrual period
	Peritoneal irritation	Sonography
	Delayed menstrual period	Pregnancy test and erythrocyte sedimentation rate
	Rebound tenderness	to rule out teratomas
	Acute abdominal pain	
	Hemoperitoneum	
Neoplastic ovarian tumor	Most are asymptomatic	Sonography
	Symptoms	Serum CA 125 titer
	Acute pain following torsion	Laparoscopy
	Increased abdominal girth	
	Pelvic pressure/congestion	
	Peritoneal irritation	
	Signs	
	Pelvic mass	
	Dull percussion sound	
	Abdominal rigidity	
	Paralytic ileus	
Endometriosis	Symptoms	Symptom triad
	Dysmenorrhea	Bimanual examination
	Dyspareunia	Normal leukocyte count and erythrocyte
	Dyschezia (difficult defecation)	sedimentation rate

TABLE 15-10 **(continued)**

Condition or Disease	*Symptoms/Signs*	*Typical Diagnostic Tests*
	Signs Small, tender nodules Cystic abdominal mass Tender, fixed adnexal mass Barb-like uterosacral ligament pain	Slightly elevated CA 125 level Sonography Laparoscopy
Dysfunctional uterine bleeding (DUB)	During years around menarche and menopause	Rule out other causes CBC Platelet count Coagulation studies Thyroid function studies Liver function studies Prolactin levels Serum FSH levels Papanicolaou smear Endometrial biopsy Sonography Hysterosalpingography Hysteroscopy D&C
Genitourinary dysfunction Pelvic organ prolapse Urinary incontinence Infections	Symptoms and signs vary with condition. All are related to support structures in the pelvic area	Bimanual examination Visual examination Urinary stress test Urethrocystoscopy Cystometrogram Sonography
Uterine cancer	Most common symptom—abnormal vaginal bleeding	Papanicolaou smear Endocervical **curettage** Endometrial biopsy
Cervical cancer	Usually asymptomatic Abnormal bleeding Vaginal discharge Abnormal Pap smear	Colposcopy Cervical conization Biopsy Endocervical curettage Schiller's test
Ovarian cancer	Usually asymptomatic Symptoms	Bimanual examination

(*continues*)

Table 15-10 (continued)

Condition or Disease	*Symptoms/Signs*	*Typical Diagnostic Tests*
	Irregular menses	Papanicolaou smear
	Pelvic congestion	Endometrial biopsy
	Abdominal pain	Endocervical curettage
	Signs	X-ray
	Solid, irregular, fixed pelvic mass	Sonography
		Barium enema
		CA 125
Vulvar cancer	Itching	Visual examination
	Visible abnormalities	Collin's test
Vaginal cancer	Usually asymptomatic	Abnormal Papanicolaou smear in a Biopsy

Table 15-11 Summary Information: Procedures in Gynecologic Surgery

Structure/Organ	*Procedure*	*Structure/Organ*	*Procedure*
Vulva and introitus	Biopsy of vulva	**Vagina and urethra**	Anterior repair—cystocele
	Excision of vulvar skin—with STSG (split-thickness skin graft)		Posterior repair—rectocele
	Wide local vulvar excision—primary closure, secondary Z-plasty		Vaginal repair—enterocele
	Vulvectomy		Vaginal suspension—sacrospinous ligament
	Vulvar injection—alcohol		Vaginal evisceration
	Vulvar excision—**LEEP** (loop electrosurgical excision procedure)		Excision transverse vaginal septum
	Vulvar injection—cortisone		Repair "double-barreled" vagina
	Excision of urethral caruncle		Sacral colpopexy
	Marsupialization—Bartholin's gland cyst		Le Fort Procedure for prolapse
	Bartholin's gland biopsy		Repair vesicovaginal fistula
	Bartholin's gland excision		Repair rectovaginal fistula
	Repair vaginal outlet stenosis		Repair urethrovaginal fistula
	Excision of vestibular adenitis		Vaginoplasty for neovagina
	Release of labial fusion		Urethral reconstruction
	Hymenectomy		Repair(s) of suburethral diverticulum
			Correction of urinary incontinence
			Sigmoid neovagina

TABLE 15-11 (continued)

Structure/Organ	Procedure	Structure/Organ	Procedure
Cervix	Biopsy	**Fallopian tubes and ovaries**	Resection—unruptured tubal pregnancy
	Endocervical curettage		Resection and hemorrhage control—ruptured tubal pregnancy (emergency)
	Cervical cone—"cold"		Ovarian biopsy
	Cervical cone—LEEP		Treatment—endometriosis Lysis of adhesions
	Abdominal excision—cervical stump		Sterilization procedures
	Correction—incompetent cervix		Salpingectomy
Uterus	Dilation and curettage		Salpingo-oophorectomy
	Dilation and curettage—vacuum		Fimbrioplasty
	Dilatation and evacuation		Tuboplasty
	Cesarean section		Wedges resection—ovary
	Myomectomy		Correction—torsion of ovary
	Correction—double uterus		Ovarian cystectomy
	Hysteroscopy—diagnostic	**Other**	Bladder and ureter (see Chapter 20)
	Hysteroscopy—intervention		Bowel, colon, abdominal wall (see Chapter 14)
	Vaginal hysterectomy		Malignant disease and special procedures
	Abdominal hysterectomy		
	Laparoscopically assisted vaginal hysterectomy		

Abdominal Incisions for Gynecologic Surgery

Incisions used in gynecologic abdominal surgery fall into three basic categories: transverse, vertical, and oblique. Although transverse incisions provide the best cosmetic result and are nearly 30 times stronger after repair, they are relatively more time consuming and hemorrhagic than vertical incisions. Transverse incisions can compromise nerves, generally involve the division of muscles, and may limit access to the upper abdomen.

Vertical and oblique incisions are discussed in detail in Chapter 14. Transverse incisions are named for the surgeons who originally developed the technique. The three most commonly used are presented here: the **Pfannenstiel**, Maylard, and Cherney incisions (Table 15-12).

Closure of these incisions commonly begins with the fascia with a running #1 or #2 polyglycolic suture. In the Cherney technique, the peritoneum may be closed separately in similar fashion. Muscles are not usually sutured in the Maylard or Pfannenstiel approaches; however, they are reunited with the rectus tendon (the original point of division) in the Cherney technique using an adequate number of nonabsorbable sutures placed in an interrupted or horizontal mattress manner. The subcutaneous tissue is generally not closed and staples or subcuticular suture is used on the skin.

Diagnostic Procedures

Laparoscopy and hysteroscopy have been in use for a long time and through the years with advances in modern technology, the procedures can be used for diagnostic and interventional purposes. Procedures 15-6 and 15-7 describe the diagnostic laparoscopy and hysteroscopy procedures.

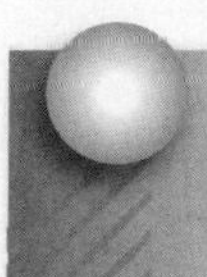

PEARL OF WISDOM

The most common cause for failure of monitors or other equipment is the failure to plug the machine into the wall socket. Develop a system for checking all equipment before you scrub.

Table 15-12 Transverse Abdominal Incisions Used in Gynecologic Surgery

Pfannenstiel	*Maylard*	*Cherney*
Gently curved incision, 10–15 cm long at any level between the umbilicus and symphysis pubis.	Less curved incision between the crests of the anterior iliac spine.	Less curved incision between the crests of the anterior iliac spine.
Skin and subcutaneous fat are incised to the level of the anterior rectus sheath.	Skin and subcutaneous fat are incised to the level of the anterior rectus sheath.	Skin and subcutaneous fat are incised to the level of the anterior rectus sheath.
Fascia is incised transversely on either side of the linea alba.	Fascia is incised transversely.	Fascia is incised transversely.
Linea alba is then divided, joining the two incisions. Rectus sheath is separated from the underlying rectus muscle by blunt dissection.	Inferior epigastric vessels are located at the lateral edges of the incision and are ligated and cut.	Inferior epigastric vessels are located at the lateral edges of the incision and are ligated and cut.
Rectus muscles are separated in the midline.	Rectus muscle is divided, usually electrosurgically.	Rectus muscle is divided, usually electrosurgically at its insertion on the symphysis pubis.
Peritoneum is opened vertically.	Peritoneum is incised transversely.	Peritoneum is incised transversely.

Procedure 15-6 Basic Laparoscopy

Surgical Anatomy and Pathology	• See previous descriptions of abdominal anatomy in Chapter 14 and surgical	procedures in this chapter.	• Pathology depends on history and physical (signs and symptoms).
Preoperative Diagnostic Tests and Procedures	• History and physical		
Equipment, Instruments, and Supplies Unique to Procedure	• Laparoscopic equipment (Figure 15-15A) • Laparoscopic instrumentation	• Laser (surgeon's preference) • Major laparotomy set available in OR	
Preoperative Preparation	• Position: Lithotomy with slight Trendelenburg • Anesthesia: General	• Patient skin prep: Abdominal with vaginal prep	• Draping: Laparoscopy (combined laparotomy and lithotomy)
Practical Considerations	• Check all equipment prior to patient entering OR.	• Surgical technologist should know how to manipulate the uterine	manipulator under the supervision of the surgeon.

PROCEDURE 15-6 (continued)

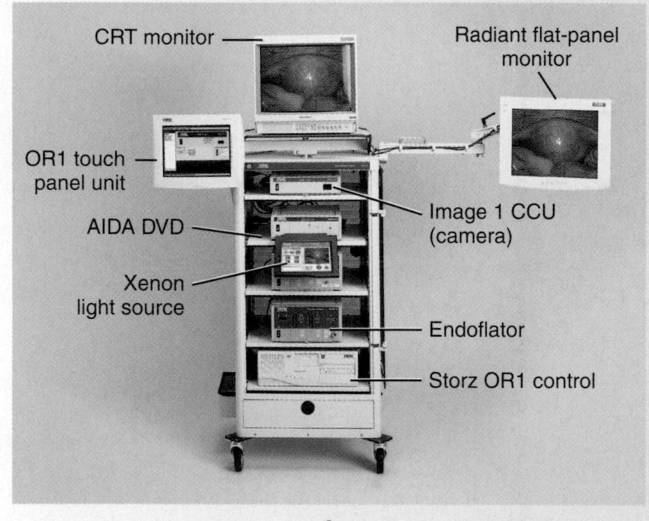

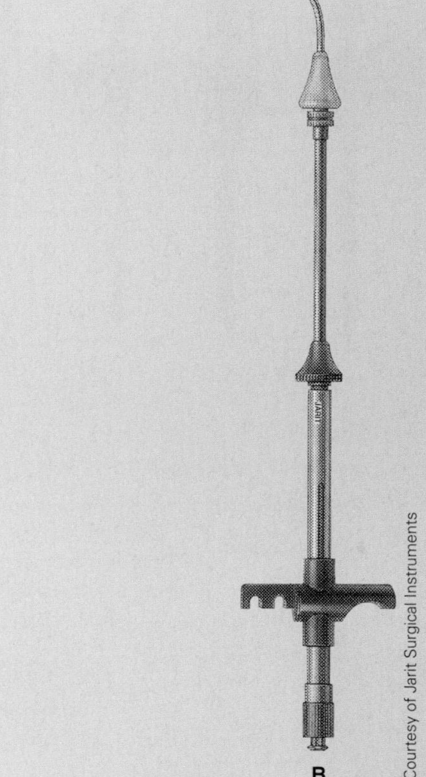

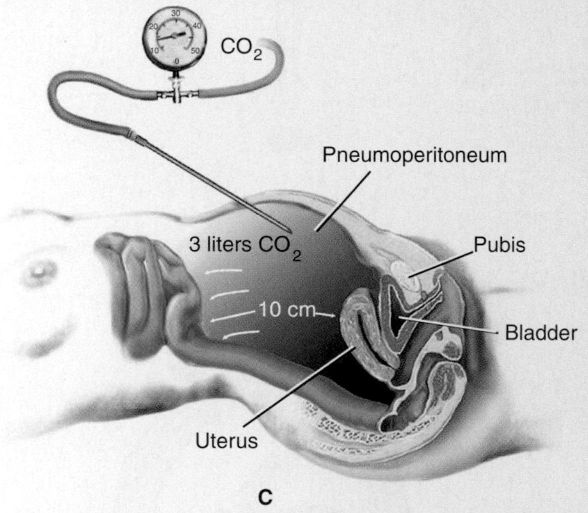

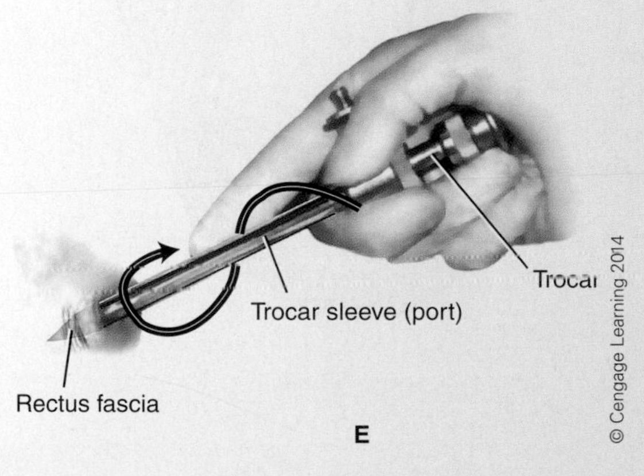

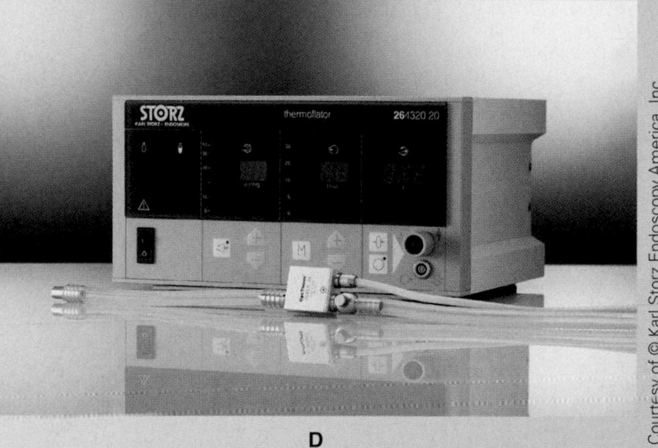

Figure 15-15 Basic laparoscopy: (A) laparoscopic tower, (B) Cohen acorn cannula, (C) effects of CO_2 and proper position of Verres needle, (D) insufflator, (E) port with trocar entering the abdomen

(*continues*)

Procedure 15-6 (continued)

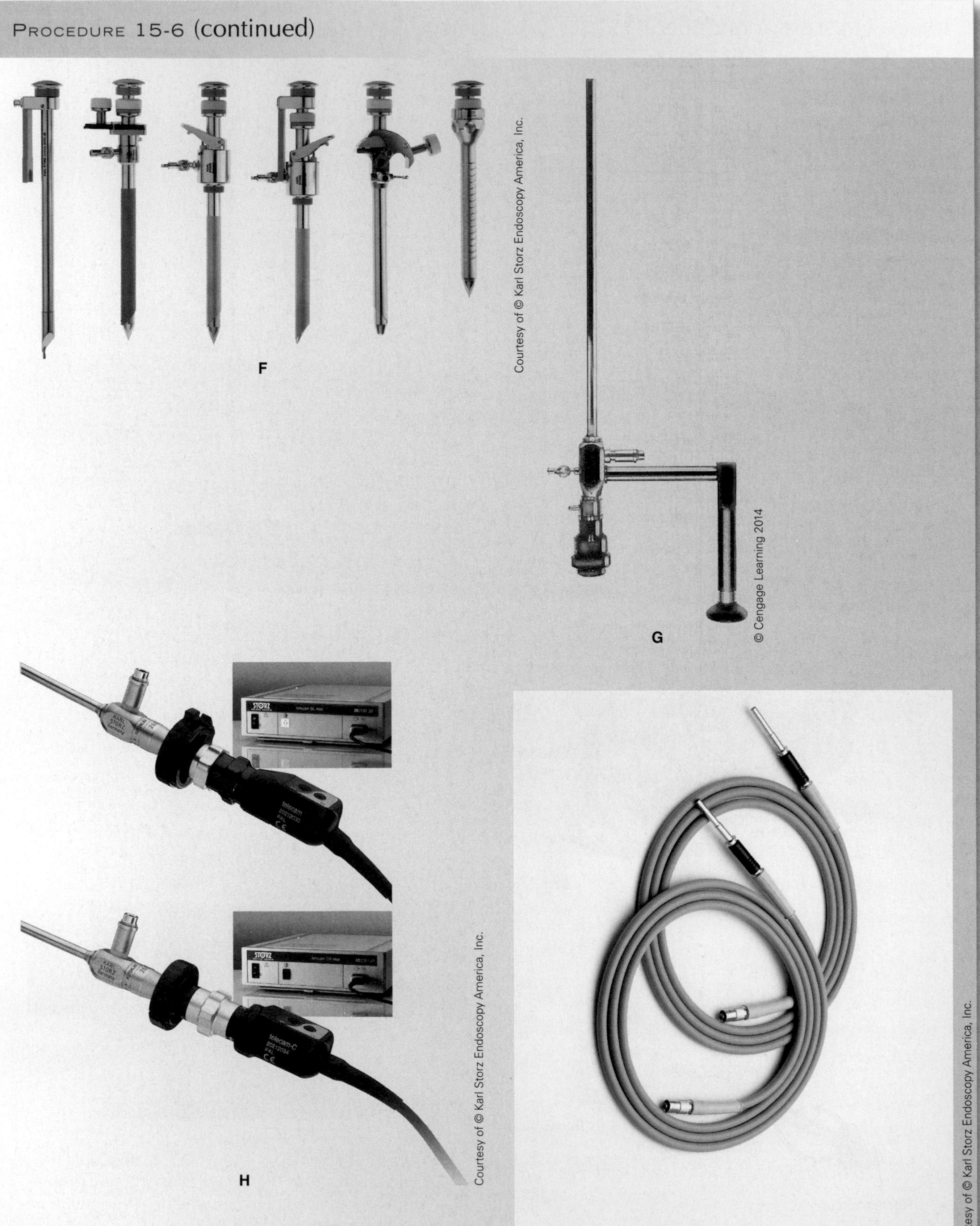

Figure 15-15 Basic laparoscopy: (F) Various types of trocars, (G) operating laparoscope, (H) camera attached to laparoscope, (I) light cord

Procedure 15-6 (continued)

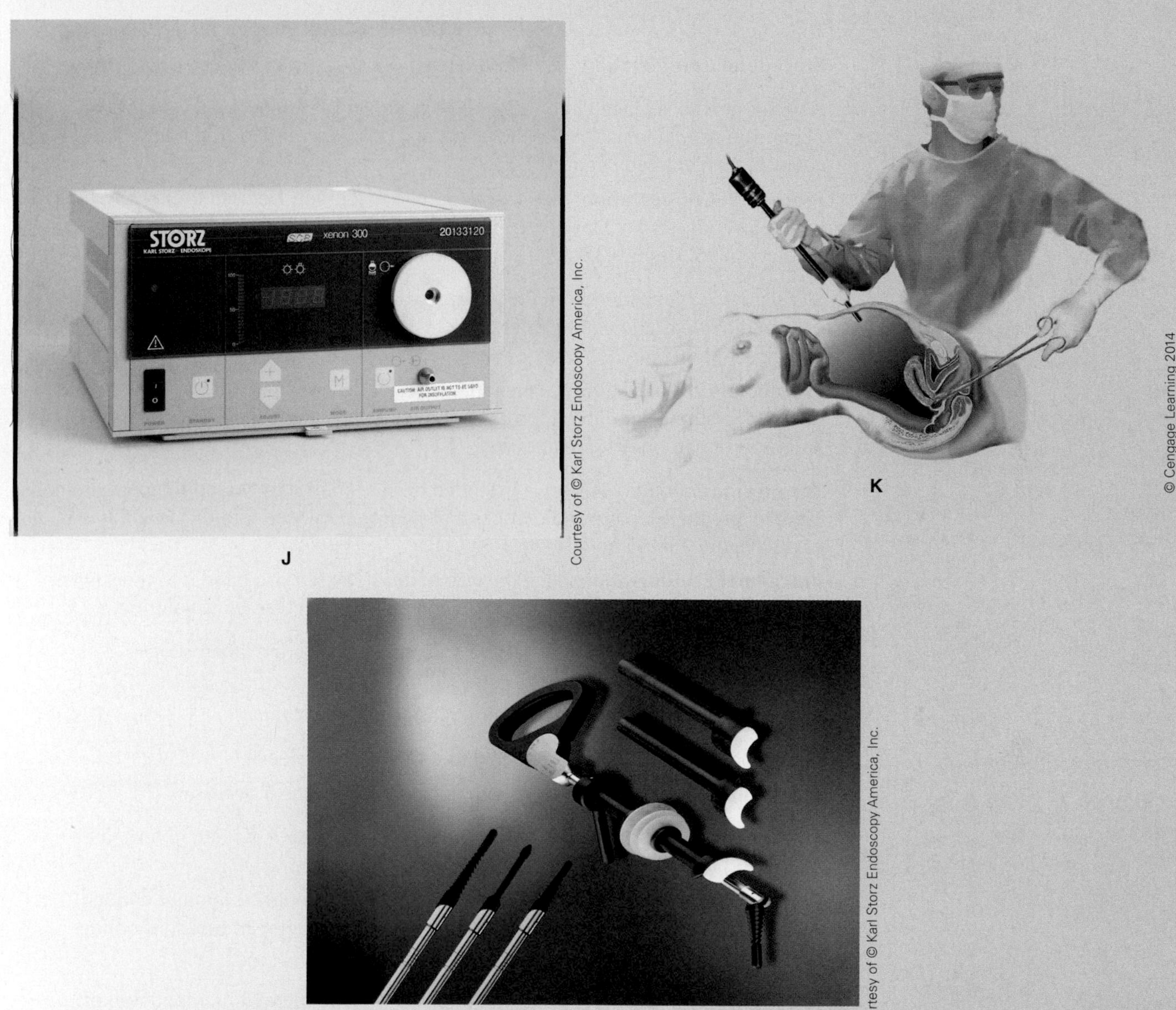

Figure 15-15 Basic laparoscopy: (J) Xenon light source, (K) use of uterine manipulator and camera, (L) Clermon-Ferrand uterine manipulator

Surgical Procedure

1. A handheld vaginal retractor is placed posteriorly in the vagina and the cervix is grasped with a tenaculum.
2. A uterine manipulator of choice is placed on the cervix. The manipulator may be covered so it can be handled by the surgeon later (Figure 15-15B).

   Procedural Consideration: The surgeon's top gloves should be removed and replaced using proper technique following the vaginal portion of the procedure. Instruments used vaginally must be isolated.

(*continues*)

PROCEDURE 15-6 (continued)

3. The anterior abdominal wall is elevated using two towel clips or hands with open raytex

   Procedural Consideration: Techniques vary from surgeon to surgeon.

4. A Verres needle is placed into the midline at an angle 90° to the elevated body plane. The needle is stopped at the fascia and position verified. The abdominal cavity is then entered (Figure 15-15C).

   Procedural Consideration: A #11 or #15 knife blade may be used to place a small nick prior to insertion. Have a syringe with saline ready to conform entrance into the abdominal cavity. Check all cords and tubes for readiness.

5. Sterile tubing is attached from the needle to a carbon dioxide CO_2 insufflator and the carbon dioxide is allowed to enter to a pressure not exceeding 15 mm Hg (Figure 15-15D).

   Procedural Consideration: If a clear flow is established, a pneumoperitoneum is produced. Pressure is monitored throughout the procedure by the circulator. Commonly 4–5 liters of carbon dioxide are used.

6. The previous midline incision is extended from a small stab wound to approximately 1 cm in length. A laparoscopic trocar and sleeve are placed into the abdominal cavity (Figure 15-15E and F).

   Procedural Consideration: State the size of the sleeve as you hand it to the surgeon. Prepare laparoscope for passage to surgeon by applying defogging solution.

7. The trocar is removed from the sleeve and replaced with the laparoscope (Figure 15-15G).

   Procedural Consideration: Assist with transfer of instruments.

8. The carbon dioxide line is connected to a valve on the sleeve.

   Procedural Consideration: Assist with transfer of CO_2 line if necessary.

9. The laparoscope is connected to a camera and light source, which, in turn, are connected to a monitor (Figure 15-15H–J).

   Procedural Consideration: The surgical technologist should be familiar enough with all the equipment and connections to assist the team with troubleshooting if there are problems.

10. If the procedure is interventional in nature or requires internal manipulation of anatomical structures, other ports will be established for operating instrumentation (Figure 15-15K and L).

    Procedural Consideration: The precise placement of these ports depends on the surgical procedure to be performed. The size of the ports depends on their use.

11. Following the operative intervention, carbon dioxide is released from the abdomen and all ports removed. Some ports may require one or two sutures to close. Band-Aids are usually applied.

    Procedural Consideration: Accept returned equipment and instrumentation. Pass prepared sutures. Prepare dressings.

Procedure 15-6 (continued)

Postoperative Considerations	
	Immediate Postoperative Care • Transport to PACU. **Prognosis** • No complications: Discharged same day of surgery; return to normal activities 2–4 days. • Complications: injury to abdominopelvic organ(s); referred shoulder pain; CO_2 embolus. • Final prognosis depends on operative findings. **Wound Classification** • Class II: Clean-contaminated due to vaginal manipulation

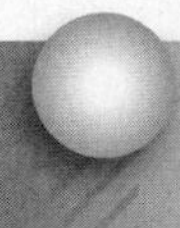

Pearl of Wisdom

Cervical intraepithelial neoplasia (CIN) or cervical dysplasia is indicated by epithelium that appears white after the application of acetic acid. Patients with CIN may present with vascular "dots" referred to as punctuation or a mosaic of capillaries lying parallel to the surface of the cervix. Increased dilation and irregularity in punctuation and mosaicism indicate atypical tissue.

Procedure 15-7 Hysteroscopy

Surgical Anatomy and Pathology	• See Procedure 15-1 page 522 for surgical anatomy of uterus.
	• The vagina is a fibromuscular tube that is continuous with the external genitalia.
	  • The vagina ascends posterosuperiorly and is close to the bladder and urethra anteriorly and the rectum and anal canal posteriorly. The ureters are also located anterior to the vagina situated lateral to the uterine arteries.
	  • Vaginal mucosa is epithelium that is supplemented by mucous from the cervix.
	  • Vaginal muscularity consists of an inner circular muscle and outer longitudinal layer that is continuous with the myometrium of the uterus.
	  • The recess created by the cervical-vaginal junction is called the fornix.
	  • Arterial supply is the vaginal, uterine, internal pudendal and middle rectal branches of the internal iliac arteries; vaginal veins drain into the internal iliac venous system.
	• Hysteroscopy is used to treat pathologies such as adhesions, polyps, and myomas.

Preoperative Diagnostic Tests and Procedures	• History and physical
Equipment, Instruments, and Supplies Unique to Procedure	• Rigid or flexible hysteroscope; size/diameter according to surgeon's preference • Endoscopic equipment • Hysteroscopic pump or insufflator for distention media • Laser (surgeon's preference) • ESU available • Vaginal instrument tray available • D&C instrument tray available

(continues)

Procedure 15-7 (continued)

Preoperative Preparation

- Position: Lithotomy
- Anesthesia: General
- Patient skin prep: Vaginal
- Draping: Lithotomy

Practical Considerations

- Surgical technologist should be familiar with the type of hysteroscope that is used, in particular the location of the ports for the insertion of surgical instruments. Under the direction of the surgeon, the surgical technologist may be responsible for inserting the instruments into and through the port(s).
- Tissue specimens may need to be kept separate; confirm with the surgeon.
- Hysteroscopy is not considered a sterile procedure; however, the best possible sterile technique should be used to prevent the patient from acquiring a postoperative SSI.

Surgical Procedure

1. A weighted speculum is placed in the vagina.
2. The cervix is grasped with a tenaculum and pulled toward the vaginal introitus.

   Procedural Consideration: Pass tenaculum with caution. The tip is pointed.
3. A uterine sound is placed into the cervical canal to determine the direction and depth of the uterine cavity.

   Procedural Consideration: Instruments are arranged in order of use, typically from left to right. It may be necessary to lubricate the tips of the sound and dilators.
4. The cervix is dilated to the required diameter.

   Procedural Consideration: Hegar or Hank uterine dilators are commonly used.
5. The hysteroscope is placed into the uterus via the cervix.

   Procedural Consideration: The hysteroscope is approximately 4 mm in diameter and may have a viewing angle of 0–30 degrees.
6. The uterus is distended with carbon dioxide, sorbitol or glycine, or dextran solution.

   Procedural Consideration: Complications are rare but fluid overload cases involving distention medium are known. Rate of flow and total fluid volume should be monitored throughout the procedure.
7. The uterus is explored visually. If biopsy or operative action is required, operative instruments will be used through the ports on the hysteroscope.

   Procedural Consideration: Operative hysteroscopic sets include flexible instruments such as scissors and biopsy punches. These should be available on all procedures.
8. At conclusion, all instruments are removed.

   Procedural Consideration: If dextran solution was used for distention purposes, instruments will need to be cleaned immediately in warm water to prevent pitting.

Postoperative Considerations

Immediate Postoperative Care

- Transport to PACU.

Prognosis

- No complications: Discharged same day of surgery; return to normal activities in 1–2 days depending on extent of what was performed during the procedure.
- Complications: Gas or air embolism; laceration or perforation of the vagina or uterus; hemorrhage; complications as related to the use of the distention medium.
- Final prognosis depends on operative findings.

Wound Classification

- Class II: Clean-contaminated

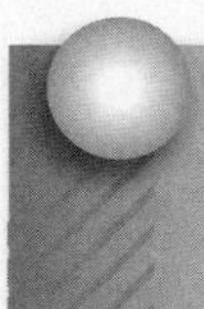

PEARL OF WISDOM

All team members need to be aware of the type of distention medium used, the proper rate of flow, the maximum volume allowed, and the outflow rate.

Surgical Procedures of the External Genitalia and Structures

PROCEDURE 15-8 Marsupialization of Bartholin's Gland Cyst

Surgical Anatomy and Pathology	• The Bartholin's glands (greater vestibular glands) are two glands that are located in the posterior third of the labia majora. Bartholin's glands secrete mucous and provide vaginal lubrication. • Distal obstruction of the duct can create painful irritation or infection, with a Bartholin's cyst developing. • Obstruction is commonly results from gonococcal infection or, most frequently, trauma. • Most cysts are asymptomatic, but an infection can lead to an abscess which causes swelling, tenderness, erythema, pain and discomfort.
Preoperative Diagnostic Tests and Procedures	• Diagnosis obtained by history and physical as well as by direct examination.
Equipment, Instruments, and Supplies Unique to Procedure	• Vaginal instrument set • Drain of surgeon's preference • Aerobic and anaerobic culture tubes
Preoperative Preparation	• Position: Lithotomy • Anesthesia: Local for incision and drainage procedure; general for marsupialization procedure • Patient skin prep: Vaginal prep • Draping: Lithotomy
Practical Considerations	• The area may be very painful to touch prior to being anesthetized. • Marsupialization, converting a closed cavity into an open pouch, may be required for second intention healing to occur.
Surgical Procedure	1. Local excision of a Bartholin's gland cyst requires an elliptical incision created in the vaginal mucosa around the duct, as close to the gland as possible. **Procedural Consideration:** The labia minor may be sutured to the skin to provide exposure. Have culture tubes on field.
	2. Dissection is begun bluntly but may require scissors to dissect the gland from its bed. **Procedural Consideration:** Blunt dissection is often accomplished with a scalpel handle. Sharp dissection: Mayo scissors or knife blade.
	3. If the cyst wall margins are unclear, it can be approached by incision into the cyst and dissection of it from the surrounding tissues. **Procedural Consideration:** Complete removal of the gland tissue adherent to the cyst wall is essential.
	4. After the cyst wall is opened, the cyst is drained (Figure 15-16A). **Procedural Consideration:** Fluid may be cultured. Have suction available.

(continues)

PROCEDURE 15-8 (continued)

5. The cavity created may be closed by approximating the vaginal wall tissues with fine, interrupted absorbable sutures.

   Procedural Consideration: Pass sutures of choice. Have drain of choice available if needed.

6. The cyst wall lining is everted and sutured to the vaginal mucosa with interrupted 2-0 absorbable sutures (Figure 15-16B).

   Procedural Consideration: Complete count. Be sure labial retraction sutures are removed. Peri-pad dressing is applied.

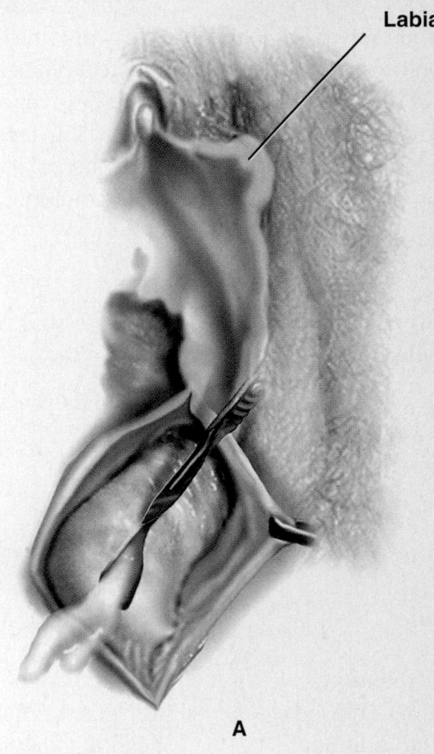

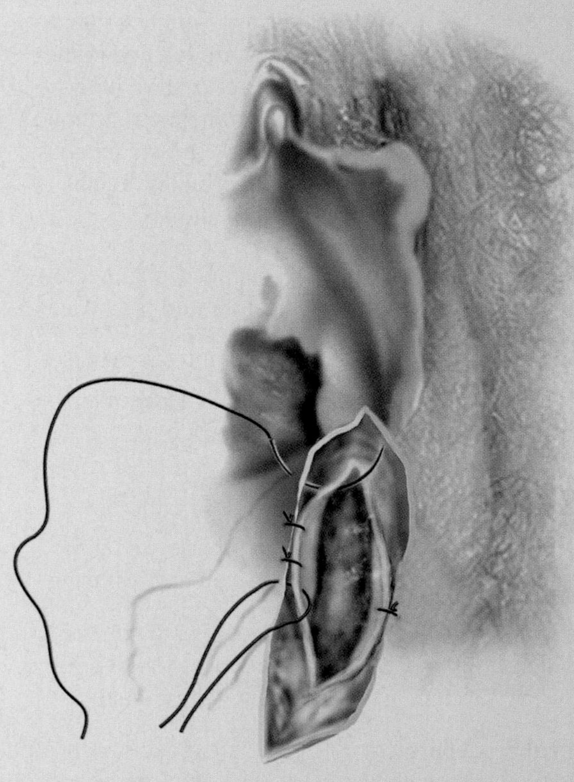

Figure 15-16 Marsupializaton of Bartholin's gland cyst: (A) Retraction of labia minora and incision into infected cyst, (B) marsupialization technique

Postoperative Considerations

Immediate Postoperative Care

- Transport to PACU.
- Apply ice if indicated

Prognosis

- No complications: Return to normal activities and discharged the same day of surgery.
- Complications: Hemorrhage; wound infection.

Wound Classification

- Class III: Contaminated
- Class IV: Dirty-infected

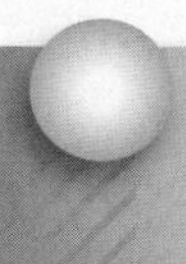

PEARL OF WISDOM

The vaginal mucosa may be closed in some cases using continuous or interrupted 3-0 absorbable stitches. When marsupialization is used, ice packs and drains are unnecessary because the created "pouch" is left open.

PROCEDURE 15-9 Simple Vulvectomy

Surgical Anatomy and Pathology	• The mons pubis is characterized by its round, slight elevation that is anterior to the symphysis pubis and superior to the vaginal opening.
	• It is formed by a collection of adipose tissue located beneath the skin.
	• It is covered with pubic hair following puberty.
	• The labia majora are two rounded longitudinal flaps extending from the mons pubis to the perineum.
	• The labia minora are two, flat cutaneous flaps lying between the labia majora.
	  • The labia minora bifurcate at the clitoris, passing below and above the clitoris.
		• The labia minora contain sebaceous glands.
		• The clitoris is an erectile structure located directly above the urethral orifice and below the mons pubis.
		  • It is covered by a hood-shaped prepuce formed by the fused ends of the anterior labia minora.
		• The **vestibule** is the cavity between the labia minora and it contains the urethral meatus as well as the Bartholin's glands.
		• The perineum is the area between the inferior vaginal opening and anus.
		  • It is supported by the levator ani, coccygeal, and deep transverse perineal muscles.
		  • The perineum is a sensitive area innervated by
			branches of the pudendal nerve.
			• Simple vulvectomy is performed for benign or premalignant conditions of the vulva.
			• Vulvectomy is performed as a last recourse when other treatments such as laser ablation and wide local lesion excision with medical therapy have failed.
			• The procedure can be performed for conditions such as condylomata and Paget's disease.
			• The lesion and small margin of tissue are excised during the procedure.
			• A radical vulvectomy involves groin exploration, removal of the lymph nodes, and a wide resection of the tissue.

Preoperative Diagnostic Tests and Procedures	• Diagnosis obtained by history and physical as well as by direct examination	• Biopsy • Computed tomography (CT) scan	• Magnetic resonance imaging (MRI)
Equipment, Instruments, and Supplies Unique to Procedure	• Vaginal instrument set	• Urinary catheter	• Aerobic and anaerobic culture tubes

(*continues*)

Procedure 15-9 (continued)

Preoperative Preparation	• Position: Lithotomy • Anesthesia: General • Patient skin prep: Vaginal and lower abdomen • Draping: Lithotomy draping
Practical Considerations	• Patient usually has a Foley catheter. • The surgical technologist should be particularly aware of the psychological trauma the patient may be experiencing and with other team members provide the appropriate support.
Surgical Procedure	1. The area to be removed is usually outlined with a skin marker. **Procedural Consideration:** The area to be excised may encompass the entire vulvar area from the mons pubis to the perineum, extending laterally from the labia majora for several centimeters, or in a "butterfly" shape, sparing the clitoris and perineum.
	2. Local injection of epinephrine may be used to reduce bleeding, but is sparingly used to avoid distorting anatomy. **Procedural Consideration:** Local is injected using a three-ring, control-tip syringe. Report amount injected.
	3. The incision with a #10 blade begins at the vaginal outlet so that the urethral borders can be identified (Figure 15-17A). **Procedural Consideration:** Be prepared to pass hemostatic instruments.
	4. The vaginal epithelium is undermined for a short distance. **Procedural Consideration:** Dissection may be sharp, blunt, or a combination of the two.
	5. The elliptical incision continues at the outer skin margins and bleeders are coagulated or ligated, including identification and ligation of the pudendal artery (Figure 15-17B). **Procedural Consideration:** Considerable bleeding can occur in the area of the clitoris due to its high vascularity, and also at the lower one-third of the vulva where the Bartholin's ducts are located. These should be controlled with hemostatic sutures.
	6. The incision is carried almost to the anal orifice; care is taken in dissection to avoid the sphincters. **Procedural Consideration:** Knife will be used repeatedly.
	7. Dissection continues into the adipose layer to facilitate closure but does not continue down to the deep fascia or muscles. **Procedural Consideration:** Various dissection techniques will be employed. Several hemostatic clamps will be used.
	8. Hemostasis is achieved, tissues are approximated in layers with absorbable suture, and the skin edges are likewise approximated. **Procedural Consideration:** Specific variation: The area may also be left open to granulate, or, if considerable excision has occurred, it can require a split thickness or myocutaneous graft. Have skin graft set available in room.
	9. A small drain is commonly placed in the lower end of the incision. **Procedural Consideration:** Drain and suture of choice are prepared in advance.
	10. The vaginal epithelium is everted over the perineum to the level of the anal orifice to allow for satisfactory coitus (Figure 15-17C and D). **Procedural Consideration:** Perform counts, if necessary. Prepare dressing.

PROCEDURE 15-9 (continued)

11. Dressing is a firm pack applied over the entire area.
    Procedural Consideration: Held in place by stretch briefs.

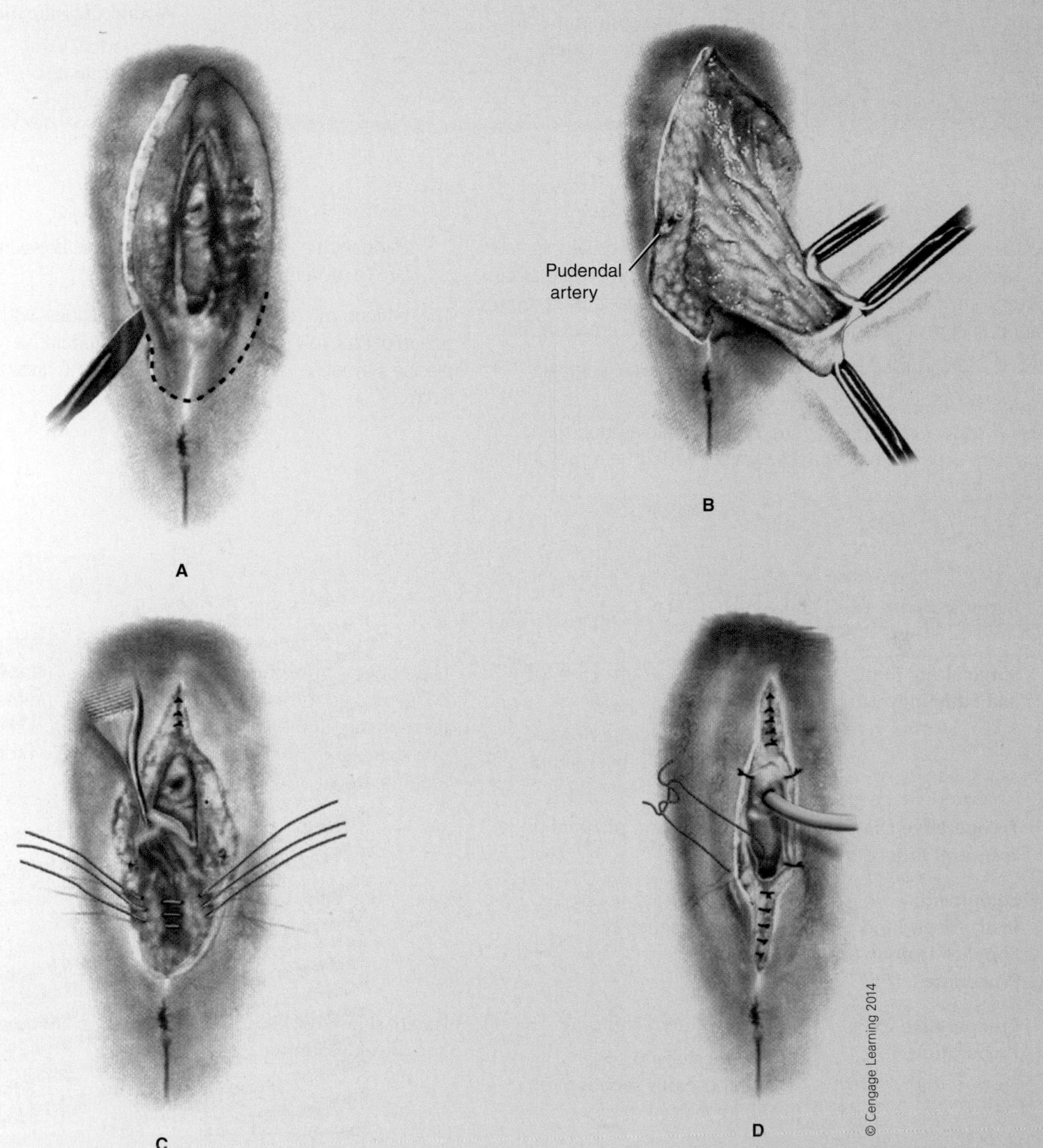

Figure 15-17 Simple vulvectomy: (A) Skin incision, (B) pudendal artery ligated and cut, (C) closure of levator ani muscles, (D) subcuticular closure (catheter in urethra)

(*continues*)

PROCEDURE 15-9 (continued)

Postoperative Considerations	**Immediate Postoperative Care** • Transport to PACU. • Indwelling or suprapubic catheter is maintained for 4–6 days.	**Prognosis** • No complications: Return to normal activities in 6–8 weeks.	• Complications: Postoperative SSI; hemorrhage; hematoma; **Wound Classification** • Class II: Clean-contaminated

Ablation of condylomata (external genitalia wart usually spread by sexual contact) is similar to the vulvectomy procedure as far as anatomy, pathology, history and physical, preoperative preparation, and postoperative considerations. The differences include:

- Preservation of the vulva and other external genitalia structures.
- A wide local excision with 5-mm margin around the lesion is performed with the scalpel with little removal of subcutaneous tissue.
- lesion with a CO_2 laser. Surgical plume is evacuated with care to prevent viral transmission.

The patient can return to normal activities within a short period of time following surgery. The postoperative care involves placing Silvadene cream on the treatment area three times a day.

PROCEDURE 15-10 Labiaplasty

Surgical Anatomy and Pathology	• See Procedure 15-9 for anatomy • Procedure is performed to correct labia minora	hypertrophy caused by congenital abnormality (genetic inheritance of oversized **labia**), or to repair tearing and	stretching due to childbirth, trauma, sexual intercourse, age, and genital piercing.
Preoperative Diagnostic Tests and Procedures	• History and physical		
Equipment, Instruments, and Supplies Unique to Procedure	• Vaginal or minor instrument tray	• Laser (surgeon's preference)	
Preoperative Preparation	• Position: Lithotomy • Anesthesia: Local, conscious sedation, or general	• Patient skin prep: Vaginal and lower abdomen	• Draping: Lithotomy drape
Practical Considerations	• Bleeding is a primary challenge when performing the procedure; the surgical	technologist will be responsible for suctioning and sponging the surgical site to	aid in the surgeon's ability to view the site.

PROCEDURE 15-10 (continued)

- There are four techniques for labioplasty:
  - Amputation: A clamp is placed across the area of labial tissue to be resected and using the scalpel the surgeon excises the excess tissue, which is then sutured.
  - Central wedge resection: A full-thickness wedge of tissue is excised from the thickest portion of the **labium** minora. A Z-plasty technique can be used for closure to avoid complications such as nerve damage that result in painful neuromas.
  - Deepithelialization: Described below; can be performed with the laser.
  - Clitoral unhooding: Labioplasty with resection of the clitoral prepuce (hood). The hood is sutured to the pubic bone in the midline, which further tightens the labia minora.

Surgical Procedure: Deepithelialization Technique

1. Using a marking pen the surgeon marks the resection pattern on each labium minora.
2. Local anesthetic is injected into the labial tissues.
3. Using the laser or sharp dissection the surgeon incises the epithelium of a central area on the medial and lateral aspects of each labium minora.
4. The surgeon may close the incision with a running buried-suture technique or Z-plasty.

Postoperative Considerations

Immediate Postoperative Care

- Transport to PACU.

Prognosis

- No complications: Discharge same day of surgery; return to normal activities in 1–2 days.
- Complications: Postoperative SSI; hemorrhage; labial asymmetry, undercorrection or overcorrection that requires revision surgery; nerve damage that can cause development of painful neuromas; Z-plasty technique presents a higher risk for necrosis of the labia minora tissues.

Wound Classification

- Class II: Clean-contaminated

Cervical Surgical Procedures

PROCEDURE 15-11 Dilation and Curettage (D&C)

Surgical Anatomy and Pathology

- See previous procedures for description of anatomy.
- Diagnostic indications for D&C include menorrhagia, metrorrhagia, dysmenorrhea, collection of cytology specimens to rule out pregnancy prior to elective sterilization, and to determine a cause for infertility.
- Therapeutic usage includes removal of suspected pathology (such as polyps), treatment of postpartum bleeding or to evacuate retained secundines (placenta), retrieval of "lost" IUD, placement of radioactive carriers for the management of cervical or uterine malignancies, and treatment of incomplete

(continues)

Procedure 15-11 (continued)

abortion, or dysmenorrhea. If the procedure is performed after the 13th week of pregnancy, it is termed dilation and evacuation (D&E) (Figure 15-18).

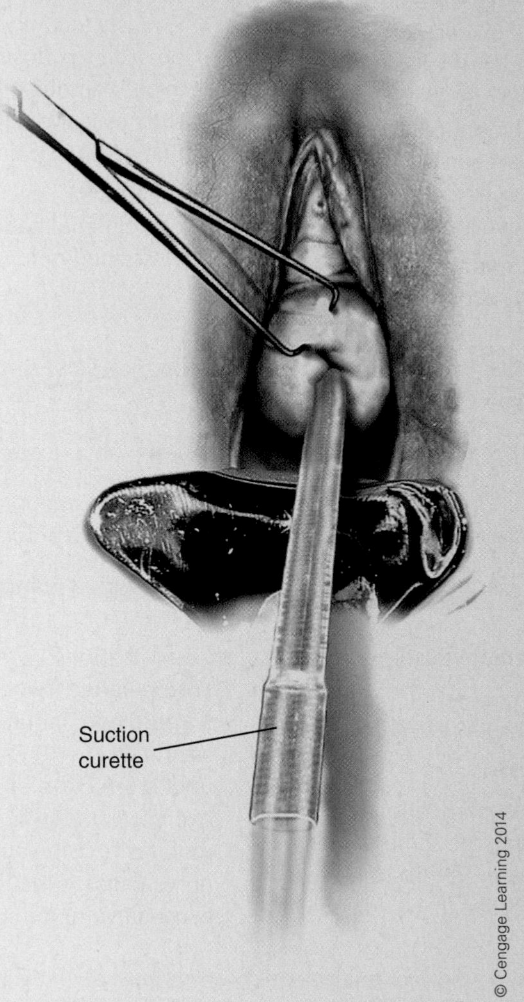

Suction curette

Figure 15-18 Vacuum aspiration of the uterus, suction curette in place

Preoperative Diagnostic Tests and Procedures	• Diagnosis obtained by history and physical as well as by direct examination. • Lab studies such as a pregnancy test or hemoglobin and hematocrit prn.
Equipment, Instruments and Supplies Unique to Procedure	• Vaginal instrument set • D&C instrument set • Telfa for specimen collection • Marking pen • Water-soluble lubricant
Preoperative Preparation	• Position: Lithotomy • Anesthesia: General preferred, but the procedure may also be performed under regional block • Patient skin prep: Vaginal • Draping: Lithotomy draping
Practical Considerations	• A preoperative sonography may be performed.

PROCEDURE 15-11 (continued)

Surgical Procedure

1. A pelvic exam is performed to determine the size, shape, and position of the uterus and to detect any masses.

   Procedural Consideration: Set up vaginal exam tray as separate tray. Reglove surgeon after examination.

2. An Auvard weighted speculum is placed in the posterior vagina and tucked under the external os of the cervix.

   Procedural Consideration: A sterile glove may be placed over the round weighted section of the speculum to catch any blood or tissue.

3. The cervix is grasped in the 12-o'clock position with a single-toothed tenaculum, and a uterine sound is placed into the external os (Figure 15-19A).

   Procedural Consideration: The surgical technologist may hold the tenaculum. Care is taken not to tear the cervix.

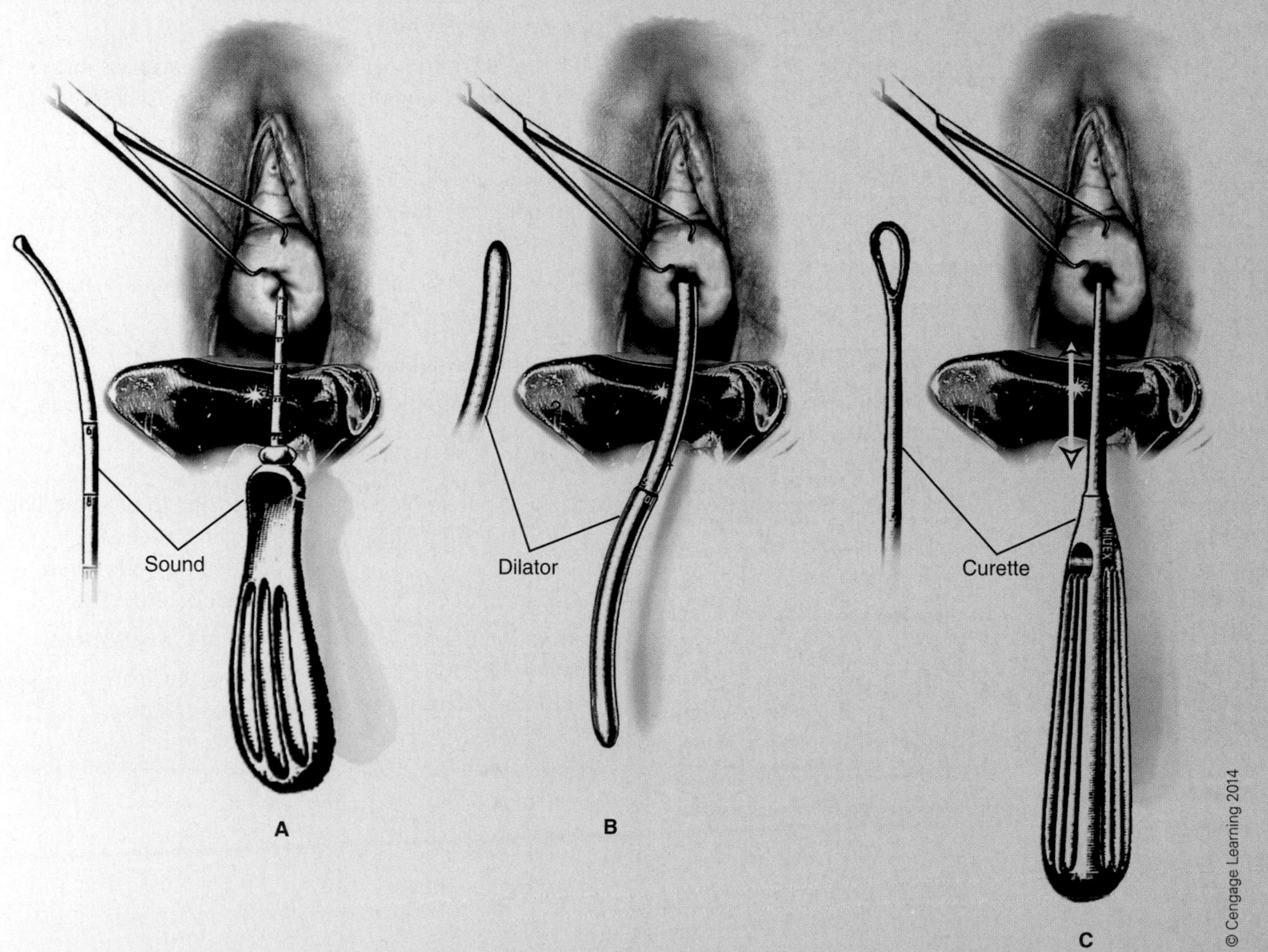

Figure 15-19 Dilation and curettage (D&C): (A) Tenaculum placement and sounding, (B) dilation of cervix, (C) curettage of uterus

(continues)

Procedure 15-11 (continued)

4. The sound is advanced through the internal os and to the fundus to determine the depth of the uterus, noted by the calibrations on the sound. After uterine depth is determined, the sound is withdrawn.

   Procedural Consideration: A piece of Telfa may be placed on the blade of the speculum to catch tissue specimens.

5. If an endocervical specimen is to be taken, a sharp narrow curette is placed into the external os and the cervical mucosa is scraped and extracted onto the Telfa.

   Procedural Consideration: Remove the Telfa and place the specimen in a predetermined container on the back table.

6. The cervix is dilated with a progressive series of dilators (Figure 15-19B).

   Procedural Consideration: Align dilators on the back table so sizes are sequential and progressive. A small amount of lubricant should be placed on each dilator before use. Provide a second Telfa for intrauterine (endometrial) specimen.

7. Randall forceps may be placed and the uterus explored for any polyps, fibroids, or remnants of pregnancy that may require removal.

   Procedural Consideration: The surgical technologist may be unable to pass instruments while providing exposure. Place instruments to allow surgeon to help him- or herself.

8. Curette of choice is advanced into the uterus and the endometrium is scraped in the same manner as the cervix; the tissue extracted onto the Telfa is handed off as endometrial specimen (Figure 15-19C).

   Procedural Consideration: Examination with Randall forceps and curettage may be repeated several times.

9. The instruments are withdrawn and the weighted speculum is removed.

   Procedural Consideration: The operative area is cleansed. A perineal pad dressing is applied.

Postoperative Considerations

Immediate Postoperative Care

- Transport to PACU.

Prognosis

- No complications: Return to normal activities; pelvic bleeding and/or cramping may occur.
- Complications: Perforation of uterus; laceration of the cervix; tear of the internal os; damage to other perlvic organs; excessive bleeding (monitored); postoperative SSI.

Wound Classification

- Class II: Clean-contaminated

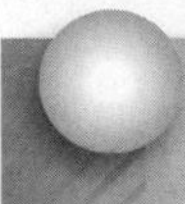

Pearl of Wisdom

Specimens may need special identification relative to location within the uterus. Have extra Telfa and specimen containers in the room. Keep a sterile marker on the back table to assist with identification. Multiple specimens require careful communication between the surgical technologist and the circulator.

A cervical biopsy is usually an office procedure that involves the use of a D&C instrument set including a Tischler biopsy forceps (Figure 15-20). The primary difference between a D&C procedure and cervical biopsy is the cervix is not dilated and curettaged. Additionally a solution such as acetic acid or Lugol's solution is used to identify the abnormal tissue or lesion. Using a cotton-tip swab the acetic acid is applied to the outer portion of the cervix to stain the abnormal tissue white. Schiller's test uses the brown-colored Lugol's solution that is a mixture of iodine and potassium iodide. When applied to the cervical tissue the tissue that remains brown in color is normal and the tissue that did not take up the stain and does not stain is the abnormal tissue. The surgeon can then identify the tissue in which to remove small pieces of abnormal cervical tissue to be sent to pathology.

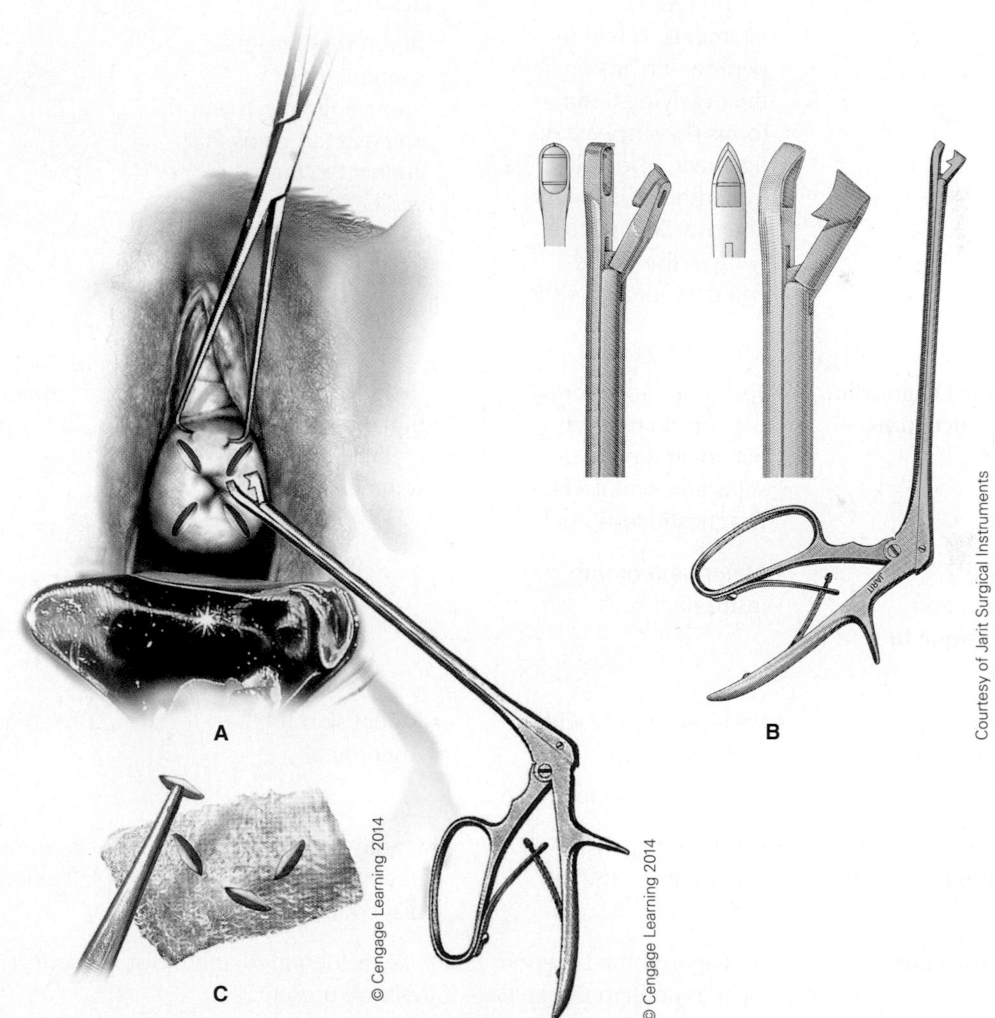

Figure 15-20 Cervical biopsy: (A) Punch biopsy, (B) Tischler biopsy forceps, (C) tissue specimen

Ovarian, Fallopian Tubes and Uterine Surgical Procedures

Procedure 15-12 Oophorectomy

Surgical Anatomy and Pathology	• The ovaries are almond-shaped structures that lie on either side of the uterus in the ovarian fossa of the lateral pelvic wall (Figure 15-8). • The ovaries are supported by ligaments. A fold of peritoneum arising near the overlying fimbria forms the suspensory ligament, also called the infundibular ligament. The ovarian ligament, lying in the broad ligament, provides the main support to the ovary. • Prior to puberty the ovaries exhibit a smooth surface, but thereafter show scarring from multiple ovulatory activities. • Blood supply is the ovarian arteries branching from the aorta and ovarian veins that connect to the inferior vena cava. • Indications for oophorectomy are ovarian malignancy, cystic disease, strangulated ovaries, infection, adhesions, and endometriosis.
Preoperative Diagnostic Tests and Procedures	• Tests and procedures depend on presenting history and physical, and signs and symptoms. Diagnostic tests could include sonography, bimanual examination, erythrocyte sedimentation rate, serum CA 125 titre, and laparoscopy.
Equipment, Instruments, and Supplies Unique to Procedure	• Major laparotomy instrument set
Preoperative Preparation	• Position: Supine with Trendelenburg • Anesthesia: General • Patient skin prep: Abdominal • Draping: Laparotomy
Practical Considerations	• Confirm diagnostic studies are in the OR. • If both ovaries are removed, they should be placed in separate specimen containers and labeled right and left.
Surgical Procedure	1. Laparotomy is performed. Ovary is identified and moist lap sponges placed around it to contain any spillage if cysts are present. 2. Using Metzenbaum scissors, tissue forceps and curved clamp, a window is created in the peritoneum of the suspensory ligament. 3. Two curved clamps are placed across the suspensory ligament and divided with scissors or electrosurgery and ligated. This is performed several times to free up the ovary. **Procedural Consideration:** When close to the ovary, the ovarian ligament is included with the suspensory ligament to free up and remove the ovary. 4. The same procedure is performed on the opposite ovary if being removed. 5. Laparotomy closure.

Procedure 15-12 (continued)

Postoperative Considerations	**Immediate Postoperative Care** • Transport to PACU. **Prognosis** • No complications: Patient discharged next day; return to normal activities in 6–8 weeks; if both ovaries removed, patient must begin hormone therapy. • Complications: Postoperative SSI; hemorrhage; peritoneal cavity sepsis due to spillage from cyst. **Wound Classification** • Class I: Clean

Procedure 15-13 Total Salpingectomy

Surgical Anatomy and Pathology	• See previous procedures for anatomy. • Performed for occlusive disease, ectopic pregnancy, acute and chronic infections, benign or malignant tumors.
Preoperative diagnostic tests and procedures; equipment, instruments, supplies; preoperative preparation; practical considerations; and postoperative considerations are the same as for Procedure 15-12.	
Surgical Procedure	1. Laparotomy is performed.
	2. Window is created in the mesosalpinx of the broad ligament between the fallopian tube and round ligament.
	3. The tube is then separated along the entire length of its broad ligament attachment by double clamping, dividing, and ligating. **Procedural Consideration:** The division of the ligament proceeds toward the uterus then the ovary until the tube is completely free.
	4. An incision is required into the myometrium of the uterus to include the cornu to facilitate removal of the tube; the incision is closed with a 0 suture using a figure-of-eight suture technique.
	5. The same procedure is performed on the opposite tube if both are being removed.
	6. The mesosalpinx is closed with interrupted 0 absorbable sutures.

Procedure 15-14 Endometrial Ablation

Surgical Anatomy and Pathology

- See previous procedures for anatomy.
- Performed as an alternative to hysterectomy to treat chronic menorrhagia.

Preoperative Diagnostic Tests and Procedures

- History and physical
- Sonography

Equipment, Instruments, and Supplies Unique to Procedure

- Depending on surgeon's preference for performing the procedure one of the following will be needed:
  - Nd:YAG, KTP, argon or diode laser; resectoscope; or balloon catheter
- Hysteroscope and equipment
- D_5W solution for balloon endometrial ablation
- Distention medium if performing hysteroscopy
- D&C instrument set if performing balloon endometrial ablation

Preoperative Preparation

- Position: Lithotomy
- Anesthesia: General
- Patient skin prep: Vaginal prep
- Draping: Lithotomy draping

Practical Considerations

- When performing a laser endometrial ablation, air or gas is not used to cool the laser fiber due to the increased risk of causing an air or gas embolism.
- If a hysteroscope is used Hyskon should not be used as the distention fluid or irrigant due to the systemic effects it can cause if absorbed through the capillaries.
- Balloon endometrial ablation does not require the use of hysteroscope.

Surgical Procedure

Due to the common use of three types of endometrial ablation procedures, the following is presented in a dialogue fashion to facilitate providing the information.

Laser Endometrial Ablation: The laser destroys the endometrial lining of the uterus, causing scarring upon healing. The two techniques used are blanching and dragging. Blanching involves holding the tip of the laser fiber at a short distance from the endometrium. The dragging technique involves direct contact of the laser fiber tip with the endometrium. The endometrium is ablated from the uterine fundus to approximately 2–4 cm above the external os.

Resectoscope: A specially designed urologic resectoscope is used as an electrosurgery device that has a rollerball electrode to resect or coagulate the endometrium. Due to the more extreme destruction of the endometrium as compared to laser treatment, the resectoscope treatment should not be used on the patient who is planning on becoming pregnant. Hyskon is usually used at the distending medium since it does not contain electrolytes.

Balloon Endometrial Ablation: The surgeon will perform a D&C to facilitate the balloon making full contact with the endometrium. The cervix is dilated 5–10 mm and the balloon catheter is inserted within the uterine cavity until the superior portion of the balloon is against the fundus. The balloon is inflated with D_5W solution, which is heated to approximately 86° C. The balloon is kept in position with the heated solution for about 10 minutes and then removed.

Postoperative Considerations

Immediate Postoperative Care

- Transport to PACU.

Prognosis

- No complications: Discharged same day of surgery; return to normal activities in 2–4 weeks.
- Complications: Postoperative SSI; uterine, bowel, and bladder injury or perforation; cervical injury; fallopian tube injury; hemorrhage; complications associated with use of distention medium.

Wound Classification

- Class II: Clean contaminated

Procedure 15-15 Myomectomy (Abdominal Approach)

Surgical Anatomy and Pathology	• See previous procedures for anatomy. • Myomectomy is the excision of uterine fibroids called myomas, but has a higher rate of morbidity and bleeding than hysterectomy.	• Pathological conditions for performing a myomectomy include: • Anemia secondary to uterine bleeding • Chronic, severe pelvic pain • Chronic secondary dysmenorrhea	• Fibroid(s) preventing evaluation of internal organs • Chronic UTIs secondary to fibroid(s) • Continued growth and/or rapid increase in size of fibroid(s) • Infertility
Preoperative Diagnostic Tests and Procedures	• Diagnosis obtained by history and physical as well as by direct examination	• Abdominal/vaginal ultrasound to locate the lesions • IVP	• CT scan • MRI • Hysterosalpingography
Equipment, Instruments, and Supplies Unique to Procedure	• Major laparotomy or hysterectomy instrument sets		
Preoperative Preparation	• Position: Supine • Anesthesia: General, spinal or epidural	• Patient skin prep: Abdominal	• Draping: Laparotomy drape
Practical Considerations	• Follow adhesion prevention procedures (see Pearl of Wisdom page 566) • Gonadotropin-releasing hormone (GnRH) may be prescribed for a 3-month period in an effort to	reduce the size of the tumors. • Myomectomy is performed when preservation of the uterus is necessary. • Myomectomy can be performed through	pelviscopy or laparoscopy, and via abdominal and vaginal approaches. Fibroid resection is usually performed through an abdominal approach.

Surgical Procedure

1. Incision may be of the Pfannenstiel or vertical midline type.

   Procedural Consideration: Adapt initial routine to incision of choice.

2. The abdominal cavity is explored. A self-retaining retractor is placed. The bowel is packed cephalad with moist sponges.

   Procedural Consideration: Balfour and O'Sullivan-O'Connor retractors are commonly used. Warm, moist sponges to pack bowel. *Note:* The best practice is to count sponges as they are placed and have circulator record the number.

3. A vertical incision into the anterior surface of the uterus is made over the **myoma**.

   Procedural Consideration: There may be several incisions depending on the number of myomas.

4. The general strategy in myomectomy is to incise the pseudocapsule of the fibroid, expose the tissue planes (controlling the edges of the capsule with Allis clamps), and use blunt dissection, scissors, electrosurgical pencil, or laser to peel the myoma from the capsule (Figure 15-21A).

   Procedural Consideration: Prepare for the specific approach to be used in advance. Use of the laser will require laser safety procedures to be in place.

(continues)

Procedure 15-15 (continued)

5. Once dissected free, the myoma is removed (Figure 15-21B).

   Procedural Consideration: Uterine bleeding is controlled with clamps and suture ligatures.

6. The uterine incision is closed with 0 or 2-0 synthetic absorbable suture (Figure 15-21C).

   Procedural Consideration: Use of several sutures may be required. Count at closure of hollow organ.

7. The abdomen is closed in the usual manner.

   Procedural Consideration: Usual closure routine. Dextran may be instilled. Counts as needed.

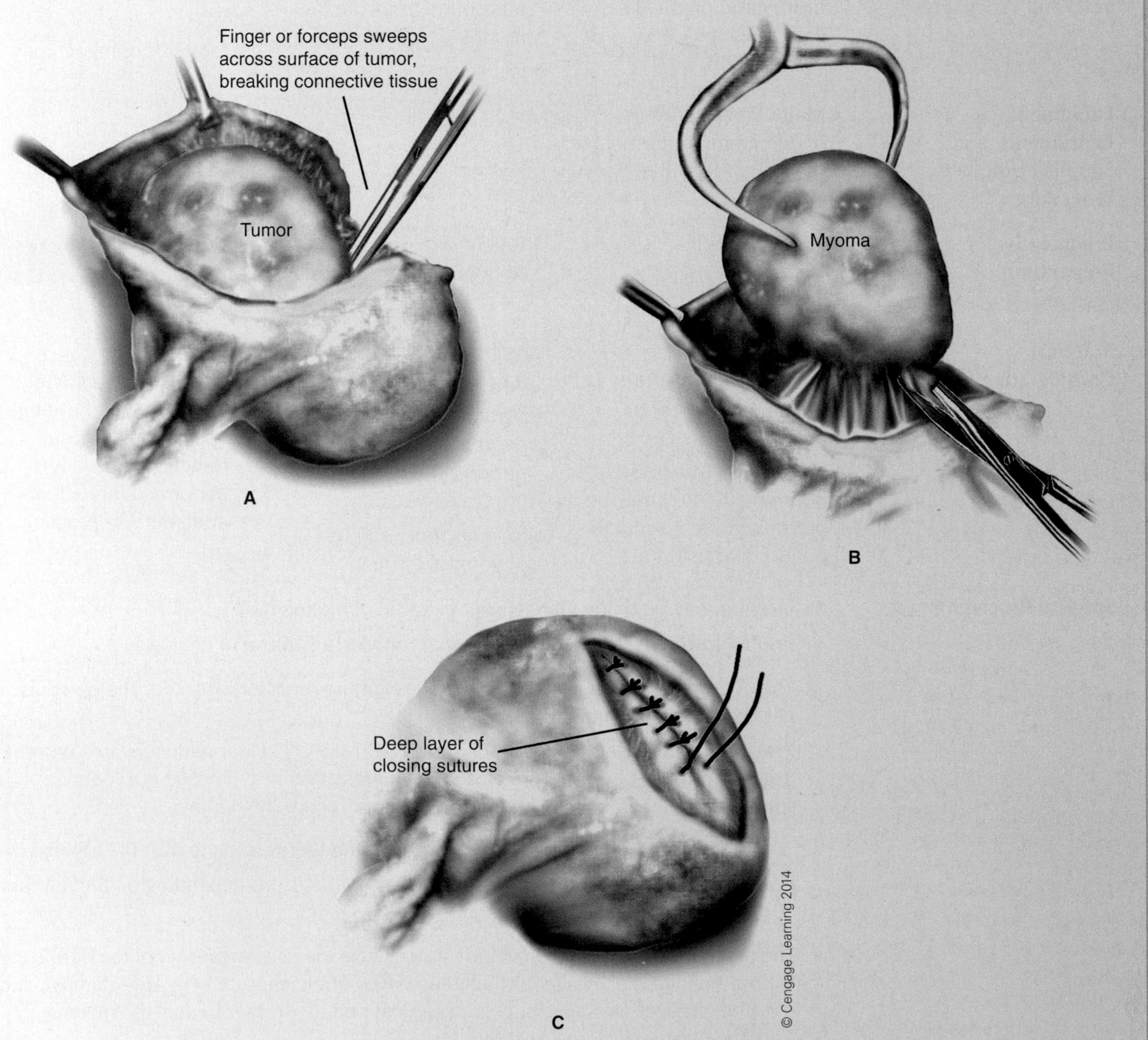

Figure 15-21 Myomectomy: (A) Longitudinal incision over myoma with blunt dissection, (B) excision of myoma, (C) uterine closure

Procedure 15-15 (continued)

Postoperative Considerations	**Immediate Postoperative Care** • Transport to PACU. **Prognosis** • No complications: Discharged from health care facility 1–2 days; return to normal activities in 6–8 weeks. • Complications: Bowel obstruction or damage; bladder injury; fallopian tube or ureter compromise; wound infection or dehiscence; approximately 20–25% of patients undergoing myomectomy will require additional pelvic surgery; infertility secondary to the procedure. **Wound Classification** • Wound Class II: Clean-contaminated

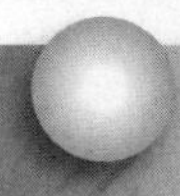

Pearl of Wisdom

The biggest problem following myomectomy is adhesion formation. This can be reduced with gentle tissue handling, removal of talc from the operators' gloves, avoiding the posterior peritoneal surface of the uterus, incorporating various uterine suspension techniques, and performing copious intraoperative irrigation with heparinized Ringer's lactate. Instillation of 100–200 mL of 10% dextran 70 can be used to provide a slippery surfactant between the organs, but is not common. Promethazine and corticosteroids, as well as intravenous Decadron (20 mg) and intramuscular Phenergan (25 mg) given every 4 hours for 48 hours, are also utilized to prevent adhesion formation postoperatively.

Procedure 15-16 Total Abdominal Hysterectomy (TAH)

Surgical Anatomy and Pathology	• A hysterectomy is the removal of the uterus and may be performed to treat many conditions that affect the uterus, such as cancer, chronic pelvic pain, abnormal uterine bleeding, uterine fibroids, endometriosis, and pelvic support problems (example: uterine prolapsed).
Preoperative Diagnostic Tests and Procedures	• Diagnosis obtained by history and physical as well as by direct examination.
Equipment, Instruments, and Supplies Unique to Procedure	• Laparotomy or hysterectomy instrument sets including self-retaining retractors and preferred hysterectomy clamps (e.g., Heaney and Heaney-Ballantine clamps) • Urinary catheter • Drain of surgeon's preference
Preoperative Preparation	• Position: Supine • Anesthesia: General • Patient skin prep: Abdominal • Draping: Laparotomy draping procedure

(continues)

Procedure 15-16 (continued)

Surgical Procedure

1. Following transverse Pfannenstiel or vertical incision into the abdominal cavity, the abdomen is thoroughly explored for any unsuspected pathology, and the uterus and adnexa are assessed (Plate 15-1).

   Procedural Consideration: Adjust according to incision selected by the surgeon.

2. A self-retaining retractor is placed and the bowel is packed cephalad with moist lap sponges.

   Procedural Consideration: Balfour, O'Sullivan-O'Connor, and Bookwalter are commonly used. Have full selection of blades available for Bookwalter. Warm, moist laps will be needed. Count lap sponges as they are placed and communicate total to circulator.

3. A tenaculum may be placed into the fundus of the uterus to facilitate control of the organ (Plates 15-2 and 15-3) (Figure 15-22A).

   Procedural Consideration: Most commonly, a multitoothed tenaculum is used to manipulate the uterus.

4. Ligament clamps are placed across the round and ovarian ligaments.

   Procedural Consideration: Some of these clamps, after division of the ligament, will be left in place to aid with elevation and deviation of the uterus during its excision.

5. The round ligaments are now divided electrosurgically or are suture ligated and cut, developing anterior and posterior "leaves" of the broad ligament (Figure 15-22B).

   Procedural Consideration: Sutures are immediately placed in area of dissection. Dissection may be sharp, blunt, or combined.

6. These are incised with Metzenbaum scissors, separating the peritoneum of the bladder from the lower uterus, and opening the retroperitoneum to expose the underlying iliac vessels and the ureters. These structures are properly identified and protected at all times for the remainder of the procedure (Plates 15-4).

   Procedural Consideration: Hysterectomies are methodical, and the same steps must be repeated bilaterally. The surgical technologist should have an adequate supply of clamps and sutures throughout the procedure.

7. The bladder is bluntly dissected from the lower uterus and cervix along an avascular plane (Plates 15-5 and 15-6).

   Procedural Consideration: Often blunt dissection may require a "sponge on a stick."

8. The peritoneal opening is enlarged to expose the ovarian suspensory ligament and uterine artery (Figure 15-22C). A curved Ballantine or Heaney clamp is placed medial to the ovary and the suspensory ligament is double ligated and divided (Figure 15-22D) (Plate 15-7).

   Procedural Consideration: Classically, a hysterectomy procedure uses the "clamp, clamp, cut, tie" method. However, the tie is usually a "stick tie," a suture with a needle on a needle holder. Heaney needle holders are often used. The jaws are curved, and the needle is loaded with the point projecting behind the convex surface. Surgeon may use electrosurgery or harmonic scalpel to divide ligaments."

9. The uterus in now retracted cephalad and deviated to one side, stretching the lower ligaments and facilitating exposure of the uterine vessels, which are then cross-clamped at the junction of the uterus and cervix, cut, and ligated (Plate 15-8).

   Procedural Consideration: Depending on the patient's pelvic anatomy, more caudal portions of the procedure may require extra-long instruments.

PROCEDURE 15-16 (continued)

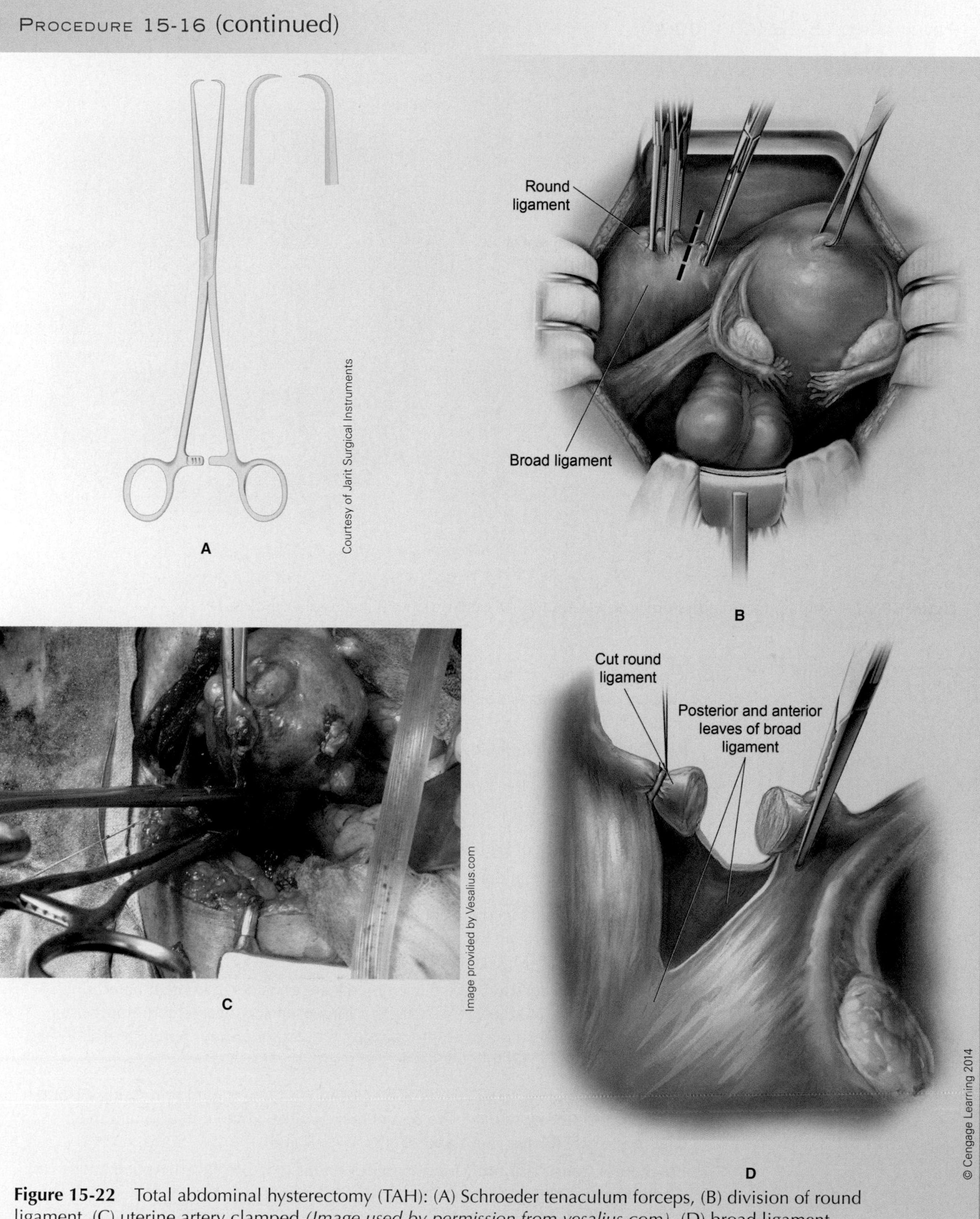

Figure 15-22 Total abdominal hysterectomy (TAH): (A) Schroeder tenaculum forceps, (B) division of round ligament, (C) uterine artery clamped *(Image used by permission from vesalius.com)*, (D) broad ligament—posterior and anterior leaves

(*continues*)

Procedure 15-16 (continued)

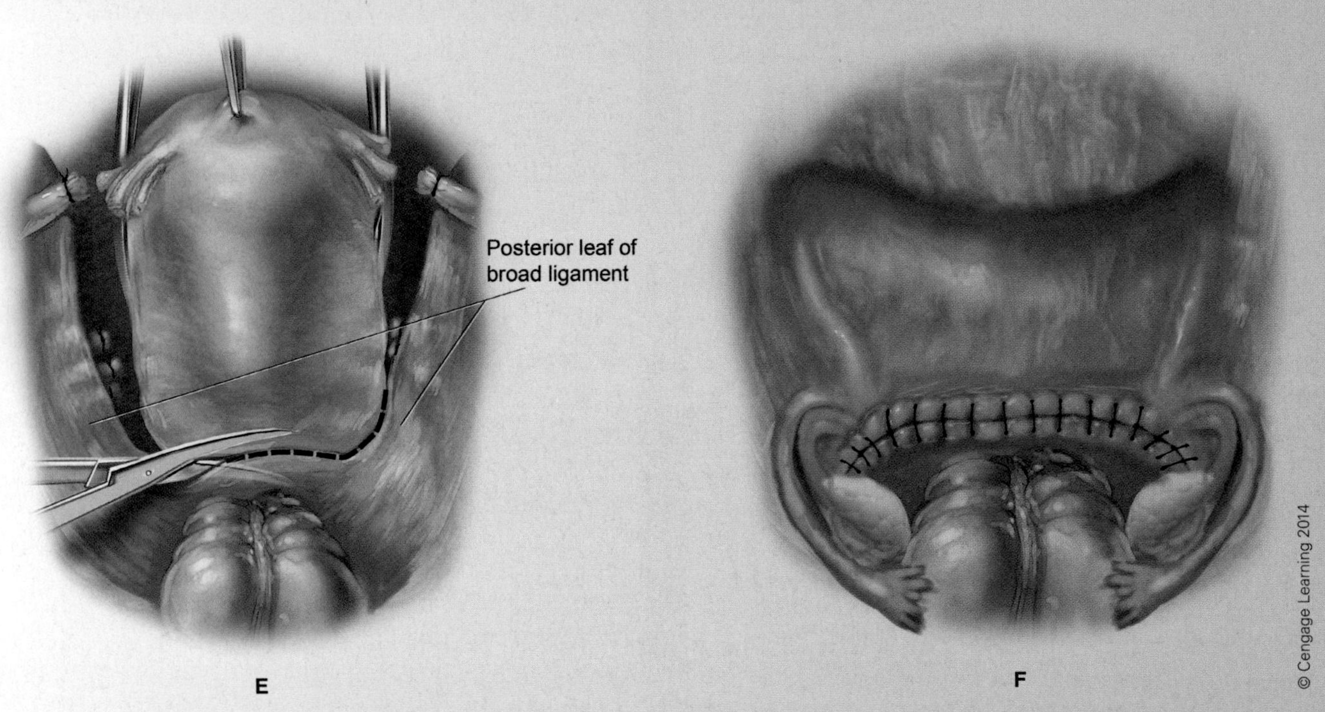

Figure 15-22 Total abdominal hysterectomy (TAH): (E) Dissection line, (F) vaginal cuff closure

10. Keeping the uterus retracted cephalad, the surgeon will use the #3 knife handle and Metzenbaum scissors to dissect the paracervical fascia to mobilize and preserve the uretus (Plate 15-9).

    Procedural Consideration: Long instruments are usually required.

11. The rectum can now be mobilized from the posterior cervix and reflected inferiorly, out of the way.

12. The cardinal ligament is clamped, divided, and ligated on both sides (Plate 15-10).

    Procedural Consideration: Follow clamp, clamp, cut, tie routine.

13. The uterus is again placed in cephalad traction and curved clamps are placed bilaterally, incorporating the uterosacral ligaments. The uterus is freed and removed (Plates 15-11 to 15-13; Figure 15-22E).

    Procedural Consideration: These instruments are considered contaminated since they may project into the vagina. Mayo or Jorgensen scissors are commonly used. Bring up a specimen container after passing the scissors. They should be isolated or removed from the field following use.

14. The resulting vaginal "cuff" can now be closed with interrupted or running #1 or 0 absorbable suture or stapled. The peritoneum is closed over it in a similar manner (Figure 15-22F) (Plates 15-14 and 15-15).

    Procedural Consideration: Various types of drains may be placed. Anticipate use of warm irrigation fluid. Prepare suture.

PROCEDURE 15-16 (continued)

15. The abdomen is thoroughly irrigated and drained and checked for hemostasis. The ureters are reassessed for position and integrity and to ensure they are not dilated. (If left behind, the ovaries may be sutured to the lateral pelvic walls.)

    Procedural Consideration: Usual closure routine. Counts as needed.

16. The abdomen is closed in the usual manner.

Postoperative Considerations

Immediate Postoperative Care

- Transport to PACU.

Prognosis

- No complications: Discharged from health care facility in 2–3 days; return to normal activities in 6–8 weeks.
- Complications: Bowel obstruction or damage; bladder injury; postoperative SSI; dehiscence; ureteral injuries; hemorrhage.

Wound Classification

- Class II: Clean-contaminated

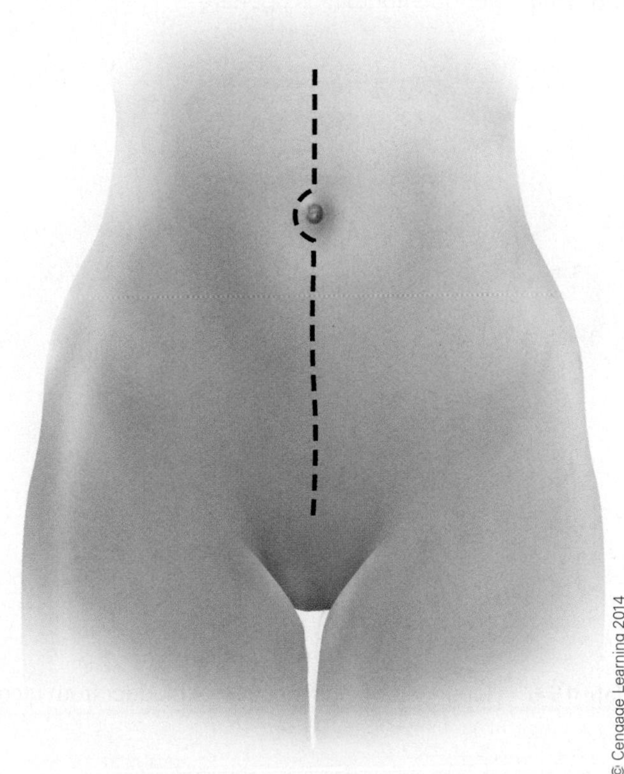

Plate 15-1 Midline incision is made

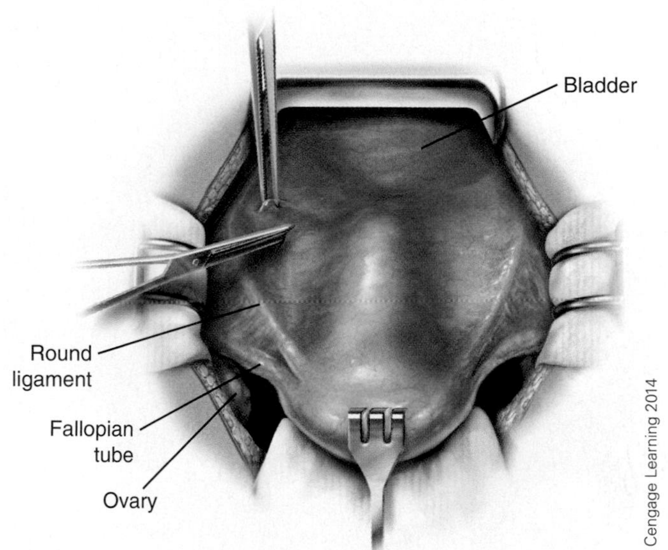

Plate 15-2 Tenaculum is placed and cut is made in broad ligament

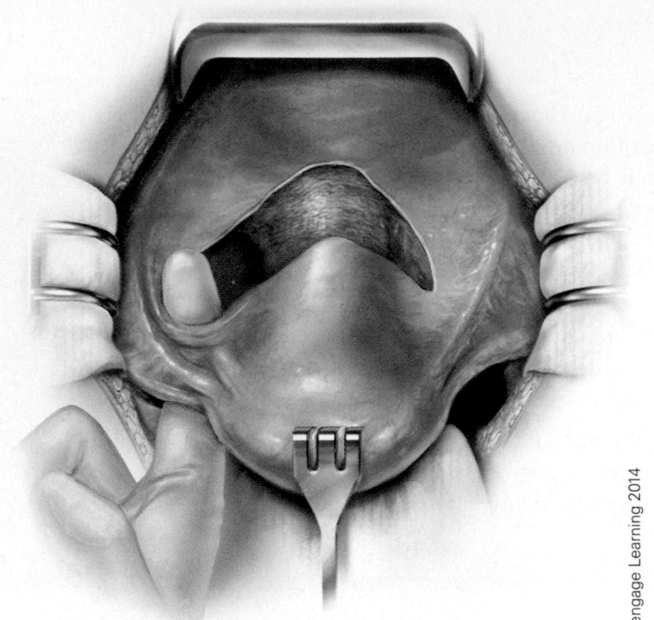

Plate 15-3 Incision in broad ligament is lengthened

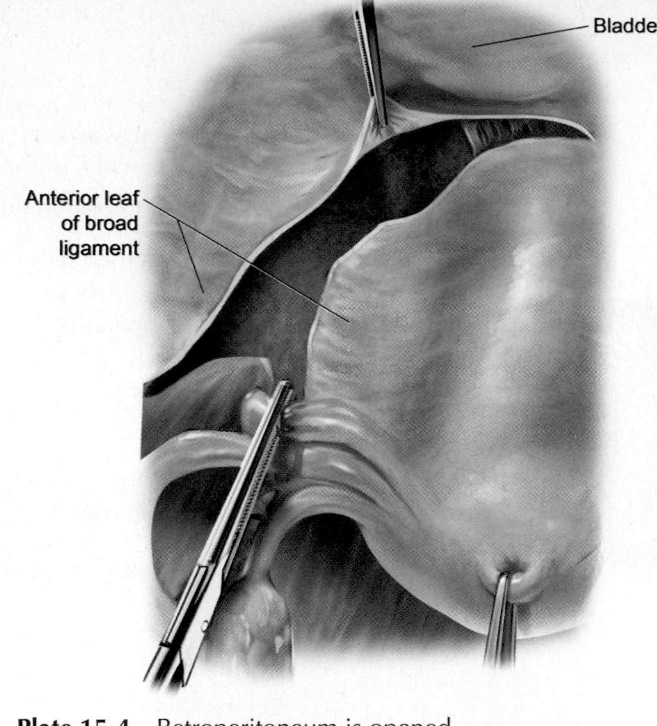

Plate 15-4 Retroperitoneum is opened

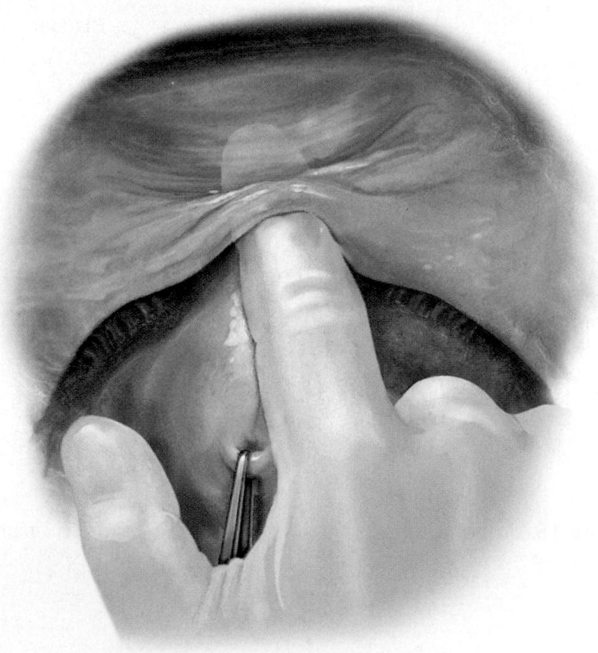

Plate 15-5 Blunt dissection of bladder from uterus

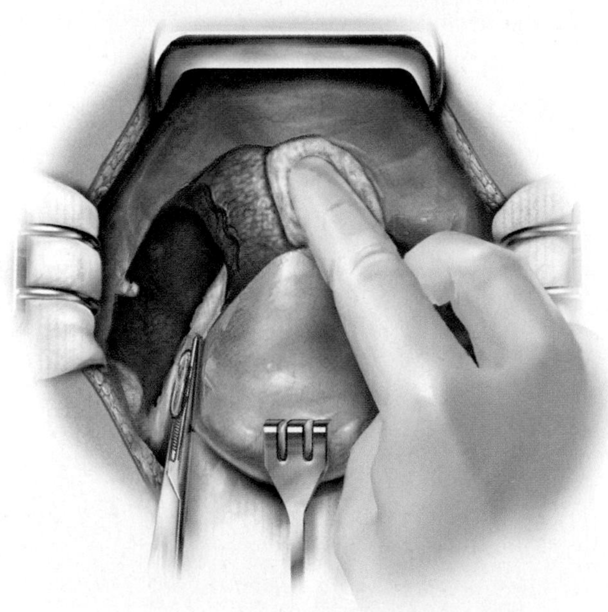

Plate 15-6 Continued blunt dissection of bladder from uterus

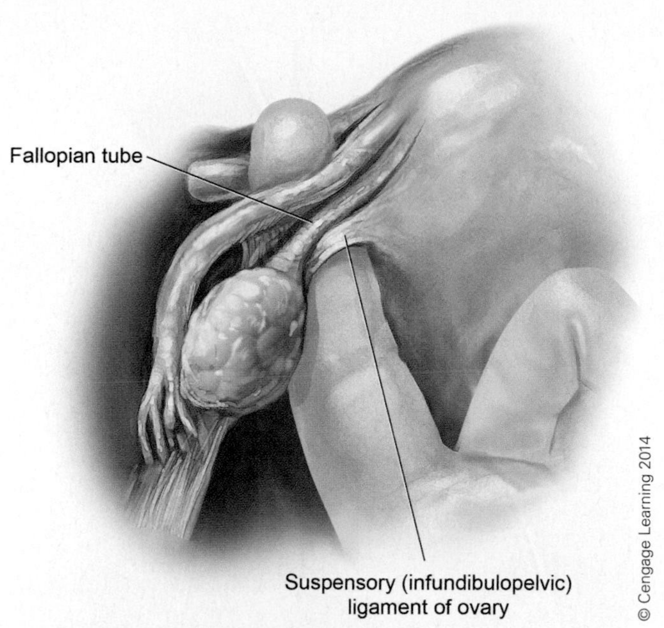

Plate 15-7 Suspensory ligament is identifed

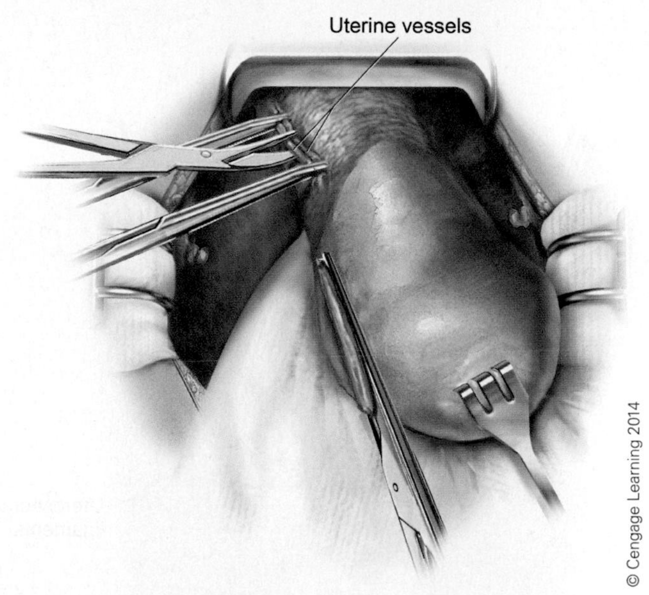

Plate 15-8 Uterine vessels are exposed, clamped, and cut

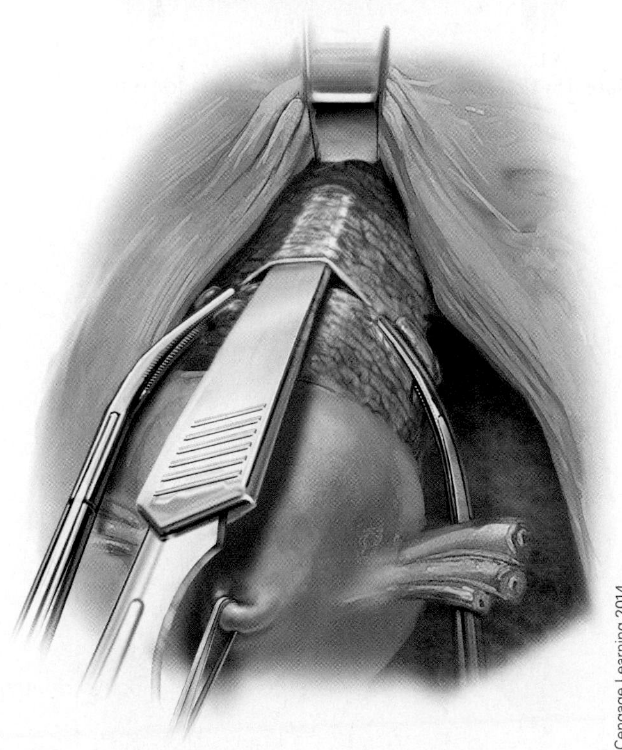

Plate 15-9 Paracervical fascia is dissected and mobilized

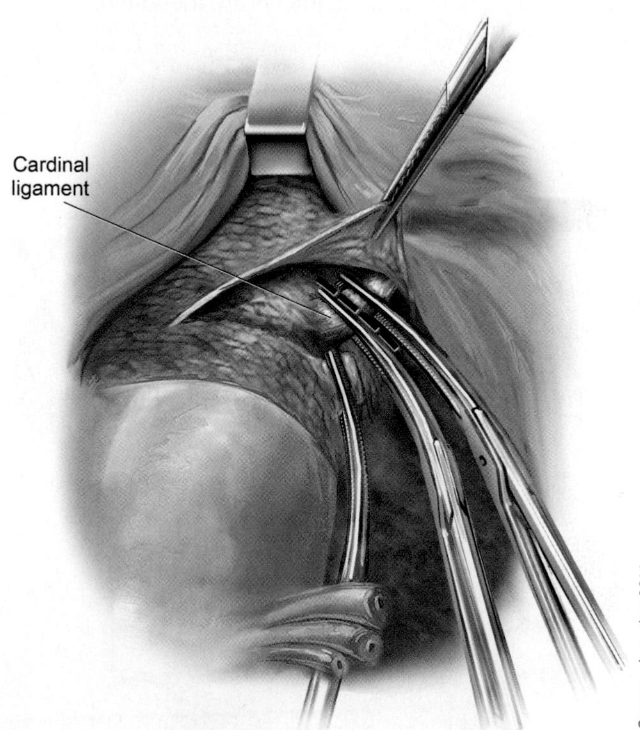

Plate 15-10 Cardinal ligament is identified, clamped, cut, and tied

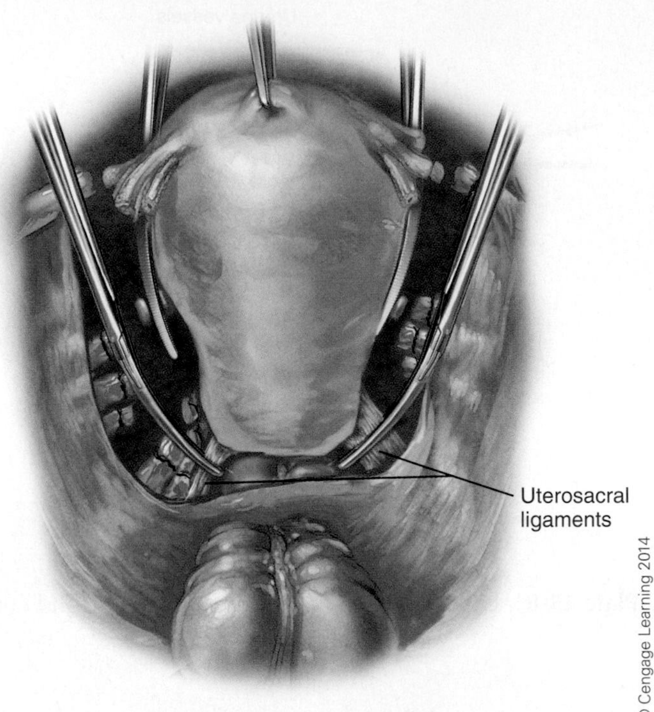

Plate 15-11 Uterosacral ligaments are identified, clamped, cut, and tied

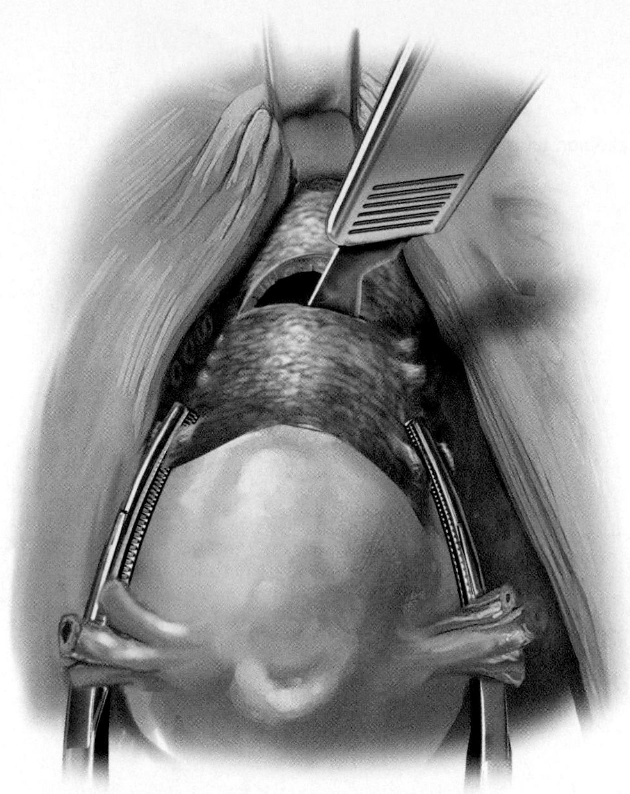

Plate 15-12 Uterus is cut in preparation for removal

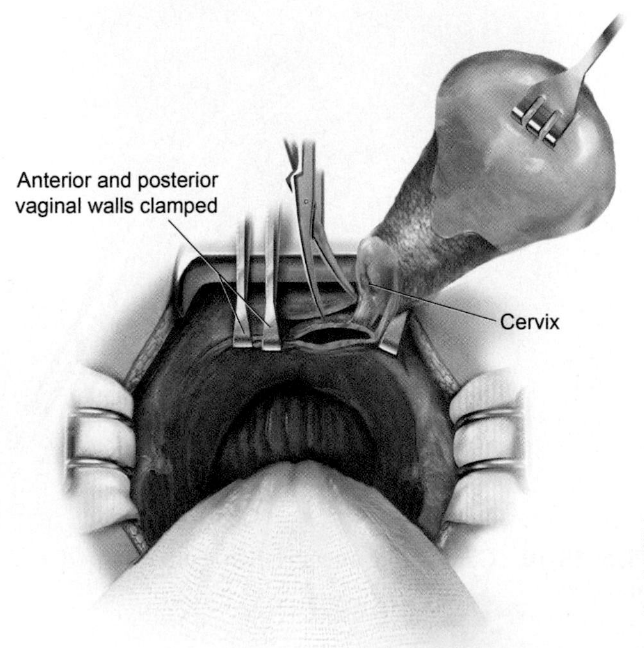

Plate 15-13 Last cut is made with Jorgenson scissors; uterus is removed

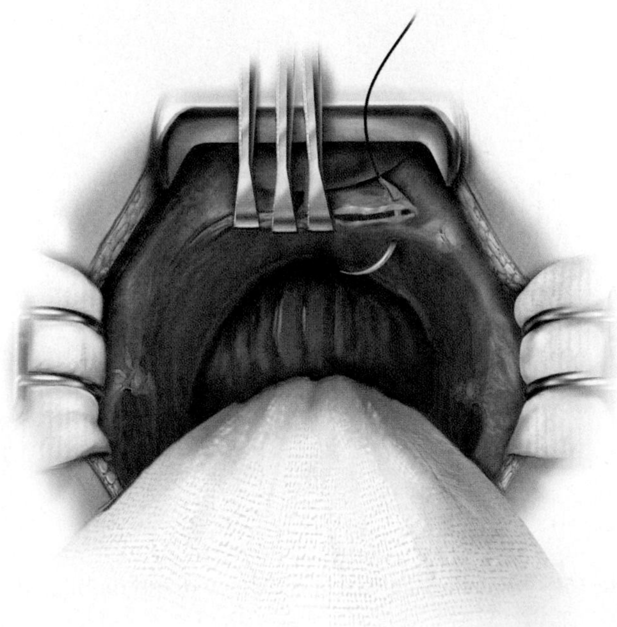

Plate 15-14 Vaginal cuff is closed

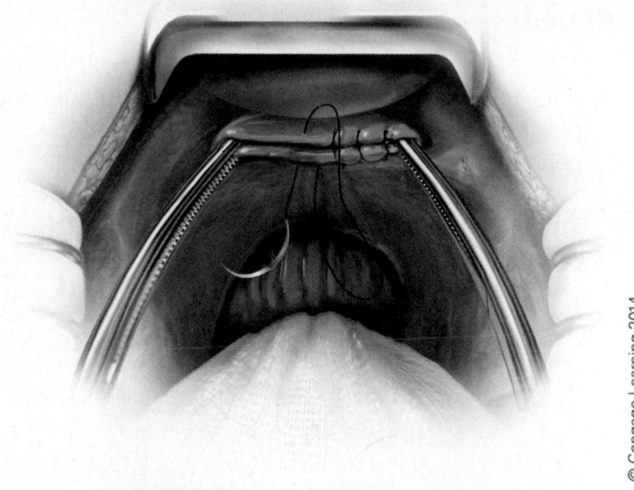

Plate 15-15 Vaginal cuff is closed

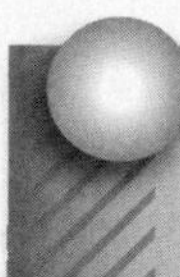

PEARL OF WISDOM

Some surgeons complete actions on one side of the uterus then move to the other side; some alternate sides as they move caudally. The surgical technologist must adjust to the pattern and be sure to have an adequate supply of hemostats.

The following hysterectomy procedures with the exception of LAVH will be presented in abbreviated fashion providing the steps of the procedures, as all other information (preoperative diagnostic tests, preoperative preparation, and postoperative considerations) is similar.

PROCEDURE 15-17 Vaginal Hysterectomy

The procedure involves the same structures as the abdominal hysterectomy. The most significant difference is that the structures are encountered in the reverse order.

1. The patient is placed in lithotomy position.
2. An Auvard weighted speculum is placed with the blade along the posterior wall of the vagina.
3. Two Heaney right-angle retractors or Deavers are inserted to retract each lateral wall of the vagina.

(*continues*)

PROCEDURE 15-17 (continued)

4. A tenaculum or Lahey vulsellum is placed through the edge of the cervix to permit placing traction and moving the organ (Figure 15-23). At this time the surgeon may perform a D&C.

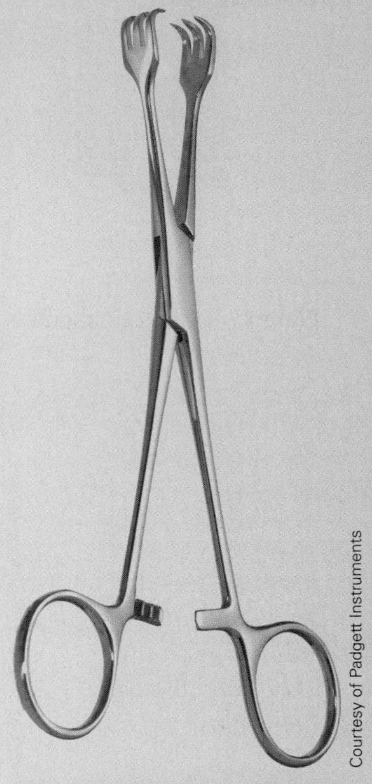

Figure 15-23 Vaginal hysterectomy: Lahey vulsellum forceps

5. Using a #15 knife blade on a #7 knife handle, the vaginal wall is incised anteriorly around the cervix. Using blunt dissection (index and middle finger with 4 × 4 sponge covering the ends of the fingers), the bladder is freed from the anterior surface of the cervix. A Deaver is placed anteriorly to elevate the bladder to protect it and allow visualization of the peritoneum of the anterior cul-de-sac. Using the #15 knife blade, an opening is made in the cul-de-sac to permit entry.
6. The peritoneum of the posterior cul-de-sac is identified and incised with the knife blade.
7. The uterosacral ligaments are doubly clamped with Heaney clamps, cut with Mayo scissors (may need to use long Mayo scissors), and ligated. The ends of the ligatures are not cut, but are left long, and each is tagged with a Crile clamp.
8. The uterus is manipulated posteriorly and the cardinal ligament on each side of the organ is doubly clamped with Heaney clamps, cut with Mayo scissors, and ligated. The same is done to the uterine arteries except the clamps will be a Kelly, Schnidt, or Pean.
9. The fundus is delivered into the vaginal canal with the use of the previously placed tenaculum or Jacob's vulsellum.

PROCEDURE 15-17 (continued)

10. If the ovaries are to be preserved, the round ligament, ovarian ligament, and fallopian tube on each side are doubly clamped with Heaney clamps and cut with Mayo scissors, and the uterine specimen is removed. The pedicles of the ligaments are then ligated.
11. The peritoneum between the rectum and vagina is approximated with a continuous absorbable suture.
12. The cul-de-sac is closed by placing sutures from the vaginal wall through the infundibulopelvic and round ligaments, and back out through the vaginal wall, and tied down on the vaginal portion of the vault.
13. The round, uterosacral, and cardinal ligaments are individually approximated and reattached to the angle of the vagina.
14. A Foley catheter is inserted, the vagina is packed, and a perineal pad is placed.

PROCEDURE 15-18 Laparoscopically Assisted Vaginal Hysterectomy (LAVH)

Use of the LAVH technique (Figure 15-24) has significant advantages: It allows potential abdominal hysterectomies to be converted to far less traumatic vaginal approaches, thereby shortening the patient's hospital stay considerably, while providing the visualization advantages of the abdominal procedure. The LAVH technique is more expensive than a traditional vaginal hysterectomy. Additionally, there is generally a longer operative time for the patient undergoing an LAVH versus the traditional vaginal hysterectomy. The surgical technologist should refer to the laparoscopy procedure in this chapter to review the initial steps of the LAVH.

Preoperative Diagnostic Tests and Procedures

- Diagnosis obtained by history and physical as well as by direct examination.

Equipment, Instruments, and Supplies Unique to Procedure

- Allen stirrups
- ESU
- SCD stockings and pump
- Video equipment
- Laparoscopic equipment
- Bipolar generator
- GYN laparoscopy instrument set
- Camera
- Laparotomy instrument set
- Abdominal hysterectomy set
- Suture, blades, and dressings per surgeon preference
- LAVH drapes and other supplies

(continues)

Procedure 15-18 (continued)

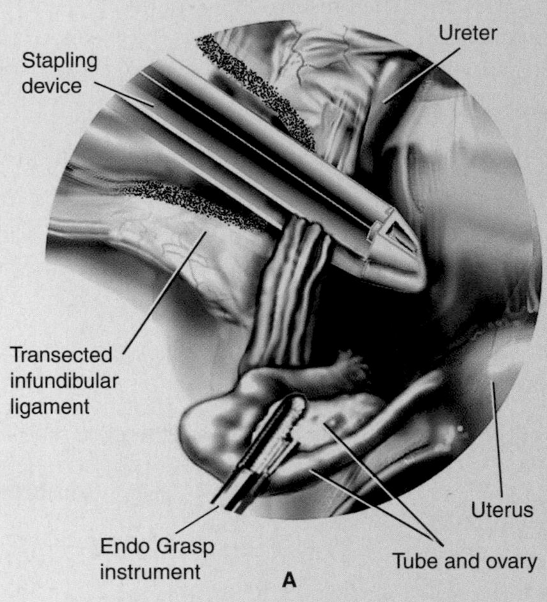

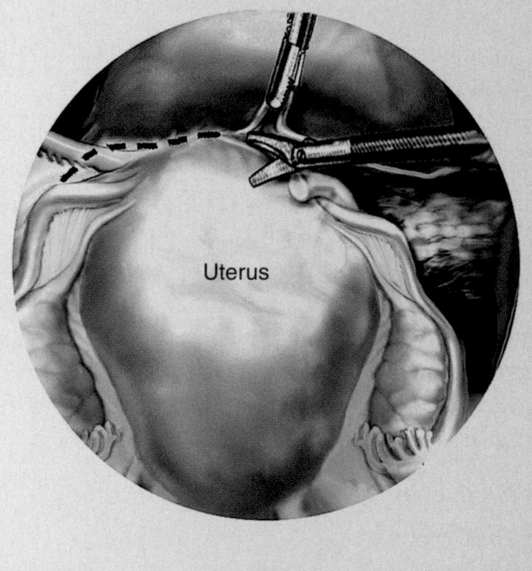

Figure 15-24 Laparoscopically assisted vaginal hysterectomy (LAVH): (A) Use of stapling device on ligament, (B) uterovesical line of dissection with endoscopic scissors

Preoperative Preparation	• Position: Low lithotomy with Trendelenburg • Anesthesia: General or spinal	• Patient prep: Abdominal and vaginal prep • Patient is catheterized • Draping: Drape sheet under the buttocks and	LAVH draping pack or supplies
Practical Considerations	• It is extremely important to check all equipment and supplies prior to the patient's arrival in the operating room.	• An examination under anesthesia is performed to assess the size and shape of the pelvis as well as the mobility and size of the uterus.	• 1% lidocaine with epinephrine may be injected in the vaginal mucosa to reduce bleeding.

PROCEDURE 15-18 (continued)

Surgical Procedure

1. Patient is placed in the low lithotomy position with Allen stirrups. Left arm may be tucked with right arm positioned on an armboard.
2. An intrauterine cannula is inserted transvaginally to assist with uterine manipulation. Pneumoperitoneum is established in routine fashion. This step may be performed prior to draping according to surgeon preference.
3. Trocars are placed in the lateral borders of the rectus muscles, inferior to the level of the umbilicus, and suprapubically (optional) in order to introduce laparoscopic instrumentation such as scissors, dissectors, and graspers.
4. The abdomen is explored.
5. The round ligaments are dissected from the pelvic wall with a stapler.
6. The infundibulopelvic ligament is dissected from the pelvic side wall if oophorectomy is being performed. The tubes and ovaries may be preserved or excised.
7. The dissection steps above may be performed using bipolar coagulation, the harmonic scalpel, ultrasound coagulation, or by placing sutures and using the extracorporal knotting technique.
8. The uterovesical fold is placed under tension by maneuvering the uterine manipulator or by direct tension.
9. The peritoneal bladder flap is dissected by using electrosurgical endoscopic scissors or by utilizing a hydrodissector.
10. Electrocircumcision of the cervix takes place and the vesicouterine space is opened.
11. The uterus is grasped and pulled in front of the vagina.

    Procedural Consideration: The surgical team now begins the cervical portion of the procedure and should not cross-contaminate by re-entering the abdomen unless gown and gloves are changed.
12. The pouch of Douglas peritoneum (rectouterine space) is opened.
13. The ureters are identified and the uterosacral and cardinal ligaments are transected.
14. The uterine vessels are tied and cut close to the uterine wall.
15. The uterus and adnexa are removed and the peritoneum and vagina are closed.
16. The trocars remain in situ during the vaginal portion of the procedure.
17. The abdomen is re-insufflated with CO_2 and the surgeon visualizes all pedicles and ensures complete hemostasis.

    Procedural Consideration: Prior to re-entering the abdomen the surgical team should change gown and gloves.
18. The pelvis is irrigated and suctioned and the pneumoperitoneum is released.
19. The trocar sites are closed with surgeon's preference of suture.

(*continues*)

PROCEDURE 15-18 (continued)

Postoperative Considerations

Immediate Postoperative Care

- Transport to PACU.
- Fluid maintenance.
- Pain relief.
- Liquid diet for 12–24 hours (nausea and slowing of gastro-intestinal activity is common in postoperative period)
- Drain bladder if spontaneous voiding does not occur.

Prognosis

- No complications: Return to normal activities after recovery period.
- Complications: Hemorrhage; failed LAVH and conversion of procedure to a laparotomy; injury to major blood vessels; bowel injury; ureteral injury; bladder injury; wound infection; hernia at trocar site; long-term complication of developing vesicovaginal or enterovaginal fistulas.

Wound Classification

- Class II: Clean-contaminated

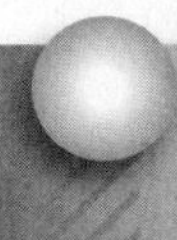

PEARL OF WISDOM

When using local anesthetics with epinephrine, be sure to state "with epinephrine" to the surgeon as you hand the medication. Be sure the anesthesia team knows that epinephrine is being given. Monitor the amount of local used.

PROCEDURE 15-19 Robot-Assisted Hysterectomy

General anesthesia is administered. The preoperative preparations are similar to those of laparoscopic surgical procedures. The surgical technologist should have the major laparotomy instrument set available in the OR in case of conversion to an open procedure.

Surgical Procedure

1. The surgeon inserts the uterine manipulator into the cervix and a vaginal balloon occluder into the vagina.
2. The initial steps of a laparoscopy are performed, including incisions at the umbilicus and other sites for the insertion of laparoscopic instrumentation.
3. The patient is placed in the Trendelenburg position.
4. The circulator positions the robotic cart with the robot arms between the legs of the patient without contaminating the sterile field.
5. The surgeon and surgical technologist position the instruments in the robotic arms and through the ports.
6. The surgeon sits at the robot console to operate the hand and foot controls. The peritoneum is opened using ESU.
7. The uterine artery and suspensory ligament are ligated with ties and divided.

PROCEDURE 15-19 (continued)

8. The broad, round, cardinal and uterosacral ligaments on both sides of the uterus are ligated and divided.
9. Using the uterine manipulator, the surgical technologist places traction on the uterus and the surgeon performs an anterior and posterior colpotomy.
10. The surgeon finishes the dissection to completely free up the uterus and cervix, which are placed in the vagina. The vaginal cuff is closed with interrupted sutures.
11. When the surgeon has completed vaginal cuff closure the specimen is removed from the vagina by the surgical technologist.
12. The surgical technologist removes the instruments from the ports and robotic arms, removes the trocars, and the circulator moves the robotic cart away from the patient.
13. The surgeon closes the fascia and Steri-Strips are used to close the skin incisions.

PROCEDURE 15-20 Uterine Radiation Seeding

Sealed radionuclide seeds are implanted temporarily or permanently to treat uterine cancer. They are useful for shrinking a tumor preoperatively, for a tumor that is non-resectable or for destroying the rest of a tumor postoperatively. Seeds can be inserted noninvasively or invasively. Surgical procedures involve the seeds strung on suture or placed in a hollow plastic tube that is sealed on both ends. Using the surgical needle, the strand of seeds or tube is pulled through into the tumor. An alternative technique is inserting empty tubes in the OR and postoperatively the seeds are placed in the tubes, referred to as post- or after-loading. A third alternative that is performed in the OR is loading the seeds into a hollow needle and, under the guidance of ultrasound, the needles are inserted into the uterus. Once needle placement has been confirmed by ultrasound the seeds are released within the uterus, the needle is removed, and any incisions are closed.

PROCEDURE 15-21 Radical Hysterectomy (Wertheim Procedure)

Surgical Anatomy and Pathology	• See previous procedures for anatomy. • Radical hysterectomy is the en bloc removal of the ovaries, fallopian tubes, uterus and ligaments, upper third of vagina, and associated lymph nodes. • Performed due to extensive malignant tumor.
Preoperative Diagnostic Tests and Procedures	• See previous hysterectomy procedures.

(continues)

PROCEDURE 15-21 (continued)

Equipment, Instruments, and Supplies Unique to Procedure	• Abdominal hysterectomy instrument set • Long and deep surgical instruments • Abdominal self-retaining retractor (surgeon's preference)	• Vessel loops • Closed-wound drainage system (surgeon's preference) • Vaginal packing • Indwelling urinary catheter	• Suprapubic indwelling catheter • Blood administration equipment
Preoperative Preparation	• Position: Supine • Anesthesia: General	• Patient skin prep: Wide abdominal skin prep (nipple line to mid-thigh)	• Draping: Laparotomy draping procedure
Practical Considerations	• Same as for abdominal hysterectomy	• Notify blood bank prior to procedure	• Diagnostic studies available in the OR
Surgical Procedure	1. Laparotomy is performed. 2. The peritoneum is incised between the two round ligaments on the anterior of the uterus. Using digital blunt dissection, the bladder surface is freed from the cervix and vagina. 3. The suspensory and round ligaments on the right side are double clamped, cut, and ligated/tied (CCCT). The external iliac artery is identified. 4. The ureters are identified and extensive dissection is completed to free them from the cervical structures in order to facilitate the removal of the uterine and vaginal ligaments. **Procedural Consideration:** The ureters will be retracted laterally with a vein retractor or loop vessels to prevent injury. If vessel loops are used, clamps will be used to clamp to the drapes to retract the ureters. 5. Extensive lymph node dissection is carried out at this point. The dissection is completed bilaterally to the bifurcation of the iliac arteries. **Procedural Consideration:** The surgeon will use long curved clamps and Lahey forceps to grasp the lymph nodes, Kitner sponges loaded on tonsil clamps and sponge sticks for blunt dissection, and long Metzenbaum scissors for sharp dissection. 6. CCCT of the uterine artery and vein is completed. 7. Using a heavy curved clamp or Lahey forceps, the surgeon grasps the uterus to position anterosuperior to facilitate using the knife to make an incision in the cul-de-sac. 8. CCCT of the cardinal and uterosacral ligaments is completed. 9. The upper third of the vagina is sharply dissected free from the surrounding paravesical and pararectal tissues. 10. Two Heaney or Ballatine clamps are cross-clamped across the lower border of the upper third of the vagina. The tissue is divided between the clamps with the long knife handle and #10 blade. The specimen is removed en bloc.		

PROCEDURE 15-21 (continued)

11. The vagina is closed with a running lock suture technique and a closed-wound drainage system of the surgeon's choice is placed.

    Procedural Consideration: The Hemovac is the most commonly used drainage system used for the procedure.

12. Continuous suture technique is used to reperitonealize the pelvis
13. The laparotomy is closed.
14. Vaginal packing may be placed. A suprapubic indwelling catheter may be inserted to assist the patient in postoperative bladder drainage if urinating is difficult after the indwelling urethral catheter is removed.

Postoperative Considerations

Immediate Postoperative Care

- Transport to PACU or ICU.

Prognosis

- No complications: Discharged from health care facility in 3–5 days; return to full normal activities will most likely not occur due to extensive nature of procedure and further medical therapy treatments (radiation and chemotherapy).
- Complications: Postoperative SSI; bladder spasms; hemorrhage; injury to adjacent organs such as ureters, bladder, and nerves; incontinence.
- Prognosis will be dependent on outcome of procedure and medical therapy.

Wound Classification

- Class II: Clean contaminated

PROCEDURE 15-22 Pelvic Exenteration

Surgical Anatomy and Pathology

- See previous procedures for anatomy.
- The en bloc removal of the rectum, distal sigmoid colon, urinary bladder and distal ureters, ovaries, fallopian tubes, uterus, cervix, vagina, pelvic lymph nodes, section of the levator muscles, pelvic peritoneum, perineum, and internal iliac vessels. Permanent ileostomy and colostomy are created.
- Procedure is performed to treat recurrent or chronic cervical cancer that is also resistant to radiation therapy.

Preoperative Diagnostic Tests and Procedures

- History and physical: A thorough history of the patient is conducted as well as determining the immediate health status of the patient and extent of the cancer in order to decide if the patient is a good candidate for the surgery.
- Additionally, the psychological state of the patient must be taken into consideration to make sure she is prepared for the physical changes that will be occurring, e.g., loss of vagina, ileostomy, and colostomy.

(continues)

Procedure 15-22 (continued)

Equipment, Instruments, and Supplies Unique to Procedure	• Two suction systems • Major laparotomy instrument set • Vascular instrument set • Kidney instrument set • GI instrument set • Abdominal hysterectomy instrument set • Abdominal self-retaining retractor (surgeon's preference) • Various sizes of hemoclip appliers and clips • Blades: #11, #10, #12, #15 • GI intestinal staplers • Two electrosurgical pencils • Kitners • Penrose drains, umbilical tapes, and/or vessel loops (surgeon's preference) • Various sizes of Robinson catheters (available in OR) • Various sizes of colostomy and ileostomy pouches
Preoperative Preparation	• Position: Lithotomy • Anesthesia: General • Patient skin prep: • Abdominal prep: nipple line to knees • Vaginal prep • Draping: Laparotomy and lithotomy draping procedure
Practical Considerations	• Pelvic **exenteration** is a lengthy procedure; the patient must be carefully positioned to prevent vascular and nerve injury to the lower back, hips, and knees. The pressure points must be identified and well padded. • Antiembolic stockings may be applied. • The surgical technologist must keep meticulous record of the amount of irrigation used throughout the procedure in order to aid in the estimate of blood loss. • The surgical technologist will need to create two instrument setups: one setup for the abdomen and the second setup for the perineum. • The surgical technologist should have extra gowns and gloves for the surgical team members as well as self. The team will need to change when moving between the abdominal portion of the procedure to perineal and back, as well as when performing the clean closure of the abdomen. Additional drapes will be needed as well. • The surgical team will need to use bowel technique when the colon or ureter is opened. Instruments that contact these open areas are contaminated and must be kept isolated from the other instruments.
Surgical Procedure	1. A midline incision is made from the upper abdomen, around the umbilicus, to the superior symphysis pubis.
	2. The surgeon explores the abdominal and pelvic cavities for signs of metastasis to the liver, other abdominal organs, and pelvic lymph nodes. Several frozen section specimens may be taken.
	3. If metastasis has not occurred, the surgeon will use several moist lap sponges to wall off and protect the small bowel. Self-retaining abdominal retractor is placed. **Procedural Consideration:** The surgical technologist must keep track of the number of lap sponges placed within the abdominal cavity.
	4. The length of the sigmoid colon is identified. Using intestinal clamps, the distal segment is cross-clamped and divided with the knife or a GI stapler is used. An opening is made in the left side of the abdomen and the proximal end is brought through the opening. An intestinal clamp is placed across the sigmoid colon to close the lumen to prevent spillage and left in place until later in the procedure when the colostomy is completed.

PROCEDURE 15-22 (continued)

5. The sigmoid mesentery is CCCT several times to include the superior hemorrhoidal vessels.

   Procedural Consideration: The surgeon will need long and deep instruments for this step of the procedure as well as any other time the procedure involves working deep in the abdominal or pelvic cavities.

6. The distal sigmoid colon lumen is closed with an inverting suture technique.

7. The sigmoid colon and rectum are freed from their sacrococcygeal attachments by blunt and sharp dissection.

8. The lateral peritoneum is incised with the knife and Metzenbaum scissors following the iliac vessels. CCCT of the ovarian arteries and veins and round ligaments is accomplished on both sides.

9. The peritoneum overlying the bladder dome is cut with the knife and Metzenbaum scissors. The bladder is freed from the symphysis pubis to the urethra.

10. The two ureters are identified and transected below the edge of the pelvis. The proximal lumen is left open for urinary drainage and the distal lumen is tied closed.

11. The internal iliac vein, superior and inferior gluteal arteries and veins, and hypogastric artery are identified and CCCT. The internal pudendal vessels are identified and CCCT. This step is repeated on the opposite side of the pelvis. The surgeon is careful to identify and preserve the obturator and sciatic nerve, and sacral plexus.

12. The surgeon now moves to the perineum and, using the knife, makes a wide elliptical incision that includes the anus and up to the clitoris. The levator muscle is exposed by an incision in the ischiorectal area and its lateral attachment cut and freed up.

13. The coccygeal muscle is cut and detached from the rectum. The levator muscles are detached laterally.

14. The last step to completely free up the en bloc specimen is sharp and blunt resection of the paravaginal and paravesical attachments to the periosteum of the symphysis pubis. The specimen is passed to the surgical technologist, who hands it off the field to the circulator (Figure 15-25).

15. The surgeon irrigates the cavity thoroughly and, using the ESU and ties, controls bleeding.

16. A closed-wound drainage system is placed and the laparotomy is closed.

17. The ileostomy is created on the right side of the abdomen by creation of an ileal pouch and the ureters attached to it. The stoma is created on the abdomen's right side.

18. A jejunostomy tube is inserted into the jejunum for postoperative bowel decompression; it is anchored to the bowel with a purse-string suture technique and brought out through the skin layer and sutured in place.

    Procedural Consideration: This step of the procedure may not always be performed. Therefore have the catheter available in the OR, but not opened unless needed.

19. A gastrostomy tube is placed into the stomach, anchored with purse-string suture and brought out through the skin layer, and sutured in place.

20. The surgeon positions the small intestine within the pelvis.

    Procedural Consideration: Lap sponges used for packing are removed; surgical technologist must count each sponge as it is removed and conform with the circulator that the correct number of sponges were removed.

(continues)

PROCEDURE 15-22 (continued)

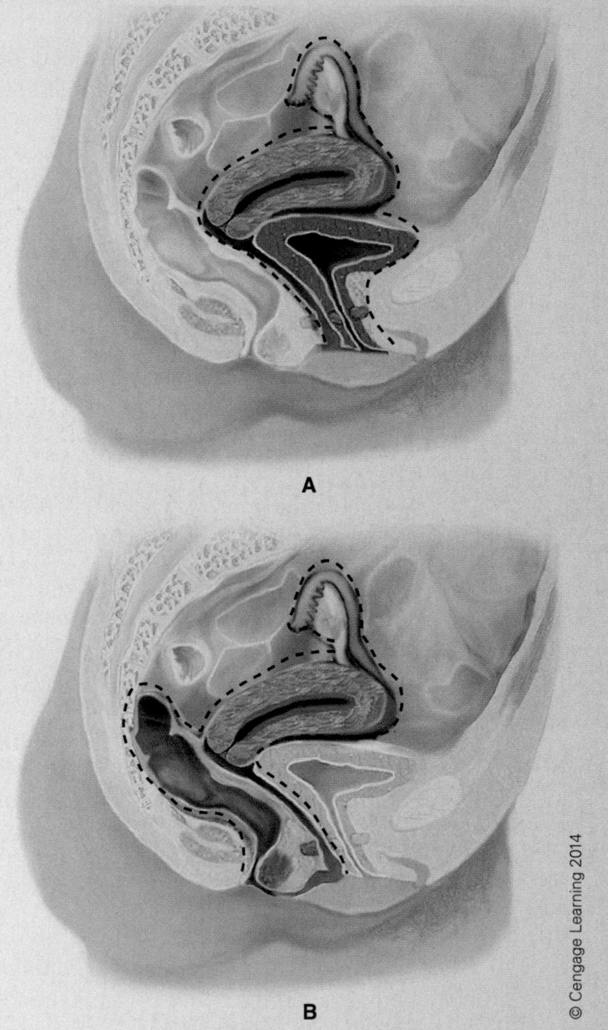

Figure 15-25 Pelvic exenteration: (A) Anterior, (B) posterior

21. The peritoneum, rectus muscles, and fascia are closed using the interrupted figure-of-eight suture technique. The skin is closed with the interrupted suture technique.

22. The colostomy is created on the left side of the abdomen; the clamp is removed and the stoma created.

Postoperative Considerations

Immediate Postoperative Care

- Transport to ICU.

Prognosis

- No complications: Discharged in 5–7 days from health care facility.
- Complications: Pelvic exenteration carries a high morbidity and mortality rate; postoperative SSI; hemorrhage; nerve damage; postoperative pain.
- Prognosis depends on outcome of procedure, ability to recover from procedure, postoperative medical therapy.

Wound Classification

- Class II: Clean contaminated or Class III: Contaminated if spillage occurs

Procedure 15-23 Anterior (Cystocele) and Posterior (Rectocele) Colporrhaphy

Surgical Anatomy and Pathology	• See Procedure 15-7 Hysteroscopy page 548 for vaginal anatomy. • A cystocele and a rectocele, herniation of the bladder and rectum into the vaginal vault, respectively, may occur after the connective tissues and musculature that support the uterus become weak. Generally, this occurs after menopause and after multiple childbirths. • Cystoceles are associated with urinary incontinence. • Both appear as bulges in the vaginal wall. • A cystocele bulge will be in the anterior vaginal wall and the rectocele bulge visible along the posterior vaginal wall.
Preoperative Diagnostic Tests and Procedures	• Diagnosis obtained by history and physical as well as by direct examination.
Equipment, Instruments, and Supplies Unique to Procedure	• Headlight/headlamp • Unless included in instrument set additional Allis clamps will be needed • Vaginal hysterectomy instrument set • Indwelling urinary catheter
Preoperative Preparation	• Position: Lithotomy • Anesthesia: General • Patient prep: Vaginal • Draping: Lithotomy draping procedure
Practical Considerations	• Place catheter drainage bag where it can be monitored. • Repair of a rectocele incorporates perineorrhaphy to restore fecal continence and sexual competency of the vagina.
Surgical Procedure	1. **Anterior repair:** a transverse incision is made at the union of the vaginal mucosa and cervix and continued down to the pubovesical cervical fascia (Figure 15-26A). **Procedural Consideration:** The labia minora may be sutured to the skin to provide exposure. Cervical traction is maintained with a tenaculum.
	2. The vaginal mucosa is dissected from the pubovesical and cervical fascia and opened in the midline (Figure 15-26B). **Procedural Consideration:** Careful positioning and manipulation of retractors are required for good visualization and tissue care.
	3. Dissection continues with the vaginal mucosa being opened in the midline until a point is reached 1 cm from the urethral meatus. The pubovesical and cervical fascia is bluntly dissected from the vaginal mucosa (Figure 15-26C). **Procedural Consideration:** Allis clamps are applied as dissection progresses. The surgical technologist should have an ample number on the field.
	4. This dissection continues until the bladder and urethra are separated from the vaginal mucosa and the urethral vesical angle is identified. **Procedural Consideration:** The technique often used is blunt dissection with gauze wrapped around the index finger. *Note:* Use radiologically detectable sponge.
	5. If a Kelly plication is performed to treat stress incontinence, a nonabsorbable suture is placed bilaterally to the urethra. A hemostat is placed so that the tissue is inverted as the suture is tied. Other sutures are placed as needed (Figure 15-26D). **Procedural Consideration:** The presence of an excessive cystocele may warrant further bladder suspension techniques.

(*continues*)

PROCEDURE 15-23 (continued)

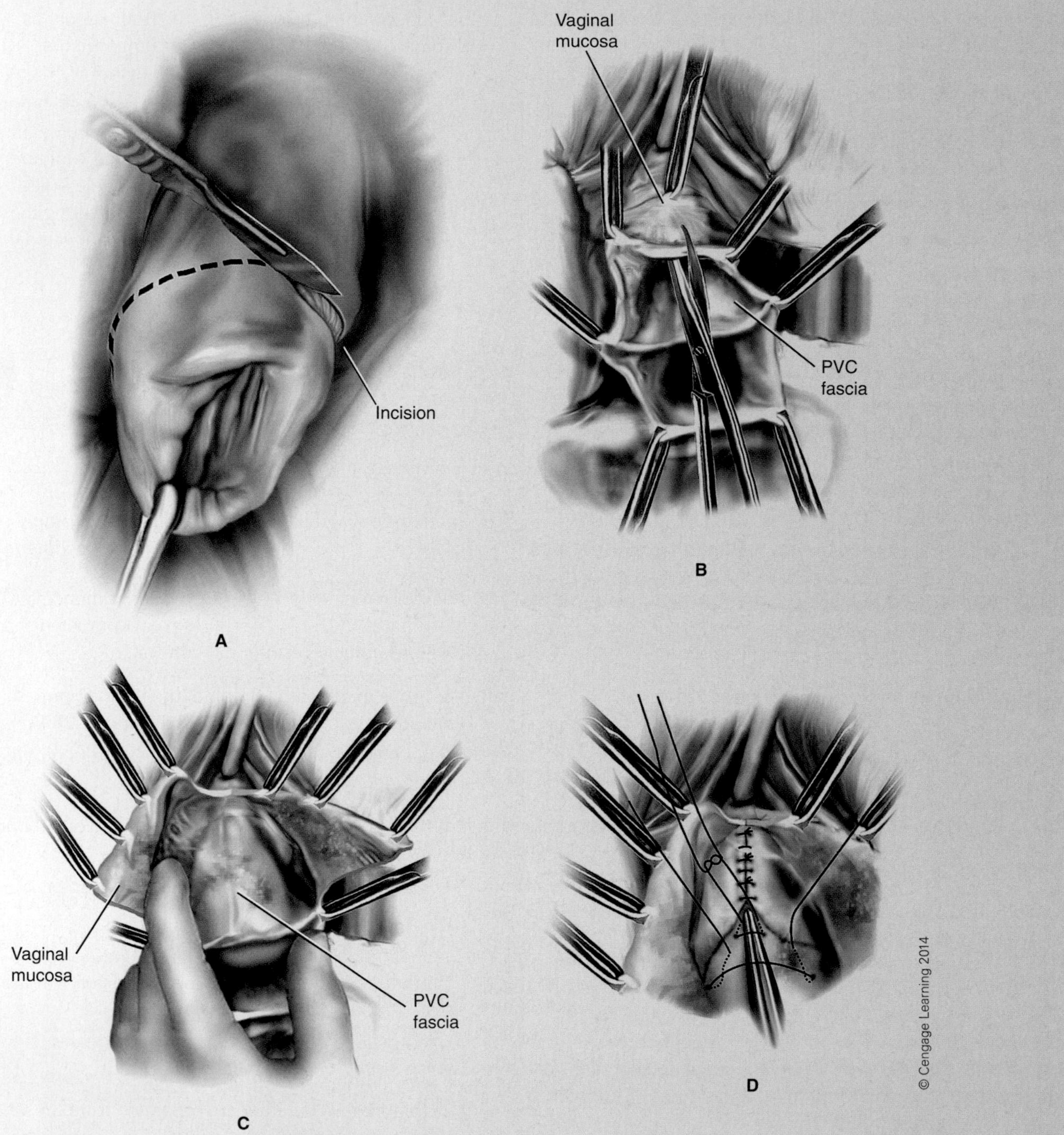

Figure 15-26 Anterior repair: (A) Transverse incision at the junction of the cervix and vaginal mucosa, (B) vaginal mucosa is dissected from the pubovesical and cervical fascia. When dissection is complete, the vaginal mucosa is incised in the midline. *Note:* Hysterectomy has been completed in this case. This is not a necessary prerequisite for anterior repair, (C) blunt dissection of vaginal mucosa from pubovesical and cervical fascia, (D) completion of Kelly plication (not always required)

Procedure 15-23 (continued)

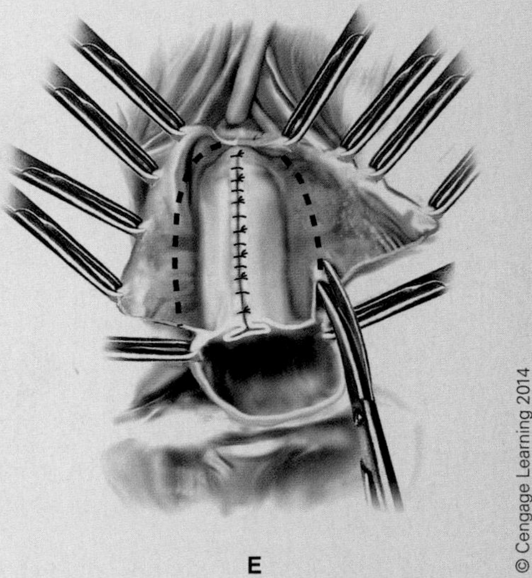

Figure 15-26 Anterior repair: (E) Excess vaginal mucosa is excised; lower portion shows vaginal cuff and plication technique used on pubovesical cervical fascia.

6. The anterior repair begins as synthetic absorbable sutures are placed in the pubovesical and cervical fascia starting 1 cm below the urethral meatus.

   Procedural Consideration: The surgical technologist should be prepared with enough sutures to complete multiple single mattress sutures.

7. The repair continues until the entire cystocele is reduced (Figure 15-26E).

   Procedural Consideration: Suture for this step is often loaded on control-release needles. Keep close track of needles.

8. The excessive vaginal mucosa is removed.

   Procedural Consideration: This will usually be done with Metzenbaum scissors.

9. The vaginal mucosa is closed in the midline with interrupted 0 synthetic absorbable sutures to the level of the vaginal cuff.

   Procedural Consideration: Pass suture of surgeon's preference.

10. The edge of the vaginal cuff is sutured with a continuous 0 absorbable suture.

    Procedural Consideration: The surgical technologist should quickly clean and reorganize instruments and be prepared to "repeat" the process posteriorly.

11. **Posterior repair:** Allis-Adair clamps are placed on the posterior vaginal mucosa and elevated to create a triangle (Figure 15-27A).

    Procedural Consideration: *Note:* Technical considerations are the same for the posterior repair.

12. An Allis clamp is placed at the top of the rectocele in the midline. A transverse incision is made at the posterior fourchette. Blunt dissection is used to separate the posterior vaginal mucosa from the perirectal fascia.

    Procedural Consideration: Pass scalpel per facility policy. Have radiologically detectable sponge for blunt dissection prepared in advance of need.

13. A V-shaped portion of the mucosa is excised as determined by extent of repair required, and the levator ani muscles are observed below (Figure 15-27B).

    Procedural Consideration: Vaginal mucosa will be sent to pathology as specimen.

(*continues*)

PROCEDURE 15-23 (continued)

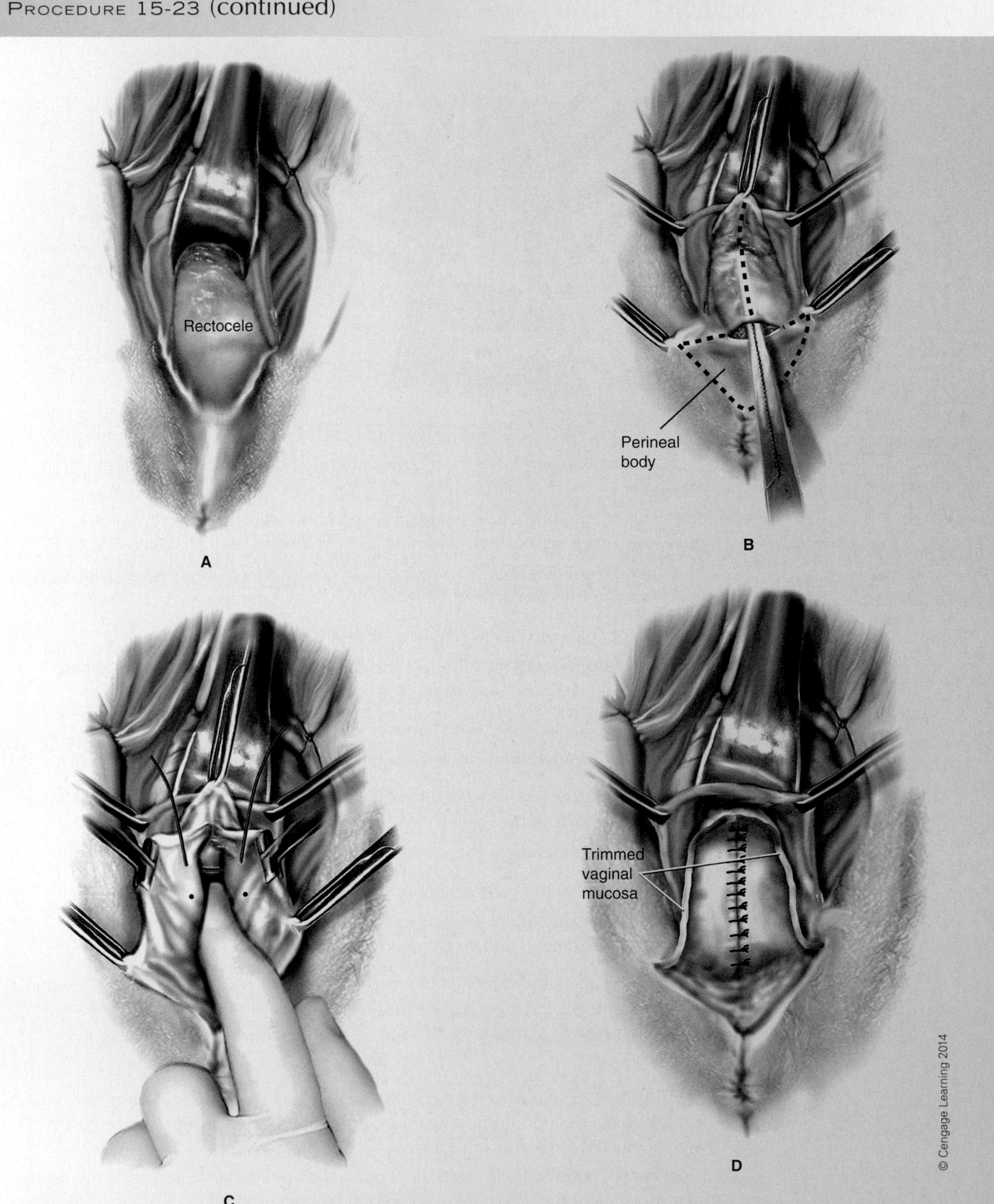

Figure 15-27 Posterior repair: (A) Elevation of posterior vaginal mucosa overlying rectocele, (B) blunt dissection of vaginal mucosa off perirectal fascia; intended incision lines noted, (C) manual reduction of the rectocele allows the margins of levator ani muscles and suture placement sites to be identified, (D) levator ani muscles sutured; excess posterior vaginal mucosa trimmed and prepared for closure

(continues)

PROCEDURE 15-23 (continued)

14. The bulbocavernosus muscle is exposed by an incision in the perineal body with removal of a triangular segment of perineal skin.

    Procedural Consideration: Sharp and blunt dissection is carried out.

15. A vertical incision is made in the posterior vaginal mucosa and the edges are retracted. The perirectal fascia is bluntly dissected from the posterior vaginal mucosa.

    Procedural Consideration: Several Allis clamps will be needed to retract the mucosal edges.

16. The rectocele is reduced with a finger, revealing the margins of the levator ani muscles. A 0 or 1 synthetic absorbable suture is placed at the margin of the levator ani to the posterior fourchette (Figure 15-27C).

    Procedural Consideration: Several of these sutures will be placed, progressively tied, and cut.

17. The excessive posterior vaginal mucosa is excised and the perirectal fascia is closed with interrupted 0 synthetic absorbable suture.

    Procedural Consideration: The surgical technologist should be prepared to supply suture for multiple stitches.

18. The posterior vaginal wall is closed to the posterior fourchette. The hymenal ring is reconstructed, as is the perineal body (Figure 15-27D).

    Procedural Consideration: Additional sutures will be needed.

19. The subcutaneous layer and skin are closed with a subcuticular suture.

    Procedural Consideration: The surgical technologist may be asked to "follow" the suture for subcuticular closure. Initiate count. Prepare dressings.

20. After closure, the repair is again assessed for integrity. The vaginal opening is reassessed to assure a two-finger-breadths space exists. Sutures are removed from the labia minora. The wound is then cleansed and a perineal pad dressing is applied.

    Procedural Consideration: A vaginal pack may be used.

Postoperative Considerations

Immediate Postoperative Care

- Transport to PACU.
- Observe color and amount of urine output in urine drainage bag.

Prognosis

- No complications: Return to normal activities in 6–8 weeks.
- Complications: Hemorrhage; hematoma; urinary tract infection; wound infection; inability to urinate or stress incontinence; shortened or narrowed vagina; rectovaginal fistula; recurrence of herniation.

Wound Classification

- Class II: Clean-contaminated

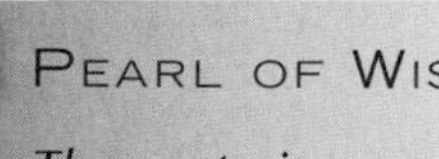

PEARL OF WISDOM

The posterior repair follows anterior because of potential contamination via the anus.

CASE STUDY Sandy, a 34-year-old female, went to see her gynecologist. She complained of a somewhat vague abdominal pain and said she "felt heavy down there." She was nulliparous and appeared to be in good health otherwise. The laboratory studies were normal. The bimanual pelvic examination revealed irregularly shaped nodules on the uterus. They felt rather firm and immobile. They moved when the uterus moved. Sonography confirmed the presence of tumors. After a period of conservative treatment, Sandy was admitted to the local facility for surgery.

1. **Sandy's symptoms are consistent with what diagnosis?**
2. **This condition is treated with what surgical procedure when the patient hopes to bear children? What other procedure could be used for treatment?**
3. **What are the common complications of the procedure Sandy will undergo?**

QUESTIONS FOR FURTHER STUDY

1. List five reasons for performing a cesarean section and state the most frequent reason for this procedure.
2. What steps performed in a traditional vaginal hysterectomy may be performed laparoscopically? What is the advantage of the laparoscopic approach?
3. Define and list the basic steps in a Pfannenstiel abdominal incision.
4. List the structures that will be removed during a total pelvic exenteration.
5. Name at least two medications that can be used to treat uterine hemorrhage following childbirth.
6. Briefly describe how the sequence of events for an emergency cesarean section (e.g., prolapsed umbilical cord, placenta abruptio) may differ from that of a planned cesarean section.

BIBLIOGRAPHY

Anderson, J. R., & Genadry, R. (2006). Anatomy and embryology. In J. S. Berek (Ed.), *Novak's gynecology* (14th ed.). Philadelphia: Lippincott Williams and Wilkins.

Association of Surgical Technologists. (2011). *Core curriculum for surgical technology* (6th ed.). Littleton, CO: Association of Surgical Technologists.

Baggish, M. S., & DeLeon, F. D. (2004). Lasers in gynecology. In J. J. Sciarra (Ed.), *Gynecology and obstetrics* (rev.). New York: Lippincott-Raven.

Brumsted, J. R., & Riddick, D. H. (2008). Menstruation and disorders of menstrual function. In J. R. Scott, R. S. Gibbs, B. Y. Karlan, & A. F. Haney (Eds.), *Danforth's obstetrics and gynecology* (10th ed.). Philadelphia: Lippincott Williams and Wilkins.

Butler, W. J. (2008). Normal and abnormal uterine bleeding. In J. A. Rock & H. W. Jones (Eds.), *TeLinde's operative gynecology* (10th ed.). Philadelphia: Lippincott Williams and Wilkins.

Chez, R. A., & Mischell, D. R. (2008). Total control of human reproduction: Contraception, sterilization, and pregnancy termination. In J. R. Scott et al.(Eds.), *Danforth's obstetrics and gynecology* (10th ed.). Philadelphia: Lippincott Williams and Wilkins.

Clarke-Pearson, D. L., Olt, G. H., Rodriquez, G. C., & Boente, M. P. (2006). Preoperative evaluation and postoperative management. In J. S. Berek (Ed.), *Novak's gynecology* (14th ed.) Philadelphia: Lippincott Williams and Wilkins.

Creasman, W. T. (2008). Disorders of the uterine corpus. In J. R. Scott et al. (Eds.), *Danforth's obstetrics and gynecology* (10th ed.). Philadelphia: Lippincott Williams and Wilkins.

Cromer, D. W. (2004). Postpartum sterilization procedures. In J. J. Sciarra (Ed.), *Gynecology and obstetrics* (rev.). New York: Lippincott-Raven.

Cruikshank, S. H. (2004). Vaginal hysterectomy. In J. J. Sciarra (Ed.), *Gynecology and obstetrics* (rev.). New York: Lippincott-Raven.

Cunningham, F. G., Leveno, K. J., Bloom, S. L., Hauth, J. C., Gilstap, L. C., & Wenstrom, K. D. (Eds.). (2009). *Williams obstetrics* (23rd ed.) New York: McGraw-Hill.

De Cherney, A. H. (2009). Infertility: General principles of evaluation. In W. J. Hoskins, C. A. Perez, R. C. Young, R. R. Barakat, & M. Markman (Eds.), *Principles and practices of gynecologic oncology* (5th ed.). Philadelphia: Lippincott Williams and Wilkins.

DeLancey, J. O. L. (2008). Pelvic organ prolapse. In J. R. Scott et al. (Eds.), *Danforth's obstetrics and gynecology* (10th ed.). Philadelphia: Lippincott Williams and Wilkins.

DeLancey, J. O. L. (2008). Surgical anatomy of the female pelvis. In J. A. Rock & H. W. Jones (Eds.), *TeLinde's operative gynecology* (10th ed.). Philadelphia: Lippincott Williams and Wilkins.

DeLeon, F. D., & Peters, A. J. (2004). Reversal of female sterilization. In J. J. Sciarra (Ed.), *Gynecology and obstetrics* (rev.). New York: Lippincott-Raven.

Del Priore, G. (2004). Vulvar intraepithelial neoplasms. In J. J. Sciarra (Ed.), *Gynecology and obstetrics* (rev.). New York: Lippincott-Raven.

DiSaia, P. J. (2008). Disorders of the uterine cervix. In J. R. Scott et al. (Eds.), *Danforth's obstetrics and gynecology* (10th ed.). Philadelphia: Lippincott Williams and Wilkins.

DiSaia, P. J. (2008). Radiation therapy in gynecology. In J. R. Scott et al. (Eds.), *Danforth's obstetrics and gynecology* (10th ed.). Philadelphia: Lippincott Williams and Wilkins.

DiSaia, P. J. (2008). Vulvar and vaginal disease. In J. R. Scott et al. (Eds.), *Danforth's obstetrics and gynecology* (10th ed.). Philadelphia: Lippincott Williams and Wilkins.

DiSaia, P. J. & Creasman, W. T. (2002). *Clinical gynecologic oncology*. New York: Mosby.

DiSaia, P. J., & Walker, J. L. (2008). Perioperative care. In J. R. Scott et al. (Eds.), *Danforth's obstetrics and gynecology* (10th ed.). Philadelphia: Lippincott Williams and Wilkins.

Dorsey, J. H. (2008). Application of laser in gynecology. In J. A. Rock & H. W. Jones (Eds.), *TeLinde's operative gynecology* (10th ed.). Philadelphia: Lippincott Williams and Wilkins.

Dorsey, J. H. (2008). Application of laser in surgery. In J. A. Rock & H. W. Jones (Eds.), *TeLinde's operative gynecology* (10th ed.). Philadelphia: Lippincott Williams and Wilkins.

Droegmueller, W. (2007). Benign gynecological lesions. In M. A. Stenchever, W. Droegmueller, A. L. Herbst, & D. Mischell (Eds.), *Comprehensive gynecology* (5th ed.). New York: Mosby.

Eifel, P. J., Morris, M., Delclos, L., & Wharton, J. T. (2004). Radiation therapy for cervical carcinoma. In J. J. Sciarra (Ed.), *Gynecology and obstetrics* (rev.). New York: Lippincott-Raven.

Elkins, T. E., & Arrowsmith, S. (2004). Repair of urogenital and rectovaginal fistulas. In J. J. Sciarra (Ed.), *Gynecology and obstetrics* (rev.). New York: Lippincott-Raven.

Estes, M. E. Z. (2010). *Health assessment and physical examination* (4th ed.). Clifton Park, NY: Delmar Cengage Learning.

Gallup, D. G. (2008). Incisions for gynecologic surgery. In J. A. Rock & H. W. Jones (Eds.), *TeLinde's operative gynecology* (10th ed.). Philadelphia: Lippincott Williams and Wilkins.

Gallup, D. G., & Hoskins, W. J. (2009). Surgical principles in gynecologic oncology. In W. J. Hoskins, C. A. Perez, R. C. Young, R. R. Barakat, & M. Markman (Eds.), *Principles and practices of gynecologic oncology* (5th Illus. ed.). Philadelphia: Lippincott Williams and Wilkins.

Goldman, M. A. (1996). *Pocket guide to the operating room* (2nd ed.). Philadelphia: F. A. Davis.

Gomel, V. (2008). Reconstructive tubal surgery. In J. A. Rock & H. W. Jones (Eds.), *TeLinde's operative gynecology* (10th ed.). Philadelphia: Lippincott Williams and Wilkins.

Grifio, J. A., & DeCherney, A. H. (2004). Myomectomy. In J. J. Sciarra (Ed.), *Gynecology and obstetrics* (rev.). New York: Lippincott-Raven.

Grimes, D. A (2008). Management of abortion. In J. A. Rock & H. W. Jones (Eds.), *TeLinde's operative gynecology* (10th ed.). Philadelphia: Lippincott Williams and Wilkins.

Grody, M. H. T. (2008). Posterior compartment defects. In J. A. Rock & H. W. Jones (Eds.), *TeLinde's operative gynecology* (10th ed.). Philadelphia: Lippincott Williams and Wilkins.

Guyton, A. C. & Hall, J. E. (2005). *Textbook of medical physiology* (11th ed.). Philadelphia: Saunders.

Hacker, N. F. (2006). Vulvar cancer. In J. S. Berek (Ed.), *Novak's gynecology* (14th ed.). Philadelphia: Lippincott Williams and Wilkins.

Hammond, C. B. (2008). Infertility. In J. R. Scott et al. (Eds.), *Danforth's obstetrics and gynecology* (10th ed.). Philadelphia: Lippincott Williams and Wilkins.

Hatch, K. D. & Hacker, N. F. (2006). Intraepithelial disease of the cervix, vagina, and vulva. In J. S. Berek (Ed.), *Novak's gynecology* (14th ed.). Philadelphia: Lippincott Williams and Wilkins.

Herbst, A. L. (2007). Principles of radiation therapy and chemotherapy in gynecologic cancer. In M. A. Stenchever, W. Droegmueller, A. L. Herbst, & D. Mischell (Eds.), *Comprehensive gynecology* (5th ed.). New York: Mosby.

Horbelt, D. V., & Delmore, J. E. (2004). Benign neoplasms of the vulva. In J. J. Sciarra (Ed.), *Gynecology and obstetrics* (rev.). Philadelphia: Lippincott-Raven.

Horowitz, I. R., Buscema, J., & Woodruff, J. D. (2008). Surgical conditions of the vulva. In J. A. Rock & H. W. Jones (Eds.), *TeLinde's operative gynecology* (10th ed.). Philadelphia: Lippincott Williams and Wilkins.

Hulka, J. F. (2004). Dilatation and curettage. In J. J. Sciarra (Ed.), *Gynecology and obstetrics* (rev.). New York: Lippincott-Raven.

Isaacs, J. H. (2004). Posterior colpoperineorrahpy. In J. J. Sciarra (Ed.), *Gynecology and obstetrics* (rev.). New York: Lippincott-Raven.

Isaacson, K. B., & Schiff, I. (2001). Surgery for infertility. In P. J. Morris & W. C. Woods (Eds.), *Oxford textbook of surgery* (2nd ed.). New York: Oxford University Press.

Kase, N. (2008). Infertility: General principles of evaluation. In J. A. Rock & H. W. Jones (Eds.), *TeLinde's operative gynecology* (10th ed.). Philadelphia: Lippincott Williams and Wilkins.

Lee, R. A. (2008). Combined compartment defects. In J. A. Rock & H. W. Jones (Eds.), *TeLinde's operative gynecology* (10th ed.). Philadelphia: Lippincott Williams and Wilkins.

Mettler, L., Ahmed-Ebbiary, N., & Schollmeyer, T. (2005). Laparoscopic hysterectomy: Challenges and limitations. *Minimally Invasive Therapy, 14*(3), 45–159.

Mischell, D. R., Jr. (2007). Family planning. In M. A. Stenchever, W. Droegmueller, A. L. Herbst, & D. Mischell (Eds.), *Comprehensive gynecology* (5th ed.). New York: Mosby.

Morley, G. W., Hopkins, M. P., & Johnston, C. M. (2008). Pelvic exenteration. In J. A. Rock & H. W. Jones (Eds.), *TeLinde's operative gynecology* (10th ed.). Philadelphia: Lippincott Williams and Wilkins.

Muckle, C. W. (2004). Clinical anatomy of the uterus, fallopian tubes, and ovaries. In J. J. Sciarra (Ed.), *Gynecology and obstetrics* (rev.). Philadelphia: Lippincott-Raven.

Nichols, D. H., & Milley, P. S. (2004). Clinical anatomy of the vulva, vagina, lower pelvis, and perineum. In J. J. Sciarra (Ed.), *Gynecology and obstetrics* (rev.). Philadelphia: Lippincott-Raven.

Nichols, D. H., & Ponchak, S. F. (2006). Anterior and posterior colporrhaphy. In J. E. Fischer, K. I. Bland, M. P. Callery, G. P. Clagett, & D. B. Jones (Eds.), *Mastery of surgery*. Philadelphia: Lippincott Williams and Wilkins.

Noller, K. L., & Wagner, A. L., Jr. (2004). Colposcopy. In J. J. Sciarra (Ed.), *Gynecology and obstetrics* (rev.). Philadelphia: Lippincott-Raven.

Partridge, E. E. (2004). Pelvic exenteration. In J. J. Sciarra (Ed.), *Gynecology and obstetrics* (rev.). Philadelphia: Lippincott-Raven.

Phillips, N. F. (2007). *Berry & Kohn's operating room technique* (11th ed.). St. Louis: Mosby.

Porges, R. F. (2004). Anterior colporraphy. In J. J. Sciarra (Ed.), *Gynecology and obstetrics* (rev.). Philadelphia: Lippincott-Raven.

Richart, R. M. (2008). Cervical cancer precursors and their management. In J. A. Rock & H. W. Jones (Eds.), *TeLinde's operative gynecology* (10th ed.). Philadelphia: Lippincott Williams and Wilkins.

Rock, J. A., & Damario, M. A. (2008). Ectopic pregnancy. In J. A. Rock & H. W. Jones (Eds.), *TeLinde's operative gynecology* (10th ed.). Philadelphia: Lippincott Williams and Wilkins.

Rock, J. A., & Keenan, D. L. (2004). Surgical corrections of uterovaginal anomalies. In J. J. Sciarra (Ed.), *Gynecology and obstetrics* (rev.). Philadelphia: Lippincott-Raven.

Sakala, E. P. (2004). *Obstetrics and gynecology, board review series.* Baltimore: Williams and Wilkins.

Schoeppel, S. L., & Lichter, A. S. (2004). The role of radiation therapy in the treatment of malignant uterine tumors. In J. J. Sciarra (Ed.), *Gynecology and obstetrics* (rev.). Philadelphia: Lippincott-Raven.

Sciarra, J. J. (2004). Surgical procedures for tubal sterilization. In J. J. Sciarra (Ed.), *Gynecology and obstetrics* (rev.). Philadelphia: Lippincott-Raven.

Scott, J. R. (2008). Early pregnancy loss. In J. R. Scott et al. (Eds.), *Danforth's obstetrics and gynecology* (10th ed.). Philadelphia: Lippincott Williams and Wilkins.

Siegler, A. M. (2004). Salpingotomy and salpingectomy: Indications and techniques for tubal pregnancy. In J. J. Sciarra (Ed.), *Gynecology and obstetrics* (rev.). Philadelphia: Lippincott-Raven.

Standring, S. (2008). Gray's anatomy (40th ed.). St. Louis: Elsevier.

Stovall, T. G. (2006). Hysterectomy. In J. S. Berek (Ed.), *Novak's gynecology* (14th ed.). Philadelphia: Lippincott Williams and Wilkins.

Stubblefield, P. G. (2006). Family planning. In J. S. Berek (Ed.), *Novak's gynecology* (14th ed.). Philadelphia: Lippincott Williams and Wilkins.

Thompson, J. D. (2008). Pelvic organ prolapse. In J. A. Rock & H. W. Jones (Eds.), *TeLinde's operative gynecology* (10th ed.). Philadelphia: Lippincott Williams and Wilkins.

Thompson, J. D. (2008). Vesicovaginal and urethrovaginal fistulas. In J. A. Rock & H. W. Jones (Eds.), *TeLinde's operative gynecology* (10th ed.). Philadelphia: Lippincott Williams and Wilkins.

Thompson, J. D., & Shull, B. L. (2008). Anterior compartment defects. In J. A. Rock & H. W. Jones (Eds.), *TeLinde's operative gynecology* (10th ed.). Philadelphia: Lippincott Williams and Wilkins.

Thompson, J. D., & Warshaw, J. S. (2008). Hysterectomy. In J. A. Rock & H. W. Jones (Eds.), *TeLinde's operative gynecology* (10th ed.). Philadelphia: Lippincott Williams and Wilkins.

Wall, L. L. (2006). Incontinence, prolapse, and disorders of the pelvic floor. In J. S. Berek (Ed.), *Novak's gynecology* (14th ed.). Philadelphia: Lippincott Williams and Wilkins.

Wallach, E. E. (2004). The mechanism of ovulation. In J. J. Sciarra (Ed.), *Gynecology and obstetrics* (rev.). Philadelphia: Lippincott-Raven.

Walton, L. A., & Van Le, L. (2004). Reconstructive surgery following treatment of female genital tract malignancies. In J. J. Sciarra (Ed.), *Gynecology and obstetrics* (rev.). Philadelphia: Lippincott-Raven.

Wells, E. C. (2004). Abdominal hysterectomy and bilateral salpingo-oophorectomy. In J. J. Sciarra (Ed.), *Gynecology and obstetrics* (rev.). Philadelphia: Lippincott-Raven.

Wright, T. C., & Ferenczy, A. (2002). Precancerous lesions of the cervix. In R. J. Kurman (Ed.), *Blaustein's pathology of the female genital tract* (5th ed.). New York: Springer.

Zaino, R. J., Robboy, S. J., Bentley, R., & Kurman, R. J. (2002). Diseases of the vagina. In R. J. Kurman (Ed.), *Blaustein's pathology of the female genital tract* (5th ed.). New York: Springer.

CHAPTER

16

Ophthalmic Surgery

CASE STUDY Heather has been referred to the ophthalmic surgeon because her symptoms have not improved after several weeks of more conservative treatment. She has been suffering pain in her left eye, and the area beneath her eye and next to her nose is red, painful, and inflamed. The area is sensitive to touch, and for several days a discharge has been present on the nasal side of the eye.

1. What must have been the diagnosis that caused the patient's doctor to refer her to a surgeon?
2. What will be the most probable surgical intervention?
3. What special anesthesia needs directly related to the particular surgical procedure will need to be met?

OBJECTIVES

After studying this chapter, the reader should be able to:

A 1. Recognize the anatomy of the eye.
P 2. Summarize the pathology that prompts surgical intervention of the eye and related terminology.
3. Determine any special preoperative preparation procedures.
O 4. Indicate the names and uses of ophthalmic instruments, supplies, and drugs.
5. Indicate the names and uses of special equipment.
6. Determine the intraoperative preparation of the patient undergoing an ophthalmic procedure.
7. Summarize the surgical steps of ophthalmic procedures.
8. Interpret the purpose and expected outcomes of the ophthalmic procedure.
9. Recognize the immediate postoperative care and possible complications of the ophthalmic procedure.
S 10. Assess any specific variations related to the preoperative, intraoperative, and postoperative care of the ophthalmic patient.

Select Key Terms

anterior chamber
balanced salt solution (BSS)
cataract
chalazion
dacryo-
diathermy
enucleation
extracapsular cataract extraction
extrinsic muscles
globe
intracapsular cataract extraction
iridotomy
kerato-
lacrimal
ocutome
posterior chamber
strabismus
trephine
tunic

INTRODUCTION TO OPHTHALMIC SURGERY

Ophthalmic surgery is considered a specialty of microsurgery since it involves the use of the microscope on the majority of procedures as well as microinstruments. The surgical technologist must have knowledge of how to set up and run the microscope, and be familiar with other specialty equipment such as the Phacoemulsification (Phaco) machine. Additionally, the surgical technologist must have fine motor skills in order to properly handle the small instruments without damaging them and to pass them to the surgeon in position of use so he or she does not have to look up from the microscope. The surgical technologist must become used to looking through the microscope to assist the surgeon during the procedure, such as irrigating the eye or cutting a small-diameter suture. This chapter will familiarize the student with the ophthalmic procedures that are commonly performed as preparation for surgical rotation.

INSTRUMENTS, ROUTINE EQUIPMENT, AND SUPPLIES

Instruments

Eye surgeons typically develop a small set of favored instruments for their own personal use, and these may be modified to suit personal tastes. Instruments for eye surgery include various microsurgical instruments. Commonly used instruments include:

Forceps

- Colibri forceps: for holding the edges of corneal and scleral incisions
- Nontoothed forceps: for holding skin edges in eyelid procedures and for holding the conjunctiva for suturing
- Bishop-Harmon iris forceps: for grasping and holding delicate eye tissue (see Figure 16-1)
- Desmarres chalazion forceps: for grasping the lower eyelid and isolating the chalazion to facilitate excision (see Figure 16-2)

Needle Holders

- Castroviejo: locking or nonlocking (surgeon's preference) needle holder (see Figure 16-3)
- Microsurgical needle holder: available with various shaped tips, locking needle holder

Scalpels

- Graefe cataract knife
- Keratomes (disposable): available in various angles

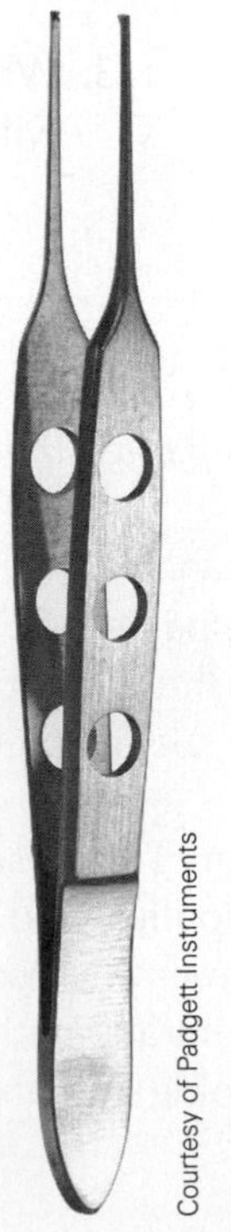

Figure 16-1 Bishop-Harmon iris forceps

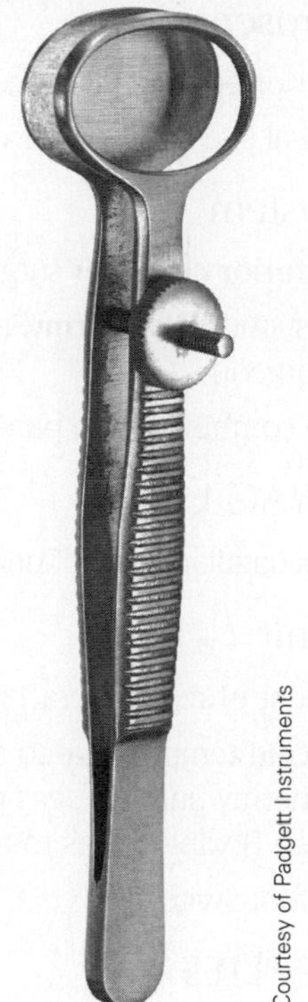

Figure 16-2 Desmarres chalazion forceps

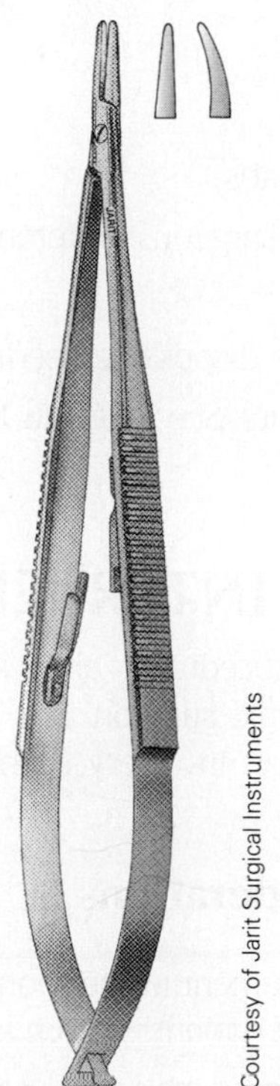

Figure 16-3 Castroviejo locking needle holder

- Razor fragments: broken from razor blades and placed in holders
- Diamond knife
- Oscillating knife

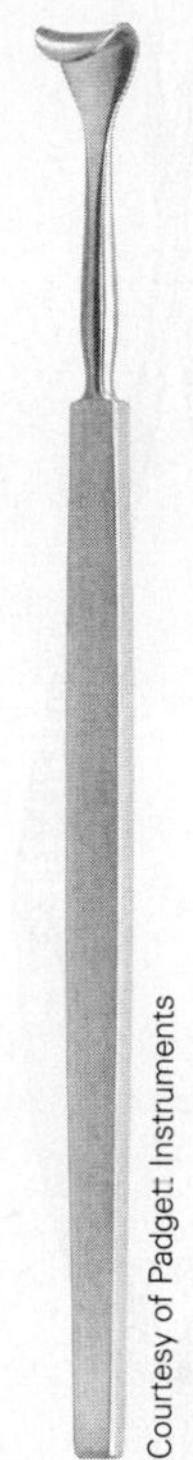

Figure 16-4 Desmarres lid retractor

- Beaver blades
- No. 15 knife blade

Hooks and Retractors

- Scleral hooks: scleral retraction
- Kilner hook: reconstructive surgery
- Desmarres lid retractors (see Figure 16-4)
- Iris retractor
- Eye speculum

Scissors

- Westcott scissors, spring-action microscissors: useful in **strabismus** and conjunctiva operations
- Small spring scissors: intraocular use
- McPherson-Vannas iris scissors (see Figure 16-5)

Miscellaneous

- Bowman probe: for probing the **lacrimal** duct (see Figure 16-6)

Routine Equipment

Routine equipment includes an ophthalmic stretcher with attachable wrist rest for the surgeon, a donut for positioning the head, and electrosurgical unit (ESU).

Special Equipment

The surgical technologist must have thorough knowledge of the operation, care and maintenance of all equipment used in ophthalmic procedures. See Chapters 6 and 10 for additional information about the equipment.

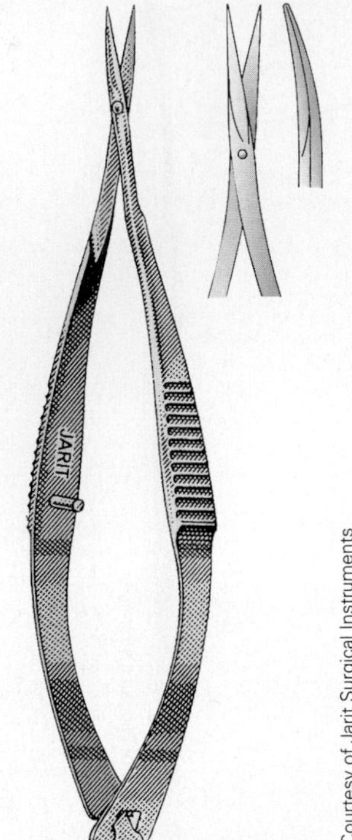

Figure 16-5 McPherson-Vannas iris scissors

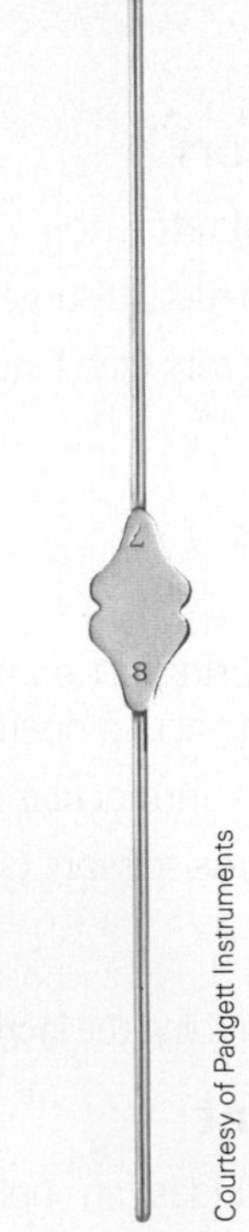

Figure 16-6 Bowman probe

Phacoemulsifier

- Used in surgical treatment of **cataracts**
- Uses ultrasonic energy to fragment the hard lens material, which then can be aspirated from the eye

Operating Microscope

- An integral part of ophthalmic surgery
- Magnifies surgical site through use of lenses

Vitreoretinal System

- Used in all **posterior chamber** surgeries
- Provides light, suction, **diathermy,** and intraoperative access to the surgeon
- System may be combined with phacoemulsification unit

Argon OR Nd:YAG Laser

- Used for photocoagulation or photodynamic therapy

Cryotherapy Unit

- Used in treatment of retinal detachment
- Uses localized cold temperature to seal tears and holes much as a diathermy unit; CO_2 gas passed is under pressure through flexible tubes to the tip of a probe
- Controlled by foot switch

ROUTINE SUPPLIES

- Prep set
- Eye or head and neck back table pack (depending on procedure)
- Wexcel sponges
- Sterile gloves
- Sterile cotton swabs
- Suture material (surgeons preference)
- BSS
- 27- and 30-gauge disposable needles, straight and angled
- Needles and suture: See Tables 16-1 and 16-2

SURGICAL INTERVENTION

Various surgical procedures and approaches are available to the ophthalmic surgeon and patient. There are elements of consistency in every ophthalmic procedure, as listed next.

Practical Considerations

- Talking and movement in the room should be kept to a minimum, as the patient is often awake.
- Nonpowdered gloves should be used; if not available, the powder should be thoroughly removed from the gloves.
- Extra care should be taken to keep lint off the instruments and sterile field to help to prevent formation of post-operative granuloma in the eye. Covering the draped Mayo stand with a clear, plastic sterile x-ray cassette cover reduces dust on the instruments as well as reduces the risk of microinstrument damage.

Table 16-1 Suture Needles for Ophthalmic Surgery

Type	*Description*	*Use*
Round bodied	Available with plain collagen and polyglactin	Conjunctival closure
Round bodied with cutting tip (taper cut)	Initially cuts like cutting needle, minimal trauma	Lacrimal sac and nasal mucosa
Reverse cutting (micropoint)	Triangular needle with third cutting edge on the outside of curvature	Eliminates possibility of outward tearing while suturing
Spatula micropoint	Fine needles with thin flat profile	Corneal and corneoscleral suturing
Spatulated	Similar to spatula	Scleral passage in strabismus correction, retinal detachment repair

Table 16-2 Suture Materials for Ophthalmic Surgery

Type	*Description*	*Use*
Nonabsorbable		
Monofilament nylon	Strong monofilament; does not support bacterial growth	Corneal incision closure
Monofilament polypropylene	Supple nonabsorbable; ties well	Intraocular lens fixation
Multifilament polyester-polybutilate coated	Multifilament braided coated with polybutilate for lubrication and smooth passage	Scleral tissue, retinal surgery
Braided silk	Tensile strength is high; tissue reaction is less than chromic gut, but more than synthetic sutures	Various
Absorbable		
Plain and chromic gut	Plain maintains tensile strength for 7–10 days; complete absorption is within 70 days. Chromic maintains tensile strength for 10–14 days, with some strength remaining up to 21 days; complete absorption is by 90 days	Various
Extruded collagen	Bovine tendon; consistent in strength; absorbs at about the same rate as plain gut	Various
Polyglactin (Vicryl)	Braided synthetic suture, less irritating than gut, absorbable coating; absorbs in 60–90 days, but retains strength for 30 days	Various

- The procedure is performed under an operating microscope; care should be taken in draping the microscope to prevent breaks in sterile technique.
- When a portable microscope is used, it should be brought over the patient from the side opposite the operative eye.

Procedural Considerations

- Avoid pooling prep solution in or near the eye.
- Periodically irrigate the eye using a bulb syringe filled with **balanced salt solution (BSS)** to prevent corneal drying.
- Trim the eyelashes before prepping if necessary.
- To protect sterility, every procedure on the **globe** requires the use of an adhesive-backed aperture drape that extends completely over the body. This will allow for proper placement of vitrector and phacoemulsification equipment. Place the opening over the operative eye and extend the drape over the patient. Make sure that the entire eye is accessible through the opening and secure the adhesive edges around the eye using sterile swabs rather than the fingers, to avoid injury to the soft tissues around the eye.
- Procedures on the eyelid or conjunctiva (chalazion, entropians, etc.) require the use of a "head drape," which usually consists of an adhesive "U" drape (or split sheet) placed around the operative site and a smaller adhesive sheet that extends across the forehead. They are placed after the towels are placed around the operative site.
- Skin prep: Prep from hairline to inferior mandibular border and from the anterior auricular border to beyond the midline. Cleanse the eyelid first, then the eyelashes, brow, and skin. Use sterile swabs soaked in prep solution to cleanse eyelashes. Rinse with sterile water. For bilateral procedures, repeat on contralateral side.

A variety of ophthalmic surgical procedures and approaches are available to the surgeon and patient. The following procedures address a variety of eye pathologies including disorders of internal structures, muscle disorders, and trauma.

Procedure 16-1 Surgical Repair of Chalazion

Surgical Anatomy and Pathology	• The meibomian glands are a type of sebaceous gland that secrete sebum from their ducts into the tears. They are located on the posterior margin and embedded in the tarsal plate (fibrous plates of cartilage that form the eyelids) of each eyelid.	• A **chalazion** is a small lump on the inner or outer surface of the eyelid. • It is caused by an inflammatory reaction to material trapped inside a meibomian gland. • A red, swollen area of the eyelid often characterizes chalazion.	• Incisional approach depends on the location of the major portion of the chalazion (e.g., transcutaneous or transconjunctival).
Preoperative Diagnostic Tests and Procedures	• Diagnosis primarily obtained from history and physical examination.		
Equipment, Instruments, and Supplies Unique to Procedure	• Chalazion eye instruments • Needle tip cautery		

Preoperative Considerations	• Position
	  • Supine
	• Anesthesia
	  • Local anesthesia
		• Skin prep
		  • As stated earlier
		• Draping
		  • As listed earlier	

Surgical Procedure: Transconjunctival Approach	1. The affected eyelid is everted with a chalazion clamp for exposure. 2. An incision is made on the inner surface with No. 11 or No. 15 blade. 3. The orbicularis muscle is incised to expose the meibomian gland. 4. The gland is incised and the lesion is curetted. **Procedural Consideration:** Clean curette with a damp Ray-Tec throughout the procedure. 5. Bleeding is controlled by cautery. **Procedural Consideration:** Irrigating the surgical site with drops of BSS shows the surgeon points of bleeding. 6. The wound is left open for drainage or approximated. 7. An eye pad is applied as dressing.		
Postoperative Considerations	**Immediate Postoperative Care** • Instruct patient not to touch the eye. • Transport to PACU.	• Prognosis of no complications: discharged same day of surgery to follow surgeon's postoperative orders.	• Complications: postoperative surgical site infection (SSI); recurrence. **Wound Classification** • Class III: contaminated

Procedure 16-2 Surgical Repair of Entropion

Surgical Anatomy and Pathology	• The eyelids consist of several layers: skin, subcutaneous, orbicularis oris muscle, tarsal plates, and palpebral conjunctiva. Additionally, there are two subunits: medial and lateral canthus tendons. The medial canthus contains the lacrimal drainage ducts and the medical canthal tendon, which is a fibrous extension of the tarsus and surrounds the lacrimal sac. The lateral canthus is located just superior to the medical canthus; fibrous extensions of the upper and lower tarsal plates join to form the lateral canthal tendon. • Entropion, abnormal inversion of the lower lid margins, causes the eyelashes to rub against the cornea, resulting in irritation, pain, and chronic tears. Usually, entropion is due to the aging process, but it can also be caused by trauma. • Involutional: This is the most common type and occurs when the canthal tendons retain their normal rigidity but the apposition of the lid to the globe has changed due to atrophy of the orbital fat, resulting in the inversion of the lower eyelid. • Congenital: This is due to hypertrophy of the oculi muscle, which causes the eyelid margin to be pushed superiorly and against the globe.
Preoperative Diagnostic Tests and Procedures	• Diagnosis primarily obtained by history and physical examination.
Equipment, Instruments, and Supplies Unique to Procedure	• Needle tip Bovie
Preoperative Preparation	• Supine position • General or local anesthesia • Bilateral skin prep: Prep both eyes as previously explained. • Draping: as previously explained
Surgical Procedure	1. A sterile marking pen is used to mark the incision to be made in the lateral canthus. 2. Using a small-gauge angled needle, local anesthetic (usually 1% xylocaine with epinephrine) is injected into the lower lid of the eye through the conjunctiva. 3. The lateral canthotomy is made with straight tenotomy scissors (Figure 16-7). **Procedural Consideration:** The surgical technologist must be ready to hold pressure and blot with Wexcel or Ray-Tec sponge while the surgeon uses electrocautery. 4. The orbicularis oculi muscle is dissected off the orbital septum with the use of the scissors. 5. The skin incision is continued across the lower lid. 6. The orbital septum is incised and the fat pockets are visualized. Extra fat is excised using the needle tip electrosurgery. Small vessels in the fat pockets are cauterized while performing this step. 7. Using smooth tissue forceps, the lower lid is gently pulled laterally toward the incision that was made in the lateral canthus to shorten the lid and correct the entropion.

(continues)

Procedure 16-2 (continued)

8. The tarsus of the eyelid is reattached to the lateral canthal tendon with 4-0 or 5-0 nonabsorbable suture, and the lower lid fascia is reattached to the orbicularis using the same type of suture.
9. Excess skin is grasped with the smooth forceps, pulled upward, and excised with the tenotomy scissors.
10. The skin incision is closed with 6-0 or 7-0 nonabsorbable suture.

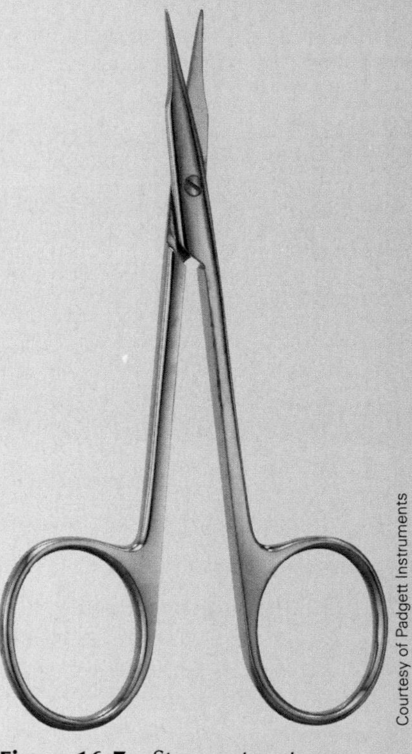

Courtesy of Padgett Instruments

Figure 16-7 Stevens tenotomy scissors

Postoperative Considerations

Immediate Postoperative Care

- Antibiotic ointment is applied to wound.
- Ice-cold compress of sterile water is intermittently applied to operative eye to reduce swelling.
- Instruct patient not to touch the eye.
- Transport to PACU.

Prognosis

- No complications: discharged same day of surgery to follow surgeon's postoperative orders.
- Complications: postoperative SSI.

Wound Classification

- Class I: clean

PROCEDURE 16-3 Iridectomy

Surgical Anatomy and Pathology	• The iris is a thin, circular membrane suspended in the aqueous humor between the cornea and crystalline lens. It is continuous with the ciliary body and connected to the cornea by the pectinate ligament. The iris divides the space between the lens and cornea into the anterior and posterior chambers. The involuntary circular smooth muscle contracts and relaxes to regulate the amount of light entering the eye through the pupil. • The **anterior chamber** is a space located between the cornea and iris. Aqueous fluid flows through the space to provide nourishment to the tissues of the eye and maintain the shape of the eye. The fluid exits the anterior chamber at the angle where the cornea and iris meet through the canal of Schlemm and the trabecular meshwork (Figure 16-8). • Iridectomy is removal of a section of iris tissue. • This is performed to reestablish communication between the anterior and posterior chambers, relieving pupillary block, and to reestablish the outflow of aqueous humor through the Schlemm canal. • Angle closure glaucoma refers to the inability of the aqueous fluid to exit the eye at the correct angle due to blockage by the iris. This places extreme pressure on the optic nerve, creating a condition called glaucoma. • Three types of iridectomy procedures are performed: peripheral, radial, and sector. The procedure is often performed at the same time as a trabeculectomy. • A laser iridectomy can be performed for treating angle closure glaucoma. The laser beam creates a small hole in the peripheral portion of the iris to connect the posterior and anterior chambers of the eye. This permits the iris to fall back away from the trabecular meshwork, opening the angle of the anterior chamber to allow the outflow of the aqueous fluid through the Schlemm canal. • Common side effects of laser iridectomy are increased intraocular pressure (IOP) and anterior uveitis.
Preoperative Diagnostic Tests and Procedures	• Diagnosis primarily obtained by history and physical examination.
Equipment, Instruments, and Supplies Unique to Procedure	• Headrest • Loupes • Ophthalmoscope • Microscope drape • Disposable eye knife • No. 57 beaver blade • 15° Super Blade • 5-Fluorouracil (5-FU)

Preoperative Preparation	• Position
	  • Supine with head on headrest
	  • Arm on operative side tucked and other arm extended on armboard
	• Anesthesia
	  • Retrobulbar block or general anesthesia (refer to Ch. 9 pp. 223–227 to review pharmacology and anesthesia as related to ophthalmic surgery)
	• Prep
	  • As previously stated
	• Draping
	  • As previously stated

(continues)

PROCEDURE 16-3 (continued)

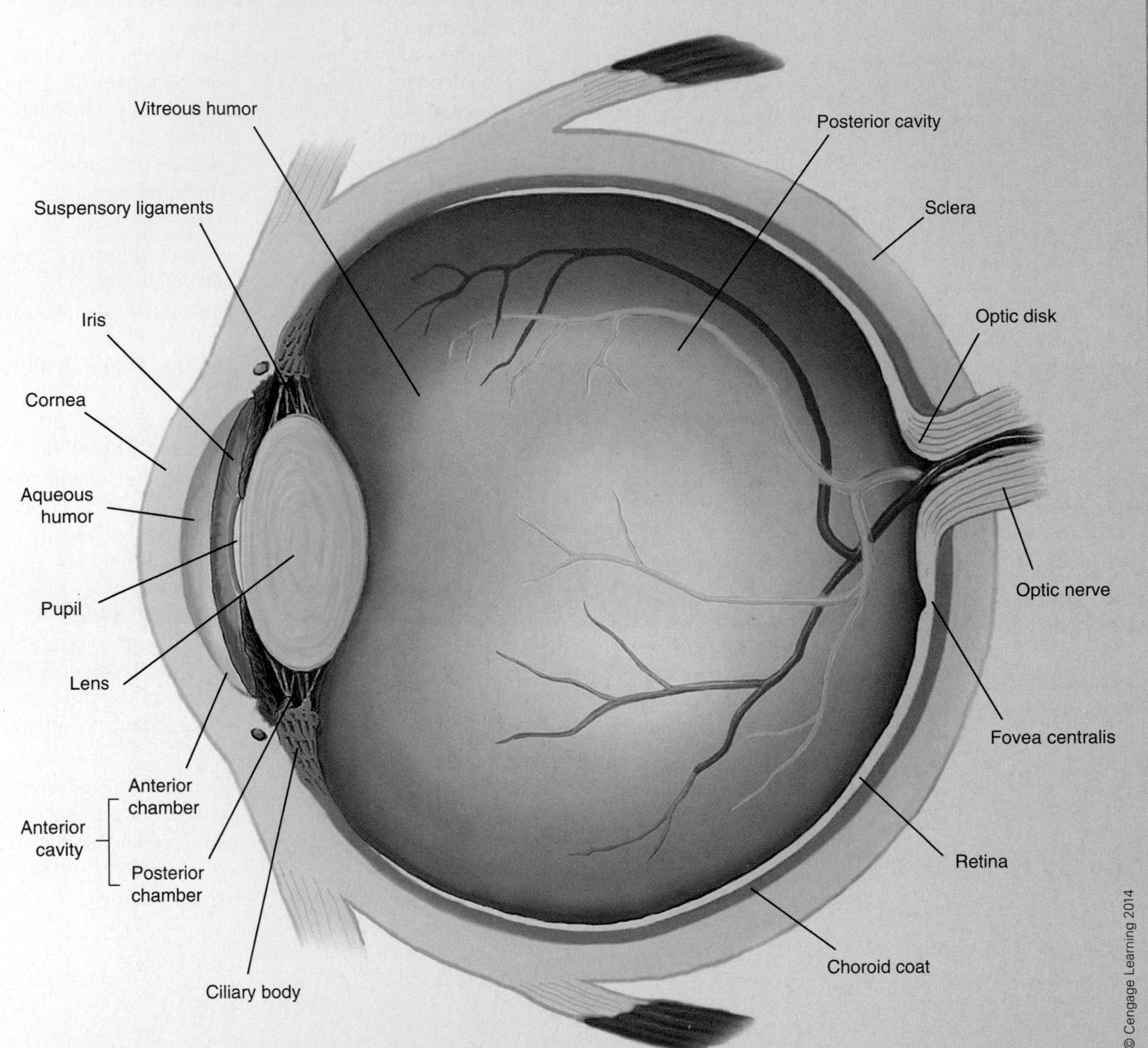

Figure 16-8 Sagittal section of the eye

Surgical Procedure

1. Before the incision is made the patient's IOP is measured with a tonometer; if too high, drugs are administered to reduce the IOP.
2. A lid speculum is placed for lid retraction (Figure 16-9).

   Procedural Consideration: Remember to periodically irrigate the eye with BSS.

PROCEDURE 16-3 (continued)

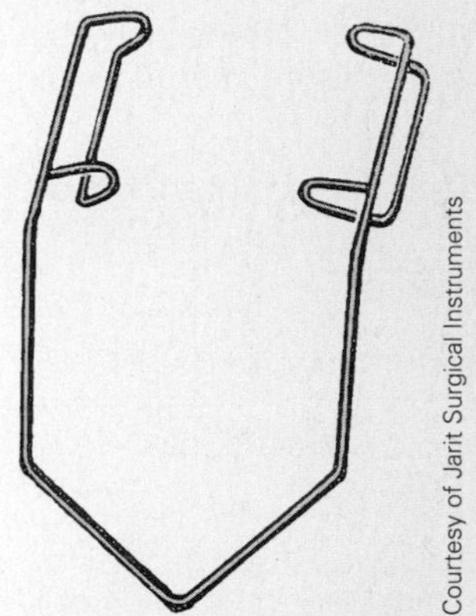

Figure 16-9 Barraquer eye speculum

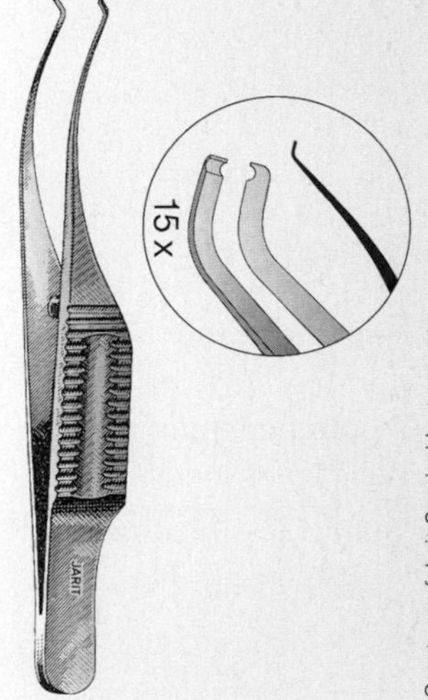

Figure 16-10 Pierse colibri forceps

3. Next, 4-0 silk sutures are placed in the superior rectus muscle for traction.

   Procedural Consideration: Using the preferred muscle hook, traction sutures are passed under the superior rectus muscle for stabilization of the eye. Free ends are tagged with a mosquito clamp or a serrafine.

4. The conjunctiva is incised using toothed Colibri forceps and knife (Figure 16-10). Tenon's capsule is dissected free from the sclera with forceps and Wescott scissors toward the limbus to create a Tenon capsule–conjunctiva flap.

   Procedural Consideration: The conjunctiva is incised with the Super Blade or a knife of the surgeon's choice. The instruments should be handed to the surgeon in such a manner that he or she does not have to look away from the microscope in order to grasp the instruments.

   A. To decrease postoperative fibrosis, the surgeon may use a sponge soaked in the chemotherapeutic agent 5-FU and mitomycin. After the Tenon capsule–conjunctival flap has been established, but before an incision is made in the sclera, the small piece of 5-FU–saturated sponge is placed between the flap and the sclera.

   Procedural Considerations: Based on surgeon's preference, the sponge is left in place 1–5 minutes and then removed. The site is thoroughly irrigated with BSS and any instruments exposed to the agents are removed from the field.

   Because 5-FU and mitomycin are antimetabolites, they must be disposed of as hazardous waste due to their toxicity. Hospital policy must be followed in the disposal of the agents and decontamination of the instruments.

   Be sure to change gloves after handling the 5-FU and mitomycin and/or contaminated instruments. It is best if the instruments can be handed off the field in a basin to the circulator but not be removed from the room until the end of the procedure.

5. Using the No. 57 beaver blade, the surgeon gently removes blood clots from the limbus. Using the disposable cautery, the surgeon marks the incision line on the sclera and, using the beaver blade, makes the incision in the sclera, creating a square or triangular scleral flap. The incision is begun at the apex of the sclera and continued upward toward the iris.

6. The scleral flap is retracted and scissors are used to remove a segment of trabecular meshwork.

   Procedural Consideration: Gently retract the scleral flap.

7. At this point in the procedure, an iridectomy is performed:

   A. A small incision is made at the superior limbus or a perpendicular incision is made in the cornea.

   B. The iris is grasped with forceps, brought up through the incision, and, using a knife or scissors, is excised.

   C. The iris is placed back into position by carefully rubbing the cornea with a blunt muscle hook (Figure 16-11).

   Procedural Consideration: Provide the muscle hook of the surgeon's preference for repositioning the iris.

   D. The corneal incision is closed with 10-0 nylon, and the limbus is closed with absorbable suture.

(continues)

PROCEDURE 16-3 (continued)

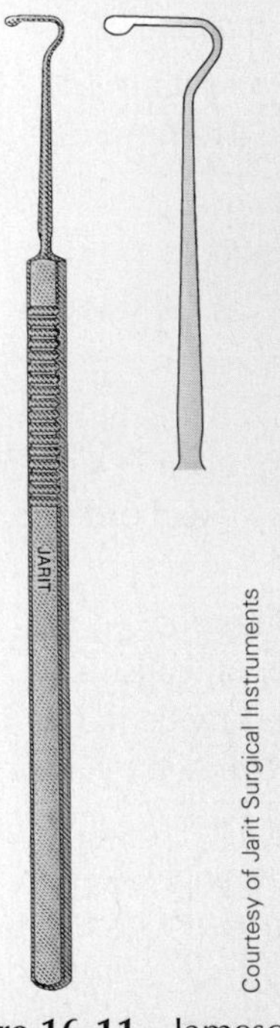

Figure 16-11 Jameson muscle hook

8. The scleral flap is closed with interrupted 10-0 nylon. Continuous 8-0 polyglactin is used to close the Tenon capsule–conjunctival flap, and the same suture is used to close the conjunctiva.

   Procedural Consideration: Follow the surgeon when the scleral flap is closed, but do not place too much tension on the suture.

9. BSS is injected into the anterior chamber.

   Procedural Consideration: Draw up the BSS and medications for injection.

10. Antibiotics and steroids are injected, and antibacterial ointment is placed into the eye.

11. Eye pad and shield are positioned over the eye.

Postoperative Considerations

Immediate Postoperative Care

- Eye patch with shield is placed.
- Transport patient to PACU.

Prognosis

- No complications: discharged same day of surgery; return to normal activities; pressure buildup is resolved due to reestablishing outflow of aqueous fluid through the Schlemm canal.
- Complications: postoperative SSI; recurrence; fluid buildup at surgical site.

Wound Classification

- Class I: clean

PROCEDURE 16-4 Strabismus Correction: Recession/Resection

Surgical Anatomy and Pathology

- The **extrinsic muscles** of the eye come from the bones of the orbit and are movable (Figures 16-12 and 16-13). Tendons attach to the eye's outer surface. Six muscles function in a coordinated fashion to move the eye in various directions, and although any eye movement may involve more than one muscle, each muscle is associated with one primary movement.

The six extrinsic muscles and function are as follows:

- Superior rectus: rotates the eye upward and medially

PROCEDURE 16-4 (continued)

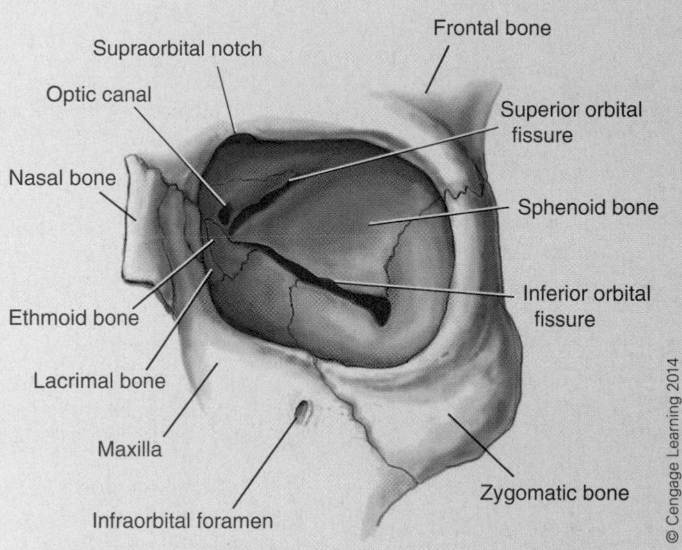

Figure 16-12 Left orbit

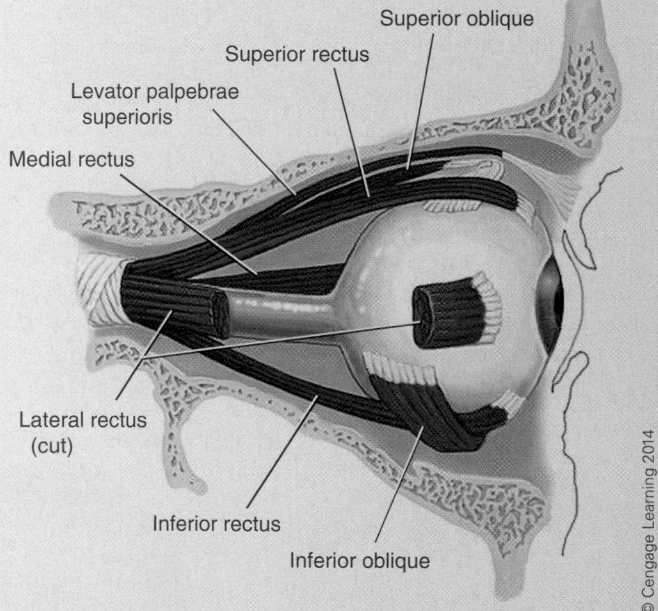

Figure 16-13 Extrinsic muscles of the eye

- Inferior rectus: rotates the eye downward and medially
- Medial rectus: rotates the eye medially
- Lateral rectus: rotates the eye laterally
- Superior oblique: rotates the eye downward and laterally
- Inferior oblique: rotates the eye upward and laterally

- The lateral and medial check ligaments limit the movement of the lateral and medial rectus. They coordinate the eyes moving together so that they are aligned when looking at something. Strabismus is a misalignment or deviation of the eyes, which normally work simultaneously to track visual objects.

(continues)

Procedure 16-4 (continued)

	• Various forms of strabismus include "crossed eyes" (esotropia) , "wall eyes" (exotropia), and "lazy eye" (amblyopic).	• Recession or resection of the muscles of the eye may be used to correct strabismus. Recession is generally more effective when	performed on the vertically acting muscles, and resection has a greater effect on the lateral rectus.
Preoperative Diagnostic Tests and Procedures	• Diagnosis primarily obtained from history and physical examination.		
Equipment, Instruments, and Supplies Unique to Procedure	• Headrest • Loupes • Disposable eye knife	• Marking pen • Xylocaine with epinephrine	• Antibiotic ophthalmic ointment

Preoperative Preparation	• Position
	  • Supine with head on headrest
	  • Arm on affected side may be tucked and the other arm
		extended on an armboard
		• Anesthesia
		  • General; sometimes local in adults
			• Skin prep
			  • As previously stated
			• Draping
			  • As previously stated

Adjustable Suture Surgery	An alternative addition to the method previously described is adjustable suture surgery. In adult strabismus, especially with diplopia, the adjustable suture technique allows more accurate alignment and placement of the field of vision is more exact. When the muscle to be recessed has been isolated, the tendon is secured with a double-armed 6-0 polyglactin suture. This suture is attached to the free end of the muscle and to the sclera; the two ends are held vertical to the eye and tied together with a knot that slides up and down the muscle sutures. The desired recession is measured and marked and the muscle is allowed to fall back into position. The knot is slipped down to the sclera. The conjunctival incision is closed using 8-0 silk, leaving the slipknot exposed for later adjustment, and the two free ends of the muscle suture are tucked into the conjunctival fornix (Figure 16-14).		

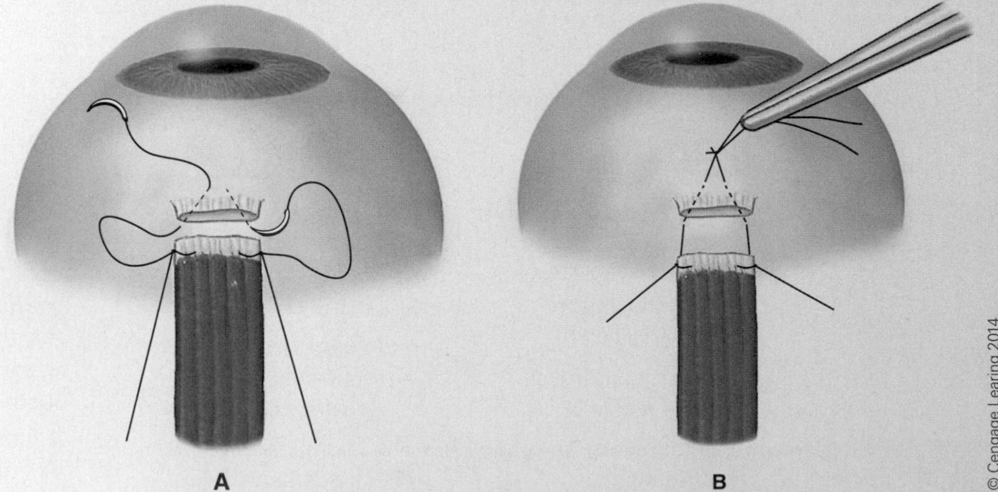

Figure 16-14 Recession by adjustable suture: (A) Suture placement, (B) adjustment

Procedure 16-4 (continued)

Surgical Procedure

1. A lid speculum is placed for lid retraction.
   Procedural Consideration: Intermittently moisten the cornea with drops of BSS.
2. Then 4-0 silk traction sutures are placed around the superior and inferior rectus muscles at the 12- and 6-o'clock positions.
   Procedural Consideration: Using the preferred muscle hook, traction sutures are passed for stabilization of the eye. Free ends are tagged with a mosquito clamp or a serrafine.
3. A radial incision is made from the limbus level with the upper border of the affected muscle.
   Procedural Consideration: Incision is made using a disposable eye knife of the surgeon's choice.
4. Westcott scissors are inserted through this incision to dissect free the conjunctiva from the limbus.
5. A second radial incision is made toward the lower border of the muscle (Figure 16-15).
   Procedural Consideration: This second radial incision forms a flap of conjunctiva–Tenon's capsule that will be dissected further to expose the upper and lower borders of the muscle.

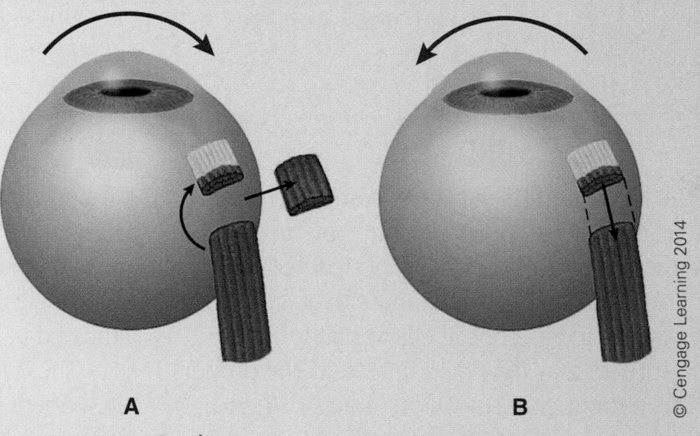

Figure 16-15 Strabismus correction: (A) Resection, (B) recession

6. A strabismus hook is introduced beneath the muscle insertion, and is swept backward, freeing the muscle from the sclera, and then forward.
   Procedural Consideration: Provide muscle hook of surgeon's preference or according to the size of the muscle.
7. Sutures are passed through the muscle for traction using 4-0 silk sutures. Disposable cautery will be needed to control bleeding at this point.
8. After this "flap" of muscle is further developed, the muscle is measured and marked at the points of recession.
   Procedural Consideration: A caliper may be used to measure the distance from the original point of insertion to the new one (Figure 16-16). The sterile marking pen may be used to mark the points of recession.

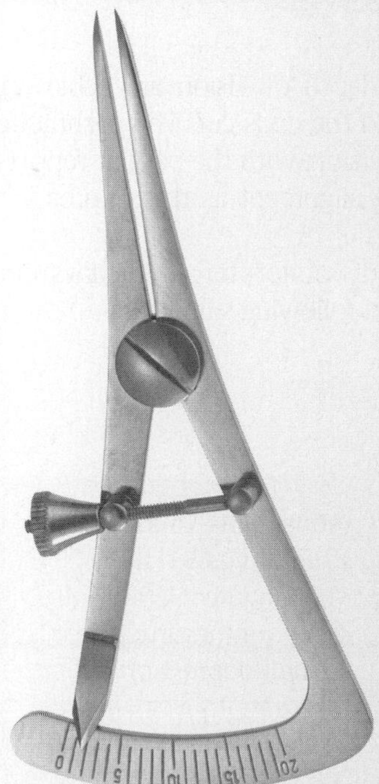

Courtesy of Padgett Instruments

Figure 16-16 Castroviejo caliper

(continues)

PROCEDURE 16-4 (continued)

9. The tendinous insertion is divided with scissors. Two absorbable sutures (6-0 polyglactin) may be placed at this point in the end of the muscles. These should be left untied with the needles attached.

   Procedural Consideration: Westcott scissors are used to divide tendinous insertion. A straight mosquito hemostat may be used to compress small blood vessels in the muscle between the suture and the insertion.

10. The muscle is reattached at the new recession point.

    Procedural Consideration: A 6-0 polyglactin suture with a needle of the surgeon's choice is used for reattachment.

11. The conjunctiva is closed using 6-0 absorbable or 8-0 silk sutures. Antibiotic drops are instilled into the eye, and usually no dressing is required.

    Procedural Consideration: Conjunctiva closed using 6-0 absorbable or 8-0 silk sutures with a needle of the surgeon's choice. Antibiotic drops may be instilled into the eye at this point.

Postoperative Considerations

Immediate Postoperative Care

- Transport to PACU.
- Eye patch dressing is placed, if the surgeon requires.

Prognosis

- No complications: discharged same day of surgery; return to normal activities; stereoscopic vision restored.
- Complications: hemorrhage; postoperative SSI.

Wound Classification

- Class I: clean

After the effects of anesthesia have completely worn off and the patient is completely awake, but not more than 24 hours after surgery, the adjustment is performed. Drops of 1% tetracaine are instilled into the conjunctival sac and a cotton applicator soaked in amethocaine is applied to the adjustment site. The sutures may now be adjusted to the proper recession while the patient reports vision status. When the proper visual alignment and depth of vision are achieved, the muscle sutures are tied and the ends cut. This technique gives the added benefit of precision, with the patient reporting proper or improper visual alignment as the sutures are adjusted.

The bulky knot may cause discomfort for several days, but the patient is usually discharged following surgery.

PROCEDURE 16-5 Scleral Buckle

Surgical Anatomy and Pathology

- The retina makes up the inner **tunic** and is the nervous membrane on which images are recorded. The outer surface is in contact with the choroid and its inner surface with the vitreous body. Posteriorly, the retina is continuous with the optic nerve. The anterior portion extends to the ciliary body. The sensory layer consists of two photoreceptors called rods and cones. Rods allow for seeing shades of gray in dim light and general shapes or outlines. Cones provide color vision and ability to see sharp images. Located in the middle region of the retina is the yellowish structure called the macula lutea. Within the center of the structure is a small depression called the central fovea, which contains only cones and is the area of highest visual acuity. Medial to the central fovea is the optic nerve; this area of the nerve contains no

Procedure 16-5 (continued)

	rods or cones; therefore vision is absent and it is referred to as the blind spot. • Retinal detachment occurs when the liquid in the vitreous cavity	passes through a retinal tear, separating the retina from the choroid. • Vision is lost wherever the retina becomes detached.	• Eventually the entire retina will detach and all useful vision in the eye will be lost.
Equipment, Instruments, and Supplies Unique to Procedure	• Retinal eye procedure instruments • Cryosurgical unit with retinal cryosurgical probe • Laser • Vitrector (if vitrectomy is indicated) • Vitrectomy set (if indicated)	• Disposable eye knife of surgeon's preference • Surgeon will select tire, band, and silicone sleeve to be soaked in surgeon's choice of antibiotic solution. • C_3F_8 (perfluoropropane) and SF_6 (sulfur hexafluoride) gas	• Indirect ophthalmoscope: 20- and 28-diopter (D) handheld lenses • Ophthalmic headlight

Preoperative Preparation	• Position
	  • Supine with donut under patient's head
	  • Arm on affected side may be tucked and the other arm extended on an armboard
		• Anesthesia
		  • Conscious sedation is used unless the procedure is expected to last for longer than 2 hours. A retrobulbar block may also be used.
			• Prep
			  • As previously stated
			• Draping
			  • As previously stated

Surgical Procedure

1. Eye speculum is inserted and conjunctiva is opened using a limbal incision.

   Procedural Consideration: Be sure to intermittently irrigate the cornea with BSS.

2. Blunt-ended scissors are used to separate the conjunctiva from the sclera.
3. An ophthalmic swab is used to clear any adherent tissue.
4. Rectus muscles are tagged using 4-0 silk sutures (or surgeon's preference suture) and sutures are secured by using a mosquito hemostat (Figure 16-17).
5. All four recti are tagged to allow the globe to be rotated in any direction during the surgical procedure.

   Procedural Consideration: The surgical technologist will be required to steady the globe in the required position by using the tag sutures.

6. The cryoprobe is used to seal any tears. Diathermy may also be used for the same purpose, but cryotherapy has become the preferred method (Figure 16-17).
7. Once cryotherapy or diathermy has been applied to all holes, an appropriately sized explant (silicone sponge or band) is selected. The explant is then sutured in place by using double-armed 5-0 nonabsorbable polyester sutures on spatulated needles. After the explant is attached, a "tire" or Silastic encircling band may be placed to support the buckle and reduce the volume of the globe, thus reducing vitreoretinal traction.
8. The strap is pulled under each rectus muscle in turn, and the free ends of the strap are positioned away from the other buckle elements.

(*continues*)

Procedure 16-5 (continued)

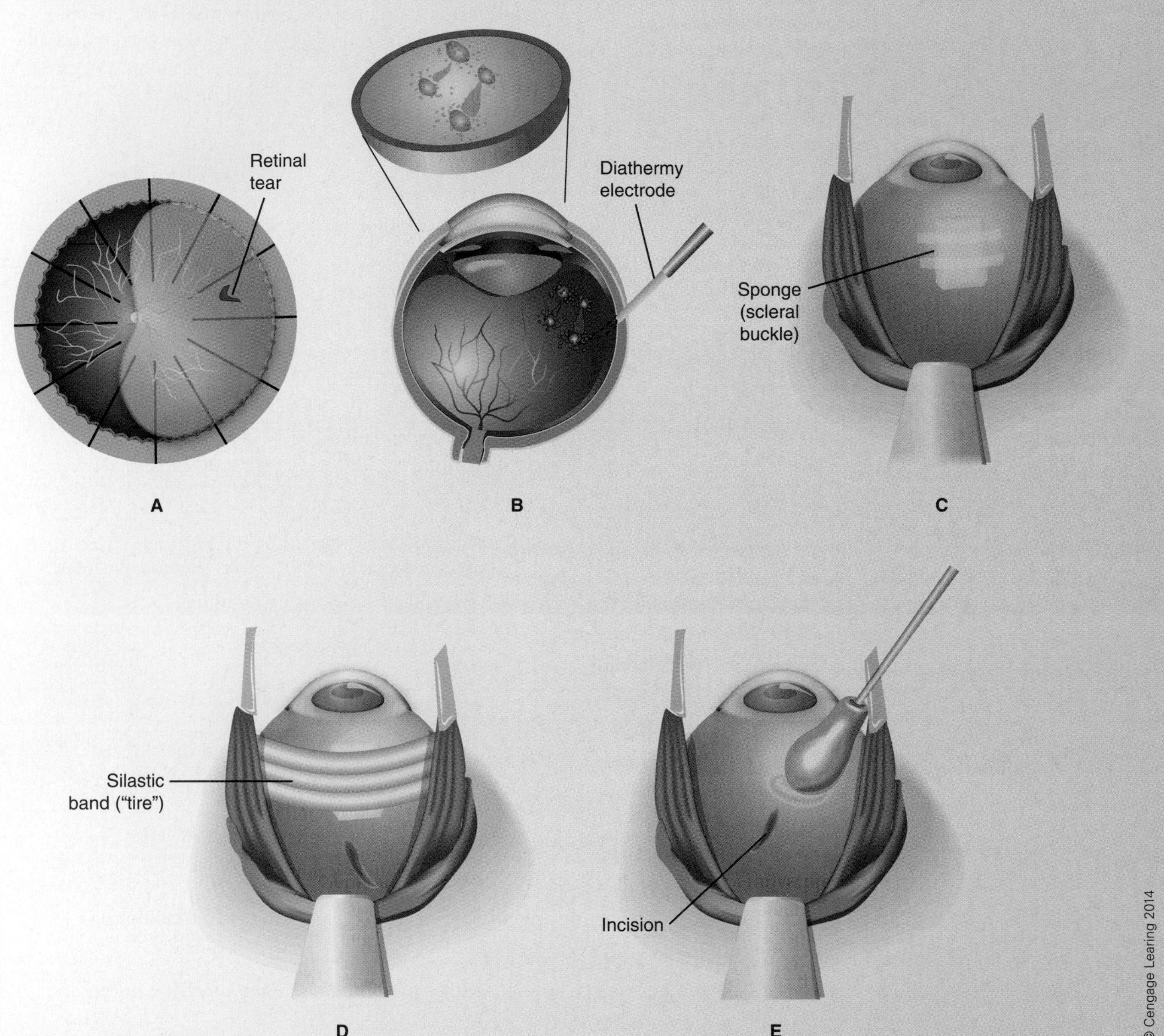

Figure 16-17 Scleral buckling procedure for treatment of retinal detachment: (A) Diagram of retinal tear, (B) diathermy used to mark area of retinal tear, (C) sponge (scleral buckle) sutured in place over retinal tear, (D) silastic band placed to support buckle, (E) incisions in sclera and choroids to facilitate drainage of subretinal fluid

9. A mattress suture is placed in each quadrant to hold the band in place.
10. During this procedure, the patient may receive an injection of intraocular gas to create pressure on the retina while subretinal fluid is reabsorbed and scars form. Gases that may be used include C_3F_8 and SF_6.
11. The gas is obtained through a handheld syringe that contains a filter. The surgeon injects the gas into the eye.

PROCEDURE 16-5 (continued)

12. An antibiotic injection of 20 mg of gentamicin may be administered subconjunctivally.
13. The eye dressing is applied.

Postoperative Considerations

Immediate Postoperative Care

- If long-acting gases were used during surgery for additional pressure on the retina, the patient must strictly maintain a special head posture to keep the gas bubble at the desired position. Patients must maintain this posture from a few days up until 2 weeks depending on the surgeon's recommendations.
- Vigorous activity must be avoided for the first month after surgery.
- Flying is contraindicated if a gas bubble is in the eye.

Prognosis

- No complications: The patient is expected to return to normal activities in 3–5 days; normal vision is restored.
- Complications: Usually there is slight immediate postoperative discomfort; extraocular infection; anterior segment ischemia; uveitis; choroidal detachment leading to glaucoma.

PROCEDURE 16-6 Dacryocystorhinostomy (DCR)

Surgical Anatomy and Pathology

- The lacrimal system consists of the lacrimal gland, which secretes the tears that keep the conjunctiva moist, and its excretory ducts, which transport the fluid to the eye surface (Figure 16-18). The fluid is carried away by the lacrimal canals into the lacrimal sac and along the nasolacrimal duct into the cavity of the nose. The lacrimal gland is located within the upper eyelid by the outer angle of the orbit, on the

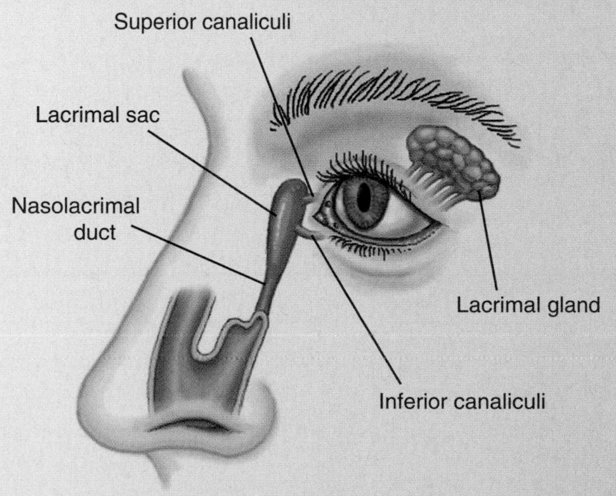

Figure 16-18 Lacrimal system

(continues)

PROCEDURE 16-6 (continued)

	inner side of the external angular process of the frontal bone. It is oval in shape and is connected by fibrous bands to the periosteum of the orbit. The surface rests on the superior and external recti muscles. Vessels and nerves enter at the posterior border and the anterior margin is located near the back part of the upper eyelid, where it is covered by conjunctiva. Six to 12 ducts exit the lacrimal gland and run at an angle beneath the	mucous membrane; they eventually separate and open through several orifices arranged in a row along the upper, outer portion of the conjunctiva. • The lacrimal canals are located at the orifices called the punctum lacrimale. There are two canals: superior and inferior canaliculi. • The lacrimal sac is the dilated segment of the nasal duct. It is positioned in a groove formed by the lacrimal	bone and nasal process of the superior maxillary bone. The superior portion of the sac is oval shaped, which narrows inferiorly at its connection with the nasolacrimal duct. • The procedure is performed when the nasolacrimal duct is obstructed by fibrous tissue or bone and has become impermeable to establish a new communication pathway between the lacrimal sac and the nose.

Equipment, Instruments, and Supplies Unique to Procedure	• Separate Mayo stand with nasal local anesthetic preparation materials
	  • Topical anesthetic: 4% cocaine
	  • Bayonet forceps
	  • Nasal speculum
	  • Packing material
	  • Medicine cup
	• Footboard, padded
	• Suction set with tubing
	• Ophthalmoscope
		• Bipolar electrosurgical unit
		• Minor set
		• **Dacryo**cystorhinostomy set
		• Kerrison rongeurs
		• Power drill with burs and cord
		• Blades: No. 15, No. 11
		• Suture: surgeon's choice, 7-0 braided silk usually used for final closure
			• Drains: catheter—10 Fr Robinson or infant feeding tube
			• Iodoform gauze packing
			• Topical anesthetic: cocaine 4 or 5% or phenylephrine 0.25% or 0.5%
			• Thrombin
			• Cautery, disposable
			• Gelfoam cut into pledgets
			• Antibiotic ophthalmic ointment

Preoperative Preparation	• Position
	  • Supine
	  • Arm on the affected side may be tucked and the other arm extended on an armboard
	  • Table in reverse Trendelenburg position; padded footboard used
	  • Head positioned with the face turned slightly away from surgeon.
		• Anesthesia
		  • Surgeon performs initial nasal preparation including the administration of local, then general anesthetic is induced.
		  • Dacryocystorhinostomy is usually performed under general anesthetic, because the procedure is often long and
			tedious due to considerable bleeding and the resultant time needed to achieve hemostasis.
			  • To minimize bleeding, hypotensive anesthesia is used.
			• Skin prep
			  • As previously stated
			• Draping
			  • As previously stated

PROCEDURE 16-6 (continued)

Surgical Procedure

1. After general anesthesia is induced, local anesthetic (tetracaine 1% with epinephrine 1:5000 two drops) is instilled into the conjunctival sac. Lidocaine 2% with epinephrine is injected at the beginning of the lacrimal crest, and lidocaine is sprayed into the anterior third of the nasal meatus. Lidocaine is injected into the mucoperiosteum after the insertion of a nasal speculum.

   Procedural Consideration: The local anesthetics help control bleeding intraoperatively and provide some pain relief in the immediate postoperative phase.

2. A curved incision is made conforming to the anterior lacrimal crest and is deepened through the orbicularis muscle to expose the entire lacrimal crest.

   Procedural Consideration: Bleeding is controlled with bipolar coagulation.

3. Retractors are inserted on each side of this incision.

   Procedural Consideration: Usually these are rake retractors.

4. Using blunt dissection, the lacrimal sac is separated from the lacrimal fossa and is retracted, and the periosteum is dissected from the lacrimal fossa.

   Procedural Consideration: A Freer elevator may be used for the dissection.

5. The anterior lacrimal crest to the entrance of the nasolacrimal duct is removed.

   Procedural Consideration: This is achieved using a Kerrison rongeur.

6. An ostium is made using either punches, a small oscillating saw, or a bur.

   Procedural Consideration: When a saw is used, the eyelids are protected with sterile gauze. Irrigation is used to keep the field clear of debris and provide cooling of the tissues.

7. A window of bone is cut and then removed using bone forceps; a mucoperiosteal elevator is used to strip the nasal mucosa within. A sphenoidal punch is used to trim the edges of this opening.

   Procedural Consideration: A sphenoidal punch will be needed to trim the edges of this opening. The surgical technologist should periodically irrigate the area (at the surgeon's request) and suction debris. Be sure to clean the tips of the punch of specimen after each use.

8. A vertical cut is made in the anterior wall of the lacrimal sac, and a probe is passed into the lumen to verify the patency of the sac.

   Procedural Consideration: Care should be taken that the probe is free of lint.

9. The wall of the sac is slit horizontally, and the nasal mucosa is incised horizontally.

   Procedural Consideration: Provide cutting instrument of surgeon's choice.

10. The flaps of the nasal mucosa and lacrimal sac are then joined.

    Procedural Consideration: Flaps are joined using 6-0 polyglactin or 9-0 monofilament nylon sutures. This is done under the microscope.

11. The incision is closed using 5-0 absorbable sutures. The skin is closed using 7-0 interrupted braided silk.

    Procedural Consideration: Bleeding is controlled using gelatin sponges. Some surgeons suture a silicone tube using absorbable sutures to the anterior wall of the sac above and a nylon suture to the nasal septum at the nares.

(*continues*)

Procedure 16-6 (continued)

Postoperative Considerations	**Immediate Postoperative Care** • The incision is sprayed with an antibiotic solution. • Eye protection is removed and an antibiotic is instilled in the conjunctival sac. • A pressure dressing is applied. • If used, the silicone tube is removed in approximately 2 weeks. **Prognosis** • No complications: The lacrimal system remains functional. • Complications: The patient will have a permanent facial scar; hemorrhage; postoperative SSI. **Wound Classification** • Class 1: clean

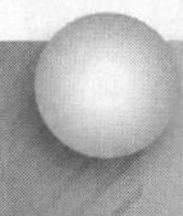

Pearl of Wisdom

Local anesthesia with epinephrine may be used during the procedure to provide additional hemostasis. The surgical technologist is expected to keep the drill and tissues cool by irrigating the area being drilled with saline. Care should be taken that all saline and bone fragments from drilling are suctioned out of the sterile field by the surgical technologist.

Procedure 16-7 Enucleation

Surgical Anatomy and Pathology	• The globe is the eyeball in its entirety that includes the conjunctiva, sclera and cornea, choroid, ciliary body, iris, retina, and crystalline lens. • **Enucleation** is excision of an eye due to malignant neoplasm, penetrating wounds, or when the eye has been so extensively damaged that no vision can be regained. • Evisceration allows the retention of the shrunken remnants of the eye. It eliminates corneal sensitivity and allows the patient to wear a prosthetic eye that will have mobility and a better cosmetic result.
Preoperative Diagnostic Tests and Procedures	• Diagnosis primarily obtained by history and physical examination. • Plain radiograph
Equipment, Instruments, and Supplies Unique to Procedure	• Enucleation instruments including cataract knife • Loupes • Headlamp • Conformer • Plastic or silicone ball • Ocular implants • Hydroxyapatite implant • Donor sclera • Chlorhexidine solution

Preoperative Preparation	• Position
	  • Supine
	  • Arm on the affected side may be tucked and the other arm extended on an armboard
	• Anesthesia
	  • General or retrobulbar
	• Skin prep
	  • As previously stated
	• Drape
	  • As previously stated

Procedure 16-7 (continued)

Surgical Procedure

1. A lid speculum is placed.
2. The conjunctiva is divided around the cornea with sharp and blunt dissection.
3. The medial lateral inferior and superior rectus muscles are divided, leaving a stump of medial rectus muscle (Figure 16-19).

   Practical Considerations: If an hydroxyapatite implant with donor sclera will be used, the four rectus muscles and two oblique muscles are identified and secured with 6-0 nonabsorbable suture to be used to reattach muscles to cut-out areas in donor sclera before muscles are divided.
4. The globe is separated from the Tenon capsule with blunt-pointed curved scissors, retractors, hemostats, and forceps. The eye is rotated laterally by grasping the stump of the medial rectus muscle.
5. The optic nerve is identified and a large, curved hemostat is passed behind the globe, and the optic nerve is clamped for 60 seconds. The hemostat is removed, the enucleation scissors are passed posteriorly, and the optic nerve is transected. The oblique muscles are severed as the eye is delivered by the stump of the medial rectus muscle (Figure 16-19).

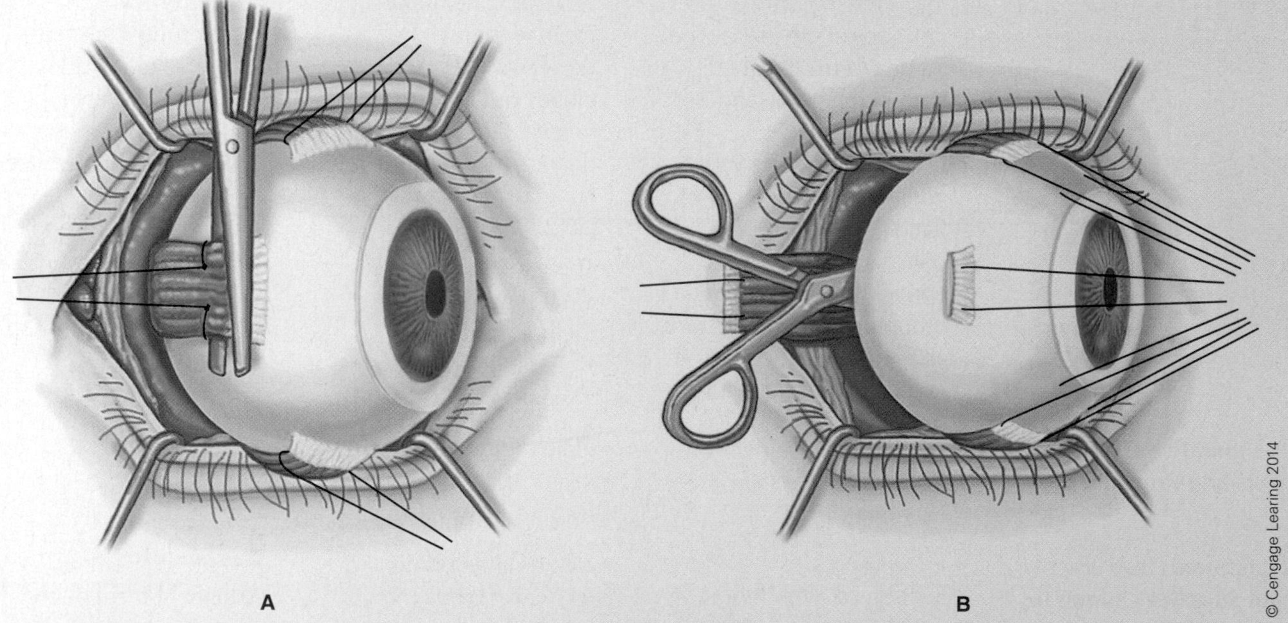

Figure 16-19 Enucleation: (A) Attachments of the globe are separated, (B) optic nerve is transected

6. The muscle cone is packed with saline-soaked sponges to obtain hemostasis.
7. The muscle cone is filled with a prosthetic sphere implant and the Tenon capsule and conjunctiva are carefully closed. Hydroxyapatite spheres, with donor sclera to reattach the muscles, are frequently placed for later use, which will allow synchronous movement.
8. A socket conformer is placed into the cul-de-sac.
9. A pressure dressing is applied.

(continues)

Procedure 16-7 (continued)

Postoperative Considerations	**Immediate Postoperative Care** • Transport to PACU. **Prognosis** • No complications: discharge same day of surgery to follow surgeon's postoperative orders. • Complications: hemorrhage; postoperative SSI. **Wound Classification** • Class 1: clean. • Class III: contaminated; fresh traumatic wound from clean source. • Class IV: dirty-infected; traumatic wound from dirty source or due to delayed treatment; presence of a foreign body.

Procedure 16-8 Keratoplasty (Corneal Transplant)

Surgical Anatomy and Pathology	• The sclera and cornea form the external tunic of the eye. Both are fibrous in structure and transparent. The sclera forms the majority of the posterior of the globe. The cornea forms the anterior sixth of the globe and is circular in shape; however, its shape varies at different periods of life, flattening out with age. It consists of four layers: epithelial cells, substantia propria, elastic lamina, and endothelial cells. The cornea allows light into the eye and bends the light rays to help the lens focus them upon the retina. To perform properly, the cornea must be clear; if not perfectly clear, vision will be decreased. Replacing cloudy or damaged corneal tissue with healthy donor tissue through a corneal transplant will correct the vision.
	• There are many causes of clouding of the cornea, including:
	  • Eye injuries that leave a dense white scar on the cornea. These injuries may be due to penetrating wounds or burns from fire or chemicals.
	  • Severe bacterial, viral, or fungal corneal infection that leads to corneal scarring (various herpesviruses are known to cause such scarring).
	  • Corneal dystrophies
	  • Inherited diseases of the cornea
	  • Cataract or other eye surgery

Preoperative Diagnostic Tests and Procedures	• Diagnosis primarily from history and physical examination • Plain radiographs
Equipment, Instruments, and Supplies Unique to Procedure	• Headrest • Suction set with tubing • Ophthalmoscope and drape • Basic eye set • Corneal procedures set (includes trephine and/or Cottingham punch) • No. 15 knife blade; No. 64 beaver blade; No. 30 Super Blade • Antibiotic ophthalmic ointment • Antibiotic solution to wash donor corneal button • Petri dish to store donor corneal button • Betamethasone

Preoperative Preparation	• Position
	  • Supine
	  • Arm on the affected side may be tucked and the other arm extended on an armboard
	• Anesthesia
	  • General
	  • Tetracaine drops may be instilled after general anesthesia is induced

PROCEDURE 16-8 (continued)

	• Skin prep
	  • As previously described
		• Draping
		  • As previously described	

Practical Considerations	• During corneal transplant surgery, only the central part of the cornea is replaced. • Corneal tissue comes from donors. An eye bank procures the tissue, examines it, and stores it until needed. The eye bank provides the donor	tissue as either a whole eye from which the cornea can be excised or prepared and sized cornea buttons. • The donor tissue is screened and tested for the presence of communicable diseases	such as hepatitis, HIV, or Cruetzfeldt-Jakob disease. • The donor cornea is sized 0.1 mm larger than the recipient opening to ensure proper fit. The surgeon may request a separate sterile table for donor cornea preparation.

Surgical Procedure

1. The medium is poured into a sterile medicine glass and the donor tissue is placed on a punching block with a concavity that conforms to the anterior corneal curvature. Calipers are used to verify the correct size of the donor cornea.

   Procedural Consideration: A portion of the medium is sent as a specimen for bacterial culture.

2. The endothelial surface is placed facing upward. The donor cornea is punched using a Cottingham punch to the correct size for placement. A punch of slightly greater diameter than the punch used for the patient's host eye is used for the donor cornea.

   Procedural Consideration: The donor cornea is stored in a safe place on the sterile field for later use.

3. The eyelids are retracted and 4-0 silk traction sutures are placed at the insertions of the superior and inferior rectus muscles and clamped to the surgical drape using a mosquito.

   Procedural Consideration: These sutures are used to fix and steady the eye while the graft bed is prepared. If a cataract is present, the surgeon can remove it in addition to the corneal transplant operation. If an artificial lens is already in place and it is believed to be responsible for the clouding of the cornea, the artificial lens can be replaced with a type of lens less likely to irritate the donor cornea tissue.

4. A **trephine** is placed on the cornea and is used to make the corneal cut around the cornea and into the anterior chamber (Figure 16-20).

   Procedural Consideration: If the trephine cut is complete, the cornea is removed; if incomplete, corneal scissors or a diamond knife is used to finish the cut.

5. The edge of the donor corneal disc is slid from its silicone base, laid in the trephine opening, and placed in position.

   Procedural Consideration: In some cases, temporary indirect sutures will have been placed prior to this step; they are now tensioned to hold the graft in place.

6. The transplant is gently held in place while 10-0 polyamide sutures are used to suture the graft in place.

   Procedural Consideration: The surgical technologist may be asked to wet the suture with saline prior to passing it to the surgeon.

7. After the graft is sutured in place, BSS or acetylcholine solution is injected into the anterior chamber through a fine cannula at the graft margin.

   Procedural Consideration: This cannula is used to ensure that the wound is watertight.

(continues)

Procedure 16-8 (continued)

8. Antibiotic drops are instilled and the traction sutures removed. The eye is covered with antibiotic-impregnated gauze, an eye pad, and a shield.

   Procedural Consideration: Medication of choice and dressing are prepared in advance.

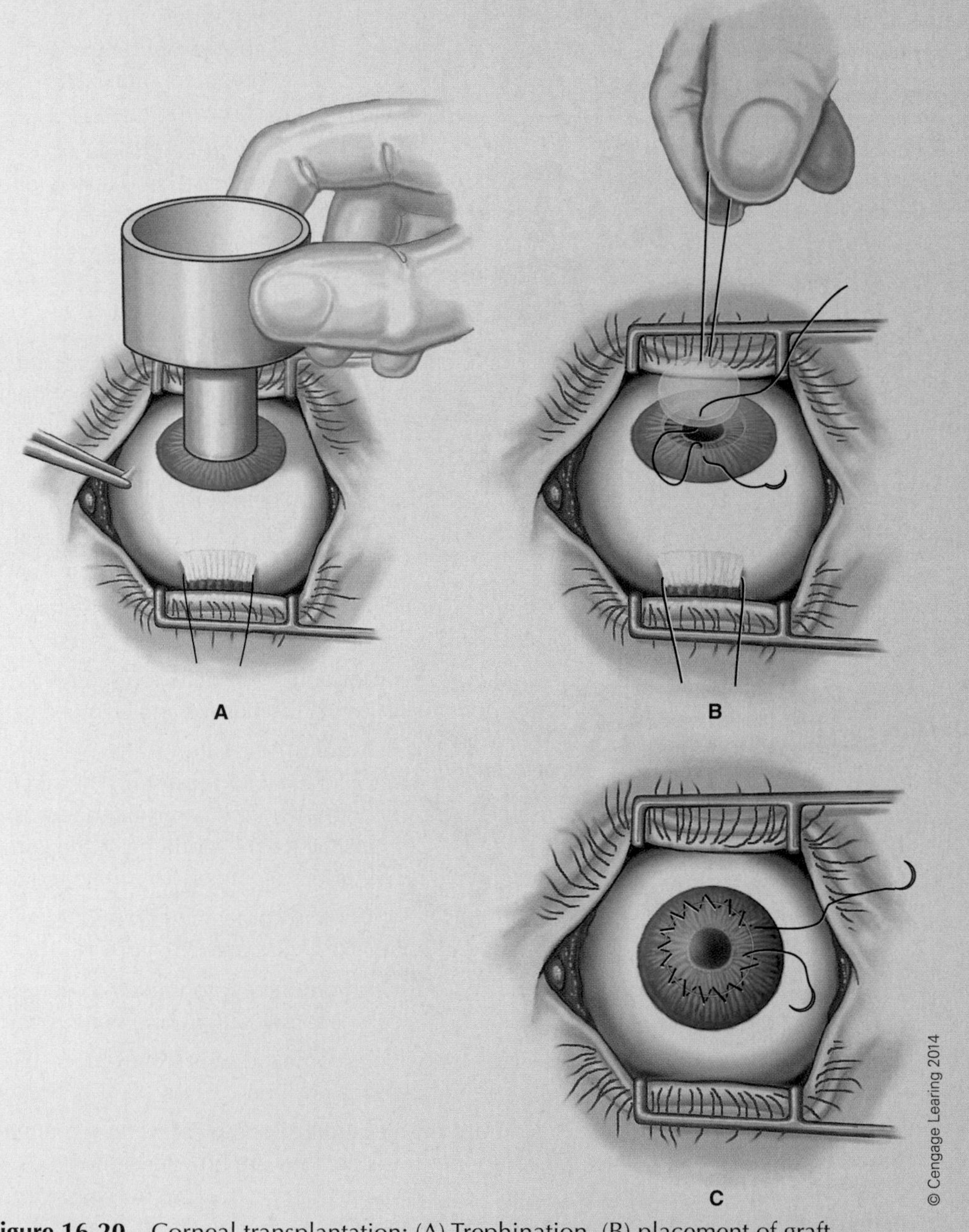

Figure 16-20 Corneal transplantation: (A) Trephination, (B) placement of graft, (C) graft sutured on position

PROCEDURE 16-8 (continued)

Postoperative Considerations

Immediate Postoperative Care

- Transport to PACU.
- The eye is patched overnight and examined the next day.

Prognosis

- Usually there is little or no discomfort after surgery.
- Occasionally, further surgery may be required to minimize residual astigmatism.
- The success of transplantation surgery is often related to the original cause of the underlying corneal disease process. Transplant procedures resulting from abnormally shaped corneas due to **kerato**conus or for corneal clouding following cataract surgery typically have very high success rates. Conversely, transplants due to scarring of the cornea from infections, such as herpes, typically have a lower success rate.
- Although risks are present, the success rate of corneal transplantation is very high. It enjoys the highest success rate of any transplant procedures commonly performed.
- Corneal graft rejection rarely occurs within 2 weeks and may occur as late as 20 years following corneal transplant. Pain, light sensitivity, redness, and decreasing vision are warning signs of corneal tissue rejection and indicate the need for immediate medical attention. When started at the first signs of tissue rejection, steroids (drops, injections, and/or pills) may be effective in halting the rejection process. If the rejection process continues, the donor tissue becomes cloudy, resulting in blurry vision. Often, a repeat transplant may be performed.
- Complications: hemorrhage; infection; rejection of transplanted tissue; impairment or permanent loss of vision; scarring; glaucoma; retinal swelling; cataract formation; swelling of the graft.

Wound Classification

- Class I: clean

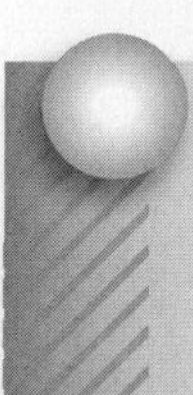

PEARL OF WISDOM

Prior to the induction of anesthesia, the surgical technologist should always confirm that the donor cornea has arrived.

Cataract Extraction

Two methods of cataract extraction are commonly used. **Extracapsular and intracapsular cataract extraction** methods are available for removal of the opaque lens. With either method, an artificial lens may be inserted.

PROCEDURE 16-9 Extracapsular Cataract Extraction

Surgical Anatomy and Pathology

- The lens is a transparent, biconvex structure that is situated behind the pupil anterior to the vitreous body. It is encircled by the ciliary processes and encapsulated in a transparent, elastic, delicate membrane. Anteriorly, the lens contacts the border of the iris forming the posterior chamber of the eye. It is held in position by the suspensory

(continues)

Procedure 16-9 (continued)

	ligament. The central points of its anterior and posterior surfaces are known as its anterior and posterior poles. • The word "cataract" is used to describe a lens that has become opaque. Cataracts are a condition affecting the eye, not a disease. As the lens gradually clouds, less light is able to pass	through, blurring and distorting images received by the retina. Vision is gradually impaired; if untreated, a cataract can cause needless blindness. • Cataracts are usually white but may take on a yellow or brown color. • The development of cataracts is usually due to the normal part of the	aging process, but they can develop due to other reasons, including traumatic cataracts resulting from an injury or blow to the eye, use of certain drugs, exposure to harmful chemicals, exposure to excessive sunlight, and congenital cataracts.
Preoperative Diagnostic Tests and Procedures	• Preoperative diagnosis obtained from	history and physical examination	
Equipment, Instruments, and Supplies Unique to Procedure	• IOP reducer cuff • Disposable cystotome • Headrest • Ophthalmoscope and drape • Phacoemulsification unit, disposable attachments, and handpiece	• Irrigator/aspirator unit • Cataract extraction tray • Intraocular lens implant (IOL) • Blades: No. 15, No. 64 disposable beaver blade, No. 30 Super Blade • Antibiotic ophthalmic ointment	• Anesthetic for retrobulbar block: lidocaine 2% with epinephrine • Anti-inflammatory agent: betamethasone drops • Viscoelastic agent such as Healon

Preoperative Preparation	• Position
	  • Supine
	  • Arm on the affected side may be tucked and the other arm extended on an armboard
		• Head may be supported on a headrest
		• Anesthesia
		  • Local with retrobulbar block
			• Skin prep
			  • As previously explained
			• Draping
			  • As previously explained

Practical Considerations	• Intracapsular cataract extraction involves a large incision and the entire capsule is removed; suturing is required for closing the incision. • Extracapsular cataract extraction is performed through a small incision and only the lens is removed; incision is self-sealing with no sutures required. • IOLs are small prescription lenses placed inside the eye for clear lens replacement surgery.	IOLs may be foldable or hard. Foldable lenses are made of silicone or acrylic and can be rolled up and placed inside a tube that is inserted through the small incision, or folded by locking forceps, and once inside the eye the IOL unfolds. Hard plastic lenses are rarely used and must be inserted through a larger incision. • Phakic lenses are a type of IOL that are implanted without removing the eye's natural lens.	• Phacoemulsification is a variation of the irrigation/aspiration technique. The tip of the phaco handpiece is inserted through the small incision and ultrasonic energy fragments the lens while simultaneously irrigating and aspirating the fragments. After the nucleus of the lens is removed, the irrigating/aspirating unit is used to remove the remaining pieces of cortex.

Procedure 16-9 (continued)

Surgical Procedure

1. The lid is retracted.

   Procedural Consideration: Provide retractor of choice. Prepare bridle suture.

2. A superior rectus bridle suture, as in the previous procedures, is placed for manipulation of the globe.

   Procedural Consideration: Suture is clamped and attached to surgical drape with a mosquito. Depending on the type of extraction method the surgeon prefers, step 2 may be eliminated.

3. An incision is made, either corneoscleral or corneal.

   Procedural Consideration: A corneal incision is self-sealing.

4. The anterior chamber is entered with the knife.

   Procedural Consideration: Beaver blade preferred by surgeon will be needed.

5. The corneal incision is followed with **iridotomy** or iridectomy if the posterior capsule is not intact.

   Procedural Consideration: Iridotomy is preferred.

6. The anterior capsule is incised and the lens is expressed using method of surgeon preference.

7. Pass sharps carefully. The surgeon may not be willing to look away from the microscope. This is one situation in which the surgical technologist may be required to accept sharps from the surgeon. The specimen may not be required to be sent to pathology according to facility policy.

8. An intraocular implant may be inserted below the iris.

   Procedural Consideration: The surgeon will select a lens prosthesis prior to surgery; the preselected lens is opened and prepared when requested.

9. Acetylcholine solution is injected into the anterior chamber to constrict the pupil, pulling the iris back into position.

   Procedural Consideration: Syringes are preloaded and labeled. Do not cover increment markings on the syringe with the label.

10. Sterile air is injected into the anterior chamber to maintain the shape of the chamber.

    Procedural Consideration: Be certain that correct syringe is passed. The room may be darkened to enhance the microscopic view.

11. A previously placed 12-o'clock suture is tied, and two interrupted sutures are placed in the cornea.

    Procedural Consideration: If possible, prepare suture in advance. This may not be possible if the surgeon prefers a nonlocking needle holder.

    Note: Steps 12 and 13 may be eliminated if the phacoemulsification process is used.

12. The remainder of the incision is closed with continuous or interrupted 10-0 sutures.

    Procedural Consideration: Prepare Miochol according to manufacturer's instructions. Miochol must be mixed on the field by the surgical technologist immediately prior to use.

13. Air in the chamber is replaced with Miochol, and the wound is checked for leaks.

    Procedural Consideration: Air extraction syringe will be used first, followed immediately by the Miochol.

14. Antibiotic drops are instilled, and the superior rectus retention suture is removed.

15. The speculum is removed and the eye dressed with antibiotic-impregnated gauze, an eye pad, and a shield.

(continues)

PROCEDURE 16-9 (continued)

Postoperative Considerations	**Immediate Postoperative Care** • Patient is transported to PACU. • Patient is discharged same day.	**Prognosis** • No complications: Patient returns to normal activities in 1–3 days. Vision is expected to be markedly improved and corrective glasses are not needed.	• Complications: hemorrhage; postoperative SSI. **Wound Classification** • Class I: clean

PROCEDURE 16-10 Vitrectomy

Surgical Anatomy and Pathology	• The posterior cavity of the eye is larger than the anterior cavity, since it occupies all of the space posterior to the lens, suspensory ligaments, and ciliary body. The posterior cavity contains a substance, with a consistency similar to soft gelatin, called vitreous humor. Vitreous humor helps maintain sufficient pressure inside the eye to prevent the eyeball from collapsing. The hyaloid membrane encloses the whole of the vitreous humor. • The incision into the globe is through the pars	plana. The pars plana is one of the three layers of the eye located near the point where the iris and sclera join, which is a section of the uvea, also called the vascular tunic. • The vitreous humor may opacify secondary to retinal hemorrhage, endophthalmitis, trauma, and formation of adhesive bands after cataract surgery. • When a retinal tear occurs, blood vessels may also be torn and a vitreous hemorrhage may occur. Because of the tear, a detachment may also occur. A vitrectomy	is performed to remove the blood so the surgeon can view whether there is a detachment. • Traction retinal detachment is another pathology that involves the vitreous humor. When vitreous humor pulls on scar tissue, the retina may detach. When the detachment involves the macula, central vision is lost. Scar tissue may wrinkle the retina and also cause visual loss. The vitreous humor and scar tissue are removed from the surface of the retina, releasing the traction.
Preoperative Diagnostic Tests and Procedures	• Diagnosis obtained by history and physical examination; however, as	previously stated, a vitrectomy procedure will be performed in order for	the surgeon to see whether a retinal tear or detachment occurred.
Equipment, Instruments, and Supplies Unique to Procedure	• Headrest • Ophthalmoscope and drape • Prism vitrectomy lens (available in O.R. varying degrees, e.g. 20°, 30°, 50°) • Vitreoretinal system and sterile accessories • Vitrectomy handpiece	• Endoilluminator—light source, handpiece, cable—provides fiberoptic microillumination for intraocular use • Endocoagulator (bipolar or wetfield)—handpiece, cable—low-current cautery for use inside or	outside the eye; different tips are used for each • Argon laser equipment and probe if indicated—endo or indirect capability • **Ocutome**—instrument with which the vitreous is cut and aspirated; variable cut and aspiration rates are

Procedure 16-10 (continued)

	controlled from the main panel • Fragmatome—ultrasonic instrument with aspiration; used to remove cloudy lens, which obstructs the view of the retina • Retinal procedures tray • Vitrectomy instruments including caliper, vitreous scissors, membrane pick, foreign body forceps,	curved and straight McPherson Lister, Pierse-Hoskins, scleral plug forceps • Membrane peeler/cutter (MPC)—microscissors used to cut and peel membranes from the retina; it has aspiration capability • Blades: vitrectomy blade, No. 15 • Cryoprobe and cable	• Infusion cannula • Antibiotic ophthalmic ointment • Betamethasone • Healon • Acetylcholine with filter • Mydricaine No. 2 • Aerobic and anaerobic cultures • Sclerotomy plugs

Preoperative Preparation	• Position
	  • Supine with slight reverse Trendelenburg with neck extended and supported on a roll sheet
	  • Arm on the affected side may be tucked and
		the other arm extended on an armboard
		  • Head may be supported on a headrest
		• Anesthesia
		  • Local; should include a retrobulbar block
			• Skin prep
			  • As previously stated
			• Draping
			  • As previously stated

Practical Considerations	• Since reverse Trendelenburg is used antiembolic hose should be used. • Vitrectomy handpiece is attached to sterile tubing by the surgical technologist who hands off the end to the circulator to attach to the ocutome unit. • Equipment should be tested before the procedure starts, including testing the cutting function of the vitrector. • The surgeon may want to cultures taken of the vitreous washings. • The infusion cannula should be primed with the solution of the surgeon's preference and confirm air bubbles have been removed.	• The vitrector unit rates (infusion, cutting, aspiration) should be set according to surgeon's preference prior to the start of the procedure. • *Intraocular gases:* Usually either C_3F_8 or SF_6; when mixed with sterile air, these gases have the property of remaining in the eye for extended periods of time (up to 2 months). The eye's own natural fluid eventually replaces them. Gas is useful for flattening a detached retina and keeping it attached while healing occurs. Gas injection is also used to close macular holes. It is frequently necessary for the patient to maintain a certain head position following surgery when gas is used. Possible	complications of intraocular gas include progression of cataracts and elevated IOP. • *Silicone oil:* This is sometimes used instead of gas to keep the retina attached postoperatively. Silicone remains in the eye until it is removed (often necessitating a second surgery). The technique is advantageous when long-term support of the retina is required. Unlike what they experience with gas, patients are still able to see through clear silicone oil. Positioning is less critical with silicone oil; therefore, it may be used with patients who are unable to position themselves appropriately postoperatively. Like gas, silicone oil may promote

(continues)

PROCEDURE 16-10 (continued)

cataracts, cause glaucoma, and damage the cornea.

- *Endophotocoagulation:* This technique uses a laser to treat intraocular structures. This modality is often used to treat retinal tears in the setting of retinal detachment and is frequently used to treat proliferative diabetic retinopathy as well.
- *Lensectomy:* Lensectomy is the removal of the eye's crystalline lens during a vitrectomy procedure. This is sometimes performed when there is a cataract, which prevents the surgeon from adequately visualizing the internal structures. A lensectomy may also be necessary to gain access to and remove scar tissue during complicated retinal detachment or diabetic retinopathy procedures. The natural lens can be replaced with a clear lens implant at a later date or during the same surgical procedure. Lensectomy is usually performed using high-frequency ultrasound.

Surgical Procedure

1. The eyelids are retracted with a speculum and mydricaine No. 2 is injected subconjunctivally to dilate the pupil.

   Procedural Consideration: Provide lid retractor of surgeon's choice. Medication should be prepared and labeled in anticipation of need.

2. A small incision is made in the conjunctiva to expose the sclera.

   Procedural Consideration: Provide beaver blade of surgeon's choice. A 5-0 suture is typically placed in advance to eventually support the infusion cannula.

3. A sclerotomy is made under the microscope.

   Procedural Consideration: A 20-gauge microvitreoretinal blade may be used for the sclerotomy.

4. This sclerotomy is placed 3–4 mm from the limbus. The blade is inserted until it is seen through the pupil; it is withdrawn and the infusion cannula is inserted through this sclerotomy (Figure 16-21).

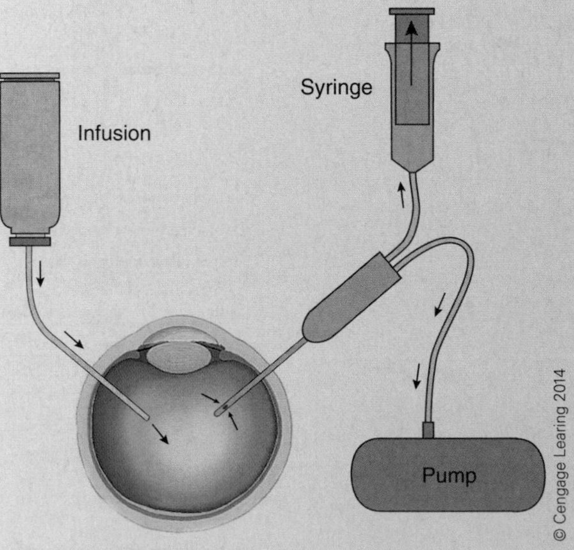

Figure 16-21 Vitrectomy

Procedure 16-10 (continued)

Procedural Consideration: The infusion cannula must be primed with solution of the surgeon's choice and air bubbles must be removed. The previously inserted suture is tightened hold this cannula in place.

5. Two more sclerotomies are made, one at the upper border of the lateral rectus muscle and one at the medial sides of the lateral rectus muscle. The endoilluminator is inserted through one of these sclerotomies, and the ocutome probe or other instruments is inserted through the final sclerotomy.

   Procedural Consideration: An irrigating contact lens may be placed on the eye. The surgical assistant moves this lens with the globe as the surgeon moves the globe. At this point, the surgical technologist will have tested the suction vacuum and assessed the cutting function of the vitrector, and also ensuring that the unit rates have been set for proper infusion, cutting, and aspiration according to the surgeon's preference.

6. The vitrectomy is performed using the maximum cutting speed on the instrument.

   Procedural Consideration: The surgeon controls the vitrector via a foot switch. Be sure it is in a comfortable, easy-to-access location. Other instruments, such as intraocular scissors or foreign body forceps, may be introduced through the same sclerotomy to accomplish the surgical objective. Prior to removal of instruments from the eye, infusion should be stopped.

7. When the procedure is complete, the instruments are withdrawn and sclerotomy plugs are inserted if necessary.

   Procedural Consideration: The surgeon may request that cultures of the vitreous washings be sent to pathology.

8. The sclerotomies are closed using 9-0 nylon sutures, infusion site last. The conjunctiva is closed with 6-0 polyglactin suture.

   Procedural Consideration: Suture should be prepared in advance of need.

9. A subconjunctival injection of betamethasone and gentamicin may be given.

   Procedural Consideration: Medications and dressing materials are ready for use. Assist with dressing application as needed

Postoperative Considerations

Immediate Postoperative Care

- An eye patch may be placed at the surgeon's request. The patient should not strain or cough, as this may increase IOP.

Prognosis

- No complications: Vision is expected to improve; return to normal activities in 1–2 weeks; discharged the same day of surgery.
- Complications: hemorrhage; postoperative SSI.

Wound Classification

- Class I: clean

Procedure 16-11 Repair of Traumatic Eyelid Laceration

Surgical Anatomy and Pathology	• See previous description of anatomy. • Traumatic laceration of the eyelid can be due to blunt and penetrating trauma, including dog bites, penetration by a small tree limb, hit by human fist, and cut by glass such as during a vehicle accident.
Preoperative Diagnostic Tests and Procedures	• History and physical examination and presenting traumatic wound
Equipment, Instruments, and Supplies Unique to Procedure	• Headrest (if adult patient) • Basic eye procedure tray • Eyelid and conjunctival instruments • Veirs rod: 10-mm-diameter rod made of stainless steel • Blades: No. 11 and/or No. 15 • Topical anesthetic, such as tetracaine, of surgeon's preference • Local anesthetic of surgeon's preference (often xylocaine 2% with epinephrine) • Antibiotic ophthalmic ointment

Preoperative Preparation	• Supine
	  • Arm on operative side may be tucked in at the patient's side and the other arm extended on an armboard
	• Local or general anesthesia
	  • Local anesthesia will include instillation of tetracaine drops
	• Skin prep
	  • As previously described; however, prep must be very gentle in order to prevent further damage to laceration.
	• Draping
	  • As previously described

Practical Considerations	• Repair of the wound is meticulously performed in order to line up the skin lines in order to preserve eyelid function and bunching of the skin. • Confirm with the surgeon if the canaliculus is involved in the wound; if involved the Veir rod will be needed.
Surgical Procedure	1. Canaliculus not involved: a. Lateral canthotomy is performed in order to prevent traction and tension on the wound closure. b. Sutures are placed through the lid margins restore stability. c. The tarsal plate is approximated with absorbable sutures. d. Skin and canthus are approximated with nonabsorbable sutures. 2. Canaliculus involved a. Veirs rod is placed through the laceration and the canaliculus is approximated with nonabsorbable suture around the rod. b. The rod is removed. c. The subcutaneous layer and skin are closed with nonabsorbable suture.
Postoperative Considerations	**Immediate Postoperative Care** • Transport to PACU. **Prognosis** • No complications: Depending on age of patient and extent of wound, patient may be hospitalized overnight and discharged the next day. • Complications: hemorrhage; postoperative SSI **Wound Classification** • Class II: clean-contaminated • Class III: contaminated • Class IV: dirty infected

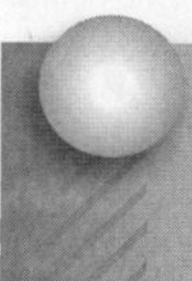

PEARL OF WISDOM

Many pieces of complex equipment are required. Always check equipment function before the procedure begins.

CASE STUDY John is a 73-year-old man. His vision has become progressively darker and more cloudy in his left eye. He has suffered no pain during this slow loss of vision and states that the loss of vision has occurred equally across his entire left field of vision. John is diagnosed with a cataract in his left eye.

1. What surgical intervention will be performed?
2. What special large piece of equipment will be required in order to perform this procedure?
3. Why must powder be meticulously removed from the gloves for this procedure?

QUESTIONS FOR FURTHER STUDY

1. What type of energy is used during phacoemulsification?
2. List two possible complications of intraocular gas injection.
3. What is meant by the term *retrobulbar* block?

BIBLIOGRAPHY

Albert, D. M., and Brightbill, F. S. (Eds.). (1999). *Ophthalmic surgery: Principles and techniques.* Malden, MA: Blackwell Science Inc.

Association of Surgical Technologists. (2011). *Core curriculum for surgical technology* (6th ed.). Littleton, CO: Association of Surgical Technologists.

Azar, D. T., Gatinel, D., and Hoangxuan, T. (Eds.). (2006). *Refractive surgery* (2nd ed.). St. Louis: Mosby.

Chignell, A. H., and Wong, D. (1998). *Management of vitreo-retinal disease: A surgical approach.* New York: Springer.

Folk, J. C., and Pulido, J. S. (1997). Laser photocoagulation of the retina and choroid. *Ophthalmology Monographs,* 11.

Goldman, M. A. (2007). *Pocket guide to the operating room* (3rd ed.). Philadelphia: F. A. Davis.

Henderson, B. A. (Ed.). (2007). *Essentials of cataract surgery.* Thorofare, NJ: SLACK Incorporated.

Phillips, N. F. (2007). *Berry and Kohn's operating room technique* (11th ed.). St. Louis: Mosby.

Stallard, H. B. (1989). *Stallard's eye surgery.* St. Louis: Elsevier Science.

CHAPTER

17

Otorhinolaryngologic Surgery

CASE STUDY Theodore, a 16-month-old male, has been brought by his father to the otorhinolaryngologist's office. The parent states that Theo has a cold and is suffering from a runny nose. The discharge is yellow and has a foul odor. Theo was uncooperative during the exam, but the physician was able to visualize a foreign object lodged between the middle and superior turbinates in his left nostril. Surgical removal of the object is scheduled for the next morning at the local surgery center.

1. Theo's surgery is considered urgent rather than emergent. Why?
2. Why is surgical removal of the object necessary?
3. What special equipment and supplies will be required for the procedure? Will the surgical technologist be required to employ sterile technique for the procedure?

OBJECTIVES

After studying this chapter, the reader should be able to:

A 1. Recognize the relevant anatomy of the ear, nose, and upper **aerodigestive tract.**

P 2. Summarize the pathology that prompts otorhinolaryngologic surgical intervention and the related terminology.

3. Determine any preoperative otorhinolaryngologic diagnostic procedures/tests.
4. Determine any otorhinolaryngologic preoperative and intraoperative preparation procedures.
5. Indicate the names and uses of otorhinolaryngologic instruments, supplies, and drugs.
6. Indicate the names and uses of special otorhinolaryngologic equipment.

O 7. Summarize the surgical steps of the otorhinolaryngologic procedures.

8. Interpret the purpose and expected outcomes of the otorhinolaryngologic procedures.
9. Recognize the immediate postoperative care and possible complications of the otorhinolaryngologic procedures.

S 10. Assess any specific variations related to the preoperative, intraoperative, and postoperative care of the otorhinolaryngologic patient.

SELECT KEY TERMS

aerodigestive tract	dynamic equilibrium	laryngo-	polysomnography
apnea	epiglottis	myringo-	rhino-
carina	epistaxis	olfaction	-sclerosis
cholesteatoma	Gelfoam	oropharynx	SMR
chondroradionecrosis	glottis	oto-	T&A
congenital	hypertrophy	polyp	UPPP

INTRODUCTION TO OTORHINOLARYNGOLOGIC SURGERY

Otorhinolaryngologic surgery ranges from simple procedures such as a **myringo**tomy to complex procedures such as laryngectomy. The specialty involves treating diseases and trauma as well as plastic surgery procedures that often include microsurgery on very small structures. The surgical technologist must be familiar with not only the surgical procedures but also the large number of specialty instruments and equipment. This chapter will present the commonly performed surgical procedures in order to familiarize the student with otorhinolaryngologic surgery.

EAR PROCEDURES

Many surgical options are available to correct deformities of the ear and restore function.

Diagnostic Procedures/Tests for the Ear

The tuning fork is a small two-pronged metal device that emits a clear tone of a fixed pitch when tapped. The tuning fork is used as a diagnostic tool to perform an initial assessment of a patient's level of hearing, and may be used intraoperatively on a patient under local anesthesia to determine improvement in his or her condition.

Audiometry is a more sophisticated method of testing a patient's hearing. The audiometer is a machine capable of emitting a tone at several different pitches and volumes. The patient indicates to the examiner which sounds are heard. The patient must be of an age and mental capacity to cooperate with the examiner. The patient may wear headphones for this examination or be placed in a soundproof room to eliminate distractions. The audiogram can be helpful in determining the amount of damage to the sound conduction system, and very valuable in determining the type of hearing aid that will be most helpful to the patient. The results are generally reported in graph form.

The otoscope is a handheld, lighted instrument for viewing the external auditory canal (Figure 17-1). A speculum is inserted in the patient's ear by placing gentle traction on the pinna to straighten the canal. Many conditions of the middle ear may also be visualized with the use of the otoscope. The translucent tympanic membrane is regarded as a window to the middle ear. With very few exceptions, diseases of the middle ear manifest themselves with alterations in the color, position, and integrity of the tympanic membrane.

Computed tomography (CT) scans, also known as computed axial tomography (CAT) scans, and magnetic resonance imaging (MRI) are two specialized noninvasive methods of viewing the inside of the body. CT scans are very accurate in defining bony structures; MRI more accurately defines the soft tissues.

A tympanogram measures the vibrations of the eardrum by placing a probe against the tympanic membrane.

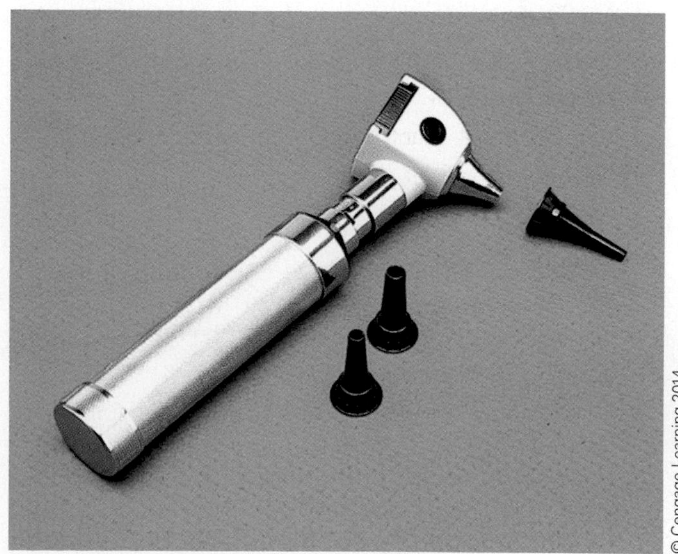

Figure 17-1 Otoscope

Electronystagmography (ENG) is an exam that tests the balance mechanism in the inner ear. Cool, then warm liquid is introduced into the ear canal. The sudden temperature changes stimulate rapid eye movements that, when recorded, indicate the functioning of the balance mechanism.

Routine Instruments, Equipment, and Supplies

Delicate microscopic instrumentation should be handled carefully. When expecting a microscope to be used, the oculars and controls should be adjusted in advance according to the surgeon's preference. The use of specially designed sterile drapes or sterile handles may be employed. It may be helpful for the surgical technologist to guide the instrumentation into the surgeon's field of vision under the microscope. A basic ear procedure instrument tray will include the following instruments:

- House elevator
- Alligator forceps
- Hartman forceps
- House curettes
- Rosen needle
- Caliper
- Chisels
- Stapedial knife
- Baby Metzenbaum scissors
- House alligator scissors
- Adson smooth and tissue forceps
- Jansen bayonet forceps
- Mosquito clamps
- Crile clamps
- Allis clamps
- Webster needle holders
- Joseph skin hooks
- Senn retractors, sharp and dull
- U.S. Army retractors
- Weitlaner retractor
- Mastoid retractor
- Ear speculums
- Frazier, Baron, Rosen, and House suction tips
- Roller knife, Sickle knife, Flap knife
- Myringotomy instrument set that includes the following (Figure 17-2):
  - Myringotomy knife (some surgeons use disposable knife)
  - Sexton ear knife (Figure 17-2F)
  - Iris scissors (Figure 17-2A)
  - Adson bayonet dressing forceps (Figure 17-2E)
  - House alligator ear forceps (Figure 17-2I)
  - Ear curettes, straight and angled (Figure 17-2D)
  - Brown applicator (Figure 17-2C)
  - Frazier and Baron suction tips, various sizes (Figure 17-2G, H)
  - Ear speculums (Figure 17-2B)

Routine supplies include the following:

- Suction system
- Sterile microscope hand grips (if available)
- Microscope drape
- Ear prep set
- Ear back table pack
- Basin set
- Ear drapes: bar drape; U-drape or fenestrated ear drape
- Bone wax
- **Gelfoam**
- Bulb syringe
- No. 10 and No. 15 knife blades
- Micro instrument wipes
- Ear dressing material (addressed within specific procedures; ear dressings range from simple to complicated)
- Nitrogen tank (if power is used)

The argon laser is especially useful in the middle ear for stapedectomy and stapedotomy procedures.

A speculum holder may be used to free the surgeon's hands. The speculum holder attaches to the rail at the side of the operating table for stability.

A nerve stimulator should be available for identification of the facial and vestibulocochlear nerves.

Powered instruments, such as a rotating drill (osteon, ototome), may be used. It may be powered electrically or pneumatically. These complex instruments involve several components. All parts should be inspected and tested prior to use. A variety of burs (cutting and diamond or polishing) should be available for selection by the surgeon. A continuous irrigation system may be needed in addition to the power equipment for cooling the tissue and removal of debris.

Practical Considerations

The operating room and equipment are prepared prior to the arrival of the patient. For procedures on pediatric patients, the temperature of the operating room may be raised and specialized anesthesia equipment employed.

If the use of a microscope is planned, the following preparatory steps should be taken:

1. Clean according to facility standards.
2. Transport to operating room (OR) from storage area.
3. Arrange eyepiece configuration according to the surgeon's preference.
4. Apply the proper magnification lens.
5. Position in advance.

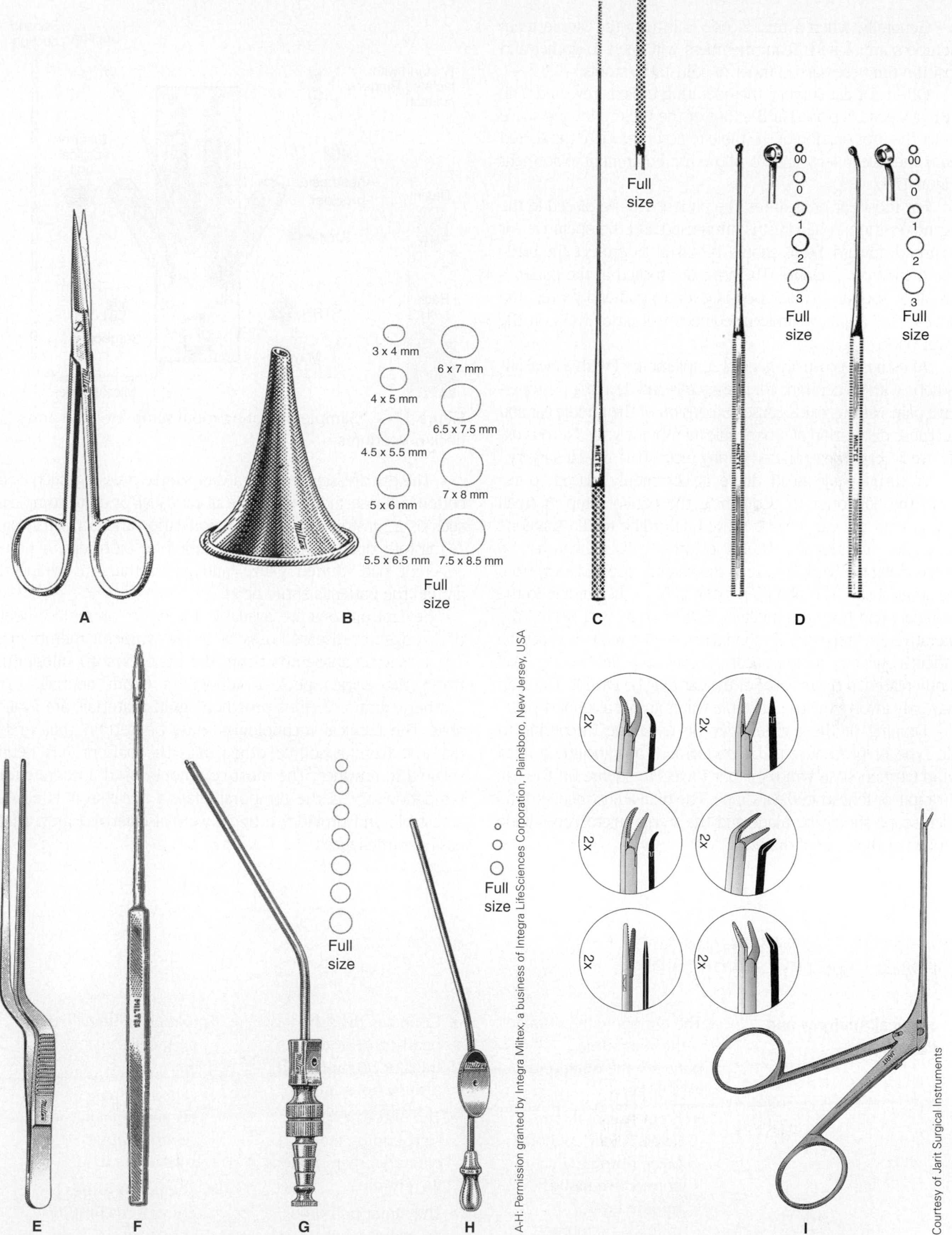

Figure 17-2 Myringotomy instrumentation: (A) Iris scissors (straight), (B) Farrior ear specula, (C) Brown applicator, (D) Buck ear curettes (straight and angled), (E) Adson bayonet dressing forceps, (F) Sexton ear knife, (G) Frazier-Ferguson suction tip, (H) Baron suction tip, (I) House alligator ear forceps

Generally, when a microscope is in use, the sterile team members are seated. Team members will need to gather and position the necessary number of adjustable stools.

Often, for ear surgery, the operating table is reversed. The patient's head is placed at the foot of the table, allowing space under the foot portion of the table to accommodate the seated team members' legs and to allow for equipment placement (Figure 17-3).

For most ear procedures, the patient will be placed in the supine position. A headrest is often used and the operative ear is turned upward. Steps should be taken to protect the unaffected ear from pressure. The arms are tucked at the patient's side after special consideration is given to pad and protect the ulnar nerve. A pillow under the knees will ease stress on the lower back.

Anesthesia is usually general supplemented with a local anesthetic with epinephrine for hemostasis and decrease postoperative pain. Nitrous oxide causes expansion of the middle ear and can cause dislocation of a tympanic membrane graft. Nitrous oxide use is therefore restricted during reconstructive ear surgery.

A turban-style head drape is commonly placed to restrain the hair prior to performing the patient prep. A small area around the ear may be shaved according to the surgeon's preference. Additionally, Vaseline or other gel/ointment may be wiped along the hairline to keep the hair in place and away from the surgical site. The skin prep extends from the hairline to the shoulders and from the midline of the face to well behind the operative ear. Prep solution should not be allowed to contact the patient's eyes or pool in or near the eyes and ears (a cotton ball gently placed in the exterior of the ear may be useful). The prep may only involve the use of sterile water and/or alcohol wipes.

Draping of the patient may be extensive (according to the type of procedure to be performed) and include a head wrap (turban-style wrap) or four towels to square off the ear, U-drape, or fenestrated ear drape. The final adjustments to the microscope should be made and the sterile microscope drape applied at the time of draping.

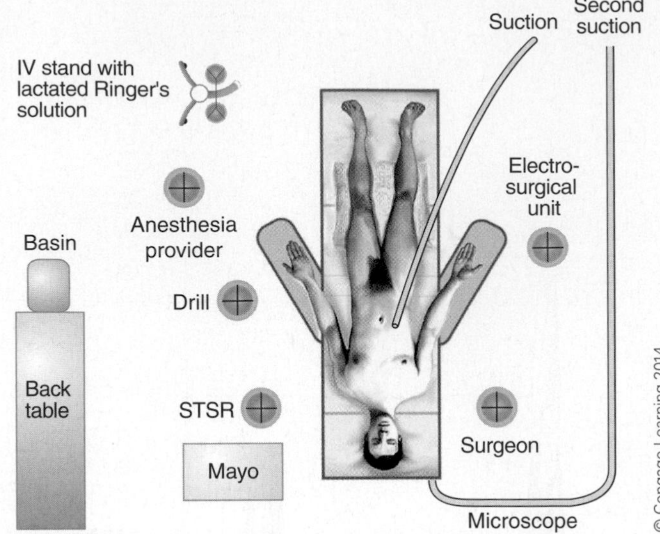

Figure 17-3 Sample operating room setup for head and neck procedures

The ear dressing may be a very simple dressing, such as a cotton ball inserted in the external ear canal; or quite complex, such as a mastoid (Shea or a modification thereof) dressing. A mastoid dressing consists of antibiotic ointment, a nonadherent pad, fluffed gauze, and gauze that are wrapped around the patient's entire head.

Several options are available for repair or replacement of damaged or diseased ossicles or the tympanic membrane. These may be autografts (from the same person), allografts (from the same species), xenografts (from animals), or synthetic grafts. Various prosthetic graft materials are available. The surgical technologist must be certain that graft material from a source other than the patient has been secured in advance. The most commonly used autograft for tympanoplasty is the temporalis fascia because it is easily accessible and provides a thick, well-vascularized graft that easily epithelializes.

Procedure 17-1 Myringotomy

Surgical Anatomy and Pathology

- The tympanic membrane is the separation between the outer and middle ear.
  - It consists of three layers: outer epithelial layer, fibrous connective tissue middle layer, mucous membrane inner layer.
  - Concave, disk-shaped; pearly gray in color, translucent, and with a shiny appearance
  - The fibrous ring surrounding the tympanic membrane is the annulus.
  - The major portion of the membrane is fibrous tissue called the pars tensa.
  - The superior portion is called the pars flaccida because it lacks the central fibrous connective tissue.
  - The umbo is the point of maximum concavity.

PROCEDURE 17-1 (continued)

- A branch of the facial nerve that carries taste impulses from the tongue passes along the inner surface of the membrane.
- The tympanic membrane can easily rupture.
- The perforation can be caused by either external trauma or excess pressure from within the middle ear.
- Otitis media is a very common acute inflammation of the middle ear, usually caused by blockage of the eustachian tube causing an accumulation of fluid that normally drains into the nasopharynx. The primary symptom of otitis media is severe ear pain. The main sign observed through the otoscope is an inflamed tympanic membrane.
- The infection may require a myringotomy to remove the accumulated fluid and insertion of a pressure-equalizing (PE) tube to allow for additional drainage and maintain the pressure equalization (Figure 17-4).

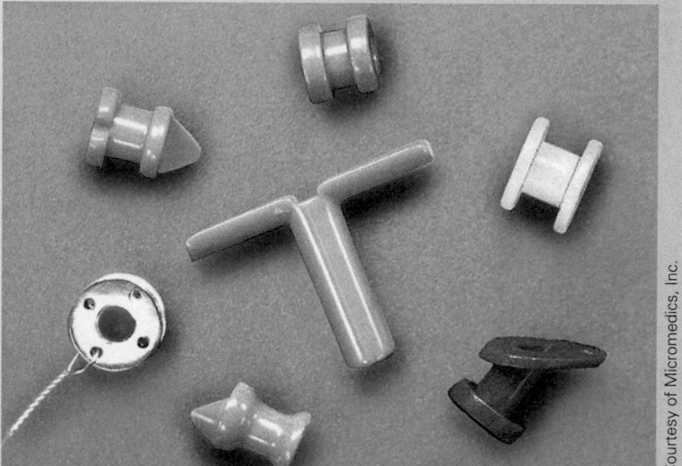

Courtesy of Micromedics, Inc.

Figure 17-4 Tympanostomy tubes

Preoperative Diagnostic Tests and Procedures	• History and physical examination (otoscope examination)		
Equipment, Instruments, and Supplies Unique to Procedure	• Hydrogen peroxide to loosen cerumen in ear	• PE tubes of various sizes (Figure 17-4)	• Disposable myringotomy knife
Preoperative Preparation	• Position, skin prep, and draping as previously described for ear procedures	• Anesthesia: Anesthetic is often delivered to the pediatric patient by mask	
Practical Considerations	• The PE tubes are considered implants and must be documented in the patient chart according to health care facility policy as well as federal regulations for medical devices. • Myringotomy is not a sterile procedure, but best sterile technique should be used. Sterile gloves are donned using the open glove technique, but a sterile gown is not worn. • Only a Mayo stand is needed for the procedure.		

(continues)

PROCEDURE 17-1 (continued)

Surgical Procedure

1. Following placement of a fenestrated drape, a speculum is placed in the external auditory canal. Any visible wax accumulation will be removed with a curette.

   Procedural Consideration: Assess the diameter of the patient's ear canal and present the surgeon with the appropriate-size speculum. The surgical technologist should be prepared to clean the wax curette with gauze between uses.

2. An incision is made in the inferior posterior portion of the tympanic membrane with a disposable myringotomy knife.

   Procedural Consideration: Prepare to pass myringotomy knife. The surgeon may not be willing to look away from the operative site, so it may be helpful for the surgical technologist to guide the surgeon's hand into the field of vision. Fluid may be collected for culture and sensitivity. Suction will be used to remove excess fluid. Keep the suction apparatus patent by suctioning water through it or using the stylet. The fluid from the middle ear is thick.

3. A PE tube is placed into the tympanic incision.

   Procedural Consideration: The surgical technologist will grasp the PE tube in the jaws of an alligator forceps or appropriate applicator (without touching it to prevent powder contamination) and carefully pass it to the surgeon.

4. Final positioning of the tube is achieved (Figure 17-5).

   Procedural Consideration: An instrument, such as a pick, may be used to aid in the final positioning of the tube.

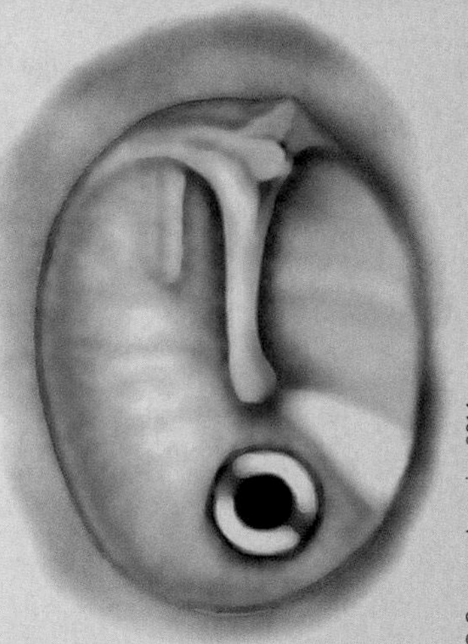

Figure 17-5 Myringotomy incision with PE tube in place

5. The speculum is removed. If desired, antibiotic/antiinflammatory solution or suspension, such as Cortisporin, may be placed in the canal and the canal may then be packed with cotton.

   Procedural Consideration: Have antibiotic solution and/or cotton ready for use. Count may not be necessary, according to facility policy.

6. If the procedure is planned to be bilateral, the patient's head will be repositioned, the surgical team members will switch sides, and the sequence is repeated.

   Procedural Consideration: Prepare to switch sides of the table with the surgeon if bilateral myringotomy is planned.

Procedure 17-1 (continued)

Postoperative Considerations

Immediate Postoperative Care

- Transport to PACU; patient is expected to be released from the health care facility within 1 hour after the procedure is completed.
- Ear canal must be kept dry until PE tubes fall out or are removed and the tympanic membrane is healed.

Prognosis

- No complications: Patient is expected to return to normal activities within a few hours; hearing is expected to return to normal in short period of time.

Complications: Recurrent infection; occasionally, a patient may require a second procedure to remove a retained tube.

Wound Classification

- Class II: Clean-contaminated

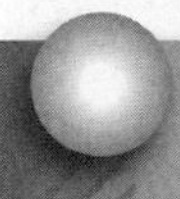

Pearl of Wisdom

Be sure that the microscope has been set up in advance of the procedure to the surgeon's specifications. The surgical technologist may have to change the lens and/or the eyepieces. In addition, the oculars may need to be adjusted specifically for the surgeon's eyes.

Procedure 17-2 Tympanoplasty

Surgical Anatomy and Pathology

- The middle ear (tympanic cavity) is an air-filled chamber located within the temporal bone.
  - The cavity is lined with mucous membrane, which is a continuation of the inner layer of the tympanic membrane.
  - There are two openings in the wall of the middle ear: tympanic antrum that opens into the mastoid sinus; eustachian tube that connects the middle ear to the nasopharynx.
  - The auditory ossicles are located in the middle ear, lateral to medial: malleus (hammer), incus (anvil), and stapes (stirrups). The ossicles are synovial joints, and ligaments connect them to the wall of the middle ear and two tiny skeletal muscles control their movement. The short process of the malleus rests against the tympanic membrane and the head articulates with the body of the incus. The incus is connected to the head of the stapes and the footplate of the stapes rests against the oval window.
- Tympanoplasty is performed to treat a variety of conditions affecting the tympanic membrane and the ossicular chain. There are five classifications for tympanoplasty, which are determined by the extent of damage to the

(*continues*)

PROCEDURE 17-2 (continued)

	tympanic membrane and middle ear: • *Type I:* The damage is limited to the tympanic membrane. All contents of the middle ear are intact. A soft tissue graft is used to replace or repair the damaged eardrum. • *Type II:* The destructive process extends beyond the damaged tympanic membrane to include the malleus. The entire malleus or the diseased portion is removed. The tympanic membrane graft is placed directly against the remaining portion of the malleus or the incus. • *Type III:* In addition to the damaged tympanic	membrane, both the malleus and incus have been affected. The replacement tympanum is placed directly against the intact stapes, permitting the transmission of sound to the oval window. • *Type IV:* All of the ossicles are affected, in addition to the perforated tympanum. The only remaining natural structure of the middle ear is the intact and mobile footplate of the stapes. Only an air pocket remains as protection for the round window, as the graft rests directly on the stapes	footplate. The ossicular chain may be reconstructed. • *Type V:* This situation is similar to type IV with one exception. The remaining footplate of the stapes is fixed. All ossicles are completely removed. A window is made into the horizontal semicircular canal and the tympanic graft seals off the middle ear and provides protection for the oval window. • Often the disease affecting the middle ear has extended into the mastoid sinus, which requires a combination procedure of tympanoplasty and mastoidectomy.
Preoperative Diagnostic Tests and Procedures	• CT and MRI		
Equipment, Instruments, and Supplies Unique to Procedure	• Ear drill if mastoidectomy is planned	• All other items as previously described for ear procedures	
Preoperative Preparation	• Position, anesthesia, skin prep, and draping as previously described for ear procedures		
Practical Considerations	• Local anesthetic with epinephrine for vasoconstriction and postoperative pain		
Surgical Procedure	1. The surgeon may choose either a transaural or a retroauricular (postauricular) approach. If a mastoidectomy is also planned, or the possibility of a temporalis fascia graft exists, the retroauricular approach is preferred. **Procedural Consideration:** Communicate with the surgeon about the specific variances for this particular patient. Assist with draping the patient and equipment. Assist with placement of sterile equipment. Be sure that powder is removed from the gloves of all team members. Once seated, remain seated.		

PROCEDURE 17-2 (continued)

2. If the surgeon is planning to use an autograft, the specimen is taken at the beginning of the procedure, so that the sometimes-lengthy graft preparation process can begin.

   Procedural Consideration: Pass No. 15 blade for postauricular incision. Electrosurgery and Senn retractors will be utilized next. The surgical technologist will likely be expected to hold the retractors. Have the scissors and tissue forceps in a position such that the surgeon can "help himself or herself" to facilitate the dissection. Once secured, the graft will need special attention according to surgeon's preference. Graft tissue, when allowed to air dry, becomes thin and light (like tissue paper). Be sure that it is in a secure location so that an air current does not carry it to the floor!

3. The tympanic membrane and the ossicular chain are assessed. A variety of micro instruments may be necessary for the exploration and dissection.

   Procedural Consideration: Provide the appropriate-size ear speculum. Install the speculum holder if its use is intended. Instrumentation for the middle ear is often stored in a rack. The rack is also designed for intraoperative use. This is an advantage for the surgical technologist, in that it keeps the Mayo stand organized, but it also presents a hazard, as the tips of the instruments are pointed upward. Use extreme caution. Take great care when handling the delicate micro instrumentation. Use a micro wipe to clean the instruments rather than gauze to keep the items free of lint.

4. Diseased tissues and damaged ossicles are removed.

   Procedural Considerations: The room is often darkened to enhance the surgeon's view of the operative site—keep safety measures in mind. Keep the most used micro instruments on the Mayo stand in the rack and *always* return them to their original location for organizational purposes. *Suggestion:* Use alphabetical order to organize the "ringed" instruments (e.g., "a" alligator, "b" Bellucci scissors, "c" cupped forceps). To save time, use one hand to take the used instrument from the surgeon and the other to pass the requested instrument. It may be helpful for the surgical technologist to guide the instrumentation into the surgeon's field of vision. Removed ossicles may be repositioned. Do not pass them off the field until the end of the case.

5. If necessary, the mastoidectomy would be performed at this point.

   Procedural Consideration: The ear drill and suction/irrigation system should be connected, turned on, and tested. Be sure that an adequate amount of irrigation fluid is constantly available during drilling to prevent bone necrosis. Bone wax may be requested. A variety of cutting burs for the drill will be necessary. Typically, the surgeon starts with a large bur and progressively changes to smaller sizes as the nerve is approached. Diamond burs are used for smoothing and reducing bleeding. The surgical technologist should be able to change the bur quickly and efficiently. Use the safety mechanism on the drill to prevent injury. Epinephrine may be instilled to reduce bleeding.

6. Ossicular reconstruction using materials of the surgeon's choice is performed, if possible.

   Procedural Consideration: A previously removed ossicle may be reinserted (it may be necessary to refashion it with the drill). An ossicle holder will be necessary. Other types of reconstruction materials may be implanted.

(*continues*)

PROCEDURE 17-2 (continued)

7. Small Gelfoam pledgets may be packed into the tympanic cavity to temporarily stabilize the contents of the middle ear and to make a bed on which the new tympanic membrane may rest.

   Procedural Consideration: Gelfoam is packaged in a large sheet; pledgets will need to be cut and possibly compressed. It may be used dry or moistened with saline, antibiotic solution or thrombin.

8. The graft is placed under the remnant of the existing eardrum. Additional packing of Gelfoam or Vaseline gauze may be placed in the external auditory canal. The retroauricular wound, if used, is sutured.

   Procedural Consideration: The graft is fragile. Handle with caution. Small scissors may be needed to tailor the graft to fit the ear canal. More packing will be needed. Suture should be ready—pass with an Adson tissue forceps. Suture scissors next. Count.

9. A protective dressing is applied.

   Procedural Consideration: Application of the dressing can be a complex process. The surgical technologist will likely be asked to hold the patient's head while the surgeon applies the dressing. Have all supplies laid out in the anticipated order of use. Be certain that the patient's airway is not disturbed when manipulating the head.

Postoperative Considerations

Immediate Postoperative Care

- Transport to PACU.
- Patient is instructed not to blow his or her nose forcefully until healing has occurred.
- Patient is instructed to keep ear dry.

Prognosis

- No complications: Patient may resume normal activity in about 2 weeks; patient expected to regain full hearing.
- Complications: Postoperative SSI; hemorrhage; failure to restore full hearing.

Wound Classification

- Class I: Clean

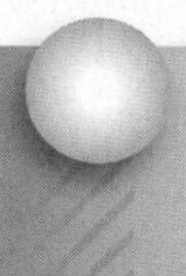

PEARL OF WISDOM

DO NOT disturb the microscope or operating table once the procedure has begun. Do not use it as a footrest or armrest.

PROCEDURE 17-3 Mastoidectomy

Surgical Anatomy and Pathology

- The mastoid process is a projection from the mastoid portion of the temporal bone (Figure 17-6).
- It is located posterior to the external acoustic meatus and lateral to the styloid process.
- It serves as a point of attachment for several muscles, including the capitis, digastric

PROCEDURE 17-3 (continued)

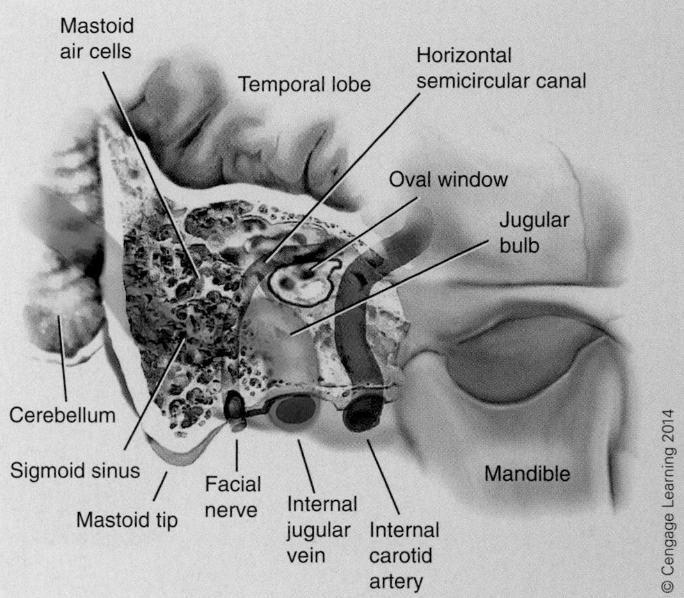

Figure 17-6 Mastoid sinus and related structures

posterior belly, and sternocleidomastoid.

- Mastoiditis is a complication of acute otitis media.
  - Signs and symptoms: severe earache, purulent discharge from the external auditory canal that generally develops 10–14 days following acute otitis media, fever, inflammation of the mastoid process.
  - Infection that has not been cleared from the middle ear may be forced into the mastoid air cells through the antrum, causing destruction of the mastoid bone.
  - Mastoiditis that extends beyond the mastoid sinus can lead to meningitis or encephalitis.
  - Mastoidectomy is performed if antibiotic therapy has failed.
- **Cholesteatoma** is a benign cyst or tumor that fills the mastoid cavity and erodes the mastoid air cells. This process can also damage the ossicles.
  - Cholesteatoma is formed when epithelial cells that would normally be shed through the eustachian tube are unable to migrate out of the middle ear cavity due to a blockage of the auditory tube.
  - Earache, headache, purulent discharge from the ear, hearing loss, dizziness, and weakness of the facial muscles due to damage to the seventh cranial nerve are evidence of cholesteatoma (Figure 17-7).
  - Mastoidectomy is the only option to correct this condition. If the disease has damaged the ossicles, ossicular reconstruction may be performed to restore auditory function.

(*continues*)

Procedure 17-3 (continued)

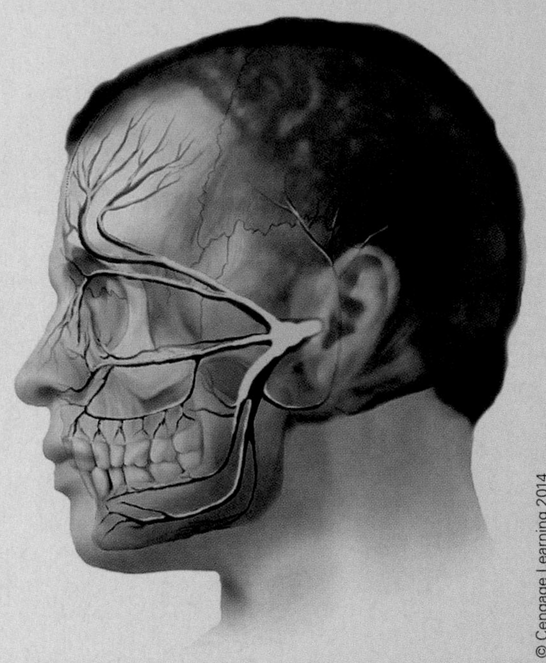

Figure 17-7 Seventh cranial nerve

Preoperative Diagnostic Tests and Procedures	• CT and MRI	
Equipment, Instruments, and Supplies Unique to Procedure	• Nitrogen tank • Power drill • Various sizes of cutting burs	• Suction irrigator • Skin graft instruments • Gelfoam
Preoperative Preparation	• Position, anesthesia, skin prep, and draping as previously described	
Practical Considerations	• Test all power equipment prior to use.	• Examine the burs for cracks, pitting, and sharpness.

Surgical Procedure

1. The ear is injected with lidocaine with epinephrine using the 27-gauge 1½"-needle and 5-mL syringe. The small postauricular skin graft is taken prior to the ear prep and draping.

   Procedural Consideration: Skin graft is removed with No. 15 knife blade and Adson smooth forceps.

2. Using the No. 15 knife blade, a postauricular incision is made.

   Procedural Consideration: Electrosurgery and Senn retractors will be used. The surgical technologist will be responsible for holding the retractors.

3. The temporalis fascia is harvested (see Procedure 17-2 for details concerning the harvesting of the temporalis fascia).

   Procedural Consideration: Once the graft is taken it will need to be secured and gently handled; place the graft on a sponge and place it in a secure location as it dries. Be careful! The graft is thin and when dry can easily be carried to the floor by an air current.

PROCEDURE 17-3 (continued)

4. Using the power drill and bur, the mastoid bone is drilled; the suction irrigator is used throughout to remove smoke plume and bone tissue and prevent charring of the bone.

   Procedural Consideration: While the surgeon is using the power drill and bur, the surgical technologist should frequently use the suction irrigator.

5. The surgeon will use a Rosen needle or pick to assess the mastoid antrum and identify surrounding structures. The surgeon will also remove the ossicles at this point of the procedure.

   Procedural Consideration: The surgical technologist should have a variety of bur sizes available; the surgeon may frequently change the size. The surgeon will typically start with a large bur; as he or she approaches the nerve it will be necessary to change to smaller burs. The surgical technologist should be able to change the bur quickly and efficiently. When changing the bur, use the safety mechanism on the power drill to prevent inadvertent activation of the drill.

6. Using a Rosen needle and pick, the cholesteatoma is removed.

   Procedural Consideration: Take great care in the handling of micro instrumentation. Protect the tips. Use micro wipes (not sponges) to clean the instrumentation. Confirm with the surgeon the ossicles and cholesteatoma tissue as specimens.

7. The surgeon places the fascia graft (again refer to Procedure 17-2 for details concerning this step) and then the skin graft is placed over the fascia.

   Procedural Consideration: Handle the fascia graft with caution; it is very fragile.

8. Using an alligator forceps, Gelfoam is cut into small squares, soaked in saline, and packed into the mastoid cavity.

   Procedural Consideration: Cut the Gelfoam into small 1 × 1 mm squares, soak it in saline, antibiotic solution, or thrombin, and hold it for the surgeon to grasp with an alligator forceps.

9. The incision is closed in layers with absorbable suture.

10. The skin is closed with 4-0 or 5-0 suture.

11. Using the alligator forceps, the surgeon packs the external auditory canal with Gelfoam squares soaked in saline or antibiotic solution.

12. Dressing usually consists of fluffed gauze ("fluffs") placed around the ear.

    Procedural Consideration: Assist with the placement of the dressing.

Postoperative Considerations

Immediate Postoperative Care

- Patient is transported to PACU.
- Patient is instructed not to blow her or his nose forcefully until healing has occurred.
- Patient is instructed to keep ear dry.

Prognosis

- No complications: Patient may resume normal activity in approximately 2 weeks.
- Complications: Damage to the facial nerve; postoperative SSI; hearing loss; vertigo; meningitis.

Wound Classification

- Class I: Clean

Procedure 17-4 Stapedectomy

Surgical Anatomy and Pathology	• See previous description of auditory ossicles. • Oto**sclerosis** occurs when there is a bony overgrowth of the stapes. This progressive disease is hereditary, affecting women more than men. • Eventually the footplate of the stapes becomes fixed to the oval window, preventing the normal sound vibrations from entering the inner ear.
Preoperative Diagnostic Tests and Procedures	• Tuning fork exam • Audiometric exam
Equipment, Instruments, and Supplies Unique to Procedure	• Power drill with burs • Bulb syringe • Prostheses
Preoperative Preparation	• Position, skin prep, and draping as previously described • Local anesthetic preferred so surgeon may immediately assess hearing restoration using voice commands or a tuning fork.
Practical Considerations	• Test all power equipment prior to patient's arrival in the OR. • Prosthesis packaging should not be opened until surgeon determines the exact type and size. • If graft is needed, verify donor site prior to starting skin prep. • Remember to keep room quiet and conversations to a minimum if local anesthetic is used.
Surgical Procedure	1. A graft may be harvested from the ear, hand, or a portion of the abdomen prior to the start of the procedure. The graft will be used to cover the oval window. **Procedural Consideration:** A fat, perichondrium, vein, or fascia graft may be utilized. The surgical technologist must place the graft in a safe place on the back table until needed; it should also be kept moist by placing it on a wet sponge.
	2. The external ear canal is injected with local anesthetic.
	3. The operative microscope is used to visualize the middle ear.
	4. The external ear canal is irrigated and suctioned with a 7-Fr Frazier suction for further visualization.
	5. Surgeon inserts an ear speculum, starting with a small speculum and advancing to a larger one. Once the appropriate-size speculum is inserted, the universal ear speculum holder is applied to stabilize the speculum during the course of the procedure. **Procedural Consideration:** The surgical technologist should have the universal ear speculum holder assembled and ready for immediate use.
	6. The surgeon may elect to suction with a 5- or 7-Fr Frazier or microsuction tip to remove any fluid from the ear. **Procedural Consideration:** The surgical technologist should have a variety of sizes of Frazier suction tips available for use.
	7. The tympanomeatal flap is created by using a roller knife, sickle knife, or flap knife. **Procedural Consideration:** The surgical technologist must know how to properly hand the specialty knives to the surgeon without him or her having to look away from the microscope.

PROCEDURE 17-4 (continued)

8. The tympanic membrane is elevated and the posterior bony ledge removed using a House knife, duckbill elevators, or a drum elevator.

   Procedural Consideration: Once the tympanic membrane is elevated, the surgeon is able to visualize the ossicular chain.

9. If the surgeon is unable to visualize the ossicles due to a bony ledge, a drill may be used to remove enough bone for proper visualization.

10. The surgeon may elect to measure the distance from the incus to the stapes footplate or may wait until after the stapes is removed. The surgeon measures with a depth gauge to ensure the proper prosthesis.

    Procedural Consideration: The surgical technologist must remember the measurement in order to reconfirm with the surgeon later in the procedure when requesting the correct prosthesis to be opened by the circulator.

11. The incudostapedial joint is disarticulated using a House or Guilford-Wright joint knife. Laser may be used to perform this step of the procedure. The stapedial tendon is severed with Bellucci scissors.

    Procedural Consideration: The surgical team must take all necessary safety precautions if the laser will be used, including eye protection.

12. A fine Rosen needle and micro cupped forceps are utilized to fracture the stapes superstructure.

13. The surgeon may ensure hemostasis by using tiny sponges that have been soaked in epinephrine.

    Procedural Consideration: The surgical technologist must keep track of the number of sponges that are inserted/used.

14. The surgeon creates an opening in the footplate with a laser, drill (such as a Skeeter), or sharp footplate pick. Half of the footplate is removed with a Hough hoe, footplate hook, or footplate pick.

15. The surgeon inspects the oval window and the graft is placed with an alligator forceps.

    Procedural Consideration: The surgical technologist should present the graft in such a manner as to assist the surgeon with loading onto the alligator forceps.

16. The prosthesis is introduced into the middle ear on alligator forceps to be positioned so it rests against the oval graft.

17. The wire is positioned over the incus by using a Hough hoe, picks, or footplate hooks. Once the surgeon is satisfied with the position, the wire is crimped onto the long process of the incus (Figure 17-8).

18. At this point the surgeon may test the patient's hearing (if using local anesthesia) by whispering to the patient. If the patient is under general anesthesia, the surgeon may touch the malleus with an ear pick to observe the mobility of the stapes, incus, and malleus prosthesis.

    Procedural Consideration: The surgeon may also need a sterile tuning fork to test the hearing.

(*continues*)

PROCEDURE 17-4 (continued)

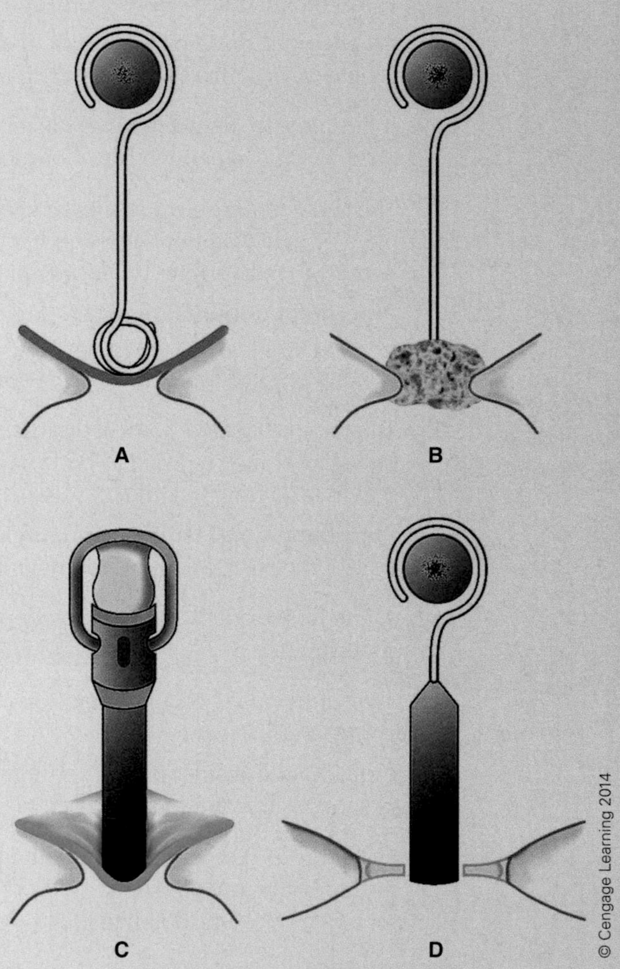

Figure 17-8 Stapes prosthesis in place: (A) Wire and absorbable sponge, (B) wire and fat graft, (C) piston-type and vein or fascia graft, (D) piston-type without graft

19. Moistened gelatin squares may be placed around the site of the prosthesis for stability.
20. The tympanomeatal flap is replaced using a duckbill elevator, Rosen needle, or drum elevator.
21. The external ear canal may be packed with moistened gelatin sponge, antibiotic gel, or antibiotic ointment.
22. Cotton is placed in the concha of the ear and the graft site is dressed.
23. A Glasscock or mastoid dressing may be utilized.

Procedure 17-4 (continued)

Postoperative Considerations

Immediate Postoperative Care

- Stapedectomy is usually an outpatient procedure but patient may remain in the hospital overnight if he or she has nausea or dizziness.
- Patient is advised not to make any sudden movements to prevent symptoms of nausea or dizziness.
- Patient should avoid loud noises until the ear retrains itself to hear sounds properly.
- Patient should avoid getting the ear wet until it is completely healed. Patient should also avoid putting pressure on the ear for a few days following surgery (blowing his or her nose, lifting heavy objects, swimming, flying).

Prognosis

- No complications: Patient is expected to return to normal activities within 2 weeks.
- Complications: Vertigo; tinnitus; postoperative SSI; taste disturbances; loss of hearing; eardrum perforation; temporary weakness of the facial muscles.

Wound Classification

- Wound Class I: Clean

Procedure 17-5 Cochlear Implant

Surgical Anatomy and Pathology

- The inner ear, or labyrinth, consists of two main sections: bony and membranous labyrinth located in the temporal bone.
  - Perilymph fluid fills the spaces of the bony labyrinth. The bony labyrinth is also lined by a thin membrane that contains endolymph fluid. The three compartments of the bony labyrinth are the vestibule, semicircular canals, and cochlea.
  - The vestibule separates the cochlea from the semicircular canals.
  - Three semicircular canals make up the lateral portion of the bony labyrinth. The membranous labyrinth extends inside each canal referred to as semicircular ducts. The base of each canal has a small swelling called the ampulla. Each ampulla contains ampullary crests that have sensitive hair cells called cristae; **dynamic equilibrium** is controlled by the cristae.
  - The principal organs of equilibrium are the vestibule and semicircular ducts. The vestibular branch of the vestibulocochlear nerve (cranial nerve VIII) carries the information related to equilibrium to the cerebral cortex.
  - The organs of Corti are contained within the cochlea, a coiled portion of the bony labyrinth. The organs of Corti consist of a series of hair cells that directly contact the fibers of the cochlear nerve, which is also a branch of the vestibulocochlear nerve that conducts sound impulses to the auditory cortex of the temporal lobe of the brain.
- Sensorineural deafness, also called nerve deafness, involves the cochlea and acoustic nerve. Treatment is limited; however, cochlear implants are providing some progress and hope for patients.

Preoperative Diagnostic Tests and Procedures

- History and physical examination
- Hearing exams

(*continues*)

Procedure 17-5 (continued)

Equipment, Instruments, and Supplies Unique to Procedure

- Cochlear implant (Figure 17-9)
  - The device has two components: (1) the internal component that has several electrodes, which are placed inside the cochlea; the electrodes are implanted under the patient's skin behind the ear; (2) the second part is the external microphone and connecting cables.
  - The microphone is a speech processor that converts sound into electrical impulses. The electrodes receive the electrical impulses that are transmitted to the cochlea, which activates the fibers of the vestibulocochlear nerve to transmit the signal to the brain for interpretation.
- All other items are the same as for the mastoid procedure.

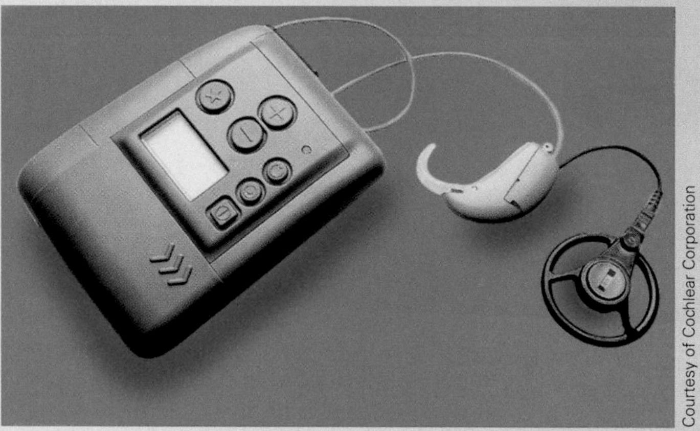

Courtesy of Cochlear Corporation

Figure 17-9 Cochlear prosthesis

Preoperative Preparation

- Position, anesthesia, skin prep, and draping as previously described

Practical Considerations

- Test power drill prior to patient entering the OR.

Surgical Procedure

1. A postauricular incision is made using the No. 15 knife blade.

   Procedural Consideration: The surgical technologist should have electrocautery, sponge, and suction with Frazier tip ready for immediate use once the skin incision has been made. The scalp can bleed profusely.

2. The temporalis muscle is gently elevated to expose the temporal bone.

   Procedural Consideration: The surgeon will use small retractors such as Senn retractors to elevate the temporalis muscle.

3. A mastoidectomy will be performed.
4. The surgeon places the receiver in the temporal bone and, through an incision in the cochlea, inserts the electrodes. The receiver and electrodes may be kept in place with the use of a small piece of temporalis fascia.
5. The surgeon closes the wound. After the surgical wound has healed in 3 to 4 weeks, the external microphone is attached.

PROCEDURE 17-5 (continued)

Postoperative Considerations

Immediate Postoperative Care

- Transport to PACU.
- Cochlear implant is usually an outpatient procedure, but patient may remain in the hospital overnight if he or she has nausea or dizziness.
- Patient is advised not to make any sudden movements, to prevent symptoms of nausea or dizziness.
- Patient should avoid getting the ear wet until it is completely healed. Patient should also avoid putting pressure on the ear for a few days after surgery.

Prognosis

- No complications: Patient expected to return to normal activities in 1–2 weeks.
- Complications: Postoperative SSI; eardrum perforation; damage to the facial nerve; vertigo; meningitis.

Wound Classification

- Class I: Clean

NASAL PROCEDURES

The nose is a facial feature that serves as the organ for the sense of smell and as the upper portion of the respiratory system. Paired nasolacrimal ducts enter the nasal cavity near the inferior meatus and are part of the tear drainage system. The nose and paranasal sinuses are prone to suffer several types of pathological conditions, which will be reviewed as well as we present the procedures performed to treat the pathologies.

Nasal Diagnostic Procedures/Tests

Diagnostic approaches to nasal and paranasal sinus pathology include direct vision, mirror examination, and radiography.

Direct Vision

The most common and highly effective method of examining the interior of the nose is direct vision. Excellent illumination is imperative. This is often accomplished with the use of a lamp affixed to the examiner's head. The direction and the intensity of the light beam are adjustable on most of these devices. A nasal speculum may be used to spread the nares.

Mirror Examination

Another approach is mirror examination of the nasopharynx and posterior nasal cavity. The patient is instructed to open the mouth and the tongue is gently retracted. A small mirror is warmed or treated with a commercial antifog preparation to prevent fogging, inserted into the **oropharynx**, and directed upward. With good illumination, the examiner is able to view the posterior nares, the turbinates, the posterior end of the vomer bone, and the outlet of the maxillary sinus.

Radiography

Standard radiography is still a very valuable tool in diagnosing nasal and sinus disorders. Simple radiography can easily show fractures and occluded sinuses. Four basic views make up a "sinus series": the Waters view, Caldwell view, lateral view, and submental view. Each is specifically valuable in viewing the four main sinuses.

CT is rapidly replacing the use of standard radiography. CT scanning makes a very clear delineation between bony and soft tissue structures. The computer-generated views are able to produce projections of otherwise inaccessible anatomical structures. MRI does not clearly define the bony structures; for this reason, it is of little value in diagnosing sinus disorders.

Angiography is used to demonstrate blood flow. This can be useful in determining the exact location of hemorrhage in case of traumatic injuries or **epistaxis.**

Routine Instruments, Equipment, and Supplies

Instrumentation for **rhino**plasty (often considered "plastic surgery") differs from the instrumentation for internal nasal and sinus surgery. Endoscopic sinus surgery requires specialized instrumentation and auxiliary equipment, for which special care and handling will be necessary. A sample nasal instrument set is shown in Figure 17-10 and its components are listed Table 17-1.

Routine equipment for most nasal procedures includes the following:

- Headlamp
- Electrosurgery unit (ESU)
- Power drill

TABLE 17-1 Basic Nasal Set

Item	Qty	Item	Qty
No. 3 and No. 7 knife handles (Figure 17-10B, C)	1 ea.	Joseph double hook, 2 mm and 7 mm (Figure 17-10V)	1 ea.
Cartilage knife	1 ea.	Farrel applicator (Figure 17-10X)	1 ea.
Joseph knives (sharp and blunt)	1 ea.	Vienna nasal speculum, various sizes (Figure 17-10Y)	
Joseph button-end knife	1 ea.	Killian septum speculum (Figure 17-10Z)	1 ea.
Ballenger swivel knife	1 ea.	Cottle septum speculum (Figure 17-10AA)	1 ea.
Freer mucosa septum knife (Figure 17-10D)	1 ea.	Aufricht nasal retractor-speculum (Figure 17-10R)	1 ea.
McKenty knife	1 ea.	Coakley angled nasal curettes, various sizes	
Mayo dissecting scissors, 5½" curved	1 ea.	Maltz nasal rasps, various sizes (Figure 17-10BB)	
Metzenbaum scissors, 5½" curved (Figure 17-10G)	1 ea.	Cottle rasp (Figure 17-10CC)	1 ea.
Metzenbaum scissors, 7" curved (Figure 17-10H)	1 ea.	Nasal antrostomy rasp, various sizes	
Plastic surgery scissors (Figure 17-10E)	1 ea.	Nasal saws, right and left	1 ea.
Joseph nasal scissors, 5¾" curved (Figure 17-10F)	1 ea.	Chisels, guarded, right and left	1 ea.
Joseph nasal scissors, 5¾" straight (Figure 17-10F)	1 ea.	Gouges, 2 mm	1 ea.
Knight nasal scissors (Figure 17-10J)	1 ea.	Osteotomes, 2 mm	1 ea.
Fomon upper lateral scissors (Figure 17-10I)	1 ea.	McKenty septum elevator (Figure 17-10DD)	1 ea.
Adson tissue forceps with teeth, angled (Figure 17-10K)	2 ea.	Freer septum elevator (Figure 17-11 A)	1 ea.
Graefe tissue forceps, 4¾" (Figure 17-10L)	1 ea.	Joseph periosteal elevator	1 ea.
Wilde nasal dressing forceps (Figure 17-10M)	1 ea.	Takahashi nasal cutting forceps (Figure 17-11 B)	1 ea.
Jansen bayonet with and without teeth	1 ea.	Knight polyp forceps, various sizes	
Halsted mosquito clamps (Figure 17-10N)	6 ea.	Jansen-Middleton septum forceps (Figure 17-10EE)	1 ea.
Baby Allis clamps, 5" (Figure 17-10W)	2 ea.	Kerrison rongeur, various sizes	
Halsey needle holder, 5" (Figure 17-10P)	2 ea.	Antrum trocar and stylet	1 ea.
Crile needle holder, 6"	2 ea.	Nasal antrostomy rasp (Figure 17-13)	1 ea.
Backhaus towel clamp (Figure 17-10O)	4 ea.	Nasal polyp snare (Figure 17-12)	1 ea.
Senn retractor, sharp (Figure 17-10S)	2 ea.	Frazier suction tips, various sizes (Figure 17-10Q)	
U.S. Army retractor (Figure 17-10T)	2 ea.	Yankauer suction tip (Figure 17-10A)	1 ea.
Joseph skin hook (Figure 17-10U)	1 ea.	Mallet	1 ea.

- Insulated ESU with suction attachment
- Bipolar unit

Routine supplies include the following:

- Basic back table pack
- Bar drape
- U-drape
- Prep set
- Basin set
- Gloves
- No. 10 and No. 15 knife blades
- ESU pencil
- Bipolar forceps
- Suction system

Practical Considerations

The patient is placed in the supine position with the head placed in a donut or foam headrest, or a roll is placed under the scapular region, to slightly tilt the head back. The head of the OR bed may be slightly elevated to reduce bleeding and prevent edema. The arms are tucked at the patient's sides with the ulnar nerves well padded and the fingers protected. A pillow placed under the knees will aid in reducing lumbar strain.

If a local anesthetic is planned, and an anesthesia provider will not be in attendance, the presence of a second circulator may be requested for patient monitoring. The patient may be given a local anesthetic in addition to a general anesthetic to help provide hemostasis, shrink the nasal mucosa, and minimize postoperative pain.

The use of a small table (prep stand) or second Mayo stand may be requested to hold the supplies necessary for

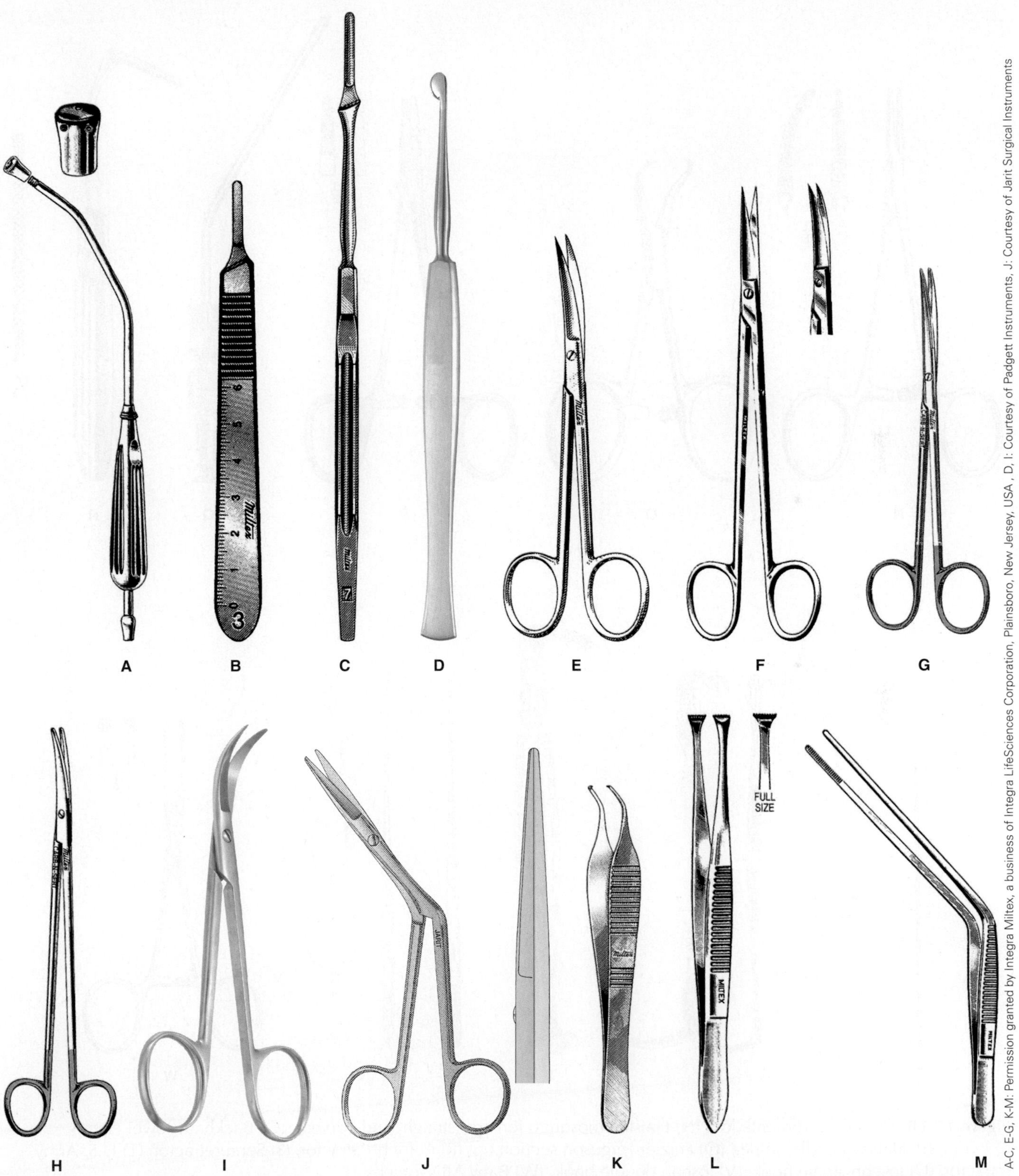

A-C, E-G, K-M: Permission granted by Integra Miltex, a business of Integra LifeSciences Corporation, Plainsboro, New Jersey, USA , D, I: Courtesy of Padgett Instruments, J: Courtesy of Jarit Surgical Instruments

Figure 17-10 Nasal instrumentation: (A) Yankauer suction tip, (B) #3 scalpel handle, (C) #7 scalpel handle, (D) Freer mucosa septum knife, (E) plastic surgery scissors (curved—sharp point), (F) Joseph nasal scissors (straight and curved—sharp point), (G) Metzenbaum scissors (delicate pattern 5 ½ in.), (H) Metzenbaum scissors (delicate pattern 7 in.), (I) Fomon upper lateral scissors, (J) Knight nasal scissors, (K) Adson tissue forceps (with teeth angled), (L) Graefe tissue forceps, (M) Wilde dressing forceps

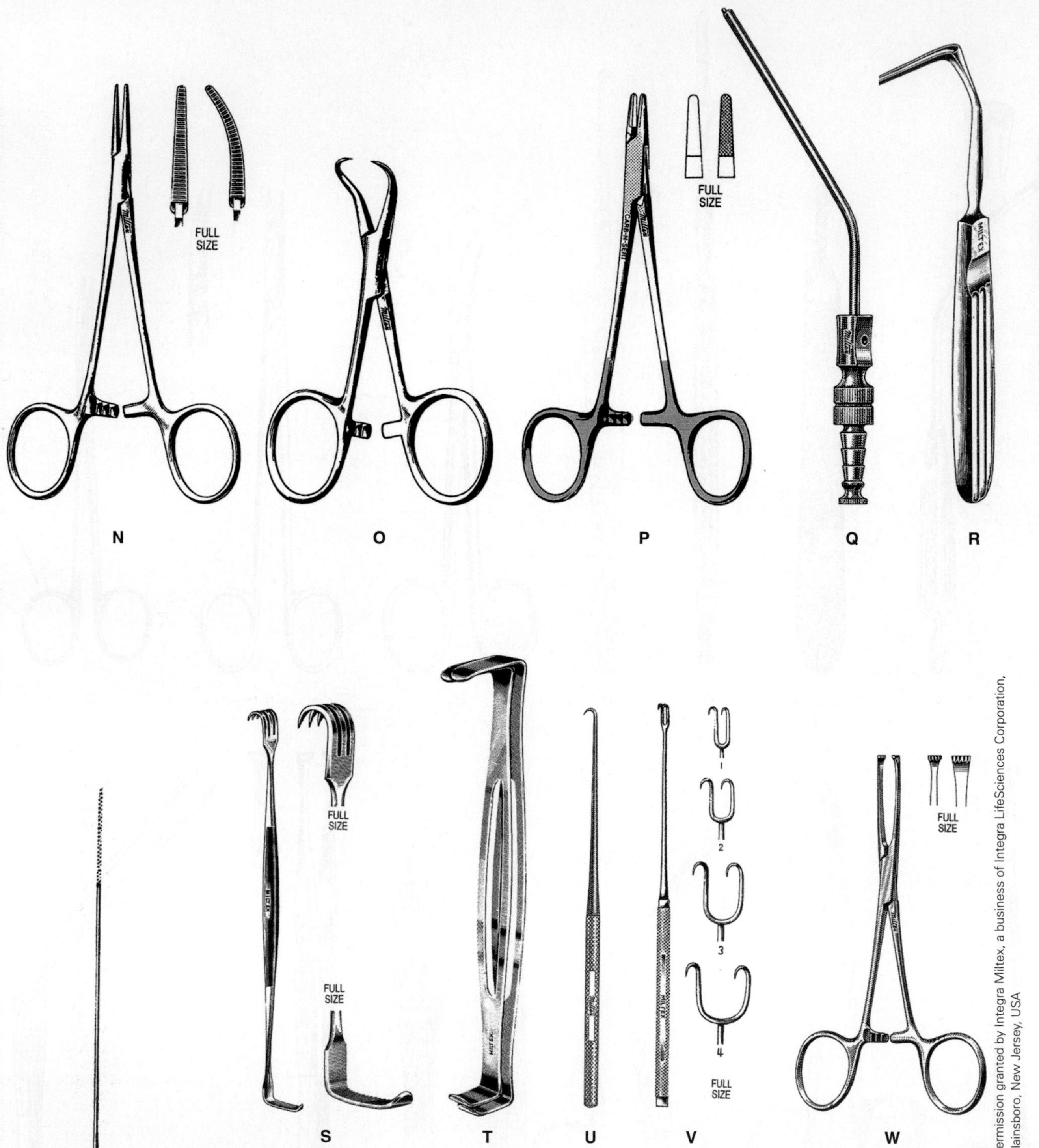

Figure 17-10 Nasal instrumentation: (N) Halsted mosquito forceps (straight and curved), (O) Backhaus towel clamp (3 ½ in.), (P) Halsey needle holder, (Q) Frazier-Ferguson suction tip, (R) Aufricht retractor, (S) Senn retractor, (T) U.S. Army retractor, (U) Joseph single hook, (V) Joseph double hook, (W) Baby Allis forceps

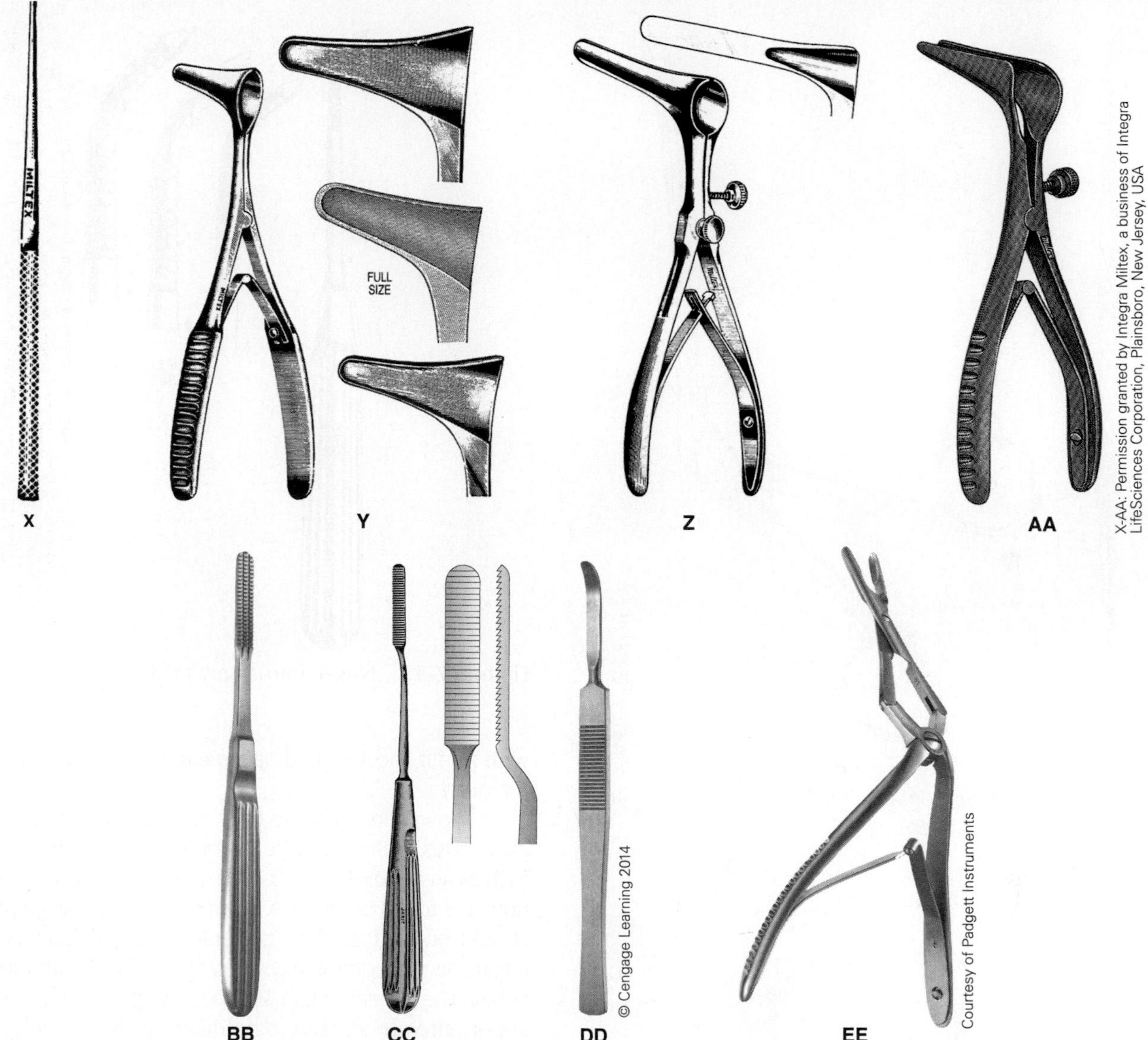

Figure 17-10 Nasal instrumentation: (X) Farrel applicator, (Y) Vienna nasal speculum, (Z) Killian septum speculum, (AA) Cottle septum speculum, (BB) Maltz nasal rasp, (CC) Cottle rasp, (DD) McKenty septum elevator, (EE) Jansen-Middleton septum forceps

administering the local anesthetic. Suggested supplies for this "clean" setup include:

- Two medicine cups
- Two local (Luer-Lok, control) syringes
- Two 25- or 27-gauge × 2"-needles
- Long cotton-tip applicators
- Packing material (½" gauze strips, cotton, or ½" × 3" cottonoids)
- Local anesthetic, with or without epinephrine
- Topical anesthetic (cocaine 4%)
- Nasal speculum
- Bayonet forceps
- Small scissors for trimming nasal hair, if necessary

Provisions to protect and prevent drying of the patient's eyes should be made. Protective eyewear should be available for the patient. The eyewear may be sterile, allowing an awake patient to open his or her eyes during the procedure without danger of injury. It should also adhere and conform to the patient's face so that fluids are restricted from entering and damaging the eye. A cooperative patient may have ointment instilled into the eyes to provide moisture, then be asked to keep the eyes closed during the procedure.

Removal of facial hair is usually not necessary. The prep, if requested, should begin at the upper lip and extend to the hairlines and beyond the chin. Caution must be used not to allow prep solution to enter the patient's eyes or ears.

Draping may include a turban-style wrap to restrain the hair. Three wound towels may be placed in a triangular arrangement, then a bar sheet placed across the forehead,

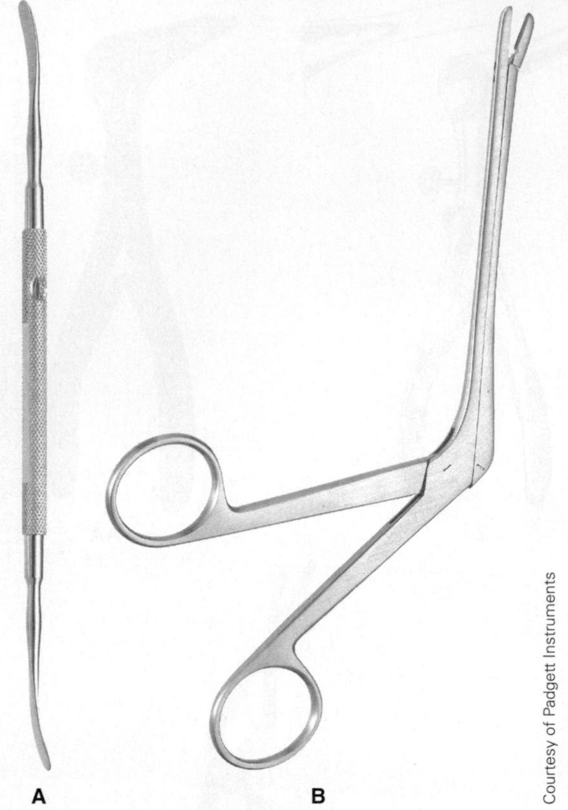

Figure 17-11 SMR/Septoplasty: (A) Freer septum elevator, (B) Takahashi cutting forceps

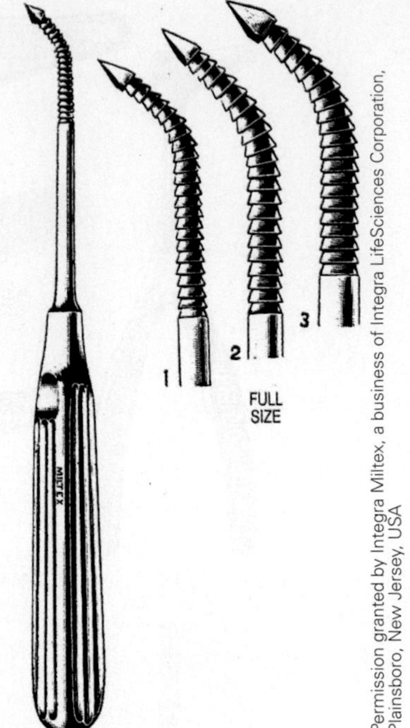

Figure 17-13 Nasal antrostomy rasp

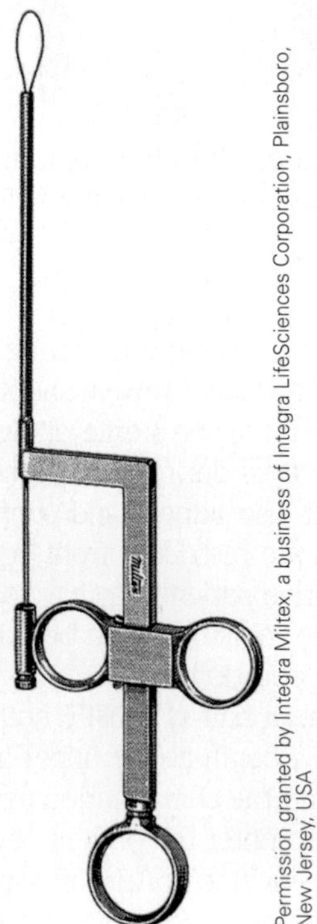

Figure 17-12 Polyp snare

with a split sheet or U-drape encircling the face and covering the body.

Following nasal procedures, the nose may be packed with gauze. This packing may be dry or impregnated with ointment, such as an antibiotic or Vaseline, to prevent crusting and infection, and to aid in removal. Internal and external splint materials may be used as well. The patient is usually provided with a mustache-style dressing that may be secured with tape or tied behind the patient's head. Preoperative patient teaching is very important with all nasal procedures. In this instance, patients should be forewarned that nasal packing will be inserted as part of the procedure. The packing may be uncomfortable and will require breathing through the mouth.

Nose and sinus surgery is generally done on an outpatient basis. Patients should be instructed to have a responsible person available to drive them home and to stay with them for the next 24 hours. A visit to the doctor's office on the first or second postoperative day is usually necessary for removal of the packing.

Procedures performed through the nose are not considered sterile procedures. However, great care should be taken to use the best possible technique to prevent introducing an infectious agent to the area.

SUBMUCOUS RESECTION (SMR)

As the name implies, submucous resection **(SMR)** indicates that the mucous membrane lining the nasal cavity will be incised and the underlying perichondrium or periosteum lifted.

The structures underlying the mucous membrane will be removed to help restore normal breathing. The mucous membrane is then laid back into position and held there with nasal packing material. An absorbable suture may be placed at the incision site.

SMR/SEPTOPLASTY

Septoplasty is most often done to straighten a deviated nasal septum (Figure 17-14). It is also used to repair a perforated septum or one damaged by trauma (Procedure 17-6). A submucosal approach is used. The cartilaginous or osseous portion of the septum causing nasal obstruction is removed, readjusted, or reinserted. Care must be taken not to perforate the septum or cause a weakness of the septum that could lead to a future deformity. Internal nasal splints may be inserted and sutured in place. Septoplasty is often done in conjunction with rhinoplasty.

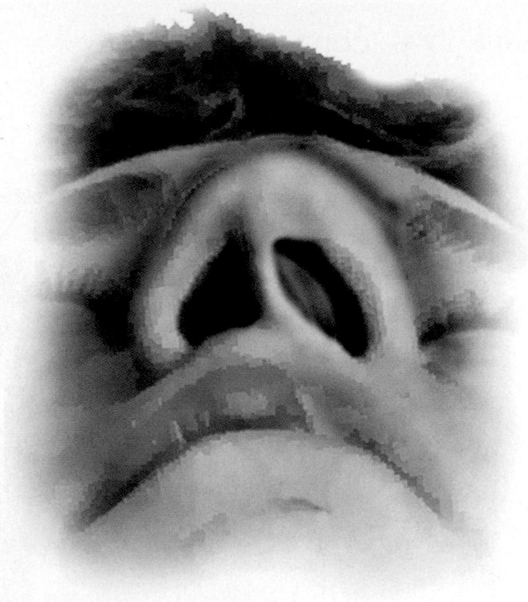

Figure 17-14 Deviated nasal septum

Procedure 17-6 SMR/Septoplasty

Surgical Anatomy and Pathology	• The nasal cavity is divided into two chambers by the nasal septum (Figure 17-15). • Anteriorly, the septum is cartilaginous; posteriorly, the septum has bony attachments to the ethmoid and vomer bones. The septal cartilage is also known as the quadrilateral cartilage. • The nasal septum is typically straight at birth. During aging, the septum tends to deviate to one side or the other. The septum may also become deviated due to trauma. • A deviated nasal septum is seen during visual examination (Figure 17-14). • The septal defect alone does not cause the patient to be symptomatic. There is no related pain, unless soft tissue damage occurs in conjunction with trauma. • If the deviation is severe, the patient may experience difficulty breathing due to the obstruction. The patient may also suffer sinusitis because of ostium blockage, resulting in failure of the affected sinus to drain. • If the septum has been traumatically displaced, it may be manually reduced.
Preoperative Diagnostic Tests and Procedures	• Radiographs • Sinuscopy
Equipment, Instruments, and Supplies Unique to Procedure	• See previous information.

(continues)

PROCEDURE 17-6 (continued)

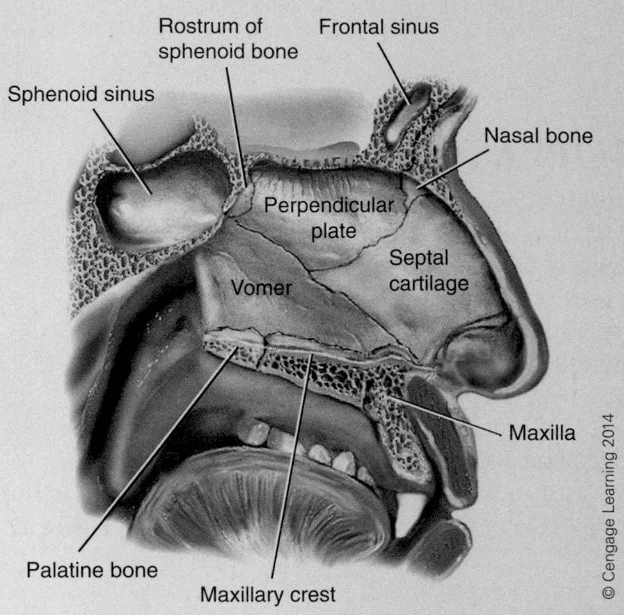

Figure 17-15 Nasal septum and related structures

Preoperative Preparation	• Position, anesthesia, skin prep, and draping as previously described
Practical Considerations	• If local anesthetic used, patient may be awake—keep noise and conversations to a minimum. • Keep drapes away from the face of an awake patient to minimize feeling of claustrophobia and facilitate respirations. • Advise the awake patient to remain still and to anticipate vibrations caused by bone remodeling (e.g., mallet and osteotome).
Surgical Procedure	1. Cocaine-soaked cottonoids placed preoperatively are removed. **Procedural Consideration:** Speculum and bayonet will be needed to remove preoperative packing. Count cottonoids to be sure all have been removed.
	2. Nostril on affected side is opened with a speculum and incision made in mucous membrane and perichondrium. **Procedural Consideration:** Provide surgeon with nasal speculum of appropriate size. Cottle clamp may be used to aid in incision process. Use No. 15 blade on No. 7 knife handle for incision.
	3. Cartilage is incised and mucous membrane is elevated. **Procedural Consideration:** Provide suction as needed. Freer elevator has a sharp and blunt end—most likely the sharp end will be used.

PROCEDURE 17-6 (continued)

4. Deviated structures or bone spurs of the septum, vomer, and/or ethmoid are reduced or removed.

   Procedural Consideration: Continue to provide suction as needed. A chisel and mallet may be used. The surgical technologist may be asked to "tap" the chisel held by the surgeon with the mallet. Bayonet or Takahashi forceps will be needed to extract tissue remnants. Bone and cartilage may be refashioned and reinserted in the nasal cavity to provide strength to weakened areas.

5. Hemostasis is achieved.

   Procedural Consideration: Have suction, hemostatic agents, and/or electrosurgical pencil available.

6. The incision may be sutured or the tissue replaced and held in position with packing material.

   Procedural Consideration: Provide suture or packing according to surgeon's preference. Count.

7. Internal splints may be used.

   Procedural Consideration: Have splint material ready. Splint may need to be cut to fit the individual patient. Heavy scissors will be needed. The splint may be sutured into place.

8. Dressing that may include an external splint is applied.

   Procedural Consideration: Provide "mustache" dressing and external splint if requested.

9. Secretions are removed from the pharynx to reduce the risk of aspiration.

   Procedural Consideration: Provide Wieder retractor and Yankauer suction tip.

Postoperative Considerations

Immediate Postoperative Care

- Transport to PACU.
- The patient should be aware in advance that nasal packing will prevent breathing through the nose.
- Bruising and swelling around the nose and eyes are expected. Advise application of ice packs.

Prognosis

- No complications: Patient is expected to return to normal activities in approximately 7 days; patient will have the packing removed in the surgeon's office 1–3 days postoperatively; full restoration of nasal function is expected.
- Complications: Postoperative SSI; hemorrhage.

Wound Classification

- Class II: Clean-contaminated

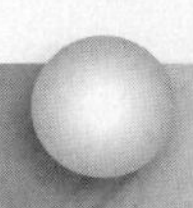

PEARL OF WISDOM

If any cocaine is left at the end of the procedure, be sure that it is irretrievably discarded. For legal reasons and accountability, the surgical technologist should ask the circulator to observe the discard process.

Procedure 17-7 Turbinectomy

Surgical Anatomy and Pathology

- Each nasal cavity has a series of four bony projections called turbinates (also called conchae).
  - The turbinates are osseus ridges on the lateral walls of the cavity.
  - Their names indicate location: supreme, superior, middle, inferior.
  - The orifice of each eustachian tube enters the nasal cavity posterior to the turbinates.
- Hypertrophied turbinates may occur as a result of chronic rhinitis.
  - Because of recurring inflammations, the turbinate loses its normal elastic ability. This can be severe enough to cause nasal obstruction.
- Preoperative diagnostic tests and procedures; equipment, instruments and supplies unique to procedure; preoperative preparation; immediate postoperative care; prognosis and wound classification are the same as for septoplasty.

Practical Considerations

- Turbinectomy usually is performed to remove the inferior hypertrophic turbinate, though it may occasionally be performed on other turbinates. It may be performed in conjunction with other nasal procedures such as septoplasty, rhinoplasty, or sinus surgery.
- There are many methods for reducing the size of the turbinate, including use of electrocautery, sclerosing agents, radiofrequency ablation, cryosurgery, argon plasma surgery, and laser turbinectomy. The history and physical examination including condition of the turbinate will determine the type of procedure that is performed, as well as the surgeon's preference. The surgical technologist will need to be familiar with the method(s) used at the health care facility.

Surgical Procedure

The following provides brief descriptions in paragraph form, as a turbinectomy is similar to a septoplasty.

Inferior Turbinectomy

A submucosal approach is used; the nasal mucosa along the edge of the affected turbinate is incised. A periosteal elevator is placed underneath the turbinate, elevating and fracturing it medially (referred to as infracturing). Angled scissors and rongeur are used to excise the bone and soft tissue of the turbinate. Insulated electrocautery is used for hemostasis and suction followed by nasal packing.

Microdebrider Turbinectomy

A small tube is inserted through a small submucosal incision within the nose and the microdebrider is inserted into the turbinate. A CT-guided imaging system is used to assist the surgeon in viewing the surgical site. The microdebrider is activated with the use of a foot pedal and it quickly and accurately removes the turbinate without damaging surrounding tissue.

Laser Turbinectomy

The lasers commonly used are carbon dioxide, Nd:YAG, and diode lasers. A defocused laser beam or optical fiber delivery is used. Through the submucosal incision, the tissue is vaporized along the anterior inferior aspect of the turbinate to approximately one-half of its length.

The complications of a turbinectomy include hemorrhaging (primary complication), postoperative dryness and crusting, postoperative SSI, formation of adhesions, and conchal bone necrosis.

Procedure 17-8 Polypectomy

Surgical Anatomy and Pathology

- The nasal cavity is the most interior chamber of the nose and is lined with mucous membrane.
  - Its two outside openings, or nostrils, are referred to as the external nares (Figure 17-16).
- The internal nares are the openings from the nasal cavity into the pharynx.
- The hard and soft palates, respectively, form the anterior and posterior floor of the nasal cavity (Figure 17-17).
- **Polyps** are growths that originate from mucous membrane (Figure 17-18). Often the polyps arise from the walls of the sinuses or the ostia and protrude into the nasal passageway.
  - Most often, nasal polyps develop in patients suffering from allergic rhinitis. The recurrent inflammatory process eventually causes a small swelling that enlarges with each subsequent episode.
- The polyp is connected to the mucous membrane by a pedicle.
- Polyps can be multiple and, in some cases, the size and number may cause complete obstruction of the nose. The sense of **olfaction** is often impaired.

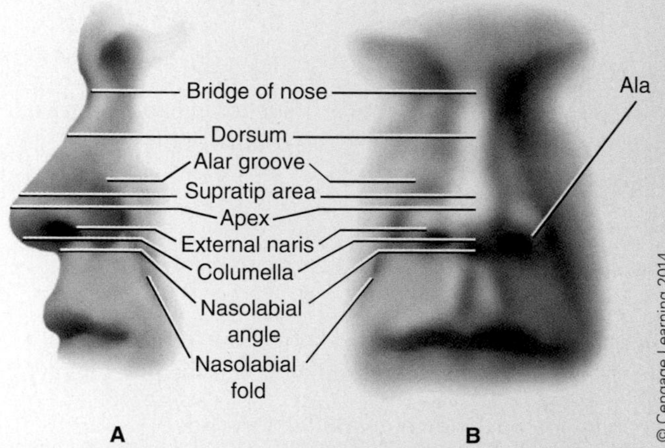

Figure 17-16 External nose: (A) Lateral view, (B) anterior view

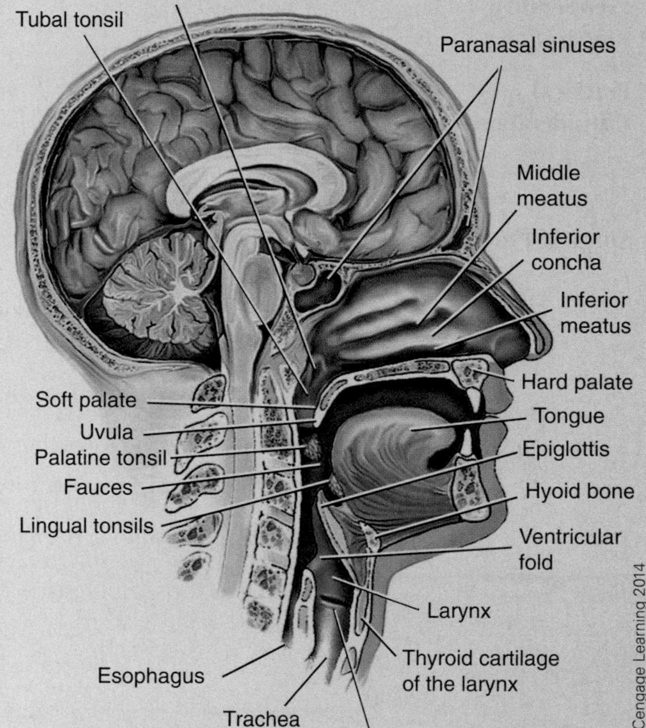

Figure 17-17 Internal anatomy of the oral cavity, nose and throat

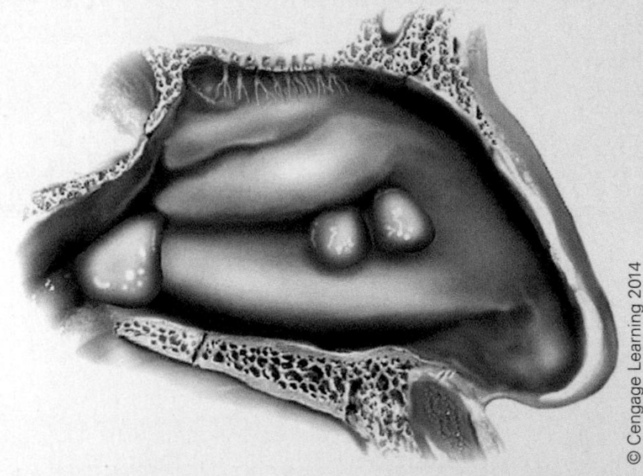

Figure 17-18 Nasal polyps

(*continues*)

PROCEDURE 17-8 (continued)

	• Polyps often reoccur following treatment. • Conservative treatment with steroids can cause temporary shrinkage, but surgical removal usually becomes necessary.
Preoperative Diagnostic Tests and Procedures	• Direct visual examination
Equipment, Instruments, and Supplies Unique to Procedure	• Polyp forceps • Polyp snare • Wires for the polyp snare
Preoperative Preparation	• Same as for septoplasty
Practical Considerations	• A microdebrider may be used for removal of the polyps, providing the advantage of dividing the polyp into small pieces (morcellate) for easy removal by suctioning and improved control of bleeding.
Surgical Procedure	1. The polyp is identified and the wire from the polyp snare is encircled around the polyp. **Procedural Consideration:** The surgical technologist must know how to load the wire onto the polyp snare. The wire should be loaded when setting up for the procedure.
	2. The polyp is grasped with the polyp forceps and gently pulled forward.
	3. The surgeon closes the polyp snare and amputates the polyp. **Procedural Consideration:** Polyps are a specimen to be sent to pathology.
	4. ESU is used to achieve hemostasis.
Postoperative Considerations	• Same as for septoplasty

PROCEDURE 17-9 Choanal Atresia Repair

Surgical Anatomy and Pathology	• See previous descriptions for surgical anatomy. • Choanal atresia is a **congenital** defect caused by the failure of the nasopharyngeal septum to rupture during embryonic development. • The result is the bony or membranous occlusion of the passageway between the nose and pharynx.
Preoperative Diagnostic Tests and Procedures	• Rhinography • CT scan • When an 8-Fr catheter cannot be inserted choanal atresia is suspected due to blockage of the nasal passage • Absence of fog on a mirror when it is placed under the nostrils • Stethoscope to listen to breath sounds

PROCEDURE 17-9 (continued)

Equipment, Instruments, and Supplies Unique to Procedure	• Instrumentation similar to septoplasty • Power drill and burs (depending on procedure that is performed) • Microdebrider (depending on procedure that is performed) • 4-mm, 30-degree angled endoscope (depending on procedure that is performed)
Preoperative preparation is the same as for septoplasty	
Practical Considerations	• The surgical technologist will need to be familiar with all the various types of procedures that are performed for choanal atresia. • The standard precautions and care for pediatric patients will need to be taken.
Surgical Procedure	The following provides brief descriptions in paragraph form, as the procedure is similar to other nasal procedures. The transnasal puncture is not described because it is rarely performed due to its high failure rate. *Transseptal Technique* This technique consists of making an incision in the septum in order to visualize the bony and/or membranous obstruction; a microscope is used by the surgeon. The obstruction is then removed by powered burs or microdebrider. *Endoscopic Technique* The 4-mm endoscope is inserted endonasally with its angle directed inferiorly. The surgeon will use powered burs and/or a microdebrider to repair the choanal atresia.
Postoperative Considerations	**Immediate Postoperative Care** • Transport to PACU. • Patient usually sent home same day of surgery as long as normal respirations are confirmed. • Parents are taught to watch child closely for any signs in difficulty in breathing. **Prognosis** • No complications: Patient returns to normal activity in less than a week. • Complications: Postoperative SSI; hemorrhage; reoccurrence; palatal fistula; maxillofacial growth disturbance. **Wound Classification** • Wound Class II: Clean-contaminated

PROCEDURE 17-10 Functional Endoscopic Sinus Surgery (FESS)

Surgical Anatomy and Pathology	• A series of ducts called *ostia* lead to the paranasal sinuses, which are air cavities in the bone surrounding the nasal cavity. • The sinuses are lined with mucous membrane that is continuous with the lining of the nasal cavities. • There are four pairs of paranasal sinuses; each is named by location according to the bone that encloses it (Figures 17-19 and 17-20): frontal, ethmoid, sphenoid, and maxillary. • Frontal sinuses are located within the frontal bone behind the

(continues)

PROCEDURE 17-10 (continued)

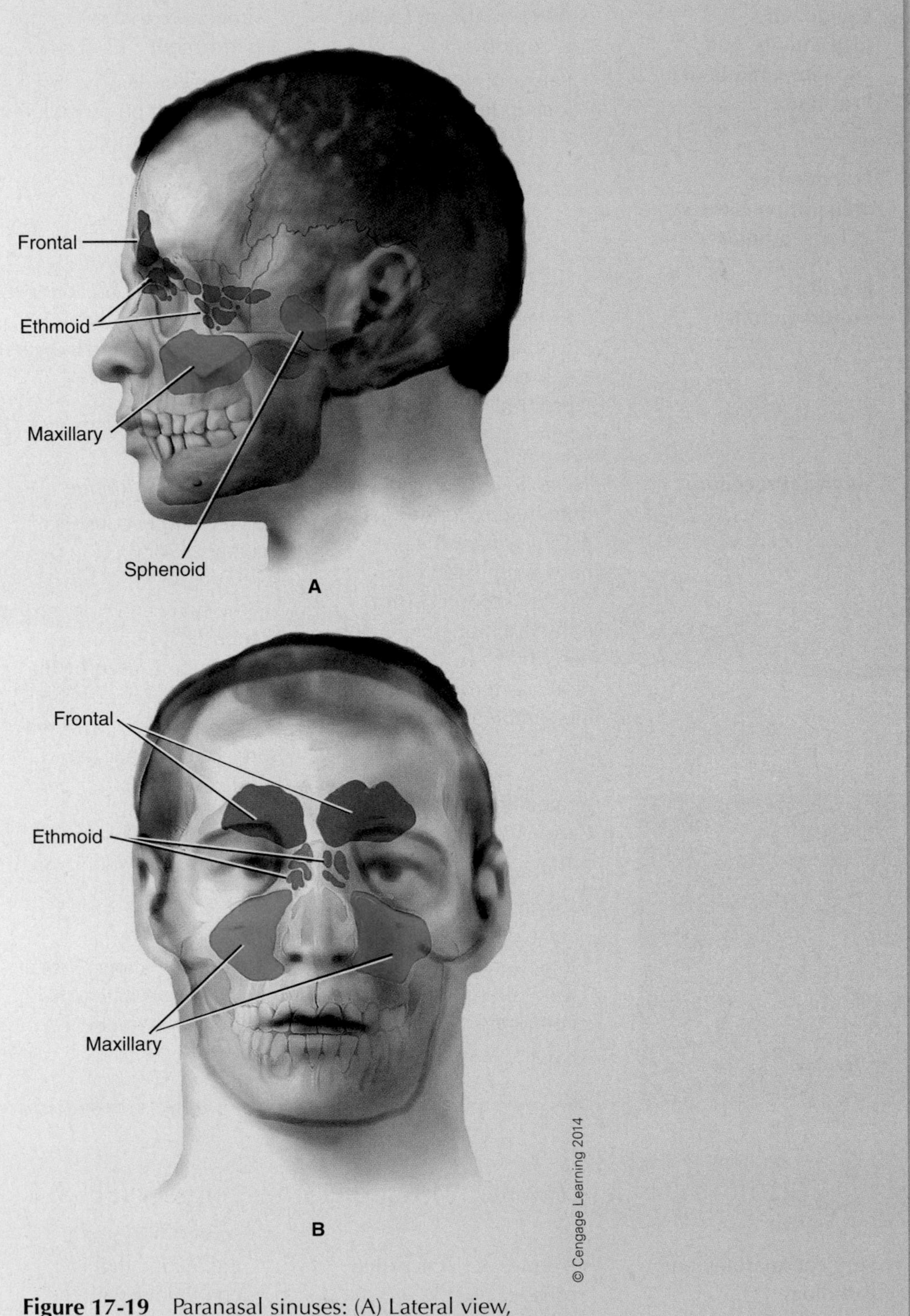

Figure 17-19 Paranasal sinuses: (A) Lateral view, (B) anterior view

PROCEDURE 17-10 (continued)

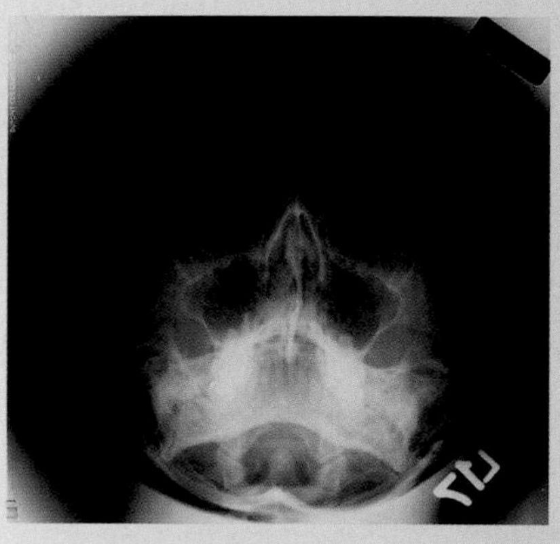

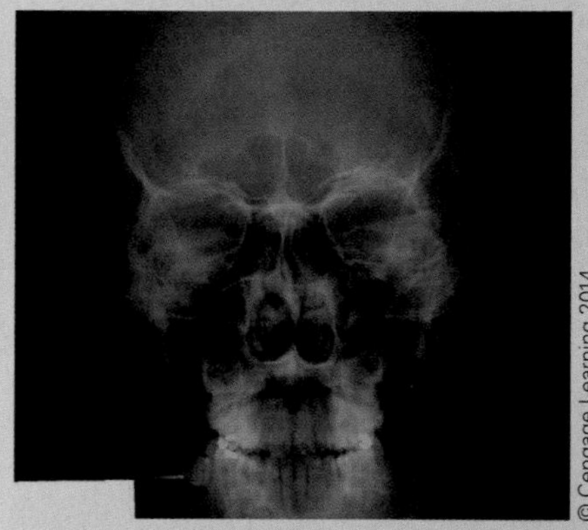

Figure 17-20 Radiographic views of sinuses: (A) Waters, (B) Caldwell

	eyebrows and may be one cavity or divided. • Ethmoid sinuses, numbering 10–15, are located between the eyes and have a honeycomb appearance. • Sphenoid sinuses are located directly behind the nose at the center of the skull and may be one cavity or divided.	• Maxillary sinuses are located below the eyes and lateral to the nasal cavity. • FESS is performed as a diagnostic procedure and/or used to treat a variety of sinus disorders, anatomical defects, and inflammatory conditions such as chronic sinusitis.	• The goal of FESS is to reestablish normal breathing and the ability of mucus to be cleared from the sinuses. Due to the inflammation, the mucus cannot be cleared and is trapped within the sinus, which can result in the formation of a mucocele and sinus infection.
Preoperative Diagnostic Tests and Procedures	• History and physical examination	• CT scans	
Equipment, Instruments, and Supplies Unique to Procedure	• Basic nasal set • Endoscopic instruments: scissors; biopsy forceps; cutting forceps; suction tips; endoscopic shavers	• Endoscopic video equipment: monitors, light source • Camera • Sinuscope light cord • 4- or 5-mm sinuscopes (Figure 17-21)	• 0-, 30-, 70-, 90-, and 120-degree lenses • Antifog for lenses • Suction-irrigation system • Navigational system
Preoperative Preparation	• Position, skin prep, draping as previously described for nasal procedures	• General anesthesia or monitored anesthesia care (MAC)	
Practical Considerations	• CT scans are available in the OR. • Test all equipment prior to the arrival of the patient in the OR.	• The surgeon may want the endoscope attached to the camera or use the eyepiece of the endoscope for viewing.	The surgical technologist should know the surgeon's preference. • The surgical technologist should be very familiar

(continues)

PROCEDURE 17-10 (continued)

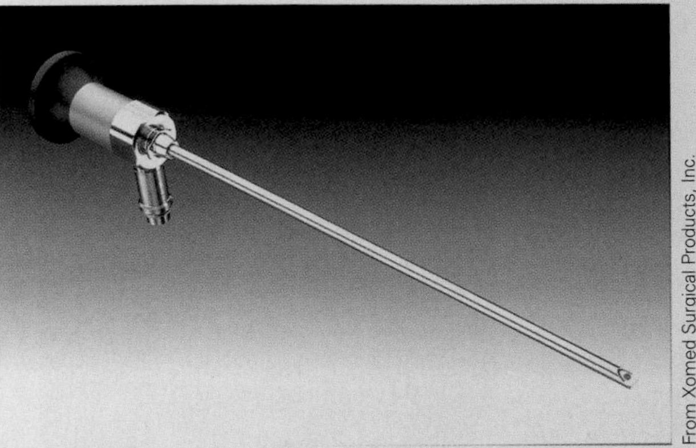

Figure 17-21 SharpSite™ AC autoclavable endoscope for sinus endoscopy

with all the specialized endoscopic equipment, endoscope, instrumentation, and navigation system.

- The surgical technologist should know how to carefully change out the lenses on the endoscope, in particular if the surgeon will be working on more than one sinus cavity. The cavity being worked on determines the angled lens that is required.
- There are several types of navigational systems available on the market. The surgical technologist should be familiar with the system used at the health care facility, including setup, testing, intraoperative trouble-shooting, and downloading the CT scans into the system.
- As with all endoscopic procedures, the surgical technologist should pass instruments in such a manner that the surgeon does not have to look away from the endoscope lens or video monitor.
- The surgical technologist should be able to help the surgeon in identifying the patient's eyes on the monitor and maintain visualization of them during the duration of the procedure to avoid injury.
  - If the surgeon identifies an intraorbital hematoma, it will need to be immediately treated.
  - If the orbit is accidentally entered, it can be confirmed by the presence of the yellow orbital fat on the monitor. If any member of the surgical team views this on the monitor, the surgeon should be immediately told.
- The topical/local anesthetic should be set up on a separate Mayo stand.

Surgical Procedure

1. The surgeon applies the topical anesthetic and injects the local anesthetic.

   Procedural Consideration: The surgical technologist should confirm the endoscope lens that will be used and if necessary change the lens.

2. The endoscope is introduced into the nose.

   Procedural Consideration: Prior to insertion of the endoscope, the lens should be wiped with the antifog wipe. The process is repeated every time the endoscope is extracted and reinserted.

3. The ostia of the sinus to be worked on is visualized and enlarged to facilitate drainage.

   Procedural Consideration: The suction-irrigation device will be used as needed. An antrum punch, spoon, or probe will be used to enlarge the ostium.

PROCEDURE 17-10 (continued)

4. The diseased tissue is visualized and excised.

   Procedural Consideration: Straight or angled Blakesley forceps will be used to remove the diseased tissue. Continue to provide suction-irrigation as needed. Maintain patency of suction device by irrigating suction tip or using a stylet.

5. Biopsy may be performed and polyps, if present, are excised.

   Procedural Consideration: Provide biopsy forceps or polypectomy instruments, or endoscopic shaver of surgeon's preference. Suction with a collection bottle, such as a Lukens tube, may be used to collect several specimens.

6. An ethmoidectomy may be performed to create one large sinus cavity to promote improved drainage.

   Procedural Consideration: The surgeon may require a different angled lens; use caution when changing the lens and use the antifog wipe before the endoscope is reinserted. The surgeon will insert the endoscope into the ethmoid sinus and will alternate between using the Blakesley forceps to cut small bits of bone and suction to remove the bone. This can be a long and tedious step of the procedure, especially in a darkened room—remain alert.

7. The surgeon may perform a sphenoidectomy if diseased bone was identified on the CT scan.

   Procedural Consideration: The sphenoidectomy is performed just like the ethmoidectomy.

8. Endoscope is removed; antibiotic ointment is placed.

   Procedural Consideration: Have antibiotic ointment drawn up in a syringe for internal application. Count may not be necessary; follow health care facility policy.

9. Mustache dressing is applied.

   Procedural Consideration: Have dressing materials prepared.

Postoperative Considerations

As previously described for nasal procedures

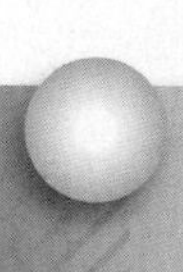

PEARL OF WISDOM

Once FESS has been performed, a second FESS becomes more difficult because the anatomical landmarks may be destroyed.

Intranasal Antrostomy

Antrostomy is performed to treat sinusitis or remove recurrent polyps that originate from within the maxillary sinus. Intranasal antrostomy is an opening into the maxillary sinus through the nasoantral wall of the maxilla just below the inferior turbinate. The incision is made over the inferior turbinate. The mucosa is elevated and the wall of the nasal cavity is punctured with an antrum trocar or an antrum rasp that has a trocar tip. The opening into the sinus may be enlarged with the use of a small rongeur. The cavity is inspected under direct vision. Purulent material is aspirated and possibly cultured. Any polyps or diseased tissue is removed with antrum curettes that are specifically angled for exactly this purpose. It may be necessary to irrigate the sinus with saline or antibiotic solution. The small defect in the maxilla is not repaired. The mucosa is returned to the normal location and is held in place with packing material. If greater exposure is needed, a Caldwell-Luc procedure may be necessary.

Procedure 17-11 Caldwell-Luc

Surgical Anatomy and Pathology	• Surgical anatomy as previously described for sinus surgery • Pathology as previously described for sinus surgery	• The Caldwell-Luc procedure is a more radical type of antrostomy and is performed when intranasal antrostomy alone does not provide adequate visualization.	• The purpose of the procedure is to remove diseased portions of the antral wall, evacuate sinus contents, and establish drainage through the nose.
Preoperative Diagnostic Tests and Procedures	• CT scan		
Equipment, Instrumentation, and Supplies Unique to Procedure	• Caldwell-Luc retractor	• Insulated ESU	• Power drill available if needed to open maxilla
Preoperative Preparation	• Position, skin prep, and draping as previously described for nasal procedures	• General anesthesia • Lidocaine with epinephrine injected for	hemostasis and postoperative pain control
Practical Considerations	• CT scans should be in the OR.	• Caldwell-Luc is contraindicated in pediatric patients prior to the descent of the permanent teeth.	

Surgical Procedure

1. The gingiva above the canine tooth and second molar is incised (Figure 17-22).

   Procedural Consideration: Provide the Caldwell-Luc retractor and the No. 15 blade. Provide suction as needed.

2. The periosteum of the inferior wall of the maxilla is elevated and the infraorbital nerve is identified and carefully retracted.

   Procedural Consideration: Have electrocautery available for hemostasis. Freer elevator will be needed for the periosteal dissection. Observe incisional site for nerve. Caldwell-Luc retractor will be repositioned.

3. The bone is perforated with an osteotome or a small drill bit.

   Procedural Consideration: Present drill or osteotome and mallet.

4. The opening into the maxillary sinus is enlarged with a small rongeur.

   Procedural Consideration: Have Kerrison rongeur ready. Continue to provide suction. Suction apparatus is easily clogged by purulent diseased material; prepare to change suction tips frequently and clean with water or stylet as needed.

5. The sinus is evacuated of any purulent matter and polyps or diseased tissue is removed.

   Procedural Consideration: Coakley curettes or Takahashi nasal cutting forceps will be needed to remove tissue. All tissue removed is saved as specimen.

PROCEDURE 17-11 (continued)

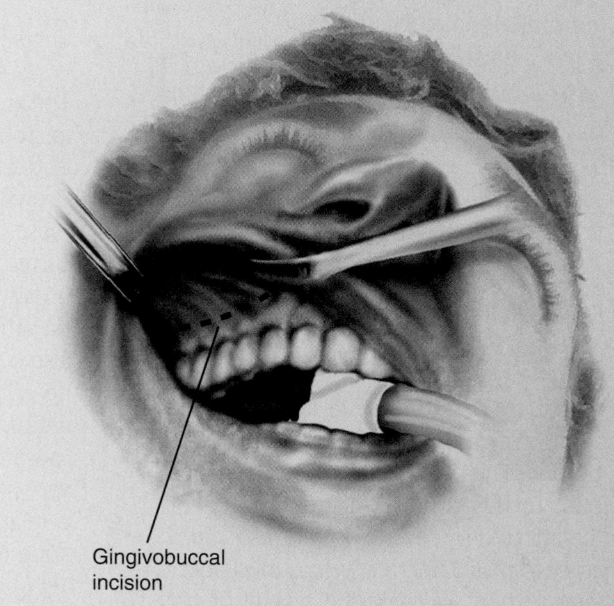

Figure 17-22 Caldwell-Luc

6. If necessary, an opening is made into the nasoantral wall below the inferior turbinate.

   Procedural Consideration: Antrum trocar/rasp will be needed to create nasoantral window. Anticipate the use of the antral suction tip and place on tubing.

7. Hemostasis is achieved and the nose and sinus may be packed.

   Procedural Consideration: Have hemostatic agents or insulated electrosurgical suction apparatus ready. Prepare packing material according to surgeon's preference.

8. The gingiva is sutured with absorbable suture material.

   Procedural Consideration: Pass suture loaded on needle holder and tissue forceps followed by suture scissors. Count.

Postoperative Considerations

Immediate Postoperative Care

- Transport to PACU.
- Bruising and swelling inside the mouth, on the upper lip, and around the nose and eyes are expected. Advise application of ice packs and soft diet.

Prognosis

- No complications: Patient is expected to return to normal activities within 7 days. Normal respiratory function is expected, but may take several weeks.
- Complications: postoperative SSI; hemorrhage.

Wound Classification

- Class II: Clean-contaminated

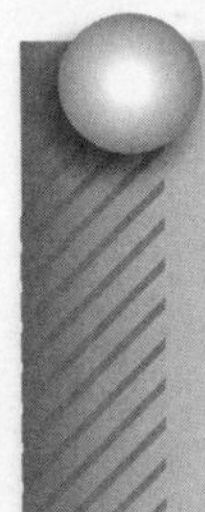

PEARL OF WISDOM

The Caldwell-Luc retractor is a specialty retractor that may need to be sterilized prior to the case. Be sure this and all other necessary instruments are available.

ORAL CAVITY AND THROAT PROCEDURES

The oral cavity and throat consists of several individual and specialized structures that work in harmony to facilitate respiration and ingestion of food. The pharynx, larynx, trachea, and esophagus all contribute to this complex anatomical region. These structures can be affected by several conditions ranging from minor inflammatory to malignancy as well as mechanical disorders. The following section will describe several of the basic procedures.

Diagnostic Procedures/Tests for the Oral Cavity and Throat

Any patient assessment should include a full history given by the patient, if possible. Any medication allergies should be noted. This should include any symptoms that the patient is experiencing and any exposure to disease that the patient may have recently had. The examiner should take the patient's temperature, as this can be a reliable indicator of an inflammatory process under way. The physical exam should include special attention to the suspected target of the disorder, but should not be limited. Nearby lymph nodes should be palpated for any abnormalities.

Direct Visualization

Direct visualization is the most efficient method of examining the pharynx. The examiner uses direct lighting, which may be in the form of a flashlight, headlamp, or gooseneck lamp. The patient is asked to open his or her mouth for the examination. A tongue blade maybe used for soft tissue manipulation.

Indirect Visualization

In addition to direct visualization, the use of a mirror can be employed to view the nasopharynx and laryngopharynx. The mirror should be treated with a commercial antifog preparation or warmed to prevent fogging. A light is directed toward the mirror and refracted into the area to be viewed. The image of the structures is revealed in the mirror. If the vocal cords are visible, the patient may be asked to imitate certain sounds so that the examiner can better view the vocal cords and assess the quality of the sound produced.

Laboratory Tests

The following laboratory examinations are useful in the diagnosis of disorders of the throat:

- *Culture and sensitivity:* If the presence of a microorganism is suspected, any tissue or body fluid can be cultured. The area of the body that is suspected of hosting a microorganism is rubbed with a sterile swab. The collected fluid is placed in a culture medium and incubated. Growth of the invading organism is encouraged under these circumstances. When sufficient growth has occurred, the organism can be identified. Cultures are usually obtained to determine the presence of bacteria, although tuberculosis, fungi, and some viruses can also be identified this way. Once the infective agent has been identified, the susceptibility (sensitivity) to various antibiotics can be evaluated so that eradication of the causative organism will be achieved. A throat culture is very common and takes only a few seconds to obtain. It is relatively painless. If *Streptococcus* is suspected, a rapid strep test may be performed.
- *Blood count:* A complete blood count may be ordered. This is useful in determining anemia, a tendency to bleed, and the presence of infection. The white blood cells (WBCs) are the cells that usually fight infection. The normal range for WBCs is from 4,000 to 10,000. A WBC count over 10,000 may indicate the presence of an infection.

Radiologic Examinations

The following radiographic examinations are useful in the diagnosis of disorders of the throat:

- *X-rays:* Routine radiographic examinations are very useful in determining pathology of the larynx and trachea. The only bony structure in the larynx is the hyoid, but the cartilaginous structures of the upper respiratory tract are clearly visible on radiography, as are some of the more dense soft tissue structures, such as the **epiglottis**. Contrast media, such as barium, may be introduced into the area to enhance visualization. The use of barium is especially helpful in determining pathology of the esophagus. Great care must be taken to prevent aspiration of the liquid. Fluoroscopy may be helpful in tracking the flow of the barium.
- *CT scans:* CT allows comparison of the soft tissue structures of the neck to the other structures. Gross changes in the structure can be detected with CT.
- *MRI:* MRI provides superb viewing of the soft tissue structures of the neck.

Videostroboscopy

Videostroboscopy is used for precise analysis of endolaryngeal tissue during speech. The strobe equipment is introduced into the larynx via a flexible **laryngo**scope. The exact movement of the vocal mucosa can be studied and pathological changes easily noted.

Polysomnography

Polysomnography is an examination used to diagnose sleep **apnea** and determine its severity. The test is used to record vital body functions such as heart rate, respiration, air flow, and blood oxygen levels during sleep, as well as brain activity, eye movement, and muscle activity.

Multiple Sleep Latency Test (MSLT)

The MSLT measures the amount of time that it takes an individual to fall asleep. The average time is 10–20 minutes. Those who fall asleep in less than 5 minutes are considered to have some type of sleep disorder.

Routine Instruments, Equipment, and Supplies

Some health care facilities may have a specialty neck instrument tray. However, for the most part, instrumentation used for oral cavity and throat procedures will be a general surgery major instrument tray with add-ons such as skin hook retractors. The exceptions are the tonsillectomy and adenoidectomy, and tracheostomy instrument trays that have instrumentation specific to those procedures.

TABLE 17-2 Tonsillectomy and Adenoidectomy Instrument Tray

Instrument	Quantity
No. 7 knife handle	1 ea.
Metzenbaum scissors	1 ea.
Mayo scissors, straight	1 ea.
Schnidt (tonsil) clamps	2 ea.
Allis forceps, straight	2 ea.
Allis forceps, curved	2 ea.
White tonsil seizing forceps (Figure 17-24D)	1 ea.
Sponge clamp, straight	1 ea.
Sponge clamp, curved	1 ea.
Needle holder, 6"	1 ea.
Davis mouth gag with blades of various sizes (Figure 17-24B)	
McIvor mouth gag with blade (Figure 17-24A)	1 ea.
Lothrop uvula retractor (Figure 17-23A)	1 ea.
Cheek retractor (Figure 12-23B)	1 ea.
Weider tongue depressor (Figure 12-24C)	1 ea.
Hurd dissector and pillar retractor	1 ea.
Sage tonsil snare with wire (Figure 17-24F)	1 ea.
Fisher tonsil knife (Figure 17-24E)	1 ea.
Adenoid punch	1 ea.
La Force adenotomes, small, medium, and large	1 ea.
Barnhill adenoid curettes of various sizes	

The following is a list of routine equipment and supplies:

- Gowns
- Gloves
- Basin set
- Suction system
- No. 10 and No. 15 knife blades

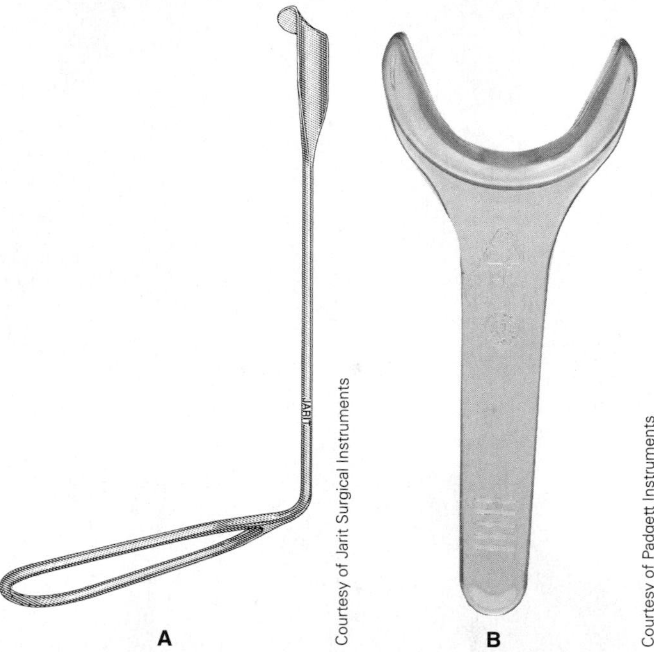

Figure 17-23 Pharyngeal instrumentation: (A) Lothrop uvula retractor, (B) cheek retractor

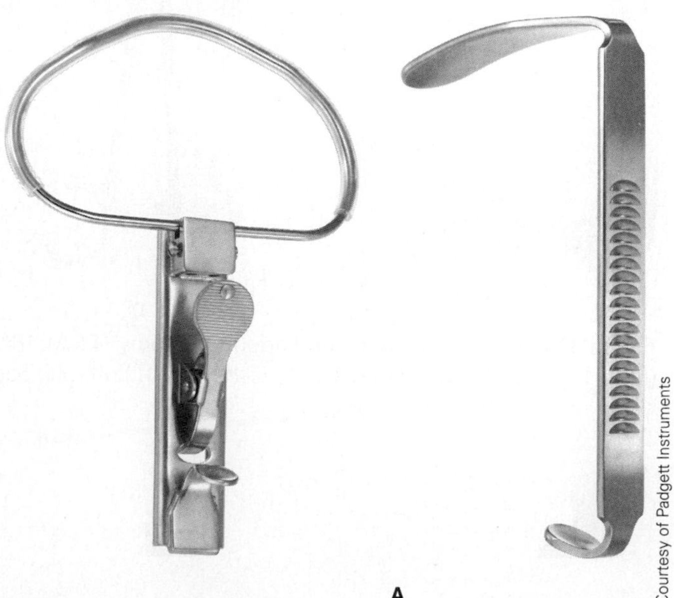

Figure 17-24 Tonsillectomy and adenoidectomy (T&A): (A) McIvor mouth gag with blade

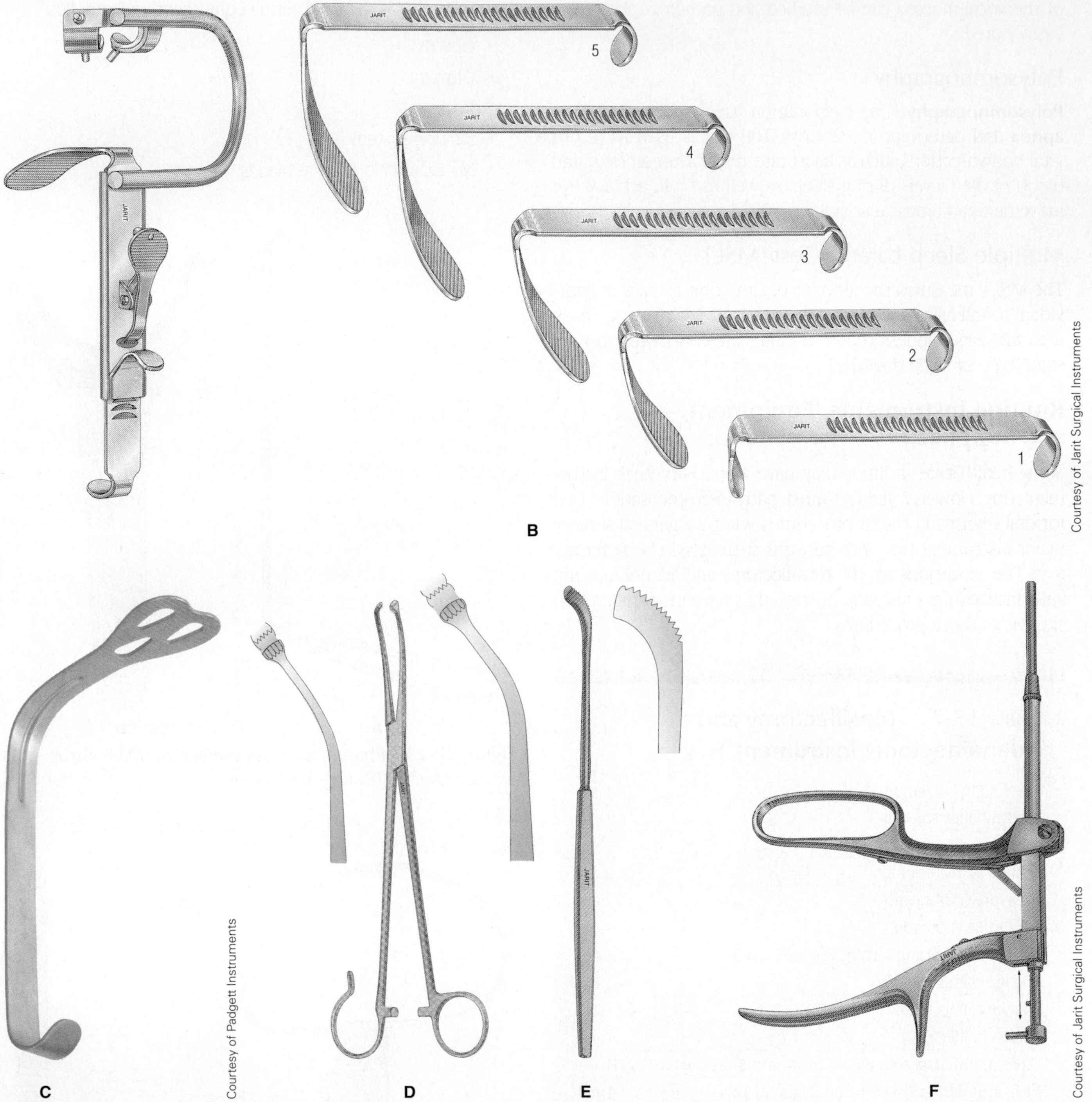

5

4

3

2

1

B

Courtesy of Jarit Surgical Instruments

C

Courtesy of Padgett Instruments

D

E

F

Courtesy of Jarit Surgical Instruments

Figure 17-24 Tonsillectomy and adenoidectomy (T&A): (B) Davis mouth gag with blades, (C) Weider tongue depressor, (D) White tonsil seizing forceps, (E) Fisher tonsil knife, (F) Sage tonsil snare

Table 17-3 Tracheostomy Instrument Tray

Item	Quantity
No. 3 knife handles	2 ea.
No. 11 and No. 15 knife blades	1 ea.
Metzenbaum scissors	1 ea.
Mayo scissors, curved	1 ea.
Mayo scissors, straight	1 ea.
Mosquito clamps, curved	4 ea.
Crile clamps, curved	4 ea.
Allis forceps	2 ea.
Needle holder	2 ea.
Adson forceps with teeth	1 ea.
Tissue forceps with teeth	1 ea.
Yankauer suction tip	1 ea.
Frazier suction tip	1 ea.
U.S. Army retractors	2 ea.
Senn retractor, sharp and blunt	2 ea.
Tracheostomy hook	2 ea.
Trosseau tracheal dilator (Figure 17-25A)	1 ea.
Jackson tracheal tube with obturator, several sizes (Figure 17-25B)	

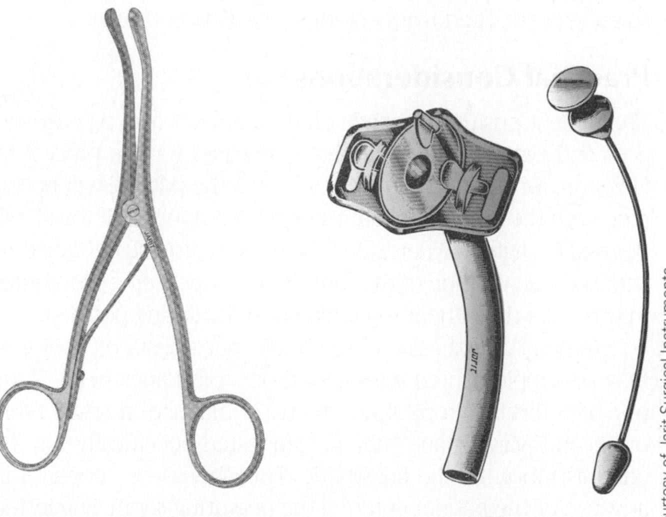

Figure 17-25 Tracheotomy: (A) Trosseau tracheal dilator, (B) Jackson tracheal tube with obturator

- ESU
- Insulated ESU with suction attachment
- Head and neck back table pack
- Kitners
- 4 × 4 radiopaque sponges
- Bulb syringe
- Marking pen
- Vessel loops
- Microscope
- Microscope drape
- Laser for specific procedures
- Sitting stools
- Lukens tube
- Endoscopic equipment and instrumentation for endoscopy procedures

The operating microscope is a critical part of laryngeal surgery (Figure 17-26). Great care should be used when relocating the microscope. The microscope should be brought into the operating room and set up in advance of the surgery. An f = 400 lens is commonly used. For laryngeal procedures, a sterile microscope cover is not usually used. A laser may be attached to the microscope to enhance microlaryngeal surgery.

Laser surgery is becoming very common in procedures involving the larynx and oropharynx. The most popular laser for this application is the carbon dioxide laser. The carbon dioxide laser can be used in conjunction with the operating microscope to focus the beam.

As with any surgical procedure, proper illumination is essential. A variety of illumination devices are available. Each surgeon will have a preference for the type of device that he or she finds most effective.

Sitting stools should be available, especially when the use of a microscope is anticipated.

A No. 12 knife blade is often used in oropharyngeal surgery. The special feature of the No. 12 knife blade is that it is curved with the cutting surface on the inner aspect of the curve. Because of its extended length and slim handle, the No. 7 knife handle is often used as well.

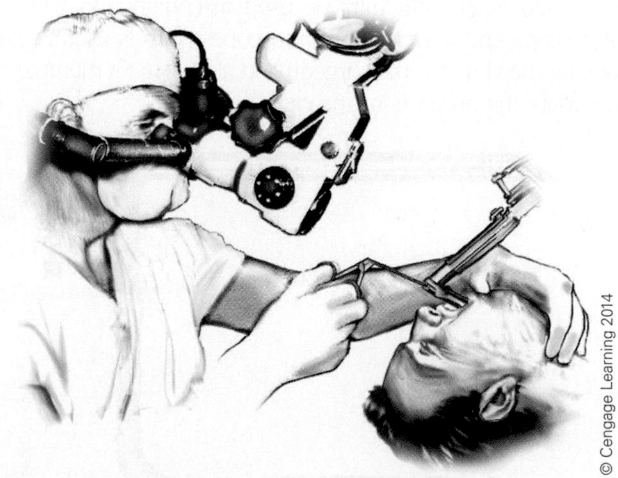

Figure 17-26 Operating microscope set up for microlaryngoscopy

Various endoscopes are used for oral or transnasal endoscopy. These instruments may be flexible or rigid. Each structure to be viewed has its own set of specialized scopes and correlating instrumentation.

There are three common varieties of laryngoscopes:

- An L-shaped, battery-operated laryngoscope is the instrument of choice for endotracheal intubation. The battery is located in the handle of the instrument. Various interchangeable oral blades are available to assist with intubation of patients of all sizes and shapes.
- Flexible laryngoscopes are available for assisting with a difficult intubation, diagnosis, or may be used for obtaining a biopsy.
- Rigid U-shaped laryngoscopes are used for biopsy, removal of a foreign body, or vocal cord procedures (Figure 17-27). The rigid laryngoscope is often suspended on a holding apparatus to maintain its position and to free the surgeon's hands. Microscopic and laser procedures are performed using the rigid laryngoscope.

Bronchoscopes are also available in flexible and rigid styles and come in a variety of sizes for use in infant, pediatric, and adult patients. A rigid bronchoscope can be differentiated from the rigid esophagoscope because the distal portion is relatively straight and it houses the ventilation holes. Flexible bronchoscopes are small in diameter and are longer than laryngoscopes. If the patient will require oxygen therapy, a special adapter must be used to make the connection with the oxygen source.

The esophagoscope, as with the other styles of endoscopes, may be either flexible or rigid. Because the esophagus is a collapsible structure, the rigid esophagoscope is flared at the distal end for better visibility (Figure 17-28). Often the flexible gastroscope is used when the esophagoscopy is performed as part of a more comprehensive procedure called esophagogastroduodenoscopy, or EGD, where the gastroenterologist inspects not only the esophagus, but the stomach and duodenum as well. There is a flexible esophagoscope available but it is not often used alone.

Video equipment may be used in conjunction with the microscope and a variety of endoscopes. This is useful in enhancing the view for the surgeon and allows team members to anticipate the progress of the case.

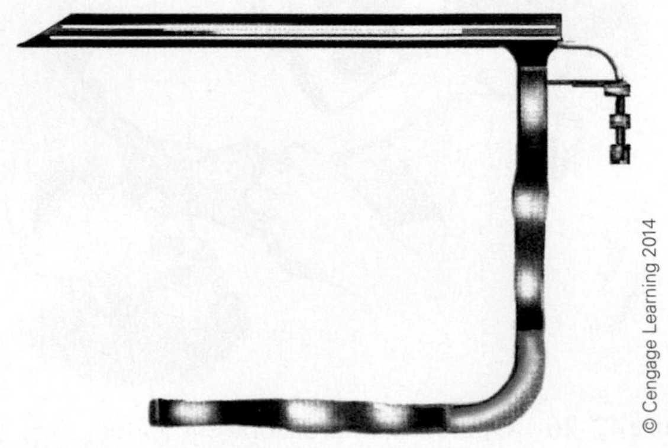

Figure 17-27 U-shaped rigid laryngoscope

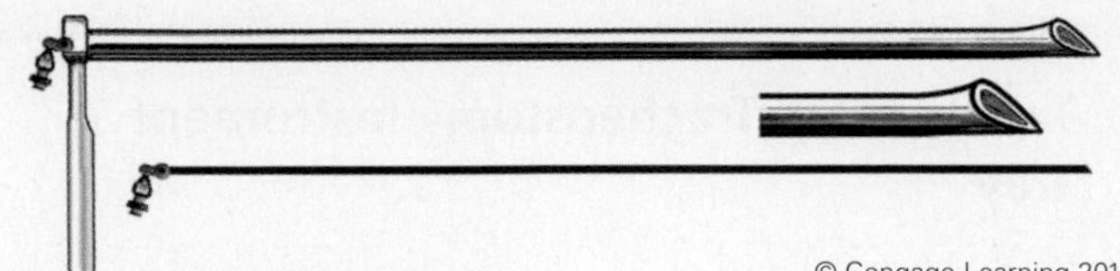

Figure 17-28 Rigid esophagoscope

An insulated electrosurgical device with a suction attachment may be used. The suction device is a flexible modification of a neuro suction tip. It is insulated and may have a thumb control for the suction. The active electrode is at the very tip of the instrument and is usually controlled with a foot pedal. It is capable of suction and coagulation at the same time. The length of the instrument makes it very useful in the pharynx.

A histological stain may be used to differentiate abnormal cells. This is especially useful in the esophagus and larynx. An example of one of these stains is toluidine blue.

Topical anesthetics may be used for oral endoscopy. The anesthetic agents may include Cetacaine spray or cocaine. Local anesthetics may be used for tonsillectomy on the adult patient. Lidocaine or bupivacaine, with or without epinephrine, may be used. The patient may be sedated.

The Lukens tube, sometimes referred to as the Lukens trap, is incorporated into the suction apparatus by attaching it between the suction tip and the suction tubing. It uses gravity to capture fluid (secretions or fluid instilled to obtain cell washings) to be sent for laboratory analysis. The tube must be maintained in the upright position during specimen collection to prevent the fluid from entering the suction tubing.

Practical Considerations

The patient position depends on the patient's age, type of surgery, and type of anesthetic that is planned for the procedure. However, for the majority of procedures the patient will be supine with the arms tucked at the side. A scapular roll towel will be used to slightly hyperextend the neck to provide better exposure and visualization of the surgical site. Endoscopic procedures may require the patient to be placed in the sitting position.

General anesthesia is usually the anesthesia of choice. It may be supplemented with a local or topical anesthetic. If the use of a local or topical anesthetic is planned, a small table or second Mayo stand may be requested specifically for the administration of the anesthetic. This should be prepared in advance of the patient entering the operating room. Suggested supplies for this "clean" setup are:

- Medicine cups
- Syringes and needles
- Cotton tip applicators
- Anesthetic of choice
- Atomizer
- Tongue blades
- Laryngeal mirror

- Small basin of warm water for defogging the mirror
- Gauze sponges

The skin prep and draping varies according to the surgical procedure. They will be discussed within the surgical procedures that are presented.

Other items of importance to the surgical team include the following:

- If only a local anesthetic is planned, and an anesthesia provider will not be in the OR, a second circulator may be requested for patient monitoring purposes.
- If the patient is expected to rest the voice following the procedure, it should be communicated to him or her in advance what type of communication will be used postoperatively.
- Many procedures of the oral cavity are performed on an outpatient basis. The patient should make arrangements in advance for transportation and assistance for at least the first 24 hours.
- The surgical technologist may work directly from the back table instead of using a Mayo stand for some oral cavity procedures, such as endoscopic procedures.
- The surgical technologist will have the responsibility of coordinating with the surgical team handling the surgical specimens and communicating the correct information to the circulator; multiple specimens may be taken during the procedures.
- The surgical technologist should know how to guide the instrumentation into the endoscope when assisting with endoscopic procedures.
- Although procedures performed through the oral cavity are not considered sterile, sterile technique should still be practiced to prevent a postoperative SSI.

Procedure 17-12 Tonsillectomy and Adenoidectomy

Surgical Anatomy and Pathology

- The pharynx is a tubular structure that serves the respiratory tract by receiving air from the nose and mouth, and the digestive system as a passageway for food and liquids (Figure 17-29).
  - The pharynx begins at the internal nares and terminates posterior to the larynx at the level of the esophagus.
  - The pharynx is lined with mucous membrane and is contiguous with the nose superiorly and the larynx and esophagus inferiorly. It lies anterior to the vertebrae in the midline of the neck.
  - It is divided into three regions: nasopharynx, oropharynx, and laryngopharynx.
  - The nasopharynx is the most superior portion of the pharynx, located posterior to the nasal cavity.
  - Beginning at the posterior nares, the nasopharynx extends inferiorly to the uvula.
  - The eustachian tubes enter the nasopharynx, and it houses the pharyngeal tonsils.
  - The pharyngeal tonsils are a single mass of lymphatic tissue embedded in the mucous membrane of the posterior wall of the nasopharynx. When the pharyngeal tonsils are enlarged, they are referred to as the adenoids. The tonsils provide protection against pathogens entering the nose. The lymphatic tissue of the tonsils usually begins to shrink in size after about age 7.
- The oropharynx is the middle portion of the pharynx, located posterior to the oral cavity, and it houses the palatine and lingual tonsils.
  - The oropharynx begins at the uvula, communicates superiorly with the nasopharynx, and extends to the level of the hyoid bone. The anterior opening is the mouth (refer to Plate 6 in Appendix A).
  - The palatine, or faucial, tonsils are the two oval masses of lymphoid tissue commonly called the "tonsils." The palatine tonsils are located at each edge of the fauces with the folds of two bands of tissue that descend from the soft palate to the base of the tongue called the tonsillar pillars. Each tonsil has an anterior and posterior pillar. Behind each posterior tonsillar pillar is a pink band of lymphoid tissue called the lateral

(continues)

PROCEDURE 17-12 (continued)

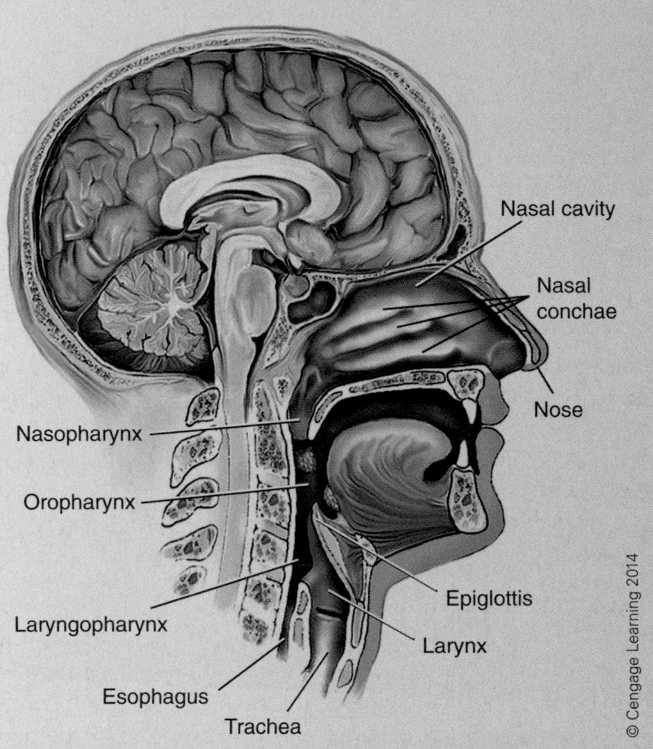

Figure 17-29 Three sections of the pharynx and related structures

pharyngeal band. The tonsils produce lymphocytes. Each tonsil contains 10–20 crypts that help trap bacteria (Figure 17-17).

- The lingual tonsils are a pair of lymphoid areas located on the posterior surface of the tongue near the base.

- Tonsillitis may affect the pharyngeal, palatine, and lingual tonsils. It usually refers to the palatine tonsils.
  - Tonsillitis of the palatine tonsils may be acute or chronic. Most often it is caused by a streptococcal organism. Acute tonsillitis is an inflammation of the tonsils and their crypts. On visual examination, the tonsils appear enlarged and dusky in color. Purulent matter may be seen in the tonsillar crypts. The tonsils may enlarge to the point of being obstructive. Repeated attacks of acute tonsillitis may indicate that removal is necessary. Chronic tonsillitis is evidenced by a persistent sore throat, foul breath, and enlarged cervical lymph nodes. Removal may become necessary. Failure to treat chronic tonsillitis can lead to peritonsillar abscess formation.
  - Peritonsillar abscess formation results from failed antibiotic therapy or chronic tonsillitis. The abscess forms between the tonsil and the fascia covering the pharyngeal constrictor muscle and is visible upon examination of the oral cavity (Figure 17-30). The patient is in extreme pain and may experience difficulty breathing and referred pain to the ear on the affected side. Antibiotics may be

Procedure 17-12 (continued)

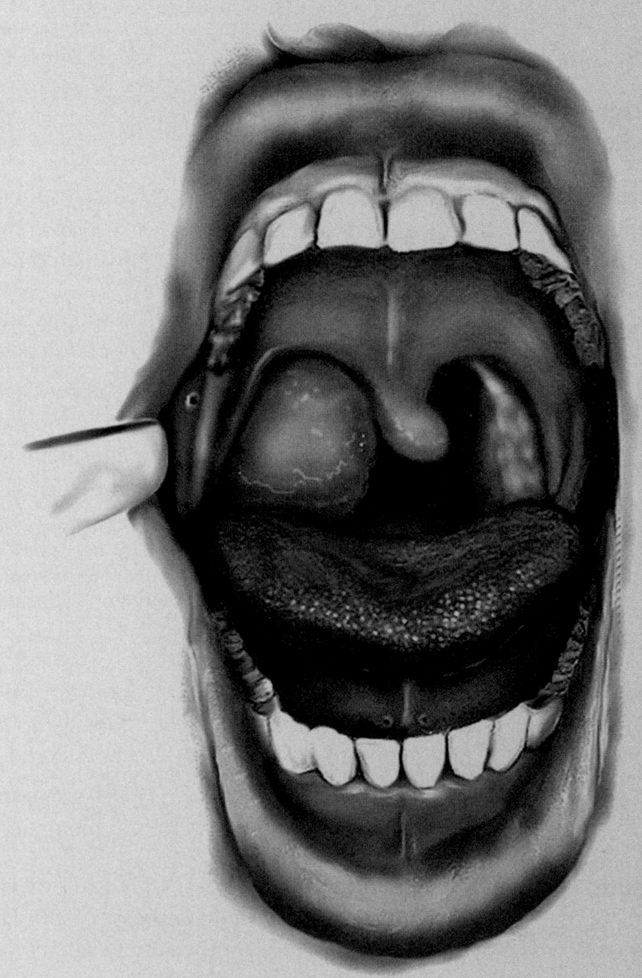

Figure 17-30 Right peritonsillar abscess

helpful, but surgical intervention may be necessary. An incision and drainage (I & D) is performed. The tonsils are usually excised when all evidence of infection has cleared. The infection from the abscess may quickly spread throughout the neck and chest, causing complications such as pericarditis, which can be fatal.

- Adenoiditis is inflammation of the pharyngeal tonsils. This is usually bacterial, although it can be viral or due to allergies. Recurrent adenoiditis can lead to **hypertrophy**. The hypertrophic tissue can cause snoring due to nasal obstruction or hearing impairment due to eustachian tube blockage. Antibiotics may be helpful, but surgical excision is often necessary.
- The palatine tonsils and adenoids are excised during a tonsillectomy and adenoidectomy **(T&A)** procedure.
- The lingual tonsils are also at risk of becoming infected. Antibiotics and saline irrigations are recommended initial treatments. If the

(*continues*)

PROCEDURE 17-12 (continued)

	infection is recurrent, lingual tonsillectomy	can be performed. This is often accomplished	with the use of the carbon dioxide laser.
Preoperative Diagnostic Tests and Procedures	• History and physical examination		
Equipment, Instruments, and Supplies Unique to Procedure	• Headlamp • ½ sheet × 2	• Tonsil sponges • No. 12 knife blade • Insulated ESU	• Suction cautery • 8-Fr Robinson catheter
Preoperative Preparation	• Position: Supine with neck hyperextended for pediatric patients. For the comfort of the surgeon and easier access to the surgical site, pediatric patients may be positioned close to the side of the OR table where the surgeon will be	standing. Sitting position for adult patients. • Anesthesia: General for pediatric patients; local anesthetic for adult patients. • Skin prep: Not required • Draping: one or two ½ or ¾ sterile sheets	placed on patient. Adult patients the surgeon will wrap two turban's around the patient's head held in place with a perforating towel clip to isolate the hair. Pediatric patients the hair will be isolated with a hair cover.
Practical Considerations	• Surgeon preference will dictate the order of the procedure. In a combination procedure some surgeons prefer to	perform the tonsillectomy first and then the adenoidectomy. • The surgeon may stand at the patient's side or sit	at the head of the table. Make the necessary equipment adjustments and arrange the OR accordingly.

Surgical Procedure

1. The mouth is held open with a self-retaining mouth gag. The tongue is retracted with a Wieder tongue depressor. An 8-Fr Robinson catheter may be inserted through the naso-oral cavity to retract the uvula from the operative site.

   Procedural Consideration: If using a Jennings mouth gag, it will be necessary for the anesthesia provider to disconnect the endotracheal (ET) tube from the anesthesia circuit for insertion of the retractor and then reconnect it. The anesthesia provider will position the oral ET tube on the nonoperative side. Be sure ET tube is not dislocated or occluded with the retractor. The surgical technologist will likely hold the tongue depressor after placement by the surgeon and provide suction. Have all other supplies within reach of the surgeon.

2. The tonsil is grasped and the mucosa of the anterior pillar is incised.

   Procedural Consideration: A tonsil tenaculum or long Allis will be needed to put tension on the tonsil. Pass the scalpel and follow with the electrosurgical pencil or scissors.

3. The tonsil is dissected free of its mucosa.

   Procedural Consideration: Pass the pillar dissector and continue to provide suction.

4. The tonsil may be amputated with a snare or a guillotine, or electrosurgically removed from its fossa.

   Procedural Consideration: If the use of a snare is planned, it should be loaded in advance.

5. Once the tonsil is amputated, pressure may be applied to the fossa with a tonsil sponge for a few minutes.

   Procedural Consideration: The tonsil sponge is loaded on a long instrument for temporary placement in the tonsil fossa.

PROCEDURE 17-12 (continued)

6. Hemostasis is achieved.

   Procedural Consideration: Hemostasis is usually achieved electrosurgically. Have tonsil hemostats and suture available if hemostasis is not achieved electrosurgically.

7. The procedure is repeated contralaterally.

   Procedural Consideration: The anesthesia provider will move the ET tube to the contralateral side of the mouth. Quickly reorganize the supplies to facilitate removal of the second tonsil. The surgeon generally does not switch sides.

8. The uvula is retracted to expose the nasopharynx.

   Procedural Consideration: The soft palate retractor is positioned by the surgeon and held in position by the surgical technologist. Provide suction as needed.

9. Adenoids are removed with an adenotome or curette.

   Procedural Consideration: Provide instrument of choice.

10. Pressure is applied to control bleeding.

    Procedural Consideration: Provide tonsil sponge loaded on a long instrument.

11. Hemostasis is achieved electrosurgically.

    Procedural Consideration: Provide pillar retractor and electrosurgical pencil to surgeon. Suction as needed. It may be necessary to change from electrosurgical pencil to the electrosurgical device with the suction attachment.

12. The nasopharynx may be irrigated to be sure all clots and tissue have been removed.

    Procedural Consideration: Have irrigation supplies ready according to surgeon's preference. Surgical technologist may be asked to instill irrigation fluid through the nose.

13. A final inspection of all sites is performed and hemostasis verified.

    Procedural Consideration: Continue to provide retraction and suction as needed. Count.

14. Retractors are removed.

    Procedural Consideration: Anesthesia provider will disconnect ET tube if necessary for retractor removal. Do not dislocate ET tube. Clean patient's face if needed.

Postoperative Considerations

Immediate Postoperative Care

- Once extubated, the patient should be placed on his or her side to prevent aspiration.
- Elevate the head of the bed slightly to reduce postoperative swelling.
- Provide cold fluids to aid in comfort and prevent swelling.
- Transport to PACU.

Prognosis

- No complications: Patient is expected to return to normal activities in 2 weeks. Incidence of sore throats and infections should be greatly reduced.
- Complications: Bleeding is the most common postoperative complication and can occur up to 10 days after surgery; postoperative SSI.

Wound Classification

- Class II: Clean-contaminated

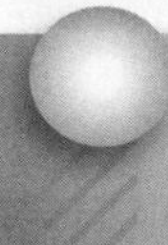

PEARL OF WISDOM

The tonsils and adenoids may be sent to pathology in the same container per facility policy. If it is necessary to distinguish the right from the left, the surgical technologist should make the necessary adjustments.

PROCEDURE 17-13 Parotidectomy

Surgical Anatomy and Pathology	• Saliva is secreted by the three pairs of salivary glands that are situated outside the oral cavity: parotid, submandibular, and sublingual glands.
	  • The saliva they secrete is transported to the cavity via ducts.
	• The parotid gland is the largest of the three glands located on the lateral sides of the face anterior to the external ear.
	  • The excretory duct is called Steno's duct, and its orifice is on the inner surface of the cheek opposite the second molar tooth of the upper jaw.
	  • A significant concern when performing surgery on the parotid gland is the course of the facial nerve, because it travels through the gland, dividing the superficial portion from the deeper portion.
	• A parotidectomy is the excision of a portion or all of the parotid gland.
	  • A common disorder is the formation of stones that block Steno's duct. The number and type of stones can vary from one or two large stones to several small stones located in the gland itself or the duct. Surgery is performed to clear the ducts or, if too many stones are present, to remove the gland.
	  • The gland may also have to be partially or fully excised due to a benign or malignant mass. Most tumors occur in the superficial lobe; tumors located in the deeper lobe usually are indicative of a malignant mass.

Preoperative Diagnostic Tests and Procedures	• History and physical examination • CT scan • MRI
Equipment, Instruments, and Supplies Unique to Procedure	• Headlamp • Thyroid instrument set in addition to major instrument set • Extra right-angle clamps • Nerve hooks • Nerve stimulator • Extra single and double skin hooks
Preoperative Preparation	• Position: Patient is supine with head turned and operative side facing up; arms tucked at sides. Donut or headrest is used. • Anesthesia: General • Skin prep: Prep the entire side of the face slightly beyond the midline including the ear, extending from the hairline to the axilla. Prevent prep solution from entering the ear by gently placing a cotton ball. • Draping: Turban-style wrap with towels to cover the hair; bar drape across the forehead and opened superiorly to cover the head; U-drape or split sheet: U or split portion placed along bottom of neck using clavicles as a landmark and the tails placed upward along the middle of the clavicles medial to the shoulder joints, and bottom portion of drape opened to cover the body.

Procedure 17-13 (continued)

Practical Considerations	• OR table may be turned to facilitate access to the surgical site. • Imaging studies should be in the OR. • Surgeon may sit for the procedure.
Surgical Procedure	1. The surgeon makes a skin incision starting anterior to the ear and continuing downward toward the neck, stopping just below the mandible. **Procedural Consideration:** Position instruments near the surgeon and in such a manner that he or she can safely grab them from the Mayo stand (if standing for procedure) or back table (if sitting for procedure).
	2. Skin flaps are established and elevated with skin hooks. **Procedural Consideration:** The surgical technologist will be responsible for holding the skin hooks to elevate the skin flaps.
	3. The gland is identified and dissected free from the sternocleidomastoid muscle (SCM) with Metzenbaum scissors, electrocautery, and DeBakey forceps. **Procedural Consideration:** The surgical technologist's movements must be as careful and meticulous as those of the surgeon to prevent damage to the facial nerve and its branches.
	4. Next, the gland is dissected free from its attachments to the external auditory canal. The surgeon performs this portion of the dissection carefully because it will reveal the facial nerve and the temporal, zygomatic, mandibular, and cervical branches for identification. **Procedural Consideration:** Pass the vessel loop to the surgeon attached to the tip of the jaw of a right-angle clamp to facilitate passing the loop around the nerve. Clamp the ends of the vessel loop with a mosquito clamp and gently retract the nerve to one side.
	5. Dissection is continued with a mosquito hemostat and electrocautery along the facial nerve and its branches until the superficial lobe is excised. **Procedural Consideration:** If both the superficial and deep lobe are removed, ask the surgeon if he or she prefers to keep the specimens separate.
	6. If the deep lobe must be excised, the facial nerve is gently retracted with a vessel loop. The mandible is retracted with the use of Kocher clamps. **Procedural Consideration:** Assist the surgeon in the placement of the dressing materials.
	7. The nerve branches are dissected from the deep lobe using the mosquito clamp and electrocautery. To preserve the nerve, care is taken with all of the dissection and the procedure is not hurried.
	8. The gland is dissected from of its attachments to the masseter muscle with the Metzenbaum scissors, electrocautery, and Debakey forceps. Allis clamps are applied to the deep lobe to provide countertraction and facilitate the dissection.
	9. The dissection is completed and the deep lobe is removed.
	10. The wound is thoroughly irrigated and suctioned and checked for bleeding.
	11. A closed-wound drainage system is placed.
	12. The wound is closed in layers and a bulky dressing is placed.

(*continues*)

Procedure 17-13 (continued)

Postoperative Considerations

Immediate Postoperative Care

- Patient is transported to PACU.
- Elevate the head of the stretcher to aid in reducing postoperative swelling.

Prognosis

- No complications: Patient should be able to return to normal activities in 2–3 weeks.
- Complications: Postoperative SSI; hemorrhage; facial nerve weakness or paralysis, temporary or permanent.

Wound Classification

- Class I: Clean

Procedure 17-14 Uvulopalatopharyngoplasty (UPPP)

Surgical Anatomy and Pathology

- The roof of the mouth consists of two segments that are collectively referred to as the palate (Figure 17-17).
  - The anterior segment is referred to as the hard palate and is supported by extensions of the maxillary and palatine bones.
  - The soft palate is posterior and consists of connective tissue and muscle. The soft palate terminates with a projection of lymphoid tissue called the uvula.
  - During swallowing the nasopharynx is protected by the soft palate, which moves upward to seal off the nasopharynx, directing food and liquids downward.
- **UPPP** is performed to treat patients who suffer from sleep apnea.
  - Sleep apnea patients suffer numerous, brief interruptions in respiration during sleep, leaving the patient feeling sleepy during the day.
  - All age groups and genders suffer from sleep apnea, but it is more common in males.
  - Sleep apnea patients often have a family history of the disorder, are overweight, snore, have high blood pressure, and may have a physical abnormality of the upper airway. Drug and alcohol use increases the frequency and duration of episodes.
  - Sleep apnea is a potentially life-threatening disorder that has been linked to serious complications, including dysrhythmias, high blood pressure, heart attack, and stroke.
  - It has two known causes. Central sleep apnea is the less common type and occurs when the brain fails to signal the muscles controlling respiration.
  - The second type, obstructive sleep apnea, occurs when a problem with the upper respiratory tract prevents movement of air through the nose or mouth during respiration. The structural problems causing the airway obstruction can be varied. A natural relaxation of the muscles of the throat and tongue can cause the tongue and soft palate to sag into the airway, causing obstruction. The supine position assumed during rest periods can also be a contributing factor. In obese individuals, an excess amount of tissue in the upper airway can cause obstruction.

Preoperative Diagnostic Tests and Procedures

- Polysomnography
- Multiple Sleep Latency Test

Procedure 17-14 (continued)

Equipment, Instruments, and Supplies Unique to Procedure	• Headlamp • CO_2 laser (surgeon's preference if performing UPPP as a laser procedure)	• ½ or ¾ sheet × 2 • Tonsil sponges • No. 12 knife blade • Suction cautery	• Tracheotomy instrument tray and supplies available in the OR
Preoperative Preparation	• Position: Supine with neck hyperextended; donut or foam headrest; arms tucked at sides	• Anesthesia: General • Skin Prep: Not required	• Draping: Head turban to keep hair controlled; ½ or ¾ sheets placed to cover patient's body
Practical Considerations	• If the patient is obese, it will be necessary to pre-plan the needed positioning equipment, including size of the OR table, instrumentation, and supplies. • A tracheotomy may be performed prior to the start of the UPPP to	ensure a patent airway. If the patient is obese, an extra-long tracheostomy tube may be needed. • If a tracheotomy is not performed, the possibility of an emergency tracheotomy exists. All equipment and supplies	should be available in the OR. • The patient may be difficult to intubate; be prepared to assist the anesthesia provider. • T & A will be performed in conjunction with UPPP if the tonsils and adenoids are present.

Operative Procedure

1. Self-retaining mouth gag is inserted.

   Procedural Consideration: The ET tube should not be dislocated or occluded with the retractor. Provide suction as needed.

2. An outline of the tissue to be resected may be made with a scalpel or the electrosurgical pencil (Figure 17-31A).

   Procedural Consideration: Provide No. 12 blade on a No. 7 knife handle or electrosurgical pencil.

3. Tonsils, if present, will be included in en bloc dissection.

   Procedural Consideration: Provide tonsil tenaculum or Allis clamp. Metzenbaum scissors, electrosurgical pencil, or laser and tissue forceps will be used for dissection.

4. Dissection progresses to include the soft palate on the operative side, uvula, and continues with the soft palate on the contralateral side. It is completed with the second tonsil, if present.

   Procedural Consideration: Dissection will continue with instrument of surgeon's choice. Continue to provide suction as necessary.

5. The specimen will be extracted and hemostasis will be achieved (Figure 17-31B).

   Procedural Consideration: Prepare to accept the tissue specimen. Tonsil clamps and suture may be needed for hemostasis. Prepare to switch back and forth between the electrosurgical pencil and the electrosurgical device with the suction attachment or the laser.

(*continues*)

PROCEDURE 17-14 (continued)

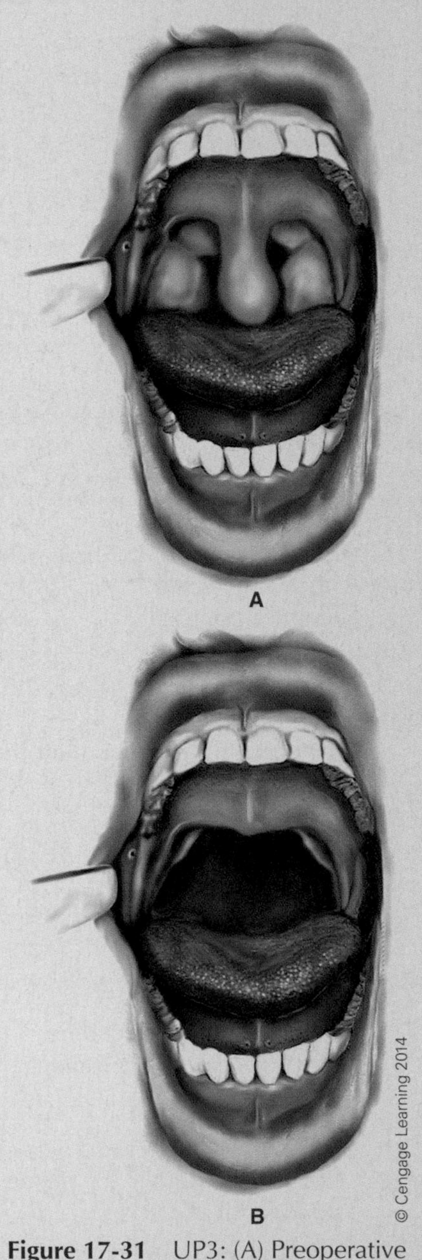

Figure 17-31 UP3: (A) Preoperative view–redundant tissue (fauces, tonsils, and soft palate, (B) postoperative view

6. Oral cavity and pharynx are irrigated to remove blood clots or tissue remnants.

   Procedural Consideration: Bulb syringe should be prefilled with irrigation solution. Suction is necessary.

7. The mucosal edges are sutured with a running stitch.

   Procedural Consideration: Provide absorbable suture according to surgeon's preference and long tissue forceps. Suture scissors as needed.

PROCEDURE 17-14 (continued)

8. Adenoidectomy is performed if necessary.

   Procedural Consideration: Refer to Procedure 17-8 for technical considerations.

9. Mouth gag is removed.

   Procedural Consideration: Count. Do not dislocate ET tube.

Postoperative Considerations

Immediate Postoperative Care

- When fully awake, the patient may be provided with cold liquids for comfort and prevention of swelling.
- The patient should be instructed not to use a straw for fluid intake.
- Tracheotomy may become necessary, if not already implemented.

Prognosis

- No complications: Patient may remain hospitalized for several days and is expected to return to normal activities in 2 weeks. Sleep disorders and episodes of hypoxia should be reduced or eliminated.
- Complications: Postoperative SSI; hemorrhage; airway obstruction due to swelling

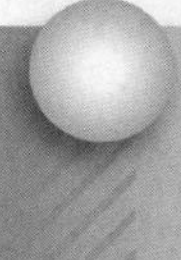

PEARL OF WISDOM

A tongue blade should not be used for postoperative inspection of the surgical site to prevent disruption of the suture line.

PROCEDURE 17-15 Laryngectomy

Surgical Anatomy and Pathology

- The larynx is located between the pharynx and trachea (Figure 17-32). Nine laryngeal cartilages and hyoid bone form its rigid framework. Muscles and ligaments connect the cartilages to one another. The larynx has ligamentous attachments to the hyoid bone.
  - There are three pairs of cartilages: arytenoid, corniculate, cuneiform; three individual cartilages: thyroid, cricoids, and epiglottis. All the cartilages, except the epiglottis, are formed of hyaline cartilage; the epiglottis is elastic cartilage.
  - The largest and most superior of the single cartilages is the thyroid cartilage. It consists of a pair of shield-like plates fused in the front, projecting forward to form what is commonly known as the Adam's apple.
  - The cricoid cartilage is the only cartilage in the upper respiratory tract to form a complete circle and is located at the base of the larynx. It is the most inferior of the laryngeal cartilages and attaches to the trachea.
  - The epiglottis is an elongated leaf-like structure. The base of the epiglottis is attached inferiorly to the thyroid cartilage; the posterior aspect is located in the laryngopharynx.
  - The arytenoid cartilages are the largest of the paired laryngeal cartilages. They are pyramid shaped and attach to the superior posterior

(*continues*)

PROCEDURE 17-15 (continued)

edges of the cricoid cartilage. They also attach to the posterior ends of the vocal folds and move them during sound production.

- The smaller cuneiform and corniculate cartilages attach to the arytenoids. The cuneiform is the attachment of the arytenoid cartilages to the epiglottis.
- The superior opening into the larynx is the **glottis.** Two pairs of ligaments extend to the posterior surface of the thyroid cartilage from the arytenoid cartilages. The uppermost are called the false vocal cords. The lower pair is the true vocal cords (Figure 17-33).
- Laryngeal neoplasms may be benign or malignant.
  - Evidence of neoplasms include changes in voice quality and pain.

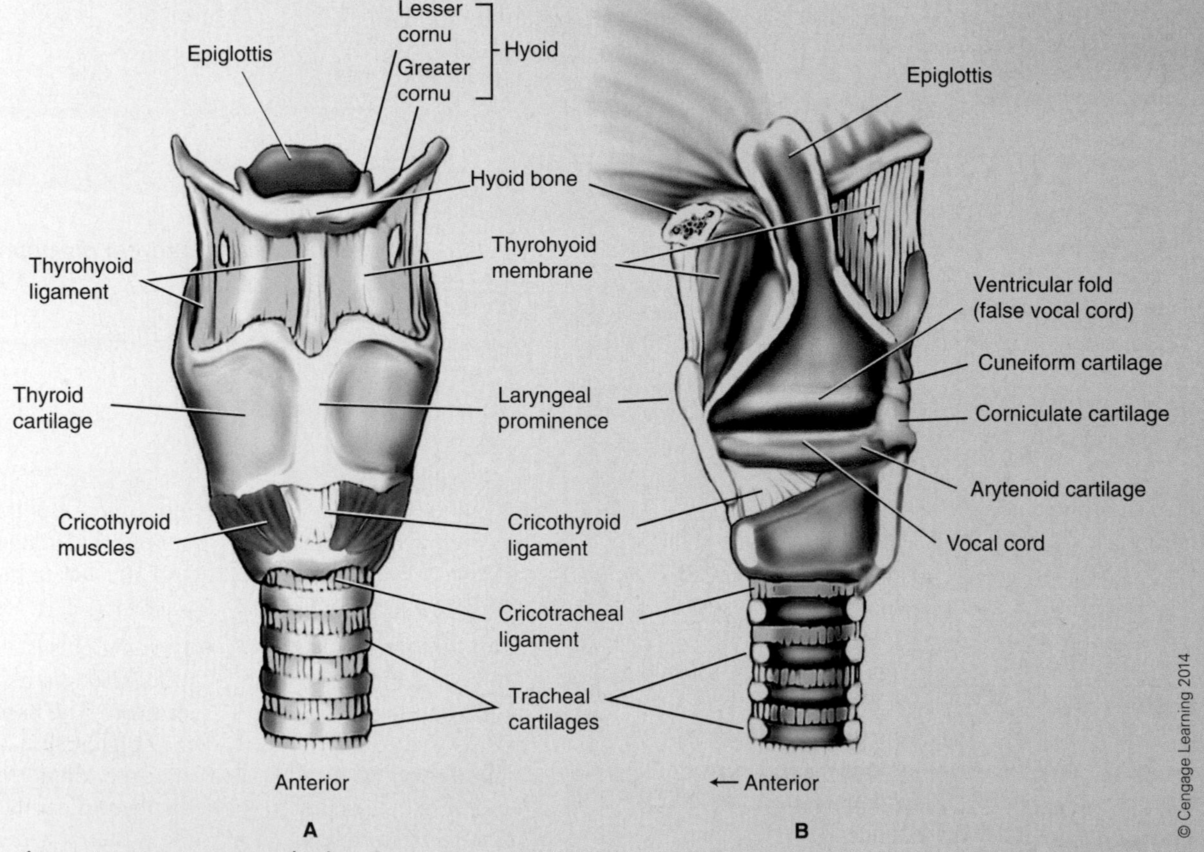

Figure 17-32 Larynx and related structures: (A) Anterior view, (B) lateral view

- The neoplasm may arise from any structure within the larynx and is not limited to the vocal cords.
- Persons who smoke are a greater risk for developing laryngeal neoplasms.
- Several types of benign neoplasms have been identified. Most of these can be treated laryngoscopically; the use of the carbon dioxide laser is common.

Procedure 17-15 (continued)

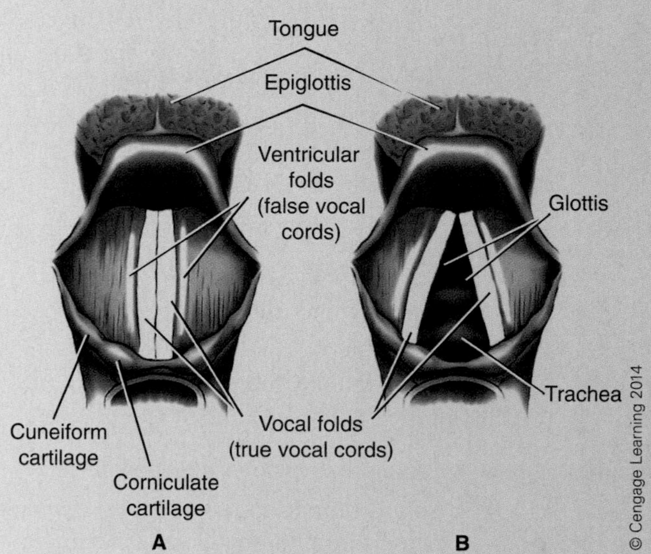

Figure 17-33 Vocal cords and related structures: (A) Closed, (B) open

- Malignant neoplasms are classified according to their anatomic location
- Supraglottic: extends from epiglottis to and including the false vocal cords
    - Glottic: extends from the floor of the false vocal cords to and including the true vocal cords
    - Subglottic (or infraglottic): extends from below the true vocal cords to the cricoid cartilage
    - Transglottic: extends from above the false vocal cords and subglottically
- Malignant tumors require extensive procedures such as laryngectomy, the partial or total excision of the larynx. In rare instances, laryngectomy may be performed when the larynx is severely damaged by a violent accident or trauma such as a gunshot wound or motor vehicle accident. Additionally, a laryngectomy may be performed as diversion for total separation of the digestive and respiratory tract or due to **chondroradionecrosis** of the laryngeal structure, a condition that occurs due to radiation treatments. Partial laryngectomy is removal of a section of the larynx. Total laryngectomy is performed when cancer is in advanced stages; it involves removal of the larynx, strap muscles, hyoid bone, and pre-epiglottic space. If the lymph nodes in the neck are involved a radical neck dissection will also be performed.

Preoperative Diagnostic Tests and Procedures	• History and physical examination	• CT scan • MRI	• Laryngoscopy with biopsy
Equipment, Instruments, and Supplies Unique to Procedure	• Thyroid instruments and tracheotomy tray in addition to major instrument set • Tracheostomy tubes of various sizes	• Kitners • Umbilical tape and/or vessel loops • Extra right-angle clamps • Extra single and double skin hooks	• Small bone clamps • Extra silk and Vicryl ties • Magnetic instrument pad • Closed wound-drainage system (surgeon's preference)

(*continues*)

PROCEDURE 17-15 (continued)

Preoperative Preparation	• Position: Supine with arms tucked at sides; donut, foam, or Mayfield headrest may be used; scapular roll to hyperextend the neck. • Anesthesia: General • Skin prep: Begins at inferior auricular border, including entire neck region to nipple line and bilaterally to sides. • Draping: The neck region is squared off with three or four towels; bar drape is placed on forehead of patient and opened superiorly to cover the hair; a transverse fenestrated drape is placed with the opening of the neck region.
Practical Considerations	• Imaging studies should be in the OR. • A tracheostomy tube is inserted until postoperative edema decreases (usually 48 hours) and it is then replaced with a laryngectomy tube.
Surgical Procedure	1. The skin incision is made by the surgeon. **Procedural Consideration:** For laryngectomy with neck dissection, the incision is made from mastoid to mastoid; for laryngectomy only, the incision is SCM to SCM.
	2. Skin flaps are formed and elevated with the use of skin hooks. **Procedural Consideration:** If necessary, neck dissection is performed.
	3. The strap muscles are divided on each side using Mayo scissors, blunt dissection, and ESU, and the muscles are retracted laterally.
	4. The suprahyoid muscles are divided from the hyoid bone and the bone is divided with bone-cutting forceps. **Procedural Consideration:** The surgical technologist will be responsible for cleaning the tip of the forceps with a lap sponge when the surgeon presents it for cleaning as he or she divides the bone.
	5. The carotid sheath is bluntly dissected free and gently retracted laterally using vein retractors. **Procedural Consideration:** The surgeon may use kitners loaded on Schnidt clamps for blunt dissection.
	6. The thyroid gland is now removed; the gland is divided by cutting the isthmus between two clamps with ESU. Each lobe is dissected free from the trachea medially to laterally using the ESU and Metzenbaum scissors. During dissection the inferior thyroid artery and recurrent larnyngeal nerve are identified, double clamped, cut, and ligated.
	7. Using a cricoid hook placed on the right side of the larynx (Figure 17-34A), the larynx is rotated, and the inferior pharyngeal constrictor muscle is removed from the thyroid cartilage with the ESU. The hook is placed on the left side (Figure 17-34B), and the same is performed.
	8. Using ESU, the surgeon removes the muscular attachments of the base of the tongue from the hyoid bone and stabilizes the bone by grasping it with a small bone clamp. Using the Mayo scissors, the rest of the attachments to the hyoid bone are dissected. **Procedural Consideration:** Due to the heavy use of the ESU, the surgical technologist should keep the electrosurgery tip clean using a scratch pad and place the scratch pad where the surgeon can easily access it.

PROCEDURE 17-15 (continued)

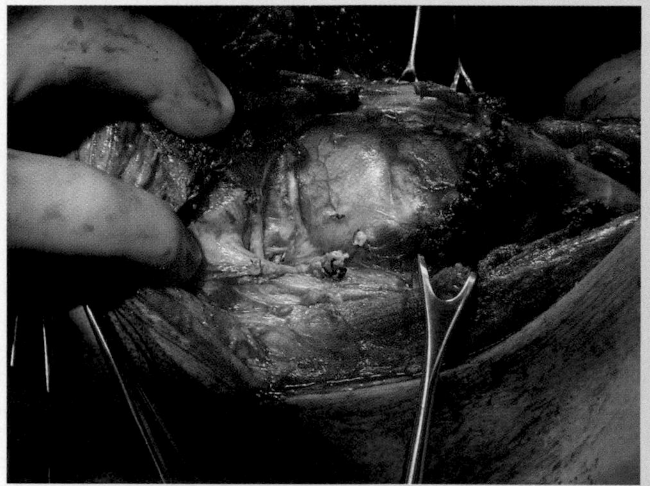

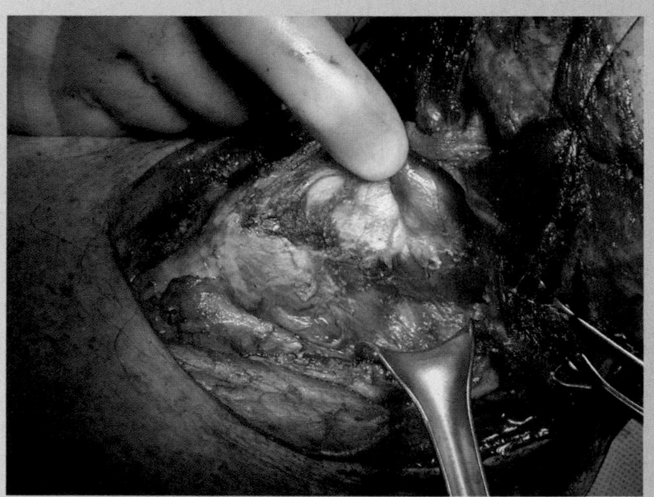

A B

Figure 17-34 Laryngectomy: (A) Right side of larynx, (B) left side of larynx

9. The tracheotomy is now performed and the tracheostomy tube placed.
10. Using Mayo scissors, an incision is made in the hypopharynx and the incision is widened with a Crile hemostat.
11. The epiglottis is exposed and grasped with an Allis clamp or small Kocher clamp and removed from the larynx.
12. The larynx is incised with the No. 10 knife blade, and the trachea is dissected free from the anterior esophageal wall. Any remaining attachments to the larynx are cut and the larynx is removed.
13. Closure begins by closing the pharynx in two layers with interrupted sutures.
14. The suprahyoid muscles are sutured to the incised edges of the inferior constrictor muscle.
15. A stoma is created by the surgeon closing the anterior tracheal wall to the inferior skin flap and the posterior tracheal wall to the superior skin flap.
16. The wound is irrigated and checked for bleeding, and a closed wound-drainage system placed. The deep cervical fascia, platysma muscle, and skin are separately closed.
17. A cuffed tracheostomy tube is placed. A dressing may or may not be placed according to surgeon's preference. Some surgeons prefer not to have a dressing in place so they can visualize the skin flaps postoperatively.

(*continues*)

Procedure 17-15 (continued)

Postoperative Considerations	**Immediate Postoperative Care** • Transport to PACU. • Patient may require intensive care and remain hospitalized for several days. • Patient will need instruction on care of the tracheostomy, as there is a risk for infection as well as water or foreign materials entering the stoma.	• The patient with a stoma will no longer be able to communicate via normal speech. Several alternate methods of vocal communication can be learned with the support of a speech pathologist. **Prognosis** • No complications: Depending on diagnosis, patient may need more	extensive treatment such as radiation therapy. Patient will not be able to return to all normal activities. • Complications: Postoperative SSI; hemorrhage; recurrence of cancer. **Wound Classification** • Class I: Clean

Procedure 17-16 Radical Neck Dissection with Mandibulectomy

Surgical Anatomy and Pathology	• See previous procedures for surgical anatomy. • Procedure is performed to treat metastatic	squamous cell carcinoma; also performed in conjunction with	mandibulectomy for metastatic cancer of the mouth and jaw.
Preoperative Diagnostic, Tests and Procedures	• History and physical examination	• CT scan • MRI scan	• Laryngoscopy with biopsy
Equipment, Instruments, and Supplies Unique to Procedure	*Team A and B* • Headlamp • Power drill • Microdrill with burs and sagittal saw • Mini-driver *Team A* • Major instrument tray • Tracheotomy tray • Dental instrument tray • Synthes facial fracture set • Head and neck back table pack with drapes • Anode endotracheal tube • Tracheotomy tubes of various sizes	• Several No. 15 knife blades • ESU pencil tips–needle and blade • Facial nerve stimulator • Large number of silk and Vicryl ties of various sizes • Several 10-mL syringes with 25-gauge, ½" and 1" hypodermic needles *Team B* • Minor instrument set • Orthopedic instrument set • Micro instrument set • Vascular instrument set • Variety of bone-holding clamps	• Microscope • Basic back table pack • Medium-large stockinette • Impervious U-drape • Extremity drape • Several No. 10 knife blades • Vessel loops • Large number of silk and Vicryl ties of various sizes • 7-0 and 8-0 Prolene or nylon for vascular anastomosis • 3-, 5-, and 10-mL syringes with heparin needles • Microscope drape

Procedure 17-16 (continued)

Preoperative Preparation	• Position: Supine with arms tucked at sides; head turned to expose operative side with donut or foam headrest; scapular roll to hyperextend neck • Anesthesia: General • Skin prep: Both sites require skin prep; see laryngectomy for skin prep of neck. • Draping: Team A: Neck draping procedure; Team B: Extremity draping procedure
Practical Considerations	• Radical neck dissection is usually performed unilaterally. The cervical lymph nodes, jugular vein, and SCM are removed. • For both psychological and physiological reasons, the ensuing defect caused by the extensive resection requires immediate reconstruction with the use of a composite graft. Several body structures make viable composite grafts for mandibular reconstruction, including the fibula and its adjoining vessels. • Two teams working concurrently are often used. This includes two surgical technologists, one assigned to each team who is responsible for one surgical site. The team that is working in the oral cavity is not considered sterile. Therefore, the two surgical teams should be diligent in preventing contamination of the sterile areas of the operative fields (e.g., no passing instruments, power equipment, or supplies between the two operative fields). • For the purposes of presenting the steps of the procedure, "Team A" will be considered the nonsterile team and "Team B" will be considered the sterile team responsible for the graft procurement. • Ordinarily, once the graft is harvested and the donor site sutured and dressed, there is no need for the second team.
Surgical Procedures	1. Team A will start by creating a tracheotomy. Once the opening is made into the trachea, the anesthesia provider will slowly remove the endotracheal tube. **Procedural Consideration:** Follow procedural guide for tracheotomy discussed later in chapter.
	2. As the ET tube is withdrawn, the surgeon will begin inserting the anode tube into the trachea. On satisfactory placement, the proximal end is connected to the anesthesia circuit (and is thus considered contaminated). The tube is then stabilized by inflating the balloon cuff at its distal end within the trachea with a 10-mL syringe, and held in place by suturing the external segment to the chest with a 2-0 silk. **Procedural Consideration:** Prepare anode tube in advance—be certain that balloon is patent. Provide anode tube and syringe for balloon inflation at appropriate time. Pass 2-0 silk on needle driver and tissue forceps followed by suture scissors.
	3. To aid in hemostasis, the surgeon may start by injecting the operative site with a local anesthetic (e.g., bupivacaine) containing epinephrine. **Procedural Consideration:** Solution for injection should be drawn up in advance. Notify anesthesia provider of epinephrine injection.

(continues)

PROCEDURE 17-16 (continued)

4. The neck dissection is initiated. The incision begins at the mastoid tip below the ear, and continues distally to approximately 2 cm inferior to the mandible, and around to the area immediately below and lateral to the chin.

   Procedural Consideration: The intended incision line may be outlined with a sterile marking pen. Pass No. 15 scalpel blade on No. 7 knife handle. Anticipate the use of the electrosurgical pencil. Provide instruments for retraction; a Green retractor is commonly used.

5. The subcutaneous tissues are separated from the underlying structures, creating a flap, which is anchored out of the way by folding it over and tacking it with a 2-0 silk suture.

   Procedural Consideration: Metzenbaum scissors and tissue forceps will be used for the dissection. Have peanut sponges loaded on clamps for blunt dissection. Provide suction as needed. Be sure fresh 4 × 4s are available throughout—expect the use of several packages. Blood vessels will be coagulated or double clamped, cut, and ligated. Prepare retraction suture in advance. Pass suture and tissue forceps when needed; follow with suture scissors.

6. Through careful and tedious dissection, the internal neck structures are identified. The nerve stimulator is used frequently in an effort to identify—and preserve—vital nerves, such as the lingual and hypoglossal.

   Procedural Consideration: The nerve stimulator should be ready for intermittent use; sharp component requires caution. Dissection will continue with Metz and tissue forceps or electrosurgical pencil. Hemostasis will be achieved as vessels are encountered.

7. Continuing the dissection, the sternocleidomastoid (SCM) muscle is divided at the point of its inferior insertion.

   Procedural Consideration: The electrosurgical pencil will likely be used to divide the SCM.

8. The internal jugular vein is located and subsequently ligated with a 0 silk stick tie. Smaller vessels are ligated with either a 2-0 or 3-0 silk or a 2-0 or 3-0 Vicryl-free tie.

   Procedural Consideration: Provide two clamps for the jugular vein. Prepare 0 silk in advance—vessel may be ligated prior to separation. Vessel will be cut. Any peripheral vessels will be clamped, cut, and ligated, or hemoclips may be applied and then the vessel cut.

9. The nodes along the cervical lymph tree are then freed from the surrounding tissues, and the entire contents of the neck dissection are removed en bloc.

   Procedural Consideration: Prepare to accept and process the first specimen. The surgeon may request that the pathologist verify that the margins are cancer free, possibly requiring a frozen section.

10. The mandibulectomy is initiated. The original incision, which terminated at the contralateral submental area, is extended superiorly over the chin, through the midline of the bottom lip, bisecting it.

    Procedural Consideration: The skin knife will be needed again. Anticipate use of the electrosurgical pencil.

PROCEDURE 17-16 (continued)

11. The soft tissues are retracted with double-prong skin hooks as the surgeon continues the incision through the oral mucosa and gingiva, along the superior aspect of the affected portion of mandible. If there are any teeth remaining in this section of the mandible, they are extracted at this time.

    Procedural Consideration: Provide skin hook retractors; use caution—tips are pointed. Scissors and tissue forceps or the electrosurgical pencil will be needed to continue the dissection. Have tooth extraction tools available.

12. Finally, once the mandible is exposed, the bone is cleaned of soft tissue with a periosteal elevator, and the involved section is excised, using a sagittal saw. *Note:* To maintain function of the jaw following reconstruction, excision of the mandible will ordinarily stop short of the temporomandibular joint.

    Procedural Consideration: Provide periosteal elevator. Anticipate the use of the sagittal saw and prepare in advance. Provide irrigation fluid to cool bone. Prepare to accept final specimen. Follow physician's orders concerning specimen care; it may be needed as a template to tailor the graft.

13. While Team A is completing the neck dissection and mandibulectomy, Team B will begin work on harvesting the fibular composite graft. First, a linear incision is made on the lateral aspect of the leg, beginning approximately 5 cm distal to the knee, and continuing to approximately 5–10 cm proximal to the ankle. (The exact length of the incision will be determined by the length of fibula needed for reconstruction.)

    Procedural Consideration: Pass the skin knife. Anticipate the use of the electrosurgical pencil. Provide retractors as needed.

14. The dissection continues through the subcutaneous tissues, fascia, and muscle layers, until the fibula is exposed.

    Procedural Consideration: Scissors and tissue forceps or the electrosurgical pencil may be used for dissection.

15. At this point, the dissection becomes slow and deliberate, in order to identify and preserve the blood vessels supplying the fibula. Some of these vessels are quite small, necessitating the use of a microscope.

    Procedural Consideration: If use of microscope is anticipated, drape and position in advance of need. Switch to more delicate instrumentation if necessary.

16. Once adequate venous and arterial conduits are located, the vessels are cannulated with a small-gauged angiocatheter and heparinized to prevent thrombus formation. (Sometimes papaverine is also used, to prevent vasospasm.)

    Procedural Consideration: Provide heparinized saline in syringes with angiocatheter attached. Have other pharmaceuticals on the field, labeled, and prepared for use.

17. A small vascular clamp, such as a bulldog, is applied proximal to the cannulation point, and the vessel is then ligated with an appropriate-sized free tie. This process is repeated for each vessel.

    Procedural Consideration: Pass the vascular clamp and appropriate suture or clips for ligation. Prepare to repeat this process as many times as necessary.

(*continues*)

Procedure 17-16 (continued)

18. Once the integrity of the fibular blood supply is preserved, the section of fibula is removed by using the sagittal saw. The proximal and distal stumps of the remaining fibula may need to be filed, in order to prevent any rough edges from damaging the surrounding tissues.

    Procedural Consideration: Prepare sagittal saw in advance. Rasp may be needed.

19. The donor site is then closed using 2-0 Vicryl for the deep layers; 3-0 Vicryl for the subcutaneous layers, and staples for the skin.

    Procedural Consideration: Have wound irrigation ready if requested. Follow closure routine including count. Be sure wound is dressed prior to introduction of mandibular template onto field.

20. The composite graft will be prepped for transplant. Using the excised section of mandible as a template, the bony portion of the graft is contoured with a micro bur to approximate size and shape.

    Procedural Consideration: A work space should be set aside for preparation of the graft. Anticipate the necessary instrumentation and have it available at the work space.

21. Under the microscope, the venous and arterial vessels of the fibula are anastomosed to their counterparts in the graft site, with the 7-0 and 8-0 Prolene or nylon.

    Procedural Consideration: The graft is transferred to Team A for insertion in the jaw. The microscope and micro instrumentation may be transferred to Team A to facilitate the implant of the composite graft. This completes Team B's participation in the procedure.

22. The bony portion of the graft is anchored to the remaining (unaffected) portion of the mandible, as well as the temporomandibular joint on the affected side, using plates and screws from the Synthes facial fracture set.

    Procedural Consideration: Have a variety of plates and screws available for fixation of the fibula to the mandible. Drill with appropriate size drill bits should be ready, along with any necessary guides, taps, etc.

23. The gingiva and oral mucosa are then closed with a running 3-0 chromic (or Vicryl) suture.

    Procedural Consideration: Anticipate the use of irrigation fluid. Provide the total amount of all irrigation fluid used during the procedure to the anesthesia provider. Prepare for closure by loading suture and obtaining appropriate size drains. Pass suture and tissue forceps when requested; follow with suture scissors when needed. Count.

24. A Jackson-Pratt drain is placed in the inferior portion of the neck dissection and covered by the skin flap.

    Procedural Consideration: Pass the drain. When appropriate, connect drain to suction device/reservoir.

Procedure 17-16 (continued)

25. The wound edges are then approximated and stabilized with 3-0 Vicryl sutures, placed subcutaneously. For skin closure, a staple gun can be used from the portion of the incision beginning at the mastoid tip, and extending to the submental area. However, for the area between the chin and the external portion of the bottom lip, a soft, nonabsorbable suture (such as 3-0 silk) is preferable.

    Procedural Consideration: Continue to provide closing materials and support as needed. Prepare dressing materials.

26. Following skin closure, the anode tube is removed by the surgeon, and replaced with an appropriate-sized tracheotomy tube. (*Note:* The STSR should verify patency of the balloon cuff prior to giving the tracheotomy tube to the surgeon.) The anesthesia circuit is then attached to the tracheotomy tube, and ventilation is resumed.

    Procedural Consideration: Communicate with surgeon in advance concerning preference for tracheotomy tube style and size. Obtain tube of choice. Assemble tube and ensure patency of balloon, if there is one. Assist with airway as needed—suction will be necessary.

Postoperative Considerations

Immediate Postoperative Care

- Patient may require intensive care and remain hospitalized for several days.
- Patient will need wound care instruction.
- Patient may have a tracheotomy.

Prognosis

- No complications: Depending on diagnosis, patient may need more extensive treatment. Tracheotomy, if present, may be permanent.
- Complications: Postoperative SSI; hemorrhage; recurrence of cancer; failure of graft to "take" or it is rejected by the body.

Wound Classification

- Oral cavity procedure: Class II: Clean-contaminated.
- Graft procedure: Class I: Clean

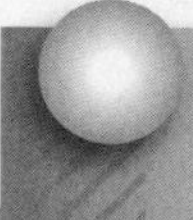

Pearl of Wisdom

Naturally, it is necessary to have at least two separate setups, as well as separate counts, for each portion of this procedure. Both surgical technologists will need to be extremely vigilant with the countable items. Extreme care must also be taken to keep the two fields separate.

Procedure 17-17 Temporomandibular Joint Arthroscopy

Surgical Anatomy and Pathology

- The largest and strongest facial bone is the mandible.
- The mandible articulates with the glenoid fossa of each temporal bone to form a synovial joint called the temporomandibular joint (TMJ).
- The TMJ contains the condylar process of the mandible and two parts of the temporal bone, the mandibular fossa, and the articular tubercle.
- TMJ arthroscopy is usually performed for

(*continues*)

Procedure 17-17 (continued)

	diagnostic purposes to confirm if temporomandibular disorder (TMD) exists. • TMD is divided into two classifications: muscle-related TMD (called	myogenous TMD) caused by chronic jaw clenching and joint-related TMD (called arthrogenous TMD) caused by malocclusion of the teeth.	• TMD is second to toothaches in the cause of facial pain.
Preoperative Diagnostic Tests and Procedures	• History and physical examination	• Standard radiographs	• CT scan
Equipment, Instruments, and Supplies Unique to Procedure	• Endoscopic equipment, including camera and light cord • Bipolar ESU • Arthroscopic shaver power unit • Fluid infusion system	• TMJ instruments • Small joint shaver • 0-, 30-, and 70-degree arthroscopes • No. 11 knife blade • Head and neck back table pack	• Incise drape with fluid collection pouch • Lactated Ringer's solution (1000-mL bag) • 18-gauge 1½" needle
Preoperative Preparation	• Position: Supine with head turned to expose operative site; donut or foam headrest; arms tucked at the sides • Anesthesia: General	• Skin prep: Head wrap/turban to restrain hair; face, chin, and neck prepped • Draping: Bar drape across forehead; U-drape or split sheet placed in	usual fashion; incise drape placed over TMJ with fluid collection pouch in correct position directly underneath the joint and the mouth and nose covered.
Practical Considerations	• TMJ arthroscopy may be performed bilaterally. Both sides of the face	may be prepped and draped. • Imaging studies should be in the OR.	• Test equipment prior to the arrival of the patient.
Surgical Procedure	1. Irrigation solution is injected into the joint space to distend the capsule. **Procedural Consideration:** Lactated Ringer's solution is preloaded in syringe with needle attached.		
	2. A small stab incision is made (Figure 17-35). **Procedural Consideration:** A No. 11 blade on the No. 7 handle will be used.		
	3. The trocar/cannula assembly is inserted, the trocar removed, and the lens inserted. **Procedural Consideration:** Trocar/cannula is preassembled. Expect return of trocar. Be prepared to assist with the connections of video equipment.		
	4. Irrigation solution is infused into the joint. **Procedural Consideration:** Lactated Ringer's solution is connected to the cannula via extension tubing.		
	5. The joint is examined. **Procedural Consideration:** Prepare to operate remote control for still photographs.		

PROCEDURE 17-17 (continued)

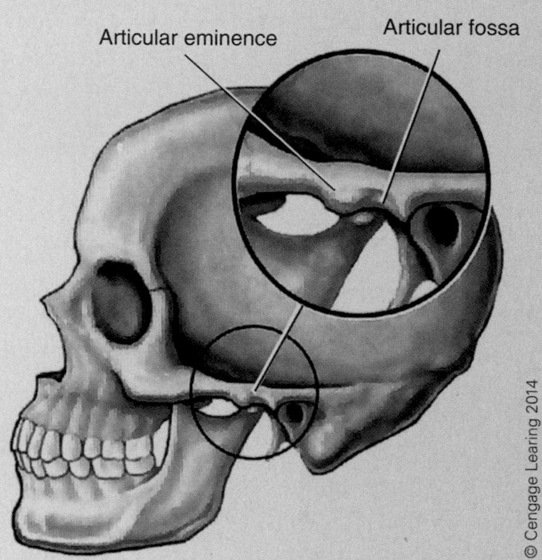

Figure 17-35 Temporomandibular joint

6. If functional surgery is required, a second stab wound is made.
   Procedural Consideration: Pass the skin knife. Prepare additional equipment (probe, shaver, or grasper may be used).
7. Final visual inspection is performed.
   Procedural Consideration: Additional photographs may be taken.
8. Cannulae are removed and excess fluid is removed.
   Procedural Consideration: Prepare for closure. Count.
9. Wound is closed and dressing is placed.
   Procedural Consideration: Pass suture of preference. Prepare dressings. Reorganize equipment and supplies if procedure is bilateral.
10. Procedure may be repeated on contralateral side.
    Procedural Consideration: Repeat previously described steps.

Postoperative Considerations

Immediate Postoperative Care

- Range of motion of the jaw may be limited. Extubation may be difficult. Suction and emergency airway supplies should be readily available.
- Application of ice may help reduce postoperative pain and swelling.
- Patient may be placed on a liquid or soft diet for several days postoperatively.

Prognosis

- No complications: Expected outcome is good; discharged same day of surgery.
- Complications: Recurrence is possible if contributing behavior is not resolved (e.g., grinding or clenching of teeth); postoperative SSI; hemorrhage.

Wound Classification

- Wound Class I: Clean

(continues)

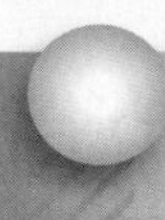

Pearl of Wisdom

This is one of those procedures where the surgical technologist may be involved in numerous activities not commonly involved with the scrub role. The activities are technology driven. The surgical technologist must understand the principles, procedures, and troubleshooting steps for all equipment involved in this procedure.

Procedure 17-18 Tracheotomy

Surgical Anatomy and Pathology

- The trachea is located anterior to the esophagus (Figure 17-35).
- The upper half of the trachea is located in the midline of the neck; as it descends, it enters the superior mediastinum.
- The trachea joins the cricoid cartilage of the larynx to the mainstem or primary bronchi leading to each lung.
- There are 15–20 C-shaped pieces of hyaline cartilage supporting the anterior and lateral tracheal walls. These cartilages keep the trachea from collapsing due to any pressure changes.
- The posterior wall of the trachea is closed with smooth muscle and connective tissue. This allows for expansion of the esophagus during swallowing.
- The most inferior tracheal cartilage is called the **carina**, which bifurcates into the two primary bronchi.
- A tracheotomy is performed for many

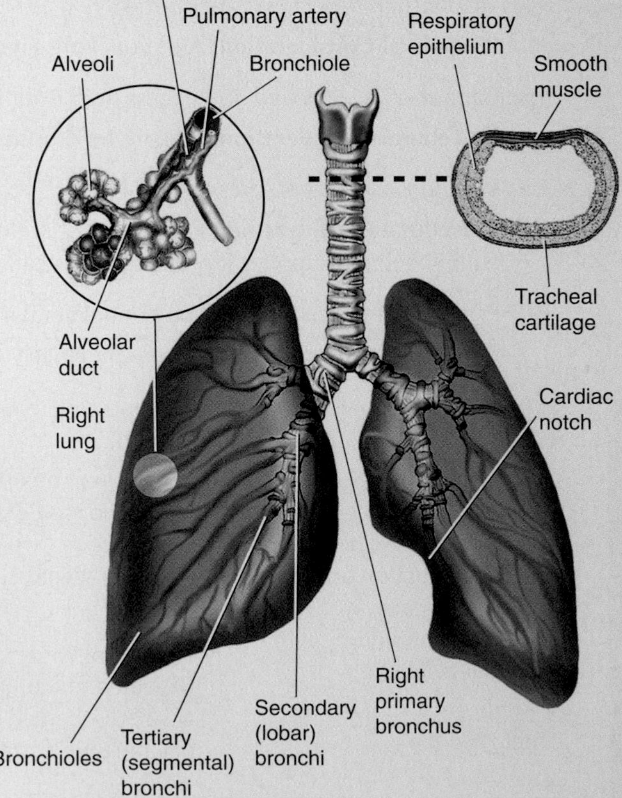

Figure 17-36 Trachea and lungs

PROCEDURE 17-18 (continued)

	reasons, including extreme emergencies. The following are indications for tracheotomy: *Upper airway obstruction with one or more of the*	*following:* Stridor, chest retractions, obstructive sleep apnea, bilateral vocal cord paralysis, previous neck surgery, throat trauma, previous irradiation to the neck	*Other:* Prolonged intubation, inability to manage secretions, facilitation of ventilation, inability to intubate, adjunct to management of head and neck surgery.
Preoperative Diagnostic Tests and Procedures	• History and physical examination		
Equipment, Instruments, and Supplies Unique to Procedure	• Tracheotomy instrument tray • Tracheotomy tubes of various sizes	• Endotracheal suction catheters • U-drape or split sheet • Basic back table pack	• No. 10 and No. 15 knife blades • Tracheotomy dressing
Preoperative Preparation	• Position: Supine with arms tucked at sides; scapular roll to hyperextend neck	• Anesthesia: General (preferred); local (emergency situation) • Skin prep: Point of chin down to nipple line and	laterally as far as possible • Draping: Head wrap/turban; bar drape; U-drape or split sheet
Practical Considerations	• The tracheotomy procedure is performed by many surgeons from various surgical specialties. • It is performed to facilitate breathing and to protect damage to other structures. • The terms "tracheostomy" and "tracheotomy" are often used interchangeably. • Tracheostomy is the creation of a tracheal stoma, usually permanent. The mucous membrane of the trachea is sutured to the skin.	• Tracheotomy is the creation of an opening in the trachea, usually temporary, for placement of a tracheotomy tube. • Have the tracheotomy tube on the back table before incision is made to ensure patency of the balloon. • Have sterile plastic suction catheter opened. • Have respirator available. • In emergency situations general anesthesia may not be able to be administered and skin prep and draping will not be able to be	completed. Tracheotomies have been performed in the field, emergency department, PACU, ICU, and on the ward. In an emergency situation the team will have to move quickly and efficiently in order to establish an airway and save the patient's life; the team will maintain sterile technique as best as possible in an emergency situation. • The procedure is described as being performed under ideal, nonemergency circumstances.
Surgical Procedure	1. A symmetrical, transverse incision is made following the Langer lines about two fingerbreadths above the clavicular head.		

(continues)

PROCEDURE 17-18 (continued)

2. The incision is extended through the subcutaneous tissues and the platysma muscle is divided.

   Procedural Consideration: Hemostasis may or may not be controlled during this step of the procedure. If performed ESU, mosquito clamps and ties will be used.

3. The strap muscles are separated and the thyroid isthmus and trachea are exposed.

   Procedural Consideration: May use U.S. Army retractors or Weitlaner retractor with blunt blades.

4. The thyroid isthmus is divided if necessary.

   Procedural Consideration: May use electrosurgical pencil to divide the isthmus.

5. A tracheal hook is placed on the tracheal ring and an incision is made into the second tracheal ring. A spreader is placed in the incision.

   Procedural Consideration: The following sequence rapidly occurs:

   - Hand tracheal hook.
   - Hand scalpel with No. 15 knife blade.
   - Hand tracheal spreader.
   - Hand tracheotomy tube with obturator in place.

6. The tracheotomy tube is placed in the incision and the obturator is withdrawn. The inner cannula is placed and secretions are removed by suction.

   Procedural Consideration: The obturator is removed. Hand the inner cannula. Hand suction to clear the tube.

7. The endotracheal balloon is inflated. The tracheotomy tube is secured. The wound is closed.

   Procedural Consideration: May suture tracheotomy tube or use umbilical tape. Count.

Postoperative Considerations

Immediate Postoperative Care

- Transport to PACU or ICU.
- Keep a clean obturator with patient at all times.

Prognosis

- No complications: Depends on response to primary condition.
- Complications: Postoperative SSI; edema; hemorrhage; damage to nearby anatomical structures.

Wound Classification

- Class II: Clean-contaminated

CASE STUDY Beth, a 26-year-old female, was involved in an automobile accident in which the air bag of her vehicle deployed. She states that she feels very fortunate that a nasal septum fracture was her only injury. Beth is scheduled for a septoplasty under local anesthesia and is fearful that she may feel pain during the procedure.

1. What is a septoplasty?
2. What steps will be taken to ensure that Beth's surgical site is adequately anesthetized?

3. What medications and supplies should the surgical technologist expect the surgeon to use to provide Beth's anesthesia?
4. What reassurances, if any, can the surgical team members offer Beth to alleviate her fears?

Questions for Further Study

1. What special preparations should be made in advance of the pediatric patient's arrival into the OR?
2. What type of anesthesia will the pediatric patient undergoing foreign body removal from the nose most likely receive? Will an IV line be necessary?
3. Outline the draping sequence for exposure of the face.
4. What position will the patient be placed in for an adenoidectomy?
5. What bone houses the tympanic cavity?
6. What is the function of the turbinates?

BIBLIOGRAPHY

Applegate, E. J. (2006). *The anatomy and physiology learning system* (3rd ed.). Philadelphia: W.B. Saunders.

Association of Surgical Technologists. (2011). *Core curriculum for surgical technology* (6th ed.). Littleton, CO: Association of Surgical Technologists.

Beckett, B. J. (2002). *Identifying surgical instruments* (3rd ed.). Thousand Oaks, CA.

Bess, F. H., & Humes, L. E. (2008). *Audiology: The fundamentals* (4th ed.). Philadelphia: Lippincott Williams and Wilkins.

Goldenberg, D., & Goldstein, B. (2010). *Handbook of otolaryngology: Head and neck surgery.* New York: Thieme.

Goldman, M. A. (2007). *Pocket guide to the operating room* (3rd ed.). Philadelphia: F.A. Davis.

Lore, J. M., & Medina, J. (2004). *An atlas of head and neck surgery* (4th ed.). Philadelphia: Saunders.

Phillips, N. F. (2007). *Berry & Kohn's operating room technique* (11th ed.). St. Louis: Mosby.

Taylor, E. J. (Ed.). (2008). *Dorland's pocket medical dictionary* (28th ed.). Philadelphia: W.B. Saunders.

Theissing, J., Rettinger, G., & Werner, J. (2010). *ENT–Head and neck surgery: Essential procedures.* New York: Thieme.

CHAPTER

18

Oral and Maxillofacial Surgery

CASE STUDY Alan is a 23-year-old male who has been admitted to the emergency department following his involvement in a motorcycle accident. Alan was not wearing a helmet at the time of his injury.

Alan is awake and alert but is having difficulty breathing. He states that he is experiencing double vision.

1. **Why may Alan be experiencing respiratory distress and what steps, if any, should be taken to protect his airway?**
2. **Which diagnostic examinations may be ordered by the team of emergency specialists treating Alan?**
3. **Is surgery a possibility in Alan's case and, if so, is it an emergency?**

OBJECTIVES

After studying this chapter, the reader should be able to:

A 1. Recognize the anatomy relevant to specific procedures in oral and maxillofacial surgery.

P 2. Summarize the pathology that prompts oral and maxillofacial surgery and the related terminology.

3. Determine special preoperative diagnostic procedures/tests pertaining to oral and maxillofacial surgery.
4. Determine special preoperative preparation procedures related to oral and maxillofacial surgery.
5. Indicate the names and uses of oral and maxillofacial instruments, supplies and drugs.
6. Indicate the names and uses of special equipment used for oral and maxillofacial surgery.

7. Determine the intraoperative preparation of the patient undergoing an oral or maxillofacial procedure.
8. Summarize the surgical steps of oral or maxillofacial procedures.
9. Assess any specific variations related to the preoperative, intraoperative, and postoperative care of the surgical patient.

SELECT KEY TERMS

alveolar process	labial	mouth prop	reduction
calvarial	malar bones	pan-	symphysis
condyle	malocclusion	ramus	TMJ
glenoid fossa	maxillofacial		

INTRODUCTION TO ORAL AND MAXILLOFACIAL SURGERY

For the patient about to undergo oral surgery, several preoperative factors need to be considered. Fear of surgery is a common patient concern. Many patients will be concerned about the aesthetic outcome of their surgery. Others will be worried about the amount of pain the procedure will produce. Each patient's concerns should be addressed properly. Patient education about the entire process from transportation to the operating room (OR) to the recovery process will help to alleviate any fears.

Many patients who come to the OR for oral procedures will have special needs. Children requiring extensive dental work may be brought to the OR. Patients already in the hospital for other concerns, such as transplant recipients, may come to the OR for dental work. The surgical team should be prepared to deal with each situation.

Each patient should be interviewed and the chart examined with specific regard to the history, physical, NPO status, allergies, and diagnostic and laboratory results. This evaluation will help the surgical team provide accurate, efficient assistance for every case. X-rays are a vital part of oral surgery, and all relevant films should be readily available to the team. Consultation with the surgeon in advance of the procedure about the specific procedural details and possible variations will help the team prepare for the wide range of possibilities.

DIAGNOSTIC TESTS

For the patient with possible **maxillofacial** defects, various diagnostic tests can be administered. To begin, a complete history should be gathered from the patient if possible. When the patient is unable to communicate, a relative, observer, or other professional (such as paramedics or emergency department personnel) should relay any vital information. This information will aid physicians and surgical team members to form an appropriate treatment plan. For example, in a trauma situation, the type of injury and direction of impact may help the physician to ascertain the extent of injuries the patient has suffered.

A physical examination should be done for the facial trauma patient. This exam should be done carefully, especially in a suspected maxillary fracture. Movement of the fracture could cause any number of repercussions, from dural tears and nerve injury to infection. Obvious signs like bleeding, bruising, lacerations, and swelling may indicate an underlying fracture. Other signs such as cerebrospinal fluid leaking from the ears (cerebrospinal otorrhea) or nose (cerebrospinal rhinorrhea) may indicate dural tears. Malocclusion could also indicate dental, alveolar, or other facial fractures.

Several types of imaging help diagnose maxillofacial fractures. Radiographic techniques involving different views highlight particular bony facial structures while obscuring others. Computed tomography (CT) scans provide important information about possible bony defects. Magnetic resonance imaging (MRI) provides details about the surrounding soft tissues of the face.

For plain films, several options are available. The suspected type of fracture dictates the type of view or views to be taken. The Waters view requires the patient to sit or stand upright and hyperextend the neck. The nose and chin are placed against the X-ray cassette while the film is taken. The facial bones are shown in best detail in this position. Specifically, the infraorbital rims, frontal and maxillary sinuses, maxillary alveolar arch, and zygomas can be observed. The Caldwell view is similar to the Waters view. Both are anteroposterior projections, but in this case, the nose and forehead are placed against the cassette (Figure 18-1). This view shows the hard palate, nasal septum, orbital floor, and zygoma. The lateral facial view is mainly used for anatomical orientation of the face. The basal view shows zygomatic fractures. A **pan**oramic X-ray shows on one film the **alveolar processes**, mandible, posterior maxillary sinuses, and the zygomas.

CT scans of the head show the facial structures in different planes. Some of the important planes for maxillofacial abnormalities are the hard palate, mid-maxillary, and mid-orbital. The hard palate plane shows the entire palate and pterygoid plates. The zygomatic arch, temporal bone, nasal septum, and turbinates can be seen in the mid-maxillary plane. Finally, the mid-orbital plane displays the globe, lens, and optic nerve.

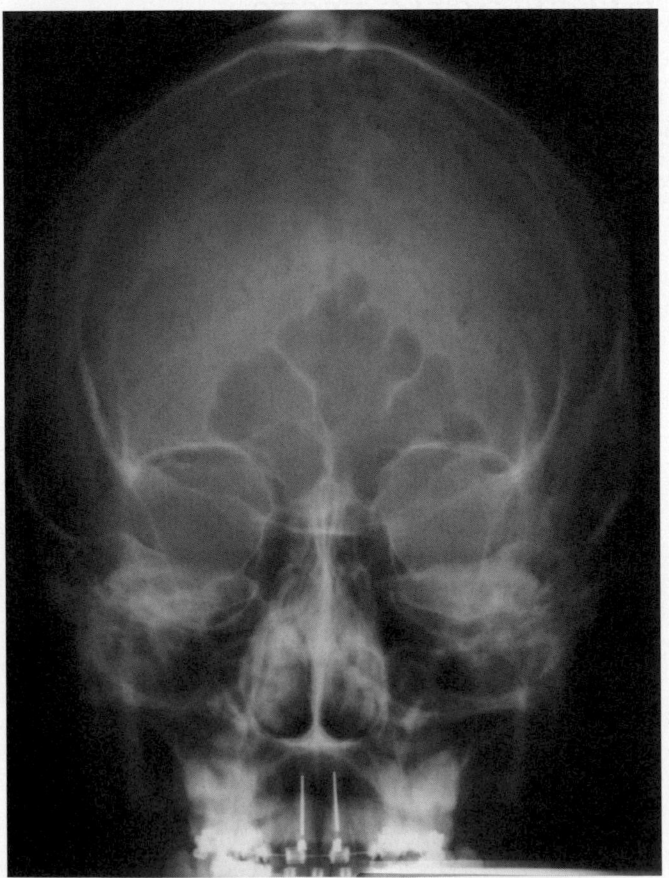

Figure 18-1 Caldwell view of the skull (anteroposterior nasal bones)

MRI best defines soft tissue injuries or congenital defects. Since an MRI image consumes a vast amount of time that a trauma victim may not have, its uses are limited to those patients who are deemed stable or receiving elective maxillofacial treatments.

Three-dimensional imaging can also be used for reconstructive procedures. The imaging involves the use of computers with three-dimensional programming and CT scans. The patient's CT scans can be projected onto the computer screen in a three-dimensional fashion. Any anatomy that interferes with viewing can be eliminated. Before and after models can be generated on the computer to aid the surgeon. This is an invaluable resource for reconstruction.

TOOTH EXTRACTION/ODONTECTOMY

Routine Instruments, Equipment, and Supplies

Most craniofacial and dental procedures use instruments from a dental instrument set and a basic plastic instrument set. Although not every instrument from each tray will be used, it is wise to have both sets available.

Routine Equipment

- Headlamp for surgeon
- Dental drill and energy source
- Suction system

Note: Often the drill, suction, and irrigation are combined into one equipment system

Routine Supplies

- Head and neck pack
- ESU
- Gloves
- #15 blades
- Drapes half-sheet × 2
- Sterile components of drill system, including an assortment of bits
- Suction tubing
- Double basin
- Irrigation fluid
- Throat pack
- Gauze sponges
- Dental rolls
- Antifog solution for mirrors
- 10-mL syringes with 25-gauge 1½-in. needles for local injection
- 20-mL syringes with 19-gauge 1½-in. blunt needles for irrigation

Table 18-1 Dental and Plastic Instrument Sets

Dental Set	Plastic Set
Mouth props—assorted sizes (Figure 18-2)	Wire twister
Plastic cheek retractor (Figure 18-3)	Wire suture cutters
Assorted periosteal elevators	U.S. Army retractors
Assorted extraction forceps	Small Richardson retractors
Mirror	Vein retractors
Gingival probe	Bone hook
Minnesota retractor (Figure 18-4)	Straight and curved iris scissors
Wieder tongue depressor	Tenotomy scissors
McGill	Metzenbaum scissors
Probe	Straight Mayo scissors
Frazier suction tips with stylet 10-Fr and 12-Fr	Sponge sticks
Yankauer suction tip	Sharp and dull rake retractors
#7 knife handle	Small malleable retractors
Needle holders	Senn retractors
Tissue forceps with and without teeth	Skin hooks
Scissors (assortment—straight and curved)	Webster needle holders
Towel clips	Mayo-Hegar needle holder
Straight and curved hemostats	Towel clips
Plastic Set	Frazier suction tip
Oschner forceps	Yankauer suction tip
Straight and curved Kelly clamps	Adson brown forceps
Straight and curved hemostats	Adson forceps with and without teeth
Straight and curved mosquito clamps	Bayonet forceps
Allis clamps	Small mallet

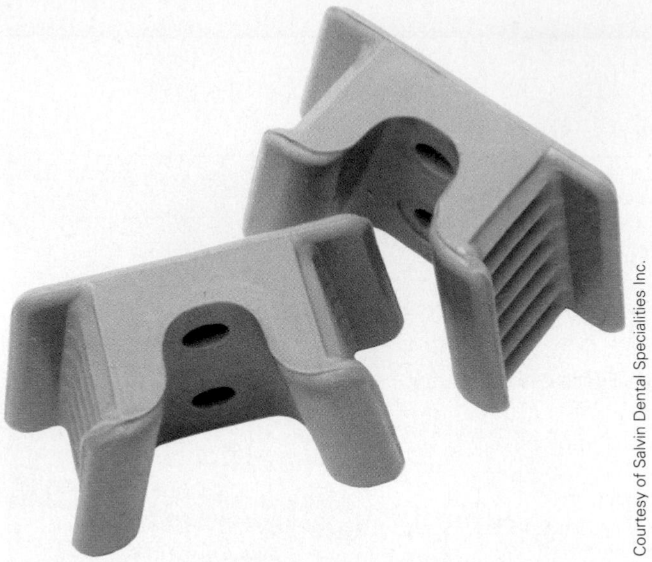

Courtesy of Salvin Dental Specialities Inc.

Figure 18-2 Mouth props

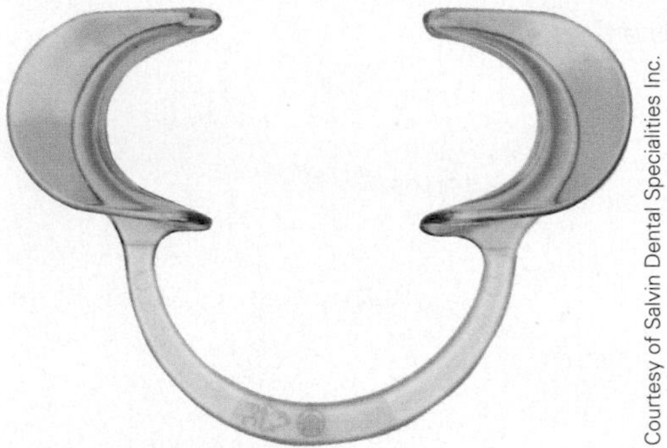

Courtesy of Salvin Dental Specialities Inc.

Figure 18-3 Plastic cheek retractor

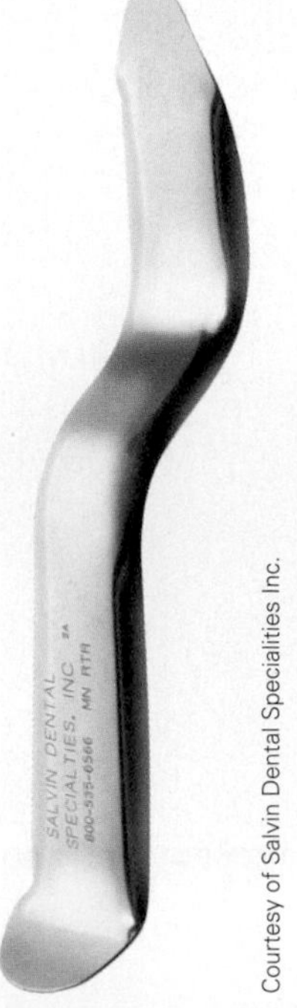

Courtesy of Salvin Dental Specialities Inc.

Figure 18-4 Minnesota retractor

Practical Considerations

- Oral procedures are not considered sterile; use the best technique possible.
- Fluoroscopy and X-ray machines should be able to enter the area without disturbing the sterile field. The OR table may be angled to allow access.
- During lengthy oral procedures, the patient's lips may dry and crack. To alleviate this problem a cream or ointment may be applied to the lips.
- Anesthesia circuits should be long enough to accommodate the position of the OR table.

Procedural Considerations

- General anesthesia is preferred.
- Lubricate and protect patient's eyes.
- Local anesthetic with epinephrine may be used alone or in conjunction with general anesthesia to reduce bleeding and minimize postoperative pain.
- Patient is supine, with head tilted back to provide exposure; a roll towel may be placed to aid in slightly extending the neck.
- A donut or foam headrest may be used for stabilization.
- Tuck arms at patient's sides; protect ulnar nerves.
- Patient prep may not be required for oral procedures. Facial procedures may require prep with mild antiseptic; the eyes and ears should be protected from contact with the prep solution.
    - Brush teeth or swab inside of mouth with an oral antiseptic.
    - Draping may not be necessary. A half-sheet may be placed across the patient's body to provide a clean surface on which to rest equipment and supplies.
        - A turban-style head wrap may be used to restrain the hair.
        - The throat pack is dampened rolled gauze that contains a radiopaque marker. It is included in the formal count. It is used to prevent oral secretions, irrigation fluid, blood, and bone or tooth fragments from becoming lodged in the pharynx. It must be removed prior to extubation.

PROCEDURE 18-1 Tooth Extraction/Odontectomy

Surgical Anatomy and Pathology	• The teeth lie in each jaw in a semicircular fashion. The side of the tooth that lies closest to the lips is referred to as the **labial**; the tongue side is lingual; cheek side is buccal. Each tooth is imbedded in a socket of the alveolar process; the alveolar maxillary process contains the upper teeth and the mandibular process contains the lower teeth. • Incisors—four front teeth used to tear food; cuspids—lateral to the incisors, used to grasp and shred food; bicuspids—distal to the cuspids, used to break up food into smaller portions; molars—flat-topped teeth also used to break up food. • Three regions of a tooth: crown—portion above the gumline; root—portion below the gumline; neck—junction of the crown and root. • The crown is covered by enamel, which is the hardest part of the tooth. Dentin forms the majority of the crown; it is harder than bone and encases the pulp. The pulp contains the blood vessels, nerves, and connective tissue. • The root is held in place by the periodontal ligament, which is made of collagenous fibers and connects the bony alveolar process and cementum of each tooth. The cementum is a bone-like substance that covers the tooth from the termination of the enamel at the neck to the thickest region at the apex of the root. • Extraction of teeth involves the removal of a tooth or teeth that cannot be salvaged by restoration, or those that interfere with occlusion. • Simple extraction is removal of the tooth from the alveolar socket with extraction forceps. • Odontectomy involves resection of the soft tissue and excision of the bone surrounding the tooth prior to removal of the tooth.
Preoperative Tests and Procedures	• Diagnosis primarily obtained from X-rays and MRI along with a visual and digital inspection of the area.
Equipment, Instruments, and Supplies Unique to Procedure	See previous information pp. 702-703.
Preoperative Preparation	• Position, anesthesia, patient prep, draping; see previous information p. 704.
Practical Considerations	• See previous information.
Surgical Procedure	1. Insert mouth prop. **Procedural Consideration:** Have appropriate-size mouth prop ready. Provide suction with Yankauer tip as needed.

(*continues*)

PROCEDURES 18-1 (continued)

2. A throat pack may be placed.

   Procedural Consideration: Prepare throat pack for use. A dressing forceps or McGill may be used to aid in the insertion of the throat pack.

3. Additional exposure is achieved.

   Procedural Consideration: Anticipate the use of the Minnesota retractor, plastic cheek retractor, or mirror for cheek/tongue retraction. Precoat mirror with antifog solution.

4. The site may be injected with a local anesthetic using a control syringe.

   Procedural Consideration: Local anesthetic should be prepared in advance according to surgeon's preference. Inform anesthesia provider of epinephrine use.

5. To determine the amount of damage to the surrounding gingiva, a probe with graduated marks is inserted into the gumline.

   Procedural Consideration: Switch suction tip to Frazier.

6. The gingiva is removed from the surface of the tooth with an elevator.

   Procedural Consideration: Periosteal elevator of surgeon's preference will be needed for gingival dissection.

7. The tooth is removed from the alveolar socket; the socket may be packed with gauze.

   Procedural Consideration: Choose extraction forceps according to the type of tooth to be removed and surgeon's preference. 2×2 gauze may be used to temporarily pack the socket.

8. The alveolar socket is inspected and irrigated to ensure that no debris remains. Direct pressure may be applied to the site for a short time and plain or chromic gut sutures may be placed as needed.

   Procedural Consideration: Irrigation fluid should be preloaded in the syringe with the blunt needle attached. Provide two irrigation systems so that one can be refilled while the other is in use. Provide suction as needed. Suture of choice is loaded on needle holder in anticipation of use. Count.

9. If the tooth scheduled for extraction is impacted, odontectomy is performed. The gumline is incised with a #15 blade.

   Procedural Consideration: A #15 blade is loaded on the #7 knife handle.

10. The soft tissue is dissected to expose the impacted tooth.

    Procedural Consideration: Provide periosteal elevator of choice.

11. A dental drill may be required to remove any bone preventing exposure of the tooth.

    Procedural Consideration: Dental drill is assembled in advance and the bit of surgeon's preference inserted and locked into position. Be sure to pass power tools with the safety mechanism in use. Suction and irrigation will be needed every time the drill is used.

12. The tooth may be removed as a whole or require splitting with the drill or an osteotome so that it can be removed in sections.

    Procedural Consideration: Provide extraction forceps of choice. Change drill bit if necessary and provide suction and irrigation. An osteotome must be accompanied by a mallet for use.

13. The area is inspected for debris, rinsed, and closed with a 4–0 chromic or silk on a cutting needle.

    Procedural Consideration: Provide suction and irrigation if needed. Suture of choice is loaded and passed. Count.

Procedure 18-1 (continued)

14. Pharynx is suctioned and throat pack removed.

 Procedural Consideration: Switch suction tip to Yankauer. Provide Wieder retractor. The instrument that was used to insert the throat pack will be needed again for extraction.

Postoperative Considerations

Immediate Postoperative Care

- The surgical team should be prepared to assist with extubation. Occasionally, reintubation is necessary and a laryngoscope and ET tube should be readily available. Additionally, a tracheostomy/tracheotomy tray should be available in the OR and transported with the patient to the PACU.
- Transport to PACU
- Bruising and swelling of the lips and cheeks may occur. The patient should be advised to apply ice.
- Outpatients must be able to tolerate a liquid diet prior to discharge.

Prognosis

- Patient is expected to return to normal activities in 3–5 days.
- No visible scarring is expected.

Complications

- Hemorrhage
- Postoperative surgical site infection (SSI)
- **Malocclusion**

Wound Classification

- Class II: clean-contaminated

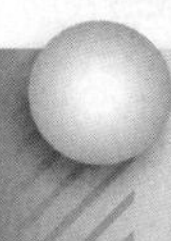

Pearl of Wisdom

The throat pack consists of rolled gauze that contains a radiopaque marker. It is moistened and any excess fluid is squeezed out prior to insertion. The throat pack should be included in the formal count. To reduce the risk of aspiration, a throat pack is used to prevent oral secretions, irrigation fluid, blood, and bone or tooth fragments from becoming lodged in the pharynx. It is imperative to provide suction to the pharynx and remove the throat pack prior to extubation.

MAXILLOFACIAL PROCEDURES: GENERAL CONSIDERATIONS

General Considerations

- Maxillofacial injuries can inhibit speech. If the patient is unable to communicate verbally, relevant information is obtained through the history and physical report, emergency personnel, observers, relatives, or with the use of a pencil and paper.
- Any facial imaging studies, dental impressions, or preoperative photographs should accompany the patient to the operating room.
- The surgeon will typically stand at the head of the OR bed. The OR bed should be reversed to create knee room if the surgery is performed in a sitting position, and the bed should be turned to allow free movement around the head close enough to accommodate the anesthesia provider.
- Maxillofacial procedures can be lengthy. Safety precautions may include the use of warming devices and insertion of a Foley catheter. Any bony areas, such as heels, elbows, sacrum, and shoulders, should be padded.
- Blood loss should be measured closely, especially in children. Blood and blood products should be ordered in advance and made available as needed.
- Maxillofacial surgery involves manipulation of the bones near the patient's airway. Both elective and traumatic procedures can endanger the airway status. Determination of the patient's NPO status is vital. Vomiting can lead to aspiration, and in the maxillofacial trauma patient, it can also lead to infection that may interfere with fracture/wound healing.
- Surgical personnel should be prepared to handle a variety of situations concerning airway management.

The trauma patient may arrive with a tracheotomy or nasal endotracheal or oral endotracheal tube already in place. If the patient requires intubation (oral or nasal), it may be difficult due to distortion of the bony anatomy and/or soft tissues as a result of congenital abnormalities, disease, or trauma. The patient may require rapid induction technique, awake intubation, or a tracheotomy.

- Because maxillofacial procedures are done in the region of the endotracheal tube delivering the oxygen to the patient, care should be taken to avoid an intraoperative fire. Sparks from the electrosurgical unit can cause ignition of oxygen from the ventilation system. A closed ventilation system, use of a fire-retardant endotracheal tube, and careful use of the electrosurgical unit can reduce the potential for fire.
- The surgical site is prepared by carefully removing any gross debris such as glass or dirt. Facial hair is removed if necessary; however, eyebrows and lashes should never be shaved or removed. The lashes may be trimmed if the surgeon deems necessary. The area is washed with the prep solution preferred by the surgeon. If trauma is present, care must be taken to avoid further soft tissue damage or dislocation of fractured bone during the skin prep.
- Maxillofacial reconstructions usually involve several procedures. Maxillofacial fractures can be treated at the same time other injuries are repaired if the patient's condition allows.
- A dural tear may be repaired by the maxillofacial surgeon by placing a suture or sealing off the cerebrospinal fluid (CSF) leak with a fat, fascia, or muscle graft. Maxillofacial fractures can be treated at the same time as other injuries are repaired if the patient's condition allows.
- Open **reduction** techniques often require the use of internal fixation devices and can involve a variety of graft materials. All implanted items must be recorded.
    - Graft materials can be used to fill defects from bone loss, fill cavities to promote osteogenesis, or support a weak reduction.
    - Autogenous bone grafts are harvested from the iliac crest, ribs, or **calvarial** bone. Refer to the craniotomy procedure in Chapter 24 for taking a bone flap.
    - Homogeneous bone is from a cadaver and is obtained from a bone bank.
    - Xenograft material, such as coral, is often used.
    - Synthetic material, such as Silastic, may be used.
- The surgical technologist may also be expected to fill the role of the surgical assistant. Be sure that the instruments and supplies are organized so that the surgeon may obtain instruments independently if the surgical technologist is using both hands to provide retraction.
- Several basic techniques will be used repeatedly: placement of arch bars, wires, and plates and screws, and/or the use of graft material. Several techniques may be used in the correction of one problem.
- Lubricate and protect patient's eyes; corneal shield may be used.
- Local anesthetic with epinephrine may be used alone or in conjunction with general anesthesia to reduce bleeding and minimize postoperative pain.
- Patient is supine, with head positioned to provide maximum exposure. A donut or foam headrest may be used for stabilization. Tuck arms at patient's sides; protect ulnar nerves.
- The operative area may be outlined with towels; place bar drape across patient's forehead, allowing the remainder of the drape to cover the head of operating table. Situate the U-drape on patient's nose. Bring the edges of the U lateral to the head. Extend the remainder of the drape to cover the patient's body.
- The controls on the power equipment must be in the "safe" position when preparing the tool for use or when it is not in operation.

Repair of Mandibular/Maxillary Fractures

Rigid fixation by plates and screws, or screws alone, is the most common repair technique for craniofacial fractures. Bone plates are available in L, Y, H, and T shapes and range in thickness from 0.5 to 3.00 mm. The screws come in diameters of 1.0 to 4.0 mm. The smaller screws are designed for the delicate facial bones; the larger-diameter screws are for placement in the mandible. Implant materials can be absorbable or nonabsorbable. Absorbable implants are of great value in pediatric cases, but other applications are limited. Nonabsorbable implants are most commonly used for facial fractures in adults. Titanium is a strong, lightweight, noncorrosive metal that is used most often in craniofacial procedures. Most fractures require a combination of plates and screws for proper fixation. For example, a four-hole 2.0-mm miniplate and four-hole 2.4-mm direct compression plates can be used together to fixate a symphyseal fracture. Two 2.4-mm lag screws, without a plate, can also be used to fixate the same fracture. The fracture and surgeon's discretion dictate how each one should be fixated.

Arch bars are used to immobilize the jaw following mandibular and/or maxillary fracture. However, the advances in rigid fixation have decreased the necessity for and/or amount of time arch bars are required.

Procedure 18-2 Application of Arch Bars

Surgical Anatomy and Pathology

- The maxillary bones meet inferior to the nasal septum to form the upper jaw; the point of connection is called the intermaxillary suture.
- The maxillary bones articulate with the following facial bones: inferior turbinate; lacrimal; nasal; palatine; vomer; zygomatic. The maxilla does not articulate with the mandible.
- The frontal and ethmoid bones articulate with the maxillary bones.
- Each maxillary bone contains a maxillary sinus, which is a cavity within the bone that is lined with mucous membrane and opens into the nasal cavity.
- The upper teeth are located in the maxillae; the alveolar portions of the teeth are located in the alveolar process in the maxilla.
- The hard palate, or roof of the mouth, is the palatine process of the maxilla.
- The infraorbital foramen, found below the eye, contains the infraorbital nerve and artery.
- The largest and strongest facial bone is the mandible.
- It articulates with the **glenoid fossa** of each temporal bone to form the synovial joint called the temporomandibular joint (**TMJ**).
- The mandible consists of three portions, the first being the body, which lies horizontally and contains the alveolar process for the lower teeth. The mental foramen is located on the body and below the first molar tooth (Figure 18-5). The mental protuberance is the chin.
- The second portion is the **ramus**. The rami project upward at an angle from the posterior part of each mandibular body. The condylar process is the posterior projection of the ramus. The TMJ contains the condylar process, portions of the temporal bone, mandibular fossa, and articular tubercle. The coronoid process is the anterior projection of the ramus. The temporalis muscle attaches here (Figure 18-6). The depression between these two processes is the mandibular notch. Located on the medial surface of the rami, the manidbular foramen contains the inferior alveolar nerve along with its vessels. The mental foramen, like the mandibular foramen, is used by dentists for the injection of anesthetics.
- The last area of the mandible is its angle. The angle connects each ramus to the body.
- Mandibular fractures can occur anywhere along the mandible (Figure 18-7). There are four categories of fractures:
- **Symphysis** and parasymphyseal fractures occur along the mandible between the bicuspid teeth. Most of these fractures do not dislocate. Hematomas can form sublingually due to damage along the floor of the mouth. They are repaired intraorally by making an incision into the anterior gingivobuccal area for reduction and placement of rigid fixation implants.
- Horizontal ramus fractures occur along the lateral portion of the mandible between the bicuspid teeth and molars. The degree of fracture dictates the type of incision, which may be intraorally or transbuccal.
- Mandibular angle fractures occur from the second molar to the

(*continues*)

PROCEDURE 18-2 (continued)

Mental
Foramen
© Cengage Learing 2014

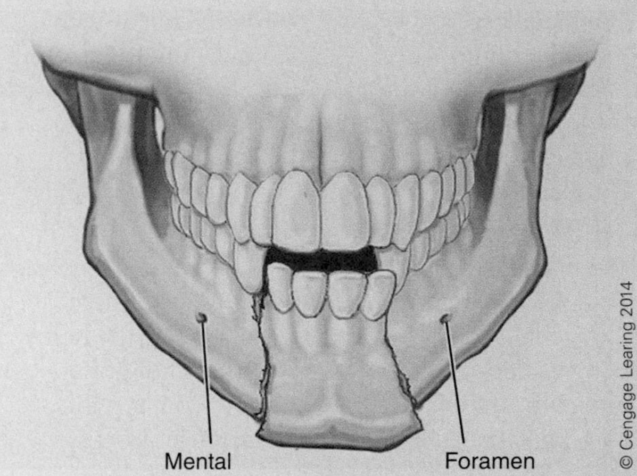

Figure 18-5 Symphysis fracture

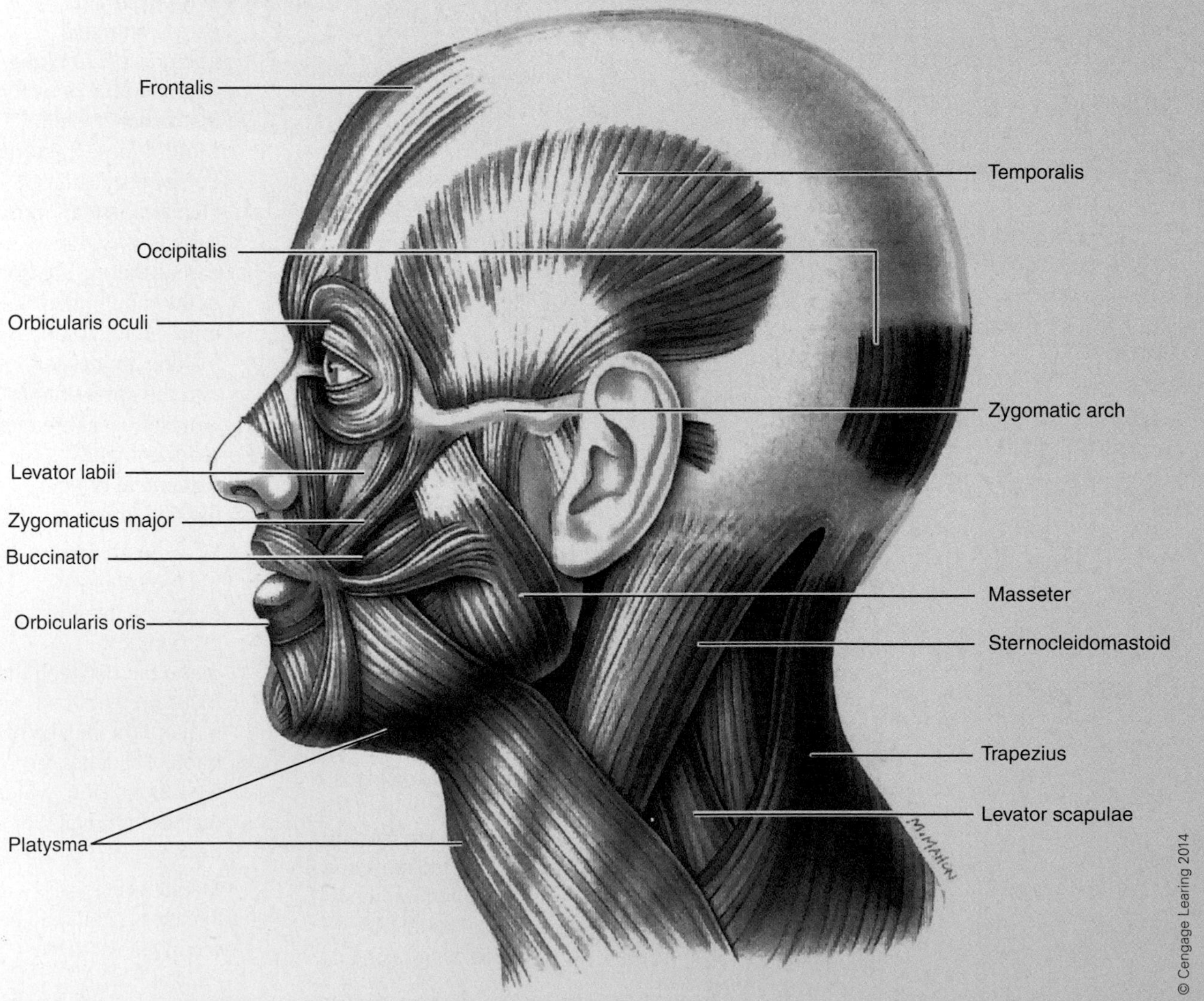

Frontalis
Temporalis
Occipitalis
Orbicularis oculi
Zygomatic arch
Levator labii
Zygomaticus major
Buccinator
Masseter
Orbicularis oris
Sternocleidomastoid
Trapezius
Levator scapulae
Platysma
McMAHON
© Cengage Learing 2014

Figure 18-6 Facial muscles

PROCEDURE 18-2 (continued)

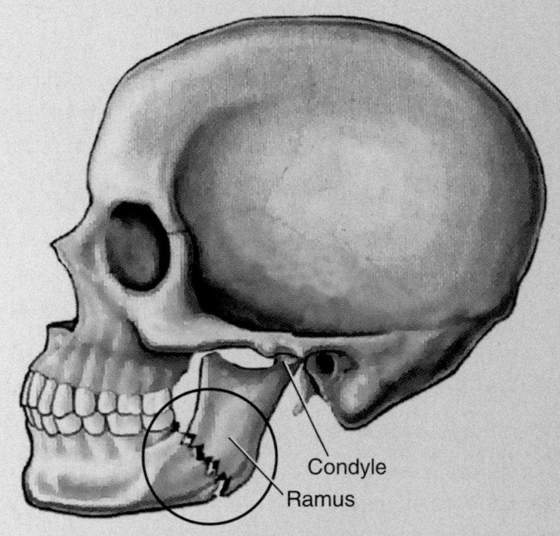

Figure 18-7 Mandibular fracture

	ascending ramus. A submandibular or preauricular incision is used. When using the submandibular incision, the mandibular branch of the facial nerve must be	preserved. Preauricular incision requires the preservation of the frontal branch of the facial nerve. • **Condyle** fractures occur within the capsular head	of the mandible, and subcondylar fractures are below the capsule. Both can be approached through submandibular and preauricular incisions, or combination of both.
Preoperative Diagnostic Tests and Procedures	• See previous information. pp. 707-708		
Equipment, Instruments, and Supplies Unique to Procedure	• Arch bar set includes pediatric- and adult-size stainless steel arch bars.	• Wire of 22 gauge (g), 23g, 24g, and 26g cut into 10-cm segments.	
Preoperative Preparation	• Position: supine (see previous information). • Anesthesia: general; nasal intubation preferred.	• Local anesthetic with epinephrine may be used alone or in conjunction with general anesthesia to reduce bleeding and	minimize postoperative pain. • Skin prep: see previous information. • Draping: see previous information.
Practical Considerations	• Wire used to attach arch bars to the teeth must be precut and prestretched to prevent stretching of the wire intraoperatively and postoperatively,	ensuring the security of the arch bars. To prepare the wire, cut segments slightly longer than needed—approximately 10 cm. Place cut ends of wire in jaws	of two wire twisters and secure. Twist each instrument half a turn and pull to stretch. Remove the instruments and trim the crimped ends. Time permitting,

(continues)

PROCEDURE 18-2 (continued)

several wires are prepared in advance. Plan to use at least one wire for each viable tooth. Allow extra in the event that some wires fall to the floor or break.

- Wire is tightened in a clockwise manner during application and removed by twisting in the opposite direction. Adherence to this method facilitates the application and removal of wires.

Surgical Procedure

1. Insert mouth prop and plastic cheek retractor.

   Procedural Consideration: Have appropriate-size mouth prop and retractor ready for insertion.

2. Insert throat pack.

   Procedural Consideration: Prepare throat pack for insertion and present instrument for insertion.

3. The arch bars are measured, shaped, and cut to size.

   Procedural Consideration: Have two (one for the mandible and one for the maxilla) appropriate-sized arch bars ready along with the wire cutter.

4. The arch bar is attached to the maxilla with prestretched wires to the individual viable teeth.

   Procedural Consideration: Prepare wire as previously instructed. Place one end of wire in jaws of wire twister and secure. Pass wire with caution—the exposed ends can easily puncture.

5. Ten-centimeter segments of wire are placed around the neck of each tooth, securing the bar to the tooth.

   Procedural Consideration: As soon as wire is passed, hand the wire twister and the V-shaped probe to position the wire during tightening.

6. A probe facilitates placement of the wires. The wire twisters are used to tighten the wires using a clockwise motion.

   Procedural Consideration: Wire cutter will be needed next. Provide suction and retraction as needed.

7. Another arch bar is secured to the mandible with wire.

   Procedural Consideration: The wire, probe, cutter sequence will be repeated until the arch bars are secured to each tooth in the mandible and maxilla.

8. If a throat pack was used, it must be removed prior to fixation of the mandible and maxilla to one another.

   Procedural Consideration: Provide bayonet to remove throat pack. Count. Anticipate use of irrigation and suction.

9. The upper and lower jaws are then stabilized to each other.

   Procedural Consideration: Additional wire or elastic bands may be used. Loops of precut, prestretched, preshaped wire may be fashioned beforehand to facilitate this step of the procedure.

10. Wire or elastic loops can now be placed over the hooks of the arch bars and tightened to immobilize the jaw (Figure 18-8).

    Procedural Consideration: Variations of mandibulomaxillary fixation are used according to the surgeon's preference and the patient's need.

PROCEDURE 18-2 (continued)

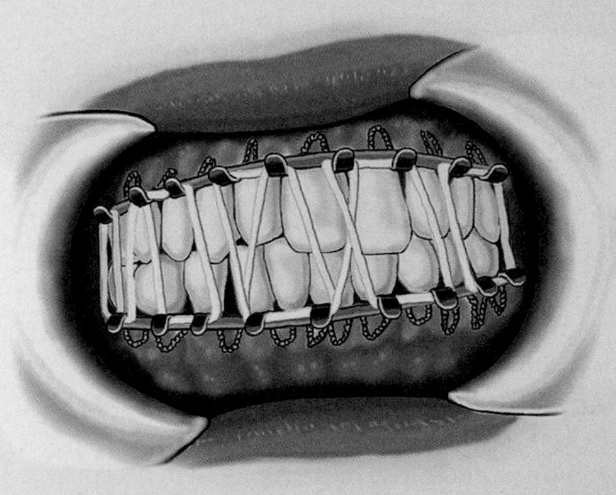

Figure 18-8 Maxillomandibular fixation

11. A final rinse of the oral cavity is performed, and all fluid and debris are removed.

    Procedural Consideration: Provide irrigation fluid and Yankauer suction tip.

12. Retractors are removed.

    Procedural Consideration: Be sure all loose wire is retrieved and disposed of properly.

Postoperative Considerations

Immediate postoperative care

- Patient transported to the PACU.
- Scissors or wire cutter should accompany the patient to the PACU. It may be necessary to open the mouth in case vomiting or respiratory distress occurs.
- Tracheotomy may become necessary secondary to airway obstruction due to swelling.
- Bruising and swelling of the lips and cheeks may occur. The patient should be advised to apply ice.

Prognosis

- No complications: bone healing is expected in 4–6 weeks. The jaw will remain immobilized for the entire time. Removal of the arch bars is usually an office procedure. Special consideration is given to the patient's nutritional needs. Patient will only be allowed liquids until fixation device is removed.
- Complications: hemorrhage; postoperative SSI; misalignment/ malocclusion.

Wound Classification

- Class II: clean-contaminated

PEARL OF WISDOM

Arch bars are thin strips of metal that have small intermittently placed hooks. The strips are malleable and the hooks should be placed pointing downward on the lower jaw and upward on the upper jaw. This placement allows for mandibulomaxillary elastic band or wire fixation.

PROCEDURE 18-3 Plate and Screw Fixation of Mandibular Fracture

Surgical Anatomy and Pathology	See application of arch bars procedure.		
Preoperative Diagnostic Tests and Procedures	• Diagnosis primarily obtained from X-rays and MRI along with a visual and digital inspection of the area.		
Equipment, Instruments, and Supplies Unique to Procedure	• Internal fixation system of surgeon's choice	• Maxillofacial instrument set	• Arch bar set (available)
Preoperative Preparation	• Position: supine • Anesthesia: general	• Skin prep: see previous information.	• Draping: see previous information.
Practical Considerations	• The procedure will be performed using sterile technique if an external incision is planned.	• Arch bars may be placed. • All implanted items must be recorded in the patient's chart.	• Notify the radiology department of the possible need for intraoperative X-rays.

Surgical Procedure

1. Local anesthetic with epinephrine is injected.

   Procedural Consideration: Local anesthetic of choice is preloaded in syringe with needle attached. Follow facility policy for passing sharps. Refill the syringe in anticipation of use on contralateral side. Notify anesthesia provider of epinephrine use.

2. An incision is made anterior to the angle of the mandible and any bleeding is controlled.

   Procedural Consideration: A #15 blade will be needed. Anticipate use of electrosurgical pencil.

3. Wound edges are retracted.

   Procedural Consideration: Retractor(s) of choice will be needed. Provide suction as needed.

4. Periosteum is stripped from the bone.

   Procedural Consideration: Periosteal elevator such as a Freer will be used.

5. Bone edges are manipulated into position and steadied by the surgical assistant or with a bone-holding clamp.

   Procedural Consideration: Stabilize patient's head during manipulation. Be sure breathing tube does not become crimped or dislocated. Bone clamp may be needed.

6. A plate of appropriate thickness, length, and design is chosen and customized for the patient.

   Procedural Consideration: Provide a variety of plates for selection. Plates can be customized to the area by curving the plate, using bending irons.

7. The plate is placed against the bone, bridging the fracture site, and secured in position.

   Procedural Consideration: Provide plate-holding clamp to secure plate to bone. Load drill with correct size bit.

Procedure 18-3 (continued)

8. A hole is drilled with the correct-diameter drill bit.

   Procedural Consideration: A drill guide may be used. Have depth gauge ready.

9. The depth of the hole is measured and tapped if necessary.

   Procedural Consideration: Present correct-size tap. Retrieve requested-size screw and load onto insertion device.

10. The proper screw is placed into the predrilled hole.

    Procedural Consideration: Reset the drill and organize insertion tools for reuse.

11. The sequence is repeated until the plate is firmly affixed to the bone.

    Procedural Consideration: Record the pertinent information about the implants for the patient's permanent operative record.

12. The procedure is repeated on the contralateral side, if necessary.

    Procedural Consideration: Reorganize tools for reuse.

13. Proper reduction/fixation is ensured by visual inspection of the area. Intraoperative X-rays may be useful.

    Procedural Consideration: Prepare to accept X-ray cassette into sterile field if requested. Prepare irrigation fluid and suture for closing.

14. The wound is irrigated and closed.

    Procedural Consideration: Count.

15. Dressings are applied.

    Procedural Consideration: Prepare dressing material for use.

Postoperative Considerations

Immediate postoperative care

- Patient transported to the PACU.
- If arch bar fixation was also performed, scissors or wire cutter should accompany the patient to the PACU.
- Bruising and swelling of the lips and cheeks may occur. The patient should be advised to apply ice.
- Patient should be observed for airway difficulties secondary to swelling.

Prognosis

- No complications: complete recovery is expected in 4–6 weeks. Bruising and swelling of the lips and cheeks may occur. The patient should be advised to apply ice.
- Complications: patient should be observed for airway difficulties secondary to swelling in the immediate postoperative period; hemorrhage; postoperative SSI; misalignment/malocclusion.

Wound Classification

- Class I: clean (external incision)
- Class II: clean-contaminated

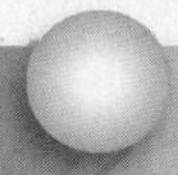

Pearl of Wisdom

The same sequence of events is employed for attachment of the plate to the bone with most fixation systems (Figure 18-9).

1. A plate of appropriate thickness, length, and design is chosen.
2. Plates can be customized to the specific anatomy by contouring the plate using bending irons provided with the fixation set for that purpose.
3. Correct-diameter drill bit is chosen and applied to the drill.

(continues)

4. A drill guide may be used.
5. The depth of the hole is then measured.
6. The drill hole may be tapped. Tap use reduces the amount of torque applied during screw placement. Self-tapping screws are available.
7. The correct screw is selected and measured by the surgical technologist and loaded onto the insertion device.
8. The screw is placed through the plate and into the predrilled hole in the bone.
9. The sequence is repeated until the plate is firmly affixed to the bone.
10. The implants are permanently recorded in the operative record.
11. Fracture reduction and prosthesis placement is verified visually or with the use of X-ray.

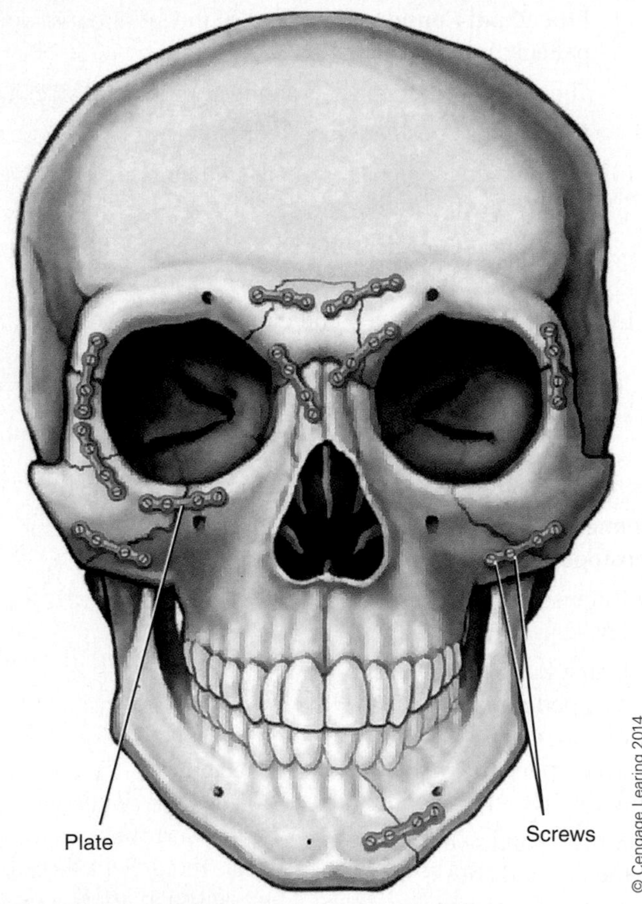

Figure 18-9 Miniplates and screws

PROCEDURE 18-4 Orbital Floor Fracture Repair

Surgical Anatomy and Pathology

- The bones of the orbit support and protect the eyes. Each orbit consists of the following seven craniofacial bones: frontal, lacrimal, ethmoid, maxilla, zygomatic, sphenoid, palatine.
- The orbit contains fat to protect the eye from shock and connective structures to retain the eyeball and allow for its motion, blood vessels, and the optic nerve (second cranial nerve).
- The orbital floor separates the eye from the maxillary sinus. The floor is a thin extension of the

PROCEDURE 18-4 (continued)

	maxillary and zygomatic bones. • Two classifications of orbital fractures—floor fractures or orbital blowouts—involve one or more of the numerous bones of the orbit (Figure 18-10). Trauma caused by auto accidents, fights, and	falls commonly results in these fractures. • Orbital fractures may appear alone, unilaterally, bilaterally, or in conjunction with other facial fractures. • Characteristics of orbital fractures: diplopia; enophthalmos; periorbital fat and muscles pinched	in the fracture line or herniated into the maxillary antrum; swelling and bruising.
Preoperative Diagnostic Tests and Procedures	• Preoperative CT scans and X-rays help in the	diagnosis of orbital floor fractures, and they should	be available for reference during surgery.
Equipment, Instruments, and Supplies Unique to Procedure	• Internal fixation system of surgeon's preference • Orbital retractors	• Corneal shield • Implant material of surgeon's preference (Teflon or Silastic sheeting	that has been washed and sterilized according to manufacturer's instructions)
Preoperative Preparation	• Position: supine • Anesthesia: general; local anesthetic	• Skin prep: see previous information.	• Draping: see previous information.
Practical Considerations	Notify the radiology department of the possible need	for intraoperative X-rays.	• All implanted items must be recorded in the patient's chart.
Surgical Procedure	1. The planned incision is marked and injected with a local anesthetic containing epinephrine. **Procedural Consideration:** Provide sterile marking pen. Medication is obtained and drawn into the syringe in advance. Notify anesthesia provider of epinephrine use.		

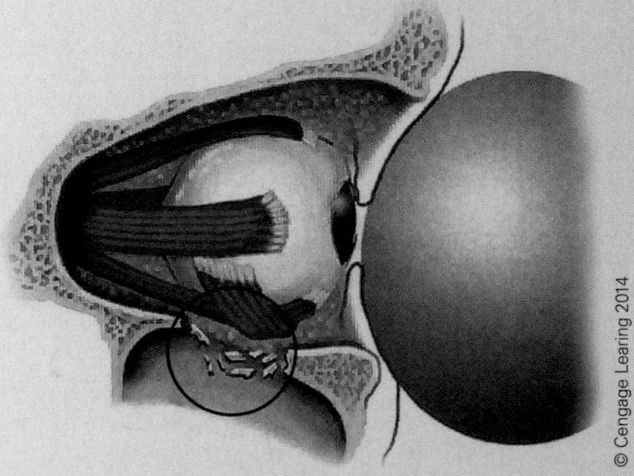

Figure 18-10 Orbital floor fracture

(continues)

PROCEDURE 18-4 (continued)

2. Incision is made with a #15 blade underneath the lower eyelid on the affected side and hemostasis is achieved.

   Procedural Consideration: Cotton swabs or Weck cell sponges are used to blot away blood and irrigation solution around the incision. Keep an ample supply readily available. Present electrosurgical pencil, if needed. Provide suction as needed.

3. A traction stitch may be placed between the lower eyelashes and incision site to aid in exposure.

   Procedural Consideration: Traction stitch is preloaded on needle holder. It may either be tied and cut or secured with a hemostat. Dull Senn or vein retractors may be needed to provide additional exposure.

4. Curved tenotomy scissors and Adson tissue forceps are used for dissection through the infraorbital fat to expose the infraorbital rim.

   Procedural Consideration: Pass scissors to surgeon's dominant hand and tissue forceps to the opposite. Electrosurgical pencil may be used intermittently.

5. The periosteum is incised with a #15 blade and elevated with the use of a Freer.

   Procedural Consideration: A new #15 blade will be needed. Pass Freer elevator. Be sure to present sharp or dull end as specified by surgeon.

6. A moistened orbital retractor or Teflon-coated malleable brain spatula may be placed to gently retract the eye, superiorly exposing the orbital floor.

   Procedural Consideration: Have premoistened retractor of choice available.

7. The periorbital fat and any other entrapped tissues are released and retracted.

   Procedural Consideration: Freer elevator or scissors and tissue forceps may be needed repeatedly.

8. The fracture site is exposed and bone fragments are manipulated into position.

   Procedural Consideration: Be sure eye is protected during reduction of bone fragments.

9. Any loose bone fragments are repositioned and the wound is irrigated.

   Procedural Consideration: Irrigation fluid of surgeon's choice is preloaded in syringe with blunt needle. Pass irrigation fluid along with Frazier tip suction. A kidney basin placed at the side of the face may be useful in containing excess irrigation fluid.

10. If the reduction is stable, Silastic sheeting may be inserted over the fracture site to prevent entrapment of the orbital contents in the fracture and support the globe.

    Procedural Consideration: Sheeting must be prepared and sterilized according to manufacturer's instructions. Sheeting will be customized—have straight scissors ready.

11. If the reduction is not stable, a rigid fixation device may be implanted, followed by the insertion of Silastic sheeting.

    Procedural Consideration: Communicate additional needs with other team members. Secure any necessary additional supplies.

12. Reduction may be verified radiographically.

    Procedural Consideration: Provide necessary supplies to facilitate X-ray.

13. Once adequate stable reduction is achieved, the traction suture is removed and the wound is closed.

    Procedural Consideration: Provide closing suture of surgeon's choice. Count.

14. If used, the corneal protector is removed and the dressing is applied.

    Procedural Consideration: Provide dressing materials. Ice may be needed.

Procedure 18-4 (continued)

Postoperative Considerations

Immediate postoperative care

- Patient transported to the PACU.
- Bruising and swelling may occur around the eyes and nose. Advise patient to apply ice.
- Patient may experience temporary vision disturbances due to swelling.

Prognosis

- No complications: a small visible scar will remain; complete recovery is expected.
- Complications: hemorrhage; postoperative SSI; vision disturbance due to trauma to the eye.

Wound Classification

- Class I: clean

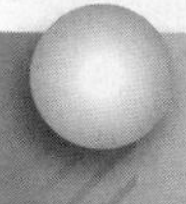

Pearl of Wisdom

The surgical technologist may also be expected to fill the role of the surgical assistant. Be sure that the instruments and supplies are organized so that the surgeon may obtain instruments independently if the surgical technologist is using both hands to provide retraction.

Procedure 18-5 Le Fort I Fracture Repair

Surgical Anatomy and Pathology

- The pair of nasal bones come together to form what is known as the "bridge" of the nose. Each nasal bone articulates with the frontal, ethmoid, maxillary, and the opposite nasal bone. In the anterior view, the nasal bones are bordered laterally by the maxilla and superiorly by the frontal bone. Cartilage attaches to the anterior portion of the small nasal bones to form the tip of the nose.
- The zygomatic (**malar**) bones form the prominences of the cheeks and a portion of the inferior and lateral wall of the orbit.
- The bones do not articulate with one another, but they do join with the frontal, sphenoid, temporal, and maxillary bones.
- Each zygomatic bone has a zygomatic arch, which is a temporal process that is located posteriorly to join the zygomatic process of the temporal bone.
- The L-shaped palatine bones articulate with each other, sphenoid, ethomoid, maxillary, inferior turbinate, and vomer.
- The horizontal plates of the bones form the anterior (hard) palate. The palate separates the nasal and oral cavities, thus forming the floor and lateral wall of the nasal cavity.
- The vomer contributes to the posterior and inferior portion of the nasal septum. It is surrounded by the sphenoid, ethmoid, both maxillary, and palatine bones. It is singular and triangular.
- A Le Fort I fracture, also called transverse maxillary, is the most common type of mid-facial fracture. The alveolar process of the maxilla is horizontally separated from the base of the skull. The upper jaw can be floating free in the oral cavity (Figure 18-11).

(continues)

PROCEDURE 18-5 (continued)

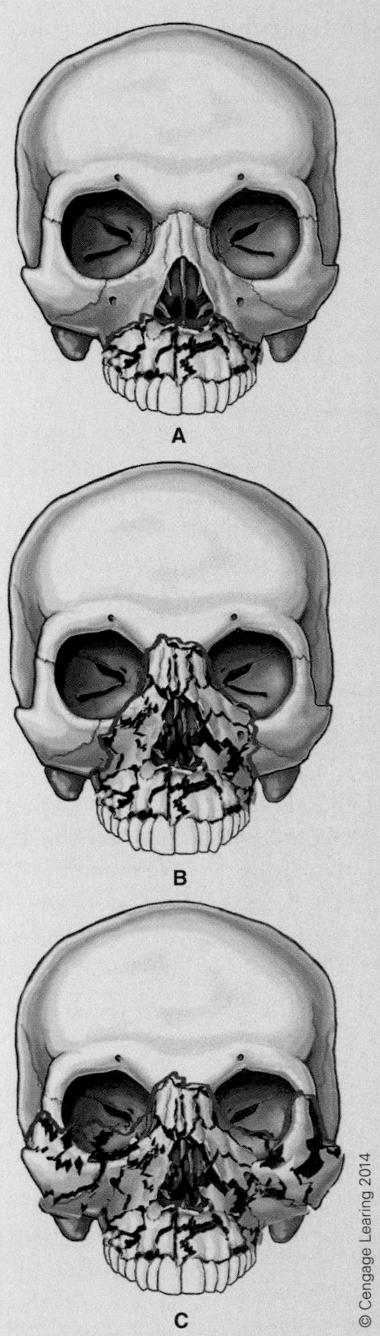

Figure 18-11 Le Fort fractures: (A) Le Fort I, (B) Le Fort II, (C) Le Fort III

- Le Fort II fractures, also called pyramidal maxillary fractures, may be triangular or pyramidal in shape. The vertical fracture line extends upward to the nasal and ethmoid bones. Le Fort II fractures can be unilateral or bilateral in nature.
- Le Fort III fractures, also called craniofacial disjunction fractures, are located high in the mid-face. The fracture line extends transversely from the zygomatic arches, through the orbits, and to the base of the nose. These fractures can exist unilaterally, bilaterally, alone, or in conjunction with other facial fractures.

PROCEDURE 18-5 (continued)

Preoperative Diagnostic Tests and Procedures	• Diagnosis of mid-facial fractures can be made through examination of X-rays and CT scans and the physical examination of the patient. • Pretrauma photographs and dental records can aid the surgeon in determining the proper placement of fractured facial bones.
Equipment, Instruments, and Supplies Unique to Procedure	• Internal fixation system of surgeon's preference • Arch bar set if required • Orbital retractor
Preoperative Preparation	• Position: supine (see previous information) • Anesthesia: general (see previous information) • Skin prep: see previous information; entire face is prepped with antiseptic. Avoid excessive pressure to minimize movement of fractured bones. • Draping: see previous information.
Practical Considerations	• Notify the radiology department of the possible need for intraoperative X-rays. • All implanted items must be recorded in the patient's chart. • Several procedures may need to be completed prior to fracture reduction and stabilization, including tracheotomy and arch bars applied. Dental impressions may be taken before the incision is made.

Surgical Procedure

1. A gingivobuccal sulcus incision provides adequate exposure of the maxilla; actual prosthesis placement will depend on the fracture site. The gingiva may be injected with local anesthetic with epinephrine prior to incising with a #15 blade. Hemostasis is achieved.

   Procedural Consideration: Anticipate retractor use for exposure of incision site. Medications are obtained in advance and prepared for use. Notify anesthesia provider of epinephrine use. Pass a #15 blade on a #7 knife handle. Anticipate the use of the electrosurgical pencil and suction with appropriate tip.

2. Exposure of the operative site is attained.

   Procedural Consideration: Retractors may be replaced or repositioned.

3. The fracture line is exposed by dissecting the gingiva from the alveolar process with a small periosteal elevator.

   Procedural Consideration: A Freer or slightly larger elevator will be used to expose the fracture site.

4. The fracture is reduced using caution not to disrupt the breathing tube.

   Procedural Consideration: Reduction of the fracture may be achieved with the use of an elevator or manually.

5. If wire fixation is anticipated, sites for the drill holes are identified.

   Procedural Consideration: Drill with appropriate-size bit is preassembled and connected to the power source.

6. A drill hole is made on each side of the fracture line.

   Procedural Consideration: Suction and irrigation fluid will be necessary to cool the drill site.

7. A single wire is passed through each hole and pulled taut, reducing the fracture.

   Procedural Consideration: Precut, prestretched lengths of wire of appropriate size are loaded onto the wire twister and passed to the surgeon.

(continues)

Procedure 18-5 (continued)

8. The wire is twisted clockwise, cut, and the ends of the wire imbedded in the drill hole. The wire technique can also be used to apply traction by simply placing the wires through the holes and pulling the impacted maxilla up and forward.

   Procedural Consideration: Anticipate the use of the wire cutter. The fracture may require placement of more than one wire for stabilization.

9. Plate and screws can also be employed to fixate the maxilla. The plate is placed over the fracture line and secured to the bone by the compressive force of the screw. Both the wiring and plating techniques can be utilized several times throughout the procedure, often in conjunction with one another.

   Procedural Consideration: Be prepared for a combination procedure that employs wire, screw, or plate and screw fixation. Refer to Procedure 18-3 for related technical considerations.

10. Fracture reduction and stabilization may be verified with the use of intraoperative X-rays (Figure 18-12).

    Procedural Consideration: Prepare to accept X-ray cassette into sterile field if requested. Anticipate closure as next step. Prepare irrigation fluid and suture.

11. The wound is irrigated and closed.

    Procedural Consideration: Count.

12. Retractor is removed.

    Procedural Consideration: Dressing is not needed with intraoral approach.

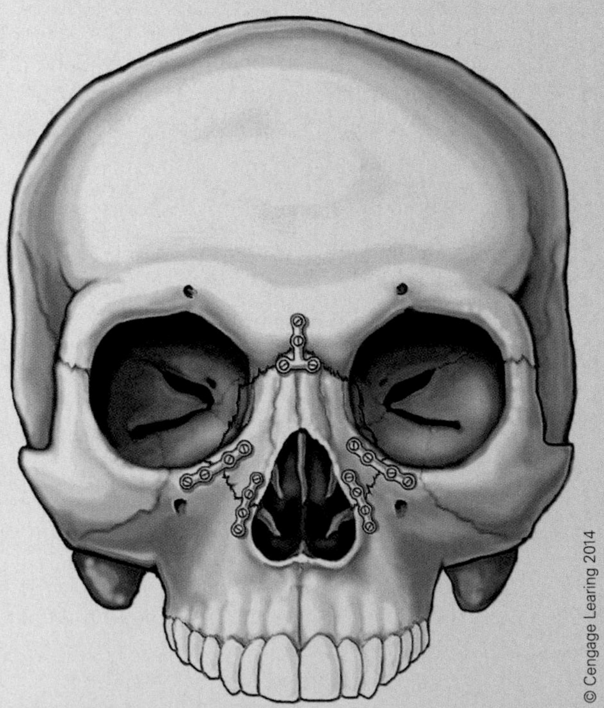

Figure 18-12 Repaired Le Fort I fracture

PROCEDURE 18-5 (continued)

Postoperative Considerations	**Immediate postoperative care** • Patient transported to the PACU. • Patency of the airway may be compromised due to postoperative hemorrhage and swelling. **Prognosis** • No complications: return to normal activities anticipated. • Complications: hemorrhage; postoperative SSI; malocclusion. Exact visual identity may not be restored. Further reconstructive surgery may be necessary. Scars will be visible. **Wound Classification** • Class I: clean

PROCEDURE 18-6 Le Fort II and III Fracture Repair

Surgical Anatomy and Pathology	Refer to Le Fort I for surgical anatomy and pathology; preoperative diagnostic tests and procedures; equipment, instruments, and supplies unique to procedure; and preoperative preparation.
Instruments Unique to Procedure	• Right and left Rowe maxillary forceps • Brown fascia needle • Sterile polyethylene buttons • Sterile small foam pad • Periosteal elevators • Rigid fixation system of surgeon's preference
Practical Considerations	In Le Fort II and III fractures, to suspend the maxillary arch to stable bones, the suspension wires are placed through holes drilled bilaterally through the zygomatic process of the frontal bone. To facilitate the wire placement, bilateral eyebrow incisions are made (similar to the incision made for a blepharoplasty).
Surgical Procedure	1. The bilateral eyebrow incisions are made to expose the edges of the infraorbital area and zygomatic frontal suture lines. Hemostasis is achieved.
	2. The Rowe forceps are situated intranasally and intraorally to reduce the maxilla.
	3. Holes are drilled into the bone on each side of the fracture along the infraorbital rim; for Le Fort III fractures holes are also drilled in the zygomatic frontal areas after the zygomatic fracture is reduced.
	4. Stainless steel wires are passed through the drill holes and using the wire twister, twisted downward in clockwise fashion to keep the reduction in place.
	5. The suspension wires are passed through the eyebrow incisions, behind the zygomatic arches and into the oral cavity using the Brown needle.
	6. A pullout stainless steel wire is looped through the suspension wire at the eyebrow incision, pulled through the skin at the hairline, and tied down over a sterile polyethylene button and foam padding. Depending on surgeon's preference, mini-compression plates, screws, and bone grafts may be used.
	7. Incisions are closed and the nasal fracture is reduced.
Postoperative Considerations	• Postoperative considerations are the same as for Le Fort I

(continues)

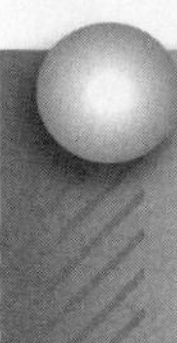

Pearl of Wisdom

The controls on the power equipment must be in the "safe" position when preparing the tool for use or when it is not in operation.

Case Study A physician in the Emergency Department notes the following during the examination of a patient who suffered facial injuries in an MVA: bruising and swelling around the left eye; diplopia; enophthalmos. The diagnosis is confirmed as an orbital floor fracture.

1. Define the following: MVA, diplopia and enophthalmos.
2. What implant material will the surgical technologist need to confirm is sterile and available for use during the repair of the fracture?
3. What instrument is often used to free up the periorbital fat that is entrapped in the fracture?
4. If the reduced fracture is not stable, what instrument set should the surgical technologist have available for the repair?

Questions for Further Study

1. Does the surgeon always stand while performing oral and maxillofacial procedures? If not, how does the choice to sit or stand affect patient positioning?
2. What is the particular danger created by operating in the area of the endotracheal tube? How is it minimized?
3. What graft materials can be used in maxillofacial surgery?
4. What intraoperative measure may be taken to prevent drying and cracking of the patient's lips?
5. Why are rubber bands applied to arch bars?

BIBLIOGRAPHY

Alling, C. C., & Osborn, D. B. (1987). *Maxillofacial trauma.* Philadelphia: Lea & Febiger.

American Association of Oral and Maxillofacial Surgeons. (1998). *AAOMS news* [Online]. Available from http://www.aaoms.org

Association of Surgical Technologists. (2011). *Core curriculum for surgical technology* (6th ed.). Littleton, CO: Association of Surgical Technologists.

Boyne, P. (1997). *Osseous reconstruction of the maxilla and the mandible: Surgical techniques using titanium mesh and bone material.* Carol Stream, IL: Quintessence Books.

Kruger, G. O. (1984). *Oral and maxillofacial surgery* (6th ed.). St. Louis, MO: Mosby.

Prein, J. (Ed.). (2002). *Manual of internal fixation in the cranio-facial skeleton: Techniques recommended by the AO/ASIF maxillofacial group.* New York: Springer.

Riden, K. (2007). *Key topics in oral and maxillofacial surgery.* Oxford, UK: Taylor & Francis.

Rothrock, J. C. (2003). *Alexander's care of the patient in surgery* (12th ed.). St. Louis: Mosby.

Shier, D. N., Butler, J. L., & Lewis, R. (Eds.). (2009). *Hole's human anatomy and physiology* (12th ed.). New York: McGraw-Hill.

Standring, S. (2009). *Gray's anatomy: The anatomical basis of clinical practice* (40th ed.). St. Louis: Elsevier

Tortora, G. J., & Derrickson, B. H. (Eds.). (2008). *Principles of anatomy and physiology* (12th ed.). Hoboken, NJ: John Wiley & Sons.

CHAPTER

19

Plastic and Reconstructive Surgery

CASE STUDY

Adriana was born just a few minutes ago. She has been diagnosed with cheiloschisis.

1. **How was the diagnosis made?**
2. **Her mother views her as a "monster." What help can be provided for the family?**
3. **How will Adriana be nourished?**
4. **Is immediate surgery necessary?**

OBJECTIVES

After studying this chapter, the reader should be able to:

A 1. Recognize the relevant anatomy and physiology of the skin and its underlying tissues.

P 2. Summarize the pathology that prompts plastic/reconstructive surgical intervention and the related terminology.

3. Determine any special preoperative plastic/reconstructive diagnostic procedures/tests.

4. Determine any special preoperative preparation procedures related to plastic/reconstructive surgical procedures.

5. Indicate the names and uses of plastic/reconstructive instruments, supplies, and specialty equipment.

6. Determine the intraoperative preparation of the patient undergoing a plastic/reconstructive procedure.

O 7. Summarize the surgical steps of the plastic/reconstructive procedures.

8. Interpret the purpose and expected outcomes of the plastic/reconstructive procedures.

9. Recognize the immediate postoperative care and possible complications of the plastic/reconstructive procedures.

S 10. Assess any specific variations related to the preoperative, intraoperative, and postoperative care of the plastic/reconstructive patient.

Select Key Terms

Abbreviated Burn Severity Index (ABSI)	cleft	poly-	sebum
aesthetic	dermatome	radial hypoplasia	STSG
arthrodesis	elliptical	replantation	syndactyly
augmentation	integumentary	rhinoplasty	synthesis
cheilo-	MPJ	-schisis	xenograft

INTRODUCTION

Plastic, or cosmetic, and reconstructive surgery refers to those procedures that have as a primary goal the restoration of appearance or function to a particular body structure. Unlike other surgical specialties that are restricted to specific anatomical systems (e.g., cardiovascular), plastic surgery encompasses a wide spectrum of many systems and structures, and often includes elements of other surgical specialties, such as vascular and orthopedics. Therefore, the surgical technologist participating in plastic/reconstructive surgery must have a strong foundation in human anatomy, as well as a working knowledge of the specialized instruments and supplies needed for the specific procedure.

DIAGNOSTIC PROCEDURES AND TESTS

Diagnosis of conditions that may require plastic/reconstructive surgery is often accomplished by visual examination. The patient may have a desire to change his or her appearance by altering physical features. A physician may recommend surgery due to a disease process or deformity that may be congenital or acquired.

Imaging studies are often used to determine the type and severity of a condition, in particular a congenital disorder. Standard X-rays, magnetic resonance imaging (MRI), and computed tomography (CT) scanning are useful in providing information regarding hand and craniofacial interventions.

INSTRUMENTATION, ROUTINE EQUIPMENT, AND SUPPLIES

The following sections list the routine instrumentation and items used for plastic and reconstructive procedures. Instrumentation, equipment, and supplies that are unique to a specific surgical procedure will be listed with the description of the procedure.

Instrumentation

Of course, instrument sets will vary from institution to institution. Variations include geographic hospital region and surgeon's specific preference. Additional instrumentation will have to be added to accommodate other body systems undergoing modification. A typical plastic set for use on the skin and immediate underlying tissues is shown in Table 19-1.

Plastic Sets

A basic plastic set is necessary for most cosmetic procedures and generally is equipped with delicate skin instruments, larger soft tissue instruments for breast **augmentation**, and some small bone instruments for nasal reconstruction. A minor orthopedic, or "hand," set is required for reconstructive hand surgery. A separate set may be required for liposuction.

Nasal Set

A nasal instrumentation set for **rhinoplasty** is tailored to suit the plastic surgeon's needs. A rhinoplasty tray will contain just the instruments used in reshaping the nose. It may be used in addition to a plastic set or may contain a modification of the previously mentioned instruments. Suggested instrumentation for a rhinoplasty set is shown in Table 19-2, and suggested instrumentation for a basic nasal set is shown in Table 19-3.

Equipment

A **dermatome** is an instrument used to cut thin slices of skin, called a split-thickness skin graft, for grafting. Several types and brands of dermatomes are available to the surgical team. These instruments vary from specialized handheld knives to powered machinery. The most common type of powered dermatome is the oscillating-blade-type dermatome (Figure 19-1).

Oscillating-Blade–Type Dermatome

Electricity or nitrogen may power the oscillating-blade–type dermatome. In either case, the surgical technologist will have a cord that will need to be partially passed from the sterile field to the circulator for connection to the power source. It is important to locate and secure the cord on the sterile field so that its presence does not interfere with either of the operative sites

TABLE 19-1 **Typical Plastic Instrumentation Set**

Clamps		*Forceps*	
4	Towel clips, 3½ in.	2	Adson tissue forceps with teeth
4	Micropoint mosquitos, curved	2	Adson tissue forceps, smooth
4	Halstead mosquitos, curved	1	Adson-Brown
2	Halstead mosquitos, straight	1	Bishop-Harmon
4	Crile hemostats	2	DeBakey, 6 in.
2	Allis clamps, 6 in.	*Retractors*	
Scissors		2	Skin hooks, double-prong, medium
1	Littler scissors	2	Skin hooks, double-prong, large
1	Iris scissors, curved	2	Skin hooks, single-prong
1	Stevens tenotomy scissors, curved	2	Senn retractors
1	Suture scissors, small	2	Spring retractors
1	Metzenbaum scissors, fine tip, 5½ in.	2	U.S. Army retractors
1	Metzenbaum scissors, blunt tip, 5½ in.	*Miscellaneous*	
1	Metzenbaum scissors, 7 in.	2	Knife handles, #3
1	Mayo scissors, straight	1	Knife handle, #7
1	Mayo scissors, curved	2	Beaver knife handles
1	Bandage scissors	2	Medicine cups
Needle Holders		2	Freer elevators
1	Regular, 4¾ in.	1	Joseph elevators
1	Padgett, 4 in.	2	Key elevators, small
2	Crile wood, 6 in.	2	Frazier suction tip, 8 Fr.
1	Crile wood, 7 in.		

(even though it will only be used at the donor site). For the safety of the surgical technologist, it is recommended that the dermatome not be connected to the power cord until the blade has been loaded. Be sure that the safety switch is engaged.

A sterile disposable blade is used for each patient, or, if several grafts are to be procured, several blades may be used for one patient. Use extreme caution when removing the blade from the package and inserting it into the dermatome so that the blade is not damaged and injury is prevented. Once the blade is positioned within the dermatome, the surface of the blade, except for the cutting edge, is covered with one of four guard plates. This guard plate retains the blade and allows for the width of the skin graft to be procured. The width of the graft is determined by a "gap" in the edge of the plate. The gaps range in size from 1 to 4 inches. The blade and the retention plate are secured with screws. A screwdriver should be provided with the dermatome.

The thickness of the graft is determined by adjusting a small lever on the side of the dermatome, which has numbered markings (in tenths of a millimeter). This will be set according to the surgeon's preference and the patient's situation. Some surgeons prefer to insert the blade and select the settings themselves.

Prior to its use, the surgical technologist should test the dermatome in a safe environment to ascertain that it is connected to the power source and functioning properly.

In addition to the dermatome, the surgeon may desire lubricant, such as sterile mineral oil, for the patient's skin. A device to stretch the skin while the dermatome is being used may also be requested. A sterile tongue blade works well for this purpose.

Other Types of Dermatomes

Three types of handheld knife dermatomes are used: Ferris-Smith, Watson, and Weck. The Ferris-Smith dermatome is used to obtain free-hand skin grafts. The depth of the graft is controlled by the surgeon. A sterile straight razor blade is used. The Watson knife has an adjustable roller for the surgeon to control the desired thickness of graft. The Weck knife also uses a straight razor blade with various sizes of guards to control

Table 19-2 Typical Rhinoplasty Instrumentation Set

Retractors	
1	Vienna nasal speculum, small
1	Vienna nasal speculum, medium
1	Vienna nasal speculum, large
2	Single-prong skin hooks
2	Cottle or Joseph double-prong skin hooks
1	Fomon retractor
1	Cottle retractor
1	Converse alar retractor
1	Cottle knife guide and retractor
1	Aufricht nasal septum retractor
Bone Instruments	
1	Cottle osteotome, 4 mm
1	Cottle osteotome, 7 mm
1	Cottle osteotome, 9 mm
1	Cottle osteotome, 12 mm
1	Cinelli osteotome, double guards, 10 mm
1	Silver osteotome, single guard, right
1	Silver osteotome, single guard, left
1	Freer septum chisel, straight, 4 mm
1	Freer septum chisel, curved, 4 mm
1	Ballenger V-shaped chisel, 4 mm
1	Ballenger swivel knife, 4 mm
1	Mead mallet, 8 oz. head
1	Joseph nasal saw, straight
1	Joseph nasal saw, bayonet, right
1	Joseph nasal saw, bayonet, left
1	Joseph rasp, cross serrations
1	Maltz rasp, double-ended, forward and backward
Miscellaneous	
1	Cushing tissue forceps with teeth, bayonet
1	Jansen bayonet dressing forceps
1	Takahashi forceps
1	Freer septum knife
1	Cottle septum elevator
1	Joseph periosteal elevator
1	Cottle cartilage crusher

Table 19-3 Basic Nasal Set

Yankauer suction tube	1 ea.
#3 and #7 knife handles	1 ea.
Mayo dissecting scissors, 5½ in. curved	1 ea.
Metzenbaum scissors, 5½ in. curved	1 ea.
Metzenbaum scissors, 7 in. curved	1 ea.
Plastic surgery scissors, 4¾ in. curved	1 ea.
Adson tissue forceps with teeth	2 ea.
Halsted mosquito forceps	6 ea.
Backhaus towel clamp, 3¾ in.	4 ea.
Halsey needle holder, 5 in.	2 ea.
Senn retractor sharp	2 ea.
U.S. Army retractor	2 ea.
Baby Allis tissue forceps, 5 in.	2 ea.
Graefe forceps, 43/8 in.	1 ea.
Farrell applicator, 6½ in.	1 ea.
Frazier suction tube, 7 French	2 ea.
Vienna nasal speculum, medium	1 ea.
Killian septum speculum, 3 in.	1 ea.
Cottle septum speculum	1 ea.
Wilde nasal dressing forceps	1 ea.
Joseph single hook	1 ea.
Joseph double hook, 2 mm	1 ea.
Joseph double hook, 7 mm	1 ea.
Aufricht nasal retractor-speculum	1 ea.
Joseph nasal scissors, 5¾ in. curved	1 ea.
Joseph nasal scissors, 5¾ in. straight	1 ea.

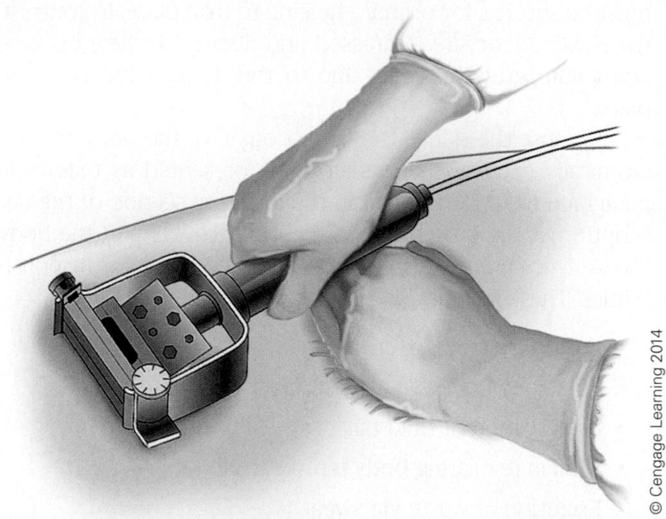

Figure 19-1 Oscillating-blade-type dermatome

the depth of graft. The Weck is primarily used to obtain small skin grafts and for debridement of burns.

Padgett and Reese drum-type dermatomes are occasionally used to obtain skin grafts. They are hand operated, not power, and consist of one-half of a metal drum in which the skin surface is fixed. A metal handle goes through the center of the drum and has an arm on each end. The arms hold the bar that contains the skin graft blade. The bar swings around the drum to cut the skin graft. The size and width of the graft are determined by the size of the drum. The knife blade moves from side to side as the drum is rotated. Sterile dermatome tape must be used with the Reese dermatome. The tape has adhesive on each side and this must be exposed by the surgical technologist by peeling the paper backing off. Remove the paper backing from one side and carefully apply the tape to the drum, making sure the edges of the tape line up with the edges of the drum. The second paper backing is removed from the other exposed side of the tape, and the drum is placed against the skin, which adheres to the adhesive. Due to the bulky size of drum-type dermatomes, their use is limited to large, flat areas of the body because they cannot follow the contours of the body.

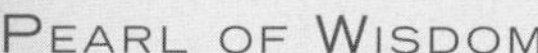
PEARL OF WISDOM

When placing the blade in an oscillating-blade-type dermatome, make sure the power, whether electrical, air, or nitrogen, is not connected to prevent inadvertent starting of the dermatome and severe injury. When handling a drum-type dermatome, always hold the blade carrier to prevent it from swinging around the drum and causing a severe injury.

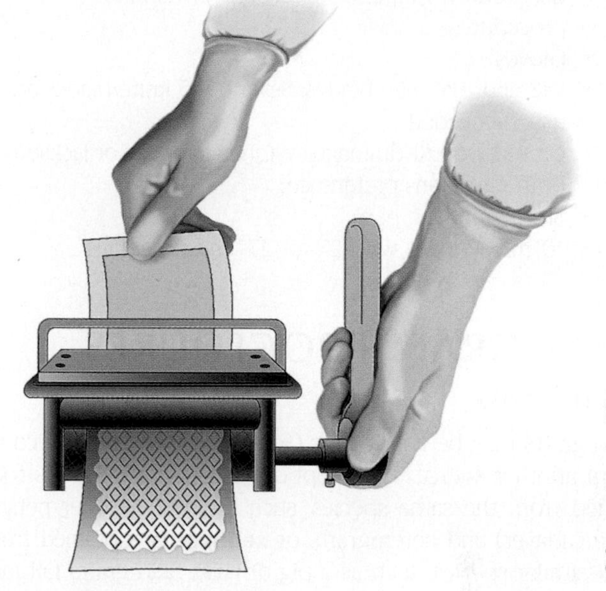

Figure 19-2 Mesh graft device with carrier for skin

A mesh graft device is often used in conjunction with a split-thickness skin graft to expand the size of the skin that has been procured. The device is a manually operated roller with sharp raised surfaces that create evenly spaced slits in the graft. The harvested skin is placed on a plastic sheet called a derma-carrier prior to insertion in the mesh graft device. The purpose of the derma-carrier is to keep the graft flat and allow it to pass through the mesh graft device. The carrier has a smooth side and a ridged side. The ridges determine the size of the slits to be placed in the skin. Derma-carriers are available in a variety of sizes, which are expressed in ratios. For example, if the packaging of the derma-carrier states that the ratio is 3:1, the expanded graft will cover three times the area that it would have prior to being meshed. When stretched, the slits in the expanded graft will take on a diamond shape resembling a fishing net (Figure 19-2).

Other routine equipment and operating room (OR) furniture used during plastic and reconstructive procedures include the following:

- Electrosurgery unit (ESU)
- Bipolar ESU
- Sitting stools
- Routine supplies:
  - Headrest for patient positioning
  - Basic back table pack for head and face, and skin graft procedures
  - Laparotomy back table pack for breast and abdominal procedures
  - Orthopedic back table pack for hand procedures
  - Head drapes for head and face procedures: bar drape; U-drape or split sheet
  - Extremity drape for hand procedures

- Laparotomy drape for breast and abdominal procedures
- Gloves
- #10 and #15 knife blades: Several #15 knife blades are usually needed
- Closed wound-drainage system: Hemovac or Jackson-Pratt (surgeons preference)
- Sterile marking pen
- 10-mL syringes with 25- or 27- gauge needles

SKIN GRAFT PROCEDURES

Skin Grafts

Skin grafts may be autologous (from one's self) or may come from another source. These options include homografts (obtained from the same species, such as from another person or a cadaver) and heterografts or **xenografts** (obtained from a dissimilar species, such as a pig or calf). Skin grafts fall into two different categories: full-thickness skin grafts (commonly abbreviated as FTSG) and split-thickness skin grafts (**STSG**). Both types of grafts, if done autologously, involve the use of a donor site, the place where the tissue to be moved is taken from. The site of the defect that is to be covered is referred to as the recipient site. Several factors are involved in the determination of which type of grafting method is to be used. Some of the determining factors are the location of the defect to be covered, the amount of surface area to be covered, the depth of the defect and involvement of underlying tissues, and the cause of the defect (trauma, disease, or heredity).

As the names suggests, an FTSG is composed of the epidermis and all of the dermis. Because of the depth of this type of graft, its use is restricted to covering relatively small defects, such as those created when excising lesions of the skin, like squamous cell or basal cell carcinoma.

STSG involves removing the epidermis and approximately half of the dermis for relocation to another part of the body. This type of graft is used when a relatively large surface area needs to be covered, such as in the case of a burn. The surgeon's choice of the donor site is influenced by many factors, including:

- Age, sex, and general health of the patient
- Location of the wound to be grafted
- Size of surface area to be covered
- Condition of potential donor sites

Ideal donor sites include:

- Abdomen
- Back
- Chest
- Lateral and ventral aspects of the thighs

The donor site when FTSG is performed does not heal by itself because no dermis is remaining. The donor site wound must be sutured for primary healing to take place. In contrast, the STSG donor site is dressed and allowed to heal because epithelium growth occurs due to the dermis that is left in place.

Because the skin is the largest organ of the body and anatomically extensive, the anatomy is presented as follows in paragraph form rather than in the anatomy section of the description of the procedure. As the outer covering of the body, the skin, or cutaneous membrane, has several major responsibilities. These include:

- Protection from external forces, such as ultraviolet rays
- First line of defense against disease and infection
- Preservation of fluid balance
- Vital in regulating body temperature
- Excretion of waste via sweat
- Sensory input through receptors for temperature, pain, touch, and pressure
- **Synthesis** of vitamin D

Thus, whenever the integrity of the skin is compromised the homeostasis of the body is threatened.

The **integumentary** system consists of two main layers. The outer layer is called the epidermis and the inner is called the dermis (Figure 19-3). Depending on the location of the body, the epidermis consists of four or five layers called strata. The epidermis consists entirely of epithelial cells and contains no blood vessels or nerves. From innermost to outermost the layers are:

1. *Stratum basale:* This is the reproductive layer that derives its nourishment by diffusion from the capillaries of the dermis. Melanin, the pigment responsible for skin and hair color, is produced in this layer.
2. *Stratum spinosum:* This layer receives the daughter cells produced by mitosis in the stratum basale. These cells have a spiny or prickly appearance.
3. *Stratum granulosum:* As the spiny cells move toward the outer surface of the body, they begin to flatten and take on a granular shape. The process of keratinization begins in this layer. Keratin is a hard, fibrous, waterproof protein that is found in the hair, nails, and epidermis.
4. *Stratum lucidum:* This layer is present only in thick skin areas such as the palms of the hands and soles of the feet.
5. *Stratum corneum:* This layer consists of approximately 20 layers of cells in various stages of disintegration. As the cell dries and becomes scaly, the keratin remains. The cells of the stratum corneum are pressed tightly together; as they reach the body surface they are shed or sloughed.

The epidermis is constantly proliferating and shedding. The newly formed epithelial cells are pushed to the body surface

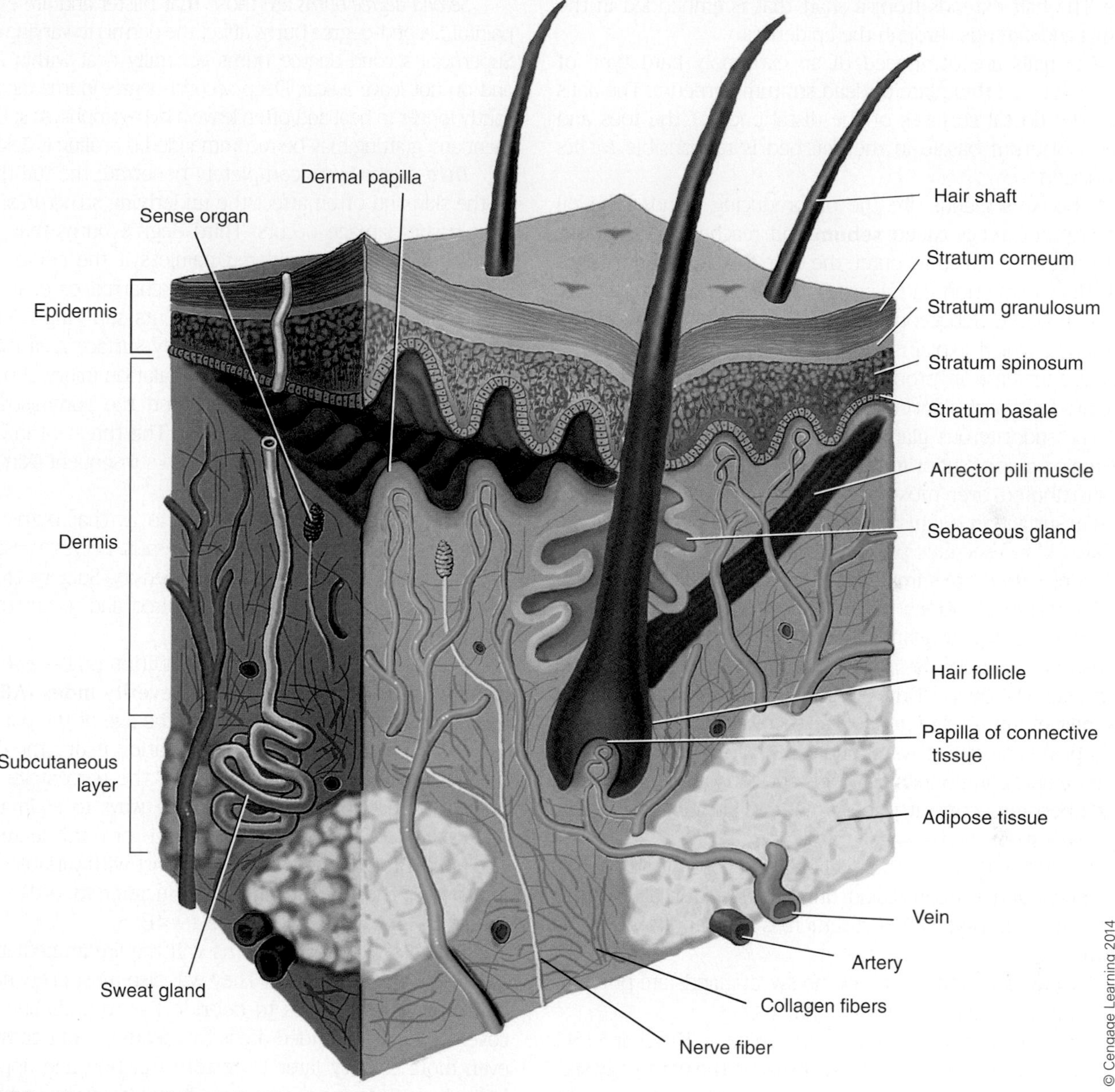

Figure 19-3 Structure of the skin

and shed by the thousands each day. The entire process takes approximately 5 weeks.

The dermis, or stratum cornium, is connective tissue that is located under the epidermis. The nerves and blood vessels that supply the skin, along with hair follicles, nails, and certain glands, are embedded in the dermal layer. The dermis has two distinct divisions:

1. *Reticular layer:* This is the thick, deep layer that provides collagen for strength and elastin for pliability of the skin.
2. *Papillary layer:* This layer is named for its papilla, or projections, which are the groundwork for fingerprints.

The subcutaneous layer is not actually considered part of the skin, but serves to anchor the skin to the underlying structures. The subcutaneous layer, or hypodermis, consists of adipose (fat) and loose connective tissue providing insulation and protection to the internal organs.

The hair, nails, and certain glands are referred to as accessory structures to the integumentary system. They all are derived from the stratum basale of the epidermis and are found embedded in the reticular layer of the dermis.

Hair is found on most body surfaces. The exceptions are the palms of the hands, soles of the feet, distal portions of the fingers and toes, parts of the external genitalia, nipples, and lips. The hair itself is made up of dead keratinized epithelial cells. The hair extends from a shaft that is embedded in the dermis and extends through the epidermis.

The nails are composed of an extremely hard type of keratin that is a thin plate of dead stratum corneum. The nails cover the dorsal surfaces of the distal ends of the toes and fingers. Stratum basale in the nail bed is responsible for its production.

Sebaceous glands are the oil-producing glands. The oil that is produced is called **sebum** and reaches the skin surface through ducts that enter the hair follicle. Sebum helps with fluid regulation and also acts to keep the skin and hair soft and pliable. Sebaceous gland activity is stimulated by sex hormones, which explains the lack of sebum in children, the dramatic increase in production at puberty, and the gradual decrease that occurs during the aging process.

The sudoriferous glands are the sweat glands. There are two main types of sudoriferous glands. Merocrine sweat glands are distributed over most of the body and open directly to the skin surface through small openings called pores. This type of sweat gland secretes primarily water with some salts. The merocrine glands are stimulated to produce sweat or perspiration by heat or emotional stress.

Apocrine sweat glands are larger than the merocrine glands; their location is limited to the external genitalia and the axillae. The ducts of the apocrine glands open through the hair follicles into these regions. The secretion from this type of sweat gland consists of water and some salts, but also includes some organic compounds (proteins and fatty acids). Apocrine glands become active at puberty and are stimulated by pain, emotional stress, and sexual arousal.

The third type of sweat gland, the ceruminous gland, is a specialized version found only in the external auditory canal. The secretion, called cerumen, is commonly known as earwax.

The few locations that have no sweat glands are portions of the external genitalia, nipples, and lips.

Burns are a major cause for performing an FTSG or STSG. Information is presented here rather than in the pathology section of the procedural description, as it is important for the surgical technologist to have an understanding of the pathology and complications of burns in order to assist the surgeon in a knowledgeable manner.

A burn is an injury that can be derived from several sources. Heat, radiation, chemicals, gases, or electricity may cause tissue damage. The depth of a burn is classified according to degree (Figure 19-4A).

First-degree burns affect just the epidermis. They are characterized by erythema (redness of the skin) but do not blister. Healing takes place in about 1 week and no scar tissue formation is expected. The patient may desire to treat the affected area with a topical ointment to help control the mild pain and keep the area from drying.

Second-degree burns are those that blister and are extremely painful. Second-degree burns affect the dermis to varying degrees. Superficial second-degree burns generally heal within 2 weeks and do not leave a scar. Deep second-degree burns take significantly longer to heal and often leave a hypertrophic scar. Debridement and grafting may be recommended if healing is delayed.

Third-degree burns completely penetrate the full thickness of the skin and often affect the underlying structures. Permanent tissue damage occurs. Third-degree burns may be very painful or may be considered painless if the nerves are destroyed. Third-degree burns appear charred or pearly white; they are referred to as *eschars*. Patients suffering from third-degree burns that cover a large body surface area may need respiratory support if there is an inhalation injury, shock management with fluid replacement, and the administration of narcotic analgesics for pain control. The threat of infection is great. Debridement of the eschar and subsequent skin grafting are usually necessary.

Fourth-degree burns are referred to as char burns. Fourth-degree burns often damage blood vessels, nerves, muscles, and tendons and can even affect bone density. Surgery to remove necrotic tissue is almost always required and reconstruction is extensive.

The severity of the patient's condition is also assessed according to the **Abbreviated Burn Severity Index (ABSI)**. The five criteria for this assessment are the age of the patient, the sex of the patient, presence of inhalation injury, the depth of the burn (according to degree), and the percentage of total body surface burned. There are two ways to estimate body surface area (BSA) affected by second- or third-degree burns. The Lund-Browder method uses a chart with variables according to age. The rule of nines uses increments of 9% BSA, as shown in Table 19-4 and Figure 19-4B.

Patients with severe burns will require immediate intensive therapy to sustain life. They will also most likely need several surgical procedures to debride the wounds and provide coverage to the denuded areas by means of skin grafting, and even more surgery later to restore function and appearance. Individuals suffering from severe burns may also benefit from long-term physical and psychological therapy.

Table 19-4 Rule of Nines

Head and neck—9%
Anterior and posterior trunk—18% each
Upper extremity—9%
Lower extremity—18%
Perineum—1%

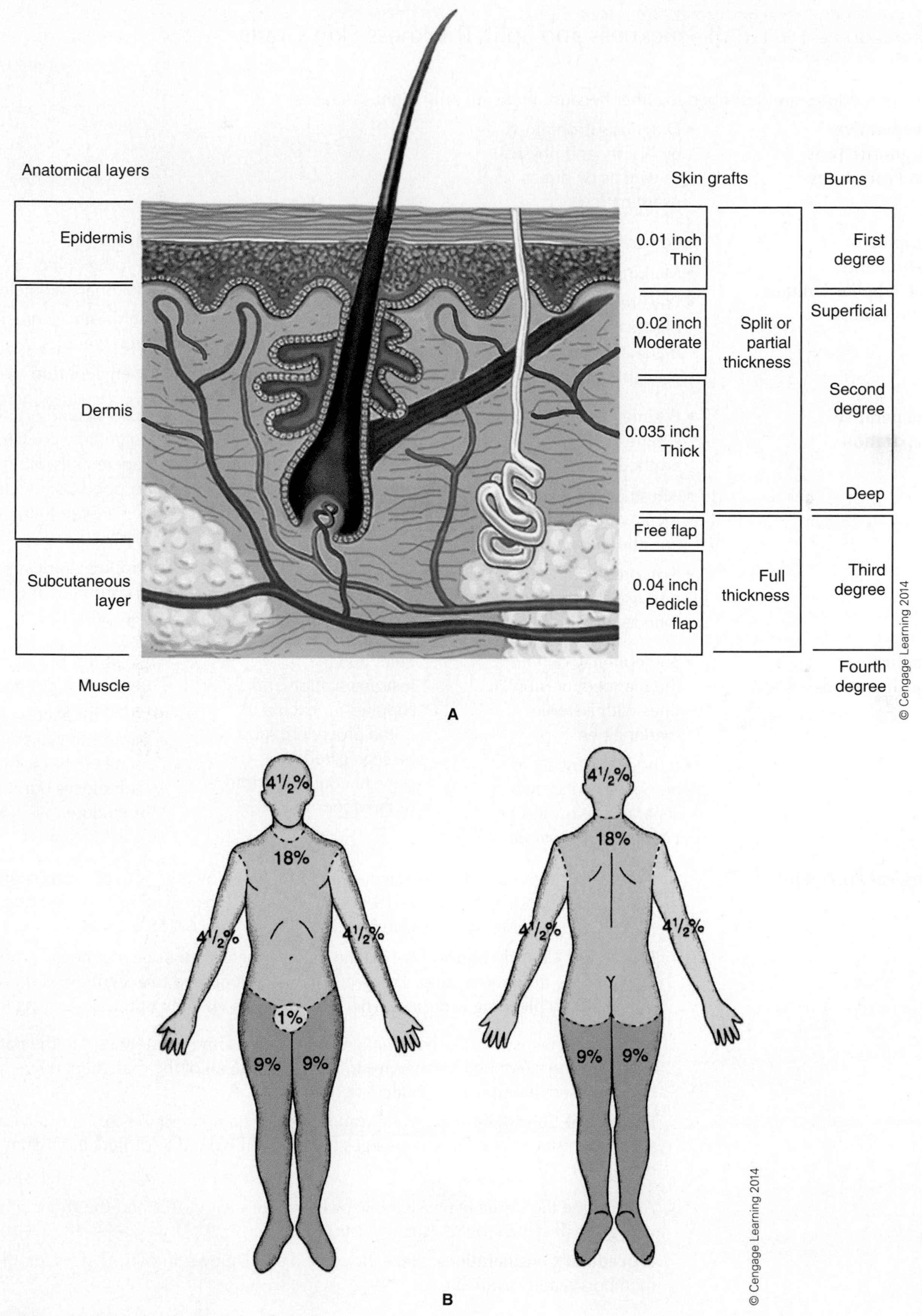

Figure 19-4A (A) Burn depth, (B) rule of nines

PROCEDURE 19-1 Full-Thickness and Split-Thickness Skin Grafts

Both procedures are described together because there are only slight variations.

Preoperative Diagnostic Tests and Procedures

- Diagnosis is obtained by history and physical as well as by direct examination.

Equipment, Instruments, and Supplies Unique to Procedure

- Powered dermatome
- Marking pen
- Powered dermatome blades (open one blade and have others available in the OR)
- Knife dermatome
- Mesh graft device
- Derma-carrier
- ESU pencil needle-tip
- Extra prep tray
- Mineral oil or chlorhexidine gluconate (Hibiclens)
- Antibiotic (surgeon's preference)
- Phenylephrine

Preoperative Preparation

- Position: Usually supine; arms on armboards
- Anesthesia: General or local with monitored anesthesia care (MAC)
- Skin prep: Hair removal is carried out if necessary; both areas are prepped according to procedure for prepping that particular area of the body; normally the donor site is prepped first and is considered to be "clean"; the recipient site, if it is an open wound or potentially contains cancer cells, is prepped last and is considered to be "dirty."
- Draping: Varies according to the body parts affected.

Practical Considerations

- Surgeon may outline the planned incision lines with a sterile marking pen.
- If the recipient site is an open wound, two separate areas must be created on the sterile field, and the instrumentation and supplies for each part of the procedure must be segregated to prevent contamination of the donor site or "seeding" of cancer cells at the donor site.
- It will be necessary for the sterile team members to change their gloves during the procedure.

Surgical Procedure

1. If necessary the recipient site may need to be readied by excision of a benign or malignant lesion, or irrigation and debridement (I & D). The excision is carried out using a #15 scalpel blade, Adson tissue forceps and tenotomy or iris scissors.

   Procedural Considerations: I & D is the removal of foreign bodies or necrotic and infected tissue from the wound. This prepares the wound bed to accept the graft. Minimal capillary bleeding is desirable because it shows viability of the underlying tissue.

2. If the specimen is considered a malignant lesion it is immediately sent to the pathology lab to be examined for margins to ascertain that all of the malignant tissue has been excised, along with a "buffer" of normal tissue.

   Procedural Considerations: While waiting for the pathologist's report, it is advisable to place saline-moistened 4 × 4 sponges on the open wound to protect the tissues from drying out.

3. At this time the sterile team members will change their gloves and the surgical technologist will switch to the "clean" instruments.

   Procedural Considerations: Have the second set of gloves in correct sizes for all team members readily available.

PROCEDURE 19-1 (continued)

4. a. **FTSG:** The next step is to excise the FTSG from the donor site using technique similar to that used for preparing the recipient site. The surgeon will use either the #15 knife blade or knife dermatome. Remember, FTSGs tend to be much smaller than STSGs.

   Procedural Considerations: Following removal, the graft is wrapped in moistened gauze and stored in a safe place on the back table.

   b. **STSG:** Prior to removing the tissue from the donor site, the area may be lubricated with sterile mineral oil or chlorhexidine gluconate (surgeon's preference). This serves to reduce friction and helps to provide a smooth surface. While the surgical technologist provides traction on the skin to be harvested, the surgeon activates the dermatome and guides it along the skin surface area. Using two smooth Adson forceps, a second surgeon or surgical technologist will grab the edges of the harvested skin as it comes through the dermatome and keep slight tension on the skin to keep it from curling up. Once the graft is taken the surgeon will use a #15 knife blade to sever the skin from the patient. Depending on the size of the recipient site, this may be performed multiple times in order to acquire the amount of tissue needed. It may be necessary for the surgical technologist to change the dermatome blade if it becomes dull. The harvested skin should be placed in body-temperature saline while awaiting meshing or application to the recipient site.

5. **FTSG:** If necessary to decrease tension on the wound edges, the subcutaneous tissue immediately surrounding the incision may be undermined using Metzenbaum or tenotomy scissors.

   Procedural Considerations: Again, the instruments should be from the second setup.

6. **FTSG:** The donor site is sutured closed and the sterile dressings are applied.

   Procedural Considerations: Suture and dressings of surgeon's choice are used.

   STSG: Following removal of the graft, topical epinephrine, thrombin, or phenylephrine is often applied to the donor site to aid in hemostasis. Once hemostasis is established, the donor site dressing is placed; nonadherent gauze such as Adaptic or Xeroform and 4 × 4s, or OpSite or Tegaderm are used.

7. **FTSG:** The graft and recipient site may each be modified in shape for proper "fit." If any subcutaneous tissue is present on the graft it is removed with tenotomy or iris scissors. The graft is positioned and secured with suture or stapled in place.

   Procedural Considerations: Any dressing used here must be dry.

   STSG: If meshing of the graft is performed, the skin is placed on the derma-carrier and inserted into the mesh graft device. After the graft has been meshed, it is applied to the recipient site and sutured or stapled into position. If the graft is sutured in place, the sutures are left long in order to tie over a stent dressing. A dry sterile dressing is applied to aid in preventing movement of the newly applied skin graft.

   Procedural Consideration: If a meshed graft will not be immediately used, it must be kept on the derma-carrier to keep the graft from rolling up and kept moist by placing a saline-soaked sponge over the graft. If more than one graft is taken and meshed, each graft should be placed on a new derma-carrier. The newly applied skin will receive its blood supply from the capillary ingrowth from the recipient site; any disruption may cause the graft to be shed (sloughed off); therefore, careful placement of the dressing is important.

(*continues*)

PROCEDURE 19-1 (continued)

Postoperative Considerations

Immediate Postoperative Care

- Patient is transported to the PACU.
- Depending on how extensive of a procedure was performed, the patient may be discharged on the day of surgery or require several days in the hospital (e.g., burn victims).
- Protect the surgical site to prevent movement of the dressing.

Prognosis

- No complications: The patient is expected to have full function at both operative sites; however, outcome often depends on the procedure that was performed and the patient may require physical therapy to help regain maximum function. Burn victims with a large area of skin grafting will have a long recovery period, possibly with subsequent surgical procedures.
- Complications: Postoperative surgical site infection (SSI); formation of scar tissue at both locations is expected, which can lead to contractures; hemorrhage. Not a complication, but if the graft was meshed, this will leave the skin with a "waffle-like" appearance.

Wound Classification

- Donor Site: Class I: Clean
- Recipient Site: Class II: Clean-contaminated

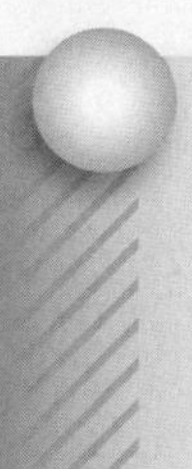

PEARL OF WISDOM

When switching from the "dirty" setup to the "clean" setup, it is very important that the surgical technologist change gloves first, or the gloves of all successive team members will be contaminated.

SCAR REVISION

Scar revision procedure is a type of aesthetic surgical procedure in which the patient wishes for an improved appearance so that the scar is not as conspicuous as previously. A simple scar revision involves the surgeon using Adson tissue forceps with teeth to grab the end of the scar, slightly elevate and use a #15 knife blade to cut underneath the length of the scar, and perform a plastic/primary closure of the skin edges. However, for thicker and/or longer scars, a Z-plasty scar revision procedure is one of the most commonly performed.

PROCEDURE 19-2 Z-Plasty Scar Revision

Surgical Anatomy and Pathology

- See previous description of skin anatomy.
- Individuals with scars, acquired through a traumatic accident or surgically, can opt to have a plastic surgeon perform the scar revision procedure.
- The goal of the procedure is to reduce the scar, realign the wound edges, and perform a closure in which, once healed, the cosmetic appearance will be improved.

PROCEDURE 19-2 (continued)

Preoperative Diagnostic Tests and Procedures	• History and physical examination		
Equipment, Instruments, and Supplies Unique to Procedure	• Plastic instrument set • Marking pen		
Preoperative Preparation	• Position, skin prep, and draping: Depends on location of scar	• Anesthesia: General or local depending on extent of procedure	
Practical Considerations	• Several techniques are used such as W-plasty, M-plasty, and Y-V-plasty; however, the Z-plasty is the most frequently used technique.	• Z-plasty allows the surgeon to make the Z-shaped incision in the same direction of the natural skin line, thus promoting healing and	making the scar less noticeable.
Surgical Procedure	1. Using the marking pen, the surgeon marks the Z-plasty incision.		
	2. As previously described for a simple scar revision, the scar is excised. **Procedural Consideration:** The scar tissue may or may not be sent to pathology as a specimen; surgeon's decision.		
	3. The Z incision is made with the primary angled incision directly over the previous scar. The straight top and bottom incisions are made in equal length (just like when writing the letter "Z") and are at right angles to the primary incision (Figure 19-5A).		
	4. The two skin flaps are slightly rotated (transposed), thus reversing the flaps, and are sutured into place (Figure 9-5B, C).		
	5. The surgeon may or may not apply a dressing depending on the extent of the procedure.		
Postoperative Considerations	**Immediate Postoperative Care** • Patient is transported to the PACU. • Patient is usually discharged on the day of the surgery.	**Prognosis** • No complications: Cosmetic appearance is improved; patient resumes normal activities.	• Complications: Postoperative SSI; scar contracture; cosmetic appearance is not improved or worsened.

(continues)

PROCEDURE 19-2 (continued)

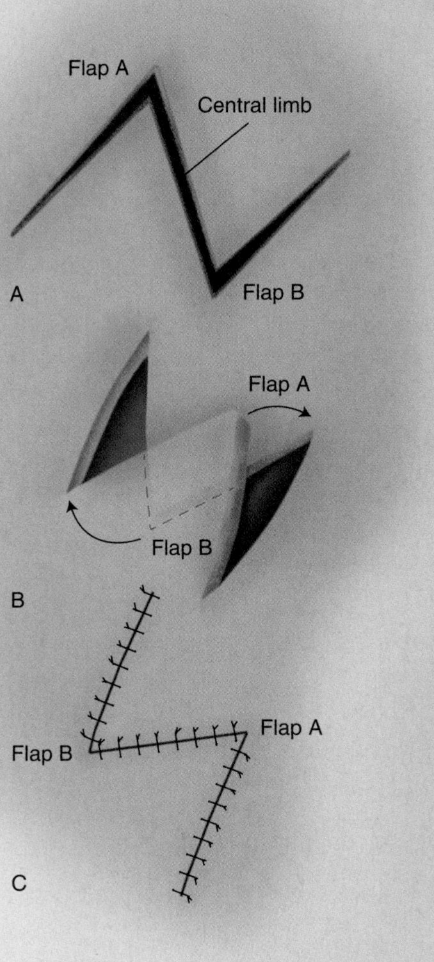

Figure 19-5 (A) Z incision, (B) skin flaps rotated and (C) sutured into place

HEAD AND FACE PROCEDURES

Obviously, being one of the most prominent features of the body that attracts everyone's attention, most individuals are very self-conscious of how their face looks to the public, in particular the "Hollywood" crowd. However, trauma and congenital defects can also cause facial features that the affected person would like to be cosmetically improved. Additionally, congenital defects such as cheiloschisis and palatoschisis can cause problems with, for example, speech development and swallowing. The following are common plastic and reconstructive procedures performed on head and face structures.

PROCEDURE 19-3 Blepharoplasty

Surgical Anatomy and Pathology	• When a blepharoplasty is performed, the anatomical structures of importance are the muscles. • The muscle that closes the eyelids is the orbicularis muscle that encircles each eye. • The primary muscle that opens the eyelids is the levator muscle. It begins deep in the eye socket and continues over the top of the eye. Its tendon, the levator aponeurosis, connects the muscle to the eyelid. • Posterior to the skin and orbicularis muscles is the thin cartilage called tarsus or tarsal plate that gives shape to the eyelid. The tarsal plate is connected to the orbital rim by a tendon on each side called the medial canthal tendon and the lateral canthal tendon. This eyelid support system is called the tarsoligamentous sling. • The orbital septum is a fibrous membrane that cushions the eyeball; in the upper eyelid, it connects at the top of the tarsal plate and extends to the rim of bone superior to the eye. • Posterior to the orbital septum is the upper orbital fat that lies in front of the levator aponeurosis. • Dermachalasis is relaxation and hypertrophy of the eyelid skin. Often in association with dermachalasis is the relaxation of the fascial bands that connect the skin to the orbicularis muscle, causing a "bag." This disorder has been linked to sun exposure and age. It can be the cause of restricted vision or the patient may just want a cosmetically improved appearance. • Signs of aging are seen throughout all body systems but are externally noticeable primarily on the skin and especially on the face. As the patient ages, elastic fibers decrease in number and adipose tissue is lost, causing wrinkling and sagging; collagen fibers are lost, slowing healing; the mitotic activity of the stratum basale slows and the skin becomes thinner; and glandular production of sweat and sebum decreases, causing drying. Patients complain of several problems. The four main complaints are loose skin, fine lines, exaggeration of normal features, and bagginess around the eyes.
Preoperative Diagnostic Tests and Procedures	• History and physical examination
Equipment, Instruments, and Supplies Unique to Procedure	• Headlamp • Plastic instrument set • Marking pen • Bipolar or monopolar ESU (surgeon's preference) • Cellulose sponges (Weck-Cel spears) • Ointment for eyes
Preoperative Preparation	• Position: Supine with arms tucked at sides; foam headrest • Anesthesia: Local with MAC • Skin prep: Begin at eyelids and include entire face, extending from hairline to the clavicles and bilaterally as far as possible; the prep solution must be prevented from entering the patient's eyes. • Draping: Headwrap/turban; U-drape or split sheet

(continues)

Procedure 19-3 (continued)

Practical Considerations

- The word *blepharoplasty* means surgical repair of the eyelid; the procedure is performed to remove excess skin or fat deposits of either the upper or lower eyelids and is usually a bilateral procedure.
- The eyes must be kept from drying out; ointment may be instilled into the eyes prior to the start of the procedure.

Surgical Procedure

1. Surgeon uses a marking pen to indicate the incision lines prior to the injection of the local anesthetic.

   Procedural Consideration: If the anesthetic were injected first the anatomy would be distorted.

2. Using the #15 knife blade an **elliptical** incision is made along the ciliary margin following the natural curve of the eyelid.
3. Using the jeweler's forceps and Westcott scissors, a skin flap is developed and any redundant tissue, including the medial and central fat pads, is removed.

   Procedural Consideration: Great care is used to prevent damage to the levator muscle.

4. Hemostasis is achieved with the use of cauterization.

   Procedural Consideration: The surgical technologist is responsible for gently dabbing the small bleeders in the incision with the use of the Weck-Cel spears, providing the surgeon with a dry visual field, and ability to identify the bleeders to cauterize.

5. A second incision is made to create a wedge of skin to be excised. It is arched above the primary incision and connected at the medial and lateral edges.

   Procedural Consideration: A caliper may be used to ensure that the incisions on both eyelids are equal in length and size and to prevent removal of too much tissue, which could cause a permanent inability for the patient to close the eyelids (Figure 19-6).

6. Using the Castroviejo needle holder, the surgeon closes the wound. The wound edges are brought together and sutured. The underlying tissue will be sutured with absorbable suture. The skin is closed with monofilament nonabsorbable suture;

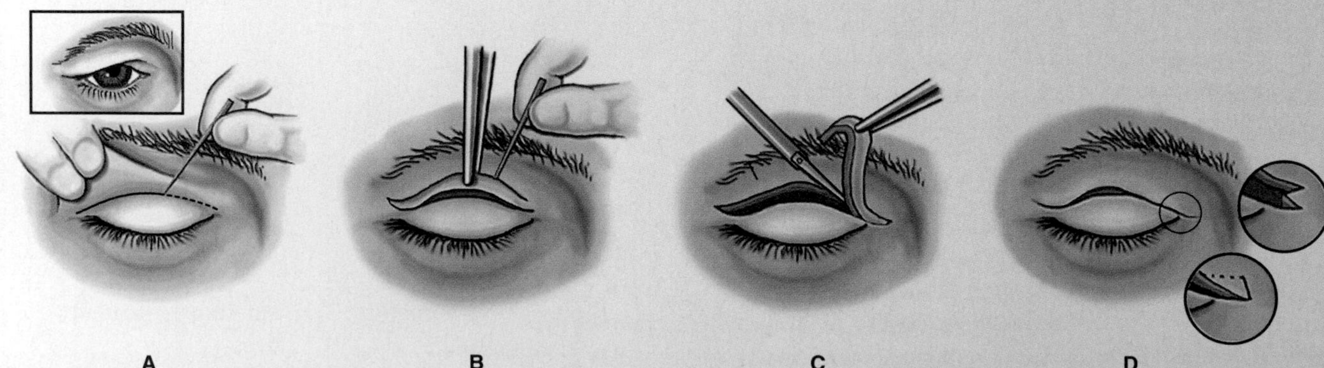

Figure 19-6 Blepharoplasty: (A) Inferior incision line is marked, (B) superior incision line is marked, (C) wedge of redundant tissue removed, (D) closure

Procedure 19-3 (continued)

Prolene is frequently used because its blue color differentiates it from the eyelashes at the time of removal.

7. The procedure is repeated on the opposite eye.
8. No dressing is applied, but antibiotic ointment may be applied.

Postoperative Considerations

Immediate Postoperative Care

- Patient is transported to the PACU.
- Patient is discharged the same day of surgery.
- Bedrest with the head of the bed elevated is recommended to the patient, as well as cold compresses applied to the eyelids to reduce swelling and provide comfort.
- OTC oral analgesics

Prognosis

- No complications: Patient is expected to fully recover and can resume normal activities the day after surgery; some bruising around eyes may occur; female patients should not wear makeup for 7–10 days postoperatively; sutures are removed in 3–5 days.
- Complications: Postoperative SSI; too much tissue removed and patient cannot close eyes; imbalance between eyes due to unequal size in incisions.

Wound Classification

- Class I: Clean

Procedure 19-4 Endoscopic Brow Lift

Surgical Anatomy and Pathology

- The procerus is a small pyramid-shaped muscle located between the two eyebrows extending slightly downward on the superior portion of the nose covering the nasal cartilage.
    - It is inserted into the skin over the lower part of the forehead between the two eyebrows on either side of the midline and merges with the frontalis muscle.
    - It is responsible for pulling the skin between the eyebrows downward, causing horizontal wrinkles.
- The corrugator muscle is situated superior to the orbit.
    - It arises medially from the frontal bone and inserts on the skin of the medial half of the eyebrow.
    - It is the muscle that pushes the skin between the eyebrows into vertical folds and draws the brow medially and inferiorly.
- Brow lift is performed to reduce or eliminate the permanent horizontal and vertical wrinkles that occur on the forehead primarily due to aging.

Preoperative Diagnostic Tests and Procedures

- History and physical examination

(continues)

PROCEDURE 19-4 (continued)

Equipment, Instruments, and Supplies Unique to Procedure	• Plastic instrument set • Minor orthopedic instrument set with periosteal elevators, nerve hooks • 5-mm 30° endoscope • Endoscopic equipment • Endoscopic facial procedure instrumentation: dissectors, up-cutting periosteal dissectors, grasping forceps and scissors • Tumescent fluid (200 mL saline, 1 amp epinephrine, 25 mL 1% lidocaine) • 60-mL syringe • 18-gauge needle • Carbon dioxide laser (surgeon's preference) • Mitek anchor, titanium screws, or absorbable screws (surgeon's preference) • Bone screw insertion instrument set • Power drill
Preoperative Preparation	• Position: Supine with arms tucked at sides; patient positioned as close as possible to side of OR table where surgeon will be standing for easy access to brow region and manipulation of endoscopic instrumentation. • Anesthesia: General (preferred) or local with MAC • Skin prep: Hairline to clavicle, entire face and bilaterally as far as possible; prep solution must be prevented from entering the patient's eyes. • Draping: Standard facial draping; see blepharoplasty procedure.
Practical Considerations	• A short method for remembering the procedure is that it is performed in three general steps: dissection, muscle elimination, and fixation. • The surgical technologist will need to know how to set up endoscopic equipment and instrumentation for the procedure as well as orthopedic instrumentation and equipment. All equipment should be tested prior to the patient entering the OR. • Due to the number of drugs on the back table, it is essential that the surgical technologist label all of them.
Surgical Procedure	1. Surgeon injects tumescent solution beneath the periosteum with the 60-mL syringe and 18-gauge needle.
	2. Small transverse incision is made in the forehead and the endoscope is inserted (Figure 19-7).
	3. Three to five small radial or transverse incisions are made behind the hairline. **Procedural Consideration:** Radial incisions in the anterior scalp tend to avoid transsection of the branches of the supraorbital nerve. Incisions in the temporal region may be either radial or vertical. In patients who are balding or have a high hairline, transverse incisions are made on the forehead.
	4. The forehead is dissected free from the skull at the periosteal level. The periosteum is separated to completely free the brow and allow access to the corrugator and procerus muscles. Supraorbital nerve and multiple small veins are located just lateral to the middle of the orbit; the nerve must be identified and preserved.

PROCEDURE 19-4 (continued)

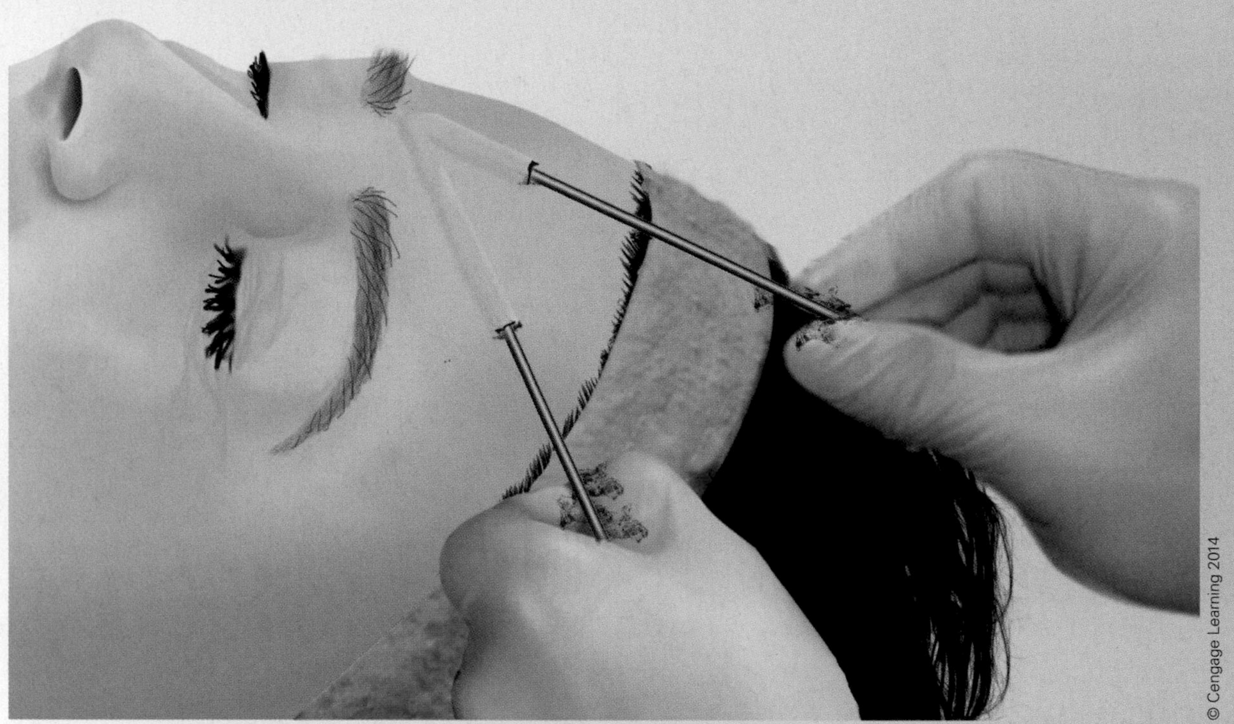

Figure 19-7 Endoscope inserted through transverse incision in forehead

5. The corrugator muscle is either separated, avulsed, or resected according to surgeon's preference.

   Procedural Consideration: The surgical technologist should know the surgeon's preference in order to have the proper instrumentation and equipment available for use. Blunt avulsion of the muscle is rarely performed because of uneven effectiveness in decreasing the corrugator function. Resection of the muscle is more effective, but overresection can cause surface indentations in the skin. The best method is ablation of the muscles with the use of the carbon dioxide laser.

6. The surgeon performs either temporary or permanent fixation.

   Temporary: Titanium screws are placed posterior to the hairline. See Chapter 21 for the screw placement procedure. Staples or sutures are placed around them to anchor the elevated brow in place for 10–14 days.

   Permanent: Permanent fixation is achieved with use of Mitek anchors and suture or short permanent titanium screws. See Chapter 21 for placement of Mitek anchors.

7. The small incisions are closed with nonabsorbable suture, interrupted technique.

8. 4 × 4s are placed for dressing and kept in place for 1–2 days.

(*continues*)

Procedure 19-4 (continued)

Postoperative Considerations	**Immediate Postoperative Care** • Patient is transported to the PACU. • Patient is usually discharged the day of surgery. • Patient is kept under close observation at home for the first day postoperatively. **Prognosis** • No complications: Swelling and bruising is minimal; ice pack may be applied; OTC analgesic medication; patient may experience moderate to severe headache. Temporary fixation screws removed in surgeon's office after 10–14 days when forehead structures have healed and are in place. After permanent fixation the sutures or staples are removed 5 days postoperatively. • Complications: Complications are rare, but include malpositioning or shaping of the brow, recurrence of brow ptosis due to ineffective procedure, alopecia, scarring, temporary or permanent paralysis of the frontalis muscle, and forehead and scalp numbness caused by edema and stretching of the supraorbital nerve, but resolves within short period of time. **Wound Classification** • Class I: Clean

Procedure 19-5 Malar Implants

Surgical Anatomy and Pathology	• The zygomatic bones (also called the malar bones) form the prominences of the cheeks and form the lateral walls and floors of the orbits. They join with the frontal, sphenoid, temporal, and maxillary bones. Each zygomatic bone has a temporal process that articulates posteriorly with the zygomatic process of the temporal bone called the zygomatic arch. • The masseter muscle is one of the primary muscles of mastication. It is a thick, flat muscle of which the origin is the zygomatic arch and the ramus of the mandible is the insertion. The masseter closes the jaw. • Submalar augmentation is performed in patients who have a deficient bone structure or severe atrophy of overlying soft tissue. The deficiency can also be due to trauma or facial surgical procedures, such as cancer of the mandible.
Preoperative Diagnostic Tests and Procedures	• History and physical examination: Surgeon analyzes the size and shape of the patient's face and approximate placement of implant as well as assesses the condition of the soft tissue structures. • Standard X-rays
Equipment, Instruments, and Supplies Unique to Procedure	• Plastic instrument set • Implant sizers, various sizes • Implants, various sizes: The submalar implant is made of silicone formed into a three-dimensional anatomical design that contours to the midfacial bone

PROCEDURE 19-5 (continued)

	structure. The permanent implant should not be opened until the surgeon	has communicated the needed size. • Bipolar ESU	• Marking pen • Dental rolls × 2
Preoperative Preparation	• Position: Sitting position for outlining incisions with marking pen; supine with arms tucked at sides for procedure	• Anesthesia: Local with MAC • Skin prep: Hairline to clavicle, entire face,	bilaterally as far as possible • Draping: Headwrap/turban; U-drape or split sheet
Practical Considerations	• Have imaging studies in the OR • Confirm implants of various sizes are available and in the OR	• Submalar augmentation is usually performed before and in conjunction with rhytidectomy.	

Surgical Procedure

1. A small gingivobuccal sulcus incision over the canine fossae is made.
2. The periosteum is incised and elevated, superiorly off the anterior surface of the maxilla. The infraorbital nerve is identified in order to preserve.
3. Using the Joseph's elevator and periosteal elevator, a pocket is created to expose the entire anterior surface of the maxilla to the lateral portion of the zygoma. The inferior surface of the zygoma, including the tendinous insertion of the masseter, is also exposed.

   Procedural Consideration: The tendinous insertions of the masseter muscle are left in place and not incised. The pocket is made large enough to prevent compression of soft tissues on the implant.
4. The implant sizers are inserted to decide upon the correct-size submalar implant.
5. When the correct implant size is chosen, it is placed on the anterior skin surface, and, using the marking pen, the surgeon outlines the implant to indicate the position for the permanent implant. The positions of the two medial fenestrations of the implant are also marked on the skin.
6. The permanent implant is inserted into the pocket over the anterior surface of the maxilla and manipulated into the desired position.

   Procedural Consideration: The surgical technologist should confirm the size of implant with the surgeon and communicate the information to the circulator, who will open the sterile implant to facilitate transfer to the sterile field. The central portion of the implant is positioned over the anterior surface of the maxilla and the tapered lateral extension fits around the zygomatic arch and rests on the superior tendinous attachments of the masseter muscle.
7. The implant is removed and 2-0 or 3-0 nonabsorbable suture is placed around the posterior surface and through the openings of the implant. The surgeon places the suture through the pocket and exits at the external markings on the skin. While placing the suture the implant is "pulled" into the pocket and again manipulated into the correct anatomical position.

(*continues*)

Procedure 19-5 (continued)

Procedural Consideration: The surgical technologist will be responsible for controlling and guiding the implant into the pocket while the surgeon places the suture.

8. The implant is held in position when the surgeon ties the sutures externally over a bolster (dental roll).
9. The steps of the procedure are repeated on the opposite side of the face.
10. The wounds are gently irrigated and checked for hemostasis. The incisions are closed in two layers; the first layer is closed with absorbable suture and the skin with nonabsorbable suture.
11. 4 × 4 compression dressing is placed to further stabilize the implants.

Postoperative Considerations

Immediate Postoperative Care

- Patient is transported to the PACU.
- Patient is discharged the same day of surgery.
- Patient is instructed to guard against movement of the dressing, avoid clenching of teeth, and eat soft foods that do not require a lot of jaw movement.

Prognosis

- No complications: 4 × 4 dressing is removed first or second postoperative day and replaced with stretch plastic bandage strips over the bolsters to prevent implant slippage. Fixation of the implants to the tissues occurs by the third or fourth postoperative day; the skin sutures and bolsters are removed.
- Complications: Postoperative SSI; wrong size of implant with less-than-desired cosmetic results; slippage of the implant requiring reoperation.

Wound Classification

- Wound Class I: Clean

Procedure 19-6 Mentoplasty

Surgical Anatomy and Pathology

- The mandibular symphysis, better known as the chin, is the region inferior to the labiomental fold, the groove that separates the lower lip from the chin.
  - Several muscles cover the chin, including the mentalis, orbicularis oris, quadratus labii inferioris, triangularis, and small superior portion of the platysma. The anterior middle portion of the digastric muscle and the genioglossus and geniohyoid muscles attach along the posterior and inferior surface of the chin.
  - The mental nerves are situated on either side of the chin.
- Mentoplasty is performed for purely cosmetic reasons, correcting micrognathia, a condition characterized by the underdevelopment of the jaw, in particular the mandible, or restoring post-traumatic facial disfigurement.
  - The chin-to-nose relationship is an

PROCEDURE 19-6 (continued)

	important consideration when evaluating the patient and discussing	options. A small chin has the effect of making the nose look larger. Additionally,	chin implantation will have an effect on the jaw line and contour.
Preoperative Diagnostic Tests and Procedures	• History and physical examination	• Photographic evaluation	• Standard X-ray
Equipment, Instruments, and Supplies Unique to Procedure	• Plastic instrument set • Bipolar ESU • Marking pen	• Implant sizers, various sizes • Implants, various sizes	
Preoperative Preparation	• Position: Supine with arms tucked at sides or Fowler's position • Anesthesia: Local with MAC; general	• Skin prep: Beginning at chin, include entire face to the hairline down to the clavicles and bilaterally as far as possible.	• Draping: Headwrap/turban; U-drape or split sheet
Practical Considerations	• Prevent skin prep solution from entering the ears and eyes. • Various types of implant materials are available, including silicone, Teflon, GoreTex, polyethylene, nylon, Supramid, Mersilene,	autografts, and injectable materials including collagen, liquid silicone, and Alloderm. • Prior to the administration of anesthesia, the surgeon uses the marking pen to indicate the anatomical	landmarks and skin incision. • There are two surgical approaches: external and intraoral. The external approach is used most often and is the procedure that is described.
Surgical Procedure	1. Using a #15 knife blade, the surgeon makes a short submental transverse incision in the middle of the chin.		
	2. The incision is carried down to the periosteum; the periosteum is incised along the inferior mandibular surface on both sides of the midline.		
	3. The periosteum is elevated off the bone using a small periosteal elevator such as a Key elevator. **Procedural Consideration:** The mental nerves must be identified and kept from injury.		
	4. The periosteum is gently retracted with Senn retractors, creating a subperiosteal pocket. **Procedural Consideration:** The pocket is slightly larger than the implant to facilitate insertion. The surgeon may place an implant sizer over the chin and outline it on the skin as an aid in creating a pocket that is not excessively large.		
	5. Implant sizers are used to determine the correct size of permanent implant.		
	6. The permanent implant is placed in the subperiosteal pocket. The implant must be placed inferior to the mental nerves. The surgeon moves the implant into the correct position according to the previously marked anatomical landmarks and visualization of the patient's face.		

(*continues*)

Procedure 19-6 (continued)

Procedural Consideration: The surgical technologist should confirm the size of implant with the surgeon and communicate the information to the circulator who will open the sterile implant to facilitate transfer to the sterile field.

7. To prevent slippage of the implant, the surgeon fixes it in place with an absorbable mattress suture to the periosteum or soft tissue at the lower border of the mandible in two places.
8. The wound is thoroughly irrigated with antibiotic solution.
9. The periosteum is closed with 3-0 or 4-0 absorbable suture and the skin closed with 5-0 or 6-0 nonabsorbable suture. Then 4 × 4s are placed for dressing.

Postoperative Considerations

Immediate Postoperative Care

- Patient is transported to the PACU.
- Patient is discharged the same day of surgery.

Prognosis

- No complications: Patient is instructed to elevate head of bed at home, do not touch or manipulate the chin area, no use of toothbrush on lower central incisors, antibiotics for 1 week, OTC analgesic, no strenuous activity for 2 weeks. Skin sutures removed 5–7 days postoperative. Patient is expected to have full recovery with good cosmetic results.
- Complications: Postoperative SSI; hemorrhage; hematoma formation; mental nerve injury; implant malposition. Late complications include implant migration or extrusion; bone resorption; postinfection deformity.

Wound Classification

- Wound Class I: Clean

Procedure 19-7 Otoplasty

Surgical Anatomy and Pathology

- The pinna (external ear) is a framework of cartilage that is covered by a thin layer of skin that consists of the auricle and external auditory meatus.
  - The auricular sulcus is the depression behind the ear next to the scalp.
  - The outer edge of the pinna is called the helix and it arises from the crus that is just superior to the tragus; the crus extends horizontally right above the auditory canal. At the superior portion of the helix, it is folded over and, as it travels downward, is no longer folded over, leading into the cauda helices (tail of the helix) and ending in the lobule (earlobe).
  - The antihelix gives form to a large part of the external ear. It is a symmetric Y-shaped structure in which the folded crest of the bottom portion of the antihelix continues upward and separates into the

PROCEDURE 19-7 (continued)

	superior crus and inferior crus ("Y" portion of the antihelix). The bottom portion (root) of the antihelix forms the lateral edge or rim of the concha. The right "Y" or inferior crux forms the superior rim of the concha as well as separates the concha from the triangular fossa. The superior crux is the branch of the "Y" that is to the left of the triangular fossa. Therefore, the triangular fossa is the space located between the branches of the "Y" shaped antihelix. • The scapha is the elongated depression that lies between the helix and antihelix.	• The concha is a slight depression located next to the ear canal. The narrow superior portion is called the cymba conchae and the larger inferior portion is called the cavum conchae. • The last three structures are the tragus (auditory canal lobule), intertragal notch, and antitragus. The tragus is a small projection that is located medial to the ear canal. It is separated from the antitragus by a depression called the intertragal notch. The antitragus is the small curved portion that is connected to and superior to the lobule.	• There are many ear defects and deformities that are corrected by surgery. The pathology to be corrected determines the otoplasty procedure to be performed. The two pathologies being addressed are microtia and prominent ears. • Microtia is the congenital absence of part or all of the ear. • Prominent ears is a term used to describe pinnae that abnormally protrude from the sides of the head most often due to an inadequate folding or absence of the antihelix. This causes the scapha and helical rim to protrude.
Preoperative Diagnostic Tests and Procedures	• History and physical examination • Standard X-rays • Using a standard X-ray film or some type of transparent sheet, the	surgeon places it over the nonoperative ear to trace an outline to serve as a template for the new ear. The template must be delivered to the	Central Sterile Supply Department to be sterilized and must be available on the day of surgery.
Equipment, Instruments, and Supplies Unique to Procedure	*Otoplasty for Microtia and Prominent Ears* • Plastic instrument set • Minor orthopedic instrument set • Headrest • Marking pen • ESU *Extra Items Needed for Microtia* • Thoracotomy instrument set	• X-ray film • Bulb syringe • Pediatric chest tubes, various sizes • Chest drainage system available • Power drill • Burs, various sizes • Topical thrombin • Local anesthetic with epinephrine	*Extra Items Needed for Prominent Ears* • 25-gauge needles • Methylene blue • Cotton-tipped applicators • Mineral oil

(continues)

Procedure 19-7 (continued)

Preoperative Preparation	• Position: Supine with arms tucked at sides; head placed in headrest/donut with the patient's head turned with the affected side up; adequate padding of the nonoperative ear must be ensured because the procedures can be long, in particular the procedure for treating microtia (6–8 hours). • Anesthesia: General for pediatric patients; local with MAC for adult patients • Skin prep: Carefully prep the external ear and area around the ear, down the neck to the shoulder, and laterally as far as possible. If bilateral procedure, prep both ears. • Draping: Headwrap/turban that leaves the ear(s) exposed; fenestrated ear drape or head drape, U-drape or split sheet
Practical Considerations	• The goal of otoplasty is to anatomically position the ear(s) or reconstruct the ear(s) so that they appear naturally proportionate and contoured with little to no evidence of surgery having been performed. When performing otoplasty for prominent ear the goal of the procedure is to create an antihelical fold that brings the external ear back against the side of the head in a normal anatomical position. • The ideal time to perform surgery is between ages 4 and 10, but preferably before the child starts school. • The microtia surgical procedure is performed as either a one-stage procedure or sequence of multistage procedures depending on the severity of the defect. The follow-up procedures can include creating an earlobe, separating the reconstructed pinna from the side of the head, creating the tragus, and sculpting the ear by creating the folds in the outer ear with the use of skin flaps that are sutured into place. The description of the surgical procedure will discuss the first phase of the procedure. • For the microtia procedure, if a costal cartilage graft will be used the surgical technologist will create two setups, one for the primary procedure and the other for removing and forming the costal cartilage graft. • The surgical technologist should set up a space on the back table or place a drape on a separate small table for the surgeon to form the costal cartilage graft using the power drill and burs. The drape should be reinforced by placing green towels on top to prevent a puncture. • When performing the skin prep prevent the prep solution from entering the eyes and ear(s). A small cotton ball can be gently inserted into the ear canal and removed once the prep is completed. • Make sure the sterilized template has been opened onto the sterile field.
Surgical Procedure	*Otoplasty for Microtia* 1. Using a marking pen the site for taking the costal cartilage graft is marked at the sixth, seventh, eighth, or ninth intercostal space. 2. Using a #15 knife blade the surgeon makes an incision over the intercostal space . 3. Using the template, the rib segment is removed while the perichondrium is preserved.

PROCEDURE 19-7 (continued)

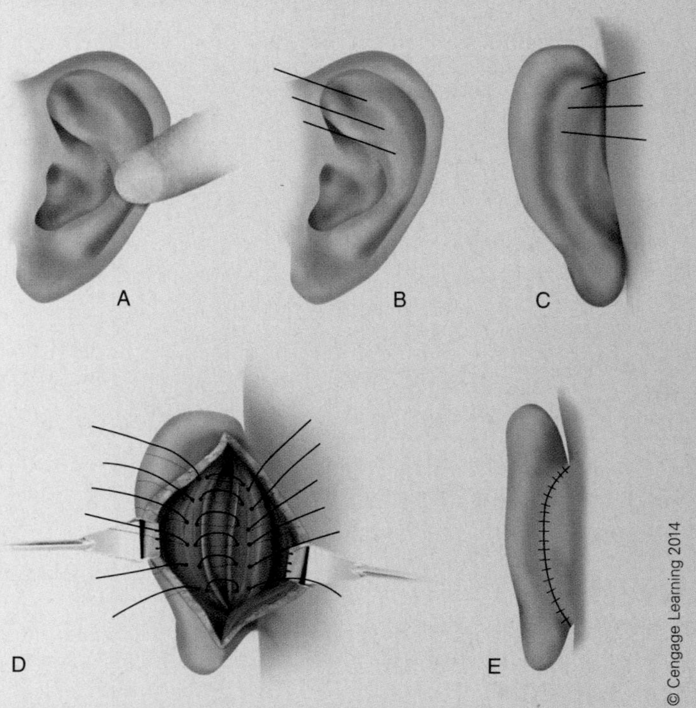

Figure 19-8 (A) Surgeon using finger to bend ear backward to identify antihelical fold, (B and C) antihelical fold position is marked several times using 25-gauge needle, (D) cartilage is incised, and (E) posterior skin incision closed

4. The pleura is assessed to make sure it is intact.

   Procedural Consideration: The surgical technologist provides the surgeon with a bulb syringe filled with saline that is instilled into the wound. If bubbles appear the surgical technologist must immediately receive a chest tube of the size requested by the surgeon for insertion and attachment to a chest drainage system. If no bubbles appear, the wound is closed.

5. The surgeon uses the template to form the graft with the power drill and burs.

   Procedural Consideration: The graft will not be immediately used. To keep it from drying out, the surgical technologist should wrap it in saline-soaked sponges and put on the back table in a safe place until needed.

6. Using the #15 knife blade, the surgeon makes a postauricular incision.

7. The temporoparietal fascia is elevated and the graft is inserted.

8. The flap is pulled over the graft and sutured in place.

   Procedural Consideration: Throughout the procedure hemostasis is achieved with the use of ESU, topical thrombin, and injection of local anesthetic with epinephrine.

(continues)

Procedure 19-7 (continued)

9. A bulky dressing is placed.

   Procedural Consideration: The dressing will consist of petrolatum gauze and several fluffs held in place with rolled gauze.

Otoplasty for Prominent Ears Due to Absence of Antihelical Fold

1. The surgeon will use a finger to bend the ear backward, which creates an antihelical fold (Figure 19-8A).
2. The antihelical fold position is marked by placing the 25-gauge needle through the ear, anterior to posterior, marking the tip of the needle with methyelene blue, and withdrawing the needle to stain the cartilage. This is performed three or four times.

   Procedural Consideration: The surgical technologist may be responsible for marking the tip of the needle by dipping a cotton-tipped applicator in the methylene blue (Figure 19-8B, C).
3. Using the #15 knife blade, the surgeon excises an elliptical portion of skin from the posterior of the ear.
4. The cartilage is incised near what will be the new antihelical fold and the anterior surface is scored to allow the cartilage to bend backward (Figure 19-8D).
5. The surgeon places several sutures to hold the cartilage in its new anatomical position (Figure 19-8D).
6. The posterior skin incision is closed with suture and a bulky dressing is placed over the incision (Figure 19-8E).

   Procedural Consideration: The dressing will consist of petrolatum gauze and several fluffs held in place with rolled gauze.

Postoperative Considerations

Immediate Postoperative Care

- Patient is transported to the PACU.
- Patient will be in hospital for 1–2 days under close observation.

Prognosis

- No complications: Patient expected to return to full activities. The bulky dressing is worn for several days, during which time the patient must avoid excessive pressure upon the ear. After removing the dressing the patient wears a loose headband when sleeping for 3–6 weeks. The purpose of the headband is to keep the operative ear from being pulled forward when the patient moves in his or her sleep. Further operations will be performed after the initial microtia otoplasty, such as placement of tissue expanders to stretch the skin surface to cover the newly formed ear and sculpting the ear by creating folds in the outer ear with the use of skin flaps that are sutured in place.
- Complications: Postoperative SSI; hematoma; overcorrection or unnatural contour when correcting prominent ear; suture complications such as suture extrusion that may or may not be associated with granulomas.

Wound Classification

- Class I (both procedures): Clean

PROCEDURE 19-8 Rhinoplasty: External Technique

Surgical Anatomy and Pathology	• See Chapter 17 for anatomy of the nose. • Rhinoplasty is reshaping of the nose. • It is considered a plastic surgery procedure because no functional changes are made to the interior nasal passageways. However, it may be performed in conjunction with other nasal procedures to repair the nose in the post-trauma patient.
Preoperative Diagnostic Tests and Procedures	• History and physical examination as well as by direct examination • Standard X-rays
Equipment, Instruments, and Supplies Unique to Procedure	• Headrest with donut • Headlamp • Nasal instrument set (some facilities have a specific septorhinoplasty set) • Nasal packing for administration of cocaine and instruments (nasal speculum, bayonet forceps) • Nasal splint
Preoperative Preparation	• Position: Supine with arms tucked at sides, or Fowler's position with hands placed in lap • Anesthesia: Local anesthesia with mild sedation; general anesthesia • Skin prep: Check with the surgeon to see if he or she requires a prep to be completed; starting at the nose, prep the entire face and neck, extending bilaterally as far as possible. • Draping: Headwrap/turban with U-drape or split drape to cover the body
Practical Considerations	• Often mentoplasty and rhinoplasty are performed together to improve the patient's overall appearance. • If rhinoplasty is performed in conjunction with another procedure, the sterile procedure should be done first. • Rhinoplasty may be performed in the hospital setting, ambulatory surgery center, or the physician's office. • Rhinoplasty may be performed as an internal procedure where the incisions are made within the nasal cavity, or as an external procedure where the skin is incised along the base of the nasal columella and one nostril. • Several aspects of the nose may be altered or restored, including increase or reduce overall size (hump may be removed or size and shape altered using a variety of techniques); remodel shape of tip or bridge; change span between nostrils; change angle between nose and upper lip; tissue may be removed, relocated, or reshaped; synthetic implants may be placed. • OR table may be turned to facilitate access to the operative site. • Even when general anesthesia is planned, the local anesthetic is still administered to aid in hemostasis, reduce the size of the nasal membranes, and aid in reducing immediate postoperative pain. • Rhinoplasty is considered a clean, not sterile, procedure.

(continues)

Procedure 19-8 (continued)

- A male patient with a mustache is generally allowed to retain it. It may have to be trimmed.
- The surgeon will often administer the topical and local anesthetic prior to the skin prep and draping to allow the medication to take effect. The surgeon may perform this in the preoperative holding area or OR. It is performed with a separate setup; the surgical technologist should have the following items available for the surgeon to use on a separate clean table or Mayo stand:
  - Nasal speculum
  - Bayonet forceps
  - Local anesthetic with epinephrine (usually 1% lidocaine)
  - 10-mL Luer-Lok syringe with 25-gauge needles
  - Cocaine (crystallized form)
  - ½-in. × 3-in. cottonoid sponges
  - Medicine cups
  - Cotton-tipped applicator
- The surgeon will inject the local anesthetic into the nose and turbinates, and then will pack the nose with the cottonoids with cocaine.

Surgical Procedure

1. The nose packing is removed. Using a #15 blade, the surgeon makes the skin incision along the base of the columella and upward along the outside of one nostril (Figure 19-9A).

   Procedural Consideration: Minor bleeding is controlled with the use of suction ESU.

2. A double-pronged skin hook is used to retract the skin upward at the apex of the nose.

   Procedural Consideration: The surgical technologist will be responsible for holding the skin prong retractors.

3. The skin is undermined using the Freer or Cottle elevators and tenotomy scissors.

   Procedural Consideration: The surgical technologist will be responsible for suctioning blood from the nose and incision site with a Frazier suction tip.

4. The periosteum and perichondrium are elevated and freed with the use of the elevators, scissors, and chisel.

5. Using the #15 blade and tenotomy scissors, the upper lateral cartilage is trimmed. If a hump is present, it is removed with a chisel and hammer and then smoothed with a rasp. Bony spurs can be removed in the same manner.

   Procedural Consideration: While the surgeon holds the chisel in place, he or she may have the surgical technologist tap the chisel with the mallet.

6. At this point the surgeon may perform a septoplasty.

7. Once the septoplasty is done, if necessary, the edges of the cartilage are trimmed with the tenotomy scissors.

8. Using his or her fingers, the surgeon molds the cartilage and bone, and if necessary places a cartilage or bone graft to mold the nasal tip.

9. As a final step, the surgeon performs lateral osteotomies using the chisel and mallet to further straighten the nose.

10. The skin is closed with a 4-0 absorbable suture (Figure 19-9B).

PROCEDURE 19-8 (continued)

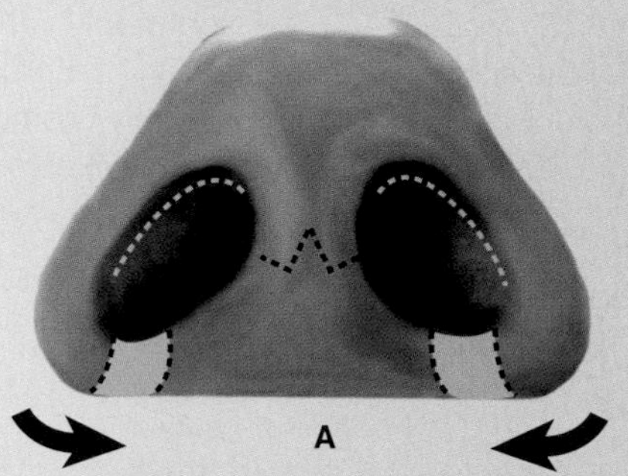

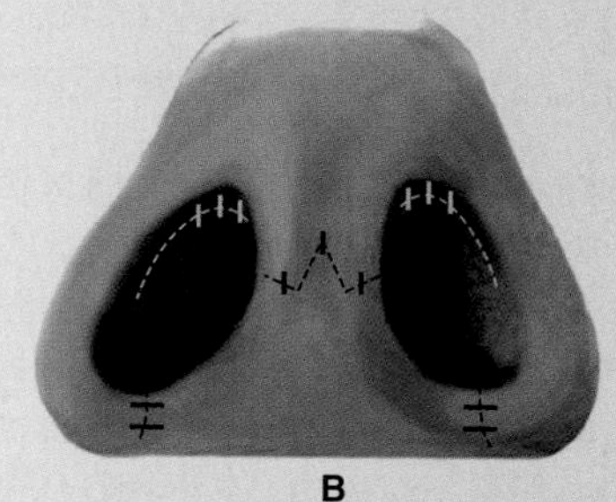

Figure 19-9 Rhinoplasty: (A) Preoperative, (B) postoperative

11. A metal or fiberglass nasal splint is placed and a small piece of gauze may be carefully taped over the nares to absorb any drainage.

    Procedural Consideration: The surgical technologist should make sure to have the correct type of nasal splint available according to the surgeon's preference.

Postoperative Considerations

Immediate Postoperative Care

- Patient is transported to the PACU with the head of the bed elevated.
- Patient is usually released the same day.
- A small ice pack may be gently applied to the nose to reduce swelling and pain.
- Patient is instructed to remain in bed for the first day with the head elevated.
- Oral analgesics are usually sufficient for pain control.
- Patient is instructed to avoid nose blowing and vigorous face washing for 1 week.

Prognosis

- No complications: Patient is expected to have full recovery. Nose will assume a normal aesthetic look in several weeks.
- Complications: postoperative SSI; bruising; swelling; nasal stuffiness; minor pain

Wound Classification

- Class II: Clean-contaminated

Procedure 19-9 Rhytidectomy

Surgical Anatomy and Pathology	• See Chapter 17 for anatomy of the skin and face. • Commonly called a facelift, the procedure is purely cosmetic to remove excessive facial skin folds and subcutaneous tissue to eliminate wrinkles and fatty deposits.
Preoperative Diagnostic Tests and Procedures	• History and physical examination as well as by direct examination
Equipment, Instruments, and Supplies Unique to Procedure	• Headrest • Bipolar unit with bayonet bipolar forceps • Plastic instrument set • Deaver retractors, 2 small • Drains: Hemovac or Jackson-Pratt (optional—surgeon's preference) • Sterile skin marking pen with ruler • Electrosurgical pencil with needle electrode
Preoperative Preparation	• Position: Patient is supine; arms may be tucked at the sides or on padded armboards. • Anesthesia: Local anesthesia with MAC preferred; general anesthesia may also be used. • Skin prep: Entire face, ears, and neck are cleansed from the hairline to the shoulders, and bilaterally as far as possible. • Draping: Headwrap/turban; bar drape; U-drape or split sheet
Practical Considerations	• Surgeon may outline the planned incision lines with a sterile marking pen. • Facial nerve must be avoided when placing and holding retractors.
Surgical Procedure	1. Incision is initiated within the hairline in the temporal region of the scalp, approximately 5 cm above the ear (Figure 19-10). **Procedural Consideration:** The surgeon uses a #15 scalpel blade for the initial incision.
	2. The incision is continued to just below the earlobe and then back up and around the ear. **Procedural Consideration:** Incision follows natural creases in the skin to camouflage scarring.
	3. The subcutaneous tissue in the preauricular area is undermined. **Procedural Consideration:** Tenotomy scissors are used for this step.
	4. Moving inferiorly to the jaw line and superiorly to the lateral aspect of the nose, the subcutaneous tissue is separated (dissected) from the platysma below. **Procedural Consideration:** The surgical technologist or surgical assistant uses double-prong skin hooks and progresses to larger retractors, as the situation allows, to hold tension along the wound edges and facilitate dissection.
	5. Wound edges of the developed flap are pulled taut to determine the amount of redundant skin to be excised. The opposite side of the face will be referred to during this stage to maintain symmetry and create a natural appearance.

PROCEDURE 19-9 (continued)

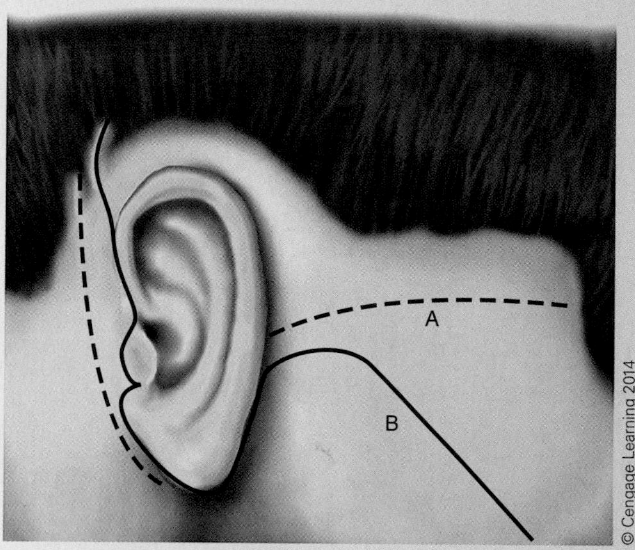

Figure 19-10 Rhytidectomy incision options: (A) Primary, (B) secondary

Procedural Consideration: "Tacking" sutures may be placed temporarily to hold the skin in place until the desired level of tension is achieved.

6. Redundant tissue is excised and wound is closed using suture of surgeon's choice. A Jackson-Pratt drain may be placed to help eliminate dead space and reduce the risk of hematoma.

   Procedural Consideration: Excision is done with new #15 scalpel blade.

7. This process is duplicated contralaterally.

   Procedural Consideration: Reorganize and repeat steps.

Postoperative Considerations

Immediate Postoperative Care

- Patient is transported to the PACU.
- Patient is discharged the same day of surgery.
- Antibiotic ointment may be placed on the incisions.
- A dressing is usually not applied.
- Patient should keep the head elevated and apply cold compresses to the area.
- Patient will return to the physician's office in 3–5 days for suture removal, and should avoid the use of makeup for 7–10 days postoperatively.

Prognosis

- No complications: Swelling and bruising are expected; recovery is usually fairly quick; patient expected to fully recover with improved cosmetic appearance.
- Complications: postoperative SSI; hemorrhage; hematoma; scarring

Wound Classification

- Class I: Clean

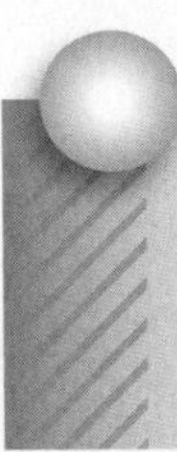

PEARL OF WISDOM

Even if the patient is under general anesthesia, the operative site will most likely be infiltrated with the local–epinephrine combination to cause vasoconstriction, which will aid in hemostasis.

PROCEDURE 19-10 Cleft Lip Repair—Rotation Advancement Technique

Surgical Anatomy and Pathology

- The function of the palate is to separate the nose from the mouth, which is important in swallowing and speech.
  - The anterior portion of the palate is the hard palate that consists of the palatine processes of each maxilla and the palatine bones. It is covered with mucous membrane.
  - The posterior portion is the soft palate and is composed of muscle, fat, and mucous membrane. It terminates with the uvula at the fauces.
- To understand the pathology, fetal development of the nose and mouth must be understood. The fetal development occurs during the first trimester of intrauterine life. The grooved middle portion from below the nose to the upper lip called the philtrum and the middle curve called Cupid's bow are formed by the joining of the frontal nasal prominence. Bilaterally the lips are formed by the maxillary prominences. The palate is formed from the joining of the central nasal prominence to the right and left maxillary prominences (Figure 19-11).

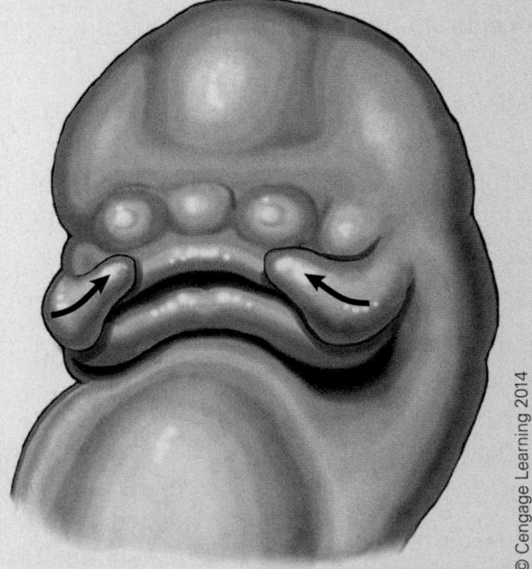

Figure 19-11 Development of the face

- A **cleft** is a split or a gap between two structures that are normally joined. **Cheilo**schisis (cleft or hare lip) and palato**schisis** (cleft palate) are two congenital deformities

PROCEDURE 19-10 (continued)

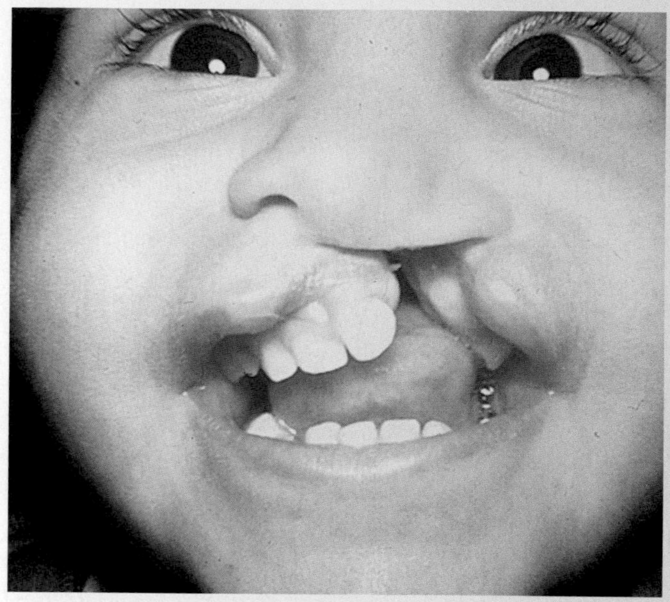

A

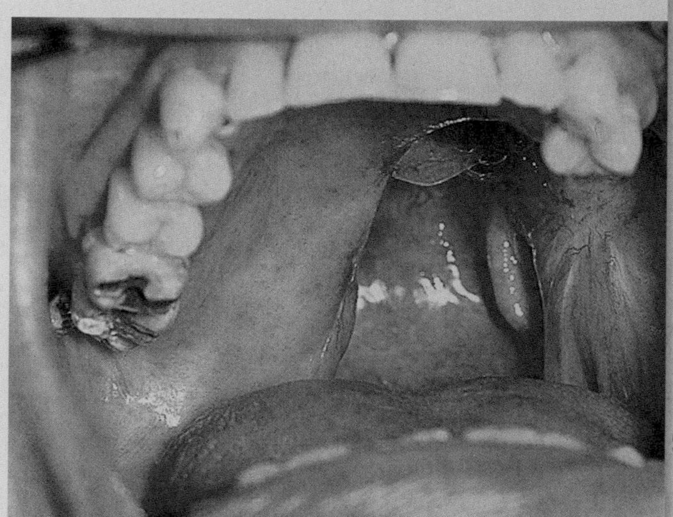

B

Courtesy of Dr. Joseph L. Konzelman, School of Dentistry, Medical College of Georgia

Figure 19-12 Cleft lip and palate: (A) Unilateral cleft lip, (B) unilateral cleft palate

	that can occur individually or are often seen in conjunction with one another (Figure 19-12). • The cleft can be unilateral or bilateral. When a disruption in normal fetal development causes the three prominences that should fuse to form the midface remain separated, a "cleft" occurs. The cleft	may affect just the upper lip, just the palate, or a combination of both structures, depending on which stage of fetal development was affected. There are four categories of cleft lip: • Unilateral incomplete cleft and nasal deformity • Unilateral complete cleft and nasal deformity	• Bilateral incomplete cleft • Bilateral complete cleft on one side and incomplete on the other side • The infant with these deformities may suffer from difficulty sucking, swallowing, and eventually forming proper sounds.
Preoperative Diagnostic Tests and Procedures	• History and physical examination as well as by direct examination		
Equipment, Instruments, and Supplies Unique to Procedure	• Headrest • Hyper/hypothermia blanket • Bipolar ESU with bayonet bipolar forceps • Plastic instrument set	• Beaver knife handle with #64 and #65 Beaver blades • Foment retractor • Brown lip clamps • Calipers	• Ruler • Marking pen • #11 and #15 blades • Logan's bow

(continues)

Procedure 19-10 (continued)

Preoperative Preparation

- Position: Supine with headrest; arms tucked at sides
- Anesthesia: General; local anesthetic with epinephrine is used for hemostasis.
- Skin prep: Beginning at the upper lip, the entire face, neck, and shoulders bilaterally as far as possible
- Draping: Headwrap/turban; bar drape; U-drape or split sheet

Practical Considerations

- The optimal age to perform the surgery is not well established, but it is usually performed between 3 and 18 months of age.
- Cheiloplasty and palatoplasty are often performed in combination. Often the lip and anterior palate defects are corrected at the same time, with the posterior palate repair done later.
- Two methods of cleft lip repair are commonly used.
  - The first and more commonly used technique is called "rotation advancement" (procedure that is described here).
  - The second and less common used repair is called the "triangular flap" method. It imitates the Z-plasty technique used in other types of plastic surgery. This method provides for additional height and length of the lip if there is a minimum of tissue available. Incisions are made on either side of the defect and the medial tissue is removed. Following closure of the mucous membrane layer and the muscle tissue, the skin flaps are overlapped and interlocked to close the defect.
- OR table may be turned to facilitate the surgeon standing or sitting at the head of the table to perform the surgery.
- The anesthesia provider will be at the patient's side.
- Prior to the skin prep the surgeon will mark the anatomical landmarks and incision using calipers and ruler.
- The surgeon may inject the local anesthetic prior to the skin prep or may inject it just before making the skin incision.
- The temperature in the OR should be increased prior to bringing the patient into the room.
- When setting up the back table and Mayo stand (if used), the surgical technologist should try to be as quiet as possible while the patient is awake. Talking should be kept to a minimum and a low tone of voice should be used.
- This is considered a clean, rather than a sterile, procedure because the aerodigestive tract is entered. Nonetheless, sterile technique must be used to reduce the risk of postoperative SSI.

Surgical Procedure

1. Using either a #11 or #15 blade, the first incision is made along the superior vermilion border, extending to the midline of the cleft into the nose.
2. Skin hooks are used for retraction; the surgeon uses curved tenotomy scissors to dissect the mucosa off the orbicularis oris muscle.

   Procedural Consideration: The main role of the surgical technologist (besides anticipating the needs of the surgeon) will be retraction.
3. A second incision is made extending from the cleft to the midline to dissect the medial lip free from the maxilla.
4. Using either a #11 or #15 blade, a Z-plasty incision is made to create three flaps; however, they are not necessarily rotated in order.

PROCEDURE 19-10 (continued)

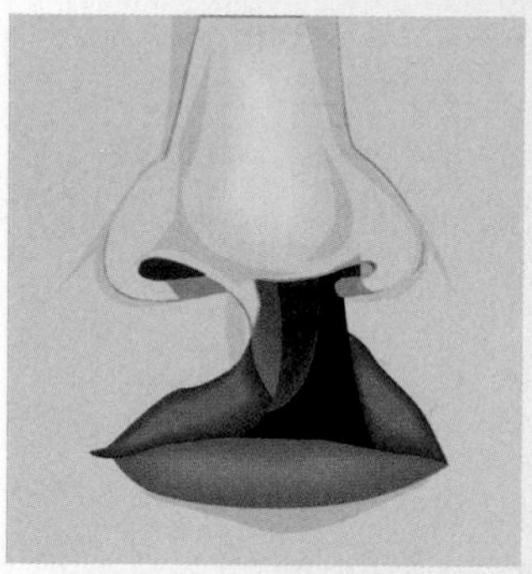
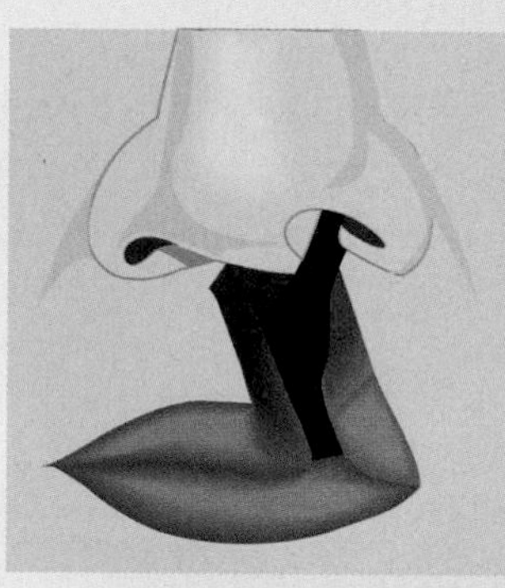
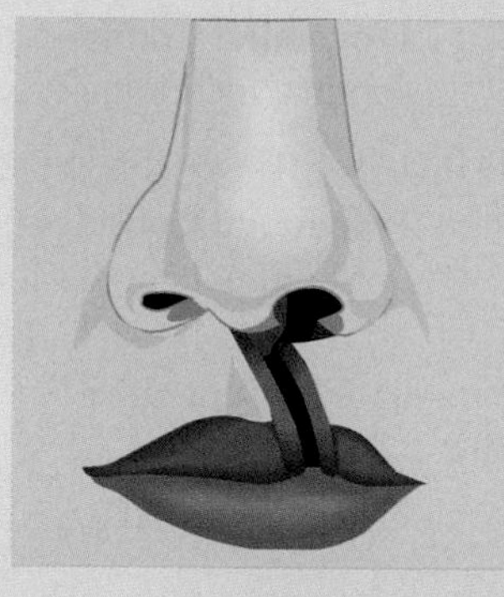
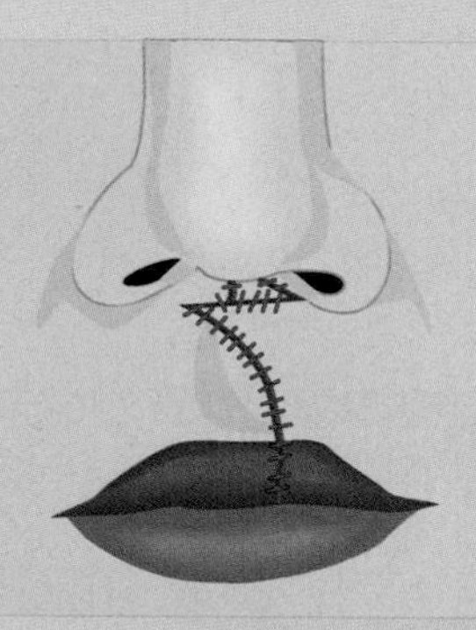

A B C D

Figure 19-13 Rotation-advancement procedure to correct unilateral cleft lip: (A) Incision marked to show rotation of Cupid's bow and philtrum into normal position; flap will advance into columella to form nostril; (B) Cupid's bow–philtrum rotated down and flap advanced into columella; (C) flap advanced into gap left by rotation-advancement procedure to correct unilateral cleft lip; (D) closure of flaps

a. First flap: Rotation incision made in such a manner that the flap is rotated down to form Cupid's bow and philtrum groove (Figure 19-13A).

b. Third flap: Rotated into columella and forms lower portion of nostril (Figure 19-13B).

c. Second flap: Advanced into the gap left by the rotations and skin used to form Cupid's bow (Figure 19-13C).

5. Closure is as follows:

 a. Mucous membrane of the upper lip is closed first with interrupted absorbable sutures.

 b. Next, the orbicularis oris muscle is closed with absorbable sutures.

 c. Skin is closed last, with every attempt made to create Cupid's bow; absorbable suture is used (Figures 19-13D and 19-14).

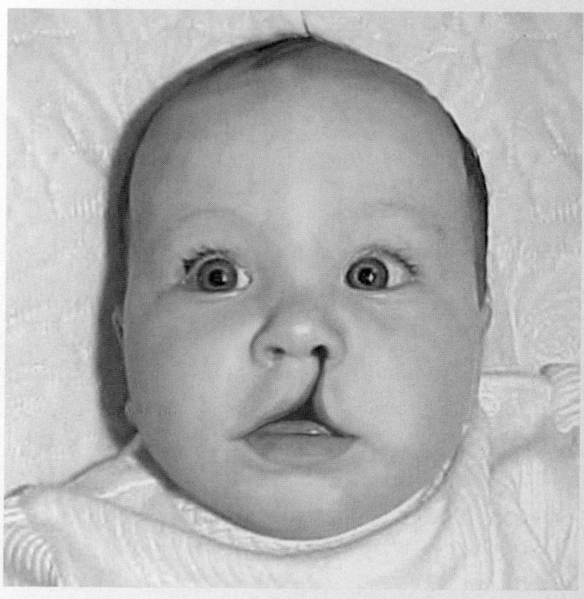
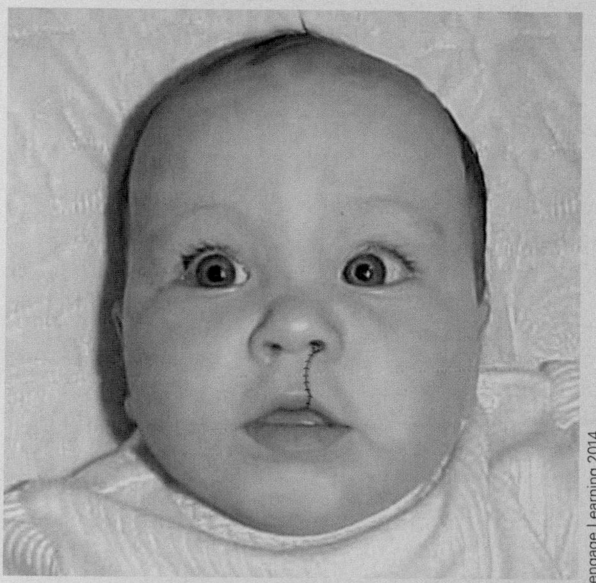

A B

Figure 19-14 Cleft lip repair-rotation advancement technique: (A) Defect, (B) closure

(*continues*)

PROCEDURE 19-10 (continued)

Procedural Consideration: Due to the small size of the needles and suture, the surgical technologist will need to carefully keep track of the suture.

6. Dressing is a small mustache type with a small 2 × 2 sponge and tape.

   Procedural Consideration: Do not break down the back table and/or Mayo stand until the patient has left the room for transport to the PACU.

Postoperative Considerations

Immediate Postoperative Care

- Patient is transported to the PACU.
- Hospital stay should only be 1–2 days.
- Padded arm restraints may have to be used on the infant to prevent touching, rubbing, or removing the dressing and causing wound disruption.

Prognosis

- No complications: The patient is expected to have good aesthetic and functional results from cheiloplasty and palatoplasty, but this is by no means the end of the treatment. Speech therapy, orthodontia, and nasal reconstruction are all options to be considered for the future. Both types of cleft lip repair leave a permanent exterior scar that will partially fade over time. Adult males may choose to grow a mustache to conceal the scar.
- Complications: Postoperative SSI; hemorrhage; scarring; edema. Closely observe patient during immediate postoperative period for hemorrhage and edema. Occasionally, edema can become severe and obstruct the airway.

Wound Classification

- Class II: Clean-contaminated

PROCEDURE 19-11 Cleft Palate Repair: V-Y Palatoplasty Technique

Surgical Anatomy and Pathology

- See Procedure 19-10.

Preoperative Diagnostic tests and Procedures

- History and physical examination as well as by direct examination

Equipment, Instruments, and Supplies Unique to Procedure

- Donut headrest
- Hyper/hypothermia blanket
- Bipolar ESU with bayonet forceps
- Nitrogen tank for power drill
- Power drill
- Plastic instrument set
- Beaver knife handle with #6910 Beaver blade
- Drill bits, various sizes
- Dingman mouth gag, assorted size of blades
- Blair palate hook and elevators
- Freer elevator
- Cottle elevator
- Fomon lower lateral scissors
- #11, #12, and #15 blades

Procedure 19-11 (continued)

Preoperative Preparation	• See Procedure 19-10.
Practical Considerations	• The Mayo stand will be used for attaching the self-retaining mouth gag. • The surgical technologist should not break down the back table or Mayo stand until the patient has left the OR for transport to the PACU. • See Procedure 19-10 for all other considerations.
Surgical Procedure	1. After the patient is positioned the surgeon inserts the Dingman mouth gag and attaches the other end to the Mayo stand.
	2. A throat pack consisting of sponges may be inserted to absorb blood and prevent it from draining into the throat. **Procedural Consideration:** The surgical technologist should assist the surgeon with irrigation and suctioning of the operative site throughout the procedure.
	3. The palatal flaps are outlined and the local anesthetic with epinephrine is injected (Figure 19-15A).
	4. Using a #15 blade, the surgeon makes a V-shaped incision along the mucosal borders.
	5. The incision is extended with the #15 blade and palate blade through the oral mucosa, muscle, and nasal mucosa.
	6. On both sides of the cleft, the surgeon uses Freer and Cottle elevators to dissect the nasal mucosa from the muscle (Figure 19-15B).
	7. Next, using the same elevators, the oral mucosa is dissected from the muscle, thus creating the three layers to be closed.
	8. During the tissue dissection, the surgeon identifies the greater palatine vessels in order to prevent them from being injured.
	9. Holes may be drilled in the hard palate to facilitate suture placement. **Procedural Consideration:** The surgical technologist should be prepared to set up the drill with the drill bit to facilitate placement of the sutures.
	10. A Y-shaped closure in three layers is achieved that closes the cleft and lengthens the palate (Figure 19-15C). The closure is as follows: a. Nasal mucosa are closed first with 4-0 or 5-0 absorbable suture. b. Muscle is closed second with the same type of suture. c. Palatal mucosa is closed last over the other layers, using the same type of suture.
	11. Area is irrigated and checked for bleeding, throat pack is removed, mouth gag is removed, and patient is extubated and transported to the PACU. The anesthesia provider must be very careful during extubation to avoid injuring the repaired palate. The surgical team should be prepared to treat the patient for airway obstruction. **Procedural Consideration:** As mentioned earlier, the surgical technologist should be ready to assist the team in treating a patient who experiences airway obstruction upon extubation. The surgical technologist should not break down the back table and Mayo stand until the patient has left the OR.

(continues)

PROCEDURE 19-11 (continued)

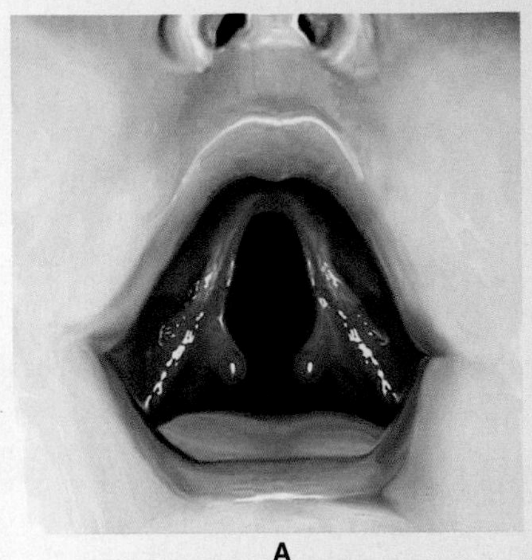

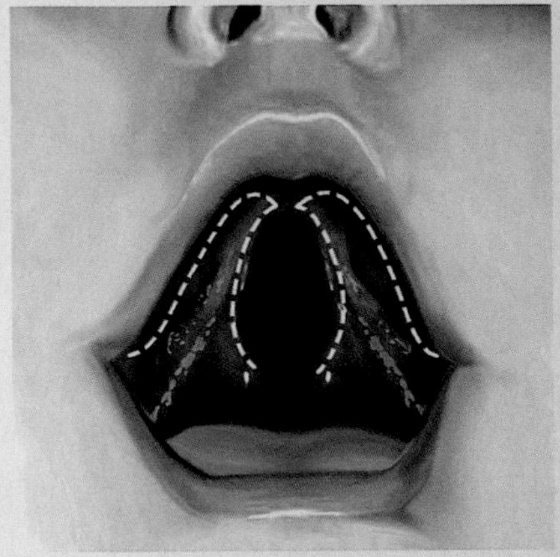

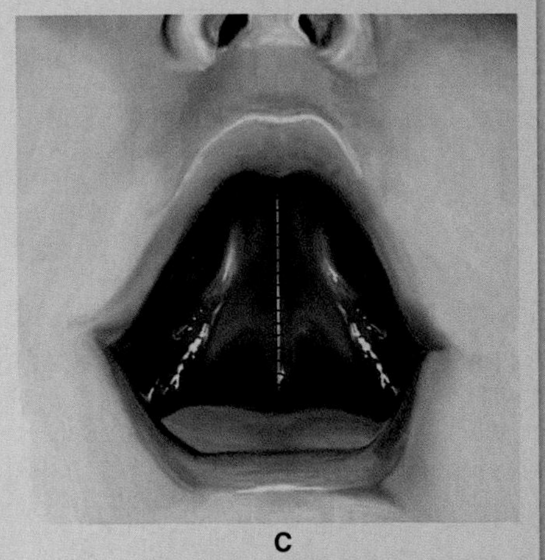

Figure 19-15 Palatoplasty: (A) Bilateral defect, (B) dissection palatoplasty, (C) closure

Postoperative Considerations	
	Immediate Postoperative Care • Patient is transported to the PACU. • Hospital stay should be 1–2 days. • Padded arm restraints may have to be used for infants. **Prognosis** • No complications: Patient should have good aesthetic and functional results. However, speech therapy, orthodontia, and nasal reconstruction may have to be considered for the future. • Complications: Postoperative SSI; hemorrhage; edema with airway obstruction **Wound Classification** • Class II: Clean/ Contaminated

HAND PROCEDURES

Due to the extensiveness of the hand anatomy, it is presented in paragraph form rather than bulleted format in the description of surgical procedures. The hand is made up of three regions: the wrist, the palm, and the fingers. Specific directional terms are also used in reference to the hand. Using the anatomical position, palms forward, the terms are as follows:

- *Volar surface:* palm of the hand
- *Dorsal surface or dorsum:* back of the hand
- *Radial:* refers to thumb side of the hand
- *Ulnar:* refers to the medial side of the hand

Eight carpal bones compose each wrist, or carpus. They are arranged in two rows (proximal and distal) consisting of four bones each. From lateral to medial, the scaphoid, lunate, triquetral, and pisiform bones compose the proximal row. Listed from lateral to medial, the bones in the distal row are the trapezium, trapezoid, capitate, and the hamate. Proximally, the carpal bones articulate with the distal radius and the distal radioulnar joint, commonly known as the wrist (Figure 19-16).

The metacarpals are the bones of the palm, or metacarpus. There are five metacarpal bones in each hand. They are numbered I through V, the first correlating with the thumb. The metacarpals are long, cylinder-shaped shafts. The proximal end is referred to as the base and the distal portion forms the head.

Each digit, or finger, is made up of a series of phalanges. There are 14 phalanges in each hand. Each digit has three phalanges, with the exception of the thumb, which only has two. The phalanges are named according to the order of their placement. The phalanx closest to the metacarpal is called the proximal, next is the medial, and the farthest is referred to as distal. As with the metacarpals, the digits are numbered, with the thumb being called the first digit.

The head of each metacarpal articulates with one of the phalanges. These joints are considered *diarthroses*, or freely movable joints, and are synovial hinge-type joints called

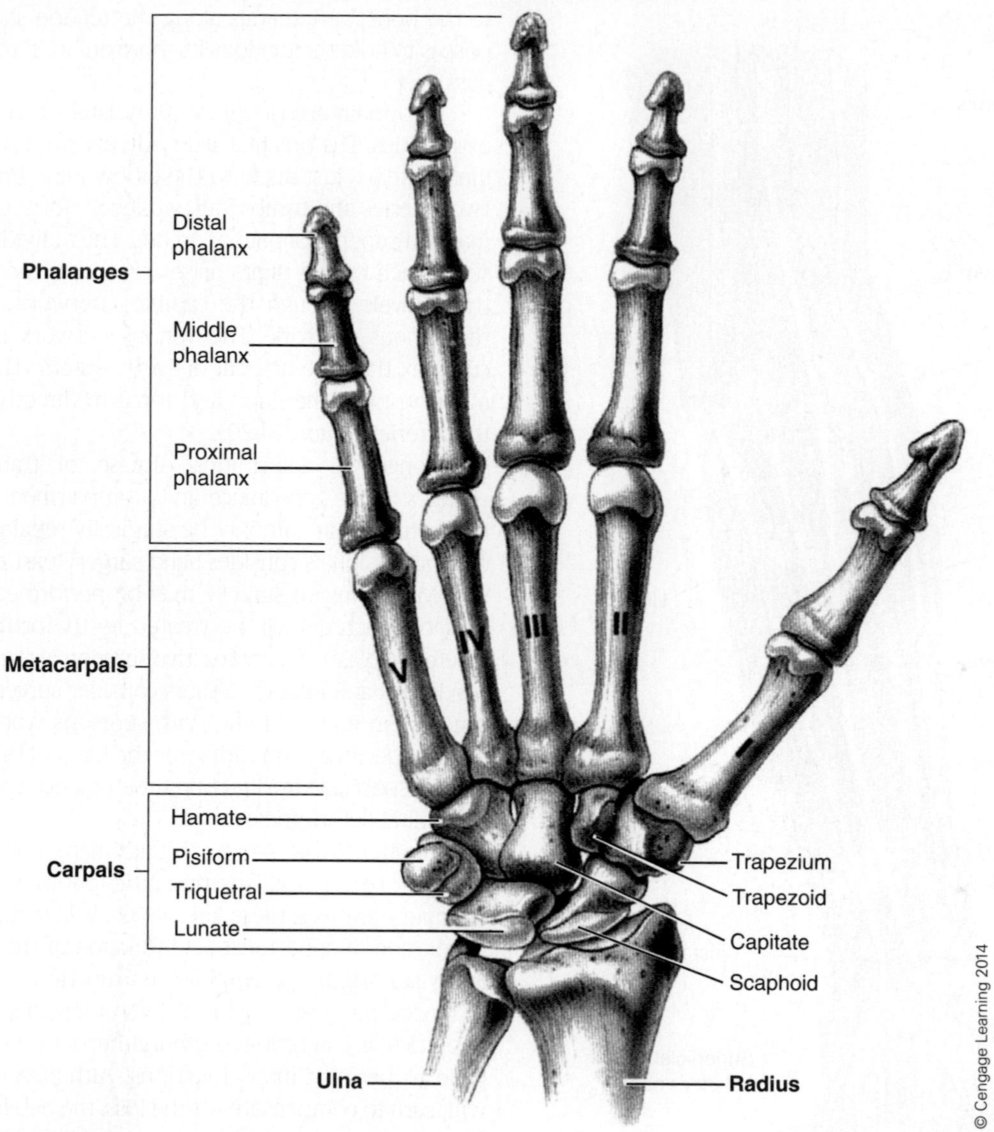

Figure 19-16 Bones of the hand

metacarpophalangeal joints (**MPJs**). The same type of joint is formed between the phalanges and is called an interphalangeal joint (IPJ). Refer to Chapter 21 for a complete description of the types of joints.

The nerves that serve the forearm and the hand are all branches of nerves from the brachial plexus. The three nerves that we will be concerned with are the radial, median, and ulnar (Figure 19-17).

The radial nerve travels along the radius and provides feeling to the skin of the hand. The median nerve branches into two main sections that innervate the skin of the lateral two-thirds of the hand and several intrinsic muscles of the hand. The ulnar nerve provides feeling to the skin of the medial third of the hand and some of the flexor muscles of the hand and wrist.

Almost 40 muscles and their coordinating tendons are responsible for movement of the wrist, hand, and fingers. Most of the muscles on the anterior aspect of the hand are responsible for flexion; those located posteriorly control extension (Figure 19-18).

On the anterior, or palm, side of the hand there is one main compartment or tunnel. This is the passageway in the wrist that is surrounded on three sides by the carpal bones and covered anteriorly by the transverse carpal ligament. Nine flexor tendons and the median nerve pass through this tunnel (Figure 19-19).

Dorsally, there are six compartments. The tendons for the muscles that extend the fingers and thumb and dorsiflex the hand separate and pass through these tunnels. The compartments are lined with synovial membrane. The synovium

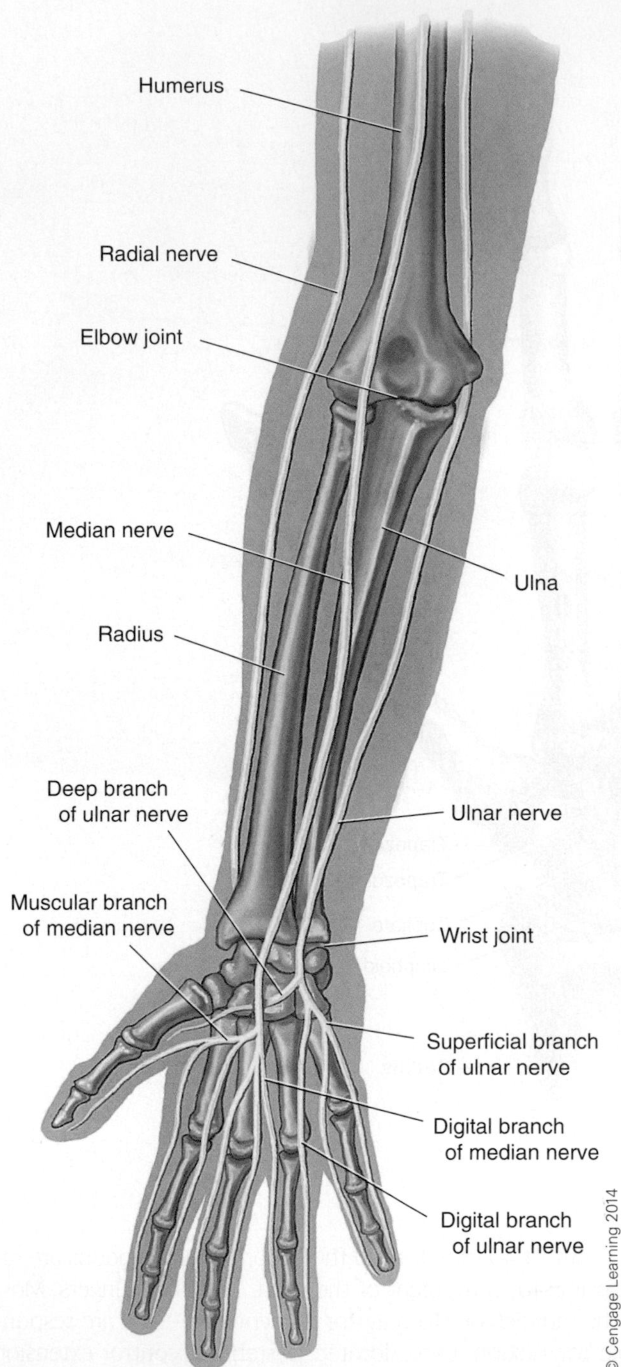

Figure 19-17 Innervation of the hand

secretes a fluid that lubricates the compartment to reduce friction. The *dorsal carpal ligament* collectively covers the compartments.

The tendons of the fingers and thumbs are contained in a protective covering called a tendon sheath. The tendon sheaths are lined with synovium. Pulleys or annular bands are attached to the bones at intervals along the tendon sheath. Their purpose is to hold the tendons in approximation to the bones they pass over.

Two main arteries serve the distal portion of the upper extremities. The brachial artery divides to form the radial and ulnar arteries just distal to the elbow joint. Branches of these two arteries anastomose at two levels, forming the deep palmar and superficial palmar arches. The individual arteries that serve each of the digits arise from these arches. The blood then travels through the capillary network and returns via the venous network. The venous network is slightly more complex than the arterial delivery system. The names of the major veins in the hand and forearm directly correlate with the arteries (Figure 19-20).

Congenital deformities, disease, or trauma may cause changes to the appearance and/or impairment of the function of the hand that can only be surgically repaired. Some health care professionals consider hand surgery part of many specialties. Median nerve surgery may be performed by the neurosurgeon, fractures will be treated by the orthopedic surgeon, whereas a plastic/reconstructive surgeon is required for certain conditions and injuries. Others consider surgery of the hand a specialty in its own right, with surgeons who focus their expertise specifically on caring for the hands. Hand surgeons may further specialize by directing their practice toward those with congenital deformities.

Trauma to the hand can take many forms: cuts, sprains, fractures, burns, crush injuries, or amputation. No matter what the injury involves, there are two goals in surgical intervention: restoration of appearance and function of the hand to its preinjury state, with the emphasis on function.

Accidents resulting in the loss of any digit, and the thumb in particular, can have a profound impact on the ability of the hand to perform many functions. Although most individuals will learn to compensate for the loss, the debility can be significant. **Replantation** of the severed digit carries the best chance for restoration of full function. Several factors will affect the viability of replantation, including:

- Type of injury (clean cut vs. crush or avulsion)
- Location of the amputation on the affected structure
- Extent of damage to underlying structures (blood vessels, nerves, tendons)
- Care of the severed part (immediate access to ice)
- Time elapsed between accident and initiation of replantation

Recent improvements in the area of microvascular techniques makes this a very hopeful time for those who have suffered severe injury to their hands. Such advancements have allowed for the replantation of severed digits, toe-to-hand transfers for lost digits, and even complete hand transplants. While revascularization is vital for the survival of a severed digit, it has been the advancements in microneuroplastic techniques that have restored function.

Flexor carpi radialis
Brachioradialis
Flexor digitorum superficialis
Flexor pollicis longus
Abductor pollicis brevis
Flexor pollicis brevis
Adductor pollicis
Lumbrical (1st)
Lumbrical (2nd)
Flexor digitorum superficialis
Palmaris longus
Flexor digitorum profundus (tendon)
Flexor carpi ulnaris
Abductor digiti minimi
Flexor digiti minimi brevis
Opponens digiti minimi
Lumbrical (4th)
Lumbrical (3rd)
A

Extensor digitorum
Extensor carpi ulnaris
Extensor retinaculum
Abductor digiti minimi
Extensor carpi radialis brevis
Extensor carpi radialis longus (tendon)
Abductor pollicis longus
Extensor pollicis brevis
Extensor pollicis longus
Dorsal interossei
B

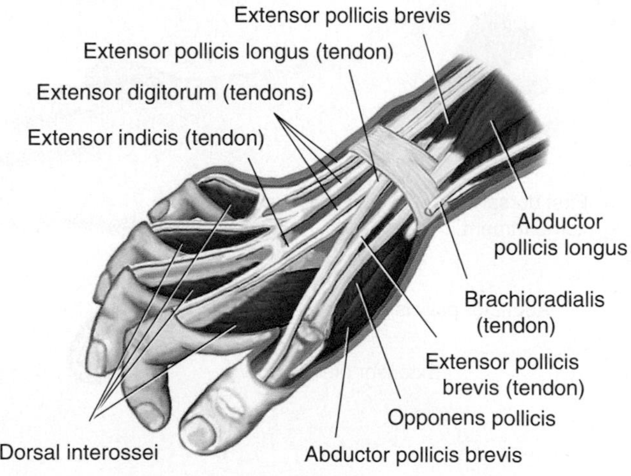

Figure 19-18 Muscles of the forearm and hand: (A) Anterior view, (B) dorsal view, (C) posteromedial view

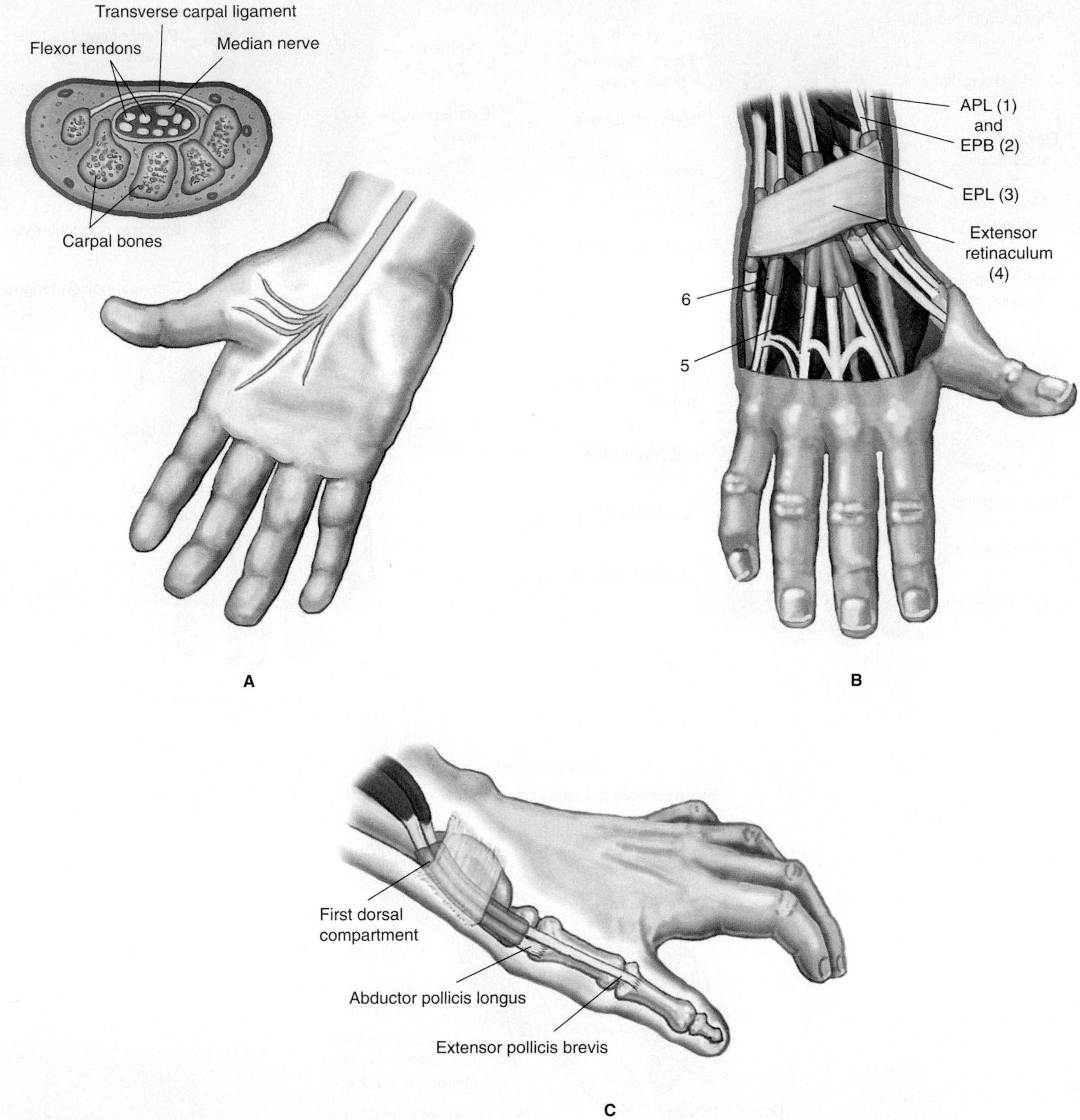

Figure 19-19 Compartments of the hand: (A) Anterior compartment with transverse section, (B) dorsal compartments, (C) first dorsal compartment

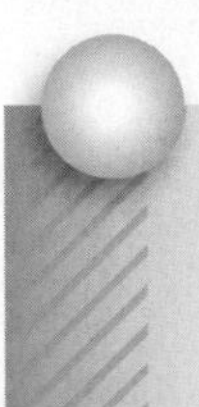

PEARL OF WISDOM

The surgical technologist must often function in the role of the surgical assistant during a hand case. This requires an extra measure of concentration and skill. The surgical technologist must anticipate not only the instrument needs of the surgeon but also the need to provide retraction, follow suture, and so on.

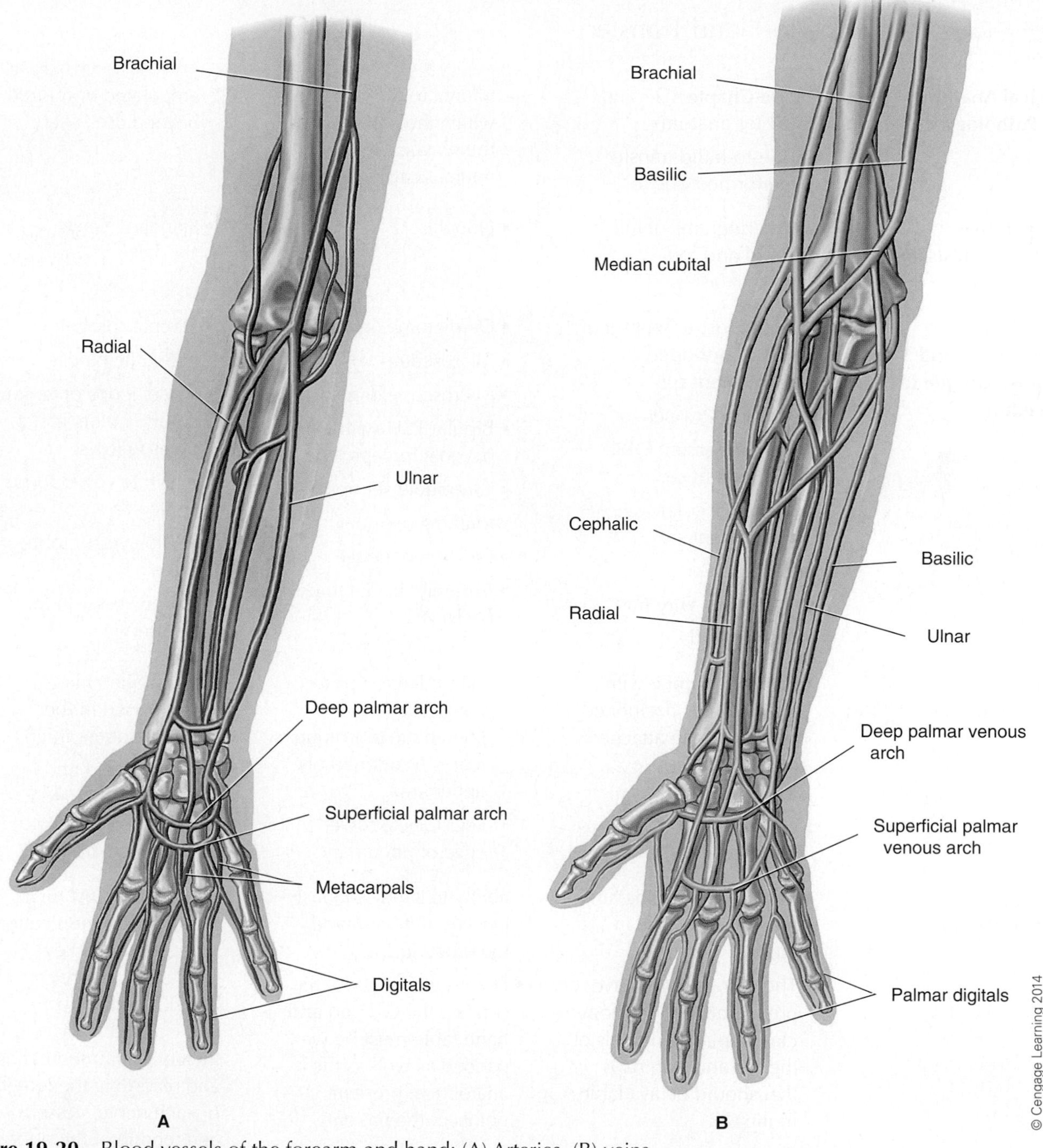

Figure 19-20 Blood vessels of the forearm and hand: (A) Arteries, (B) veins

Replantation of a digit involves the implementation of every type of procedure that would be used to correct any traumatic injury to the hand. Therefore, it will be used here to illustrate:

- Tenorrhaphy
- Neurorrhaphy
- Restoration of vasculature
- Bone approximation

The following is a general procedural description of replantation of a traumatically amputated digit. The toe-to-hand replantation is given in more detail (Procedure 19-13). Due to the detail of the structures involved, the process of replantation is tedious and can take upward of 12 hours to complete. This procedure is usually performed under general anesthesia because of the length of time required.

Procedure 19-12 Toe-to-Hand Transfer

Surgical Anatomy and Pathology	• See Chapters 21 and 23 for anatomy. • Toe-to-hand transfer is performed due to	trauma to the hand in which the patient's thumb was traumatically	amputated or injured beyond use.
Preoperative Diagnostic Tests and Procedures	• Arteriograms of the hand and foot	• Doppler	• Standard X-rays

Equipment, Instruments, and Supplies Unique to Procedure	• Hand instrument set or major orthopedic instrument set
	• Tendon stripper
	• Mini-fragment ORIF instrument set
	• Microvascular instrument set
	• Wire driver
	• Kirschner wire tray
	• Power drill
		• Dermatome (available)
		• Microscope
		• Microscope drape
		• Bipolar ESU with bayonet forceps × 2
		• Tourniquet set ups × 2
		• Marking pen
		• Esmarch bandage
		• Extremity back table packs × 2
			• Doppler probe
			• #15 knife blades
			• Vessel loops of various colors. Colors match up as follows:
			  • White vessel loop: Nerves
			  • Blue vessel loop: Vein
			  • Red vessel loop: Artery

Preoperative Preparation	• Position: Supine with affected arm positioned on hand table attached to OR table • Anesthesia: General • Skin prep:	• Hand: Fingertips to lower edge of pneumatic tourniquet that is positioned on upper arm • Leg: Toes to lower edge of pneumatic	tourniquet that is positioned in the middle of the thigh • Draping: Hand and leg are draped separately. See Chapter 12 for draping an extremity.
Practical Considerations	• X-rays and arteriograms must be available in the OR. • The surgeon may have preoperatively developed clay or plaster models of the toe and skin flaps that should be available in the OR. • The length of surgery is 12–16 hours; therefore, tourniquet time must be carefully monitored and communicated to both surgical teams. • The patient must be positioned and draped to allow both teams the	ability to simultaneously perform the hand and toe procedures. • Due to the length of the surgery, the OR bed and hand table must be well padded as well as the anatomical pressure points of the patient. • The surgical wounds must not be allowed to dry out and kept moist with saline. • The procedure involves two surgical teams: one for the foot and the other for the hand.	• Both teams must be in constant communication in regard to the key structures that are identified, mobilized, and isolated. This includes communicating and recording the length of each nerve, vessel, and tendon of the donor toe and hand. The team dissecting the hand should measure, record, and communicate the required length of each structure before any structures are divided in the foot to ensure

PROCEDURE 19-12 (continued)

adequate length is achieved.

- The order of anastomosis is as follows: Bone-to-bone to keep ischemia time to a minimum; tendons; arteries; veins; nerves.
- To be a successful transplant, at least one artery and two veins must be anastomosed.

Surgical Procedure

Toe Procedure

1. A lateral triangular incision is made on the foot as far back as the dorsal medial aspect to expose the saphenous vein, dorsalis pedis artery and branches, and short extensor muscle.
2. Using the Metzenbaum scissors, the short extensor muscle is divided.
3. The dorsalis pedis artery and its branch, the communicating artery, and communicating vein from the saphenous vein are mobilized from the dorsum of the foot distally into the toe.
4. The long extensor tendon is dissected free from its attachment back to the dorsum of the foot to provide an excellent length of tendon.
5. The deep peroneal nerve is identified and dissected free; it will be used to anastomose to the superficial radial nerve in the hand to provide sensation to the dorsum of the transplanted toe.
6. The proximal communicating vein and artery at the base of the first web space are clamped, cut, and ligated to complete freeing up the dorsalis pedis artery.
7. On the medial side, the long flexor tendon and medial digital nerves are isolated, dissected free, and transected.

   Practical Consideration: The white vessel loop is used to gently retract the deep peroneal nerve superiorly out of the surgical site, the red vessel loop is used to superiorly retract the dorsalis pedis artery, and the blue vessel loop is used to medially retract the saphenous vein.
8. The toe is placed in an angulated medial position and, using the #15 knife blade, the joint capsule is incised and disarticulated through the metatarsal joint.

   Procedural Consideration: The long flexor tendon must be distally retracted to protect it from injury.
9. All structures except for the arteries and veins have been divided. The tourniquet is released and bleeders are cauterized or ligated.
10. Microvascular vessel clamps are placed on the dorsalis pedis artery and saphenous vein and the vessels are tied and divided, freeing the toe from the foot.

    Procedural Consideration: At this point the vessels, tendons, and nerves that are included with the transplant are dorsalis pedis artery, saphenous vein, extensor hallucis longus tendon, flexor hallucis longus tendon, lateral digital nerve, and medial digital nerve.
11. The skin flaps are positioned and sutured over the donor defect of the foot.

    Procedural Consideration: During the surgical amputation of the toe, the surgeon ensures that there is an adequate amount of skin tissue left to cover the defect. Closure of the donor defect can create serious postoperative problems such as delayed healing if too much tissue is transferred with the toe. It is advised to take less tissue from the foot and, if necessary, cover open areas on the hand with a split-thickness skin graft (STSG).

(continues)

Procedure 19-12 (continued)

Hand Dissection and Implantation of Toe Transplant

1. A dorsal coronal incision is made in the midline of the amputated area of the stump of the thumb, exposing the median nerve and its branches. The flexor pollicis longus tendon is identified at the base of the metacarpal, which will be used as a bone peg for insertion into the proximal phalanx of the toe transplant.

   Procedural Consideration: This creates an adequate web space in order to restore an adequate grip and pinch to the patient's hand.

2. The toe is fixed into position with the use of a Kirschner wire and the use of a bone peg on the hand fitted into a hole that has been created in the proximal toe phalanx.
3. A screw from the mini-fragment set is transversely positioned.
4. The metacarpophalangeal joint of the thumb is reconstructed to provide additional movement to the transplant.
5. The extensor pollicis longus tendon and extensor hallucis longus are sutured together.
6. The flexor hallucis longus tendon and flexor pollicis longus tendon are anastomosed in the wrist.

   Procedural Consideration: The surgeon uses a figure-of-eight suture technique to anastomose the tendons.

7. The dorsalis pedis artery is anastomosed end-to-end to the dorsal radial artery.
8. The saphenous vein is anastomosed end-to-end to the cephalic vein.
9. The digital nerves from the toe are anastomosed to the digital nerves in the thumb.

   Procedural Consideration: The microscope is brought up to the surgical field to be used by the surgeon when anastomosing the arteries, veins, and nerves.

10. The skin flaps are sutured into place on the lateral and medial aspects of the thumb. If the skin flaps cannot be sutured in place without creating tension, an STSG will be placed directly over the anastomosis.

    Procedural Consideration: The surgical technologist must make sure there are plenty of sutures of the correct size available. Interrupted suture technique is used by the surgeon to secure the skin flaps.

11. A nonadherent bulky dressing is placed that allows for exposure of the fingertips.

Postoperative Considerations

Immediate Postoperative Care

- Patient is transported to the PACU.
- Arm is elevated on a pillow.
- Fingertips are frequently assessed for adequate blood flow.
- Patient will stay in hospital 3–4 days before discharge.

Prognosis

- No complications: Patient is expected to regain most of the original function of the hand, including gripping and pinching. However, extensive physical therapy will be necessary.
- Complications: Postoperative SSI; transplant does not "take"; hemorrhaging; vessel spasms

Wound Classification

- Class I: Clean

The surgical technologist will need all of the supplies listed for Procedure 19-12 to prepare for this type of surgery.

The affected limb is positioned, prepped, and draped in the routine fashion described for Procedure 19-12.

If the availability of personnel allows, two workstations are set up simultaneously within the sterile field. While one surgeon is debriding the proximal stump and identifying the structures to be anastomosed, another is doing the same on the severed part. This is frequently done with the use of loupes or under the operating microscope. The structures to be anastomosed are often "tagged," meaning marked with suture or other materials. Tagging serves two main purposes: it eases future identification of the tendons, blood vessels, and nerves planned for reconnection and it prevents retraction of the structures into the deeper tissues. If two surgeons are not available, the severed part is kept cold and the surgeon first deals with the stump (Figure 19-21). In some unfortunate situations, a determination will be made that the stump will not be able to receive the severed part and the wound is closed at this point. Once the stump has been prepared, the severed digit is removed from the ice and the processes of debridement and identification are repeated. Often, it is necessary to trim the ends of the structures to facilitate anastomosis.

Replantation begins with bone-to-bone attachment. The bone ends are shortened with the use of bone cutters to eliminate tension on the reanastomosed veins, artery, and nerves. The bone is stabilized using K-wires or plates and screws; K-wires are used on the small bones of the hands and feet, and plates and screws are used on larger bones such as the radius, ulna, humerus, tibia, etc. The tendons are reconnected next by suturing the proximal and distal ends together. Following stabilization of the supportive structures, reanastomosis of the blood vessels is performed. Heparin may be used to irrigate the vessels prior to anastomosis to ensure patency. Because of the size of the vasculature, it is often necessary to perform this step under a microscope; it involves the use of microsuture and microinstrumentation. The repair of at least one artery and two veins will be necessary for viability. Papaverine may be used to prevent vasospasm. The final structures to be repaired are the nerves. In some situations nerve grafting may be necessary.

Prior to final closure, the wound may be irrigated with antibiotic solution. To allow for expected edema and to prevent ischemia of the underlying structures, the soft tissues and skin are closed with a loose nonabsorbable suture. Drains may be placed if necessary. The dressing will most likely begin with a nonadherent gauze and progress to a bulky restrictive bandage. The use of a splint may be used. If possible, the fingertips should remain exposed so that they may be checked for circulation and feeling. The arm should be kept elevated postoperatively to minimize edema. Frequent inspections should be made to ensure that proper circulation is maintained. The first few postoperative hours are critical to the success of the replantation.

Complications of digit and limb replantation include:

- Failure of the reattachment (usually due to poor vascularity), causing tissue necrosis
- Decreased nerve function, causing reduced motor function
- Digit or limb deformity

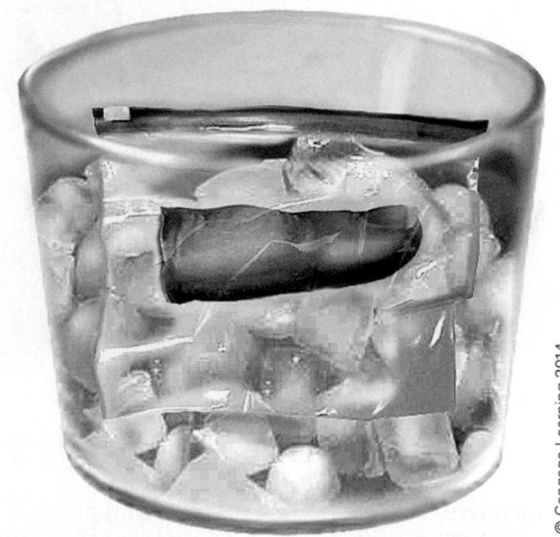

Figure 19-21 Preservation of a digit for replantation

PROCEDURE 19-13 Subtotal Palmar Fasciectomy for Dupuytren's Contracture

Surgical Anatomy and Pathology

- See previous description of anatomy.
- Dupuytren's contracture may present itself in one of three ways: a nonpainful nodule in the palm of the hand near the fourth or fifth digit; a dimpling or pit in locations just described; or finally as a longitudinal fibrous band or cord extending from the palm toward the fingers (Figure 19-22).

(continues)

PROCEDURE 19-13 (continued)

- All of these primary signs are caused by contraction of the palmar fascia. The contraction causes deformity and contractures of the dermis and/or digits. Occasionally the patient may experience tenderness over an existing nodule.
- When the contracture causes restricted movement and impaired function, surgery is indicated. The surgery is variable depending on the extent of the pathology; it can range from simple nodule excision to very complex in which restoration of full function and normal appearance may not be possible.

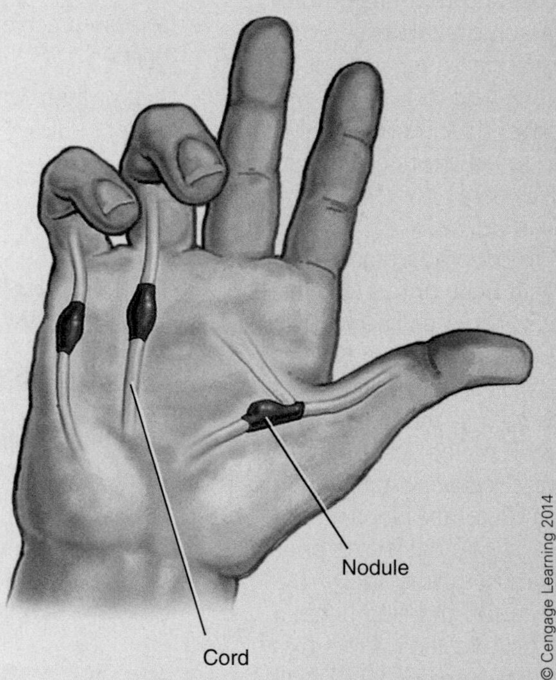

Figure 19-22 Dupuytren's contracture

Preoperative Diagnostic Tests and Procedures	• History and physical examination as well as by direct examination	• Standard X-rays	
Equipment, Instruments, and Supplies Unique to Procedure	• Plastic instrument tray • Minor orthopedic instrument tray (available) • Dermatome (available)	• Hand table attachment to OR table • Lead hand • Tourniquet and insufflator	• Impervious stockinette • Esmarch bandage • Marking pen • #15 knife blades × 3 • ESU pencil with needle tip

Procedure 19-13 (continued)

Preoperative Preparation	• Position: Supine with affected arm positioned on attached armboard • Anesthesia: Bier block preferred; general • Skin prep: Beginning at incision site on palm and moving outward to include fingertips up to axillary region • Draping: Three-fourths sheet laid over armboard table; impervious stockinette placed over arm and unrolled up to axillary region; extremity drape
Practical Considerations	• Have X-rays in OR. • If a skin graft is anticipated to be taken, the surgical technologist should confirm the donor site with the surgeon. • Test power equipment prior to the patient entering the OR. • Surgery team must remember the patient is sedated but conscious; keep conversations and noise to a minimum.
Surgical Procedure	1. The surgeon may or may not use the lead hand to keep the hand in place. If not used, the surgical technologist will be responsible for holding the hand and digits in place.
	2. The surgeon marks the incision(s) with the marking pen.
	3. If a free skin graft will be used it is first taken. **Procedural Consideration:** The graft is often taken from the medial region of the arm. The surgical technologist must keep the graft moist by wrapping saline-soaked sponges around it until needed.
	4. Using the #15 knife blade, the surgeon will make one or more incisions on the volar or palmar surface of the hand according to the extent of the disease (Figure 19-23). For extensive contractures, a Z-plasty incision may be used so that the existing tissue can be used to cover the palm. **Procedural Consideration:** The surgeon may use several #15 knife blades; make sure to frequently change the blades to avoid the surgeon using a dull blade.
	5. The incision is carried down to the palmar fascia, taking care to avoid injury to digital nerves and tendons.

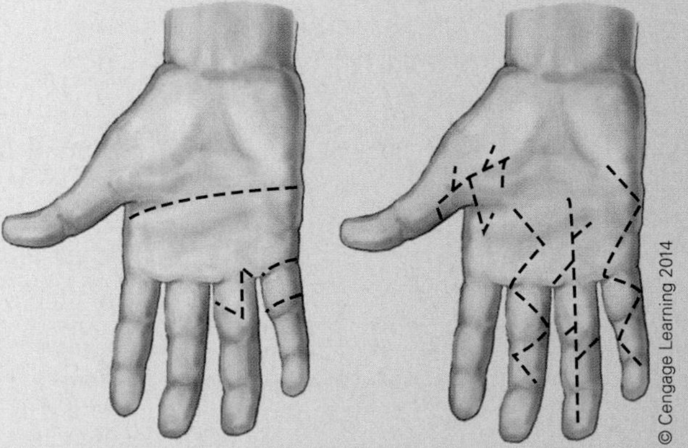

Figure 19-23 Possible incisions for treatment of Dupuytren's disease

(continues)

Procedure 19-13 (continued)

6. Using Adson tissue forceps and curved tenotomy scissors, the surgeon dissects the contracted fascia away from the underlying nerves, blood vessels, and tendons.

   Procedural Consideration: This dissection can be very tedious and time consuming if the contracture is advanced. The surgical technologist must remain alert throughout the procedure.

7. If being used, the skin graft is placed at this point of the procedure.

8. Wound closure may be performed as primary closure. Numerous stitches may be required to successfully stretch the existing skin to add the length necessary for closure.

   Procedural Consideration: If a skin graft cannot be taken to cover a small surface of the palm, the wound may be left open to heal by second intention.

9. Nonadherent dressing such as petrolatum gauze is placed with fluffs and an elastic bandage to hold the dressing in place for several days. A splint may be placed depending on surgeon's preference.

Postoperative Considerations

Immediate Postoperative Care

- Patient is transported to the PACU.
- Elevate arm on pillow.
- Patient will be discharged the same day of surgery.

Prognosis

- No complications: Some pain and swelling will occur; OTC analgesics; ice applied; arm should be kept elevated when walking and by the use of a pillow in bed; physical therapy that can be short term or last several months depending on extent of repair.
- Complications: Postoperative SSI; wound disruption (minor wound disruptions are not uncommon, forcing the patient to wear a dressing for an extended period of time); recurrence of palmar fasciectomy

Wound Classification

- Class I: Clean

Procedure 19-14 Centralization of Radial Dysplasia

Surgical Anatomy and Pathology

- See previous description of hand anatomy and Chapter 21.
- **Radial** dysplasia or **hypoplasia** is a congenital defect commonly referred to as "clubhand" and is often seen in conjunction with deformities of the thumb ranging from hypoplasia to complete absence of the radius. Due to the failure of the radius and adjacent soft tissues to fully develop, the hand is medially deranged. The degree of derangement is determined by the size or absence of the radius.
- There are four classifications based on the degree of deformity (Figures 19-24 and 19-25A).
  - Type I: Elbow and proximal radius are normal; distal radius physis is deficient

PROCEDURE 19-14 (continued)

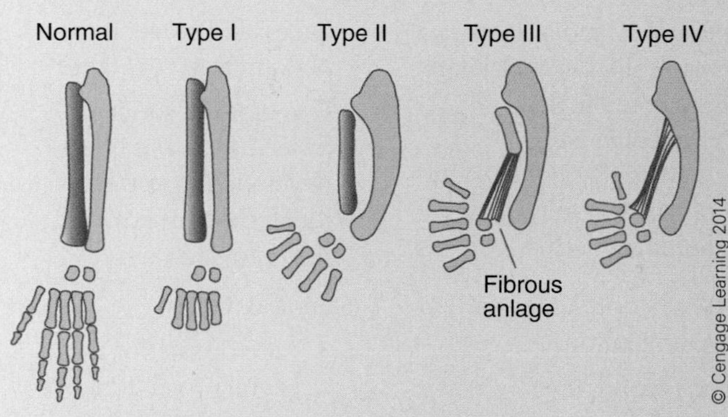

Figure 19-24 Radial dysplasia

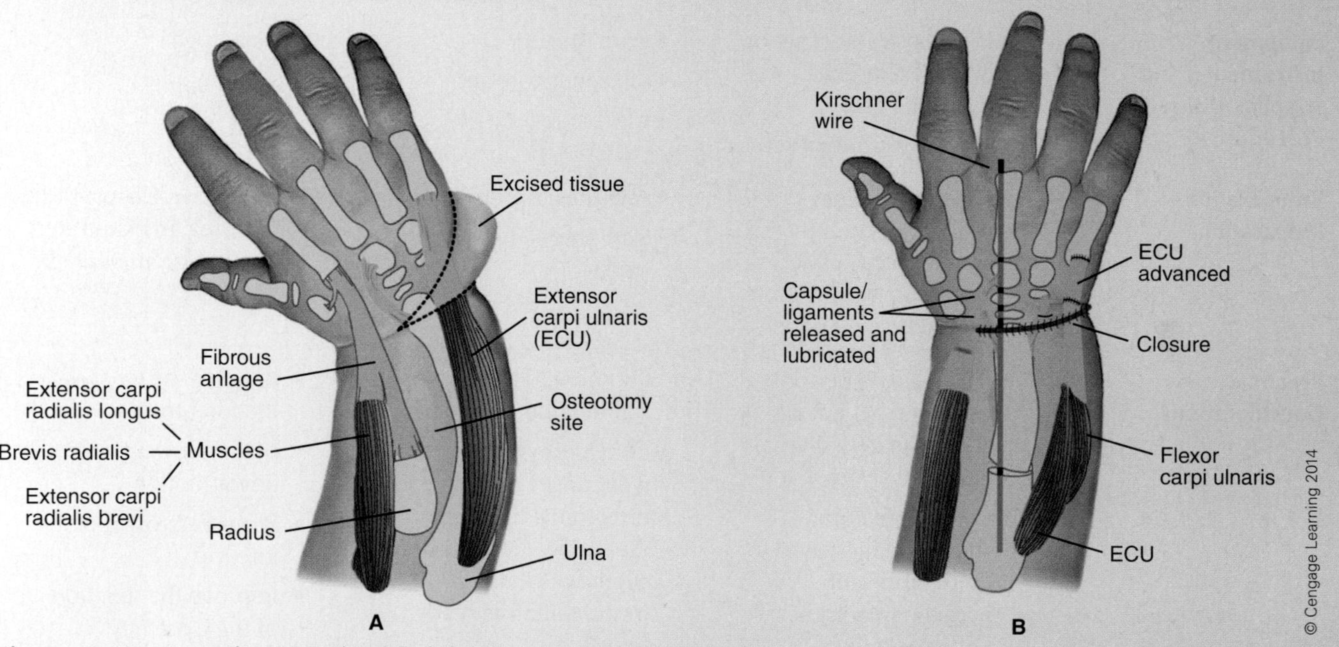

Figure 19-25 Centralization of a radial dysplasia: (A) Defect, (B) correction

and radius is abnormally short; soft tissue contractions limit motion; thumb may show varying degrees of hypoplasia.

- Type II: Hypoplastic radius; unstable wrist and radially deviated
- Type III: Partial absence of radius
- Type IV: Most common type; complete absence of the radius often accompanied by absence of the radial carpi and first and second metacarpals; elbow may be stiff; severe soft tissue contractures on the radial and volar side of the wrist and, if not treated, the contractures worsen with age and growth.

(continues)

PROCEDURE 19-14 (continued)

	• Repair of radial dysplasia, also called clubbed hand, is a complicated procedure and, depending on the extent of the deformity, may require an orthopedic and plastic surgeon to perform the procedure. • Five types of surgical procedures have been developed to correct radial dysplasia: soft tissue release; centralization (procedure performed most often and described here); replacement of the deficient radius; tendon transfer; **arthrodesis**.

Preoperative Diagnostic Tests and Procedures	• History and physical examination
	  • Preoperative measurements of the degree of active and passive motion of the digits and wrist recorded.
	Standard X-rays
	  • Anteroposterior and lateral projection, including the elbow and hand
	  • Degree of ulnar bow is calculated from the lateral X-ray.
	Angulation of more than 30° requires planning of corrective osteotomy when performing the centralization procedure.

Equipment, Instruments, and Supplies Unique to Procedure	• Hand instrument set or major orthopedic instrument set • Plastic instrument set • Wire driver • Kirschner wire set • #15 blades × 3–4 • Marking pen • Casting supplies (available)
Preoperative Preparation	• Position: Supine; procedure can be somewhat lengthy; therefore, the OR table should be well padded • Anesthesia: General • Skin prep: Fingertips to axilla • Draping: See Chapter 12 for draping an extremity; pediatric extremity drape will be used

Practical Considerations	• Procedure is performed when the patient is approximately 1 year of age.
	• OR temperature should be increased to help to prevent hypothermia in the pediatric patient.
	• Conversation and noise should be kept to a minimum when the patient is brought into the room to avoid startling the child.
	• Bony correction will consist of an osteotomy; therefore, the surgical technologist should have the instrumentation ready for use.
	• The goals of the procedure are to:
	  • Correct the radial deviation of the wrist
	  • Balance the wrist on the forearm
	  • Maintain wrist and finger motion
	  • Promote growth of the forearm
	  • Improve the function of the extremity

Surgical Procedure	1. Using the #15 knife blade, the surgeon makes a radial Z-plasty incision along the fold between the hand and forearm. **Procedural Consideration:** The incision allows for Z-plasty closure of the skin.
	2. The median nerve is identified and preserved at the skin fold at the wrist.
	3. Using the #15 knife blade and/or tenotomy scissors, the contracted fibrous bands are released to allow passive correction of the carpus that are centered over the ulna.

PROCEDURE 19-14 (continued)

4. A second incision is made beginning dorsally at the midline of the wrist and continues ulnarly in a transverse direction to the volar midline.

   Procedural Consideration: This incision exposes the carpus and allows the surgeon to excise the redundant ulnar tissue.

5. The flexor carpi ulnaris muscle and ulnar nerves are identified in order to avoid injury to the structures.

6. The carpus is exposed by a transverse arthrotomy with the #15 knife blade and extra fibrous tissue is excised from the ulnocarpal joint.

7. The distal ulna is squared off using the #15 knife blade and rasp, and inserted into a rectangular notch that has been created on the radial side of the carpus for centralization.

   Procedural Consideration: If the centralization cannot be achieved, the surgeon will examine the surgical site for additional contracted radial tissue to be excised. In severe cases of deformity, to affect centralization the surgeon may need to perform carpectomy and shave some bone off the distal ulna epiphysis but avoid damage to the growth plate.

8. Soft tissue stabilization is performed by distal advancement of the extensor carpi ulnaris insertion and transfer of the flexor carpi ulnaris to the dorsum.

9. A Kirschner wire (K-wire) is inserted through the carpus and third metacarpal into the ulnar shaft to reduce the wrist and hold it in position (Figure 19-25B).

   Procedural Consideration: If the ulnar bowing is more than 30°, a diaphyseal osteotomy is performed at the top of the deformity and the position of the osteotomy is maintained by the same K-wire used to maintain the centralization. The surgeon may need to use additional K-wires to aid in stability.

10. The surgical wound is thoroughly irrigated and the skin closed with interrupted sutures. The patient is placed in a restrictive dressing that may include a splint or cast.

Postoperative Considerations

Immediate Postoperative Care

- Patient is transported to the PACU.
- Patient will remain in hospital 1–2 days.
- Immediate active and passive digital motion is started.

Prognosis

- No complications: K-wire(s) are removed at least 8–10 weeks after the procedure; some surgeons may not remove until 6 months postoperative. The patient is fitted with a splint that is removed for physical therapy exercises with gradual decrease in wearing it over a 4- to 6-week period. The expectation is the patient will recover with an improvement of arm function.
- Complications: Postoperative SSI; infection at site of K-wire insertion; recurrence (most common procedural failure); fracture of regenerated bone; digital stiffness; vascular thrombosis of the microsurgical anastomosis

Wound Classification

- Wound Class I: Clean

PROCEDURE 19-15 Release of Syndactyly

Surgical Anatomy and Pathology

- See previous descriptions of hand anatomy.
- **Syndactyly**, or webbed digits, occurs when the digits of the hands or feet fail to separate.
    - Any combination of two or more digits may be partially or completely connected by a web of skin. It most often occurs in the hand and often bilaterally. The middle and ring finger are the most frequently affected digits of the hand. It may be a simple connection to the skin, or it may be more complex, involving conjoined bone and fingernails (Figure 19-26). But each finger contains its own blood vessels, tendons, bones, and nerves.

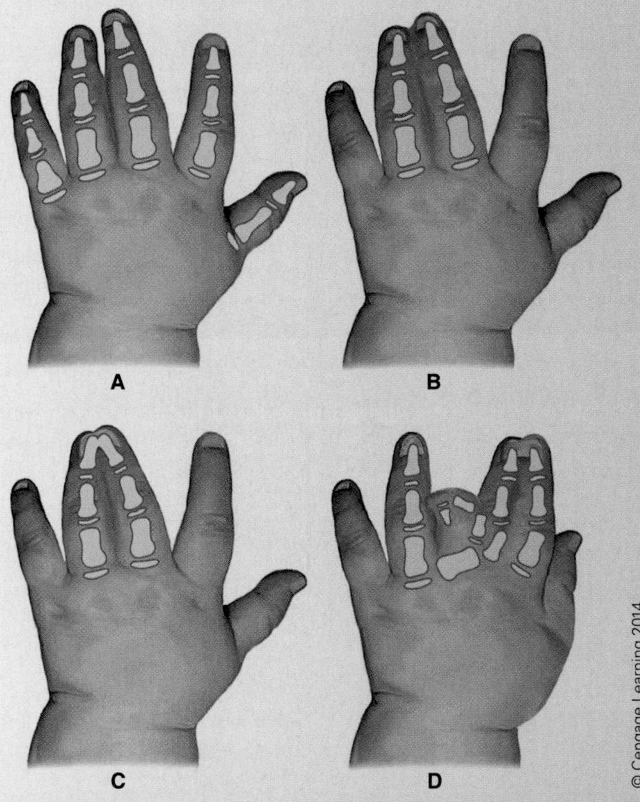

Figure 19-26 Syndactyly: (A) Simple, incomplete, (B) simple, complete, (C) complex, (D) complicated

Preoperative Diagnostic Tests and Procedures

- History and physical examination
- Standard X-rays

Equipment, Instruments, and Supplies Unique to Procedure

- Hand instrument set or orthopedic instrument set
- Plastic instrument set
- Dermatome (available)
- Skin graft supplies (available)
- Esmarch bandage
- #15 knife blades × 2–3
- ESU pencil with needle tip
- Bulb syringe
- Marking pen
- Pediatric tourniquet and insufflator
- Hand table attachment
- Pediatric hand/extremity drape
- Sterile unexposed X-ray film

Procedure 19-15 (continued)

Preoperative Preparation

- Position: Supine with arm extended on hand table attached to OR table
- Anesthesia: General
- Skin prep: Starting at site of syndactyly to include fingertips up to lower edge of tourniquet
- Draping: See Chapter 12 for draping an extremity.

Practical Considerations

- Procedure can be performed at any age, but usually after 1 year of age and before starting school.
- Surgical technologist should be prepared for a full-thickness skin graft (FTSG) to be taken. Site of skin graft is surgeon's preference, but often taken from wrist or forearm.
- Have X-rays in the OR.

Surgical Procedure

1. The surgeon marks the Z-plasty incisions with the marking pen on the volar and dorsal side of the hand.
2. Using a #15 knife blade, the surgeon makes a Z-plasty incision in the interdigital space on the volar and dorsal side of the hand (Figure 19-27A, B).

   Procedural Consideration: The Z-plasty incision allows for maximizing the size of the skin flaps for full coverage of the separated digits in order to reduce the future risk of developing contractures.

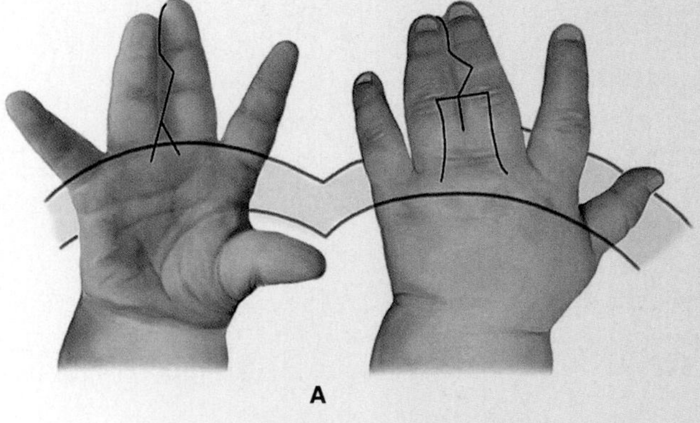

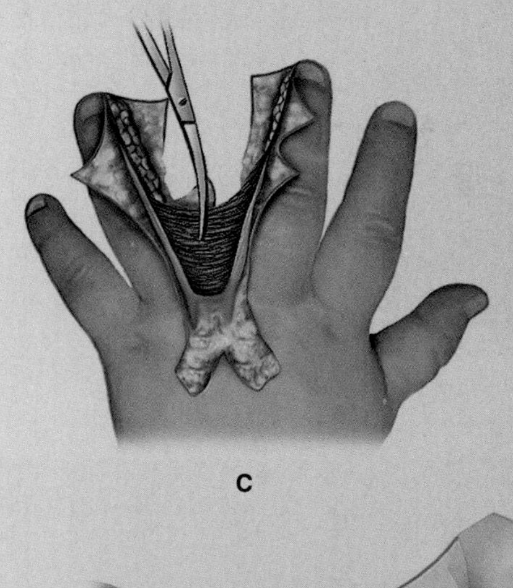

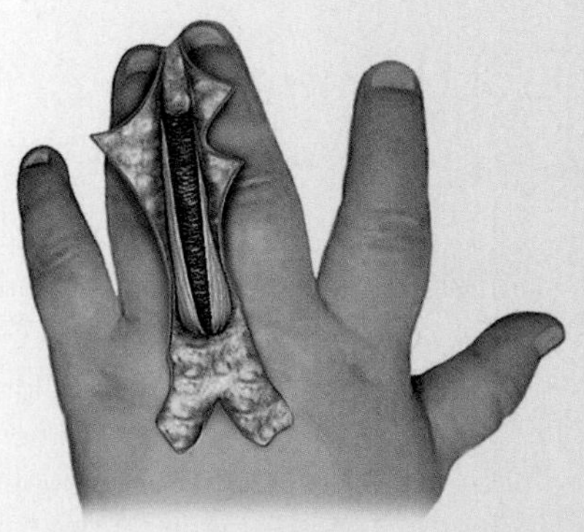

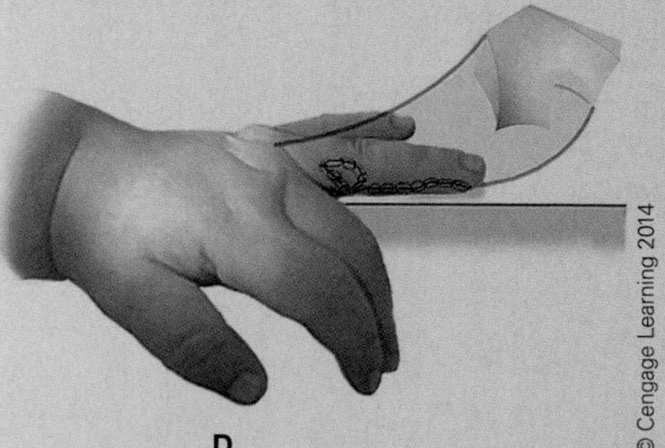

Figure 19-27 Release of syndactyly: (A) Planned incision, (B) dissection, (C) separation, (D) closure

(*continues*)

Procedure 19-15 (continued)

3. The neurovascular bundles are identified and prevented from injury.
4. Using the Metzenbaum or tenotomy scissors, the interdigital fibrous band of tissue is cut and excised, fully separating the digits (Figure 19-27C).

   Procedural Consideration: Hemostasis is achieved with the use of the ESU pencil with needle tip.
5. The full-thickness tissue flaps are slightly undermined with the tenotomy scissors to free up and form large enough flaps to fully cover the digits creating a new interdigital space.
6. The flaps are sutured into place using interrupted sutures (Figure 19-27D).
7. If the flaps do not fully cover the digits, an FTSG will be taken and sutured into place.

   Procedural Consideration: The surgeon will use the sterile unexposed X-ray film as a template to place on the exposed area of the digit(s) and draw an outline. The outline is used to cut the FTSG into the shape needed to cover the defect. The fat must be trimmed from the FTSG prior to being sutured into place.
8. Stent dressings are placed over the FTSGs.
9. A bulky dressing and splint are applied to the arm or a long arm cast.

Postoperative Considerations

Immediate Postoperative Care

- Patient is transported to the PACU.
- Patient's arm is kept elevated by a pillow.
- Patient is discharged same day of surgery.

Prognosis

- No complications: Patient is expected to gain full use of involved digits; dressing or cast is removed within 4–6 days and movement of the digits is encouraged.
- Complications: Postoperative SSI; contracture(s); recurrence

Wound Classification

- Class I: Clean

Procedure 19-16 Ablation of Radial Thumb and Collateral Ligament

Treatment for Polydactyly of Hand (Procedure Performed for Type III–VI Bifid Thumbs)

Surgical Anatomy and Pathology

- See previous descriptions of hand anatomy.
- Duplication of the digits is referred to as **poly**dactyly.
  - This can be a partial or complete additional digit or digits; it may affect the hands and/or feet and it may be unilateral (more common) or bilateral.
- The condition usually involves just the phalangeal bones.
- Fifth-finger duplications are the most common type (Figure 19-28).
- The procedure described here is for treating duplication of the thumb called bifid thumb. The duplication can be complete or partial.

PROCEDURE 19-16 (continued)

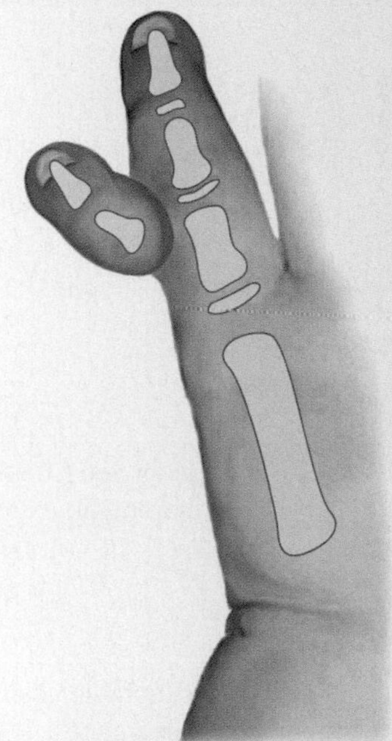

Figure 19-28 Polydactyly

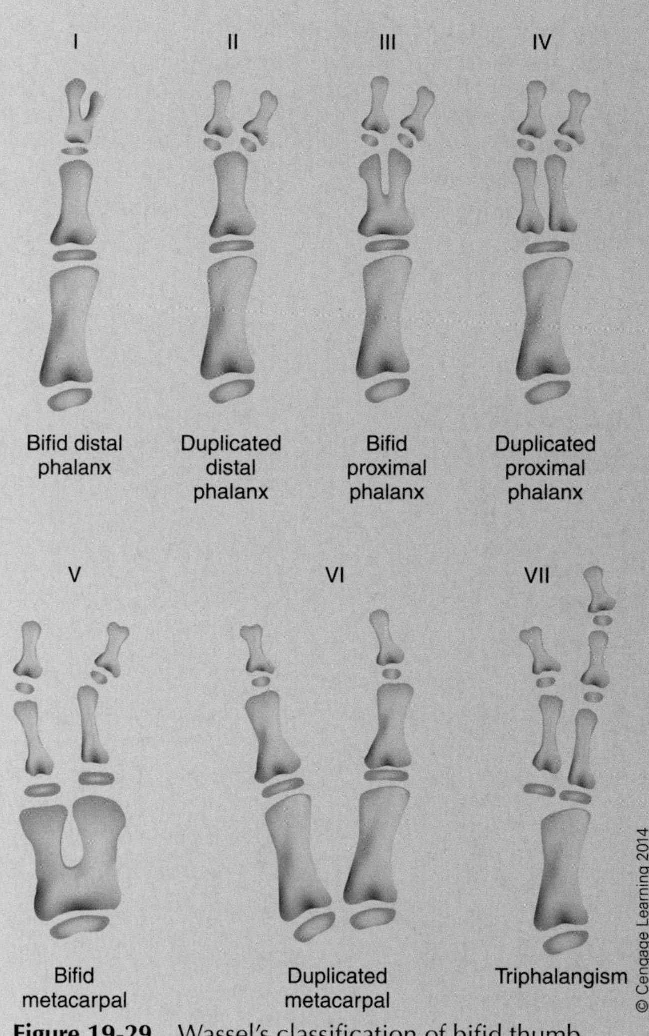

Figure 19-29 Wassel's classification of bifid thumb

- The cause of bifid thumb is unknown.
- The Wassel classification of bifid thumb is the most commonly used classification (Figure 19-29):
  - Type I: partial duplication of the distal phalanx and same epiphysis
  - Type II: complete duplication including epiphysis of distal phalanx
  - Type III: duplication of distal phalanx and bifurcation of the proximal phalanx
  - Type IV: most common type; complete duplication of the distal and proximal phalanges
  - Type V: Type IV with bifurcation of the metacarpal
  - Type VI: Type IV with duplication of metacarpal
  - Type VII: Varying degrees of duplication associated with triphalangeal thumb
- There is usually some hypoplasia of both thumbs, commonly worse in the thumb on the radial side, which is desired because this allows for preserving the all important ulnar collateral ligament when the radial-side thumb is removed. The nail may be one conjoined nail or each thumb has a nail.

(continues)

Procedure 19-16 (continued)

Preoperative Diagnostic Tests and Procedures	• History and physical examination	• Standard X-rays: Anteroposterior and oblique	
Equipment, Instruments, and Supplies Unique to Procedure	• Hand instrument set or orthopedic instrument set • Esmarch bandage • #15 knife blades × 2–3 • ESU pencil with needle tip	• Wire driver • K-wires • Bulb syringe • Marking pen • Pediatric tourniquet and insufflator	• Hand table attachment • Pediatric hand/extremity drape • Casting supplies
Preoperative Preparation	• Position: Supine with arm extended on hand table attached to OR table • Anesthesia: General	• Skin prep: Starting at site of polydactyly to include fingertips up to lower edge of tourniquet	• Draping: See Chapter 12 for draping an extremity.

Practical Considerations	• Procedure performed usually at 1½ years of age, but before the age of 5.
	• OR temperature should be increased to help to prevent hypothermia in the pediatric patient.
	• Conversation and noise should be kept to a minimum when the
		patient is brought into the room to avoid startling the child.
		• Have X-rays in the OR.
		• Goals of the procedure are:
		  • Restoration of normal hand function
		  • Unrestricted growth of the extremity
			• Acceptable cosmetic appearance
			• The parent(s) or guardian(s) of the child should be preoperatively told that the remaining thumb on the operative side will always be slightly hypoplastic as compared to the nonoperative thumb.

Surgical Procedure

1. The surgeon marks the incision with the marking pen.
2. Using the #15 knife blade, the surgeon makes the skin incision over the dorsal aspect of the radialmost thumb.
3. The incision exposes the abductor pollicis brevis tendon where it inserts into the proximal phalanx of the radialmost thumb; this tendon must be preserved. The incision also exposes the intrinsic tendon and radial and ulnar collateral ligaments (Figure 19-30A).
4. The radial collateral ligament is detached distally from the phalanx that will be excised (Figure 19-30B).
5. The radialmost thumb is removed with part of the metacarpal.
6. The remaining thumb is centralized over the articular surface and the radial collateral ligament and intrinsic tendon are sutured to the base of the proximal phalanx (Figure 19-30C).
7. A K-wire is placed across the joint to hold the alignment in place (Figure 19-30D).

PROCEDURE 19-16 (continued)

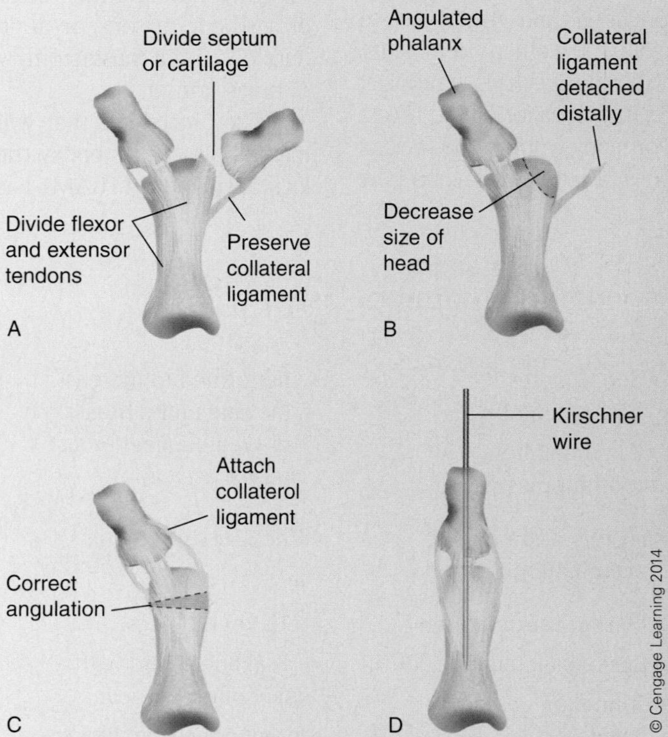

Figure 19-30 (A) Initial incision; (B) detachment of radial collateral ligament; (C) thumb centralized; ligament and tendon sutured in place, and (D) K-wire in place

8. The positions of the extensor and flexor tendons are confirmed to ensure they are in a central position along the thumb. If the position is not correct, the surgeon will resect and move the distal ends of the tendons to establish centralization and stability of the thumb.

   Procedural Consideration: The abductor pollicis brevis tendon can be advanced to the level of the extensor tendon and sutured in place with 5-0 Vicryl to achieve centralization and stability of the thumb.

9. The wound is thoroughly irrigated and the skin closed with 6-0 nylon interrupted sutures. A short arm thumb spica cast is applied.

Postoperative Considerations

Immediate Postoperative Care

- Patient is transported to the PACU.
- Arm is kept elevated on pillows.
- Patient will stay in hospital 1–2 days.

Prognosis

- No complications: Thumb is immobilized for about 4 weeks. At 4 weeks the K-wire is removed and a splint worn for 3–4 weeks. Patient is anticipated to have full restoration of normal hand function. Short-term physical therapy may be required.
- Complications: Postoperative SSI; infection at site of wire insertion; full function of hand not achieved; late angular deformity and instability; scar contracture; joint stiffness; narrowed first web space

Wound Classification

- Class I: Clean

BREAST PROCEDURES

The primary function of the female breast is to produce milk, which provides nutrition and vital immunities to the newborn and infant. In most cultures throughout time, this ability to lactate has been intimately linked to a woman's femininity. Today, however, especially in Western society, this symbol of femininity has less to do with the functionality of the breast than with its **aesthetic** qualities. For many women, the societal perception of what constitutes physical perfection—and how they measure up to that standard—has a profound impact on self-esteem. Thus surgery to improve the appearance of the breasts can have great psychological importance. The patient may desire to have the size of her breasts changed for medical or aesthetic reasons, or desire a breast reconstruction procedure because a mastectomy was performed for the treatment of breast cancer.

The procedures that will be discussed are augmentation mammoplasty, mastopexy, transverse rectus abdominis musculocutaneous flap (TRAM), and nipple reconstruction.

PROCEDURE 19-17 Augmentation Mammoplasty

Surgical Anatomy and Pathology	• See Chapter 14 for breast anatomy. • Augmentation mammoplasty is	performed to increase the size of the breast or create a new breast post-mastectomy.	
Preoperative Diagnostic Tests and Procedures	• History and physical examination	• Chest measurements	
Equipment, Instruments, and Supplies Unique to Procedure	• Plastic instrument set • Basic back table pack • Tunneling device (available) • Temporary implant sizers • Permanent implants • Endoscopic equipment (surgeon's preference) • 0° endoscope • Transverse chest drape	• #15 knife blades • Local anesthetic with epinephrine • Syringes and needles for local • Antibiotic to be mixed with saline irrigation fluid • Syringes and saline solution to fill implants	• Fiberoptic retractor set • ESU • ESU pencil with needle tip • Marking pen • Bulb syringe • Dressings, including postsurgical bra
Preoperative Preparation	• Position: Supine with arms placed on armboards • Anesthesia: Local anesthesia with mild sedation	• Skin prep: Neck to umbilicus to include entire chest; bilaterally as far as possible	• Draping: Four towels to square off both breasts; chest drape
Practical Considerations	• The two types of implants available are saline and silicone-gel filled. Saline-filled implants are still used slightly more often than the silicone gel–filled implants. • The implant is a bag composed of materials	that are inert to the body—the materials do not activate the body's defense mechanisms. • The implants are available in teardrop or round shape as well as various sizes. The implants are introduced into the body empty and	filled to a predetermined size by injecting saline (measured in cubic centimeters) through a port that the manufacturer has provided in the prosthesis. • Incision options are designed to minimize or

PROCEDURE 19-17 (continued)

completely hide the surgical scar. The options include the periareolar line, inframammary fold, axillary crease, or the umbilicus. The procedure is open or endoscopic.

- Prior to surgery, the surgeon should collaborate with the patient in developing realistic expectations regarding the size of the implant to be used, incision, and the planned outcomes.
- The procedure should not prevent a woman to breastfeed, although it should be kept in mind that there was minimal breast tissue present originally (except in the case of mastectomy, in which all breast tissue is absent).
- It should be noted that breast implants may distort radiographic studies, such as mammography, making accurate diagnosis of breast cancer more difficult.

Surgical Procedure—Periareolar Incision

1. The surgeon marks the circumferential incision with the marking pen.
2. The local anesthetic is injected.
3. The incision is made along the inferior border of the areola with the #15 knife blade.
4. The subcutaneous tissue is dissected toward the inferior border of the breast.
5. The pocket for the implant is created just under the existing breast tissue or beneath the pectoralis muscle. The subpectoral pocket may provide better long-term support of the prosthesis (Figure 19-31).

   Procedural Consideration: The surgeon may use the fiberoptic retractor during this step of the procedure. Steps 1–5 are repeated on the opposite breast.
6. The implant sizers are inserted into the pockets and inflated with saline to determine the final size of implants. The circulator will elevate the OR bed to raise the patient into a sitting position to allow the surgeon to evaluate the appearance and identify adjustments that should be made to the implants and/or pocket.
7. The implant sizers are removed and pocket adjustments made if necessary.
8. The surgical technologist confirms the size of implants with the surgeon and communicates the information to the circulator who facilitates transfer of the implants to the sterile field with the surgical technologist.

   Procedural Consideration: While the implants are being transferred to the sterile field, the surgeon will irrigate the pocket with the saline–antibiotic irrigation solution using the bulb syringe.
9. The surgeon rolls up the implant, inserts into the pocket, unrolls, and positions it. The surgical technologist provides the surgeon with a saline-filled syringe to fill the implant.
10. The inferior border of the breast tissue is sutured to the pectoralis fascia and the periareolar incision is closed using a subcuticular running stitch.
11. 4 × 4 dressing sponges are placed and postsurgical bra is used to provide support.

(continues)

PROCEDURE 19-17 (continued)

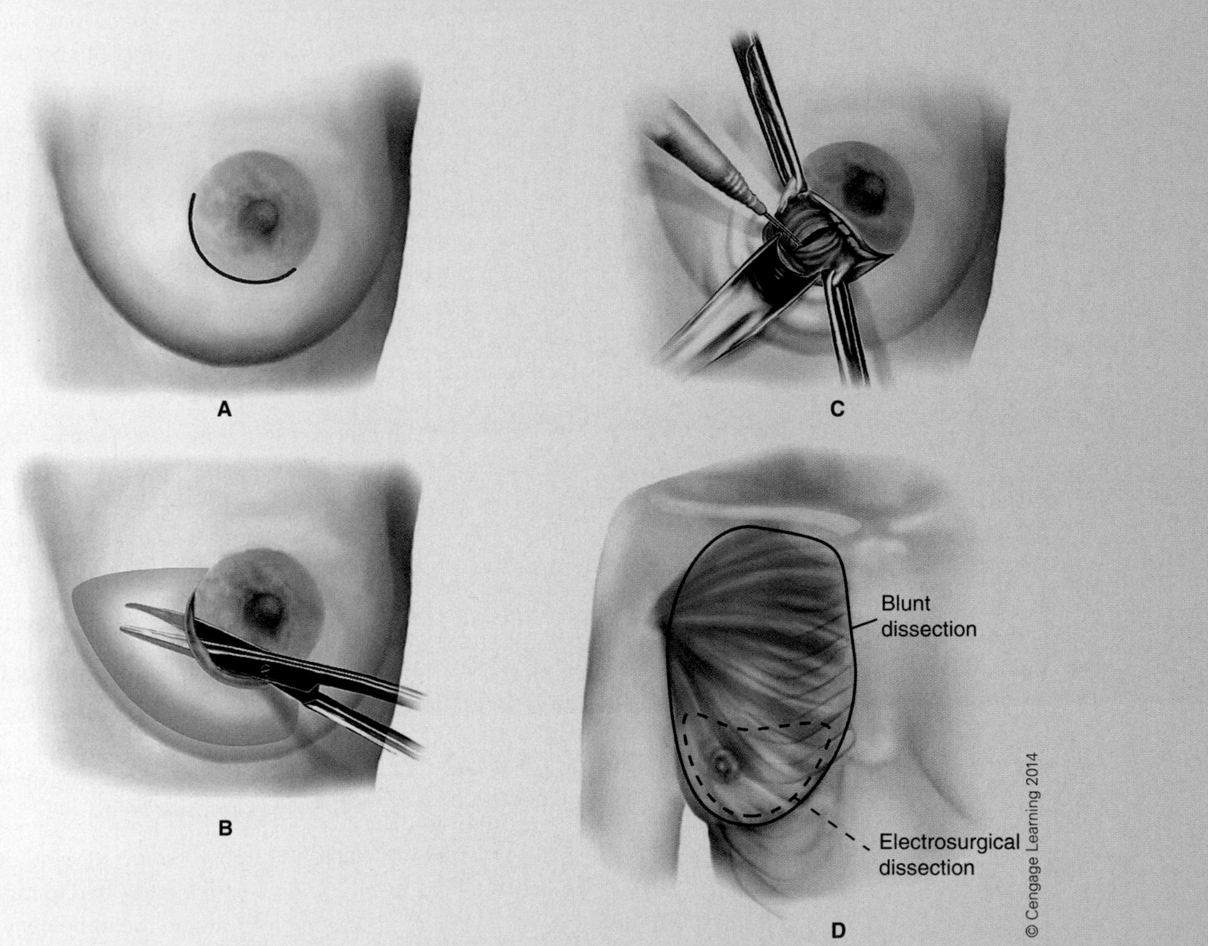

Figure 19-31 Augmentation mammoplasty: (A) Areloar incision, (B) creation of pocket, (C) pectoral muscle incision, (D) implant position

Postoperative Considerations

Immediate Postoperative Care

- Patient is transported to PACU unless procedure was performed in surgeon's office.
- Patient is discharged same day.
- OTC analgesics

Prognosis

- No complications: Patient is expected to have a full recovery with excellent cosmetic results; return to full normal activities in 5–7 days.
- Complications: Postoperative SSI; less-than-desired cosmetic results; visible scar

Wound Classification

- Class I: Clean

PROCEDURE 19-18 Transverse Rectus Abdominis Musculocutaneous Flap (TRAM)

Surgical Anatomy and Pathology

- See Chapter 14 for description of breast anatomy.

The following is provided in paragraph format to facilitate the presentation of the information.

Breast removal due to cancer or other disease may be one of the most psychologically devastating procedures that a woman may have to endure. Along with dealing with the diagnosis of cancer, many women feel that they have been stripped of their womanhood. Reconstruction mammoplasty can help to restore a woman's appearance, positive self-image, and quality of life.

For some patients, breast restoration may begin at the same time that the mastectomy is performed. The reconstructive process can involve more than one procedure. The nipple and areolar reconstruction is often the final stage. Some patients may choose to have surgery performed on the otherwise unaffected breast to gain symmetry. For patients with advanced malignancies, reconstruction may not be recommended.

A description of the different types of mastectomy can be found in Chapter 14. Several options for breast reconstruction exist, depending on the type of mastectomy that has been performed. These options include:

- *Implant reconstruction:* If the patient has enough remaining tissue, the surgeon may insert an implant similar to those used for augmentation mammoplasty under the existing muscle. Otherwise, a temporary device called a tissue expander is inserted in the same location that the final implant will be located. This temporary device allows for fluid to be gradually added at intervals to stretch the existing tissue. When the desired result is achieved, the permanent implant is substituted.
- *Flap reconstruction:* Flap reconstruction involves transferring tissue from one part of the body to another. The tissue may be taken from the abdomen, back, buttocks, or thigh. Two types of flap surgery exist.

1. *Free flap reconstruction* involves totally removing the tissue to be transferred from its original location and transplanting it to the chest. The blood vessels must be microscopically reconnected at the new site. The patient will not experience any sensation to the grafted area.
2. *Pedicle flap reconstruction* allows the tissue to be transferred to remain attached to its blood supply. It is relocated via a tunnel under the existing skin. The flap consists of the skin (if necessary), fat, and muscle. The flap may be used to create a pocket to accept an implant, or the tissue itself may create the new breast mound. The latissimus dorsi musculocutaneous flap and the TRAM flap techniques are the two most commonly used pedicle flaps (Figure 19-32).

Pedicle flap reconstruction using a TRAM flap will be used to illustrate breast reconstruction. Patients who are excessively overweight or those who have previously undergone abdominal surgery may not be good candidates for this type of reconstruction. In addition to the items previously mentioned, the surgical technologist should consider the following:

- If the reconstruction is to be performed at the same time as the mastectomy, it may be necessary for the sterile surgical team members to use a new set of sterile supplies for the reconstructive portion of the procedure to prevent the spread (seeding) of cancer cells.
- Tissue repair material such as synthetic mesh may be needed to reinforce the donor site.

(*continues*)

PROCEDURE 19-18 (continued)

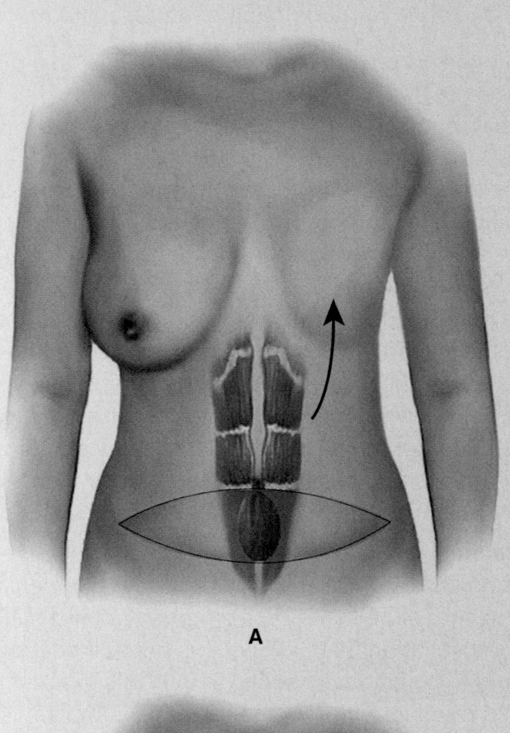

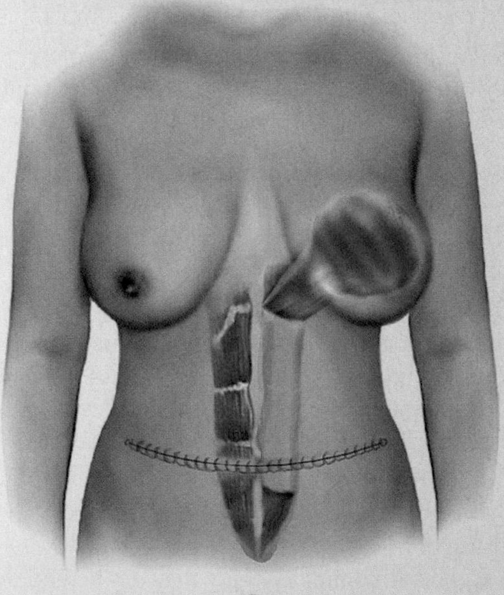

Figure 19-32 TRAM flap reconstruction: (A) Abdominal incision, (B) TRAM flap rotated into position

- Closed wound drainage systems may be used at both surgical sites.
- A Doppler with a sterile probe should be available to identify the location of the major blood vessels serving the flap.

Breast reconstruction often immediately follows mastectomy and the patient remains under general anesthesia. The initial prep and draping should be done to

PROCEDURE 19-18 (continued)

accommodate the secondary procedure. Therefore, the entire chest and abdomen should be exposed. The exposed area should include the natural breast to use for comparison. The general surgeon and the plastic surgeon will have collaborated prior to the mastectomy regarding the type of mastectomy to be performed and the planned breast incision. Often, the general and plastic surgeons work together for the entire procedure, changing roles as primary surgeon and assistant as the case progresses. The general surgeon terminates the mastectomy portion of the procedure following removal of the breast and axillary contents. Hemostasis is achieved and the wound is left open and covered with a sterile towel. At this point the TRAM procedure is performed.

Preoperative Diagnostic Tests and Procedures	• Diagnosis obtained by history and physical as well as by direct examination		
Equipment, Instruments, and Supplies Unique to Procedure	• ESU • Doppler with sterile probe • Basic laparotomy set • Basic plastic instrument set	• Skin graft instrumentation (if nipple–areolar reconstruction is performed at the time of TRAM)	• Basic laparotomy back table pack • #10 and #15 blades • Synthetic mesh • Surgeon specific suture, drains, and dressings
Preoperative Preparation	• Position: Supine with arms placed on armboards • Anesthesia: General	• Skin prep: Neck to mid-thigh and bilaterally as far as possible	• Draping: Drapes are placed in a wide fashion to allow exposure of entire chest and abdomen.
Practical Considerations	• If the TRAM immediately follows a mastectomy procedure, the surgical technologist will need to prepare two procedural setups. • The surgical technologist should confirm with the surgeon if nipple reconstruction will be done as part of the	procedure or performed at a later date. • After the flap is positioned over the mastectomy site, the surgeon will trim excess skin with subcutaneous tissue. The surgical technologist should save this skin and	subcutaneous tissue for possible later use. • Due to the wide area of the surgical site, the surgical technologist should keep the operative site free of instruments and aid in maintaining the control of the suction tubing and electrosurgical pencil.

Surgical Procedure

1. Using a #10 blade, the surgeon makes an elliptical incision from iliac crest to the other iliac crest. The superior incision includes the umbilicus and the inferior incision is just above the symphysis pubis.
2. Using blunt dissection and long Metzenbaum scissors, the surgeon creates a subcutaneous tunnel from the abdominal incision to where the mastectomy was performed (Figure 19-33).

(continues)

Procedure 19-18 (continued)

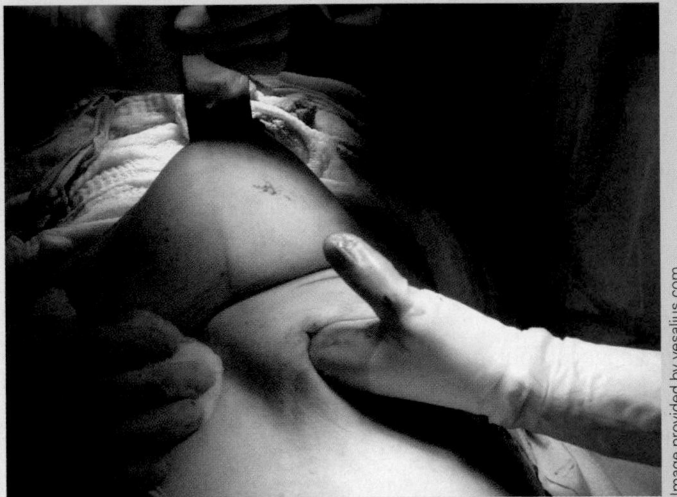

Figure 19-33 Tunnel dissection

Procedural Consideration: The surgical technologist should keep clean moist lap sponges on the field at all times during the dissection and tunneling phase of the procedure.

3. The surgeon dissects down to the anterior rectus sheath with the use of electrosurgery and Metzenbaum scissors.

   Procedural Consideration: The surgical technologist should also keep the cautery tip clean. Due to the frequency of its use during the procedure, in particular when the surgeon is dissecting down to the anterior rectus sheath and incising the sheath, the tip may become clogged with charred tissue. If it is not kept clean, the effectiveness of the tip will diminish.

4. A transverse incision is made into the anterior rectus sheath and the inferior edge of the rectus abdominis muscle is transected.

5. Using the sterile Doppler probe, the superior and inferior epigastric arteries are identified. The superior vessels are preserved in order to provide continual perfusion to the flap. The inferior epigastric artery is double clamped, cut and ligated with the surgeon's preferred suture.

   Procedural Consideration: The surgical technologist should have the sterile Doppler probe available for use throughout the procedure.

6. Dissection continues superiorly, developing the pedicle of rectus muscle up to the costal level.

7. Using his or her hands, the surgeon passes the flap through the subcutaneous tunnel in a superior direction and positions it on the mastectomy site. The surgeon performs this step of the procedure in such a manner as to preserve the arterial and venous supply to the newly created breast. Any compromise in circulation could cause the flap to become ischemic and slough.

Procedure 19-18 (continued)

8. Using Metzenbaum scissors and a #15 blade, the surgeon trims excess skin with subcutaneous tissue from the flap. The surgeon shapes the breast, using the nonoperative exposed breast as a template to achieve as much symmetry as possible.

   Procedural Consideration: The surgical technologist should save the excess skin because the surgeon can use the subcutaneous tissue as an aid in adding more tissue to the breast mound and shaping it.

9. The abdominal wound is closed. The anterior rectus sheath is closed with absorbable suture. The skin is closed with a subcuticular closure or skin staples. The first closed wound drainage system is placed.

   Procedural Consideration: The surgical technologist should have synthetic mesh available for use in closure of the abdominal wound.

10. The surgeon visually inspects the vascular status of the flap for color and gently touches it to check for warmth. The surgeon may perform further shaping of the breast.

    Procedural Consideration: The surgeon may use the sterile Doppler probe as an aid in assessing the vascular status of the flap prior to closure.

11. The flap is secured to the chest wall with synthetic absorbable suture and the skin flaps are closed with a nonabsorbable suture. The second closed wound drainage system is placed in the wound and the distal end of the drain is brought out at the lateral edge through a stab wound.

12. The abdominal wound dressing is placed. A loose fluff-style dressing is placed on the chest. A postsurgical bra may be used for support.

    Procedural Consideration: The fluffs should be carefully applied to the chest to prevent placing any unnecessary pressure on the wound that might compromise the circulation to the flap. A Montgomery strap may be used to keep abdominal dressings in place.

13. This completes the first stage of reconstruction. Rarely is nipple–areolar reconstruction planned as part of this first stage. If performed at this time, an FTSG is taken from the postauricular area and used to create the areola. An FTSG is taken from the labia to create the nipple (see Procedure 19-19, Nipple Reconstruction).

Postoperative Considerations

Immediate Postoperative Care

- Patient is transported to the PACU.
- A pillow should be available for the patient to splint the abdominal wound for protection and comfort when coughing. The patient should be educated on the use of the splint when in bed and when ambulatory.
- The patient is expected to remain hospitalized for several days.
- Narcotics will be needed for initial pain relief.
- Ambulation will be painful but should be encouraged.
- The patient should be educated on wound and drain care. The drains will be removed 10–14 days postoperatively.

Prognosis

- No complications: Patient is expected to return to normal activity in 4–6 weeks. There will be permanent visible scars on the abdomen and breast. However, most patients are aesthetically satisfied with the results of the breast reconstruction.
- Complications: Postoperative SSI; hemorrhage; blood supply to flap is compromised, causing necrosis and sloughing of tissue; dehiscence or evisceration of the abdominal wall

Wound Classification

- Class I: Clean

Procedure 19-19 Nipple Reconstruction

Surgical Anatomy and Pathology	• See Chapter 14 for anatomy. • See Procedure 19-18 for pathology.
Preoperative Diagnostic Tests and Procedures	• See Procedure 19-18.

Equipment, Instruments, and Supplies Unique to Procedure	• Dermatome
	• Sterile tattoo equipment and needle
	  • Disposable needle or nondisposable stainless steel needle that would need to be sterilized according to manufacturer's instructions.Tube (also called a grip): The needle is inserted into the tube and held by the surgeon to perform the tattooing. The tube can be disposable or stainless steel.
	  • Tattoo machine: Connects to the tube; part of the pathway for delivering electricity; nondisposable.
	  • Clip cord: Power cord (nondisposable); clip cord and tattoo machine sterilized according to manufacturer's instructions
	  • Power supply
	• Sterile tattoo supplies, including ink of various colors
	• Marking pen
	• #15 blades × 3

Preoperative Preparation	• See Procedure 19-18.
Practical Considerations	• Nipple reconstruction may be performed at the time of breast reconstruction. However, some surgeons prefer to wait until the breast tissue from the reconstruction procedure has healed, swelling has disappeared, and reconstructed breasts are in normal anatomical position. The procedure is usually performed 8–10 weeks post-reconstruction. • The surgical technologist should confirm the graft site with the surgeon. An FTSG will be taken. • The surgical technologist must be familiar with the tattooing equipment in order to correctly set it up and troubleshoot malfunctions.
Surgical Procedure	1. Surgeon outlines the incision with the marking pen. The nipple design is composed of two wing flaps and a central flap (Figure 19-34A). **Procedural Consideration:** The width of the two wing flaps determines the length of projection of the new nipple and the diameter of the central flap determines the diameter and top of the new nipple. The wing flap design permits primary closure and the central flap for forming the tip of the nipple as well as providing a circular site for wrapping the wing flaps into place. The base of the central flap must not be divided since the blood supply to this flap is from the underlying subcutaneous tissue.
	2. Using the #15 knife blade, the wing flaps are elevated from the subcutaneous tissue (Figure 19-34A). **Procedural Consideration:** Some fatty tissue is left on the underside of the wing flaps.
	3. The donor sites are closed, leaving the wing and central flaps on the outside.

Procedure 19-19 (continued)

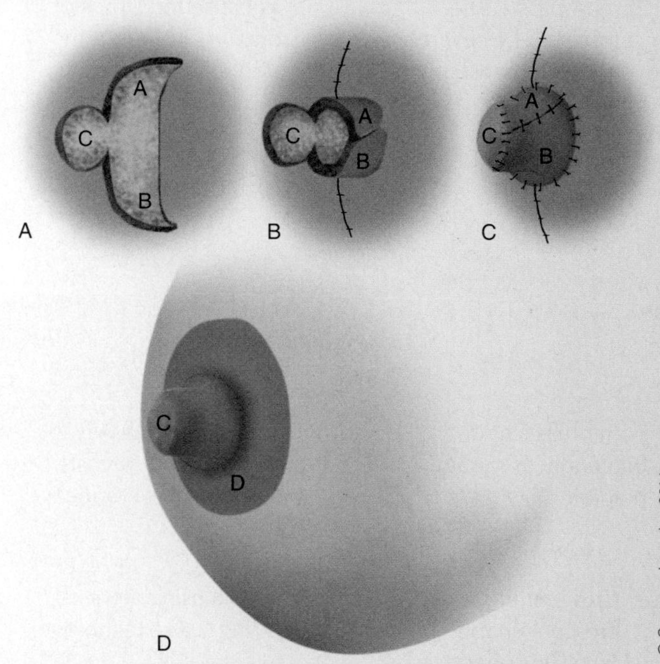

Figure 19-34 (A) Surgeon outlines and makes incision to elevate the wing flaps, (B and C) wing flaps are wrapped around central flap to create nipple, (D) circumference of the areola is marked

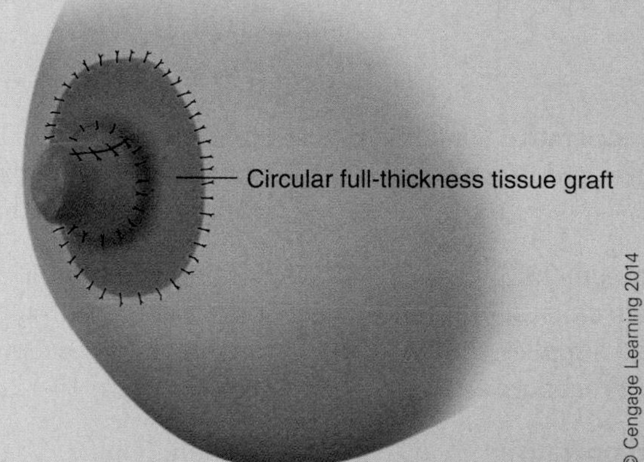

Figure 19-35 Areolar skin graft held in place with sutures

4. The wing flaps are wrapped around the central flap, creating the nipple (Figure 19-34B, C).
5. A paper template of the nonoperative breast's areola circumference is prepared. The template is centered on the new nipple and the circumference marked (Figure 19-34D).
6. The inner portion of what will be the new areola is deepithelialized from the areolar border to the center toward the new nipple using the #15 knife blade.
7. Using the dermatome knife, an FTSG is taken from the upper inner thigh or labial fold.
8. The graft is cut to size and secured using interrupted sutures (Figure 19-35).
9. The surgeon mixes the tattoo ink to achieve the desired color and, using the tattoo equipment, creates the areolar tattoo.
10. The graft is held in place with a nonadherent dressing.

Postoperative Considerations

Immediate Postoperative Care

- Transport to PACU and discharge; procedure may be performed in surgeon's office and the patient is also immediately discharged.

Prognosis

- No complications: Patient is expected to have good cosmetic results. Dressing is removed on postoperative day 6. Patient is followed for 6 months to monitor nipple healing, projection, pigmentation, sensation, anatomical position, and patient's level of satisfaction.
- Complications: Postoperative SSI; FTSG does not take; patient's level of satisfaction with results is not achieved

Wound Classification

- Class I: Clean

Procedure 19-20 Mastopexy: Anchor Technique

Surgical Anatomy and Pathology	• See Chapter 14 for anatomy. • Mastopexy is performed to correct breast ptosis. The ptosis can be severe enough to cause lower back problems as well as cause the straps of braziers to indent the skin, causing chronic discomfort.
Preoperative Diagnostic Tests and Procedures	• History and physical examination as well as by direct examination
Equipment, Instruments, and Supplies Unique to Procedure	• Routine equipment, instruments, and supplies for a plastic procedure; see Procedure 19-17.
Preoperative Preparation	• Position: Supine • Anesthesia: General • Skin prep: Neck to umbilicus to include both breasts and bilaterally as far as possible • Draping: Four towels to square off both breasts; transverse chest drape
Practical Considerations	• The skin incision and breast lift technique to be used depend on the degree of ptosis and the extent of the procedure. The surgical technologist should confirm with the surgeon the surgical plan for the patient to ensure all needed instrumentation is available. The procedure discussed here is a full mastopexy using the anchor technique, which is the most commonly used. • Crescent lift: A crescent-shaped piece of tissue superior to the areola is excised and the tissue is reapproximated higher, thus lifting the breast. • Benelli lift: A periareolar incision is made removing a doughnut-shaped piece of tissue and the surrounding tissue is reapproximated to the areola using a purse-string suture technique. • Benelli-lollipop lift: Similar to the Benelli lift, a keyhole incision is made that involves a periareolar incision that extends in a straight line from under the middle of the areola to the mammary crease. • Often augmentation mammoplasty is performed at the time of the mastoplexy procedure.
Surgical Procedure	1. The surgeon marks the planned incision with the marking pen on both breasts (Figure 19-36).

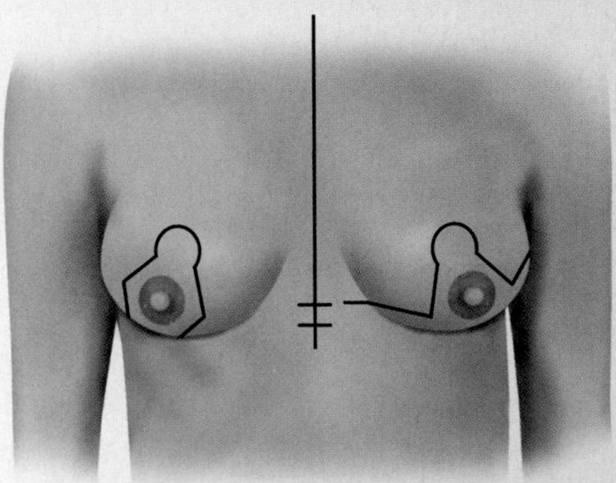

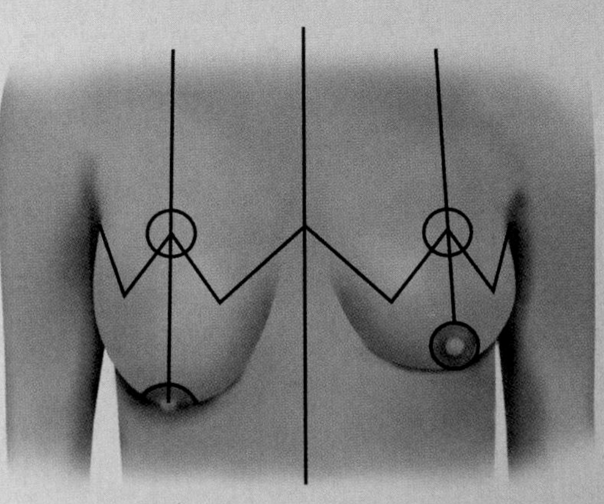

Figure 19-36 Surgeon marks the planned incisions on both breasts

PROCEDURE 19-20 (continued)

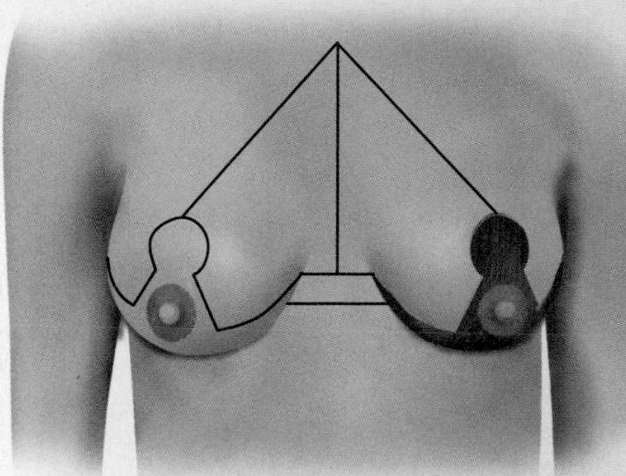

A

Full mastopexy. Anchor-shaped pieces of breast envelope removed.

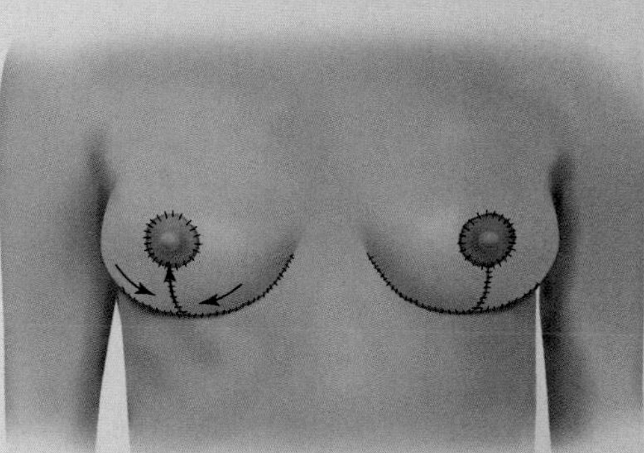

B

Breast envelope is pulled and sutured together.

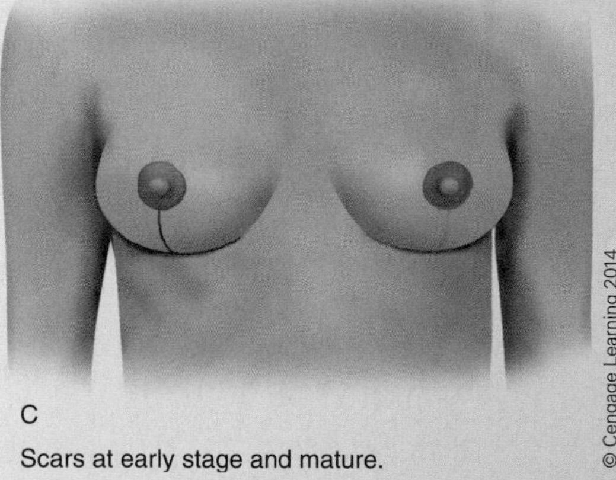

C

Scars at early stage and mature.

Figure 19-37 (A)Anchor-shaped incision made with #15 knife blade, (B) skin is drawn together and reapproximated to lift the breast, (C) example of scars on left at early stages of healing and scars on right side at late stages of healing

Procedural Consideration: The incision may have been marked in the preoperative holding area.

2. Using the #15 knife blade, the surgeon makes an anchor-shaped incision that starts at the base of the areola and extends at an angle vertically on both sides and upward to form the boundaries of where the nipple will be relocated (Figure 19-37A).

   Procedural Consideration: The nipple is removed and relocated when performing a full mastopexy.

3. The excess dermal tissue is excised from within the borders of the incision including removal of the nipple.

4. The skin is drawn together and reapproximated, lifting the breast to a new position, and the nipple repositioned (Figure 19-37B).

   Procedural Consideration: If augmentation mammoplasty is indicated, it is now performed.

5. Fluffs are used for the dressing and a postsurgical bra is used to hold the dressings and breasts in position while healing takes place.

(continues)

Procedure 19-20 (continued)

Postoperative Considerations	**Immediate Postoperative Care** • Patient is transported to the PACU. • Patient will be discharged the same day of surgery. • The head of bed should be slightly elevated as patient recovers from anesthesia to help in reducing swelling.	**Prognosis** • No complications: Sutures will remain in place for approximately 10 days. Patient will need someone at home to provide care during the first 48 hours after surgery. Patient is expected to have a full recovery and return to normal activities as well	as excellent cosmetic results (Figure 19-37C). • Complications: Postoperative SSI; stretching of scars over time due to tension, large implant, improper support during healing phase, poor tissue elasticity due to age or illness. **Wound Classification** • Class I: Clean

ABDOMINAL PROCEDURES

Plastic abdominal procedures are performed to enhance the patient's image of his or her body. The procedures should not be confused with panniculectomy, which is removal of the apron of abdominal fat in the formerly obese patient who lost a large amount of weight. The two commonly performed procedures are liposuction and abdominoplasty.

Procedure 19-21 Tumescent Liposuction

Surgical Anatomy and Pathology	• See previous procedures for anatomy and Chapter 14 for abdominal anatomy. • Liposuction is performed for the	removal of subcutaneous fat deposits to provide the patient with a pleasing cosmetic appearance. It provides a means of contouring those areas of the body that have	not responded to changes in diet and exercise. The procedure may be performed on virtually any area of the body.
Preoperative Diagnostic Tests and Procedures	• History and physical examination as well as direct observation		
Equipment, Instruments, and Supplies Unique to Procedure	• Minor instrument tray • Large-bore suction tubing • Mercedes suction cannulae, various sizes 3–10 mm • Marking pen	• High-pressure vacuum/ liposuction unit (Figure 19-38) • 30-mL syringes × 2 • 25-gauge needles × 2 • Medications and solutions to mix tumescent solution:	saline, 0.5% lidocaine with epinephrine, Wydase • Abdominal girdle • Laser (surgeon's preference) • Ultrasound machine (surgeon's preference)

PROCEDURE 19-21 (continued)

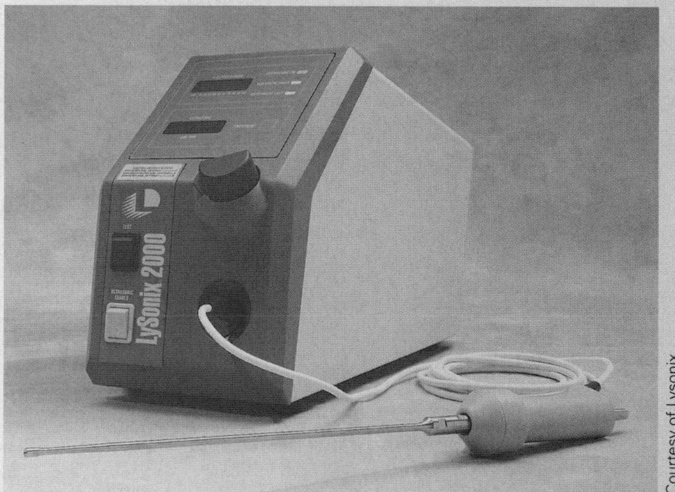

Figure 19-38 Liposuction equipment

Preoperative Preparation	• Position: Supine; keep in mind that if the procedure requires multiple incision sites, the patient may need to be repositioned.	• Anesthesia: Traditional liposuction–general; tumescent liposuction–local with mild sedation	• Skin prep: Nipple line to mid-thigh and bilaterally as far as possible • Draping: Square off entire abdomen with four towels; laparotomy drape.
Practical Considerations	• Other procedures may be performed along with liposuction, such as abdominoplasty. • Liposuction requires minimal preparation time for the surgical technologist and utilizes very few instruments. • Test all equipment prior to the patient entering the OR. • The surgical technologist should mix the	tumescent solution when preparing the instrumentation and equipment: 250 mL saline, 75 mL lidocaine with epinephrine, 2 mL Wydase. The 30-mL syringes should be used to draw up the solution and kept filled throughout the procedure. • The presence of the local anesthetic may	allow the patient to be awake with mild sedation rather than under general anesthesia and may provide some immediate post-operative pain control. The vasoconstrictive properties of the epinephrine provide intraoperative hemostasis. The mixture liquefies the fat to make suctioning easier.

Surgical Procedure

1. The surgeon marks the area to be suctioned with a nonerasable marker (Sharpie).

   Procedural Consideration: This may be done in the preoperative holding area.

2. The surgeon injects the tumescent solution and waits a few seconds for it to take effect.

   Procedural Consideration: The surgical technologist must keep close track of the amount of solution that is injected.

(continues)

Procedure 19-21 (continued)

3. Using the #15 knife blade, the surgeon makes the smallest possible incision in the lower abdomen following a crease and skin lines.
4. The smallest-diameter cannula is inserted and maneuvered forward. The liposuction machine is turned on and the surgeon begins to suction out the adipose tissue by making several jabbing passes parallel to the skin.

   Procedural Considerations: This blunt dissection technique contributes to further loosening the fat globules, which are then removed by the suction through the openings at the distal end of the cannula. Depending on the situation, the surgeon may request a larger suction cannula as the procedure progresses.

   If using laser liposuction, the laser probe is inserted through the cannula and vaporizes rather than extracts the adipose tissue.

   Ultrasonic liposuction uses ultrasound waves applied with a titanium probe to break down the walls of the fat cells, liquefying them for easier removal with the suction. Both of these methods may decrease the patient's risk for hemorrhage and reduce postoperative pain, swelling, and bruising.
5. When the surgeon is satisfied with the amount of tissue that has been removed, the cannula is removed and the wound closed.

   Procedural Consideration: The suctioned material is collected in a graduated canister. Close monitoring of the volume of adipose extracted is very important because excessive suctioning (greater than 1000 mL) can cause hypovolemia and other fluid/hemodynamic complications.
6. According to the amount of tissue that has been removed, the dressing may be as simple as a self-adherent bandage. A more complex pressure dressing may be applied to reduce dead space and decrease postoperative edema.

   Procedural Consideration: The surgeon may want the patient to wear an abdominal girdle over the dressings to provide additional pressure. The girdle is opened on the stretcher and the patient transferred from the OR table onto it. The girdle is then wrapped around the patient and hooked or snapped together.

Postoperative Considerations

Immediate Postoperative Care

- Patient is transported to the PACU.
- Patient is expected to be discharged the same day of surgery.

Prognosis

- No complications: Moderate pain (controlled by OTC analgesics), swelling, and bruising are expected. Mild edema may be persistent for several weeks. Patient is expected to have good cosmetic results.
- Complications: Postoperative SSI; hemorrhage; severe edema

Wound Classification

- Class I: Clean

Procedure 19-22 Abdominplasty

Surgical Anatomy and Pathology

- See previous procedures for description of anatomy and Chapter 14 for abdominal anatomy.
- Abdominoplasty is performed to thin the upper abdominal fat, tighten the abdominal muscles, and remove excess subcutaneous fat and skin from the mid- to lower abdomen.

Procedure 19-22 (continued)

Preoperative Diagnostic Tests and Procedures	• History and physical examination as well as direct observation		
Equipment, Instruments, and Supplies Unique to Procedure	• Plastic instrument set • Extra Crile hemostats and Kocher clamps • Fiberoptic retractor set • Sterile umbilical template	• ESU pencil with long blade tip • Large number of laparotomy sponges • Marking pen • Several #10 knife blades	• Closed wound drainage system (surgeon's preference) • Abdominal girdle
Preoperative Preparation	• Position: Supine • Anesthesia: General • Skin prep: Pubic hair should be removed. Beginning at site of low	abdominal transverse incision, prep should extend to nipple line to mid-thighs and bilaterally as far as possible.	• Draping: Entire abdomen outlined with 4 towels and laparotomy drape
Practical Considerations	• A woman planning to bear children should delay undergoing this procedure until all pregnancies are complete.	• Full abdominoplasty is considered a major surgery and can take 2–5 hours to complete.	• Test the fiberoptic retractors prior to the patient arriving in the OR.

Surgical Procedure

1. The surgeon marks the incision using the marking pen.
2. A low transverse incision in the shape of a "W" is made down to the level of the rectus sheath. A small inferior flap is created (Figure 19-39).

   Procedural Consideration: The incision is made low enough so the scar will be hidden by the patient's undergarment or bathing suit as well as by the regrowth of the pubic hair. Bleeding is controlled with cautery.
3. Next, dissection begins on the superior flap that extends beyond the level of the umbilicus.

   Procedural Consideration: Much of the initial dissection may be accomplished with the use of electrosurgery in either the cut or blend mode. The surgical technologist should keep the pencil tip clean with the use of a scratch pad and/or position the pad near the surgeon to be used.
4. A second incision is made around the umbilicus using the sterile template, commonly called the "cookie cutter," to ensure that the incision is a perfect circle. The umbilicus is freed from the skin and subcutaneous tissue, allowing it to remain attached to its pedicle, or base.
5. The flap dissection continues superiorly to the level of the outline of the ribs bilaterally.

   Procedural Consideration: A variety of retractors is used as the dissection continues. The fiberoptic retractor may be used according to the surgeon's preference.

(*continues*)

PROCEDURE 19-22 (continued)

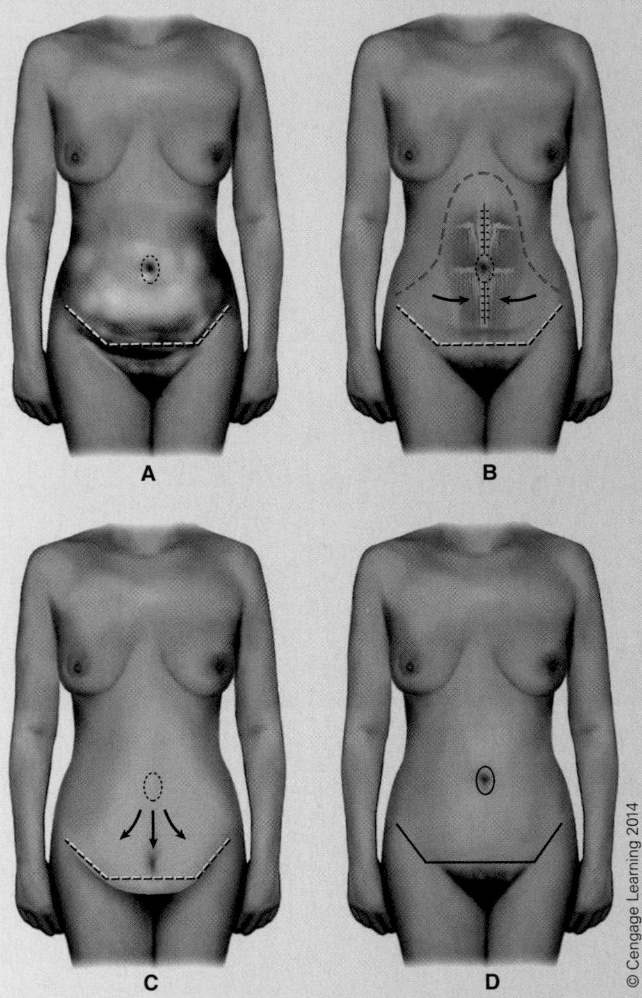

Figure 19-39 Abdominoplasty: (A) Primary incisions, (B) dissection and muscle tightening, (C) secondary incisions—panniculectomy, (D) closure, final effect

6. The superior flap is retracted to reveal the rectus abdominis muscle. The muscle, along with its fascia, or sheath, is pulled together and sutured to firm the abdominal wall and accentuate the waistline.
7. The skin flap is then pulled down, the new location for the umbilicus is marked, and the excess tissue is removed.
8. An opening is created for the umbilicus using the "cookie cutter" template and the structure is sutured into position.
9. The wound is now closed in layers. One or two closed wound drainage systems may be placed, with the tubing exteriorized through the lateral wound edges. Staples may be used to close the skin layer.
10. A small dressing is placed over the umbilicus and a pressure dressing over the transverse incision. The surgeon may request an abdominal girdle placed on the patient.

PROCEDURE 19-22 (continued)

Postoperative Considerations

Immediate Postoperative Care

- Patient is transported to the PACU.
- Patient's bed should be slight flexed for comfort.
- Patient will be hospitalized overnight.
- Hypodermic injections of narcotic pain medication are given for the first 24 hours.
- Although it will be difficult for the patient to stand erect, ambulation is encouraged as soon as possible.

Prognosis

- No complications: Drain(s) remain in place for 2–3 weeks after patient is discharged from the hospital. Patient education regarding wound and drain care is necessary. The patient should have an appointment with the surgeon approximately 1 week postoperatively to have the external sutures or staples removed and another week or two later for taking out the drains. It may take several weeks for the patient to return to normal activities.

Complications: Postoperative SSI; hemorrhage; severe edema; less-than-desired cosmetic results

CASE STUDY Selena had a modified radical mastectomy for breast cancer. She has completed her treatments and the wound is healed. It appears that she will survive this malignancy, and she has asked for a breast reconstruction.

1. **What are the options for breast reconstruction for Selena?**
2. **Will implants or muscle be used?**
3. **What instruments will be required?**

QUESTIONS FOR FURTHER STUDY

1. **What are the steps in a facelift procedure?**
2. **Why is the term *plastic* used to define this field of surgery?**
3. **What types of suture are typically used to close incisions or wounds on the face?**
4. **What are the reasons for the use of sterile mineral oil when preparing to take a split-thickness skin graft?**
5. **Describe the most commonly used technique for performing a cheiloplasty, referred to as the "rotation advancement."**
6. **What are the purposes of using cocaine when a rhinoplasty is performed?**

BIBLIOGRAPHY

Association of Surgical Technologists. (2011). *Core curriculum for surgical technology* (6th ed.). Littleton, CO: Association of Surgical Technologists.

Borowitz, K. C., & Williams, C. (1998). Children's Medical Center, University of Virginia. Available at http://avery.med.virginia.edu/medicine/clinical/pediatrics

Indiana Hand Center. (1997). The Indiana Hand Center. Bloomington: MANUS. Available at http://www.indianahandcenter.com

Kozin, S. H. (2009). Radial clubhand treatment and management. Available at http://emedicine.medscape.com/article/1243998-treatment

Muller, C., & Quinn, F. B., Jr. (2004). Chin and malar implants. Available at http://www.utmb.edu/otoref/grnds/chin-aug-2004-0331/chin-aug-2004-0331.htm

Neuman, J. F. (1997). Evaluation and treatment of gynecomastia [Online]. *American Family Physician 55*. Available at http://www.aafp.org

Phillips, N. F. (2007). *Berry & Kohn's operating room technique* (11 th ed.). St. Louis: Mosby.

Rothrock, J. C. (2007). *Alexander's care of the patient in surgery* (13th ed.). St. Louis: Mosby.

Thorne, C. H., Bartlett, S. P., Beasley, R. W., Aston, S. J., and Gurtner, G. C. (Eds.). (2006). *Grabb and Smith's plastic surgery* (6th ed.). Philadelphia: Lippincott Williams & Wilkins.

Torre, J. (2008). Endoscopic brow lift treatment and management. Available at http://emedicine.medscape.com/article/1276726-treatment

Venes, D. (Ed.). (2009). *Taber's cyclopedic medical dictionary* (21st ed.). Philadelphia: F.A. Davis.

Wheeless, C. R. (2011). Radial club hand. Available at http://www.wheelessonline.com/ortho/radial_club_hand

CHAPTER

20

Genitourinary Surgery

CASE STUDY Homer is a 63-year-old man scheduled for a TURP.

1. What does TURP mean?
2. What is the most likely cause of Homer's bladder outlet obstruction?
3. What is the anesthetic of choice for Homer and why?
4. Homer and his wife are concerned about their marital relations following surgery. Can he expect his sexual function to be normal?

OBJECTIVES

After studying this chapter, the reader should be able to:

A 1. Recognize the relevant anatomy of the genitourinary system.

P 2. Recognize the pathology that prompts genitourinary system surgical intervention and the related terminology.

3. Assess any special preoperative genitourinary diagnostic procedures/tests.
4. Assess any special preoperative genitourinary preparation procedures.
5. Indicate the names and uses of genitourinary instruments, supplies, and specialty equipment.
6. Determine the intraoperative preparation of the patient undergoing the genitourinary procedure.

O 7. Summarize the steps of the genitourinary procedures.

8. Determine the purpose and expected outcomes of the genitourinary procedures.
9. Assess the immediate postoperative care and possible complications of the genitourinary procedures.

S 10. Recognize any specific variations related to the preoperative, intraoperative, and postoperative care of the genitourinary patient.

Select Key Terms

ACTH	Gerota's fascia	intravenous urogram (IVU)	stoma
Adenocarcinoma	Gibson incision	medulla	suprarenal glands
calculi	hilum	prepuce	torsion
Circumcision	hypertrophy	prostate-specific antigen (PSA)	TURP
conduit	hypospadias	retroperitoneal	UTI
cortex	incontinence		vesical trigone

INTRODUCTION

Genitourinary (GU) surgery is a surgical subspecialty that addresses a wide spectrum of diseases involving the male and female GU systems and the male reproductive system. Medical professionals that specialize in the field of urology are called urologists. Urologists diagnose, treat, and manage diseases ranging from GU malignancies and renal calculi to congenital GU defects. This chapter will address common GU surgery procedures of the kidney, ureter, bladder, prostate, testicles, and penis.

DIAGNOSTIC PROCEDURES AND TESTS

Disorders of the GU tract, whether congenital or acquired, are diagnosed through many of the standard procedures that apply to determining pathology in other body systems. Many of the usual methods of diagnosis have been thoroughly discussed in other chapters and will be only briefly mentioned as they apply to GU conditions.

History and Physical

A detailed history should be obtained from the patient or another reliable person if the patient is unable to provide the information. All men, as part of their health maintenance program, should perform routine testicular self-examination. Additionally, men over the age of 40 should have a yearly digital rectal examination to check for prostatic enlargement.

Laboratory Findings

Microscopic examination is the most accurate method for determining blood and urine composition. Chemical reagent strips are available for fast general results for some tests. The chemical reagent strips are handy for a patient needing to monitor certain blood and urine levels several times per day. These home/office test strips are not highly accurate and occasional professional testing should be performed to verify the results.

Hematology Findings

Tables 20-1 and 20-2 are intended to provide the reader with some basic information. It is important to realize that a great number of additional, more specific tests are available.

Specific hematologic examinations will require a patient to comply with certain prerequisites, such as remaining NPO for a specified period prior to the examination (Table 20-1).

Common chemistry findings are listed in Table 20-2.

One important blood value that has not been listed previously is the **prostate-specific antigen (PSA)** test, which is useful in determining cancer of the prostate. An elevated PSA result does not automatically indicate the presence of a malignant process, but should be followed up with a prostatic biopsy. Additionally, following prostatectomy for cancer, the PSA test is used as an indicator in determining the presence of metastatic processes. An increased phosphatase acid level is also an indicator for possible prostatic malignancy.

Urinalysis

Urinalysis is the single most important laboratory examination used in diagnosing problems affecting the urinary tract. Ideally, the sample should be the first of the day and should be examined as soon after collection as possible. With the exception of samples requiring culture, the sample should be refrigerated if it cannot be examined immediately.

A simple voided specimen is commonly used. The patient simply urinates into a clean container. This method is ineffective if an infection is suspected; in that case, a clean-catch midstream sample or a catheterized specimen should be obtained.

The collection of a 24-hour urine sample is useful in determining some urinary and adrenal conditions. Blood urea nitrogen (BUN), creatinine, and catecholamine concentrations are studied. The first sample of the day is discarded. All urine excreted from that time to the same time the next day is collected and chilled. The patient is provided with a collection device and one or more large storage containers for the urine. The sample is easily collected at home provided the patient is compliant. Often blood samples to measure plasma creatinine are ordered in conjunction with the 24-hour urine test.

Table 20-1 Hematology Findings

Normal Range	Conditions in Which Variations from Normal May Occur
Volume 7–9% of body weight (4000–6000 mL)	Decreased: hemorrhage, surgical shock, burns
Erythrocytes 4.5–5 million/mm^3	Increased: polycythemia, anoxia, chronic pulmonary disease, high altitudes, renal disease with increased secretion of erythropoietin, Cushing's syndrome
	Decreased: anemia, hemorrhage, leukemia
Reticulocytes 0.8–1% of red blood cells (RBCs)	Increased: hemolytic jaundice, anemia with increased bone marrow activity
Leukocytes 5,000–10,000 mm^3	Increased: infections and tissue destruction, leukemia, metabolic disorders
	Decreased: irradiation, bone marrow aplasia
Platelets 250,000–350,000	Increased: after trauma or surgery, after massive hemorrhage, polycythemia
	Decreased: thrombocytopenic purpura, lupus erythematosus, following massive blood transfusions
Hematocrit 42–47%	Increased: dehydration, plasma loss, burns, conditions in which there is an increase in erythrocytes
	Decreased: hemorrhage, anemia
Bleeding time 1–3 min	Increased: thrombocytopenia, acute leukemia, Hodgkin's disease, hemorrhagic disease of the newborn, hemophilia
Coagulation time 6–12 min	Increased: hemophilia, anticoagulant therapy
Prothrombin time 10–15 sec	Increased: treatment with anticoagulants, hemorrhagic disease of the newborn, liver disease, hemophilia

Source: Data from Burke, 1980.

Table 20-2 Blood Chemistry Findings

Normal Range	Conditions in Which Variations from Normal May Occur
Albumin 3.5–5.5 g/dL	Increased: dehydration
	Decreased: renal disease, liver disease, malnutrition
Amylase 60–160 Somogyi units/dL	Increased: pancreatitis, postgastrectomy, cholecystitis, salivary gland disease
	Decreased: hepatitis, thyrotoxicosis, severe burns, toxemia of pregnancy
Bicarbonate 21–28 mEq/L	Increased: metabolic alkalosis
	Decreased: metabolic acidosis
Bilirubin Total 0.3–1.5 mg/dL Direct 0.1–0.3 mg/dL	Increased: biliary obstruction, impaired liver function, hemolytic disease
Blood gases pH arterial 7.35–7.45	Increased: alkalosis
pH venous 7.3–7.41	Decreased: acidosis
Blood urea nitrogen (BUN) 8–18 mg/dL (adult)	Increased: fever, excess body protein catabolism, renal failure, congestive heart failure with decreased renal blood supply, obstructive uropathy
	Decreased: growing infant

TABLE 20-2 **(continued)**

Normal Range	*Conditions in Which Variations from Normal May Occur*
Calcium Ionized 2.1–2.6 mEq/L Total 4.5–5.3 mEq/L Infants 11–13 mg/dL	Increased: hyperparathyroidism, vitamin D excess, multiple myeloma, thyrotoxicosis, sarcoidosis, bone cancer, fractures
	Decreased: hypoparathyroidism, acute pancreatitis, vitamin D deficiency, steatorrhea, nephrosis, rickets, Paget's disease, malabsorption, pregnancy, respiratory alkalosis
Creatinine 0.6–1.2 mg/dL	Increased: acromegaly, renal failure
Glucose 70–120 mg/dL (fasting)	Increased: diabetes mellitus, severe thyrotoxicosis, burns, shock, stress, after norepinephrine injection, pheochromocytoma (during attack), Cushing's syndrome, pancreatic insufficiency, diuretics
	Decreased: insulin overdosage, hyperplasia of islet cells, hypothalamic lesions, postgastrectomy dumping syndrome, liver disease, Addison's disease
Iodine (PBI) 4.0–8.0 μg/dL	Increased: hyperthyroidism, exogenous iodine intake, elevated serum protein
	Decreased: hypothyroidism, low serum protein
Iron, total 50–150 μg/dL	Decreased: hypochromic anemia, hemoglobinopathies
Lactic acid Venous 5–20 mg/dL Arterial 3–7 mg/dL	Increased: lactic acidosis
Lipids (values increase with age) Total 400–800 mg/dL	
Cholesterol 150–250 mg/dL (age 35 yr)	Increased: familial hypercholesterolemia, obstructive jaundice, renal disease, pancreatic disease, hypothyroidism, pancreatitis, untreated diabetes mellitus
	Decreased: severe liver disease, starvation, uremia, hyperthyroidism, cortisone therapy, anemia
Triglycerides 10–150 mg/dL (age 35 yr)	Increased: atherosclerosis, hyperlipemia, diabetes mellitus, lipid metabolism abnormality
	Decreased: deficient bile production, liver damage, poor intestinal absorption, lipid metabolism abnormality
Phospholipids 150–380 mg/dL (age 35 yr)	Increased: hyperlipidemia, atherosclerosis, lipid metabolism abnormality, diabetes mellitus
	Decreased: severe liver disease, malabsorption
Low-density lipoprotein (LDL) 45–50% of total lipids	Increased: hyperlipidemia, coronary artery disease
Magnesium 1.5–2.5 mEq/L	Increased: administration of magnesium compounds in presence of renal failure
	Decreased: severe malabsorption
Osmolality 280–295 mOsm/L	Increased: water loss, diabetes, azotemia, sepsis, lactic acidosis, liver failure, drug intoxication
	Decreased: water excess, sodium loss
Oxygen pressure Po_2 arterial 95–100 mm Hg	Increased: administration of high concentrations of oxygen
	Decreased: hypovolemia, decreased cardiac output, chronic pulmonary disease
pH Arterial 7.35–7.45 Venous 7.3–7.41	Increased: alkalosis
	Decreased: acidosis

TABLE 20-2 (continued)

Normal Range	Conditions in Which Variations from Normal May Occur
Potassium 3.0–4.5 mEq/L	Increased: shock, crush syndrome, anuria, Addison's disease, renal failure, diabetic ketosis
	Decreased: severe diarrhea, bowel fistula, diuretic therapy, Cushing's syndrome
Protein	Increased: dehydration
Total 6.0–7.8 g/dL	Decreased: renal disease, malnutrition, liver disease, severe burns
Albumin 3.5–5.5 g/dL	Increased: dehydration
Globulin 2.5–3.0 g/dL	Decreased: renal disease, liver disease, malnutrition
	Increased: chronic infectious diseases, sarcoidosis, Hodgkin's disease
Sodium 133–143 mEq/L	Increased: steroid therapy, hypothalamic lesions, head injury, hyperosmolar states
	Decreased: gastrointestinal loss, sweating, renal tubular damage, water intoxication, Addison's disease, diuretics, metabolic acidosis, inappropriate ADH syndrome, bronchogenic carcinoma, pulmonary infections
Thyroid hormone tests (expressed as thyroxin)	Increased: hyperthyroidism
	Decreased: hypothyroidism
T_4 (Murphy-Pattee) 6.0–11.8 μg/dL	Increased: hyperthyroidism, thyrotoxicosis
T_3 (resin uptake) 25–35% uptake	Decreased: hypothyroidism
Uric acid 1.5–4.5 mg/dL	Increased: gout, gross tissue destruction, renal failure, hypoparathyroidism
	Decreased: administration of uricosuric drugs (cortisone, salicylates)

* Values depend to a certain extent on the technique used for the determination; therefore occasional discrepancies may occur when comparing different normal value charts.

Source: Data from Burke, 1980.

Visual examination of the urine prior to microscopic study is often helpful. Preliminary diagnoses are often made based on the color and consistency of urine. Particular smells are also associated with certain pathological conditions.

The normal composition of urine is shown in Table 20-3; abnormal constituents are listed in Table 20-4.

Radiologic Findings

Regular X-rays, ultrasound, CT scan, and MRI are important tools in diagnosing tumors and obstructions of the genitourinary tract.

The acronym KUB stands for kidney, ureters, and bladder. A KUB is an AP (anterior-to-posterior [anteroposterior]) radiographic view of the urinary system that provides basic information about the size, shape, and position of the organs. Certain types of calculi may be visible on a KUB.

Intravenous urogram (IVU) previously called intravenous pyelogram (IVP), is an enhancement of the KUB that involves injection of a contrast medium into the patient's vein. The radiopaque material is filtered through the kidney and excreted. The procedure takes approximately an hour and provides an excellent outline of the entire urologic system. The patient should be NPO 8–12 hours prior to the test and may be asked to use a laxative or administer an enema in preparation for the IVU.

Retrograde urogram (previously called retrograde pyelogram) serves the same purpose as IVU. However, the contrast medium must be injected into the ureters with the use of a cystoscope because an obstruction is preventing the antegrade process from occurring.

MIBG stands for metaiodobenzylguanidine and is a nuclear medicine study that is specifically designed to detect and locate pheochromocytoma, a vascular tumor of the adrenal medulla characterized by hypersecretion of epinephrine and norepinephrine.

Biopsy

Biopsy is the only accurate way to determine the presence of malignancy and the exact cell type. Tissue samples are obtained using percutaneous, endoscopic, and open methods.

TABLE 20-3 Composition of Urine

Normal Range	*Conditions in Which Variations from Normal May Occur*
Volume in 24 hr: 1200–1500 mL (varies greatly with fluid intake)	Increased: diabetes insipidus, absorption of large quantities of edema fluid, diabetes mellitus, certain types of chronic renal disease, tumors of brain and spinal cord, myxedema, acromegaly, tabes dorsalis
	Decreased: dehydration, diseases that interfere with circulation to kidney, acute renal failure, uremia, acute intestinal obstruction, portal cirrhosis, peritonitis, poisoning by agents that damage kidneys
pH 4.7–8.0	Increased: compensatory phase of alkalosis, vegetable diet
	Decreased: compensatory phase of acidosis, administration of ammonium chloride or calcium chloride, diet of prunes or cranberries
Specific gravity 1.010–1.020	Increased: dehydration, administration of vasopressin tannate, glycosuria, albuminuria
	Decreased: diabetes insipidus, chronic nephritis
Urea 20–30 g	Increased: tissue catabolism, febrile and wasting diseases, absorption of exudates as in suppurative processes
	Decreased: impaired liver function, myxedema, severe kidney diseases, compensatory phase of acidosis
Uric acid 0.60–0.75 g	Increased: leukemia, polycythemia vera, liver disease, febrile diseases, eclampsia, absorption of exudates, X-ray therapy
	Decreased: before attack of gout, but increased during attack
Ammonia 0.5–15.0 g	Increased: diabetic acidosis, pernicious vomiting of pregnancy, liver damage
	Decreased: alkalosis, administration of alkalies
Creatinine 0.30–0.45 g	Increased: typhoid fever, typhus, anemia, tetanus, debilitating diseases, renal insufficiency, leukemia, muscular atrophy
Calcium 30–150 mg	Increased: osteitis fibrosis cystica
	Decreased: tetany
Phosphates 0.9–1.3 g	Increased: osteitis fibrosa, alkalosis, administration of parathormone
Sodium 43–217 mEq	Increased: compensatory phase of alkalosis
	Decreased: compensatory phase of acidosis
17-Ketosteroids Men 5–27 mg Women 5–15 mg	Increased: Cushing's syndrome, adrenal malignancy, administration of cortisone, administration of **ACTH,** ovarian tumors
	Decreased: hypopituitarism, pituitary tumors, Addison's disease, myxedema, hepatic disease, chronic debilitating diseases
Aldosterone up to 15 μg	Increased: adrenal malignancy, conditions associated with excessive sodium loss, cardiac failure, nephrosis, hepatic cirrhosis
	Decreased: Addison's disease, eclampsia

Source: Data from Burke, 1980.

Table 20-4 Abnormal Constituents of Urine

Constituent	*Conditions in Which Variations from Normal May Occur*
Bence-Jones protein	Multiple myeloma, bone metastases of carcinoma, osteogenic sarcoma, osteomalacia
Albumin	Transient albuminuria may occur during pregnancy or prolonged exposure to cold, or following strenuous exercise; albuminuria present in nephritis, nephrosis, nephrosclerosis, pyelonephritis, amyloidosis, renal calculi, bichloride of mercury poisoning, and sometimes with blood transfusion reactions
Acetone	Diabetes mellitus, eclampsia, starvation, febrile diseases in which carbohydrate intake is limited, pernicious vomiting of pregnancy
Glucose	Unusually high carbohydrate intake, diabetes mellitus
Bilirubin	Obstructive jaundice, hemolytic jaundice, hepatitis, cholangitis
Urobilin and urobilinogen	Hemolytic jaundice, pernicious anemia, hepatitis, eclampsia, portal cirrhosis, lobar pneumonia, malaria
Erythrocytes	Glomerulonephritis, pyelonephritis, tuberculosis of kidneys, tumors of kidney, tumors of ureter and bladder, polycystic kidneys, calculi, hemorrhagic diseases, occasionally with anticoagulant therapy
Leukocytes	Increased in urethritis, prostatitis, cystitis, pyelitis, pyelonephritis (a few leukocytes are found in normal urine)
Casts	Glomerulonephritis, nephrosis, pyelonephritis, febrile diseases, eclampsia, amyloid disease, poisoning by heavy metals

Source: Data from Burke, 1980.

Endoscopy

Endoscopy allows for visualization of the affected structures; tissue and fluid samples may be collected at the same time, and/or additional tests (such as retrograde urogram) performed. Laparoscopic procedures may also be performed to diagnose and treat conditions of the genitourinary system.

INSTRUMENTATION, ROUTINE EQUIPMENT, AND SUPPLIES

The routine instrumentation, equipment, and supplies for GU surgery are similar to those for general surgery with the exception of specialty items needed for kidney, ureter, and prostate surgery.

Instrumentation

In addition to the instrumentation used for general surgery procedures, the surgical technologist should add several items to the instrumentation according to the type of procedure scheduled and the patient's individual situation. A list of suggestions follows.

General

- Laparotomy instrument set: pediatric or adult depending on procedure
- Long instrumentation set
- Self-retaining abdominal retractor
- Mixter right angles
- Potts scissors
- Vascular instruments
- Hemoclip appliers, various sizes
- Bladder and prostate retractors

Kidney

- Pedicle clamps (Figure 20-1 A, B)
- Stone/lithotomy forceps

Thoracic (Rib Resection)

- Self-retaining rib retractor (Finochietto)
- Alexander periosteotome
- Doyen rib elevator and raspatory
- Rib shears
- Sauerbruch rongeur
- Bailey rib contractor (approximator)

The instrumentation and supplies required for transurethral procedures are far more complex and unique to genitourinary surgery (Table 20-5).

Equipment

Depending on the size of the health care facility, endoscopic GU procedures are performed either in an OR in the main surgery department or a cystoscopy OR (referred to as the "cysto"

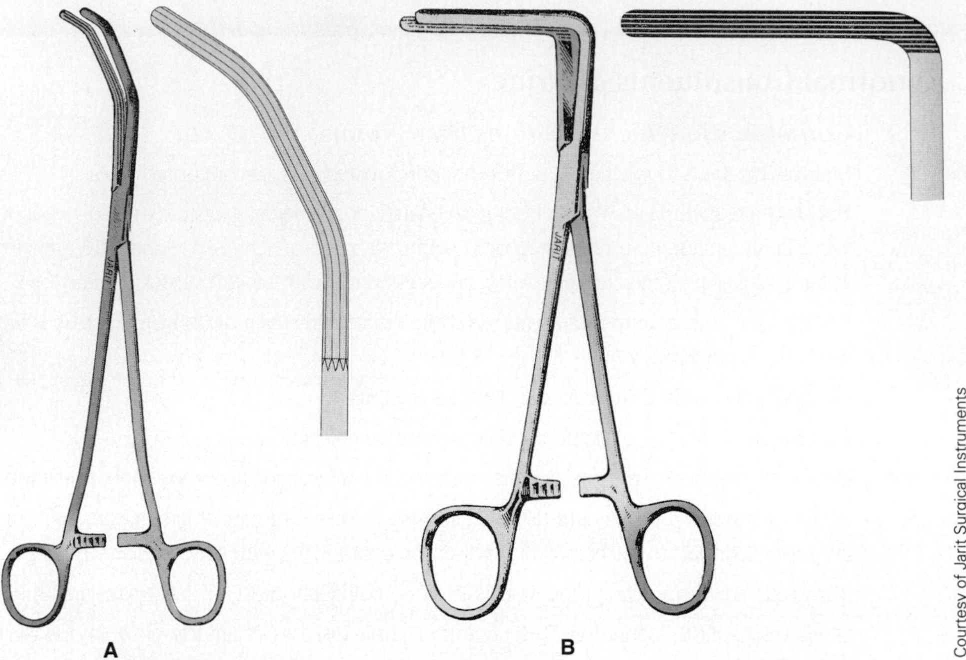

Figure 20-1 GU instruments: (A) Herrick kidney clamp, (B) Wertheim-Cullen pedicle clamp

TABLE 20-5 **Transurethral Instruments and Supplies**

Item	*Description*
Van Buren urethral sounds (dilators)	Available in male, female, and pediatric designs and a variety of French sizes (8 Fr, or 2.6 mm, to 40 Fr, or 13.2 mm) (Figure 20-2) Courtesy of Jarit Surgical Instruments **Figure 20-2** TURP: Van Buren urethral sound
Lithotrite	Designed to crush bladder stones to allow for removal

TABLE 20-5 **(continued)**

Item	*Description*
Urethrotome	Cutting instrument designed for internal urethrotomy of the male or female urethra
Penis clamp	To prevent local anesthetic gel from escaping from urethra
Flexible endoscopic instruments	Adult and pediatric: cystoscope, ureteroscope, and nephroscope, each with a variety of accessories used for irrigation, biopsy, and stone extraction purposes (Figures 20-3 and 20-4)

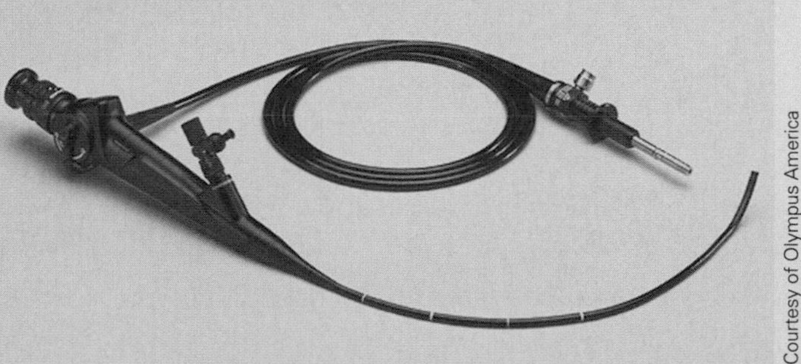

Courtesy of Olympus America

Figure 20-3 Flexible cystoscope

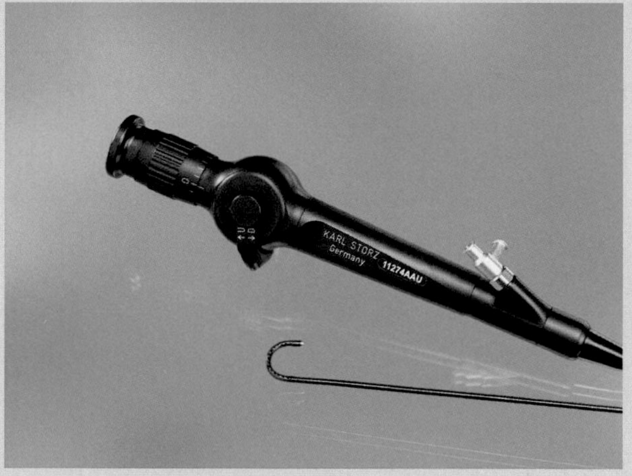

A

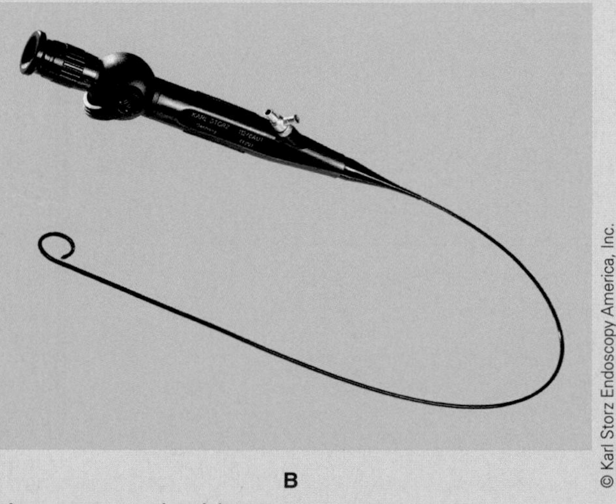

B

Figure 20-4 Flexible ureteroscope: (A) Eyepiece, (B) ureteroscope

TABLE 20-5 (continued)

Item	Description
Rigid endoscopic instrumentation	Adult and pediatric: components and accessories (Figure 20-5).
	Sheath: Hollow stainless steel tube available in a variety of sizes from 14–26 Fr. May have a port outfitted with stopcocks affixed to either side to allow for inflow and outflow of irrigation fluid.
	Obturator: Blunt tip, fits inside sheath to facilitate introduction of the sheath into the urethra without traumatizing the mucosal lining. Size of obturator corresponds to the sheath.
	Bridge: To accommodate added length of telescope. May have additional ports for introducing catheters, probes, electrodes, or forceps.
	Deflecting mechanism: May be incorporated into the bridge or may be a separate instrument. A movable deflector that extends to the end of the sheath aids in placing accessories such as catheters or probes into the ureters.
	Telescopic lens: Primary viewing component. Available with the lens angled at a variety of degrees. The surgeon will likely use the 0° or straight lens first. A 120° lens is for retrograde viewing. Has a receptacle for attachment of the fiberoptic light cord.

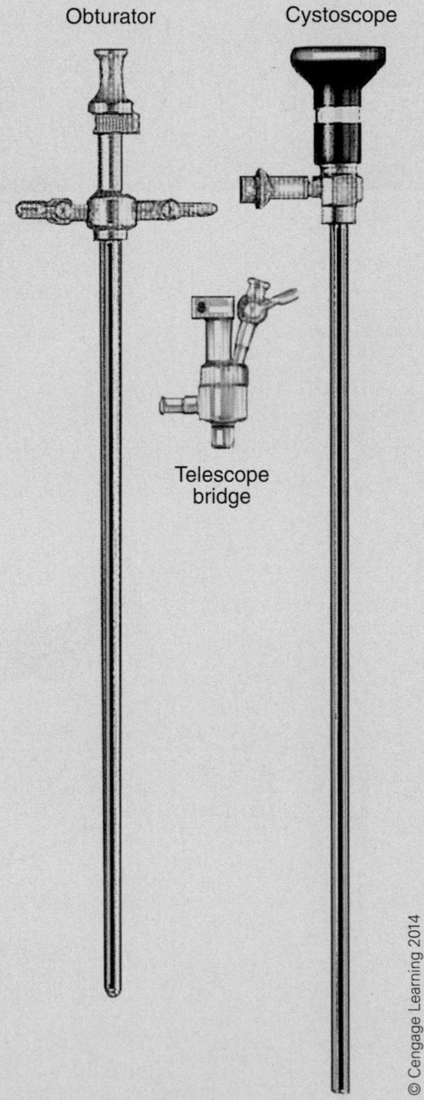

Figure 20-5 Rigid cystoscope, telescope bridge, and obturator

Table 20-5 (continued)

Item	*Description*
Resectoscope	Sheath: Range in size from 11–30 Fr. Resectoscope sheaths differ from cystoscope sheaths only in the fact that they have insulation to allow for use of electrosurgery.
	Obturator: Same as above.
	Telescopic lens: Same as above.
	Bridge: Same as above.
	Working element: Several styles available. Has receptacle for attachment of cautery cord. Receives an assortment of cautery loop, ball, and blade tips (Figure 20-6). 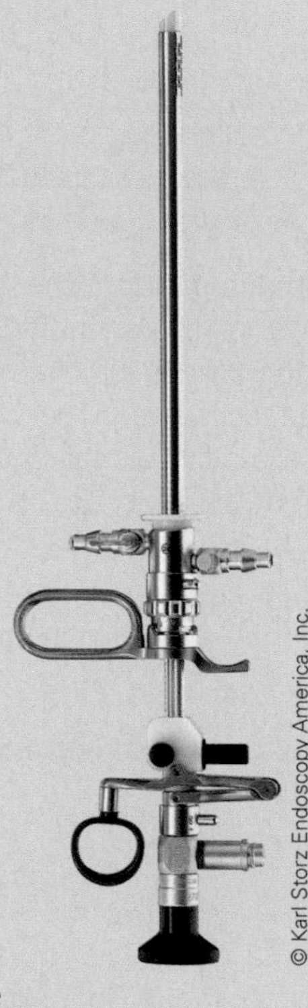 **Figure 20-6** TURP: Resectoscope
Accessories	Luer-lok stopcocks to control the flow of irrigation fluid
	Light source with cable
	Electrosurgical unit with grounding pad, cable, and assortment of tips
	Video equipment: camera, monitor, VCR, etc.
	Tubing: Inflow for irrigation fluid. May have one or more entry sites. Outflow to collection unit or floor drain Continuous-flow pump for isotonic irrigation solution
Irrigation fluid	According to surgeon's preference: 3–6 liters of water, saline, 3% sorbital, or 1.5% glycine. Use of electrosurgical unit will affect the type of irrigant used; nonhemolytic and nonelectrolytic solutions are preferred.
O'Connor shield	Disposable item that allows the surgeon to examine the prostatic urethra digitally through the rectum without contamination of the operative field.
Pharmaceuticals	According to surgeon's preference. May include antibiotics, contrast media, local anesthetic gel. Fluorescein is an intravenous illuminating agent that shows orange when exposed to a Wood's lamp. Though not a drug, sterile KY jelly lubricant is needed.

Table 20-5 (continued)

Item	*Description*
Ellik evacuator or Toomey syringe	Forcefully removes tumor segments and blood clots from the bladder.
Three-way Foley catheter	22 or 24 Fr with a 30-mL balloon, bag, and 30-mL syringe.
GU back table pack	Some facilities may have a GU back table pack or surgical technologist will open a basic back table pack and the GU drape separately. The GU drape allows for draping the patient in the lithotomy position and it has a mesh area that is placed over the drain pan of the cystoscopy OR table.

room). The cysto room contains the specialty equipment and supplies required to perform endoscopic procedures, including transurethral resection of the bladder or prostate, such as:

- Specialty cysto OR table that is fixed in position. The table top can be rotated and allows for the patient to be placed in the low lithotomy position. It has a radiolucent top to allow X-rays to be taken intraoperatively. The mesh-bottomed fluid drain pan (also called a strainer or screen pan) is attached to the end of the table; it is used to "catch" tissue specimens or stones.
- Advanced cysto rooms may have X-ray equipment in the room and it may be a permanent part of the cysto OR table.
- Adjacent darkroom for developing X-rays.
- Lead aprons and thyroid shields may be stored and available in the cysto room.
- Back table that may be semicircular in shape
- Poles to support large, multiple bags or bottles of irrigation fluid
- Drainage system built into operating table or floor drain connected to sanitary sewer
- Adjustable sitting stool for the surgeon
- Multiple X-ray view boxes
- Built-in video, illumination, and electrosurgical equipment

Equipment needed for open GU procedures, as previously mentioned, is similar to that for general surgery, including ESU and suction system. A chest tube water-seal drainage system will need to be available in the OR during some procedures, such as a nephrectomy.

Supplies

The required supplies will depend on how extensive of a procedure will be performed. The following are items used routinely in genitourinary surgery:

- Lubricant: To facilitate entry of instrumentation into urethra; must be sterile
- Foley catheter with drainage bag: Size and style according to surgeon's preference and age of patient
- Alternate catheters: For difficult catheterization; size and style according to surgeon's preference but may include Pezzer, Robinson, Coudé, whistle, and multi-eyed
- Catheter guide: Introduced into catheter lumen to facilitate insertion
- Ureteral catheters: According to surgeon's preference
- Ureteral drainage bag: Specially designed to accept unilateral or bilateral ureteral catheters and measure the drainage from each individually
- Double basin set: Usually the surgical technologist needs a double rather than single basin set for irrigating fluids and basin for soaking instruments.
- Knife blades: Usually #10 and #15
- Laparotomy back table pack: Contains laparotomy drape
- Closed wound drainage systems: Hemovac or Jackson-Pratt
- Penrose drain: Often used for testicular procedures
- Extension tip for electrocautery pencil
- Suction tubing and tip: Type of suction tip depends on surgical procedure; abdominal procedures will require the use of the Yankauer and/or Poole tips, and for pediatric procedures the Frazier suction tip will be used.
- Sponges: 4 × 4 sponges for pediatric procedures or placed on a sponge stick for abdominal procedures; pediatric or regular-size laparotomy sponges
- Kitners: Loaded onto a Kelly or Pean clamp for abdominal procedures
- Chest tubes: Various sizes will need to be available in the OR during some types of procedures, such as a nephrectomy.
- Hemoclips: Various sizes
- Dressing material: Type depends on procedure being performed

- Drugs: Type, strength, and amount depend on procedure being performed and surgeon's preference
- Suture and ties: Types, sizes, and number needed depends on procedure being performed and surgeon's preference

INCISIONAL OPTIONS

Operative approaches include inguinal, scrotal, abdominal, Gibson, flank, and lumbar incisions.

Inguinal Incision

An inguinal incision is often used to access the scrotal contents of an adult or child. Cryptorchidism is often treated through an inguinal incision. This would also be the incision of choice for radical orchiectomy. A detailed description of the inguinal incision, prep, and draping can be found in Chapter 14.

Scrotal Incision

Scrotal incisions are performed to access the scrotal contents. This may be for the purpose of vasectomy, testicular biopsy, simple orchiectomy, or orchiopexy. Tension is applied to the scrotum and a transverse incision is made through the skin and dartos muscle. The tunica vaginalis is opened, exposing the contents of the hemiscrotum. The wound is typically closed in two layers with interrupted absorbable sutures.

Abdominal Incisions

Any abdominal incision may be used by the genitourologist. Most of the abdominal incision information can be found in Chapter 14. The low transverse incision or Pfannenstiel incision is covered in Chapter 15.

Gibson Incision

The **Gibson incision** is an extraperitoneal abdominal approach that is specifically designed for access to the lower portion of the ureter (Figure 20-7). It is sometimes used for implantation of a donor kidney.

The incision begins medial to the anterosuperior iliac spine and curves downward and medially, ending slightly above the symphysis pubis. The external oblique muscle and the rectus sheath are incised, the rectus muscle is retracted toward the midline, and the internal oblique muscle and transversalis fascia are divided to expose the peritoneum. The peritoneum is retracted medially to expose the iliac vessels and the ureter. If additional exposure is needed, the inferior epigastric artery and vein can be ligated and the rectus muscle transsected. Wound closure is systematic approximation of the fascia enclosing the internal and external oblique muscles and that of the anterior rectus.

Flank Incisions

When the use of a flank incision is planned, direct access is provided to the adrenal gland, kidney, and proximal ureter; the peritoneal cavity is not entered. The flank incision usually involves cutting the muscles. Only in a very limited approach to the mid-ureter can the muscle-splitting flank incision be used. According to the exact surgical site, the flank incision may be subcostal, transcostal, or intercostal.

Subcostal flank incisions are appropriate if the preoperative radiographic studies show the kidney to be low lying or if the mid-to upper ureter is the intended target. The incision line extends from the rectus sheath around to the sacrospinalis muscle approximately 2 cm below the 12th rib. The latissimus dorsi, external oblique, and internal oblique muscles are transsected with the electrocautery. The subcostal neurovascular bundle is identified and gently retracted to prevent injury. The lumbodorsal fascia is opened, exposing the perinephric fat and the Gerota's fascia surrounding the kidney and adrenal gland. The transversus abdominis muscle may be partially split if necessary to increase exposure. The wound is held open with a self-retaining retractor. Blunt dissection is used to free the retroperitoneal contents from the peritoneum and diaphragm, allowing for anterior or posterior exposure of the renal pedicle. Wound closure is accomplished layer by layer with interrupted absorbable figure-eight stitches. The skin may be stapled or sutured.

Transcostal incisions are used to expose the entire kidney, especially if it is high in the retroperitoneal space and involves the resection of a rib. The incision is made directly over the rib selected for removal, usually the 11 th or 12th. The muscles encountered are transsected, providing exposure of the periosteum. The periosteum is incised and dissected anteriorly with the Alexander periosteotome. This maneuver also separates the intercostal muscles from the rib. The undersurface of the rib is separated from the periosteum with a Doyen rib elevator. The segment of rib to be removed is grasped with a heavy instrument, and the anterior free or "floating" edge is freed from its fibrous attachments. The rib shears is used to sever the rib posteriorly and any rough edges are smoothed with a rongeur. The diaphragm and pleura should not be disturbed. Wound closure, in addition to that previously described, involves closure of the rib bed. This is accomplished in two layers with interrupted absorbable sutures placed in the muscle or fascia.

Intercostal incisions are usually planned between the 11 th and 12th ribs and involve separation rather than resection. The dissection proceeds as described previously, with the ribs to be separated and stripped of their periosteum, and the underlying pleura bluntly dissected away from both ribs. Care is taken to protect the intercostal neurovascular structures. A self-retaining rib retractor is placed between the ribs to be separated and opened far enough to provide adequate exposure. Rib fractures often occur during this process, and this should not alarm the surgical team members. The closure of the intercostal incision will begin with the approximation of the ribs using the rib contractor. Three to four heavy absorbable sutures will be placed around the upper and lower ribs, avoiding the intercostal vessels and nerves. Once the ribs have been secured, the contractor is removed and the closure proceeds as described for the subcostal incision.

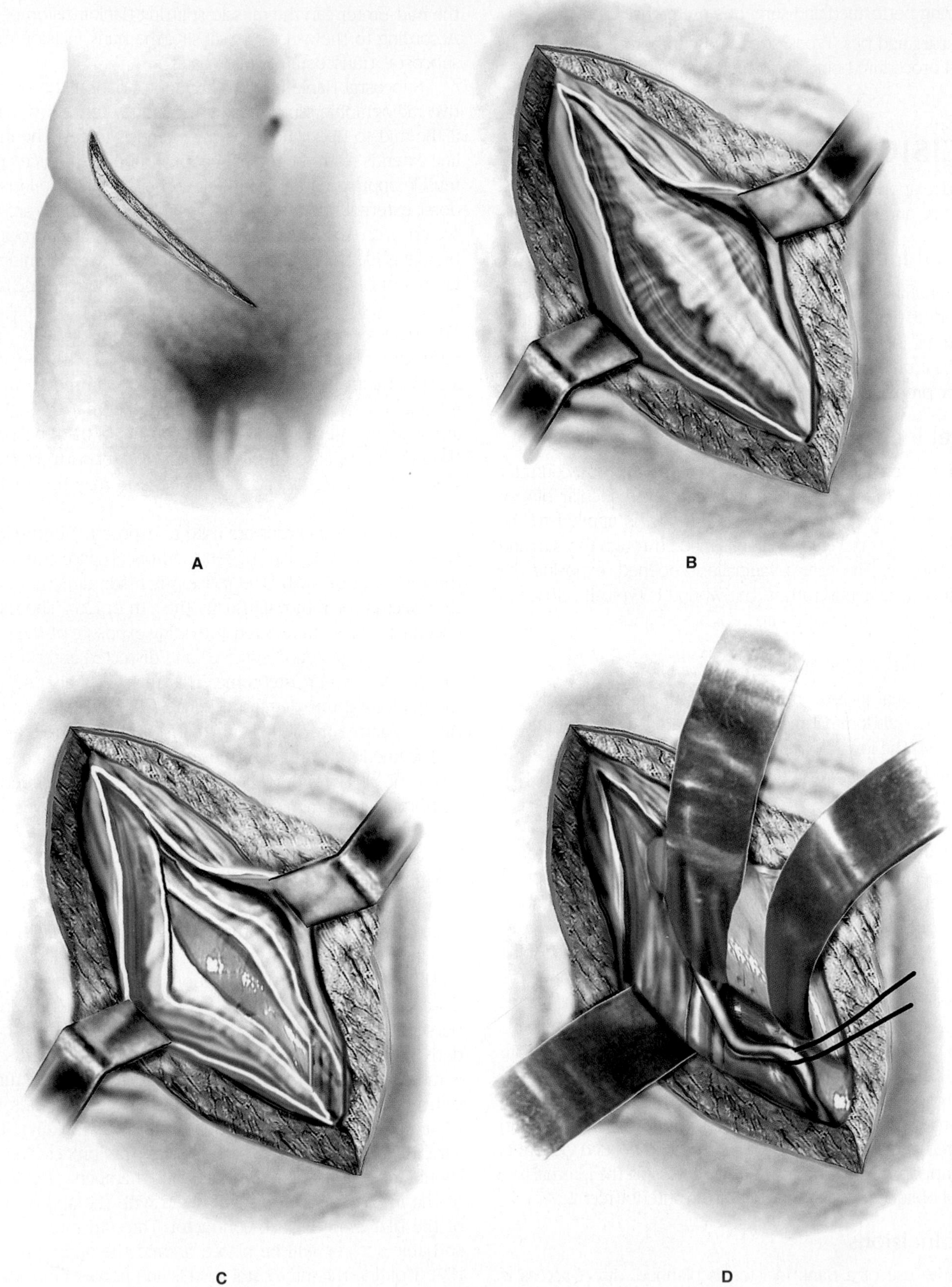

Figure 20-7 Gibson incision: (A) Location of incision, (B) internal oblique exposed, (C) transversalis fascia opened, (D) ureter isolated

Lumbar Incision

The lumbar incision provides limited exposure and is used for adrenalectomy, renal biopsy, or removal of a small low-lying kidney. This type of incision may be done with the patient in lateral or prone position; this is especially nice when there is a need for bilateral access. The incision is made below the 12th rib lateral to the sacrospinalis muscle and extends past the tip of the rib. The underlying muscles are divided with the electrocautery until the Gerota's fascia is exposed. Exposure of the retroperitoneal space can be enhanced by upward retraction of the 12th rib, which can be maintained with the use of a self-retaining retractor. The wound is closed like the subcostal flank incision.

KIDNEY, URETER, AND BLADDER SURGICAL PROCEDURES

Several procedures, both open and endoscopic, are used to treat conditions affecting the kidney, ureters, and bladder.

Procedure 20-1 Wilms' Tumor Excision

Surgical Anatomy and Pathology

- The adrenal glands (also called **suprarenal glands**) are located on the superior and medial portions of the kidneys (Figure 20-8).
  - The glands are concave and the surface of the concavity is against the top of the kidney.
  - They are enclosed in **Gerota's fascia** but separated from the kidney on the concave side by a thin fascial sheet.
  - The glands are highly vascular. Arterial supply is as follows: superior adrenal artery branch from the inferior phrenic artery; middle adrenal artery branch from abdominal aorta; inferior adrenal artery branch from the renal artery. Venous drainage: right adrenal vein drains into the inferior vena cava; left adrenal vein drains into the left renal vein or left inferior phrenic vein.
  - They are endocrine glands with a **cortex** and **medulla**. The cortex secretes steroid-type hormones essential to the control of fluid and electrolyte balance in the body. The medulla secretes the two catecholamines epinephrine and norepinephrine.
- Wilms' tumor, also called congenital nephroblastoma, is the most common pediatric tumor of the abdomen that affects the kidney.
  - Wilms' tumor is a mixed-cell tumor that originates in the kidney and eventually replaces most of the involved kidney, causing hemorrhage and eventual necrosis. The tumor also eventually affects the renal vein, causing thrombosis that can extend to the inferior vena cava.
  - The child is usually asymptomatic until the late stages of the disease, when hypertension, hematuria, and abdominal enlargement occur, sometimes with a palpable mass. The tumor is often discovered during a routine physical exam.
  - The exact cause of the tumor is unknown, but it is associated with certain birth defects such as urinary tract abnormalities.
  - The tumor can become quite large, but is usually encapsulated. However, it does have an affinity for spreading to the lungs and liver. Rarely does it occur bilaterally, but the surgeon will still explore both glands.
- The peak occurrence of the tumor is age 3 and rarely occurs after the age of 8.

(continues)

PROCEDURE 20-1 (continued)

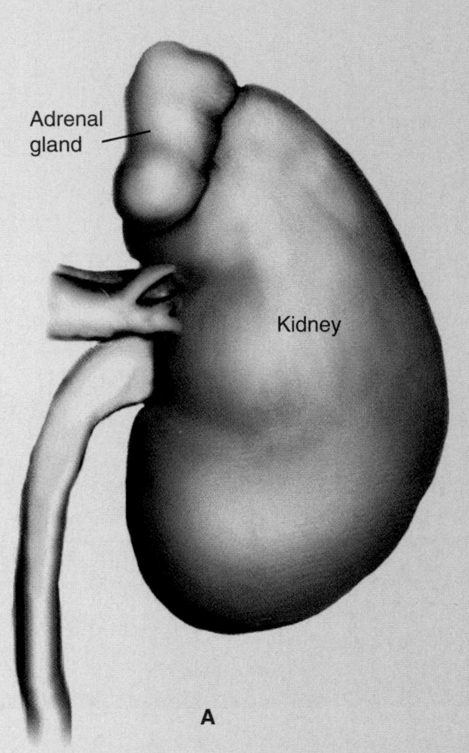

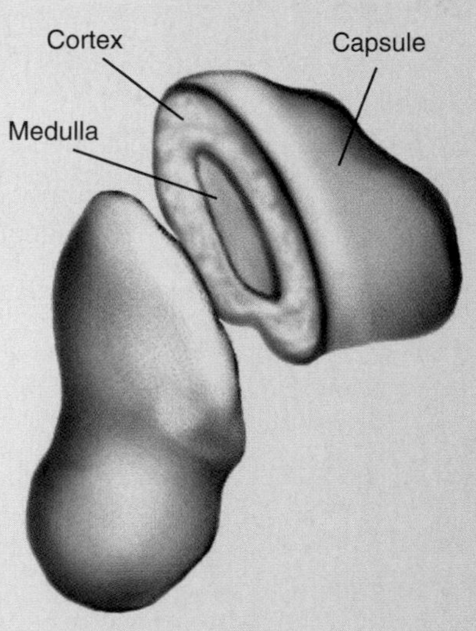

Figure 20-8 Adrenal gland: (A) Location, (B) cross section

Preoperative Diagnostic Tests and Procedures	• Ultrasound	• CT scan	• MRI

Procedure 20-1 (continued)

Equipment, Instruments, and Supplies Unique to Procedure	• Pediatric laparotomy instrument set • Thoracotomy and peripheral vascular instrument sets (available in OR) • Kitners • Pediatric hemoclips • Pediatric laparotomy sponge • 2-0 and 3-0 silk ties: Several packages
Preoperative Preparation	• Position: Supine with small roll positioned under the affected side to slightly elevate the tumor • Anesthesia: General • Skin prep: Middle of chest to symphysis pubis, bilaterally as far as possible • Draping: Pediatric laparotomy drape
Practical Considerations	Normal pediatric considerations, including increasing the OR temperature, use of a warming blanket, and noise and conversations kept to a minimum until patient is anesthetized.
Surgical Procedure	1. The transverse skin incision is made two finger-breadths superior to the umbilicus. The incision extends from the midaxillary line on the side of the tumor to the anterior axillary line on the contralateral side.
	2. Bleeding throughout the procedure is primarily controlled with the use of electrocautery. **Procedural Consideration:** The surgical technologist should use the scratch pad to keep the cautery tip clean and/or position the pad near the surgeon for his or her use.
	3. The anterior rectus sheath on the side of the tumor is incised and the incision is extended laterally through the external oblique fascia and muscle. The internal oblique fascia and muscle are also sharply incised. Retractors are placed and repositioned after each layer is incised. **Procedural Consideration:** Depending on the size of the patient, the surgical technologist should have U.S. Army or small Richardson retractors available for use.
	4. The posterior rectus sheath, transversalis fascia, and peritoneum are incised to expose the abdominal cavity. A moist laparotomy sponge is placed over the tumor to protect it from injury. The opposite side of the abdomen is opened in the same way. **Procedural Consideration:** U.S. Army or Richardson retractors will continue to be used.
	5. The umbilical vein is identified, doubly clamped with Crile clamps, divided between the clamps, and ligated with 3-0 silk ties.
	6. The surgeon completes an inspection of the abdominal cavity, including palpating the opposite kidney to rule out a second tumor. The liver is also visualized and palpated to rule out liver metastases.
	7. A large Wilm's tumor can displace the colon. If so, the left transverse and descending colon and its mesentery are dissected free medially and inferiorly from the anterior surface of the tumor by incising the lateral colonic attachment (white line of Toldt) and doubly clamping, dividing, and ligating the splenocolic and splenorenal ligaments with 2-0 silk ties or surgeon's preferred suture material.

(*continues*)

Procedure 20-1 (continued)

8. The medial aspect of the tumor is mobilized by blunt and sharp dissection and the blood supply to the kidney identified. The renal vein is palpated to rule out extension of the tumor into the venous lumen or vena cava. The renal vein is doubly ligated with 2-0 silk ties and divided close to its entrance/attachment to the vena cava.

   Procedural Consideration: Dissection to free up the tumor is carefully and meticulously performed in order to prevent damage to the kidney. The surgical technologist must remain focused on the procedure at all times in order to anticipate the needs of the surgeon and prevent his or her having to look away from the surgical site.

9. The renal artery is identified, dissected free, doubly ligated with 2-0 silk ties and one 3-0 suture ligature on the aortic side, and divided between the ligatures (Figure 20-9).

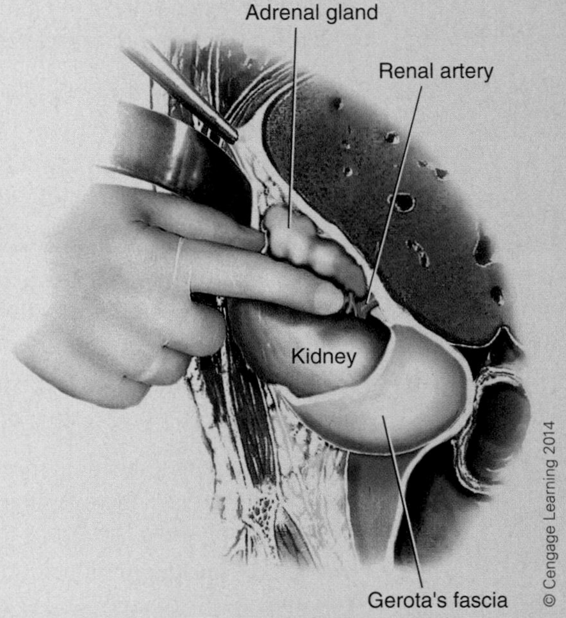

Figure 20-9 Wilms' tumor excision

10. An area/plane of dissection is established outside Gerota's fascia with curved Metzenbaum scissors and toothed forceps to facilitate the eventual removal of the tumor and adrenal gland. Vessels that enter the area from the retroperitoneal tissues are doubly clamped, ligated with 3-0 silk ties, and divided. This is carefully performed to prevent the rupture of the tumor capsule and spillage of its contents, which is associated with an increase of local tumor recurrence.

11. The spleen and pancreas are gently retracted superior and medial to the tumor to provide exposure.

12. The adrenal artery, branches, and superior adrenal vein are identified, doubly ligated with 2-0 or 3-0 silk ties, and divided.

13. The remainder of the resection involves freeing the tumor from the posterior retroperitoneal attachments of the kidney using blunt and sharp dissection while

PROCEDURE 20-1 (continued)

retracting the tumor anteromedially. The dissection is extended down to the pelvis to ligate the ureter near the bladder. The majority of the ureter is resected with the tumor.

14. Unilateral lymph node dissection begins at the aortic bifurcation inferiorly and extends in a superior direction to the superior mesenteric artery. The tumor with adrenal gland, ureter, and lymph nodes is delivered from the abdominal cavity.

    Procedural Consideration: The tissue of the specimen is friable; the surgical technologist must carefully handle it to keep the tumor intact and the other tissues from tearing.
15. The tumor bed is thoroughly irrigated and inspected for bleeding.
16. The previously mobilized colon is replaced laterally to partially fill in the space left by the tumor resection. Omentum can also be used for this purpose.
17. The peritoneum, transversalis fascia, and posterior rectus sheath are the first layer to be closed with continuous 2-0 or 3-0 polypropylene suture.
18. The internal and external oblique fascia and muscle are closed as separate layers with continuous 2-0 or 3-0 polypropylene suture.
19. The fascia is closed with interrupted 2-0 or 3-0 polypropylene suture to approximate the anterior rectus sheath.
20. The subcutaneous layer is irrigated. Scarpa's fascia is closed with continuous 4-0 polyglactin suture.
21. Subcuticular closure is accomplished with a continuous 4-0 polyglactin suture. Adhesive strips are placed to approximate the skin edges.

Postoperative Considerations

Immediate Postoperative Care

- Patient is transported to the PACU or PICU.
- Patient will be hospitalized for 3–5 days.

Prognosis

- No complications: Patient is expected to have a full recovery and eventually return to normal activities. However, the patient will most likely have to undergo postoperative radiation and chemotherapy. The cure rate is high; 90% of cases have a 5-year survival rate.
- Complications: Postoperative SSI; hemorrhage; recurrence of tumor; tumor develops on remaining adrenal gland.

Wound Classification

- Class I: Clean

Nephrectomy

Nephrectomy is total or subtotal removal of the kidney. Partial nephrectomy may be accomplished at the upper or lower pole of the kidney only (Figure 20-10). Partial nephrectomy is performed to obtain a specimen for biopsy, remove small cancers, remove calculi that have caused damage to the surrounding parenchymal tissue, or to treat a traumatic injury. A generous flank incision is used, the Gerota's fascia entered, and the entire kidney mobilized to provide access to the renal artery, which must be isolated and controlled. Control of the artery may be accomplished with the use of a vessel loop or a small vascular clamp such as a spring bulldog. The renal capsule is incised and retracted from the operative site. The superior and inferior renal segments are clearly delineated and the appropriate segmental artery is isolated, secured, transsected, and ligated. Following removal of the affected segment of the kidney, any visible intrarenal vessels should be ligated. Blood flow is slowly returned to the remaining portion of the kidney by releasing

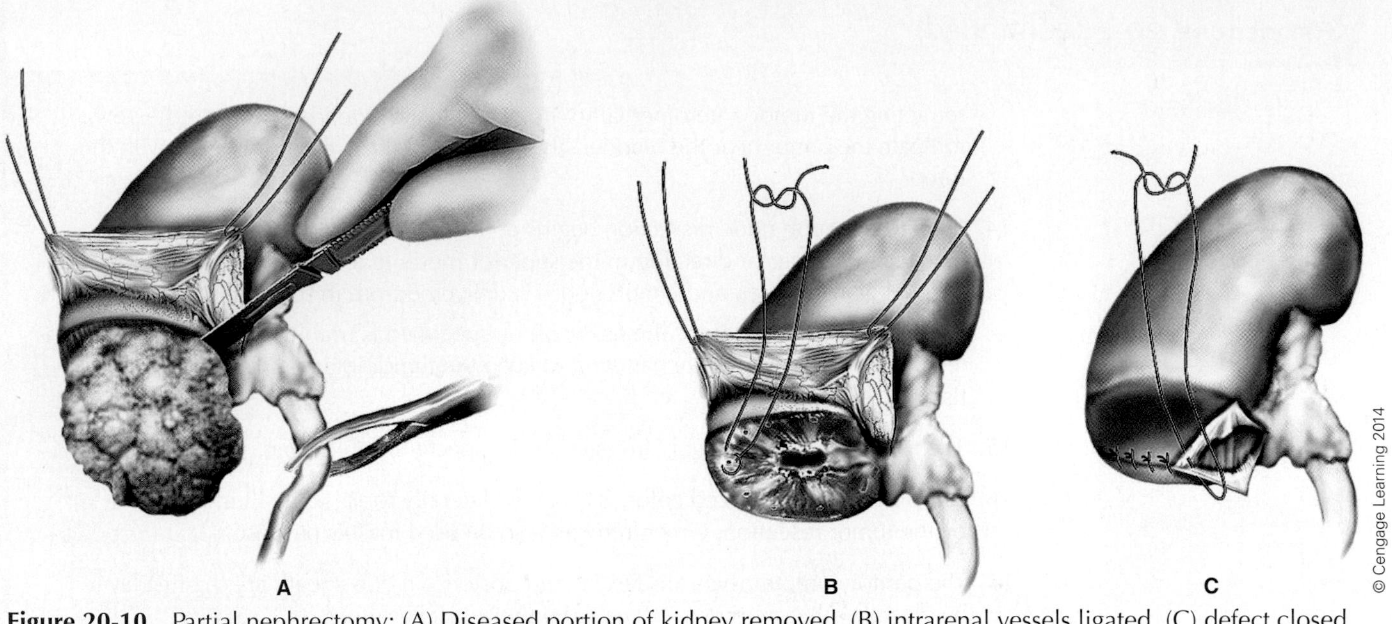

Figure 20-10 Partial nephrectomy: (A) Diseased portion of kidney removed, (B) intrarenal vessels ligated, (C) defect closed with redundant renal capsule

the tension on the vessel loop or clamp. The resulting defect is covered with a patch of peritoneum, omental fat, or the redundant renal capsule. A Penrose wound drain will likely be positioned adjacent to the renal closure, Gerota's fascia closed, and the remainder of the wound closed. *Note:* The first closure count should clearly demonstrate that the constrictive device on the renal artery has been completely removed from the patient.

Radical nephrectomy is the removal of the kidney, adrenal gland, perirenal fat, upper ureter, and Gerota's fascia, en bloc. Regional lymph nodes may be removed if the situation so dictates. Radical nephrectomy is usually accomplished through an abdominal incision with the patient in the supine position. The transperitoneal incision allows the abdominal organs to be inspected for metastases. The most direct approach to the renal vessels should be used. Keep in mind that minor anatomical variances are possible, and that the anatomy may be grossly distorted with certain types of tumors. Also, the surgical technologist should be aware that slight differences will be noticed between right and left nephrectomy. A common approach for exposure of the renal vessels is through the posterior peritoneum medial to the inferior mesenteric vein (Figure 20-11).

The vein is typically isolated first, then retracted to expose the artery. Once the renal artery is isolated, three ligatures of strong nonabsorbable sutures are applied. Two ligatures are placed as close to the aorta as possible and the third approximately 1 cm distal to the aorta. The ligatures on the renal vein are placed similarly in relation to the vena cava. The vessels are transsected between the second and third ties. If necessary, the vascular stumps can be further secured with stick ties of the same material used for the ligatures. The lower portions of Gerota's fascia are freed, exposing the ureter, which is then doubly clamped, transsected, and ligated. If possible, the superior portion of Gerota's fascia is reserved until last, allowing for the best exposure and control of the adrenal vessels. Once all vessels are secured, all remaining attachments of Gerota's fascia are freed and the specimen is removed. The renal fossa is irrigated and inspected for any residual bleeding, which will be ligated or cauterized. If lymphadenectomy is planned, it is performed following nephrectomy. It is not usually necessary to drain the renal fossa. Usual wound closure methods are used.

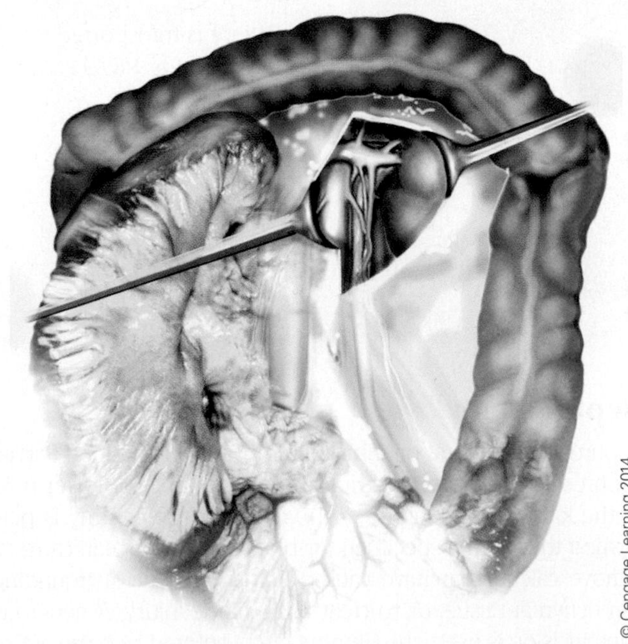

Figure 20-11 Transperitoneal exposure of renal vessels

Procedure 20-2 Open Simple Nephrectomy

Surgical Anatomy and Pathology

- The kidneys are located in the **retroperitoneal** space in the lower thoracic and upper lumbar area (Figure 20-12).
  - The kidneys are bilateral structures embedded in paravertebral gutters of fat and fibrous connective tissue formed by the positions of the vertebral column and psoas muscles. The adipose and fibrous connective tissue form distinct layers around the kidney. A membraneous sheet, the renal fascia, separates the fatty layers.
  - The left kidney is larger than the right kidney. The right kidney is located slightly lower than the left.
  - The kidneys are convex and the medial border receives the renal artery and vein at the indentation called the **hilum**. The renal pelvis is located at the hilum and becomes the descending ureter.
  - The kidneys' smooth exterior results from being surrounded by a fibrous capsule called Gerota's fascia.
    - The muscles around the kidneys are the psoas muscles medially, transverse abdominal muscles laterally, and quadratus lumborum muscles posteriorly.
  - The following are the anatomical relations of the kidneys to other organs:
    - The medial border of the right kidney is posterior to the middle portion of the duodenum. The superior portion of the right kidney is in contact with the right lobe of the liver. The inferior third of the right kidney is lateral to the right flexure of the colon and jejunum.
    - The pancreas lies across the hilum of the left kidney. The stomach and spleen contacts the superior portion of the left kidney. The left flexure of the colon lies laterally and the jejunum medially to the left kidney.
- The kidney has two regions: outer cortex and inner medulla.
  - Nephrons are the functional unit of the kidney (refer to Plate 9A, B in Appendix A). There are more than 1 million nephrons, which are subdivided into two types: juxtamedullary and cortical. The juxtamedullary nephron extends deep into the medulla and the cortical is located in the cortex. Each nephron is composed of two basic units: renal corpuscle and renal tubule.
  - Renal corpuscles consist of a network of capillaries called the glomerulus and a double-layered cup of the renal tubule called Bowman's capsule. Both of these structures are located in the cortex.
  - Bowman's capsule contains a special type of epithelial cell called podocytes. The podocytes have multiple branches that adhere to the glomerulus. The branches along with the spaces between them create a filter through which many substances must pass before entering a Bowman's capsule. This is one of series of filtration systems within the kidneys.
  - Renal tubules are the second component of the nephron

(*continues*)

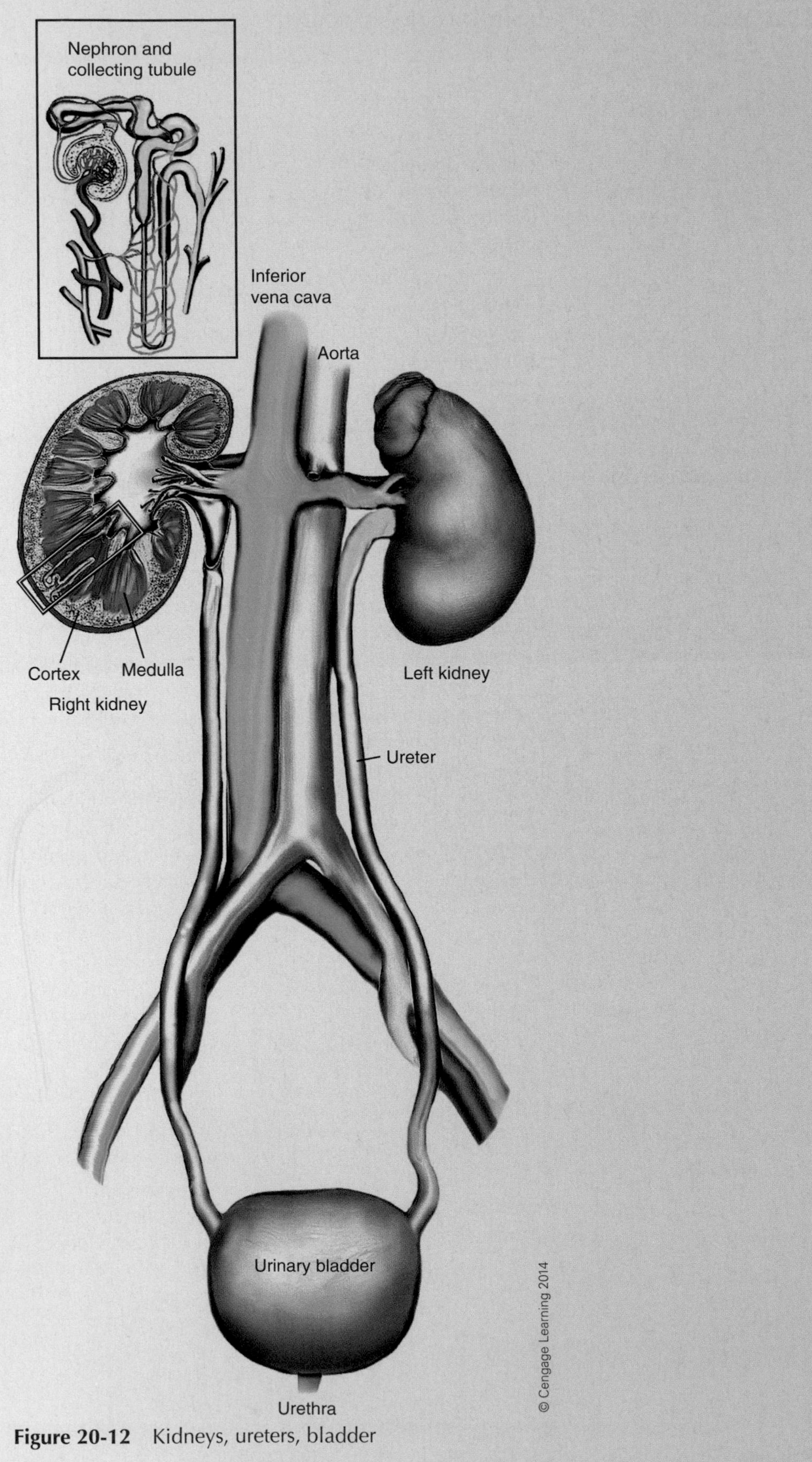

Figure 20-12 Kidneys, ureters, bladder

Procedure 20-2 (continued)

	Figure 20-12. The tubules consist of three units: proximal convoluted tubule, loop of Henle, and distal convoluted tubule.
	• The medulla, as the name implies, consists of medullary pyramids.
	  • The innermost portion of the cortex transitions in appearance to the medulla. The tubules of this portion are called the pars radiata.
	  • Between each medullary pyramid the cortex extends to the inner renal sinus called the renal columns. The renal columns are what form the medullary pyramids. Together each pyramid and column forms a lobe of the kidney.
	• The medullary pyramids taper to form 8–12 renal papillae, which enter the 4–13 minor calyces. The minor calyces empty into 2–3 major calyces. The major
		calyces drain the superior, middle, and inferior portions of the kidney into the renal pelvis. As previously stated, the renal pelvis is located in the hilum of the kidney and continues as the ureter.
		• Blood supply: The renal arteries follow a transverse course from the abdominal aorta to the hilum of the kidney. At the hilum, the arteries form multiple branches that enter the kidney sinus anterior and posterior to the renal pelvis. The arteries branch into anterior and posterior interlobar branches and extend into the renal columns. Two branches exit from the anterior and posterior sides of the kidney to form the renal vein, which empties into the inferior vena cava.
		• Simple nephrectomy is performed for small malignancies, chronic obstructive disorders, benign tumors, or removal of a kidney to be used for transplant.
			• Renal cell carcinoma, also called **adenocarcinoma** of the renal cells, is the most common type of kidney cancer.
			• Development is directly linked to cigarette smoking and heredity and often occurs in patients with end-stage renal disease who are on dialysis.
			• The cancer causes a malignant change to cells lining the renal tubule, causing hematuria, flank pain, and the presence of a palpable mass. The patient may be affected by hypertension, fatigue, and weight loss.
			• The tumor easily invades the surrounding tissues and most commonly metastasizes to the lungs. It often metastasizes prior to the detection of the tumor.
			• If the disease is caught in the early stages a simple nephrectomy may be able to be performed. However, usually a radical nephrectomy has to be performed.

Preoperative Diagnostic Tests and Procedures	• History and physical • Abdominal ultrasound	• CT scans • Angiography and/or MRI to determine metastasis	
Equipment, Instruments, and Supplies Unique to Procedure	• Antiembolism device • Laparotomy or GU instrument set • Long instrument set • Vascular instrument set	• Thoracic instrument set (available in OR) • Water-seal drainage system (available in OR) • Chest tubes (various sizes available in OR)	• Hemoclip appliers • Self-retaining abdominal retractor • Collins solution • Sterile ice slush • Lahey intestinal bag

(continues)

PROCEDURE 20-2 (continued)

Preoperative Preparation	• Postion: Lateral with affected side up • Anesthesia: General	• Skin prep: Axilla to thigh and as far anterior and posterior as possible	• Draping: Towels and a transverse laparotomy sheet
Practical Considerations	• Preoperative radiographic films should be displayed in the OR • If the kidney is intended for transplant, the living donor may be heparinized several minutes prior to removal. The artery, vein, and ureter are dissected in such a way that the maximum length is available for the implantation. The kidney is infused with cold	Collins solution, a preservative, referred to as renal cooling. • Renal cooling is a technique used to preserve renal function during an episode of planned prolonged arterial occlusion (ischemia) of a kidney or portion of a kidney that is to remain in the patient, or a kidney scheduled for transplant. Renal cooling reduces	the metabolic requirements of the kidney and lowers the possibility of tubular necrosis. The surgical technologist will need sterile ice slush along with a sheet of sterile plastic or a Lahey intestinal bag to contain the ice slush. Preparation of the slush is a task that requires additional supplies and preparation time.

Surgical Procedure

1. A subcostal flank incision is made approximately 2 cm below the 12th rib (Figure 20-13A).

   Procedural Consideration: A #10 blade on a #3 knife handle will be used. Anticipate use of cautery and suction.

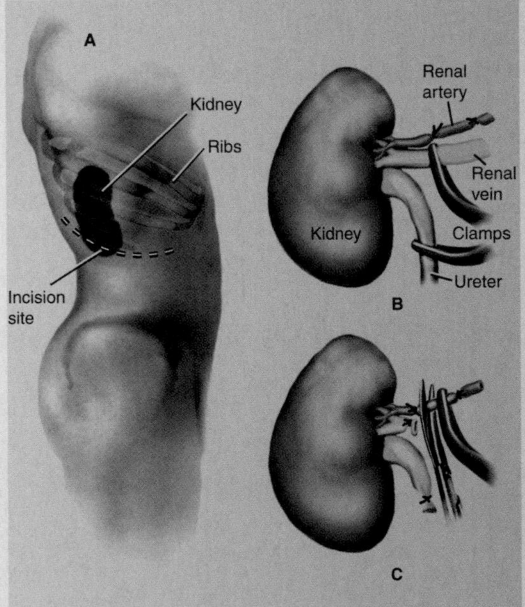

Figure 20-13 Simple nephrectomy: (A) Subcostal incision, (B) renal artery ligated first, (C) renal artery transected

2. The latissimus dorsi, external oblique, and internal oblique muscles are transected.

   Procedural Consideration: Soft tissue retraction is initially achieved with Parker or Richardson retractors. Muscle segments may be doubly clamped, cut, and ligated or transsected with the electrocautery.

Procedure 20-2 (continued)

3. The subcostal neurovascular bundle is identified and retracted.

   Procedural Consideration: A self-retaining retractor preceded by moist lap sponges is inserted. A vein retractor may be needed to retract the neurovascular bundle.

4. The lumbodorsal fascia is opened.

   Procedural Consideration: Provide new #10 blade (deep knife) followed by DeBakey tissue forceps and long Metzenbaum scissors.

5. If necessary, the transversus abdominus muscle is partially split.

   Procedural Consideration: Anticipate the use of a deeper retractor such as a Harrington at this point.

6. Gerota's fascia is opened.

   Procedural Consideration: Return scissors and tissue forceps to surgeon.

7. The renal pedicle is exposed anteriorly and posteriorly with the use of blunt dissection.

   Procedural Consideration: Surgeon may use the fingers, a peanut sponge on a long Mayo clamp, or a sponge on a stick for this step. Have all items prepared in advance.

8. Perinephric fat and the adrenal gland at the upper pole of the kidney are dissected.

   Procedural Consideration: Scissors and tissue forceps may be needed again or blunt dissection may continue. Unexpected bleeding may occur. Have hemoclips and suction available.

9. The ureter is isolated, doubly clamped, transsected, and ligated.

   Procedural Consideration: Provide two Mayo clamps, Metzenbaum scissors, and suture of surgeon's preference. Automatically provide suture scissors of appropriate length after ligatures.

10. The kidney is retracted superiorly to expose the renal artery and vein.

    Procedural Consideration: Prepare pedicle clamps.

11. Renal artery is clamped first and then the vein (Figure 20-13B).

    Procedural Consideration: Prepare heavy nonabsorbable sutures. Surgeon may request that the suture be presented at a right angle to facilitate placement around the artery and vein.

12. The vessels are doubly secured with heavy nonabsorbable sutures and transsected (Figure 20-13C).

    Procedural Consideration: Prepare at least three sutures for each vessel.

13. Any remaining attachments are released and the kidney is removed.

    Procedural Consideration: Prepare to accept the specimen. Anticipate the use of body-temperature irrigation fluid and obtain if necessary. Keep track of amount of irrigation fluid used and report to circulator or anesthesia provider at end of procedure.

14. Hemostasis is achieved.

    Procedural Consideration: Suction and cautery will be needed. Be prepared for the possibility that a suture ligature may be needed.

(*continues*)

PROCEDURE 20-2 (continued)

15. If necessary, a drain is placed and Gerota's fascia is closed.

    Procedural Consideration: Present moistened Penrose drain. Prepare and pass suture for closure.

16. The wound is closed layer by layer with interrupted absorbable figure-eight stitches.

    Procedural Consideration: Several sutures will be needed for the figure-eight suturing technique. Count.

17. The skin is stapled or closed with the surgeon's preference of suture and the drain is secured if a drain has been inserted.

    Procedural Consideration: Provide stapling device and two Adson tissue forceps with teeth for skin closure or prepare to pass the surgeon's specific suture. Prepare dressing material (additional absorbent layer material may be needed if drain has been placed).

Postoperative Considerations

Immediate Postoperative Care

- Patient is transported to the PACU or ICU.
- Intake and output are measured for 24–48 hours postoperatively.
- Respiratory effort may be decreased due to incisional pain; monitor oxygen saturation.

Prognosis

- No complications: Patient is expected to return to full activity in 6–8 weeks. However, patient may have to undergo radiation and/or chemotherapy, which delays return to all normal activities. Remaining kidney is expected to handle additional load without difficulty if not diseased.
- Complications: Postoperative SSI; hemorrhage; patient still requires dialysis.

Wound Classification

- Class I: Clean

PROCEDURE 20-3 Laparoscopic Simple Nephrectomy

Surgical anatomy, pathology, diagnostic tests, preoperative preparation, and postoperative considerations are the same as for the open procedure.

Equipment, Instruments, and Supplies Unique to Procedure

- Laparotomy instrument set (available in OR in situations where laparoscopic procedure converts to open)
- Laparoscopy instrument set
  - 5-mm trocars × 3
  - 10-mm to 12-mm trocars × 2
  - Veress needle
- 10-mm laparoscope
- Electrosurgical scissors
- Endoscopic Babcock forceps × 2
- Endoscopic graspers (curved) × 2
- 10-mm endoscopic hemoclip appliers
- 10-mm irrigator/aspirator
- Insufflation tube
- Insufflator
- Cystoscope
- 16 Fr Foley catheter with bag
- Ureteroscope
- Ureteral catheter
- Guidewires × 2
- Laparoscopic equipment (light source, video monitors)

Procedure 20-3 (continued)

- Surgical entrapment sack
- 10-mm electrical tissue morcellator
- #15 knife blade

Practical Considerations: Laparoscopic simple nephrectomy is usually performed when the tumor is benign and not a large size.

- The procedure performed is transperitoneal (most common), intraperitoneal, or retroperitoneal.
- Prior to the start of the nephrectomy a ureteroscopy will be performed to place a ureteral catheter and renal balloon catheter. The 16 Fr Foley catheter will also be inserted.

Surgical Procedure

1. Using the #15 knife blade, the surgeon makes a supraumbilical stab wound incision. The Veress needle is inserted; a 10-mL syringe with saline is placed on the Veress needle, the stopcock valve on the needle opened, and saline injected. If the saline flows through the needle the syringe is removed, insufflation tube connected to Veress needle, and abdomen inflated with CO_2.

   Procedural Consideration: When the Veress needle is being inserted the surgeon and surgical technologist will slightly elevate the abdomen on each side of the umbilicus using sponges to facilitate the abdominal organs falling away from the site of insertion. If the saline does not flow through the Veress needle, it means the needle is not in proper position and should be reinserted.

2. The Veress needle is removed and the surgeon inserts the 10-mm trocar.

   Procedural Consideration: The surgeon and surgical technologist will elevate the abdomen during insertion.

3. A second stab wound incision is made right below the costal margin using the middle of the clavicle (midclavicular line) as an anatomical point for making the incision. The 10-mm to 12-mm trocar is inserted.

4. A third stab wound incision is made approximately 1 in. below the umbilicus using the midclavicular line as an anatomical point and the first 5-mm trocar inserted.

5. A fourth incision is made in the anterior axillary line at the level of the umbilicus and the second 5-mm trocar is inserted.

6. A fifth incision is made in the anterior axillary line at the subcostal level and the third 5-mm trocar is inserted.

   Procedural Consideration: The trocars are all removed, leaving the sheaths in place.

7. Depending on which kidney is being operated upon, using the electrosurgical scissors, the ascending or descending colon is freed from its attachments and retracted medially. The scissors are also used to open the retroperitoneum.

8. The surgeon identifies the ureter and dissects it free from its attachments. The Babcock forceps is used to grasp the ureter and retract.

   Procedural Consideration: During the procedure, blood vessels will be ligated with the use of the endoscopic hemoclip applier. Depending on the size of the vessel, two to four clips will be placed distally and proximally, and the vessel divided between the clips with the use of the electrosurgery scissors. The surgical technologist should have a large number of clips of various sizes ready for use on the sterile field.

(continues)

PROCEDURE 20-3 (continued)

9. Using the electrosurgery scissors and blunt dissection, the kidney is freed of superior and lateral attachments.
10. Continuing to use the scissors, Gerota's fascia is opened and the adrenal gland freed from its attachments to the kidney in order to preserve the gland.
11. The renal artery and vein are identified and mobilized. The hemoclip applier is used to place two hemoclips near the kidney and two more medially on both vessels. The artery and vein are cut between the clips.
12. Two hemoclips are placed distally and proximally on the ureter, which is divided with the scissors between the clips.
13. The kidney is now freed from all attachments and other abdominal organs. Using Babcock forceps, the kidney is grasped and placed in the upper abdomen.
14. The surgeon inserts the surgical entrapment sack through the 10-mm to 12-mm sheath into the abdomen. When the bottom of the sack appears at the end of the sheath, a grasper is used to facilitate pulling the sack into the abdomen and the sack is unrolled.

    Procedural Consideration: The surgical technologist should provide the surgical entrapment sack to the surgeon rolled up to facilitate placement through the sheath and prevent it from sustaining a tear during insertion into the abdomen.
15. The sack is opened and the kidney with ureter is placed inside using the Babcock forceps. The drawstrings are pulled to shut the sack.
16. The drawstrings are exteriorized through the sheath of the umbilical port. The sheath is carefully removed and the neck of the sack exteriorized using a Kelly or Pean clamp.
17. The electrical tissue morcellator is placed inside the sack and the kidney morcellated using suction. Once the sack is empty it is completely removed from the abdomen.
18. The sheaths are removed. The abdomen is allowed to deflate. The fascial layer at the umbilical site where the 10-mm to 12-mm trocar was inserted is closed with a 1-0 or 2-0 absorbable suture. A 3-0 or 4-0 absorbable suture is used to perform a subcuticular closure at the 5-mm trocar sites.
19. Small dressings are applied to each trocar site.

Postoperative Considerations

Immediate Postoperative Care

- Patient is transported to the PACU.
- Postoperative recovery is usually shorter for the laparoscopic procedure as compared to an open procedure.

Prognosis

- No complications: The length of hospitalization for the laparoscopic procedure, is shorter as compared to the open procedure, often with fewer complications and less pain.
- Complications: Postoperative SSI; hemorrhage

Wound Classification

- Class I: Clean

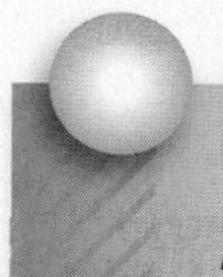

PEARL OF WISDOM

If the pleural cavity is entered (intentionally or accidentally), chest tube insertion becomes necessary. The surgical technologist should anticipate this possibility by obtaining the necessary equipment and supplies in advance. According to the patient's condition, chest tube insertion may be an urgent or emergent procedure.

PROCEDURE 20-4 Kidney Transplant

The following section will describe kidney transplant with a living and cadaveric donor. Anatomy; preoperative diagnostic tests; equipment, instruments, and supplies; and preoperative preparation and postoperative considerations are the same as described for nephrectomy. Practical considerations and surgical procedure will be presented for each procedure.

Pathology

- See Procedure 20-2 for kidney anatomy.

There are several kidney diseases in which the only choice for treatment in order for the patient to survive is a kidney transplant. The following three are common diseases that require a kidney transplant.

- Polycystic kidney disease (PKD)
  - PKD occurs when the parenchyma of the kidney is replaced by multiple fluid-filled benign cysts. The cysts begin their formation in the tubular portions of the nephrons and enlarge substantially.
  - There are three types of polycystic kidney disease:
    - Autosomal dominant PKD: Inherited form of the disease. The symptoms usually develop between the ages of 30 and 40.
    - Autosomal recessive PKD: Other inherited form and extremely rare. This type of PKD affects young children.
    - Acquired PKD: Develops in patients with long-term kidney disorders.
  - The symptoms of PKD include back and flank pain, headaches, hypertension, chronic **UTIs,** hematuria, and development of cysts in other organs such as the liver.
  - Family medical history is probably the most important factor in diagnosing PKD. The diagnosis is verified with ultrasound.
  - Medical treatment is antibiotic therapy to resolve infections and prescription analgesics. There is no cure. In the final stages of the disease, if both kidneys are affected, dialysis or transplantation will become necessary.
- Diabetic nephropathy
  - Also called diabetic sclerosis, diabetic glomerulosclerosis, and Kimmelstiel-Wilson disease.
  - Uncontrolled diabetes mellitus causes damage to many body systems, including the urinary system. The disease causes sclerosis to the glomerular apparatus of the kidney and may be accompanied by an excess of connective tissue called hyaline. As the glomeruli are destroyed, so is the kidney's capability to filter the blood.
  - Symptoms include excessive thirst and edema. Clinical signs include hypertension and proteinuria.
  - The disease is progressive, leading to chronic renal failure and continuing to end-stage renal disease within 2–6 years. Dialysis and/or kidney transplant become necessary.

(continues)

Procedure 20-4 (continued)

- End-stage renal disease (ESRD)
  - ESRD is a term that refers to the final stages of many types of kidney diseases that occur when the filtration of the kidney is no longer effective. A person is considered to be in ESRD when the kidneys are functioning at less than 10% of their normal capacity. Almost half of the population suffering from ESRD are diabetic.
  - The main symptom is severely decreased or no urine output. This is accompanied by malaise, fatigue, headache, hypertension, and decreased mental alertness. Clinical findings include increased creatinine and blood urea nitrogen (BUN) levels.
  - Death occurs from the accumulation of waste products and fluids if treatment is not started immediately. The only two treatments for ESRD are dialysis and kidney transplant.

Living Donor Procedure

Practical Considerations

- In order, the best living donors are identical twins, parents, and siblings.
- Blood type and crossmatch as well as tissue typing are completed on the living kidney donor to confirm the compatibility of the donor and recipient.
- A thorough history and physical and laboratory tests are completed, including ECG, CBC, BUN, coagulation tests, serologic tests, serum creatinine, glucose tolerance test, and titer values for viruses. The function of the kidney is determined by urinalysis and IVP.
- Imaging studies of the donor include chest X-ray, urography, and angiography.
- Two ORs will be set up: one for the donor procedure and the other for the recipient procedure. They are separated by a substerile room to facilitate the surgeon taking the donor kidney into the recipient OR.
- Surgeon's preference determines which donor kidney will be removed. Some surgeons prefer to remove the left kidney because the renal vein is longer, while others prefer the right kidney due to its smaller size in order to leave the donor patient with the larger kidney, which must now do the work of two kidneys.
- Collins solution must not be used as the perfusion solution for a living donor kidney because the residual perfusion solution could increase the serum potassium level in the recipient.

Surgical Procedure

1. A nephrectomy is performed on the donor.

   Procedural Considerations

   - The surgeon divides the ureter close to its junction with the bladder in order to obtain as long of length as possible.
   - Just before the surgeon clamps and divides the renal vessels, the anesthesia provider will heparinize the patient by administering heparin and mannitol through the IV line to promote diuresis and prevent clotting in the arteries and veins.
   - After the ureter is divided, the surgeon divides as long of length as possible of the renal artery and vein by double clamping and dividing. If the right kidney is being removed, the surgeon will work to get as long of length as possible of the renal artery. A Satinsky clamp will be placed on the inferior vena cava (IVC) to achieve partial occlusion. When the renal vein is divided, it will include a small portion of the IVC.

PROCEDURE 20-4 (continued)

- The kidney is removed from the patient. The anesthesia provider administers protamine sulfate to reverse the heparinization; administers furosemide and mannitol to promote urinary output from the donor's kidney; and increases the amount of IV fluids.

2. The harvested kidney is placed in the basin on the back table that contains the sterile ice slush and flushed with the electrolyte solution.

   Procedural Considerations

   - The electrolyte solution is either a mixture of Ringer's lactate with procaine and heparin, or the commercially purchased Chelex-treated University of Wisconsin.
   - The surgeon uses smooth vascular forceps to slightly open the end of the renal artery to facilitate placement of a needle catheter attached to IV tubing. The electrolyte solution passes through the tubing and needle into the kidney to remove the donor's blood.

3. The basin with the kidney is covered with sterile towels and the surgeon takes it to the recipient's OR.

4. Wound closure as described in Procedure 20-2 is completed and dressing applied.

Cadaveric Donor Procedure

Practical Considerations

- The cadaveric donor should have no infections or cancer of any type present.
- The donor must be kept under constant observation while waiting for the harvesting teams to arrive.
- Cadaveric donors are persons who have executed advance directives requesting that their organs be used for transplant in the event that they become brain dead, but their circulatory function can be preserved until a recipient for their organs is contacted.
- When an advance directive is not available, permission must be obtained from the family who can authorize the procurement of the organs.
- The medical examiner must declare the patient as brain dead before procurement can take place.
- A thorough medical history of the donor must be documented to discover any possible contraindications, including IV drug use or abuse; chronic disease(s) or infection and malignancies; past trauma that could have affected internal organs; HIV.
- Laboratory tests include CBC, blood typing, BUN, hepatitis B antigen, HIV antigen, serum creatinine, urinalysis, urine and blood cultures, presence of venereal disease.
- Equipment, instruments, and supplies are the same as described for nephrectomy and living donor procedures.

Surgical Procedure

1. Donor is placed in supine position, then prepped and draped for a major laparotomy procedure.

   Procedural Consideration: The patient is transported into the OR while the anesthesia provider is maintaining the mechanical respirations and cardiac status of the patient as long as is necessary. If other organs are being donated, they may be removed prior to the kidneys.

2. Using a #10 knife blade, the surgeon makes an incision through the skin, subcutaneous, fascia, and muscle layers from the xiphoid process to the symphysis pubis.

   Procedural Consideration: Bleeding is controlled with the use of electrocautery and ties. A self-retaining abdominal retractor of the surgeon's preference will be placed.

(*continues*)

Procedure 20-4 (continued)

3. The kidneys, renal vessels, and ureters are identified and examined to confirm no presence of disease, infection, or trauma. Using the Metzenbaum scissors, the surgeon mobilizes the organs and vessels.

4. Using the #15 knife blade, the surgeon incises the small bowel mesentery superiorly to the esophageal hiatus.

5. The small bowel, colon, spleen, and pancreas are mobilized by blunt and sharp dissection using the Metzenbaum scissors to allow access to the retroperitoneal area. In the process of performing this step, the surgeon ligates and divides the superior mesenteric artery.

6. The surgeon identifies the inferior vena cava and abdominal aorta below the kidneys. The surgeon places two angled vascular clamps on each vessel; the distal clamps are placed as close as possible to the bifurcation of each vessel. Then 1-0 or 2-0 silk ties are placed and the vessels are divided between the ties with the Metzenbaum scissors.

   Procedural Consideration: Branches from the two vessels are divided with the use of hemoclips.

7. The surgeon places a long curved clamp on each ureter as close to the junction with the bladder as possible. Silk ties are placed and the ureters divided with the Metzenbaum scissors.

8. The surgeon identifies the inferior vena cava and abdominal aorta above the renal vessels. The surgeon places two angled vascular clamps on each vessel near the diaphragm. The 1-0 or 2-0 silk ties are placed and the vessels divided between the ties with the Metzenbaum scissors.

9. The kidneys with ureters, renal vessels, and sections of the abdominal aorta and IVC are removed en bloc.

10. The kidneys are immediately perfused by placing in a large container of electrolyte solution (Collins solution) and sterile saline ice slush and transported out of the OR.

11. The surgeon will excise the spleen and abdominal lymph nodes to aid in tissue typing and crossmatching the donor with the recipient.

12. The abdominal incision is closed usually in one layer using interrupted suture technique, and life-support systems are terminated by the anesthesia provider.

    Procedural Consideration: The surgical technologist and circulating person may be responsible for preparing and transporting the body to the health care facility morgue.

Recipient Procedure

Practical Considerations

- A patient is not considered a good candidate for a transplant procedure if he or she has a systemic disease or infection, including cardiovascular and/or lung disease, malignancy, HIV, or HBV.
- Preoperative diagnostic tests include liver function tests; HIV, HBV, and viral screening tests.
- Imaging exams include chest X-ray, voiding cystourethrography, and abdominal ultrasound.

PROCEDURE 20-4 (continued)

- The patient will undergo dialysis just prior to the transplant procedure to be sure that his or her fluid and electrolyte balance is optimal.
- Equipment, instruments, and supplies are the same as described for nephrectomy and living donor procedures.

Surgical Procedure

1. Following dialysis, the patient is brought to the OR and placed in the supine position, the Foley catheter is inserted, the skin is prepped from nipple line to mid-thigh and bilaterally as far as possible, and the laparotomy drape is placed.
2. In an adult, the donor kidney will be placed in the right pelvis; therefore, a Gibson incision is used by the surgeon. In pediatric patients, a midline incision is used, the donor kidney is placed in the mid-retroperitoneum posterior to the colon, and the aorta and inferior vena cava are used for vascular anastomosis.
3. The self-retaining abdominal retractor is placed.
4. Using the long Metzenbaum scissors and DeBakey forceps, the surgeon mobilizes the hypogastric, external, and common iliac arteries down to the level of the aortic bifurcation and continues downward by mobilizing the internal iliac artery. Two angled vascular clamps are placed on the internal iliac artery, ligated with silk ties, and divided (Figure 20-14).
5. The internal iliac vein is mobilized by ligating and dividing its branches. Two angled vascular clamps are placed on the vein, and the surgeon uses a #11 knife blade to make a small venotomy between the clamps. The vessel is internally irrigated with heparin sodium using a bulb or Asepto syringe. The 45° Potts scissors are used to extend the incision in preparation for anastomosis with the donor kidney renal vein.
6. The surgeon or surgical technologist places the donor kidney in a stockinette that has been soaked in the electrolyte saline ice slush solution. Holes are cut in the stockinette and the renal vessels brought out through them.

   Procedural Consideration: The stockinette aids in keeping the friable kidney tissue from being injured during handling by the OR team.
7. The donor kidney renal vein is anastomosed to the recipient's internal iliac vein in end-to-side fashion using 5-0 or 6-0 double-armed polypropylene suture.

   Procedural Consideration: The suturing technique will be according to the type of anastomosis performed; interrupted sutures will be placed for an end-to-end anastomosis and continuous suturing technique will be used for end-to-side anastomosis.
8. The renal artery is anastomosed to the internal iliac artery in end-to-end fashion using 5-0 or 6-0 double-armed polypropylene suture.

   Procedural Consideration: Before the surgeon places the final stitch in each anastomosis, the surgical technologist should remind him or her to irrigate the vessels with heparin sodium using a 10-mL syringe and catheter.
9. The stockinette is carefully removed as well as the angled vascular clamps from the venous vessels. The anastomoses are gently irrigated and visualized for leaking of blood.
10. The vascular clamps on the internal iliac artery are removed and the anastomosis irrigated and visualized.

(*continues*)

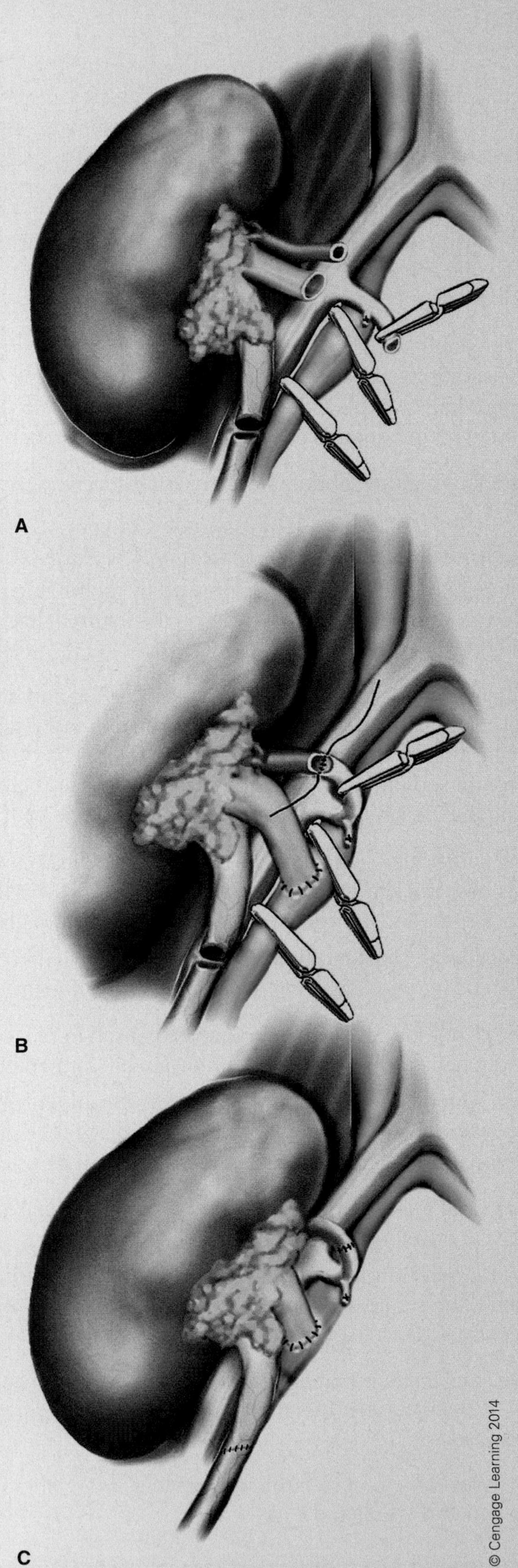

Figure 20-14 Renal transplantation (adult recipient): (A) Iliac vessels exposed, (B) renal artery and vein anastomosis, (C) donor kidney in place

PROCEDURE 20-4 (continued)

11. The final steps of the procedure involve performing a ureteroneocystostomy. Two long curved clamps are used to grasp the anterior bladder wall. Using a long #7 knife handle with a #15 knife blade, the surgeon makes a 1½-in. incision in the anterior wall.

    Procedural Consideration: The surgical technologist should have narrow but deep retractors available such as the narrow Deaver or Harrington for additional exposure of the bladder.

12. The ureter is inserted through the bladder wall. The end of the ureter is sutured to the bladder using 4-0 or 5-0 absorbable sutures, placing them in interrupted fashion; several sutures will be required.
13. A 5 Fr ureteral stent is inserted through the ureteroneocystostomy up to the renal pelvis and exteriorized through the urethra. The stent remains in place for up to 2 days to maintain the patency of the ureter during the immediate postoperative period when ureteral edema can occur.
14. The bladder is closed in three layers using 4-0 or 5-0 absorbable suture for closing the first layer in continuous technique and 2-0 or 3-0 absorbable for closing the bladder muscles in interrupted technique.
15. The ureteroneocystostomy is irrigated and visualized for leaks.
16. The abdomen is thoroughly irrigated with antibiotic solution and all anastomoses visualized one last time for leaks.
17. Retractors are removed and a closed wound drainage system is placed with the tube exteriorized through a lateral abdominal wall incision.
18. Muscle layers and fascia are closed using a 0 or 1-0 nonabsorbable suture. The subcutaneous layer is closed with 2-0 or 3-0 absorbable suture. The skin is closed with skin staples.

GU Endoscopy

Transurethral endoscopy of the genitourinary tract provides an internal view of the structures. GU endoscopy is accomplished by introducing the scope through the male or female urethra with the patient in the lithotomy position. Anesthesia may be local, regional, or general. Viewing instruments are available in a variety of sizes and styles for several purposes.

Urinary tract endoscopy is commonly referred to as *cystoscopy*, although that limited term does not begin to identify all of the procedures that can be performed endoscopically. Often the procedure encompasses all of the structures of the genitourinary tract and is not limited strictly to "viewing." The main purpose of urinary tract endoscopy is diagnosis. In addition to viewing instruments, various accessories are available to make cystoscopy an operative procedure as well. Current technological developments continue to expand the procedural capabilities of endoscopy. A brief listing of some of the procedures that are possible endoscopically follows:

- Retrograde urogram
- Visual diagnosis of a variety of genitourinary tract conditions
- Biopsy
- Bleeding tissue fulguration
- Prostate tissue removal (transurethral resection of the prostate, **TURP**)
- Removal of small bladder tumors (transurethral resection of bladder tumor, TURBT)
- Placement of ureteral stents in one or both ureters
- Calculi removal from any part of the GU tract
- Urethral enlargement

The role of the surgical technologist during the endoscopic procedure is minimal, but the responsibilities are of paramount importance.

The surgical technologist is responsible for assembling all of the necessary items according to the type of procedure scheduled and the surgeon's preference. If the health care facility does not have a designated cysto room, a major amount of equipment may need to be moved into the OR. Often the health care facility has designated a specific team of personnel that specializes in GU procedures to work in the specialty area. This, however, does not excuse the generalist from being responsible for knowledge of the equipment and procedures in case he or she is asked to fill in due to staff illness or other emergency.

Communication with the radiology department may be necessary to obtain preoperative films or arrange for intraoperative studies.

Because endoscopic equipment is extremely delicate, it is often stored in protective cases, in a nonsterile state. The surgical technologist must be able to quickly determine which instruments are suitable for steam sterilization and which must be sterilized using an alternate method. Items with lenses and electrical connections typically are not steam sterilized.

A sterile field must be created and maintained. Sterilized items must be transported to the operating suite using sterile technique. The surgical technologist is not required to "scrub in" for the endoscopy, but must organize the instruments and supplies on the sterile field for use by the surgeon. Some instruments must be assembled; all connections should be secure and fluid-tight. In many facilities it is permissible to don sterile gloves and perform the necessary tasks. Once the sterile field is prepared, the surgical technologist may leave the sterile area and deglove.

The surgical technologist may receive fluids and pharmaceuticals onto the sterile field from the circulator. These must be labeled for use by the surgeon. All irrigation fluids should be prepared in advance and placed for use.

The surgical technologist will assist the circulator with patient care once all of the components of the sterile field have been taken care of. Responsibilities may include:

- Positioning the patient for anesthesia and the procedure
- Applying the dispersive electrode if one is necessary
- Prepping the patient
- Assisting the surgeon with draping
- Receiving the nonsterile ends of the cables, cords, and tubings to be connected
- Connecting such devices as the cautery cords, light cable, video camera cord, irrigation (inflow and outflow) tubings, and so on
- Turning on and setting the devices as directed

The main role of the surgical technologist during the endoscopic procedure is to be certain that the irrigation fluid of choice is constantly available. The type of fluid used may change as the procedure progresses. Fluid inflow and outflow are monitored and should closely match.

A variety of urinary catheters should be available for insertion at the end of the procedure. The surgeon, circulator, or surgical technologist may perform this task.

Any specimens should be transferred from the sterile field to a properly labeled container for transport to the laboratory.

On completion of the procedure, several pieces of equipment must be disconnected and safely removed from the field. Drapes are then removed and discarded.

All urologic endoscopic procedures are expected to follow this basic routine. Any variances will be determined according to the patient's exact situation. Procedure 20-5 is a specific example of an endoscopic procedure.

Procedure 20-5 Ureteroscopy (male patient)

Surgical Anatomy and Pathology

- The ureters conduct urine from the kidney to the bladder.
- The ureters extend through the abdomen in extraperitoneal connective tissue and through the pelvis in the retroperitoneal space.
- They are directly anterior to the psoas muscles until they cross the bifurcation of the common iliac arteries and enter the pelvis.
- The abdominal section of the ureters' blood supply is from branches of the renal and testicular/ovarian arteries. Veins follow the arteries.
- The pelvic section blood supply is from branches of the superior and/or inferior vesical artery. Some branches may come directly from the internal iliac artery and, in the female, from the uterine artery. Veins follow the arteries.
- The ureters terminate by extending obliquely through the wall of the bladder for about 1.5 cm. The oblique course allows the bladder to prevent reflux through the muscular contraction upon the ureter.
- **Calculi**, or stones, are small solid particles that may form in one or both kidneys. One or several stones may be present and they can vary in size from that of a grain of sand to a very large mass.
  - It is possible for the stone to remain in its original location or travel through the urinary tract and become lodged at any point distal to the formation point. The presence of a stone will partially or totally obstruct the urinary tract.
  - The size and location of the calculi will

PROCEDURE 20-5 (continued)

	determine signs and symptoms, which can include painful and frequent urination, oliguria, flank pain (mild to severe with site	of pain determined by location of the stone), nausea and vomiting, UTI, and hematuria. • Urinary calculi recur in more than 50% of	those affected. Diet and lifestyle changes can reduce the possibility of recurrence.
Preoperative Diagnostic Tests and Procedures	• Blood tests • Urinalysis • Urine culture	• Standard X-ray • Ultrasound	• CT scan • IVU
Equipment, Instruments, and Supplies Unique to Procedure	• Ureteroscope • Urethral dilators • Lithotrite • Basket stone forceps • Holmium laser • Foley catheter with drainage bag	• JJ ureteral stents (various sizes) • Light source and cable • Irrigation fluid • Irrigation inflow and outflow tubings • KY jelly	• Stopcock • ESU and cautery cord • Minor procedure back table pack • 4 × 4 radiopaque sponges
Preoperative Preparation	• Position: Low lithotomy • Anesthesia: General	• Skin prep: Penis and scrotum; surgeon may not require a prep	• Draping: Cysto drape
Practical Considerations	• See information under "GU Endoscopy"	• Fluoroscopy will be needed in the OR.	

Surgical Procedure

1. The surgical technologist instills the local anesthetic jelly down the urethra of the male patient and applies the penile clamp. For female patients, the surgical technologist will use a sterile cotton applicator; the local anesthetic is squeezed out onto the tip, which is then placed in the urethral meatus.
2. Surgeon dilates the urethra if necessary.

   Procedural Consideration: Due to the small diameter of the ureteroscope the surgeon may not have to dilate the urethra.
3. The ureteroscope is inserted into the urethra and slowly advanced into the bladder and then into the ureter. The ureteroscope is advanced in the ureter up to the stone.

   Procedural Consideration: The surgical technologist may provide KY jelly lubricant on a sponge for the surgeon to place a small amount on the end of the ureteroscope. The surgeon will use fluoroscopy to visualize the ureteroscope and location of stone.
4. Depending on the size of the stone, the surgeon will:
   a. Insert a basket stone forceps down the port of the ureteroscope and advance to the level of the stone to "capture" and remove it intact.
   b. If the stone is large the surgeon may use the holmium laser to break up the stone into small pieces and remove the pieces with the basket stone forceps or grasper.
5. Once the stone or pieces of stone have been removed, a JJ stent is inserted.

   Procedural Consideration: The ureteroscope causes swelling of the ureter, which will obstruct the flow of urine to the bladder and cause reflux into the kidney. Therefore, it is necessary to insert the temporary JJ stent to maintain the patency of the ureter.

(*continues*)

PROCEDURE 20-5 (continued)

Postoperative Considerations	**Immediate Postoperative Care** • Patient is transported to the PACU. • Patient is discharged the same day of surgery. **Prognosis** • No complications: OTC analgesics for mild pain; antibiotics for 3-4 days; return to full activity and work approximately 1 week after surgery. Removal of JJ stent varies from 3 days to several weeks; removal takes place in the surgeon's office/clinic on an outpatient basis with the aid of a flexible cystoscopy under local anesthesia. However, it is important that the patient have the stent removed when scheduled by the surgeon, as an indwelling ureteral stent that is left in place for a long period of time can result in infection, ureteral obstruction, encrustation by stone debris, and loss of kidney function. • Complications: Postoperative SSI; UTI; hemorrhage; stricture of the ureter; perforation of the ureter; failure to retrieve the stone, resulting in an alternative procedure; detachment (avulsion) of the ureter from the kidney. **Wound Classification** • Class II: Clean-contaminated

PROCEDURE 20-6 Pyelolithotomy

Surgical Anatomy and Pathology	• See previous procedures for ureter and kidney anatomy and pathology. • Pyelolithotomy is the excision of a calculus from the renal pelvis.
Preoperative Diagnostic Tests and Procedures	• Same as for ureteroscopy
Equipment, Instruments, and Supplies Unique to Procedure	• Same as for nephrectomy
Preoperative Preparation	• Position: Lateral with kidney rests • Anesthesia: General • Skin prep: Axilla to mid-thigh • Draping: Transverse drape
Practical Considerations	• The position of the patient is lateral if the stone is within the renal pelvis or located in the upper part of the ureter. Supine position is used if the stone is located in the distal ureter. • X-rays should be in the OR.
Surgical Procedure	1. Using the #10 knife blade, the surgeon makes a flank incision. 2. The surgeon may have to remove the 12th rib with the rib resector in order to fully visualize the renal pelvis. 3. Vessels loops are placed around the distal ureter as close to the renal pelvis as possible and clamped to occlude the ureter. **Procedural Consideration:** This is performed to prevent the stone from traveling down the ureter if it becomes dislodged from the renal pelvis.

PROCEDURE 20-6 (continued)

4. With the help of the X-ray studies to view the location of the stone, the surgeon incises the renal pelvis over the stone using a #15 knife blade on a #7 knife handle.
5. Two traction sutures are placed lateral and medial to hold the two flaps of the incision open.
6. The surgeon uses the stone forceps to grasp and remove the stone.
7. The renal pelvis is thoroughly irrigated and inspected for additional small stones that may not have appeared on the X-rays.
8. The incision is closed with a 4-0 or 5-0 absorbable suture using interrupted technique.
9. A closed wound drainage system is placed with the tube laterally exteriorized.
10. Surgical wound is closed in layers as described for a nephrectomy.
11. Additional 4 × 4 dressings should be placed to reinforce the dressing. Urinary leakage can be expected for up to 5 postoperative days.

Postoperative Considerations

- Same as for nephrectomy

PROCEDURE 20-7 Cystoscopy with Overview of TURBT

Surgical Anatomy and Physiology

- Urine collects in the urinary bladder (henceforth referred to as bladder), which lies in the anterior half of the pelvis (Figure 20-15).
  - The bladder is located in a space bounded by the symphysis pubis anteriorly, walls of the pelvis bilaterally, and the rectovesical septum posteriorly.
  - The intimate space for the bladder is created by structures of the pelvic wall and diaphragm:
    - Inferior: levator ani muscles
    - Superior: obturator internus muscle
    - Posterior: rectum (male: Also the ductus deferens and seminal vesicles)
    - Anterior: abdominal wall
- In the male, the bladder lies on and is attached to the base of the prostate gland. In the female, the bladder lies on the pelvic diaphragm.
- The bladder is covered by endopelvic fascia. The puboprostatic ligament is an extension of the endopelvic fascia. It originates at the neck of the bladder and the base of the prostate gland and attaches to parietal fascia on the rear of the pubis and superior fascia of the pelvic diaphragm. This anchors the inferior portion of the bladder. Added stability of the bladder in both sexes results from the passage of the urethra through the structures of the perineum. The median umbilical ligament connects the bladder with the connective tissue of the umbilicus.

(continues)

PROCEDURE 20-7 (continued)

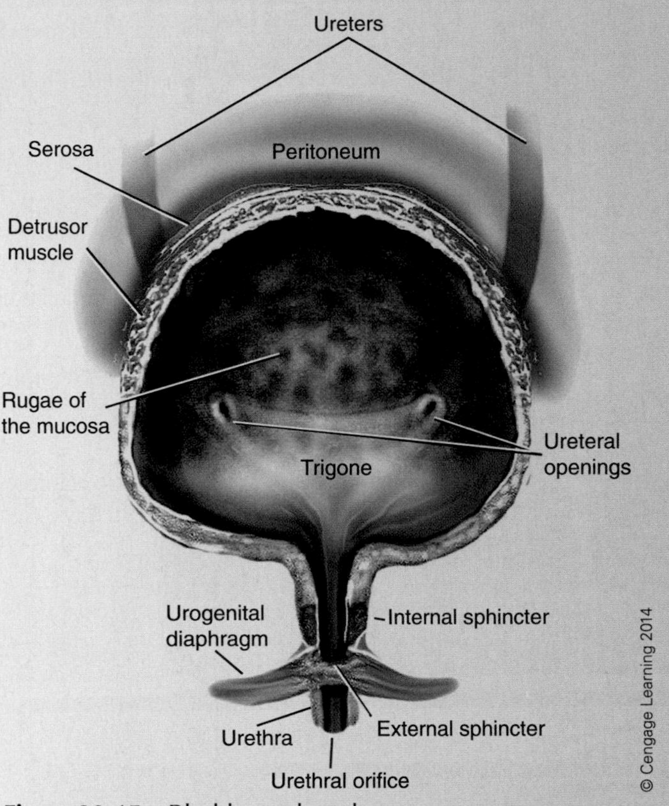

Figure 20-15 Bladder and urethra

- The detrusor muscle is responsible for both emptying the bladder and closing the bladder orifice.
- Internally, the bladder is lined with a mucous membrane that is wrinkled when the bladder is not distended. In the fundal area, the mucous membrane is smooth, making it easy to visualize. This triangular area, called the **vesical trigone**, is an important clinical landmark. The ureteral openings are found at the posterolateral angles of the triangle and the urethral aperture at the inferior angle. The ureteral openings are approximately 3 cm apart.
- Vascular supply to the bladder comes from the superior and inferior vesical arteries. These arteries arise from the anterior branch of the internal iliac artery. A plexus of veins within the endopelvic areolar tissue surrounds the neck of the bladder. The plexus extends to the point at which the ureters enter the bladder. In the male, the plexus communicates with the prostatic plexus, from which several vesical veins branch on each side. The veins empty into the internal iliac vein.
- Nerve supply extends to the bladder, lower ureter, seminal vesicle, and ductus deferens. Parasympathetic actions serve the bladder-emptying reflex (contraction of the detrusor muscle).
- Bladder tumors can be benign or malignant.
    - Benign tumors or papillomas occur only in young adults. The tumors seldom recur and follow-up care is not usually indicated.

Procedure 20-7 (continued)

	• Malignant tumors arise from the epithelial lining of the bladder and usually affect individuals over the age of 50. The tumor is often	mushroom shaped with a stalk-like attachment to the bladder wall. Bladder cancer has a tendency to recur and careful follow-up is necessary.	• Indications for performing a cystoscopy include hematuria, UTI, fistulas, urinary retention, urinary incontinence, and calculi.
Preoperative Diagnostic Tests and Procedures	• Cystoscopy itself is a diagnostic procedure, but can be performed for removing tissue biopsies,	calculi, catheters, and tumors. • Standard X-rays • CT scan	• Ultrasound • Laboratory tests: CBC, urinalysis, urine culture • IVP
Equipment, Instruments, and Supplies Unique to Procedure	• Rigid or flexible cystoscope (adult or pediatric) • Fiberoptic light source • Fiberoptic light cord • Albarran bridge (also referred to as short bridge if using a rigid cystoscope) • Foroblique telescope (if using a rigid cystoscope) • Cystoscopic instrumentation: Flexible grasping, biopsy, lithotrite (for lithopaxy procedure) and clamp forceps; flexible-stem electrode with ball,	cone, and bayonet tips available • Urethral sounds (male or female) • Ureteral catheter • Stopcock • Bags of irrigation solution (2000- or 3000-mL bags) • Cystoscopic irrigation tubing • Omnipaque or Renografin (radiopaque solutions) • Graduated pitcher to measure residual urine	• Specimen cups with lids for urine specimens • Topical local anesthetic jelly (Anestacon jelly) • Penile clamp • Sterile KY lubricant/jelly • Sterile cotton applicators • Ellik evacuators or Toomey syringes × 3 • ESU • Bugbee electrode for ESU • Fluoroscopy • Cystoscope drape • Drain pan attached to cystoscopy OR table
Preoperative Preparation	• Position: Low lithotomy • Anesthesia: Spinal or general	• Skin prep: Pubic area including scrotum and perineum	• Draping: Cystoscopy drape
Practical Considerations	• Because the patient could be in the lithotomy position for a period of time, it is important that the knees and legs of the patient are well padded and protected from pressure, in particular to relieve pressure on the popliteal region. The circulating person should check the pedal pulses	after the patient is positioned and at the end of the procedure after the drape has been removed and the patient moved back into the supine position. • The instruments and endoscopes should at least undergo high-level disinfection with	2% glutaraldehyde. However, some health care facilities may sterilize the instruments and cystoscope; the manufacturer's recommendations must be followed for sterilizing endoscopic instrumentation and endoscopes.

(*continues*)

Procedure 20-7 (continued)

- The irrigating solution should be nonelectrolytic and isotonic (e.g., glycine, sorbitol, water).
- Cystoscopy is performed to examine the urethra, bladder, ureteral orifices, and bladder neck; in the male the prostate is examined.
- The patient is requested to void just prior to transport to the OR. The volume of urine and time of urination should be documented in the patient's chart in order to confirm it is not residual urine.

Surgical Procedure

1. The surgical technologist instills the local anesthetic jelly down the urethra of the male patient and applies the penile clamp. For female patients, the surgical technologist will use a sterile cotton applicator; the local anesthetic is squeezed out onto the tip, which is then placed in the urethral meatus.
2. The urethra is dilated with urethral sounds.
3. The tip of the cystoscope is lubricated with KY jelly and inserted into the urethra and advanced into the bladder. The obturator is removed and a urine specimen may be obtained while the bladder is drained (Figure 20-16)

   Procedural Consideration: Residual urine may also be measured using the graduated pitcher.

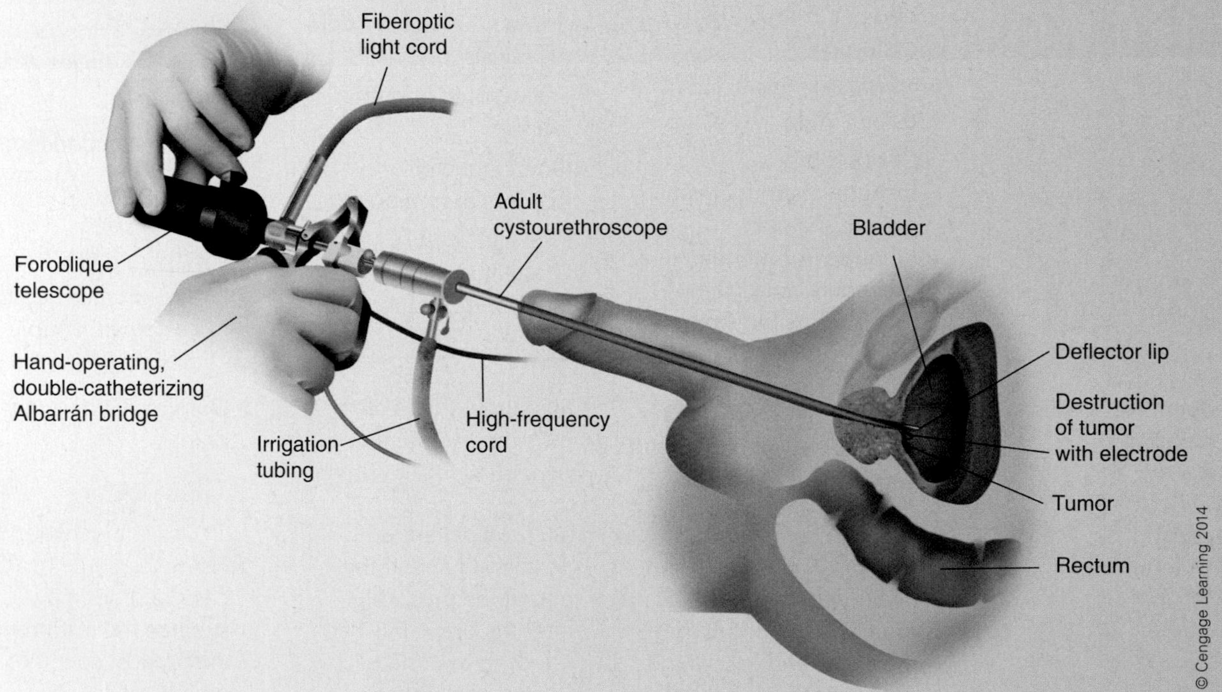

Figure 20-16 Fulguration of a bladder tumor.

4. The irrigation tubing is connected to the cystoscope and the fluid from the bags allowed to flow into the bladder.

   Procedural Consideration: The surgeon is able to control the rate of flow with the use of the stopcock on the cystoscope.

PROCEDURE 20-7 (continued)

5. To view the upper urinary tract the surgeon can insert a ureteral catheter through the cystoscope port, through the ureteral orifice of the bladder and advanced into the ureter. Omnipaque or Renografin is injected and fluoroscopy is used to view the upper urinary tract.
6. Other procedures are performed at this time if necessary, such as extraction of calculi, removal of a bladder tumor, etc.
7. The surgeon removes the cystoscope and inserts the Foley catheter with drainage bag.

Postoperative Considerations

Immediate Postoperative Care
- Patient is transported to the PACU.
- Depending on extent of procedure, the patient is either discharged the same day of surgery or hospitalized for 1–2 days.

Prognosis
- No complications: Patient expected to have ful recovery. Extent of bladder tumor determines if follow-up radiation and chemotherapy is necessary.
- Complications: Postoperative SSI; hemorrhage; urethral injury.

Wound Classification
- Class I: Clean
- Class II: Clean-contaminated

Because the transurethral resection of bladder tumors (TUBT) procedure is the same as for transurethral resection of the prostate (TURP), an overview of TURBT will be provided and the details provided in the description of the TURP procedure.

The instruments to be added to the cystoscopy setup include the resectoscope that includes the sheath and obturator, working element (also called operating element), and cutting loops. A 24 Fr rigid cystoscope will be used; therefore, the Albarran bridge and Foroblique telescope will be needed as well as a biopsy forceps to excise bladder tissue specimens from various areas of the bladder.

Sterile water will be used for irrigation. If the bladder tumor is malignant, cancer cells can be dislodged during the procedure. The cells take up water until they burst (lyse), thus preventing their reimplantation onto the bladder wall and/or systemic entry into the body.

A cystoscopy is often quickly performed; the cystoscope is removed, leaving the sheath in place. The resectoscope with sheath, obturator, and bridge is inserted down the urethra into the bladder. Irrigation tubing, fiberoptic light cord, and cautery cable are connected to the resectoscope. The obturator is removed and the working element with cutting loop and Foroblique telescope is inserted through the bridge and sheath. The tumor is removed using the cutting loop. The surgeon will often excise a small portion of the bladder muscle with the tumor for the pathologist to determine if the tumor has invaded the bladder muscle and wall. Additional tissue specimens will be taken with the biopsy forceps after the tumor is removed. The bladder is thoroughly irrigated and checked for hemostasis and the resectoscope and sheath are removed. A Foley catheter with drainage bag is inserted.

Cystectomy/Ileal Conduit

Cystectomy is removal of the bladder. Partial or segmental cystectomy may be performed to remove a single invasive bladder tumor situated in the dome of the bladder. Occasionally, the need arises for a simple total cystectomy consisting of bladder removal only. Radical cystectomy differs slightly between male and female patients. In the male, the bladder, prostate, and seminal vesicles are removed; in the female, the dissection includes the bladder, urethra, anterior vaginal wall, uterus, fallopian tubes, and ovaries. The radical procedure is for treatment of malignancies that have invaded the nearby tissues.

When the entire bladder is removed, a urinary diversion procedure must accompany cystectomy. Several surgical options are available for urinary diversion. Simple cutaneous ureterostomy is not a sound choice for long-term drainage, but may be temporarily implemented if the patient cannot tolerate a prolonged procedure. The ileal **conduit**, also called the ureteroileocutaneous diversion, is the standard procedure (Procedure 20-8). The patient wears an external stoma bag for collection of the urine. A final, more difficult to accomplish, option is the continent urinary reservoir (referred to as a Koch pouch) fashioned from reconfigured bowel to serve as the holding area for the urine. The reservoir has a capacity of 400–1200 mL and is emptied by periodic catheterization of an abdominal **stoma**. The stoma's continence is maintained by intussusception of the ileum just inside the stoma.

Procedure 20-8 Radical Cystectomy with Ileal Conduit—Male Patient

Surgical Anatomy and Pathology	• See previous procedures for anatomy of the bladder.		
Preoperative Diagnostic Tests and Procedures	• History and physical • Standard X-rays • CT scan	• MRI • Abdominal ultrasound • Laboratory blood tests	
Equipment, Instruments, and Supplies Unique to Procedure	• Extended electrocautery tip • Stoma bag • Ureteral stents of surgeon's preference (available) • Laparotomy instrument set	• Long instrument set • Bowel instrument set • Vascular instrument set • Hemoclip appliers and hemoclips (various sizes) • Stapling devices for bowel	• Self-retaining abdominal retractor (surgeon's preference) • Surgeon specific drains and catheters • #10 knife blades × 4-5 • Kitner sponges
Preoperative Preparation	• Position: Supine • Anesthesia: General	• Skin prep: Mid-chest to thigh and bilaterally as far as possible	• Draping: Four towels to square off; laparotomy drape
Practical Considerations	• Ileostomy site may be predetermined and marked. (Be sure markings are not inadvertently removed during the skin prep.) Patient or caregiver is given instructions regarding stoma care. • Preoperative radiographic films should be displayed in the OR. • Variation (according to surgeon's preference):	Patient may be placed in low lithotomy position (additional positioning aids and drapes will be necessary). The Foley catheter is inserted from the sterile field and the entire drainage system remains sterile throughout the procedure. • Patient may have already undergone a series of radiation treatments that could negatively affect	the tissue at the operative site. • Notify pathologist that frozen section specimens will be sent during procedure. • The genitourologist may request that a general surgeon assist with the procedure. For female patients, a gynecologist may be requested to assist.

Surgical Procedure

1. A long vertical incision is used to enter the abdominal cavity.

   Procedural Consideration: A #10 knife blade on a #3 knife handle is used. Anticipate use of cautery and suction.

2. The bladder is exposed and the intraperitoneal contents are palpated to be sure the area is free of unsuspected masses.

   Procedural Consideration: Warm, moist lap sponges are used as packing to retract the bowel and a self-retaining abdominal retractor is placed. The procedure may be terminated at this point if it is determined that the tumor has progressed beyond resection.

PROCEDURE 20-8 (continued)

3. The urachus, a connective tissue that forms the umbilical ligament, is clamped and transsected. The proximal end is ligated and the large clamp remains distally to be used for traction.

   Procedural Consideration: Large Mayo clamps are needed to clamp the urachus; one remains to provide bladder traction. Long, heavy nonabsorbable ties on a passer (Kelly or Pean clamp) are needed for the proximal urachus.

4. If planned, a lymphadenectomy is performed at this time.

   Procedural Consideration: A combination of sharp and blunt dissection is used. Sharp dissection: Long Metzenbaum scissors and DeBakey tissue forceps are used. Blunt dissection: Surgeon may use the fingers, a Kitner placed on the end of a long Mayo clamp, or a sponge on a stick. Several specimens may be collected.

5. The bladder is freed from its attachments to the posterior symphysis down to the level of the puboprostatic ligaments.

   Procedural Consideration: Any bleeding is immediately controlled with the cautery, hemoclips, or ligatures.

6. The bladder is retracted medially, exposing the iliac blood vessels and obturator fossa on that side.

   Procedural Consideration: Sharp and blunt dissection continues. Suction will be used almost constantly.

7. Then 8–10 cm of vas deferens is excised and the gonadal vessels are mobilized.

   Procedural Consideration: Sudden hemorrhage may occur. Long hemostatic clamps must be available at all times.

8. The dissection is repeated on the contralateral side.

   Procedural Consideration: Reorganize supplies and repeat procedural steps.

9. The pelvic peritoneum is incised and the dissection carried downward on each side of the bladder to free the superior and lateral aspects.

   Procedural Consideration: A #10 knife blade on a #15 knife handle is needed. Follow with cautery.

10. The right paracolic gutter is incised to expose the ureter. The cecum, right colon, and small intestine are mobilized and retracted superiorly. Similarly, the peritoneum lateral to the sigmoid is opened and the ureter exposed.

    Procedural Consideration: Instruments for dissection will be needed repeatedly. Observe progression of procedure and anticipate instruments for use. More warm, moist laparotomy sponges are needed as packing to retract the intestine.

11. The ureters are isolated and dissected back as far as necessary. A segment of each proximal ureter is sent for frozen section to determine if the surgical margins are free of malignancy.

    Procedural Consideration: Prepare to accept two specimens for frozen section. Be sure that each is correctly labeled.

12. The ureters are temporarily tucked into the upper abdomen until needed for the reconstruction.

(continues)

Procedure 20-8 (continued)

Procedural Consideration: Provide warm, moist lap sponges to wall off and protect the ureters. The surgical technologist must keep track of the number of laparotomy sponges that are placed within the abdominal cavity.

13. The bladder is pulled to one side with the traction clamp and the endopelvic fascia is opened and bluntly dissected inferiorly to its pedicle.

    Procedural Consideration: Reload Kitners and stick sponges as they become soiled. Provide clean lap sponges as needed throughout the procedure.

14. Dissection is repeated on the contralateral side and then both pedicles are doubly clamped, cut, and tied. The process is repeated as many times as necessary for tissue in each pedicle.

    Procedural Consideration: Provide long Mayo clamps, long Metzenbaum scissors, and ties preloaded on passers, followed by long Mayo suture scissors.

15. The cul-de-sac of the peritoneum is incised and the incision extended to the level of the existing lateral peritoneal incisions.

    Procedural Consideration: The incision may be initiated with a #15 knife blade on a #7 knife handle and extended with the long Metzenbaum scissors. Long DeBakey tissue forceps are usually needed along with the scissors for dissection.

16. The rectum and sigmoid are retracted, the bladder pulled forward, and the dissection carried toward the prostate and seminal vesicles.

    Procedural Consideration: A malleable retractor may be useful for rectal resection. Once retractors are set, dissection continues.

17. The hemorrhoidal vessels are encountered and are immediately clamped, cut, and tied.

    Procedural Consideration: Continue clamp-clamp-cut-tie routine. Suture is prepared in advance of need.

18. Mobilization continues toward the prostatic and membranous urethra. The structures affecting erectile function may be preserved with careful dissection, if this is a concern.

    Procedural Consideration: Blunt and sharp dissection continues. Provide suction and cautery as needed.

19. The Foley catheter is removed prior to clamping the membranous urethra with two clamps. The urethra is cut and tied with strong nonabsorbable sutures.

    Procedural Consideration: Syringe is needed to deflate Foley balloon. Provide clamps, scissors, and ligatures.

20. All remaining attachments are severed and the bladder is removed. Hemorrhage is controlled. If pressure is needed to control bleeding, a Foley catheter with a 30-mL balloon may be inserted transurethrally; the balloon is fully inflated, and external traction is applied.

    Procedural Consideration: Prepare to accept the bladder specimen. Suction and irrigation fluid may be used. Provide cautery or hemoclips as needed. Anticipate possible use of Foley catheter for hemorrhage control.

(*continues*)

Procedure 20-8 (continued)

21. The area is packed with moist laparotomy sponges and the diversionary procedure begun.

    Procedural Consideration: Provide warm, moist lap sponges. Prepare for intestinal portion of the procedure. Keep in mind that entry to the GI tract will change the wound classification and that certain instruments used to create the conduit will require isolation on the sterile field, and bowel technique should be implemented.

22. The conduit is fashioned from a 20-cm length of terminal ileum. The designated segment of ileum is divided between two noncrushing intestinal clamps. Stapling devices may be used according to surgeon's preference.

    Procedural Consideration: Provide bowel clamps of surgeon's choice.

23. The corresponding mesentery is divided on both sides of the segment to be used for the conduit.

    Procedural Consideration: Stapling devices may be used to divide the mesentery or the routine clamp-clamp-cut-tie system is used.

24. The remaining ileum is positioned posteriorly, continuity restored with routine small bowel anastomosis, and the mesenteric defect is closed.

    Procedural Consideration: Refer to Chapter 14 for technical considerations for bowel anastomosis. Prepare stents if use is expected.

25. Both ureters are implanted into the ileal segment (Figure 20-17). Stents may be inserted if necessary.

    Procedural Consideration: The ileum is opened sharply and suture for anastomosis is provided. The procedure is repeated for the second ureter.

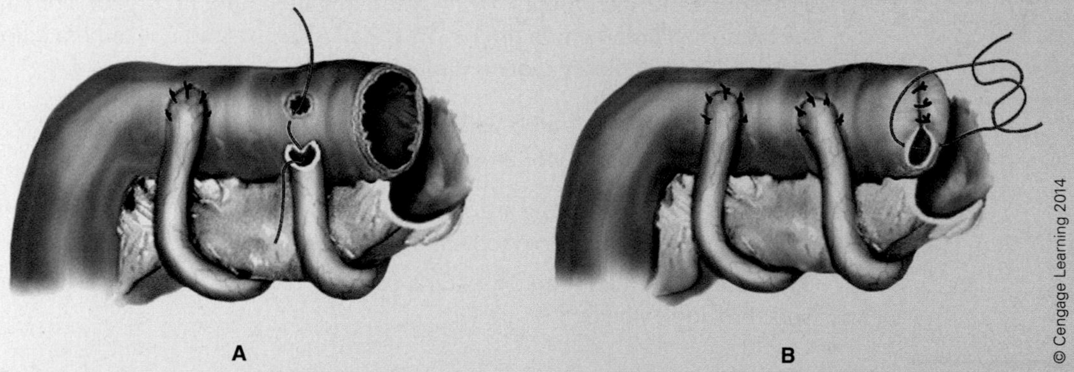

Figure 20-17 Ileal conduit: (A) Ureters implanted into ileal segment, (B) closure of proximal ileal conduit

26. The proximal end of the conduit is closed.

    Procedural Consideration: The proximal ileum may be closed with suture or staples according to the surgeon's preference.

27. The distal end of the ileum is brought through the abdominal wall at a predetermined location through a separate incision.

    Procedural Consideration: A skin knife is needed, followed by cautery. Provide a pair of U.S. Army or small Richardson retractors.

(continues)

PROCEDURE 20-8 (continued)

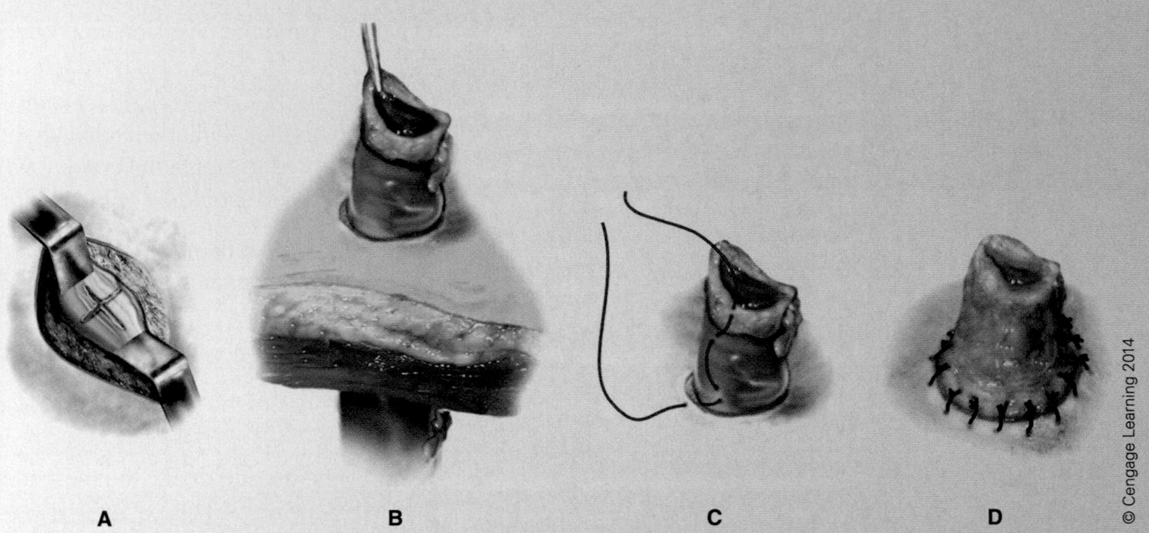

Figure 20-18 End ileostomy: (A) Abdominal incision for stoma, (B) ileum brought through abdominal wall, (C) ileal edge everted to created stoma, (D) end of ileal stoma

28. The conduit is fixed into position and the stoma created by everting the ileal edge and affixing it to the skin (Figure 20-18).

    Procedural Consideration: Sutures are needed to secure the conduit to the abdominal wall. The stoma is affixed to the skin with sutures or staples.

29. The wound is inspected, hemostasis is achieved, and wound drains are inserted if necessary.

    Procedural Consideration: Provide warm irrigation fluid of surgeon's preference and suction. The Poole suction tip may be useful. Clamps, cautery, or hemoclips may be needed. Prepare closed wound drain(s).

30. The midline incision is closed in the usual manner.

    Procedural Consideration: Provide suture for closure. Count.

31. Dressings and a stoma bag are applied. Some surgeons prefer to catheterize the stoma to prevent urine contact with the external tissues until the stoma has matured.

    Procedural Consideration: The stoma bag may be customized. Provide heavy scissors. Provide catheter if requested.

Postoperative Considerations

Immediate Postoperative Care

- Patient is transported to the PACU.
- Antibiotics and analgesics will be prescribed.

Prognosis

- No complications: Patient may be hospitalized for 5–7 days; diet should be resumed slowly and patient should have a bowel movement before discharge; patient or caregiver will be responsible for a lifetime of stoma care; additional treatment for cancer may be necessary; patient is expected to resume normal activities within 6–8 weeks.
- Complications: Postoperative SSI; hemorrhage; leakage of the small bowel or ureteroileal anastomosis; irritation around the stoma site; stenosis at the stoma site or at the ureteroileal anastomosis.

Wound classification

- Class I: Clean (bladder portion of procedure)
- Class II: Clean-contaminated (ileum and ureter portion of procedure)

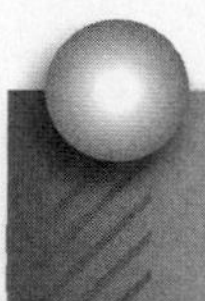

PEARL OF WISDOM

If seeding of malignant cells is of concern, the bladder may be filled with formalin solution prior to the urethral transsection. The fluid should remain in the bladder and urethra for approximately 10 minutes to decrease the viability of potentially contaminating tumor cells. After the prescribed amount of time, the fluid is drained and the urethral dissection continues.

PROCEDURES FOR STRESS INCONTINENCE AFFECTING WOMEN

Several procedural options are available to women who experience stress **incontinence**. The objectives are to restore the posterior urethrovesical angle and elevate the base of the bladder, which may have been distorted during childbirth or as the natural result of aging.

Mild stress incontinence may be reduced following an anterior colporrhaphy. Colporrhaphy elevates the base of the bladder by eliminating redundant and weakened vaginal tissue. The gynecologist often performs this procedure in conjunction with vaginal hysterectomy (refer to Chapter 15).

Significant incontinent episodes may be eliminated with suprapubic vesicourethral suspension (Marshall-Marchetti-Krantz [MMK] procedure). The MMK procedure may be performed by the genitourologist or gynecologist in conjunction with abdominal hysterectomy or as a lone procedure (refer to Procedure 20-9).

PROCEDURE 20-9 Marshall-Marchetti-Krantz Procedure

Surgical Anatomy and Pathology	• See previous procedures for anatomy of the bladder.	• See introduction to stress incontinence above for pathology.	
Preoperative Diagnostic Tests and Procedures	• History and physical	• Standard X-rays	• CT scan
Equipment, Instruments, and Supplies Unique to Procedure	• Extended electrocautery tip • Laparotomy instrument set	• Long instrument set • Heaney needle holders • Hemoclips	• Blades: #10 × 2, #15 × 1 • Kitner sponges
Preoperative Preparation	• Position: Supine with Trendelenburg or modified lithotomy (surgeon's preference) • Anesthesia: General is preferred but regional may be used.	• Skin prep: Mid-chest to thigh and bilaterally as far as possible; vulvar and internal vaginal prep is also required. • Draping: Supine position: four towels for	squaring off and a transverse laparotomy sheet; modified lithotomy position: drape sheet under buttocks, leggings, towels, and transverse sheet
Practical Considerations	• Foley catheter may be inserted by circulator preoperatively or from	the sterile field by the surgeon or surgical technologist.	

(continues)

Procedure 20-9 (continued)

Surgical Procedure

1. A Pfannenstiel incision is used to approach the retropubic space.

   Procedural Consideration: A #10 knife blade on a #3 knife handle is used to make the incision. Provide cautery and suction.

2. The bladder and urethra are freed from behind the symphysis pubis using blunt dissection techniques.

   Procedural Consideration: The surgeon may use the fingers, Kitners on a Kelly or Pean clamp, or a sponge on a stick for dissection. Prepare supplies in advance of need.

3. The endopelvic fascia is incised to allow for displacement of the bladder.

   Procedural Consideration: A #10 knife blade on a #3 or #7 knife handle may be needed, according to patient's size (depth of surgical wound).

4. The assistant will insert two gloved fingers into the vagina to elevate the base of the bladder (which is easily palpable due to the presence of the Foley catheter balloon) to facilitate suture placement and reduce tension.

   Procedural Consideration: Protect sterile field from contamination during this process.

5. Four heavy absorbable sutures are placed in strategic locations in the anterior vaginal wall bilaterally to the urethra and are secured in the posterior symphysis or Cooper's ligament (Figure 20-19).

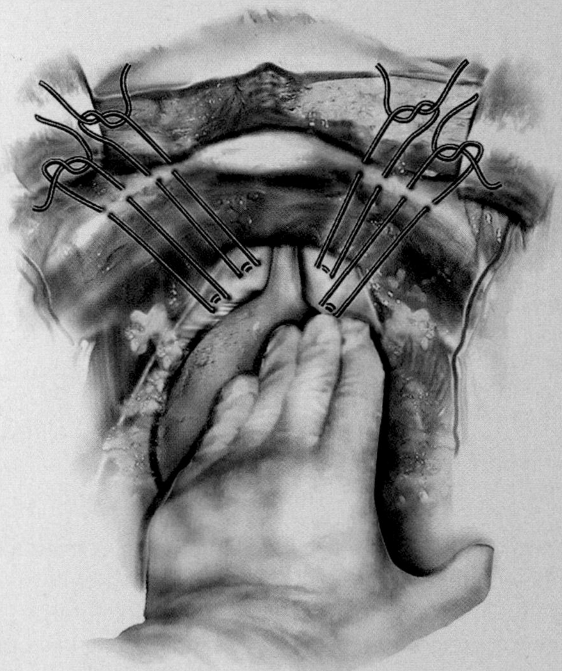

Figure 20-19 Marshall-Marchetti-Krantz procedure—suprapubic vesicourethral suspension with suture fixation to Cooper's ligament

(continues)

PROCEDURE 20-9 (continued)

Procedural Consideration: Load sutures on Heaney needle holders for placement. Anticipate the use of all four sutures sequentially. A series of curved hemostats may be required to "tag" the sutures until all have been placed and are ready for tying.

6. All sutures are positioned and then tied sequentially for optimum elevation of the bladder.

   Procedural Consideration: Provide Mayo suture scissors as needed. Assist circulator in changing assistant's gown and gloves. Provide towel to cover site following bladder elevation. Prepare closed wound drain, if requested. Anticipate wound closure and prepare suture.

7. Closed wound drain is placed. The wound is closed and dressed in the usual laparotomy fashion.

   Procedural Consideration: Count. Provide dressing material.

8. Vaginal packing may be inserted to temporarily reduce tension on the suture line.

   Procedural Consideration: Vaginal packing is inserted after the abdominal dressing is in place.

Postoperative Considerations

Immediate Postoperative Care

- Patient is transported to the PACU.
- Blood-tinged urine may be noted in the Foley drainage bag.
- The Foley catheter may be removed in the PACU; the patient is expected to void normally.

Prognosis

- No complications: The patient may remain hospitalized overnight; patient is expected to return to normal activities in 6–8 weeks and incontinence resolved.
- Complications: Postoperative SSI; hemorrhage; recurrence of urinary stress incontinence.

Wound Classification

- Class I: Clean

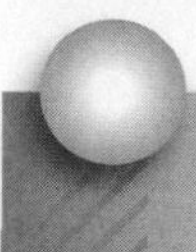

PEARL OF WISDOM

The surgical technologist should be cognizant that a potential for contamination of the field exists due to the vaginal and abdominal areas being incorporated in the same drape. The assistant will need to change gloves (and possibly gown) immediately after providing intravaginal urethral support during suturing.

Suburethral Sling (Pubovaginal Sling)

A suburethral or pubovaginal sling procedure may be recommended to women who have been unsuccessfully treated for stress urinary incontinence via surgical elevation and stabilization techniques. These particular patients have severe stress urinary incontinence, which negatively impacts their lives and daily activities. The suburethral or pubovaginal sling procedure requires that a piece of a graft strip (fascia lata) or a synthetic material be placed in the patient. The fascia lata graft may be an autograft or an allograft. The sling material is placed directly under the bladder neck (proximal urethra) or mid-urethra and acts as a support to prevent bladder neck and urethral descent during physical activity. Tension-free vaginal tape (TVT) is a polypropylene-meshed tape, which is placed mid-urethra. The TVT device includes the polypropylene-mesh tape covered by a plastic sheath and held by two stainless needles on both ends.

Many patients are discharged from the hospital following these procedures within 1–3 days. Patients receive both intravenous antibiotics and oral antibiotics. Vaginal packing is removed prior to the patient leaving the health care facility. Patients are prescribed pain medication for use after discharge from the health care facility. Potential complications include hemorrhage, infection, urethral obstruction, urinary retention, recurrence of stress urinary incontinence, and urge incontinence.

PROSTATE SURGERY

Prostatectomy is the surgical removal of all or part of the prostate. The procedure can be accomplished transurethrally or may require an open procedure. The approach will be determined primarily by the patient's pathological condition. Removal of a cancerous prostate usually requires an open procedure, whereas the patient suffering from benign prostatic hypertrophy (BPH) is most often treated transurethrally.

PROCEDURE 20-10 Transurethral Resection of the Prostate (TURP)

Surgical Anatomy and Pathology

- The male urethra passes through the prostate gland, urethral sphincter, perineal membrane, and penis.
  - It is divided into three parts: prostatic, membranous, and spongy.
  - The prostatic section passes through the prostate gland. It receives most of the ducts of the prostate gland. The ejaculatory duct opens on each side of a urethral structure called the prostatic utricle.
  - The membranous section crosses the annulus of the sphincter urethra muscle and the perimenal membrane. The bulbourethral glands enter the spongy section of the urethra.
  - The spongy section of the urethra enters the bulb of the penis just after the perineal membrane has been crossed and terminates at the urethral orifice.
- The ductus deferens, more commonly called the vas deferens, arises from the duct of the epididymis. The vas deferens ascends through the inguinal canal within the spermatic cord. It descends to the fundus of the bladder and travels medial to the ureter and seminal vesicle. It narrows just superior to the base of the prostate gland and is joined by the duct of the seminal vesicle to form the ejactulatory duct. The vas deferens has a thick muscular layer that delivers semen to the prostate urethra by peristaltic action.
- The seminal vesicles lie on the fundus of the bladder, enclosed by endopelvic fascia. The seminal vesicles narrow at the prostatic end and unit with the vas deferens.
- The thin-walled ejaculatory ducts are formed by the unification of the vas deferens and seminal vesicles. The ejaculatory ducts open into the prostatic urethra at either side of the prostatic utricle.
- The prostate gland lies under the bladder. Its apex touches the perineal membrane.
  - The boundary of the lateral surfaces of the prostate is the superior fascia of the pelvic diaphragm.
  - The rectoprostatic fascia separates and covers the posterior portion of the prostate and the urinary bladder from the rectum and covers the seminal vesicles. The fascia is composed of multiple layers that are fused together. It is also called Denonvilliers' fascia after the famous French surgeon Charles-Pierre Denonvilliers.
  - The prostate is covered with endopelvic fascia, which is a part of the puboprostatic ligament (also called Denonvilliers' ligament).
  - The urethra extends through the prostate, entering near the midbase and exiting on the anterior surface just above the apex.
  - The ejaculatory ducts enter the posterior

Procedure 20-10 (continued)

	base and open at the prostatic utricle. • The prostate gland itself is enclosed by a fibromuscular capsule. The gland is lobulated into approximately 50 lobules. • The arterial supply consists of branches of the inferior vesical and middle rectal arteries. • Veins form a prostatic plexus to the anterior and lateral portions of the gland. They empty into the sacral and internal iliac veins. • Benign prostatic **hypertrophy** (BPH) is considered to be a normal part of aging	affecting most men over the age of 50. • As a man matures, the prostate increases in size; this is thought to be due to hormonal changes that occur throughout the life span. • Eventually, the capsule surrounding the prostate prevents it from expanding and it begins to exert pressure on the urethra, which it encircles. As the urethra narrows, urination becomes more difficult, leading to urinary urgency, frequency, and	retention. Retained urine can lead to chronic UTIs. • Prostate cancer in the early stages is asymptomatic. • As the tumor grows the patient will experience the same signs and symptoms as those with BPH. • Patients in the advanced stages of prostate cancer experience pelvic pain due to the tumor mass and bone pain from metastasis. Prostate cancer has an affinity for metastasizing to the large bones.
Preoperative Diagnostic Tests and Procedures	• Digital rectal examination • PSA blood test	• Tissue biopsy • Chest X-ray	• CT scan • Bone scan
Equipment, Instruments, and Supplies Unique to Procedure	• See Table 20-5 for additional descriptions of the equipment, instruments, and supplies. • KY jelly lubricant • Fiberoptic light source • Cystoscope • Continuous-flow pump for isotonic irrigation solution • Resectoscope, including sheath, obturator, cutting loops, operating	element, Foroblique telescope, high-frequency ESU cord (Figure 20-6) • Fiberoptic light cord • 2–3 Ellik evacuators or Toomey syringes (surgeon's preference) • Strainer/screen for cystoscopy table • Penis clamp • Stopcock • Van Buren sounds (Figure 20-2)	• Hemostats • 3–6 liters of isotonic, nonhemolytic irrigant (3% sorbitol or 1.5% glycine; surgeon's preference) • Three-way Foley catheter, 22 or 24 Fr, with 30-mL balloon and bag • 30-mL syringe • Ball and/or blade style electrode tips
Preoperative Preparation	• Position: Lithotomy • Anesthesia: Regional or general	• Skin prep: Entire pubic area, including scrotum and perineum is prepped.	• Draping: Four towels and cystoscopy drape

(continues)

PROCEDURE 20-10 (continued)

Practical Considerations

- The irrigating solution should be sterile, isotonic, nonhemolytic, and at body temperature or slightly warmed.
- The surgical technologist may need to practice filling and refilling the Ellik evacuator prior to assisting a surgeon on a TURP.
- It is recommended that the surgical technologist have 2–3 Ellik evacuators available and fill them while setting up for the procedure.
- The surgical technologist should know how to efficiently assemble the resectoscope and know the connections for the irrigation tubing, light cord, and high-frequency ESU cord. There are four types of resectoscopes: Baumrucker, Iglesias, Stern-McCarthy, and Nesbit; the surgical technologist should know ahead of time which one will be used.
- The amount of time required for TURP is directly related to the size of the prostate gland and can range from 30 minutes to 3 hours.
- The surgical technologist should be aware of several intraoperative complications specific to TURP that could negatively affect the outcome of the procedure:
  - It may be impossible to enter the urethra with the resectoscope due to obstruction. Urethral dilation may be effective in opening the passage or a perineal urethrostomy may be performed to introduce the resectoscope.
  - Uncontrollable hemorrhage may obscure the visual field. The procedure may be terminated immediately and pressure applied to the area with a Foley catheter balloon under traction, or the procedure may be converted to an open procedure.
  - A sudden jerk of one of the patient's legs is an indicator that the electrical stimulation from the elctrocautery is irritating the obturateor nerve and that perforation of the prostatic capsule may be imminent. Surgical team members should report any unexpected movement by the patient to the surgeon and anesthesia provider. Modification of the technique used by the surgeon can prevent nerve injury and prevent perforation of the capsule.
    - Accidental perforation of the prostatic capsule allows irrigating fluid to escape into the space surrounding the prostate. When the sudden jerk of the leg is observed, the surgeon may immediately terminate the procedure once hemostasis is achieved and any remaining loose prostatic tissue is removed. The perforation should be documented with a urethrocystogram. If the leakage is extensive, a drain may be inserted to remove the fluid.
  - Systemic absorption of the irrigating fluid is a serious complication. The irrigant is absorbed into venous circulation and places an abnormal fluid load on the circulatory system referred to as TURP syndrome. Early signs include restlessness, confusion, nausea, and vomiting when the patient is regionally anesthetized. The diagnosis is more difficult with the patient under general anesthesia.
  - Late signs of systemic absorption of the irrigant affecting the neurological system are seizures, coma, and blindness; the respiratory and cardiovascular signs are pulmonary edema and congestive heart failure.
  - The anesthesia provider will

PROCEDURE 20-10 (continued)

	administer furosemide to help reduce the amount of intravascular fluid. The patient will be monitored for electrolyte and blood gas imbalances and a central venous pressure (CVP) monitor will be inserted. The patient will be transported to the ICU.
Surgical Procedure	1. Patient is anesthetized regionally or generally, placed in lithotomy position, prepped, and draped. A screen is part of the drape and it should be positioned over the cysto table drainage pan.
	2. The urethra is dilated with the Van Buren sounds. **Procedural Consideration:** The surgeon may want lubricant for the Van Buren sounds.
	3. The surgeon may perform a preliminary cystoscopy to determine the size of the prostate and visualize the bladder.
	4. The cystoscope is removed.
	5. The lubricated sheath with obturator is inserted into the urethra. **Procedural Consideration:** The surgical technologist should lubricate the tip of the sheath with obturator just before giving it to the surgeon for insertion into the urethra.
	6. The obturator is removed and the resectoscope with the Foroblique telescope and cutting loop is inserted through the sheath. Additionally, if a continuous-flow resectoscope is used, an outlet stopcock is connected.
	7. The irrigation tubing, light cord, and high-frequency ESU cord are connected. When a continuous-flow resectoscope is used, the irrigation tubing is connected to the outlet stopcock. The circulator opens the clamp on the irrigation fluid tubing to allow it to flow and fill the bladder. The bladder is continuously irrigated. **Procedural Consideration:** The surgical technologist will assist the surgeon in connecting the irrigation tubing, light cord, outlet stopcock, and high-frequency ESU.
	8. The surgeon examines the urethra and bladder trigone.
	9. The surgeon begins electrodissection of the prostate tissue, alternating between coagulating and cutting currents through the use of a foot pedal. A loop electrode is used to resect the tissue. The surgeon performs multiple strokes or passes with the electrode to dissect the tissue (Figure 20-20). **Procedural Consideration:** The surgical technologist should have a sterile brush or scratch pad for cleaning the cutting loop electrode.
	10. The surgeon will intermittently remove tissue fragments by removing the resectoscope and allow the irrigation fluid to flow out. Additionally, the surgeon will use the Ellik evacuator or Toomey syringe to remove resected prostatic tissue. Once the resectoscope is removed, the tip of the evacuator is attached to the sheath and the surgeon manually removes the tissue. **Procedural Consideration:** The surgical technologist must move quickly in refilling the Ellik evacuator or Toomey syringe.
	11. Once the resection of prostate tissue is complete, the bladder, protatic fossa, and urethra are inspected for debris and bleeding. A ball or blade electrode will be substituted for the loop electrode for use in coagulating bleeding vessels.
	12. The resectoscope is removed.

(*continues*)

Procedure 20-10 (continued)

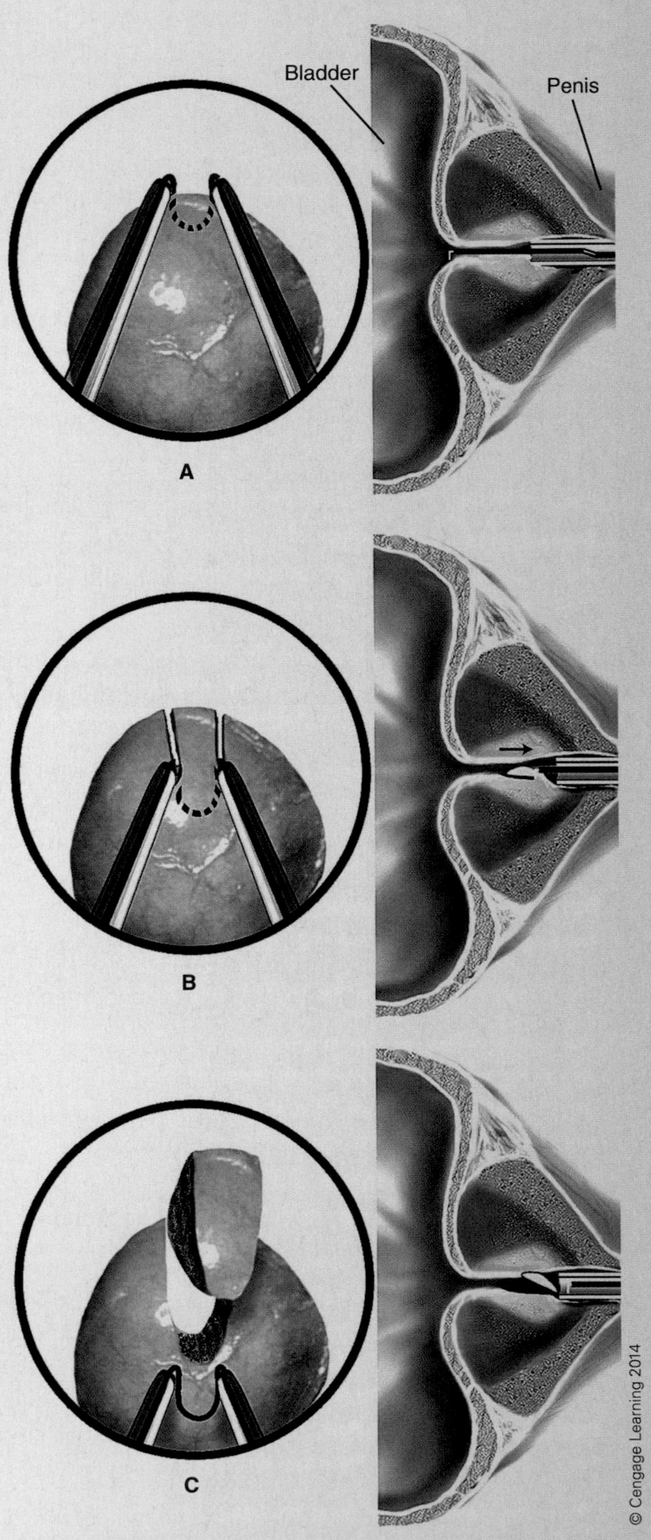

Figure 20-20 Transurethral prostatectomy: (A) Prostate gland visualized, (B) resectoscope used to remove hyperplastic tissue, (C) prostate chip separated

PROCEDURE 20-10 (continued)

13. The Foley catheter is inserted into the bladder. The catheter may be manually irrigated to assess hemostasis. Bladder drainage is expected to be clear or slightly tinged with blood. Grossly bloody drainage may be indicative of bleeding. If necessary, the surgeon will remove the catheter, reinsert the resectoscope, inspect the operative site for bleeding, and fulgurate bleeding vessels.

    Procedural Consideration: The surgical technologist should have a syringe available for the surgeon to manually irrigate through the Foley catheter. The syringe also is needed to fill the catheter balloon.

14. Once the Foley is in place and the balloon is inflated, the balloon is gently pulled against the bladder neck and the external tubing is taped to the patient's leg to provide traction, which aids in reducing bleeding.

    Procedural Consideration: The surgical technologist must gently remove the drape; he or she is responsible for removing the resected prostatic tissue from the screen because this is tissue specimen and must be sent to pathology.

Postoperative Considerations

Immediate Postoperative Care

- Patient is transported to the PACU.
- Pain medication should not be required until the regional anesthetic wears off.
- The urine in the Foley bag should be periodically visualized for indications of bleeding in the PACU and when the patient is in his hospital room.

Prognosis

- No complications: The patient remains hospitalized for several days until the urine draining from the catheter is clear, the catheter can be removed, and the patient is able to void on his own satisfactorily. Normal activity, including sexual activity, can be resumed in 4–6 weeks.
- Complications: Postoperative SSI; hemorrhage; urethral stricture; injury to the urethra; TURP syndrome.

Wound classification

- Depending on health care facility policy, a TURP procedure may be classified as Class II: Clean-contaminated or Class V: Unclassified

PROCEDURE 20-11 Laparoscopic Prostatectomy with Robot

Surgical Anatomy and Pathology

- See Procedure 20-10

Equipment, Instruments, and Supplies Unique to Procedure

- Regular laparoscopic setup and instrumentation with addition of robotic system
- 0° and 30° laparoscopes
- 12-mm trocar
- 5-mm trocars × 4
- Surgical entrapment bag

Preoperative Preparation

- Position: Low lithotomy
- Anesthesia: General
- Skin prep: Mid-chest to mid-thigh
- Draping: Four towels and laparotomy drape

(continues)

PROCEDURE 20-11 (continued)

Practical Considerations

- Laparoscopic removal of the prostate with the use of a robot is an alternative to an open prostatectomy. The advantages include reduced blood loss, reduced postoperative pain, shorter hospitalization, significantly faster recovery, less chance of sexual function being affected, and reduced possibility of postoperative urinary incontinence as compared to open procedures such as suprapubic prostatectomy (UCLA Health System, 2007).
- The surgeon will use an extraperitoneal or transperitoneal approach. The transperitoneal is used most often and is the procedure that is described.

Surgical Procedure

1. After the patient has been draped, the surgical technologist or surgeon will insert a 24 Fr Foley catheter that is left on the sterile field. Additionally, the anesthesia provider will place the patient in slight Trendelenburg position.
2. Using a #11 or #15 knife blade, the surgeon makes an umbilical stab wound incision and inserts the Veress needle to establish the peritoneum.
3. A 12-mm trocar and sheath are placed through the umbilical incision; the trocar is removed and a 30° laparoscope is inserted through the sheath.
4. Using the knife blade and visualizing the incision site with the laparoscope, the surgeon makes the second and third stab wound incisions along each side of the rectus muscle and inserts two 8-mm trocars and sheaths.
5. Using the knife blade again and laparoscope for visualization, the fourth and fifth stab wound incisions are made. An incision is made laterally just above the right anterior superior iliac spine; a 10-mm sheath is placed for retraction and passage of sutures. A medial incision is made slightly inferior to the umbilicus; a 5-mm sheath is placed for suction and irrigation.

   Procedural Consideration: A lateral incision opposite the medial incision used to be made to accommodate one more 5-mm sheath. However, when the da Vinci robotic system added a fourth arm, it eliminated the need for two scrub people at the OR table.
6. The surgical technologist places a sterile drape on the manipulators. The robot is docked and robotic instrument ports and camera port are attached to the manipulators.

   Procedural Consideration: Placement of instruments depends on surgeon's preference, but usually the bipolar cautery is placed in the left manipulator and instrumentation (scissors, hook, spatula) in the right manipulator. Grasping forceps will be attached to the fourth manipulator.
7. The surgeon breaks scrub and sits at the robotic console while the surgical technologist remains at the sterile field to connect instruments to the manipulators, reload hemoclips, load suture onto the endoscopic needle holder, operate suction, and troubleshoot malfunctions of equipment and instrumentation.
8. The 30° scope is replaced with the 0° scope. The bowel is grasped and pulled superiorly and the rectum identified.

(*continues*)

PROCEDURE 20-11 (continued)

9. The peritoneum is incised in the midline and blunt dissection is performed to identify the vas deferens and seminal vesicles. The surgeon divides the vas deferens bilaterally.

   Procedural Consideration: The surgeon is careful to stay in the midline because the ureters insert onto the bladder laterally.

10. The peritoneum is divided further in a lateral direction and the seminal vesicles are identified. The seminal vesicles are dissected free and the vessels divided bilaterally. The vas deferens and seminal vesicles are retracted superiorly.

11. The surgeon bluntly dissects the rectoprostatic fascia to the prostatic apex to create a space between the fascia and rectum.

    Procedural Consideration: The surgeon avoids lateral dissection in order to preserve the neurovascular bundles.

12. The 0° scope is replaced with the 30° scope. The transverse peritoneum is incised extending from the left to the right medial umbilical ligament and extending to the level of the vas deferens bilaterally. The umbilical ligaments are divided, allowing the bladder to fall away from the surgical site.

13. The 30° scope is replaced with the 0° scope. The prostate is retracted medially and the endopelvic fascia is incised using the cautery endoscissors or hook. The incision in the fascia is extended distally until the urethra is exposed.

14. The surgical technologist loads a 1-0 or 2-0 polyglactin suture on a CT-1 needle and the surgeon places a figure-of-eight stitch around the dorsal venous complex.

15. The surgical technologist places vertical traction on the prostatic suture. Using the endoscopic scissors, the surgeon makes an anterior incision in the bladder neck until the Foley catheter is visualized. The surgical technologist then provides countertraction by gently retracting the catheter and the surgeon makes an incision in the posterior bladder neck. Using the bipolar forceps, the surgeon grasps the incised posterior bladder neck in the midline and dissects it away from the prostate.

16. Clips are placed on the lateral pedicles at the prostate–vesicle junction as close to the prostate as possible and divided. The placement of clips and dissection continue to the puboprostatic ligaments.

17. The final steps of dissection involve the dorsal vein and the urethra. The dorsal vein complex is divided. A space is created between the urethra and dorsal vein complex to expose the anterior urethral wall; the anterior wall is transsected with scissors just distal to the apex of the prostate. The posterior wall of the urethra and rectourethralis muscle are transsected next. The prostate is now completely freed up.

18. The surgical technologist inserts a surgical entrapment bag through a sheath and the prostate is placed inside. The bag is moved slightly away from the surgical site.

19. Using 2-0 or 3-0 polyglactic or polyglicaprone suture, the surgeon completes the urethrovesical anastomosis using a continuous stitch.

    Procedural Consideration: The surgical technologist fills the bladder with 200 mL of saline irrigation solution for the surgeon to check for leaks in the anastomosis. The surgical technologist should be ready to load additional suture if the surgeon indicates leaks need to be sutured.

(*continues*)

Procedure 20-11 (continued)

20. The surgical technologist replaces the Foley catheter that has been in use during the procedure with a new Foley catheter.
21. The surgeon places the neck of the surgical entrapment bag into the umbilical sheath. Using a hemostat, the surgical technologist brings the strings of the bag through the sheath to the outside.
22. Using the #15 knife blade, the umbilical stab wound incision is lengthened by the surgeon and the surgical entrapment bag removed.
23. The rest of the sheaths are removed, and port sites are checked for hemostasis and closed by the surgeon.

Postoperative Considerations

- Immediate Postoperative Care and Prognosis are the same as for the TURP procedure.

Wound Classification

- Wound Class I: Clean

Procedure 20-12 Suprapubic Prostatectomy

Surgical Anatomy and Pathology

- See Procedure 20-10 for anatomy and pathology.
- Suprapubic prostatectomy is performed to treat adenomas that are too large to be removed endoscopically or to remove malignancy.

Preoperative Diagnostic Tests and Procedures

- See Procedure 20-10.

Equipment, Instruments, and Supplies Unique to Procedure

- Electrocautery extended tip
- Laparotomy instrument set
- GU instrument set
- Lahey clamps
- Otis urethral sounds
- Long instrument set
- Heaney needle holders
- Self-retaining abdominal retractor (e.g., Judd-Mason)
- Hemoclip appliers with hemoclips (various sizes)
- Bladder retractor
- Knife blades: #10 × 2; #11; #12; #15 × 2
- Kitners
- Lubricant
- Shoulder braces for OR table (available)
- 16 Fr Foley catheter with 5-mL balloon
- 22 Fr Foley catheter with 30-mL balloon
- Suprapubic catheter (surgeon's preference, Malecot or Pezzer)
- 1-in. Penrose drain
- Closed wound drainage system (surgeon's preference)

Preoperative Preparation

- Position: Supine with the legs placed in slight frog leg. Shoulder braces will be needed if the patient is placed in Trendelenburg position.
- Anesthesia: General
- Skin prep: Mid-chest to lower thighs and bilaterally as far as possible. Prep the perineum and anus last, discarding each used sponge after cleansing the anus and using a new sponge.
- Draping: Cuffed towel and three-quarters sheet

Procedure 20-12 (continued)

	placed under the scrotum and extended towards the feet; four towels and laparotomy	or transverse drape depending on incision; penis remains exposed.	
Practical Considerations	• Foley catheter is inserted and maintained within the sterile field.	• Prior to bladder closure, a suprapubic catheter may be inserted to supplement	bladder drainage or provide a means of bladder irrigation.

Surgical Procedure

1. A low transverse (Pfannenstiel) or vertical suprapubic incision is made down to the level of the bladder (Figure 20-21A).

   Procedural Consideration: A #10 knife blade on a #3 handle is used for the incision. Bleeding is controlled with electrocautery. Richardson retractors are initially used.

2. The peritoneum is reflected away from the dome of the bladder.

   Procedural Consideration: Blunt dissection by the surgeon's fingers or with a sponge stick is used.

3. The bladder is entered suprapubically between two stay sutures and the ureters are visualized (Figure 20-21B).

   Procedural Consideration: The two stay sutures should be prepared in advance. Tags will be needed. A #15 knife blade on a #7 knife handle is used for the cystotomy. Suction is used frequently.

4. Retraction is provided to expose the bladder outlet.

   Procedural Consideration: Provide deep retractors of choice (e.g., Harrington, Deaver). Moist lap sponges are used to protect underlying tissue.

5. The Foley catheter is removed and the mucosa surrounding the base of the prostate is incised, avoiding the ureteral orifices.

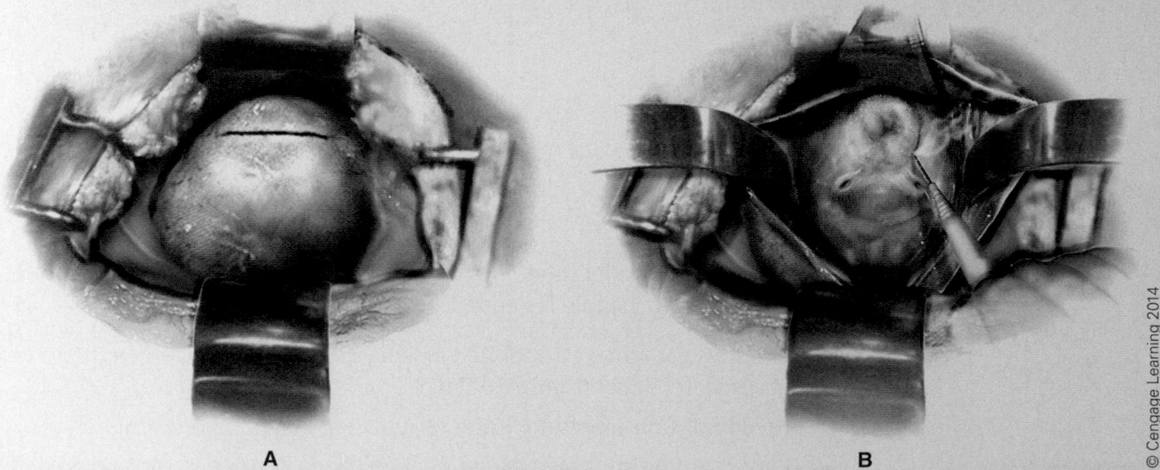

Figure 20-21 Suprapubic prostatectomy: (A) Bladder exposed through low transverse incision, (B) bladder entered,

(*continues*)

PROCEDURE 20-12 (continued)

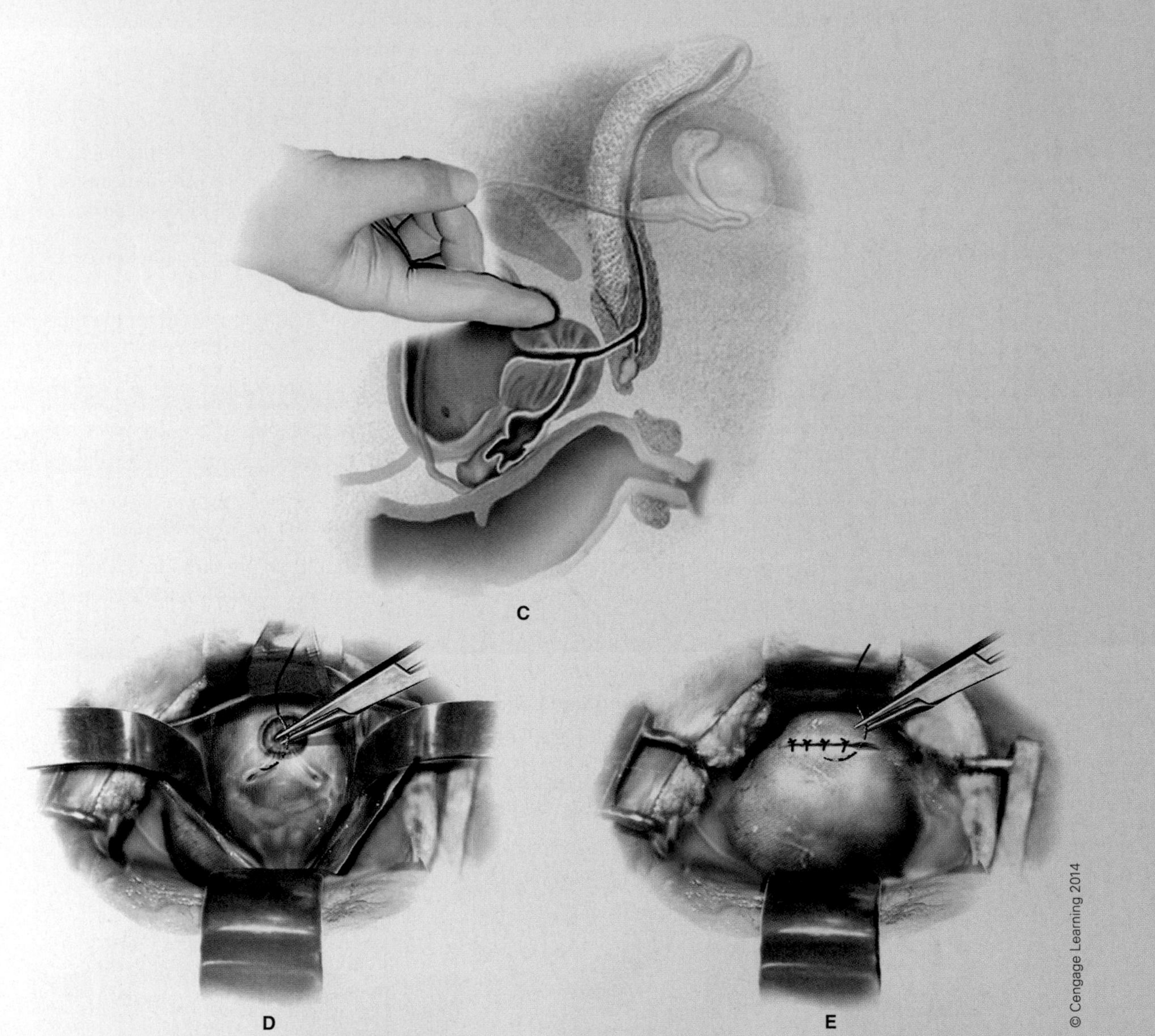

Figure 20-21 Suprapubic prostatectomy: (C) Blunt dissection of prostate, (D) postate fossa sutured to bladder mucosa, (E) bladder closure

Procedural Consideration: Provide empty syringe to deflate Foley balloon. A #10 blade on a #3L handle is needed.

6. Retractors are removed and the prostate (or lobe) is dissected circumferentially with the surgeon's finger (Figure 20-21C).

   Procedural Consideration: Retrieve retractors; prepare for reuse.

7. The tumor is delivered into the bladder and removed. Specimen may be removed en bloc or dissection may continue if the prostatic lobes have been divided for removal.

   Procedural Consideration: Prepare to accept specimen.

Procedure 20-12 (continued)

8. Figure-eight sutures are used in the prostatic fossa to control bleeding.

   Procedural Consideration: The surgeon may prefer to use the Heaney needle holder.

9. The integrity of the bladder outlet is restored by suturing the mucosa of the bladder to the prostatic fossa (Figure 20-21D).

   Procedural Consideration: Six sutures are often used to reconnect the bladder to the prostatic fossa. All sutures may be placed and tagged, then tied sequentially.

10. A 22 Fr 30-mL Foley is inserted transurethrally and the balloon is inflated. If necessary to control hemorrhage, external traction may be applied to the Foley.

    Procedural Consideration: Prepare Foley for insertion by lubricating the tip. Prepare to connect drainage bag.

11. Bleeding may be difficult to control because the suprapubic approach does not provide good visualization of the prostatic fossa and it is difficult to maneuver a needle holder into the restricted space.

    Procedural Consideration: The surgeon may choose to use electrocautery.

12. Once hemostasis is achieved, the cystotomy is closed (Figure 20-20E).

    Procedural Consideration: Provide suture of surgeon's preference. Long suture scissors may be necessary.

13. A closed wound drainage system is placed in the retropubic space and the remainder of the wound is closed.

    Procedural Consideration: Provide drain and suture as needed. Drain will likely be sutured in place. Perform counts.

14. A pressure dressing is applied.

    Procedural Consideration: Provide dressing materials.

Postoperative Considerations

Immediate Postoperative Care

- Patient is transported to the PACU.
- An epidural anesthetic may be useful in postoperative pain control.

Prognosis

- No complications: Patient is expected to remain hospitalized for several days until the urine is clear, the catheters are removed, and normal voiding occurs. The patient is expected to return to normal activities in 6–8 weeks. Sexual function and urinary continence should not be compromised. Additional treatment for malignancy may be indicated; radiation and/or hormone therapy. However, chemotherapy has not been found to be effective in the treatment of prostatic malignancy. Monitor PSA blood levels.
- Complications: Postoperative SSI; hemorrhage.

Wound Classification

- Class II: Clean-contaminated

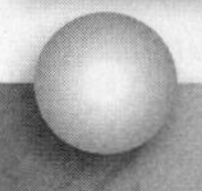

Pearl of Wisdom

If the ureters are difficult to identify when the bladder is opened, intravenous indigo carmine may facilitate locating the orifices.

Percutaneous Implantation of Radioactive Seeds in the Prostate Gland

Implantation of radioactive seeds in the prostate gland allows for a focused release of high doses of radiotherapy as compared to external radiotherapy. Additionally, due to the focused nature of the radiation release, adjacent organs are not affected. The seeds are either iodine-125 or palladium-103. Both are commercially purchased by the health care facility. Iodine-125 is transported in what are called magazines, which are rods enclosed in titanium. The magazines are sterilized prior to the start of the procedure. Palladium-103 seeds are implanted on a graphite pellet and placed in titanium tubes for transport to the health care facility. Palladium-103 seeds have a stronger radioactive effect, allowing for lower total dosing. Additionally, due to their strength, they are more effective in treating rapidly growing tumors and higher-grade prostate cancers.

Prior to the surgical procedure being performed, detailed preoperative planning is completed by the surgeon. The size of the prostate and tumor determines the number of seeds that will be required, the strength/dose of the seeds, and their placement. The surgeon will use the abdominal ultrasound to complete the preplan. A needle-guide template with a grid is produced on which the surgeon labels the placement of the seeds. The template also helps to avoid the delivery of radiation to the bladder neck, urethra, and rectum, which could result in urethrorectal fistula and scarring.

Procedure 20-13 Percutaneous Implantation of Radioactive Seeds in the Prostate Gland

Surgical Anatomy and Pathology	• See previous procedures.		
Preoperative Diagnostic Tests and Procedures	• CBC • Prothrombin time	• Activated partial thromboplastin time	• Urine culture and analysis
Equipment, Instruments, and Supplies Unique to Procedure	• Iodine-125 or palladium-103 • Geiger counter • Ultrasound transrectal transducer (also called probe) • Sterile probe cover	• Stabilizer bar • Stepping unit • Sled • Needles to implant the seeds • Cystoscope	• Foley catheters × 2 • Sterile water • Contrast medium (surgeon's preference on type of contrast solution)
Preoperative Preparation	• Position: Lithotomy • Anesthesia: Spinal or general • Skin prep: Symphysis pubis down to perineum	and anus; up to the mid-thigh on the inside • Draping: Four towels, incise drape and perineal drape; the incise drape	can be used to secure the scrotum in a superior direction away from the perineum.
Practical Considerations	• The surgical procedure will take approximately 2 hours to complete. • If the patient has undergone radiation	therapy, the implantation of the seeds is not performed until 4 weeks after the last radiation treatment.	
Surgical Procedure	1. The surgeon attaches the stabilizer bar and stepping unit to the OR bed. The "sled" that holds the ultrasound transducer in place is attached to the stepping unit.		
	2. The template with grid is attached to the ultrasound transrectal transducer (from here on simply referred to as the transducer) so the position of the needles inserted through the transducer match the position of the seeds indicated on the grid. **Practical Consideration:** The needle-guide template is placed against the perineum, leaving 1–3 cm of space between the skin and template.		

PROCEDURE 20-13 (continued)

3. The surgeon inserts a urethral catheter to drain the bladder and then fills the bladder with sterile water as an aid in visualizing the prostate. The surgeon may use contrast medium to help visualize the bladder neck.
4. The transducer is covered with a sterile probe cover that is filled with gel.

   Practical Consideration: While the surgical technologist is placing the sterile probe cover on the transducer, the surgeon is removing the urethral catheter.
5. The surgeon inserts the transducer into the rectum to visualize the prostate.
6. The anterior seeds are placed first. The radioactive seeds are loaded into the designated number of needles. Each needle is inserted through the holes in the needle-template guide into the perineum and advanced into the prostate while visualizing the prostate with the transducer. The seeds are implanted just inside the anterior prostatic capsule while avoiding placing the seeds too close to the urethra or inside the bladder.

   Practical Consideration: The surgical technologist should hand the needles to the surgeon with the bevel facing down, not up.
7. The posterior seeds are placed second just inside the posterior prostatic capsule using the next set of needles and seeds.

   Practical Consideration: During the procedure, the circulator will perform several checks of the radiation level in the OR using the Geiger counter. The information will be recorded in the patient's chart, including time radiation level was checked and the Geiger counter level.
8. The transducer is removed. The surgeon will perform a cystoscopy to view the urethra and bladder, and remove any seeds within either structure.
9. A new Foley catheter with drainage bag is inserted.
10. The surgical team, disposable trash, nondisposable supplies, and equipment must be scanned with the Geiger counter before leaving or taken out of the OR.

Postoperative Considerations

Immediate Postoperative Care

- Patient is transported to the PACU.
- Patient is discharged the same day of surgery.
- Patient teaching includes avoid contacting with and maintaining as much distance as possible from pregnant females and adolescents.

Prognosis

- No complications: Antibiotic prophylaxis for several days; Foley catheter removed in 24–48 hours; final CT scan performed 1–30 days postoperatively; patient must use a strainer when urinating to catch any seeds that are expelled through the urethra and return the seeds to the surgeon.
- Complications:
  - Perineum will be tender and bruised with slight bleeding at needle puncture sites.
  - Hematuria, dysuria, frequency, and urgency 1–2 weeks, sometimes longer.
  - Incontinence (low rate of occurrence).
  - Diarrhea and painful bowel movements.
  - Decrease in sexual function and activity with some degree of erectile dysfunction.
  - Seeds implanted too close to urethra, causing urethral stricture
  - Prostatitis.

Wound Classification

- Class II: Clean-contaminated

TESTICULAR SURGERY

A large percentage of the testicular surgical procedures is performed on pediatric patients, such as orchiopexy. However, adult males may undergo procedures such as orchiectomy as an adjunct procedure in the treatment of cancer or due to trauma. The first procedure that will be presented in the following section is hydrocelectomy.

PROCEDURE 20-14 Hydrocelectomy

Surgical Anatomy and Pathology

- The layers of the scrotum are as follows: skin, dartos muscle (contractile tissue), external spermatic fascia, cremastric fascia, internal spermatic fascia.
- The testes are paired structures that lie in the scrotum (Figure 20-22).

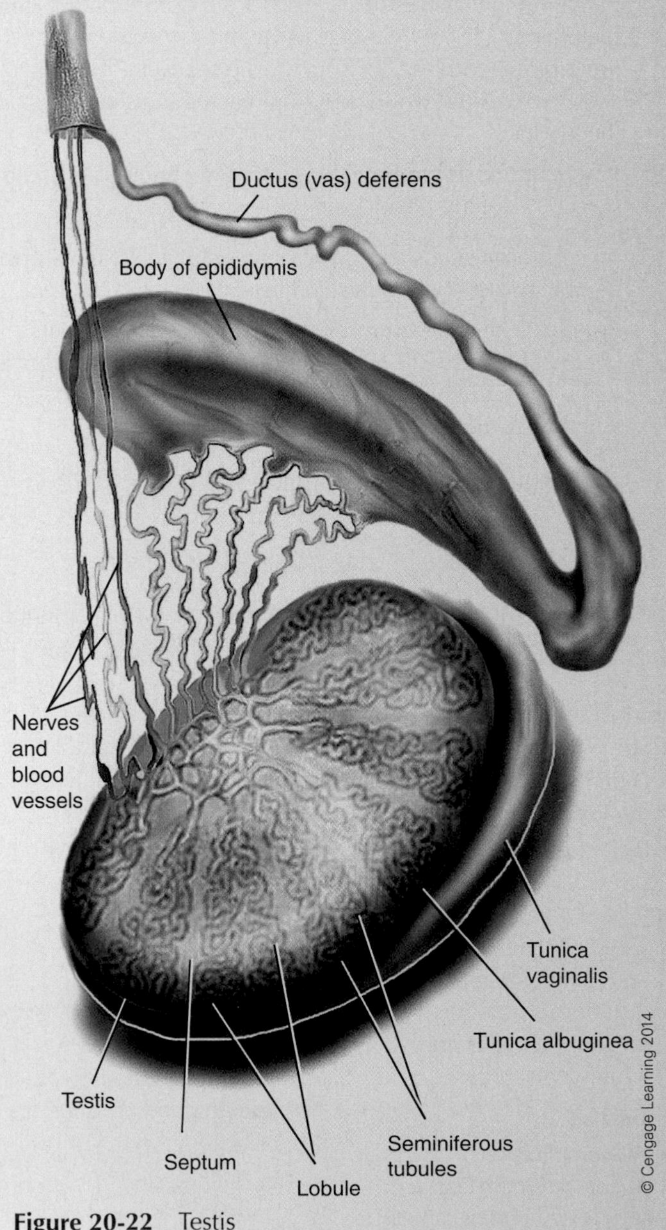

Figure 20-22 Testis

PROCEDURE 20-14 (continued)

	• The tunica vaginalis is an invaginated serous sac that covers most of the testis, epididymis, and lower end of the spermatic cord. It does not cover the posterior portion of the testis, and it is here that the blood vessels and nerves of the testis enter. • The testis has a thick external covering of white-colored connective tissue called the tunica albuginea. • On the posterior of the testis is a mass of thick connective tissue that is continuous with the tunical albuginea called the mediastinum testis. Thin dividers of connective tissue called septa extend from the mediastinum testis into the testis, dividing it into approximately 250 lobules. Each lobule contains	1–4 coiled seminiferous tubules. The seminiferous tubules are lined with a specialized stratified tissue called germinal epithelium, which produces sperm cells. • The seminiferous tubules become united to form a complex network of channels called the rete testis, which are located in the mediastinum testis. The rete testis give rise to 12–15 efferent ducts that pass through the tunica albuginea and join the epididymis. The sperm, therefore, travels from the seminiferous tubules through the rete testis into the efferent ducts and into the epididymis. • The epididymis is coiled around the outer superior portion of the testis.	• The testicular arteries exit the abdominal aorta just below the renal arteries. They descend obliquely in the retroperitoneal space. The testicular arteries cross the psoas muscles, ureters, and external iliac arteries to enter the deep inguinal rings. The testicular arteries give off ureteral branches during their course. The artery exits the spermatic cord from the inguinal ring and gives off several branches that supply the epididymis and testicles. The testicular vein is located next to the artery. • A hydrocele is an abnormal accumulation of serous fluid around the testis contained within the tunical vaginalis. The fluid buildup is often the result of trauma or infection.
Preoperative Diagnostic Tests and Procedures	• History and physical		
Equipment, Instruments, and Supplies Unique to Procedure	• Minor instrument set • #15 knife blades × 3 • Penrose drain • 30-mL syringe	• 20-gauge needle • 1% lidocaine—plain • Needle tip for electrocautery pencil	• Fluffs for dressing • Adult: Scrotal support
Preoperative Preparation	• Position: Supine with legs slightly spread apart • Anesthesia: Adult—local with MAC; pediatric—general	• Skin prep: Beginning at incision site on scrotum extending from umbilicus to mid-thigh and bilaterally as far as possible	• Draping: Cuffed towel under scrotum; four towels to square off; adult or pediatric laparotomy drape
Practical Considerations	• Usually only one testis is affected.		

(continues)

PROCEDURE 20-14 (continued)

Surgical Procedure

1. The local anesthetic is injected into the base of the scrotum.
2. Using the #15 knife blade, the surgeon makes an anterior scrotal incision near or over the location of the hydrocele.
3. Bleeding is controlled with mosquito hemostats and 3-0 or 4-0 absorbable suture ties or electrocautery with the needle tip.
4. The tunica vaginalis is exposed by incising the dartos and fascial layers.
5. With tenotomy scissors, Adson forceps, and blunt dissection, the hydrocele is dissected free.
6. The contents of the sac are aspirated with the 20-gauge needle attached to the 10-mL syringe.
7. The sac is opened with the tenotomy scissors and, using mosquito clamps, the surgeon everts the edges of the sac.
8. Using the tenotomy scissors, a pouch is created between the tunical vaginalis and internal spermatic fascia. The pouch will be used to hold the testis in place.
9. The sac is now inverted to surround the testis and epididymis.
10. If present, excess tunica vaginalis is excised using the tenotomy scissors.
11. The edges of the tunical vaginalis are sutured behind the testis using a 4-0 or 5-0 absorbable suture in interrupted technique; 8–10 stitches will be placed.

    Practical Consideration: Due to the small size of suture being used as well as the small surgical site, the surgical technologist will want to use the straight tenotomy scissors to cut the suture rather than the bulky straight Mayo scissors.
12. The testis is resituated in the pouch within the scrotal sac.
13. A Penrose drain is placed within the scrotum and exteriorized through a small stab incision in the scrotum.
14. The scrotal incision is closed in layers with 4-0 or 5-0 absorbable sutures in continuous technique.
15. A fluff dressing is applied and for adult patients a scrotal support (jockstrap) is placed to keep the dressing in place and to keep light pressure on the surgical site to aid in preventing postoperative scrotal edema.

Postoperative Considerations

Immediate Postoperative Care

- Patient is transported to the PACU.
- Adult—discharge same day.
- Pediatric—may stay overnight.

Prognosis

- No complications: Patient expected to have full recovery; return to normal activities in 7–10 days.
- Complications: Postoperative SSI; scrotal edema.

Wound Classification

- Class I: Clean

Procedure 20-15 Orchiopexy

Surgical Anatomy and Pathology

- See Procedure 20-14 for surgical anatomy.
- Cryptorchism occurs when one or both testicles fail to descend into the scrotum after the first year of life.
  - The disorder is commonly associated with premature birth and is often accompanied by an inguinal hernia.
  - The testicle may be found in the abdomen or most commonly in the inguinal canal.
- **Torsion** of the testicle is a twisting of the spermatic cord that causes extreme pain (Figure 20-23).
  - The spermatic cord contains the blood vessels that supply the testicle; twisting may reduce or obstruct the blood flow to the testicle, producing ischemia or necrosis. Immediate reduction must occur or the testicle may be permanently compromised.
  - Orchiectomy is necessary if the testicle is necrotic.

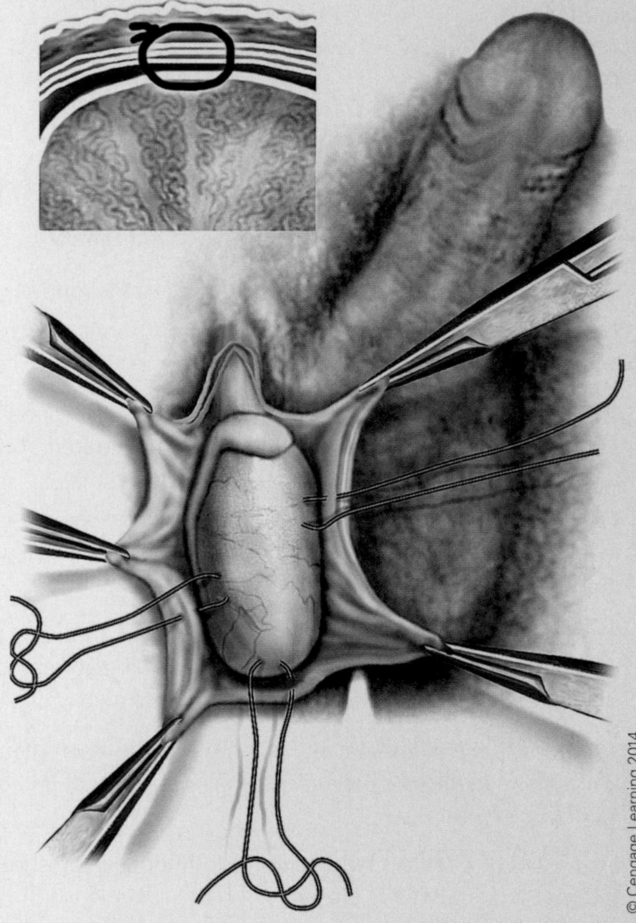

Figure 20-23 Testicular torsion

(continues)

PROCEDURE 20-15 (continued)

Preoperative Diagnostic Tests and Procedures	• History and physical • Abdominal ultrasound to locate the undescended testicle	• Testicular torsion: IV fluorescein in conjunction with a Wood's lamp or black	light may aid in diagnosis.
Equipment, Instruments, and Supplies Unique to Procedure	• Minor instrument set • #15 knife blades × 2	• Needle tip for electrocautery pencil • Small pledget	• Penrose drain • Fluffs • Adult—scrotal support
Preoperative Preparation	• Position: Supine • Anesthesia: General • Skin prep: Inguinal incision site from	umbilicus down to mid-thigh to include external genitalia	• Draping: Four towels to square off; towel under the scrotum; pediatric laparotomy drape
Practical Considerations	• If an orchiopexy procedure for cryptorchidism is necessary, it should be performed at a young age to position the testicle in its normal location to prevent infertility.	• Testicular torsion: Manual derotation is possible but is only a temporary measure; orchiopexy should be performed as soon as possible to prevent recurrence. Orchiopexy	may be performed bilaterally because the gubernaculum that secures the testicle to the scrotum may be deficient on both sides.

Surgical Procedure

1. Inguinal oblique incision is made using the #15 knife blade.

   Procedural Consideration: The surgeon and surgical technologist may gently apply tension to the skin on each side of the incision.

2. The inguinal canal is exposed by continuing the incision into the external oblique aponeurosis. The gubernacular testis is dissected free from its attachments up to the level of the internal inguinal ring.

   Procedural Consideration: The gubernaculum testis is a fibrous cord in the fetus that extends from the caudal end of the testis through the inguinal canal. It serves to guide the descent of the testicle into the scrotum.

3. The inguinal hernia sac is dissected free with blunt and sharp dissection in order to contribute to freeing up additional length of the gubernaculum testis. A clamp is placed at the base of the sac, cut, and ligated.

4. The floor of the inguinal canal is incised at the internal inguinal ring with the #15 knife blade to allow a better anatomical position of the spermatic cord and other vessels.

5. Using 3-0 or 4-0 absorbable sutures in interrupted fashion, the lateral section of the internal inguinal ring is closed.

6. Using the #15 knife blade, the surgeon makes a short transverse scrotal incision. Using tenotomy scissors, a subdartos pouch is created between the skin and dartos muscle. Using the #15 knife blade or tenotomy scissors, the surgeon makes a small incision in the dartos muscle and places the testicle through the incision into the

PROCEDURE 20-15 (continued)

subdartos pouch. One 4-0 or 5-0 absorbable suture is used to fix the testicle in position.

7. The scrotal incision is closed with 4-0 or 5-0 nonabsorbable suture in interrupted fashion. The inguinal incision is closed in layers; the skin is closed with subcuticular closure; and a collodion dressing is applied to the skin.

Postoperative Considerations	**Immediate Postoperative Care** • Patient discharged same day or overnight stay. • Pediatric patient must be watched closely to prevent touching and injuring surgical site.	**Prognosis** • No complications: Patient is expected to make a full recovery and the testicle will function normally. Return to normal activities in 7–10 days.	• Complications: Postoperative SSI; hemorrhage. **Wound Classification** • Class I: Clean

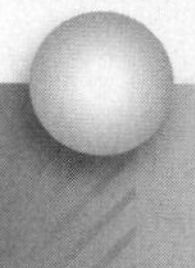

PEARL OF WISDOM

In addition to the testicular incision, an inguinal incision may be required to mobilize the testis or repair any hernia that may coexist.

PROCEDURE 20-16 Simple Orchiectomy

Surgical Anatomy and Pathology	• See Procedure 20-14 for anatomy. • Testicular cancer is often first noticed during bathing or self-examination.	• This aggressive type of cancer usually affects men between the ages of 20 and 40. Infants with cryptorchidism are at a higher risk for	developing testicular cancer. • Pain is not evident in the early stages of the disease.
Preoperative Diagnostic Tests and Procedures	• History and physical • Tests and procedures to determine metastasis:	• Chest X-ray • Ultrasound • CT scan	• Bone scan • Hematologic studies
Equipment, Instruments, and Supplies Unique to Procedure	• Same as Procedure 20-14 with addition of testicular implants		

(continues)

PROCEDURE 20-16 (continued)

Preoperative Preparation	• Same as Procedure 20-14
Practical Considerations	• In some situations, if bilateral orchiectomy will be performed, sperm can be preserved if future paternity is desired. • Testicular implants are available to provide a postoperative aesthetic appearance. The patient must be measured preoperatively and the correct-size implant ordered. The implant must be sterilized for implantation during the procedure. • If both testicles are removed, the patient will be required to be on testosterone hormone therapy for a lifetime. • The removal of one testicle is indicated for testicular cancer, trauma, or necrosis due to testicular torsion. The removal of both testicles is for endocrine control of prostatic carcinoma. • Radical orchiectomy, performed for testicular cancer, is the removal of the entire contents of the hemiscrotum, tunica vaginalis, and spermatic cord. • Simple orchiectomy is the removal of the testicle and epididymis.
Surgical Procedure	1. Using the #15 knife blade, the surgeon makes an anterolateral scrotal incision.
	2. The incision is made through all the layers of the scrotum and tunica vaginalis to expose the testicle. The testicle and spermatic cord are brought out through the incision. **Procedural Consideration:** Bleeding is controlled using the needle tip electrocautery and mosquito clamps and suture ties. Small retractors such as the Senn retractors will be used or the surgeon will place traction sutures to keep the wound edges open.
	3. Using the #15 knife blade, the surgeon incises the spermatic cord above the testicle. The structures within are identified and dissected free, and each section is doubly clamped, cut, and ligated with 0 or 1-0 nonabsorbable suture. The testicle is now free and is removed (Figure 20-24).
	4. The procedure is repeated on the other side if both testicles are being removed. **Procedural Consideration:** The surgical technologist must confirm with the surgeon if the testicles should be sent separately as right and left specimens and communicate this information to the circulator.
	5. Testicular prostheses are placed.
	6. A Penrose drain is inserted; if both testicles removed, a Penrose may be inserted on each side.
	7. Wound is closed in layers.
	8. Fluff dressing is applied with scrotal support to prevent hematoma formation.

(*continues*)

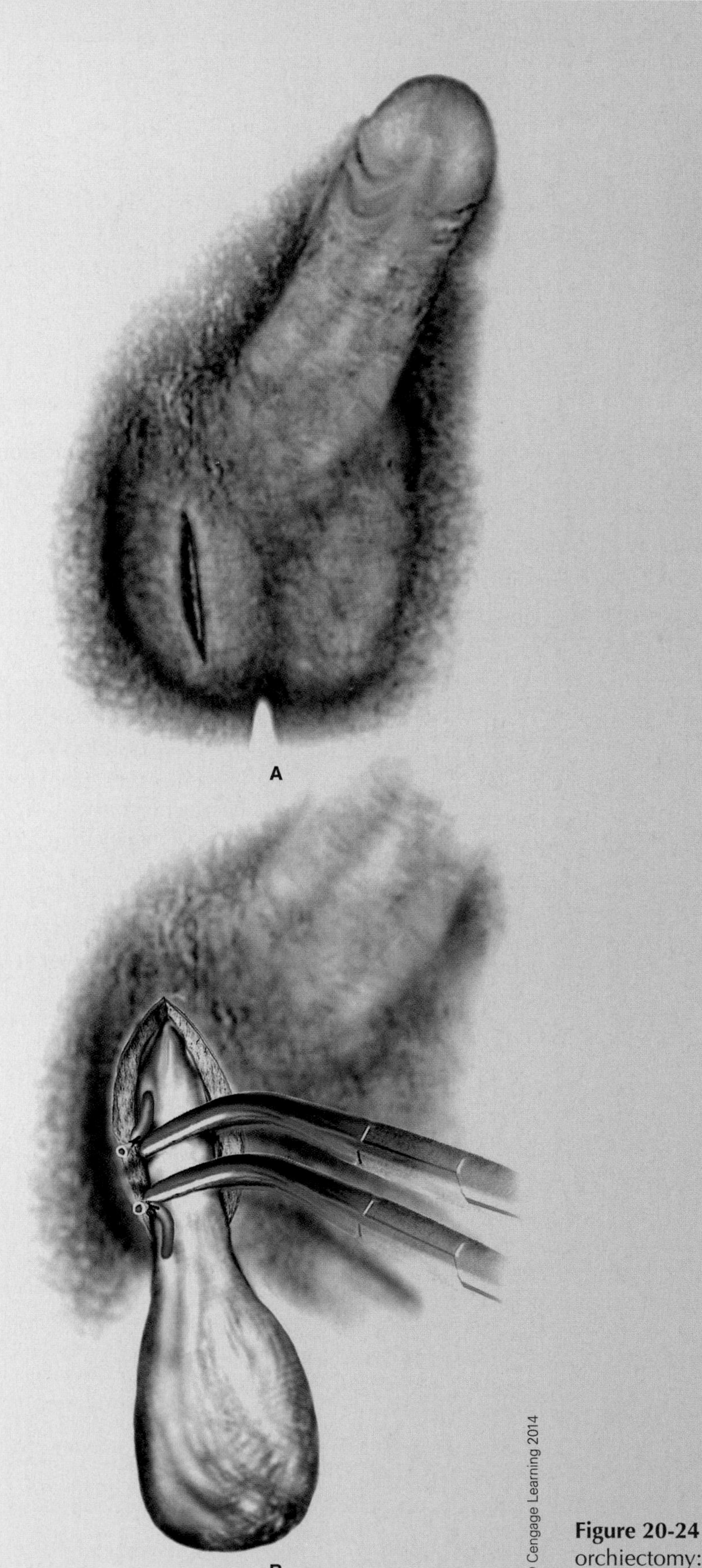

Figure 20-24 Simple orchiectomy: (A) Scrotal incision, (B) removal of testicle

PROCEDURE 20-16 (continued)

Postoperative Considerations	
Immediate Postoperative Care	• Patient is transported to the PACU. • Hospitalized overnight. • Ice applied to area.
Prognosis	• No complications: Return to normal activities in 2–4 weeks. However, depending on the reason for performing procedure, patient may have follow-up therapy such as chemotherapy and/or radiation treatments. • Complications: Postoperative SSI; hematoma.
Wound Classification	• Class I: Clean

PENILE SURGICAL PROCEDURES

Penile surgical procedures are performed to treat congenital defects, disorders, and cancer. The procedures described in the next section are **circumcision**, epispadias repair, hypospadias repair, penile implant, and penectomy.

PROCEDURE 20-17 Circumcision

Surgical Anatomy and Pathology

- The penis is a cylindrical structure composed of three cavernous tissues that are bound together by fibrous tissue and covered by skin.
  - The cavernous structures of the penis, the two corpora cavernosa, are positioned on the dorsal side of the penis and lie side by side.
  - The corpus spongiosum lies in the midline below these two structures. The corpus spongiosum expands distally, forming a conical structure, the glans penis.
  - The raised and backward-pointing margin of the glans penis is called the corona.
  - The urethra passes through the corpus spongiosum and opens to the exterior via a slit-like opening, the meatus.
  - The skin covering the penis is thin and loosely connected to the underlying structures. On the ventral surface, the skin exhibits a median penoscrotal raphe that is continuous with the raphe (seam or line of union) of the scrotum. At the distal base of the penis, the skin forms a free fold called the **prepuce** (or more commonly the foreskin) that covers the glans penis.
  - The subcutaneous connective tissue of the penis is loose areolar tissue that contains no fat. This tissue is reinforced by smooth muscle fibers from the dartos muscle of the scrotum.
  - The superficial dorsal vein passes along the dorsal midline of the penis and joins the superficial external pudendal veins near the base of the penis. A layer of deep fascia encloses the cavernous bodies of the penis and the associated nerves and vessels.
- Circumcision is the removal of the prepuce.
  - It is performed on the infant at the parent's request or religious reasons. The following paragraph describes the circumcision procedure that is performed on infants.

    The procedure may be performed in the delivery room, newborn nursery, or physician's office. A minimal prep may be done and drapes are not often used. In this situation, a guided method is frequently used. This involves placement of

PROCEDURE 20-17 (continued)

	a bell-shaped device called a Plastibell over the glans (another device called the Gomco is also frequently used). The foreskin is then pulled taut over the bell and the second part of the instrument is placed over the foreskin and connected to the base of the bell. The device is tightened, trapping the skin in position. This serves a dual purpose: it compromises the blood supply to the foreskin and provides a protective surface for the surgeon to move the scalpel along as the foreskin is	excised. The clamp is removed and sutures are placed if necessary. A frenulectomy may be performed at this time. A nonadherent dressing is loosely applied to the distal penis allowing for urination and preventing irritation by the diaper. The parents should be instructed on how to care for the wound. Pain medication if needed may be administered in the form of rectal suppository or oral liquid. Complete wound healing is expected within 7–10 days and no further care is necessary.	• It is performed to treat phimosis. Phimosis is the inability to retract the prepuce over the glans penis. It is attributed to a thin band of skin at the opening of the foreskin. Phimosis can be infantile or adult. It can be a painful condition that is often treated by performing a circumcision. • It is also performed to treat recurrent balanitis. Balanitis can occur because the individual has poor hygiene habits and does not retract the prepuce to cleanse the area.
Preoperative Diagnostic Tests and Procedures	• History and physical		
Equipment, Instruments, and Supplies Unique to Procedure	• Minor instrument set • Needle tip for electrocautery pencil • #15 knife blades × 2	• Adaptic dressing • 10-mL syringe and 25-gauge needle if local anesthetic will be used	• 1% lidocaine with epinephrine
Preoperative Preparation	• Position: Supine • Anesthesia: General is preferred but local or regional anesthesia may be used.	• Skin prep: External genitalia; retract foreskin if patient's condition allows.	• Draping: Towel over the scrotum and additional towels to square off; adult or pediatric laparotomy drape
Practical Considerations	• Prep solution may be needed on the sterile field if adequate preoperative prep was	not carried out due to phimosis. • Consider the needs of the Jewish patient for ritual	circumcision. Accommodations may need to be made to allow a rabbi into the OR.
Surgical Procedure	1. Straight hemostat is applied to the posterior midline of the foreskin to provide hemostasis as well as mark the incision. **Procedural Consideration:** Hemostat will likely remain in place 1–2 minutes.		
	2. The clamp is removed and a dorsal slit is created. Two hemostats will be placed on the skin edges of the tip of the dorsal slit and traction applied to straighten out the skin folds to facilitate the surgeon performing the next step. **Procedural Consideration:** A #15 knife blade or straight scissors are used to make the dorsal slit. Some surgeons may place a clamp on the ventral side and create a ventral slit.		

(continues)

Procedure 20-17 (continued)

3. A circumferential freehand cut around the shaft is carried out as far back as the surgeon determines appropriate (Figure 20-25). If two incisions were made, the surgeon will cut around the shaft to remove one piece of tissue and perform the second cut to remove the other piece of tissue.

   Procedural Consideration: A knife or scissors is used to remove the foreskin. It may or may not be necessary to send foreskin as a specimen. Be familiar with facility policy. Sponges and/or electrocautery will be used to remove blood from field to enhance surgeon's visualization.

4. If frenulectomy is to be performed, it may be accomplished at this time.

   Procedural Consideration: Scissors or cautery may be necessary.

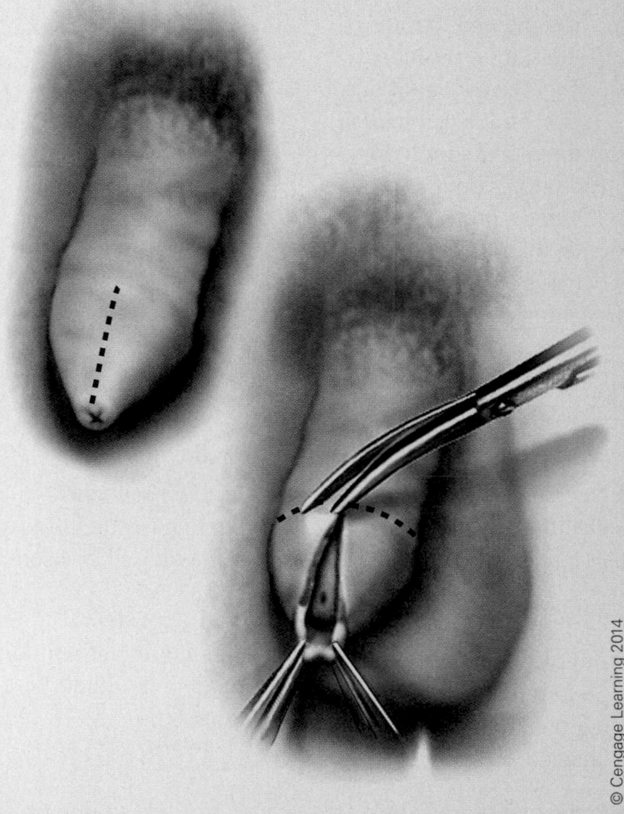

Figure 20-25 Circumcision

5. Raw edges of the small remainder of the foreskin are pulled together and sutured, leaving the glans and frenulum exposed.

   Procedural Consideration: Provide absorbable suture on short needle holder and Adson tissue forceps with teeth. Prepare to cut suture with the tenotomy scissors. Count may not be required according to facility policy.

6. Nonadherent dressing is loosely applied to the distal penis.

   Procedural Consideration: Adult patient—loosely wrap Adaptic around penis to allow for urination. Diaper, if infant patient.

PROCEDURE 20-17 (continued)

Postoperative Considerations	**Immediate Postoperative Care** • Patient is transported to the PACU; discharged the same day. • Oral analgesics should be adequate for pain control. • Apply cold packs to minimize swelling. **Prognosis** • No complications: OTC analgesics should be adequate for pain control; apply cold packs to minimize swelling; resume normal activities within 7–10 days; adult male patient should be instructed to have smelling salts available to prevent an erection. • Complications: Postoperative SSI; sutures break or torn out due to erection. **Wound Classification** • Class II: Clean-contaminated

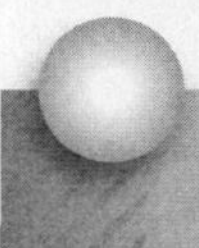

PEARL OF WISDOM

Emotional needs of the male must be considered. Provide privacy and protect patient's dignity as procedure allows.

PROCEDURE 20-18 Hypospadias Repair (male patient)

Surgical Anatomy and Pathology	• See previous procedures for anatomy.
	• **Hypospadias** is a congenital condition of the urethra.
	  • It is diagnosed when the urethral opening occurs on the underside (ventral) of the penis, anywhere along the penile shaft, on the corona, or on the perineum of the male or in the vagina of the female.
	  • The degree of chordee is determined by how proximal the urethral opening is located. Chordee is caused by fibrous bands that extend from the urethral opening to the tip of the glans.

Preoperative Diagnostic Tests and Procedures	• History and physical
Equipment, Instruments, and Supplies Unique to Procedure	• Minor or pediatric instrument set • Plastic instrument set • Lacrimal duct probes • Coban or Elastoplast as part of dressing materials • 0.9% saline solution • 10-mL syringe • 25-gauge needle • Pediatric Red Robinson catheter • Pediatric Foley catheter
Preoperative Preparation	• Position: Supine with legs placed slightly apart • Anesthesia: General • Skin prep: Start at ventral side of penis including all the external genitalia, extending from the umbilicus to mid-thigh and bilaterally as far as possible. Prep the perineum and anus last. • Draping: Cuffed towel under the scrotum; four towels to square off and pediatric laparotomy drape

(continues)

PROCEDURE 20-18 (continued)

Practical Considerations

- The procedure is usually performed between the ages of 1 and 4.
- Hypospadias procedure can be accomplished as a one-stage or two-stage procedure depending on the severity and extent of the condition.
- The goal of the procedure is to relocate the meatus to the correct anatomical location at the center of the glans.
- The repair involves three subprocedures: glanuplasty, which also involves meatoplasty; chordee repair—release of chordee to straighten the penis (also called orthoplasty); urethroplasty—reconstruction of the urethra.
- Circumcision is not performed on infants with hypospadias to preserve the skin, which is useful for the procedure.

Surgical Procedure

Meatoplasty and Glanuplasty

1. Using a #15 knife blade, a circumferential incision is made about 8–9 mm proximal to the meatus and corona. Using curved tenotomy scissors, the skin is stripped away and downward from the phallus by dissecting the subcutaneous tissue.
2. A transverse closure of the dorsal upper meatal edge to the distal glanular groove is completed with the use of continuous 4-0 or 5-0 suture.
3. The surgeon now places three traction sutures: (a) lateral region of the glans; (b) where the foreskin ends; (c) at the top of the ventral meatus.

   Procedural Consideration: Mosquito hemostats will be used to clamp the traction suture. To help the surgeon identify the three sutures, place a straight clamp on the lateral suture, curved on the foreskin suture, and another straight on the ventral meatus suture.
4. The edges of the glans are sutured together on the ventral side in a "V" shape and the excess tissue of the edges removed with tenotomy scissors. Vertical mattress sutures are placed and used to approximate the glans below the meatus.

   Procedural Consideration: Use small straight Mayo scissors or straight tenotomy scissors to cut the suture.
5. If an excess of foreskin is present, it is removed with tenotomy scissors. The skin is reapproximated with interrupted 4-0 or 5-0 nonabsorbable suture. In the presence of a ventral skin defect, a rotational skin flap closure is performed.

Chordee Repair

1. To determine the degree of curvature, artificial erection is accomplished by injecting 0.9% saline solution into the corpus cavernosum to fill both corporal bodies.

   Procedural Consideration: Solution is injected using a 10-mL syringe and 25-gauge needle.
2. Using a #15 knife blade, the surgeon makes a circumferential incision around the corona and extended distally to the urethral meatus, staying below the glans cap.
3. Dissection is carried down to the tunica albuginea of the corpora cavernosa.
4. Using the curved tenotomy or baby curved Metzenbaum scissors, the surgeon begins the dissection of the fibrous bands of tissue just distal to the glans cap. The surgeon works side to side along the entire penile shaft to the junction of the penis and scrotum (penoscrotal junction). Small skin hooks are placed and the freed portion of the fibrous tissue is retracted laterally to aid in visualization and to keep the tissue out of the way.

PROCEDURE 20-18 (continued)

5. Once the chordee is released, the glans penis is closed with 4-0 or 5-0 absorbable sutures in a circumferential manner.

6. If a urethroplasty is not necessary or will be performed at a later date, excess dorsal skin is removed with the small scissors. The dorsal incision is approximated along the midline with 4-0 or 5-0 absorbable sutures in interrupted mattress fashion.

Urethroplasty—Free Skin Graft

Note: There are many procedures that can be performed for the reconstruction of the urethra. Three of the most popular procedures are free skin graft, adjacent skin flap, and mobilized vascularized flaps. The procedure described here is the free skin graft, which is usually used with a one-stage repair.

Free Skin Graft

1. The surgeon makes a "V"-shaped incision on the glans, and the penile skin is mobilized by dissecting it free after the chordee release is completed.

2. The three points of the glans are dissected and developed and held in a triangular fashion with the use of mosquito clamps. The ventral preputial skin is used for the full-thickness free skin graft.

   Procedural Consideration: The surgical technologist will be responsible for holding the clamps upward to keep traction on the skin.

3. The skin is placed around a urinary catheter that serves as a stent.

   Procedural Consideration: The surgical technologist should have the pediatric urinary catheter available on the Mayo stand.

4. The graft is anastomosed proximal to the urethra with the suture line of the graft placed next to the corpora. The middle glans dart is sutured in interrupted fashion to the corpora.

5. A meatoplasty in the dorsal glans dart is completed and 4-0 or 5-0 absorbable sutures are placed in interrupted fashion around the meatus, glans, and down the dorsal penile shaft.

Skin Cover

1. Excess dorsal foreskin is utilized for the skin cover. Then 2–3 mosquito clamps are placed along the edge of the skin and held upward.

   Procedural Consideration: Again, the surgical technologist will be responsible for holding the clamps.

2. A small hole is made with the #15 knife blade in the midline. The glans penis is delivered through the hole.

3. The skin flap is sutured into place with 4-0 or 5-0 absorbable sutures placed in interrupted mattress fashion.

Postoperative Considerations

Immediate Postoperative Care

- Patient is transported to the PACU.
- Patient remains hospitalized 2–3 days.

Prognosis

- No complications: Patient is expected to make a full recovery with normal ability to urinate and have sexual intercourse. Return to normal activities in 7–10 days.
- Complications: Postoperative SSI; urethral fistula (repaired with little difficulty; urethral stricture (more difficult to repair).

Wound Classification

- Class I: Clean

Procedure 20-19 Epispadias Repair

Surgical Anatomy and Pathology	• See Procedure 20-18 for anatomy.
	• Epispadias is a congenital condition of the urethra.
	  • It is the developmental absence of the anterior wall of the urethra and opening of the urethra somewhere on the dorsum of the penis.
	• There are three types of epispadias:
	  • Balanic: Urethral opening is on the dorsum of the glans
	  • Penile: Urethral opening is on the shaft of the penis
	  • Penopubic: Urethral opening is on the proximal ends of the penile shaft or in the penopubic area. This is the most acute type of congenital deformity that is challenging to the surgeon to repair; the patient usually experiences extreme chordee and urinary incontinence due to lack of development of the bladder neck.

Preoperative Diagnostic Tests and Procedures	• History and physical
Equipment, Instruments, Supplies, Preoperative Preparation, and Practical Considerations	• Same as for Procedure 20-18.
Surgical Procedure	*First Stage of Repair* 1. Using the #15 knife blade, the surgeon makes a circumferential incision beginning distal to the dorsal meatus and up to the dorsal coronal margin. 2. The narrow band of dorsal urethra is dissected from the corpora cavernosa. 3. The ventral portion of the foreskin is rotated in a dorsal direction and sutured in place to cover the defect on the dorsal side that was formed when the penis was straightened. *Second Stage of Repair* 1. Using the #15 knife blade, the surgeon makes a vertical abdominal suprapubic incision. The incision is extended down to the bladder. A pediatric self-retaining retractor is placed to visualize the bladder neck. 2. A wedge incision is made in the prostatic urethra on both sides of the bladder neck and the wedges of tissue removed. 3. The top section of the membranous urethra is excised using sharp and blunt dissection. 4. The surgeon closes the incisions in the prostatic urethra using 3-0 or 4-0 absorbable suture with continuous technique. 5. A pediatric suprapubic catheter is inserted into the bladder and it is closed with 3-0 or 4-0 absorbable suture.

PROCEDURE 20-19 (continued)

6. The laparotomy is closed in layers.
7. Using the marking pen, the surgeon marks the incision site for the band of skin to be removed from the dorsal penis.
8. The rest of the procedure is performed the same as the urethroplasty and skin cover that is carried out during a hypospadias procedure.

Postoperative Considerations	• Same as for hypospadias repair

PROCEDURE 20-20 Insertion of Inflatable Penile Prosthesis

Surgical Anatomy and Pathology	• See previous procedures for anatomy. • A penile prosthesis is inserted for the treatment of male impotence. • Impotence occurs for a variety of reasons, including diabetes mellitus, pelvic trauma, damage to the nerves, penile trauma, priapism, Peyronie's disease, and vascular disease.		• The procedure facilitates the patient's ability to have sexual intercourse, but it does not cure or treat the disorder causing the impotence.
Preoperative Diagnostic Tests and Procedures	• History and physical		
Equipment, Instruments, and Supplies Unique to Procedure	• Minor instrument set • Hegar dilators • Caliper • Furlow inserter • Assembly tool • Closing tool • Connectors (various sizes)	• Penile prosthesis • Keith needles • Needle tip for electrocautery pencil • Kitners • Saline solution for penile prosthesis reservoir	• 16 Fr Foley catheter • 0.5% plain Marcaine • Penile block drugs: 1% plain lidocaine; 0.9% saline; papaverine • Keflex or kanamycin (surgeon's preference)

(*continues*)

PROCEDURE 20-20 (continued)

Preoperative Preparation

- Position: Supine
- Anesthesia: Spinal or general
- Skin prep: Begin at base of penis, including the entire external genitalia up to the umbilicus to mid-thigh and bilaterally as far as possible.
- Draping: Cuffed towel under scrotum; four towels to square off; laparotomy drape

Practical Considerations

- The most serious complication is postoperative SSI.
  - The surgical technologist should either establish an area on the back table for the implant or set up a separate Mayo stand. The implant must not come into contact with towels or drapes to avoid lint; additionally, the surgical team should thoroughly wash off the powder from gloves.
  - Implants are commercially available that have InhibiZone (combination of minocycline hydrochloride and rifampin) impregnated onto the outer surface (InhibiZone has been safely used in indwelling venous and urinary catheters). The majority of the drug is released during the initial 2–3 postoperative days and the rest over the next 2–3 weeks, and thus is primarily focused on preventing postoperative SSIs during the early stages of healing.
  - Implants without InhibiZone are usually irrigated with an antibiotic solution of bacitracin and cephalexin (Keflex) or kanamycin sulfate (Kantrex) just before insertion. Implants with InhibiZone must not be irrigated with the antibiotic solution because it would destroy the InhibiZone.
- Due to the number of drugs and solutions that will be on the sterile back table, the surgical technologist must be particularly careful when labeling the medications and not mislabel a drug. It is recommended that the surgical technologist receive one drug and apply label, receive the next drug and apply label, and so forth.
- Confirm with the surgeon the size and type of implant, but do not have it opened onto the sterile field until needed.

Surgical Procedure

Placement of Inflatable Rods

1. A 16 Fr Foley catheter with drainage bag is inserted and kept within the sterile field throughout the surgical procedure. The catheter aids in identifying the position of the urethra, and it is used to retract the urethra to the side when necessary.
2. Using a #15 knife blade, the surgeon makes a midline incision from the penile base into the scrotum.
3. The tunica albuginea of both corpora is incised and traction sutures are placed.
4. The corpora are dilated with the Hegar dilators.

   Procedural Consideration: The surgical technologist should help the surgeon in stating the size of the dilator when handing it to the surgeon; this will help the surgeon to remember to stop with the dilator that is 1 mm larger than the diameter of the implant.
5. The surgeon uses the Furlow inserter to measure the corporal length.
6. 3-0 absorbable sutures are placed along the incision of the tunica and tagged with mosquito clamps.
7. The implant package is now opened onto the sterile back table or Mayo stand. The inflatable rods are packaged by the manufacturer with traction sutures attached at the distal end. The surgeon places a suture through a Keith needle and the needle is placed into the groove of the Furlow inserter.

PROCEDURE 20-20 (continued)

8. The Furlow inserter is placed through the corporal tunnel and the plunger at the end of the inserter is pushed to puncture the glans with the Keith needle.

   Procedural Consideration: If the inflatable rods are not impregnated with Inhibi-Zone, the surgeon may have the rods irrigated with the antibiotic mixture (bacitracin, cephalexin, and normal saline). The surgeon may also want the corporal tunnel irrigated with the antibiotic solution prior to inserting the rod.

9. The needle is grasped with a needle holder and pulled through the glans, thus pulling the inflatable rod up into position for insertion. The suture is unthreaded from the Keith needle so it can be used for the next inflatable rod.
10. The Furlow inserter is removed and the inflatable rod is inserted into the corpora tunnel.
11. The procedure is repeated in the other corpora.

Placement of the Pump

1. The surgeon locates the external inguinal ring and a path bluntly formed with the fingers.
2. Metzenbaum scissors are used to separate the transversalis fascia. Cooper's ligament is located and the fluid reservoir positioned in the perivesical space. The surgical technologist provides the surgeon with saline solution and the fluid reservoir is filled and positioned within Hesselbach's triangle.

   Procedural Consideration: The surgical technologist should confirm with the surgeon how much saline is needed to fill the fluid reservoir in order to draw up that amount.

3. The pump is placed in the scrotum, usually on the patient's dominant side, lateral to the testicle in a space bluntly dissected.
4. Using the assembly tool to clamp in place, the inflatable rods and fluid reservoir are connected to the pump with the appropriate size of connectors. The inflatable rods and fluid reservoir are tested.
5. The scrotal tunica albuginea is closed over the pump with a 3-0 or 4-0 absorbable suture in continuous fashion.
6. To aid in preventing postoperative hemorrhage and promote healing, the penile prosthesis is partially inflated for 24 hours. After 24 hours, the prosthesis is deflated to allow healing of the corpora and pockets created for the pump and fluid reservoir.
7. The incision at the penile base is closed with 3-0 or 4-0 absorbable suture, subcuticular fashion.
8. The Foley catheter is left in place for approximately 24–48 hours and then removed.
9. The dressing is applied. Because the penile prosthesis is partially inflated, the penis is positioned against the patient's abdomen for comfort; the dressing and penis are kept in place with a loose scrotal support.

Postoperative Considerations

Immediate Postoperative Care

- Patient is transported to the PACU.
- Patient is hospitalized for 1–2 days.
- Placement of ice pack recommended.

Prognosis

- No complications: Patient is expected to make a full recovery and be able to engage in sexual intercourse. Return to normal activities in 7–10 weeks.
- Complications: Postoperative SSI; hemorrhage; scrotal edema.

Wound Classification

- Class I: Clean

PROCEDURE 20-21 Penectomy

Surgical Anatomy and Pathology	• See previous procedures for anatomy. • Penectomy is performed for penile cancer that is not responding to radiation and/or chemotherapy, or when the size and depth of the cancer are extensive. Depending on the extensiveness of the disease, either a partial or total penectomy is performed. • In order for the patient to be eligible for a partial penectomy, a minimum of 3 cm of nondiseased proximal penile shaft must be available. The procedure may allow the patient to be able to stand when urinating. • Anything less than 3 cm and the patient will undergo a total penectomy.
Preoperative Diagnostic Tests and Procedures	• History and physical
Equipment, Instruments, and Supplies Unique to Procedure	• Major instrument set • ¼-in. Penrose drain • Vessel loops • Needle tip for electrocautery pencil • Marking pen • Foley catheter with drainage bag
Preoperative Preparation	• Position: Supine with legs slightly apart • Anesthesia: Spinal or general • Skin prep: Starting at penile base to include entire external genitalia; extended up to umbilicus down to mid-thigh and bilaterally as far as possible; prep perineum and anus last. • Draping: Isolate the anus with towel or adhesive drape, but must leave access to the perineum; four towels to square off; laparotomy drape; small adhesive drape placed around glans penis.
Practical Considerations	• Notify pathology department prior to start of procedure tissue that specimens may be sent to determine the margin of healthy tissue.
Surgical Procedure	1. Using the marking pen, the surgeon marks the elliptical incision that will be made around the base of the penis.
	2. Using the #15 knife blade, the surgeon begins the skin incision slightly below the base of the penis in the midline of the scrotum and completes the elliptical incision around the base of the penis. **Procedural Consideration:** The surgical technologist will be responsible for holding the penis and moving it to follow the surgeon as the incision is made. Small retractors such as the Senn retractors will be placed medially and laterally.
	3. An incision is made in the deep fascia of the penis, and the urethra is dissected free and mobilized from the corpora. The suspensory ligament and dorsal vessels are clamped, cut, and tied during the dissection. A vessel loop is placed around the urethra to laterally retract while the dissection is completed proximally and distally within the penis. **Procedural Consideration:** As the name indicates, the fascia is a deep layer that surrounds the penis. It is a continuation of the suspensory ligament.
	4. The urethra is cut and pulled downward with smooth forceps. The surgeon completes the penectomy, irrigates the surgical site, and controls bleeding with electrocautery. The end of the urethra is spatulated with the curved tenotomy scissors. **Procedural Consideration:** The amputated penis is considered a specimen to be sent to the pathology department.

PROCEDURE 20-21 (continued)

5. The surgical technologist manually retracts the scrotum cephalad to expose the perineum. Using the #15 knife blade, the surgeon makes a small circular subcuticular incision in the perineum and removes the plug of skin and subcutaneous .
6. Using the Metzenbaum scissors, the surgeon creates a small tunnel through the subcutaneous layer up to the penile base.
7. The surgeon inserts a DeBakey forceps through the tunnel, grasps the urethra, and brings it through the tunnel. The urethra is anastomosed to the skin in the perineum using 2-0 or 3-0 suture; the sutures are placed in interrupted fashion.
8. A ¼-in. Penrose drain is placed horizontally in the penectomy incision. The incision is closed over the drain using 2-0 or 3-0 suture in interrupted fashion. The ends of the drain are exteriorized on each end of the closure.
9. A Foley catheter with drainage bag is inserted through the new urethral opening. A nonadherent dressing is placed on the penectomy incision and small dressing on the incision around the Foley catheter.

Postoperative Considerations

Immediate Postoperative Care

- Patient is transported to the PACU.
- Patient is hospitalized for 1–3 days.

Prognosis

- No complications: Patient expected to have full recovery and ability to urinate. Depending on extent of cancer, patient may have to undergo additional procedures such as chemotherapy, radiation, or surgery to treat metastases.
- Complications: Postoperative SSI; scrotal edema; difficulty urinating; UTI.

Wound Classification

- Class II: Clean-contaminated

CASE STUDY Raymond is 35 years old. He lives in an area that has water with high mineral and salt content. He has been admitted to the emergency department with a diagnosis of kidney stones. This is his third admission for this condition.

1. What are kidney stones?
2. What are the treatment options for Raymond?
3. If he has surgery, what procedure will most likely be performed?

Questions for Further Study

1. **What is end-stage renal disease? Is it serious?**
2. **Which kidney is preferred for live donor transplantation, and why?**
3. **What types of incisions are most common to genitourinary surgery in the male?**
4. **When a simple nephrectomy is being performed, which is clamped first—the renal artery or vein—and why?**
5. **What other purpose does the indwelling Foley catheter with balloon serve besides urinary drainage when a patient has undergone a TURP?**
6. **When a TURP is being performed, why should the surgical technologist report a sudden jerking of the patient's leg to the surgeon and anesthesia provider?**

BIBLIOGRAPHY

Association of Surgical Technologists. (2011). *Core curriculum for surgical technology* (6th ed.). Littleton, CO: Association of Surgical Technologists.

Burke, S. R. (1980). *The composition and function of body fluids* (3rd ed.). St. Louis, Mosby.

Carlson, B. M. (2004). *Human embryology and development biology* (3rd ed.). St. Louis: Mosby.

Clayman, R. V., Kavoussi, L. R., Soper, N. J., Albala, D. M., Figenshau, R. S., & Chandhoke, P. S. (2009). Laparoscopic nephrectomy: Review of the initial 10 cases. *Journal of Endourology, 6*(2), 127-132.

Clinical guideline—Varicocele management: Explanatory notes [Online] (2002, October 2). Retrieved from http://freespace.virgin.net.cd.1

Estes, M. E. Z. (2010). *Health assessment and physical examination* (4th ed.). Clifton Park, NY: Delmar Cengage Learning.

Fulmer, B. R. (2011). Laparoscopic and robotic radical prostatectomy. Retrieved from http://emedicine.medscape.com/article/458677-overview#showall

Gilbert, B. R. (2003, February 21). Microsurgical varicocele ligation—patient information [Online]. Retrieved from *http://wwwppol.com*

Guyton, A. C., & Hall, J. E. (2005). *Textbook of medical physiology* (11th ed.). Philadelphia: W. B. Saunders.

HealthAnswers.com, Inc. (1999). Medical reference library [Online]. Retrieved from http://www.healthanswers.com

HealthGate Data Corporation. (1999). [Online]. Retrieved from http://www.healthgate.com

James Buchanan Brady Urological Institute. Minimally invasive surgery: Ureteroscopy. Retrieved from http://urology.jhu.edu/MIS/lap_ureteroscopy.php

Miquel, M. E., Rhode, K. S., Acher, P. L., MacDougall, N. D., Blackall, J., Gaston, R. P., et al. (2006). Using combined X-ray and MR imaging for prostate I-125 post-implant dosimetry: Phantom validation and preliminary patient work. *Physics in Medicine and Biology, 51*, 1129-1137.

National Institutes of Diabetes and Digestive and Kidney Disease (NIDDK). (2011). [Online]. Retrieved from http://www.niddk.nih.gov

Theodorescu, D., & Krupski, T. L. (2011). Prostate cancer—brachytherapy (radioactive seed implantation therapy). Retrieved from http://emedicine.medscape.com/article/453349-overview

UCLA Health System. (2007). Robotically assisted prostatectomy uses minimally invasive tools to treat cancer. Retrieved from http://www.uclahealth.org/workfiles/documents/clinicalupdates/w6-12-robot0807.pdf

Vasavada, *S. P., Appell, R.,* Sand, P. K., & Raz, S. (eds.). *(2004). Female urology, urogynecology, and voiding dysfunction.* New York: Informa Healthcare.

Walsh, P. C., Retick, A. B., Vaughan, E. D., Wein, A. J., Kavoussi, L., Novick, A. C., et al. (2002). *Campbell's urology* (8th ed.). Philadelphia: Saunders.

WebMD. (2011). Prostate cancer: Radioactive seed implants. Retrieved from http://www.webmd.com/prostate-cancer/radioactive-seed-implants

Windson Urology. (2011). Ureteroscopy. Retrieved from http://www.windsorurology.co.uk/Clinical_Information/Kidney/Ureteroscopy.aspx

CHAPTER 21

Orthopedic Surgery

CASE STUDY Marcella works evenings at a trauma center. She was just advised that a patient will be coming to the OR with a severe Colles' fracture. She will be the surgical technologist on the case.

1. **What is a Colles' fracture?**
2. **What are the options for surgical intervention?**
3. **What equipment will Marcella need to secure?**

OBJECTIVES

After studying this chapter, the reader should be able to:

A 1. Recognize the relevant anatomy and physiology of the musculoskeletal system.

P 2. Summarize the pathology of the musculoskeletal system that prompts surgical intervention and the related terminology.

O 3. Determine any preoperative orthopedic diagnostic procedures/tests.

S 4. Determine any special preoperative preparation related to orthopedic procedures.

5. Indicate the names and uses of orthopedic instruments, equipment, and supplies.
6. Determine the intraoperative preparation of the patient undergoing an orthopedic procedure.
7. Summarize the surgical steps of the orthopedic procedures.
8. Interpret the purpose and expected outcomes of the orthopedic procedures.
9. Recognize the immediate postoperative care and possible complications of the orthopedic procedures.

Select Key Terms

abduction
AC joint
adduction
amphiarthrosis
avascular necrosis
cancellous bone
cartilage
comminuted
compartmental syndrome
compound fracture
cortical bone
delayed union
diarthrosis
distraction
epiphysis
flexion
ligament
malunion
marrow
nonunion
osteogenesis
proximal
shoulder joint
splint
valgus

BONE AND BONE TISSUE

The following is general anatomy and physiology of bone and bone tissue, including pathologies and bone healing; the student will often be referred back to Table 21-2 to review the pathology associated with a surgical procedure. Anatomical information about specific bones is provided within the surgical procedures.

Bones are living tissue that provide form and structure to the human body and are actively involved in the maintenance of homeostasis. The skeletal system comprises the bones and other structures that make up the joints of the skeleton (refer to Plate II in Appendix A). Those other structures include the **cartilage**, tendons, and ligaments that hold the skeletal framework together.

The skeleton performs the following functions:

1. It provides a framework to support the body.
2. It serves as points of attachment for muscles, which in turn move the bones.
3. It protects some internal organs from injury; for example, the ribs protect the lungs.
4. It serves as a source of red blood cells (RBCs). Because it contains the red bone **marrow**, bone is one of the hematopoietic tissues of the body.
5. It serves as a storage site and source of calcium. Calcium is a necessary component of the blood clotting sequence and is needed for the normal functioning of the muscles and nerves.

Bone Tissue

Bone is a specialized connective tissue that takes several basic forms (Figure 21-1). Bone cells are called osteocytes and the surrounding matrix is made up of calcium salts and collagen. The calcium salts give the bone the strength it needs to fulfill its supportive function. Osteocytes act as both bone-forming and bone-destroying cells. The osteocytes have the ability not only to synthesize, but also to resorb the matrix. The specific cells of bone will be discussed in more detail later.

Two types of bone tissue exist (Figure 21-2). Compact bone, or **cortical bone**, is the hard, dense tissue of bone that surrounds the marrow cavity. Found within compact bone are the haversian systems. A single haversian unit is made up of circular rings of bone matrix with implanted osteocytes that

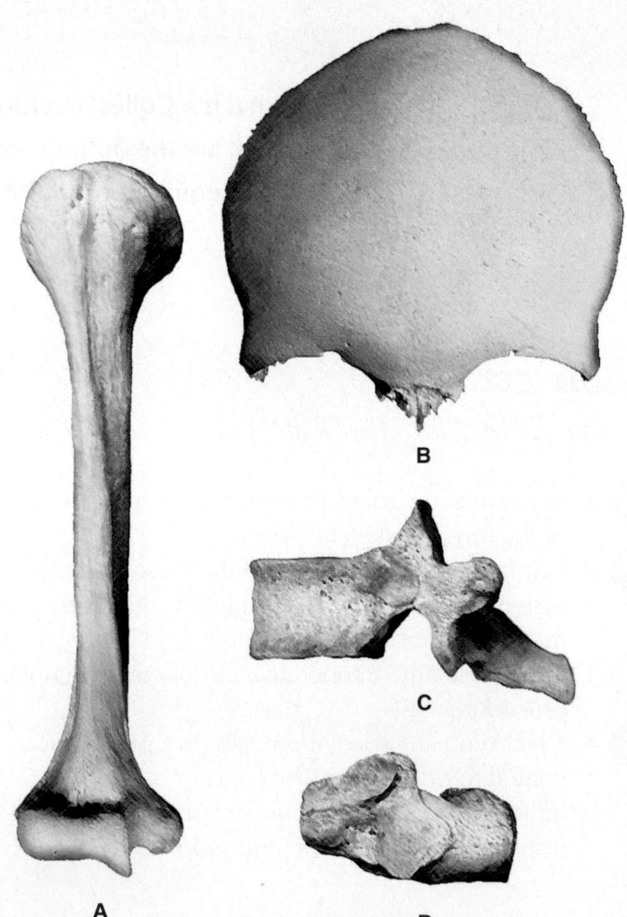

Figure 21-1 Types of bone: (A) Long bone (humerus), (B) flat bone (frontal), (C) irregular bone (vertebra), (D) short bone (cuboid)

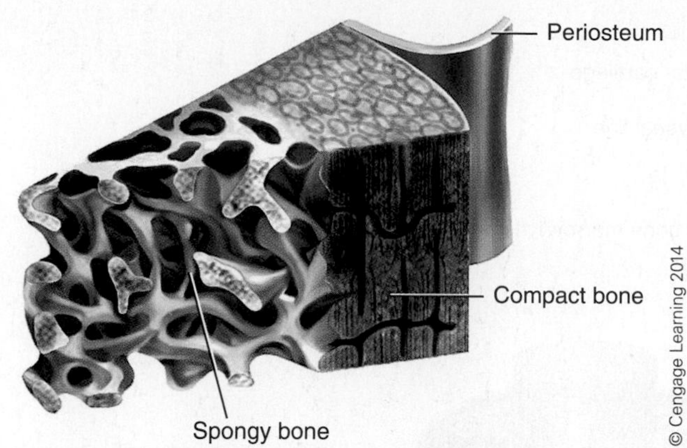

Figure 21-2 Bone tissues, microscopic view

form a canal. Traversing each canal is a single venule and arteriole, which account for the rich vascularity of bone. The haversian units are connected to make up compact bone and are not found in **cancellous bone**. Each osteocyte is found in a space, or lacuna, of the matrix and extends filament-like processes through canaliculi (microscopic channels) called Volkmann's canals to contact adjacent osteocytes' processes and the blood vessels.

Cancellous, or spongy, bone is found at the ends of bone and lining the medullary marrow cavity. Cancellous bone gives the appearance of a sponge due to its porous matrix. The name *cancellous bone* is used to describe the appearance of the bone, but does not explain the structure. The end bone structure is composed of columns of bony substance called trabeculae with large spaces interspersed among the columns, hence giving it the appearance of a sponge. The columns are well suited for adapting to load bearing due to their formation along stress lines. Cancellous bone is composed of osteocytes and matrix.

Surrounding bone is a thin, fibrous layer of tissue called the periosteum. It is composed of two cell layers. The inner cambium layer is the area where new bone cells are formed. The collagen fibers of the periosteum serve as an anchor of attachment merging with those of the tendons and ligaments that are attached to bone. The periosteum is permeated with nerves and blood vessels that nourish the underlying bone, but by itself is not capable of providing enough nourishment to the bone cortex. The periosteum also serves as a layer of defense against infection of bone.

Bone marrow is a semisolid tissue that is found in the spaces of cancellous bone. In infants, adolescents, and young adults, red bone marrow is found in the cancellous bone at the ends of the long bones, sternum, ribs, and vertebrae. The red bone marrow is essential for the production of RBCs, platelets, and white blood cells (WBCs). In long bones, a medullary cavity extends through the shaft of the bone. A fibrous layer of tissue, similar to periosteum, lines the cavity and is called endosteum. In adults, the red bone marrow in the cavity is slowly replaced by yellow bone marrow that does not produce RBCs. The blood supply in yellow bone marrow is extensive and supplies the cortex of the bone. Interestingly, the yellow bone marrow in adults will convert back to RBC-producing red bone marrow in reaction to hemorrhagic trauma. When the body's RBC count returns to normal, the marrow reconverts back to yellow bone marrow.

Types of Bones

The long bones include bones of the arm (humerus), legs (femur), hands, and feet (phalanges) (Figure 21-3). The shaft of the long bone is called the diaphysis and the ends are called **epiphyses** (singular, *epiphysis*). The diaphysis is composed of compact bone that surrounds the medullary cavity. The epiphyses are composed of cancellous bone.

The epiphyses make up the joint area of the bone. The joint surfaces are covered by cartilage called the articular cartilage, which, in turn, is covered by the synovial membrane. The combination of ligaments surrounding the joint and synovial membrane is referred to as the joint capsule. The articular cartilage and synovial membrane provide a smooth surface for the movement of joints and tendons and prevent bone from rubbing against bone during movement. Types of joints will be discussed later.

The origin of synovial fluid is the synovial membrane. Small sacs, called bursa, are located in many joints such as the shoulder. The sacs contain synovial fluid, which acts as a lubricant to aid in joint movement. The sacs also cushion the joint during weight-bearing or impact activities such as football.

At the epiphyses in growing bone there is an area under the cartilage known as the epiphyseal plate (Figure 21-4). This is the area of active bone growth. In the majority of growing bones, new bone is formed at the epiphyseal plate by the process known as endochondral ossification. When the growth of bones is complete, usually in early adulthood, the epiphyseal plate area disappears and the area is known as a closed epiphysis.

Short bones are the bones of the wrists (carpals) and ankles (tarsals). As evidenced by the wrist and ankle bones, short bones usually occur in clusters and aid in the movement of an extremity.

The ribs, scapula, sternum, and cranial bones are examples of flat bones. In adults, the majority of RBCs are manufactured and supplied to the body in the ribs and sternum. The bones of the skull and face and the vertebrae are known as irregular bones.

Sesamoid (round) bones are found within tendons. The patella is a type of sesamoid bone. Another example is the two sesamoid bones found on the head of the metatarsal in the foot forming what is referred to as the "ball" of the foot.

Types of Joints

The area where two bones meet to form a joint is called the *articulation* (articulate). Joints are classified according to the movement that is possible. The three general groups are called immovable, slightly movable, and freely movable joints.

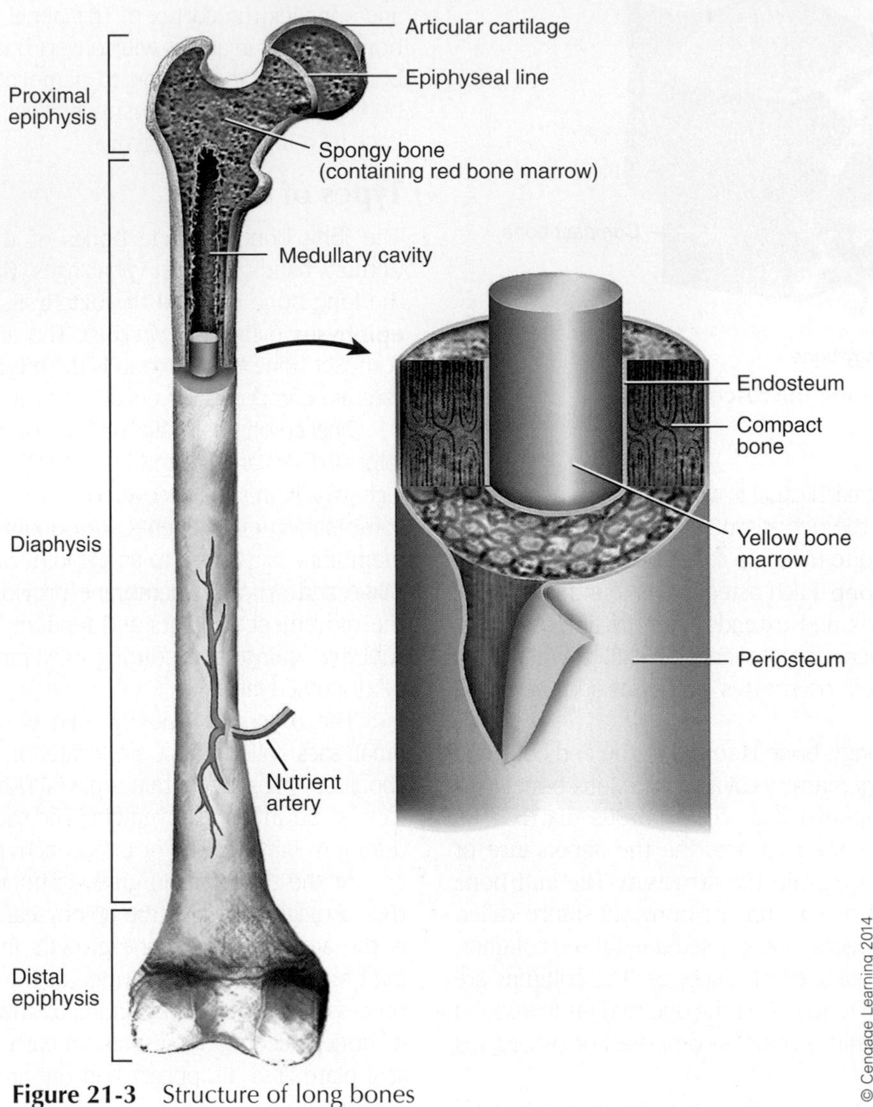

Figure 21-3 Structure of long bones

IMMOVABLE JOINTS

A synarthrosis is an immovable joint. In synarthroses, the bones are in close contact with each other and separated by a thin layer of cartilage. An example is the suture lines of the cranial bones.

SLIGHTLY MOVABLE JOINTS

An **amphiarthrosis** is a joint that is slightly movable. Lying between the bones of the joint is a disk of fibrous cartilage that connects the bones. Examples of this type of joint include cartilage that connects the vertebrae and the disk of cartilage called the symphysis pubis that connects the pubic bones. This type of joint allows some movement due to the limited flexibility of the cartilage.

FREELY MOVABLE JOINTS

A **diarthrosis** joint is a freely movable joint (Figure 21-5). All diarthroses are also referred to as synovial joints because these joints all contain a synovial membrane that secretes synovial fluid. Diarthroses are further classified according to the movements they allow (Figure 21-6).

Ball-and-Socket Joints

This type of joint allows for the widest range of motion (ROM). It consists of a bone with a ball-shaped head that articulates with the cup-shaped socket in another bone. Movement in all planes is possible, including rotational. Examples include the shoulder and hip joints.

Condyloid Joints

The condyloid joint allows for movement in only one plane with some lateral movement. The joint is composed of a condyle of one bone fitting into the fossa of another bone. An example is the temporomandibular joint in which the condyle of the mandible fits into the fossa of the temporal bone.

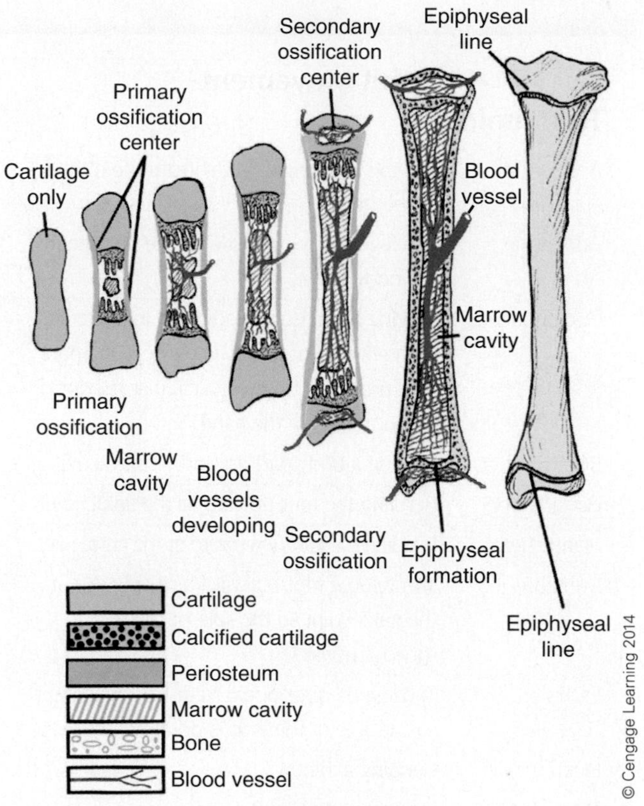

Figure 21-4 Long bone development

Gliding Joints

Gliding joints allow side-to-side and twisting movements. The articulating surfaces of the bones in the gliding joint are either flat or slightly curved. An example of a gliding joint is the carpals of the wrist joint.

Hinge Joints

The elbow is a hinge joint. This type of joint allows movement in only one plane, much like the motion permitted by the hinge on a door. The hinge joint is formed by the convex surface of one bone fitting into the concave surface of the adjacent bone.

Pivot Joints

Pivot joints allow only a rotational movement around a central axis. The joint formed at the **proximal** end of the radius is a type of pivot joint.

Saddle Joints

Saddle joints allow movement in a variety of planes. The articulating surfaces of the bones have both concave and convex regions. The surface of one bone fits into the equivalent surface of the other bone. An example is the joint formed by the trapezium of the wrist with the metacarpal of the thumb.

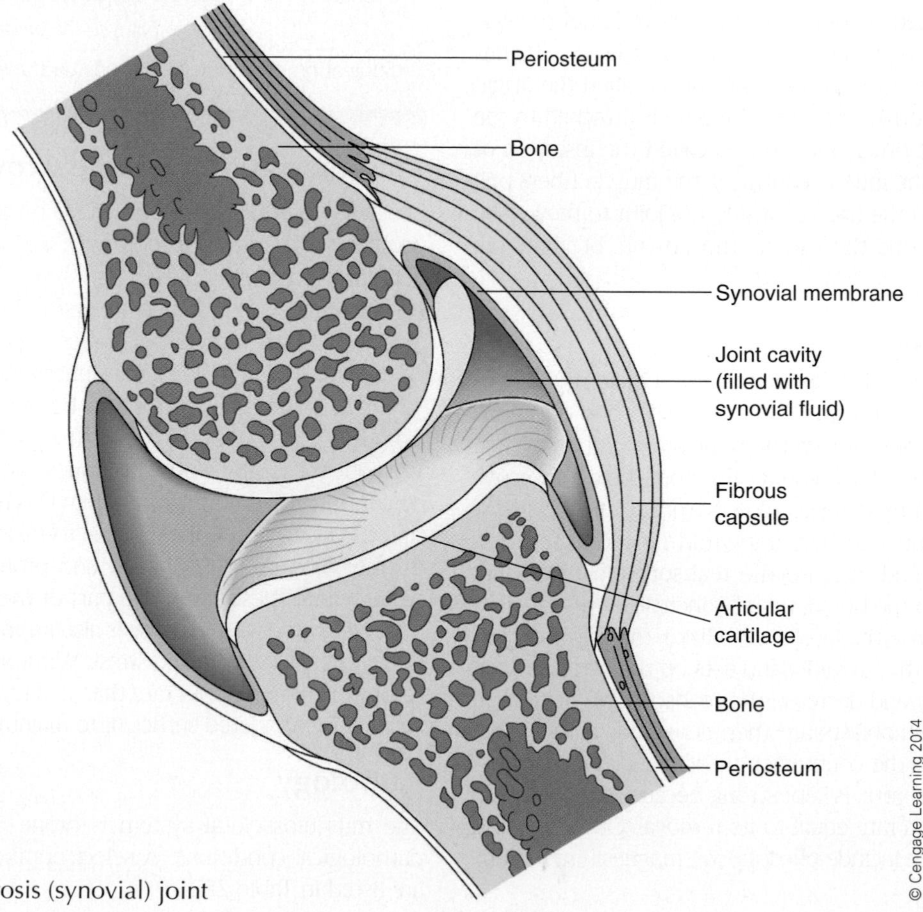

Figure 21-5 Diarthrosis (synovial) joint

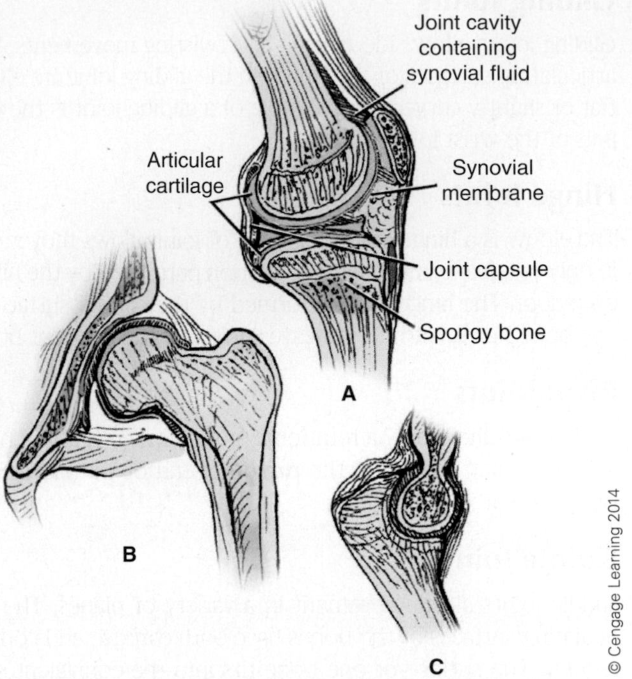

Figure 21-6 Joint types: (A) Hinge (knee), (B) ball and socket (hip), (C) hinge (elbow)

TERMS RELATED TO JOINT MOVEMENTS

The muscles attached to bone produce movements of diarthroses. Most often, one end of a muscle is attached to the immovable end of one bone of the joint; this is called the origin of the muscle. The other end of the muscle is attached to the movable end of the other bone; this is called the insertion of the muscle. When the muscle contracts, the muscle fibers pull the insertion toward the origin, causing the joint to move. The terms used to describe the various movements of joints are listed in Table 21-1.

Mineral Storage

Bone contains large quantities of calcium. Calcium is essential for many of the body's metabolic processes, and calcium is constantly being removed from the bones to maintain normal blood calcium levels. This accounts for bone being an active tissue. When the body detects a low serum level of calcium, osteoclasts are stimulated by parathyroid hormone to break down bone tissue and increase the reabsorption of calcium from the bones into the blood, thereby increasing the circulating calcium level. Once the level is stabilized, the hormone calcitonin secreted by the thyroid gland acts on the osteoclasts to inhibit their activity and decrease the reabsorption of calcium from the bones. Osteoblasts are then activated to form new bone tissue. Due to the counteraction of osteoblasts and osteoclasts, the bone matrix is kept strong because the calcium in bone is replaced at a rate equal to its removal. Other minerals stored in bone tissue include phosphorus, magnesium, sodium, and potassium.

Table 21-1 Joint Movement Terminology

Abduction	Moving a body part away from the midline of the body
Adduction	Moving a body part toward the midline of the body
Circumduction	Moving a particular body part in a circular path without moving the entire body part (e.g., moving a finger in a circular motion without moving the hand)
Rotation	Moving a body part around a central axis
Dorsiflexion	Bending the foot upward at the ankle joint
Plantarflexion	Bending the foot downward at the ankle joint
Eversion	Turning the foot outward or inside out at the ankle joint so the sole of the foot is shown outward
Inversion	Turning the foot outward at the ankle joint so the sole of the foot is pointing inward
Flexion	Bending a joint
Extension	Straightening a joint
Pronation	Pointing a body part downward (e.g., facing the palm of the hand downward)
Supination	Pointing a body part upward

Factors That Affect Bone Growth

Besides the effect hormones have on bone, three other important factors affect the growth and maintenance of bone: heredity, nutrition, and exercise.

Heredity is not a well-understood mechanism in relation to bone growth. Individuals possess a potential for height that is most likely due to the genes inherited from both parents.

Nutrition is a key factor also, because the nutrients derived from food are the raw materials from which bone is produced. Without these nutrients, the bones cannot grow normally or be continually remodeled. Vitamin D is needed for the absorption of calcium and phosphorus to take place in the small intestine. Calcium, phosphorus, and protein are needed in the diet because these become a part of the bone matrix.

Weight-bearing exercise is also important. Bones are meant to bear normal weight and stress. Without this stress, bones lose calcium at a more rapid rate than it is replaced. Exercise such as walking is considered sufficient to maintain the density of bone.

Pathology

The musculoskeletal system is prone to numerous types of pathological conditions. A select number of these conditions are listed in Table 21-2.

TABLE 21-2 Orthopedic Pathologies

Condition	*Description*
Arthropathies	
Arthralgia	Pain in a joint
Arthritis	Inflammation of a joint
	Note: The term *arthritis* is applied to rheumatoid as well as to osteoarthritis; however, it is only the rheumatoid type that shows all the signs of inflammation.
Rheumatoid Arthritis (RA)	Rheumatoid arthritis involves connective tissue throughout the entire body, but mainly involves the synovium in the joint.
	Rheumatoid arthritis is considered an autoimmune disease (abnormal response against one's own body). In the disease process, the body does not recognize its own natural antibodies as "self." Because the body thinks its own natural antibodies are foreign, it produces antibodies called rheumatoid factors (RFs) that fight against its own natural antibodies. The disease starts with a simple synovitis and can progress through several stages, the last being joint immobility. Because of the role of RF antibodies, an RF test confirms RA.
	The inflammation is initiated by RF antibodies producing an inflammatory exudate called *pannus.* Movement is difficult and painful because the thick pannus adheres to the joint surfaces, producing *ankylosis,* which is abnormal stiffness or fixation of a joint.
	Diagnostic tests may include analysis of synovial fluid, antinuclear antibody, latex fixation tests, and RFs. (For a detailed description of these and other tests, see Table 21-4.)
OsteoArthritis (OA)	Osteoarthritis is a degenerative disease of the joint and is a normal part of aging. Although the exact cause is unknown, the articular cartilage wears away, often because of overuse, exposing underlying bone. Pain is caused by the friction between the two bones as they glide across each other without the protection of the articular cartilage.
	The most effective treatment for both RA and OA is acetylsalicylic acids, such as aspirin, and nonsteroidal anti-inflammatory drugs (NSAIDs).
	Diagnosis is made by skeletal X-ray of arthritic joint.
Internal derangement of the knee joint	Disruption in the arrangement of the structure, of the knee joint which therefore affects the function of the knee.
Bucket handle tear	A bucket handle tear includes abnormalities of the internal structures of the knee joint, such as C-shaped meniscus tears on the medial or lateral edge with the opposite side still attached. The torn edge resembles a bucket handle.
Joint mice	Joint mice, so called because of loose particles within the joint, are caused by repeated trauma to the knee. Joint mice often create a constant irritation within the joint cavity, which produces an excess of synovial fluid. When a particle becomes lodged between articulating surfaces, pain or a locking of the joint may occur.

Table 21-2 (continued)

Condition	*Description*
Tendons, Tendon Sheaths, and Bursa	
Ganglion of tendon sheath	A cystic growth commonly occurring on the dorsum of the wrist. 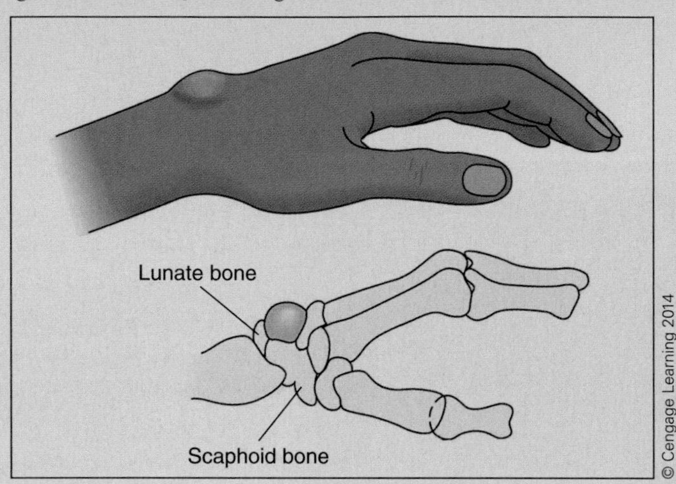
Osteopathies and Chondropathies	
Osteochondritis	Inflammation of bone and cartilage
Osteoma	Tumor of the bone
Osteomalacia	A softening of bone caused by loss of calcification of the bone matrix
	Note: The condition is a result of an inadequate amount of phosphorus and calcium in the blood for the mineralization of bone caused by a lack of vitamin D or by malabsorption of calcium and is called rickets in children.
Osteomyelitis	Inflammation and infection of the bone and bone marrow usually caused by bacteria. *Staphylococci* are the most common causative bacteria.
	Note: Osteomyelitis is caused by the presence of pyogenic bacteria, usually *Staphylococcus.* The infection can spread to the bone through the blood from a previously injured site, or the microorganism can infiltrate the bone directly following open fractures, surgical reductions, or other exposures to the air.
Osteonecrosis (Avascular necrosis)	Destruction and death of bone tissue. Occurs frequently in the head of the femur due to a disease process or trauma that obstructs or destroys the blood supply to the femoral head.
Osteoporosis	Condition of decreased bone density due to an excessive loss of calcium from bone without replacement and diminished osteogenesis—the bone becomes porous and fragile, and fractures are common.
Primary osteoporosis	Primary osteoporosis is idiopathic; however, contributing factors include reduction in calcium intake and hormonal imbalance. It is most commonly seen in postmenopausal women.
Secondary osteoporosis	Secondary osteoporosis is caused by extended drug use, particularly steroids, or by extended periods of inactivity. In general, osteoporosis is usually seen in elderly women who first come to a health care facility complaining of back pain, because the vertebral column is most commonly affected. Diagnosis is mainly through X-rays of the thoracic and lumbar vertebrae. Treatment is preventive by increasing bone mass through proper dietary consumption of calcium and vitamin D and through exercise.

TABLE 21-2 **(continued)**

Condition	*Description*
Acquired Deformities of the Toe	
Bunion	A bunion is a bony protuberance on the medial aspect of the first metatarsal. The condition is associated with hallux valgus deformity. A bony prominence projecting from a bone is called an exostosis. 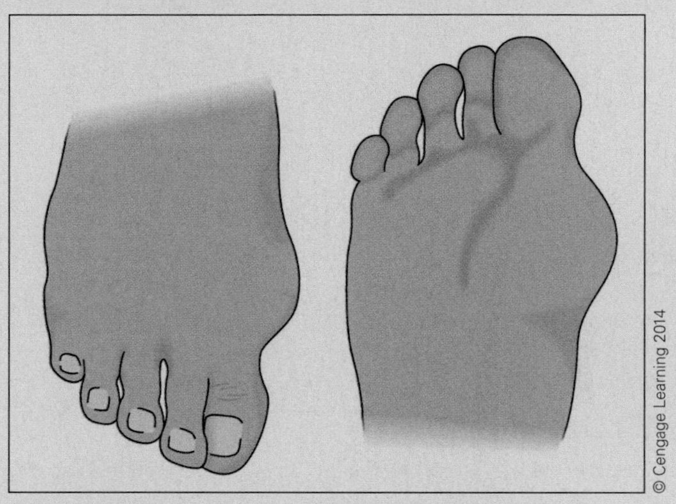 © Cengage Learning 2014
Hallux valgus	The outward turning of the great toe away from the midline
Hallux varus	The inward turning of the great toe toward the midline
Hammer toe, claw toe, mallet toe	Acquired or congenital deformities of the toes as a result of abnormal positioning of the interphalangeal joints
Acquired Deformities of the Hip	
Coxa valga	Outward turning of the hip joint
Coxa vara	Inward turning of the hip joint
Genu valgum	Knock-kneed; the knees are in close position and the space between the ankles is increased. 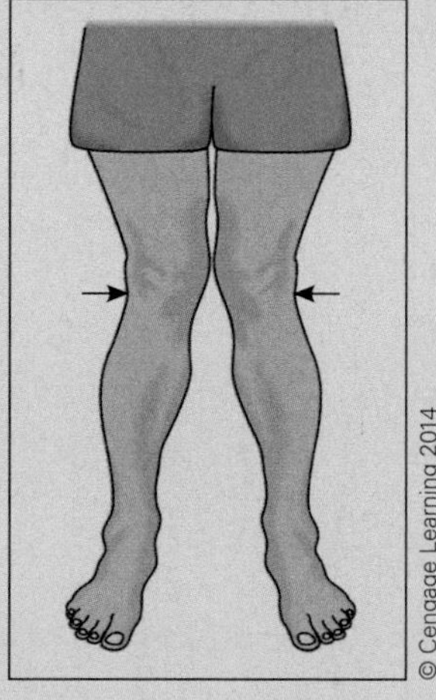 © Cengage Learning 2014

TABLE 21-2 (continued)

Condition	*Description*
Genu varum	Bowlegged; the space between the knees is abnormally increased and the lower leg bows inwardly. 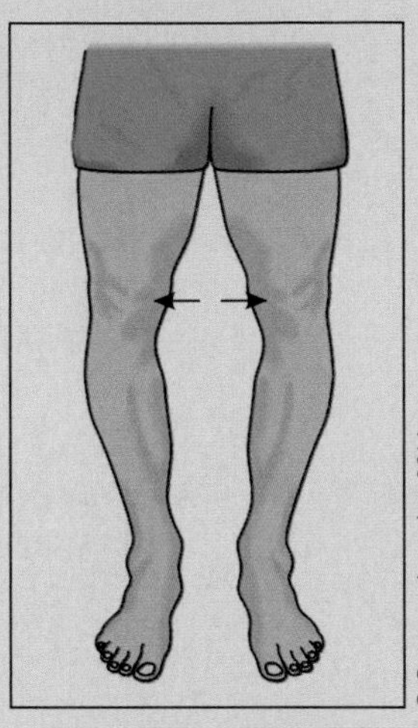
Congenital Anomalies	
Talipes valgus	Outward turning of the foot away from the midline 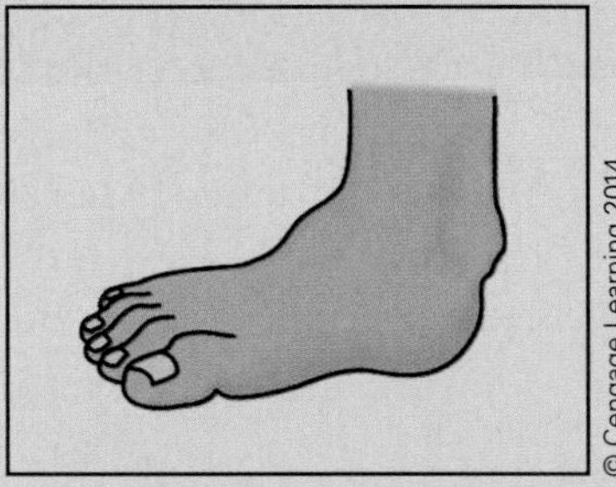
Talipes varus	Inward turning of the foot toward the midline 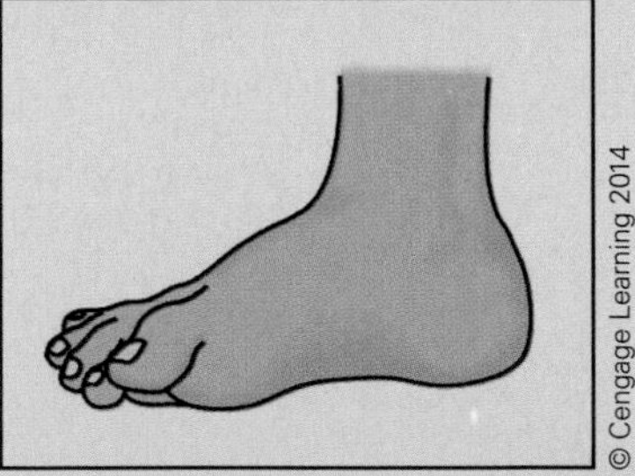 *Note:* All varieties of talipes can be acquired.
Osteogenesis imperfect a [imperfecta]	Genetic and congenital condition that involves the defective development of connective tissue resulting in deformed and abnormally brittle bones that are easily fractured
Injuries	
Dislocations	A dislocation is the displacement of bone from its socket, usually caused by trauma. The types of dislocations include compound or open, which is the complete displacement of the bone from its socket along with a break in the skin so that the joint communicates with the air; luxation, which is the complete separation of the joint with no break in the skin; and subluxation, which is the partial separation of the joint with no break in the skin.

TABLE 21-2 **(continued)**

Condition	*Description*
Fracture	Discontinuity of the normal alignment of bone
	Note: Most fractures are caused by accidents, although some are pathological (fractures caused by diseased bones).
Classification of fractures	Fractures can be grouped according to the following list: • *Whether or not the bone pierces the skin* If the bone pierces the skin, it is called a compound or open fracture. If the fracture does not pierce the skin, it is called a simple or closed fracture. Simple fractures are caused by moderate energy that continues until the bone reaches a level of tolerance, usually by direct force.
	• *Type of fracture line through the bone* If the fracture line is continuous through the bone, it is called complete. If the fracture line is not continuous through the bone, it is called incomplete or partial. A type of partial fracture is a greenstick fracture, which, like a green stick or twig from a tree, will bend on one side and break on the other.
	• *Direction of the fracture line* In a linear fracture, the line of the fracture runs parallel to the axis of the bone. A spiral fracture is where the fracture line curves around the bone. A transverse fracture is where the fracture line is across the bone. In an intra-articular fracture, the fracture line is on the joint surfaces of bone. Caused by a direct force to the joint area.
Avulsion	Bone and other tissues are pulled from normal attachments. Caused by direct force; most often extremity is bent in an abnormal manner.
Bucket handle	Dual vertical fractures on the same side of the pelvis. Caused by direct force or anterior compression of the pelvis.
Butterfly	Associated with **comminuted** type of fracture; butterfly-shaped piece of fractured bone. Cause by direct or rotational force.
Depressed	Fracture occurs when bone is driven inward; frequently seen with cranial fracture. Caused by moderate to severe direct force.
Displaced	Fracture in which bone ends are out of alignment. Caused by direct force to area.
Greenstick	Fracture that occurs in only one cortex of the bone and is not a complete break.
	Sometimes referred to as an incomplete or stress fracture.
	Cause: Minor direct energy; repetitive direct force such as jogging on a hard surface every day or jumping (basketball)
Oblique (type of linear fracture)	Fracture that occurs at an oblique angle across both cortices. Caused by direct force, possibly with some compression.
Spiral	Fracture that curves around bone Cause: Direct twisting force or distal part of bone unable to move

TABLE 21-2 **(continued)**

Condition	*Description*
Transcervical	Transverse fracture through the neck of the femur
	Cause: Direct force on bone

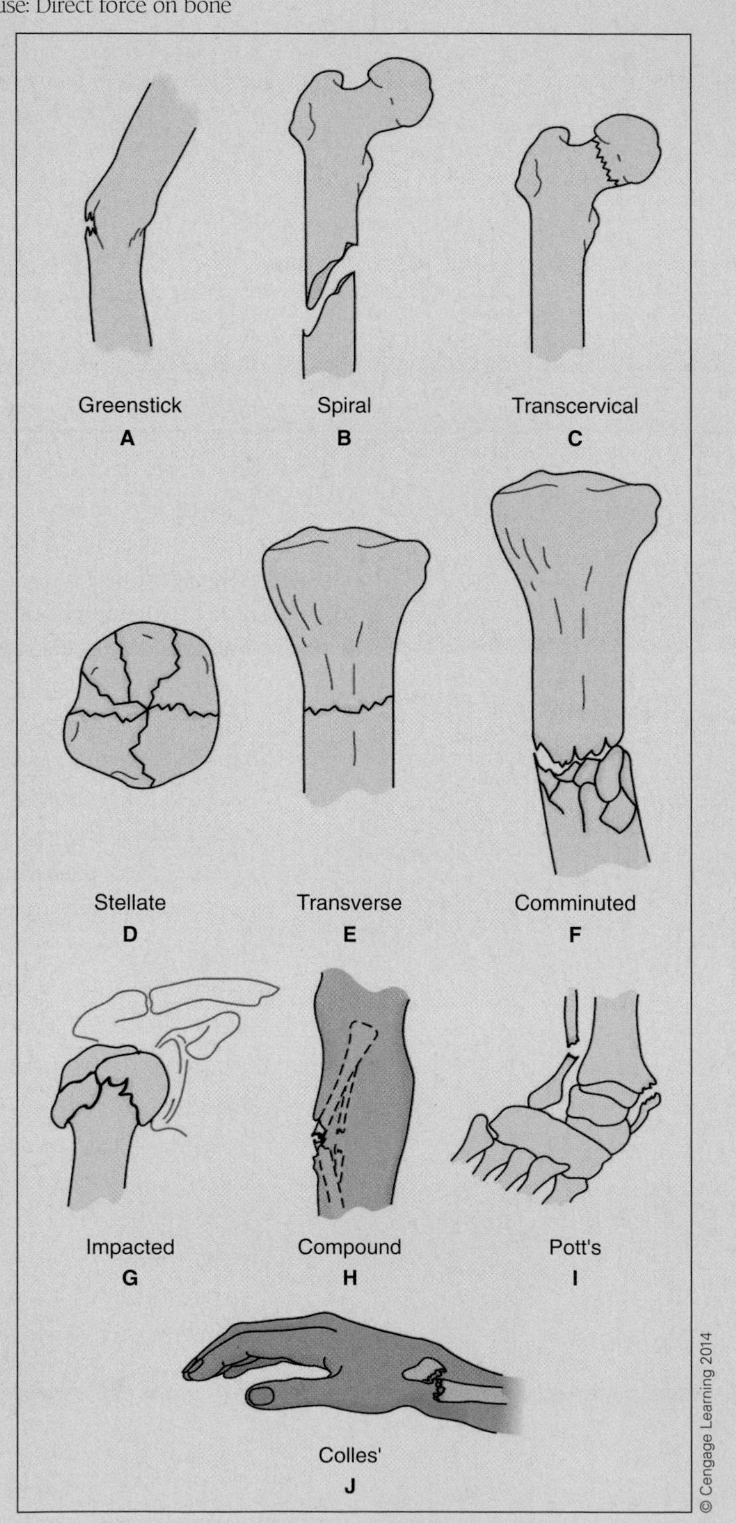

Table 21-2 (continued)

Condition	*Description*
Stellate	Fracture occurs at central point; additional breaks in bone radiate from the central point
	Cause: Direct force of moderate energy
Transverse	Horizontal fracture through the bone
	Cause: Direct force toward the bone
Comminuted (segmental)	Fracture with more than two pieces of bone fragment; may have notable amount of associated soft tissue trauma
	Cause: Direct crushing force
Impacted	The broken ends of each bone are forced into each other, usually creating many bone fragments.
	Cause: Compressive force
Compound (open)	Broken end of bone has penetrated the skin, exposing the bone. Significant damage may be present to surrounding blood vessels, nerves, and muscle; occurrence of infection is greatly increased
	Cause: Moderate to severe energy that is continuous until bone reaches level of tolerance; usually produced by direct force
Pott's fracture (old term—better known as bimalleolar ankle fracture)	Fracture of the fibula near the ankle, often accompanied by a break in the medial malleolus of the tibia and/or rupture of the internal lateral ligament
	Cause: A combination of abduction external rotation from an eversion force
Colles' fracture	A fracture of the distal radius that occurs at the epiphysis within 2.54 centimeters of the wrist joint, forcing the hand into a dorsal and lateral position
	Cause: Direct force, such as when falling and stretching out the hand to break the fall
Sprains	Injury to the joint characterized by the rupture of some or all fibers of the supporting ligament
Malignant Neoplasms	
Ewing's tumor	Malignant tumor of bone affecting mostly boys between 5 and 15 years of age; the cure rate is currently greater than 60% with proper treatment such as chemotherapy, radiation therapy, and surgery
Multiple myeloma; plasma cell myeloma	Malignant neoplasm of the marrow plasma cells resulting in bone destruction and overproduction of immunoglobulins and Bence Jones protein (see Table 21-6)
	Note: Treatment is chemotherapy
Osteogenic sarcoma; osteosarcoma	Malignant tumor of the long bones, particularly the femur, commonly metastasizing to the lungs
	Note: Treatment is chemotherapy and surgery
Benign Neoplasms	
Chondroma	Benign tumor of cartilage
Giant cell tumor	Tumor of the epiphysis of long bones, particularly the distal femur at the knee; commonly seen in the 20–40 age group
	Note: Treatment is removal of the tumor followed by bone grafting.
Osteoma	Benign tumor of bone

Source: From *Modern Medical Language* by C. E. Collins and J. J. Davies (1996). Clifton Park, NY: Delmar Cengage Learning. Reprinted with permission.

Types of Fractures

Fractures are classified according to the type of fracture and extent of damage. Fractures are either complete, in which the fracture completely interrupts the continuity of bone, or incomplete, in which the fracture is partial and some of the bone is still intact.

Normal Bone Healing

When a bone fracture occurs, complete bone healing is expected in 8–12 weeks under the right circumstances. For complete union of a fracture, the site of injury should be completely immobilized (internal or external fixation) and in proper alignment; the patient should be in good general health, well nourished, and infection free; and all physiological mechanisms to facilitate the normal process of bone healing should be intact.

The normal process of bone healing (**osteogenesis**) involves the following five stages:

1. Inflammation
2. Cellular proliferation
3. Callus formation
4. Ossification
5. Remodeling

The inflammatory stage begins at the time of injury and lasts approximately 2 days. A fracture hematoma, which is a result of the extravasation of blood caused by the injury, is formed during this time. The blood clot serves as a foundation for the subsequent cellular proliferation stage.

The cellular proliferation stage begins approximately on the second day following the traumatic event. Macrophages debride the area and allow for the formation of a fibrin mesh that seals the approximated edges of the fracture site. The fibrin mesh serves as the foundation for capillary and fibroblastic ingrowth. A soft tissue or periosteal callus is formed on the outer surface or cortex of the fractured bone by the collagen-producing fibroblasts and osteoblasts.

The callus formation stage lasts 3–4 weeks. The soft tissue growth continues and the bone fragments grow toward one another, bridging the gap. Osteoblasts form a matrix of collagen that invades the periosteal callus, bridging the fracture site and uniting the two ends of the bone. Fibrous tissue, cartilage, and immature bone stabilize the fracture site.

The ossification stage begins 2 or 3 weeks following the injury and can last 3–4 months. The matrix of osteoblasts, now called the osteoid, calcifies, firmly uniting the bone. The bone is now able to accept mineral deposits.

The remodeling stage is the maintenance state of normal bone. Following a fracture, any devitalized tissue is removed and the new bone is organized to provide maximum support and function. Osteoblastic and osteoclastic activity should be equal, constantly resorbing and reforming the bone. The process of remodeling continues throughout the life cycle and is affected by local stress on the individual bone, circulation, nutrition, and hormones. Any disruption of the homeostasis will result in a pathological condition.

Pathological Bone Healing

A disruption at any stage of bone healing or maintenance can be responsible for a variety of abnormal conditions. Fracture healing is a process that goes through stages to reach the end result. If the process is interrupted, the final result may be devastating for the individual. Interruptions of the normal path of bone healing include poor immobilization of the fracture, distraction of the bone fragments, deficient or nonexistent blood supply to the bone, infection, and interposition of soft tissue.

The majority of fractures must be immobilized to hold the bones in place in order for healing to take place. Movement of the fractured bones can cause disruption of the hematoma, thus prolonging the healing process and causing additional bleeding at the fracture site. Excellent immobilization must be achieved to assure a stable union.

Distraction is a term used to describe bone fragments that are separated so that bone contact does not occur. Distraction can be caused by too much weight applied to skeletal traction. The gap between the bone fragments created by distraction is filled with granulation tissue, which delays the healing. The excessive tension placed by distraction on the blood vessels may decrease the blood supply to the fracture site, which also increases healing time.

Distraction is linked with the complication known as interposition of soft tissues. The gap formed by distraction can allow soft tissue to grow over the ends of one or both fracture fragments. The soft tissue seals off the surface of the fractured bones, disallowing the hematoma to form and inhibiting callus formation. The result is a poor union of the fracture.

Avascular necrosis occurs when the capillary network or collateral circulation cannot be reestablished following a traumatic injury or when the vascular system is disrupted by other means. This can be pharmacological (e.g., steroid use), pathological (e.g., diabetes), or idiopathic. Decreased blood supply to the bone may lead to irreversible necrosis.

A **compound fracture** compromises the integrity of the skin and allows for the possible entry of microorganisms, which may cause infection of the bone and injury to surrounding soft tissues. Infection can delay healing and lead to serious consequences such as a generalized infection of the bone and bone marrow. Osteomyelitis, a serious infection of bone, starts as a local infection and can lead to chronic osteomyelitis.

Individuals heal at different rates, but the average time required for a fracture to heal does not ordinarily vary much from person to person. **Delayed union** is a term used to describe an increase in the healing time of fractures. The reasons for delayed healing are pathological (e.g., osteoporosis), mechanical (e.g., distraction of the fracture site or inadequate immobilization), or traumatic, referring to the type of injury sustained (e.g., comminuted fractures).

Nonunion is when the fractured bone ends do not unite. The presence of infection and movement of the fracture site are what usually cause nonunion. Infection and movement cause continual bleeding at the fracture site and a continual breakdown of the fragile hematoma. The fracture gap may increase to a point where the fracture ends have no chance of healing and a permanent nonunion exists.

Malunion occurs when the fracture heals in a position that does not resemble the original anatomical form of the bone and alters the mechanical function of the bone.

Compartmental syndrome is an increase in pressure within a closed space that usually occurs in the forearm and tibia. The fractured ends of the bone cause excess pressure that leads to neurovascular compromise. Tissue viability may be affected, increasing the risk for infection, and permanent nerve damage can occur. Other causes of compartmental syndrome are from a cast that is placed too tight or intracompartmental bleeding.

The forearm and leg are divided into compartments composed of bones, muscles, and nerves. Fascia and skin create the compartments that surround these structures. When a fracture occurs, pressure within the compartment increases due to the bleeding and swelling of tissues. The fascia can expand only so far to accommodate the swelling. When the fascia reaches its limit, the pressure is directed inward and compresses the blood vessels and nerves. Eventually the capillary circulation to the muscle stops. When the circulation is compromised the muscles become ischemic; necrosis begins in 2–4 hours and becomes irreversible in 12 hours. Nerve damage starts within 30 minutes, and after 12 hours, if the swelling is not stopped, there will be irreversible loss of muscle function.

Other soft tissues can be damaged by fractures. Tendons and ligaments are involved in avulsions. When the fracture occurs, the tendon or ligament avulses a small piece of bone to which it was attached. If left untreated, a dysfunction in the movement of the extremity may occur. Avulsions are commonly associated with fractures of the phalanges. Visceral damage may also occur from fractures. Examples of serious damage include a fracture of the pelvis in which the bladder is ruptured and the female internal reproductive organs are damaged, and a rib fracture that punctures a lung, causing it to collapse.

Casts

A cast is one of the more common methods utilized to immobilize a fracture. The complications of distraction and malalignment can be avoided with the application of a cast to the extremity. A common option is a closed reduction of the fracture with the subsequent application of a cast.

Fiberglass and plaster are the most frequently used types of casting material. Advantages and disadvantages of fiberglass are as follows:

Advantages	**Disadvantages**
Stronger than plaster	Expensive
Achieves weight-bearing strength faster than plaster	Even though it is considered waterproof, it must be dried as soon as possible after getting wet
Waterproof	
Durable	
Lightweight	

Advantages and disadvantages of plaster are as follows:

Advantages	**Disadvantages**
Inexpensive	Not waterproof
Easy to manipulate and handle when applying	Breakdown of casting material can lead to reapplication
Strong	
Rigid	

The majority of surgery departments have a cast cart that contains all the necessary supplies for application of a cast in the OR. The supplies include a disposable bucket for lukewarm water, Webril and stockinette of various sizes, plaster casting material of various widths and lengths, and heavy-duty scissors. The surgeon will first apply Webril or a stockinette to the extremity to protect the patient's skin from the cast (Figure 21-7). The casting material quickly begins to harden once wet, requiring that all the necessary materials for casting be ready.

If a **splint** is being applied, flat sheets of the casting material will be used. The surgeon will indicate how many layers thick the splint should be and the length of the splint. If necessary, the heavy-duty scissors is used to cut the material. The circulator wets the cast material and the surgeon applies it to the extremity and holds it in place until it hardens.

When applying a cast, rolls of casting material are used (Figure 21-8). These rolls are available in a variety of widths; the correct width is chosen according to the extremity or body part that requires casting. The circulator submerges the roll and holds it under the water until the bubbles stop rising to the surface, which indicates that the roll is adequately wet. Numerous types of casts can be made (Table 21-3).

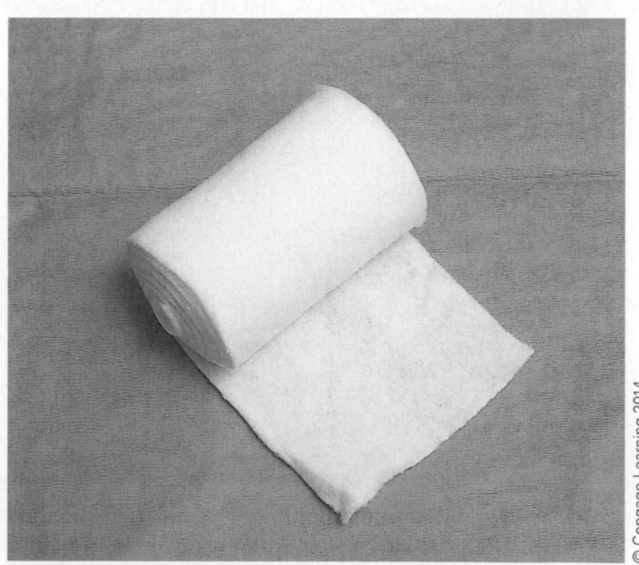

Figure 21-7 Undercasting material—cast padding

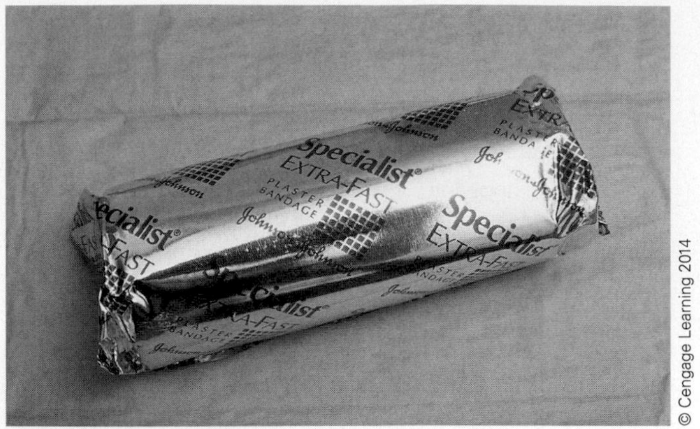

Figure 21-8 Casting material—plaster

TABLE 21-3 **Types of Casts**

Type	*Description*
Short arm cast	Applied from below the elbow to the metacarpal heads; wrist fracture
Long arm cast	Applied from axilla to metacarpal heads; fracture of forearm or elbow
Short leg cast	Applied from tibial tuberosity to metatarsal heads; ankle and foot fractures
Long leg cast	Applied from hip to metatarsal heads; fracture of femur, tibia, fibula, ankle
Cylinder cast	Applied from the groin to the ankle; required when complete knee immobilization is desired
Hip spica cast	Applied to trunk, complete leg of affected side, one-half of unaffected leg
Body jacket cast (Minerva jacket)	Applied to trunk of body to immobilize the spine

Diagnostic Procedures and Tests

Select common orthopedic diagnostic procedures and tests are presented in Table 21-4.

Radiography is frequently used during orthopedic surgery, particularly during the repair and/or reduction of fractures. The two most popular types of radiography are standard X-rays, in which the cassette is draped with a sterile cassette cover by the surgical technologist, and fluoroscopy.

Fluoroscopy provides the surgical team with the ability to view the procedure as it progresses, allowing confirmation of the fracture reduction or placement of pins, screws, and/or plates. The C-arm is a convenient fluoroscopy machine that can be directly positioned over the operative site. A sterile C-arm drape is commercially available, which allows the surgeon to adjust the C-arm's position during the procedure.

TABLE 21-4 **Diagnostic Terms and Procedures**

Term	*Description*
Range of motion (ROM)	Degree to which a joint can be moved in any range, including abduction, flexion, extension, dorsiflexion
	Note: Range is measured in degrees. For example, limited joint movement may be 55°; full-range movement, 360°.
Lachman and Drawer	Tests ligament stability of the knee
Sulcus test	Tests ligament stability of the shoulder
Laboratory Tests	
Analysis of synovial fluid	Synovial fluid is aspirated (withdrawn) and then examined. This test is used to distinguish between osteoarthritis, rheumatoid arthritis, and gout. In rheumatoid arthritis, rheumatoid factors are present in the synovial fluid.
Antinuclear antibody (ANA)	ANAs are antibodies the body produces against its own nuclear material; their presence indicates autoimmune diseases such as systemic lupus erythematosus.

TABLE 21-4 **(continued)**

Term	*Description*
Bence Jones protein	Bence Jones protein is produced by malignant plasma cells and secreted by the bone marrow in multiple myeloma. Initially, this protein is catabolized by the kidneys; however, as the disease progresses, the protein is produced in such large amounts that the kidneys are unable to cope. The excess spills over into the urine, where it can be detected by laboratory examination.
Cultures	Cultures are used to isolate and identify microorganisms causing disease. These tests are used in diagnosing infectious diseases such as osteomyelitis and septic arthritis.
Erythrocyte sedimentation rate (ESR)	This test measures the rate at which RBCs fall or settle to the bottom of a test tube. RBCs fall faster during inflammations, elevating the ESR above its normal value. This test, in conjunction with other tests, helps diagnose inflammatory conditions such as ankylosing spondylitis and rheumatoid arthritis.
Human leukocyte antigen (HLA) B27	HLAs are proteins found on WBCs. The occurrence of HLA-B27 is seen in ankylosing spondylitis.
Latex fixation tests (agglutination tests)	This test is used to diagnose rheumatoid arthritis because it detects rheumatoid factors.
Rheumatoid factors (RFs)	This test measures the quantity of RF in the blood. Rheumatoid factors are proteins present in the blood and synovial fluid of patients with rheumatoid arthritis.
Serum alkaline phosphatase (SAP)	Alkaline phosphatase is important in the building of new bone. However, increased levels indicate bone disease such as multiple myeloma, osteomalacia, osteogenic sarcoma, and rheumatoid disease.
Serum and urinary calcium and phosphorus	Calcium and phosphorus are important constituents of bone. Abnormal values are present in osteoporosis and osteomalacia.
Serum urate	Elevated amounts of serum urate are present in patients with gout.
Urinary uric acid	Elevated amounts of urinary uric acid are found in patients with gout.
Radiology and Diagnostic Imaging	
Arthrography	X-ray of a joint after injection of a contrast medium
Bone scans	A visual image of bone is displayed following injection of technetium (99mTc), a radioactive substance. This substance is picked up by bone undergoing abnormal metabolic activity and shows up as dark areas on the image. Bone scans are useful in detecting tumors and are used to distinguish between osteomyelitis and cellulitis.
Computed tomography (CT)	A CT scan is an X-ray of an organ or body detailing that structure at various depths. Multiple radiographs are taken at multiple angles, and the computer reconstructs these images to represent a cross-section or "slice" of the structure.
Magnetic resonance imaging (MRI); nuclear magnetic resonance (NMR)	This is a noninvasive imaging technique that relies on the body's responses to a strong magnetic field.
Skeletal X-rays	This simple X-ray of bone is often used to initially evaluate patient's complaints. No contrast media or radioactive substances are used.
Clinical Procedures	
Arthrocentesis (aspiration of synovial fluid)	Removal of synovial fluid for analysis in such conditions as gout, rheumatoid arthritis, hematoma, and infection

Table 21-4 (continued)

Term	*Description*
Arthroscopy	Diagnostic and therapeutic procedure used to inspect certain joint cavities. The instrument used is an arthroscope. The scope houses a video camera, and the image is projected onto a television monitor. Arthroscopy is most commonly used on the knee joint. The advantages of this procedure include the use of local anesthetic, a quick recovery time, and a reduced hospital stay. 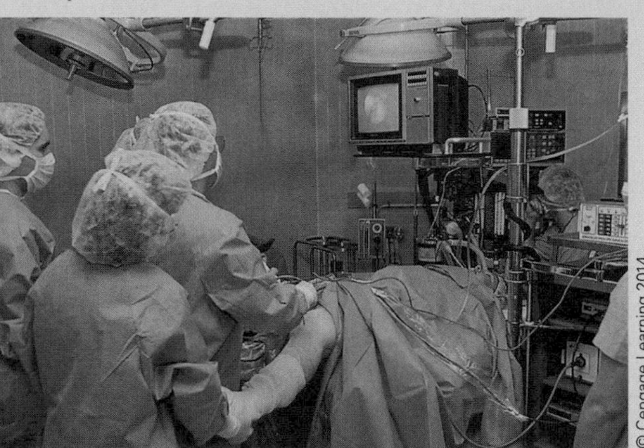 © Cengage Learning 2014 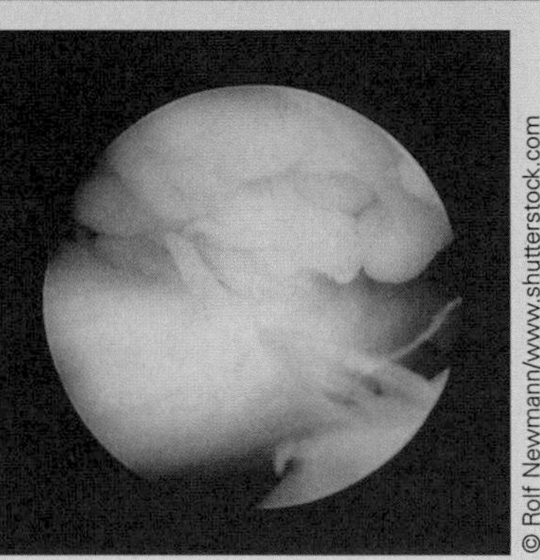 © Rolf Newmann/www.shutterstock.com
Aspiration of bone marrow	Withdrawal of bone marrow for the evaluation of bone marrow disease, such as blood dyscrasias (abnormalities) and multiple myeloma
Biopsy	Removal of a piece of bone that is to be examined by a pathologist for diagnostic purposes
	Note: This test is used to diagnose tumors and chronic infections such as osteomyelitis.

Source: From *Modern Medical Language* by C. E. Collins and J. J. Davies (1996). Clifton Park, NY: Delmar Cengage Learning. Reprinted with permission.

INSTRUMENTATION, ROUTINE EQUIPMENT, AND SUPPLIES

The following sections introduce the student to the basic orthopedic instruments, equipment, and supplies that are used for the majority of surgical procedures. Specialty items will be listed within the description of surgical procedures.

Instrumentation

Students often mention how overwhelmed they are when trying to learn orthopedic instruments due to the large number of instruments that are used and large instrument sets, including all of the specialty instrument sets (e.g., five to seven trays of specialty instruments sets for a total hip arthroplasty). The best advice is to learn the basic orthopedic instrument set that

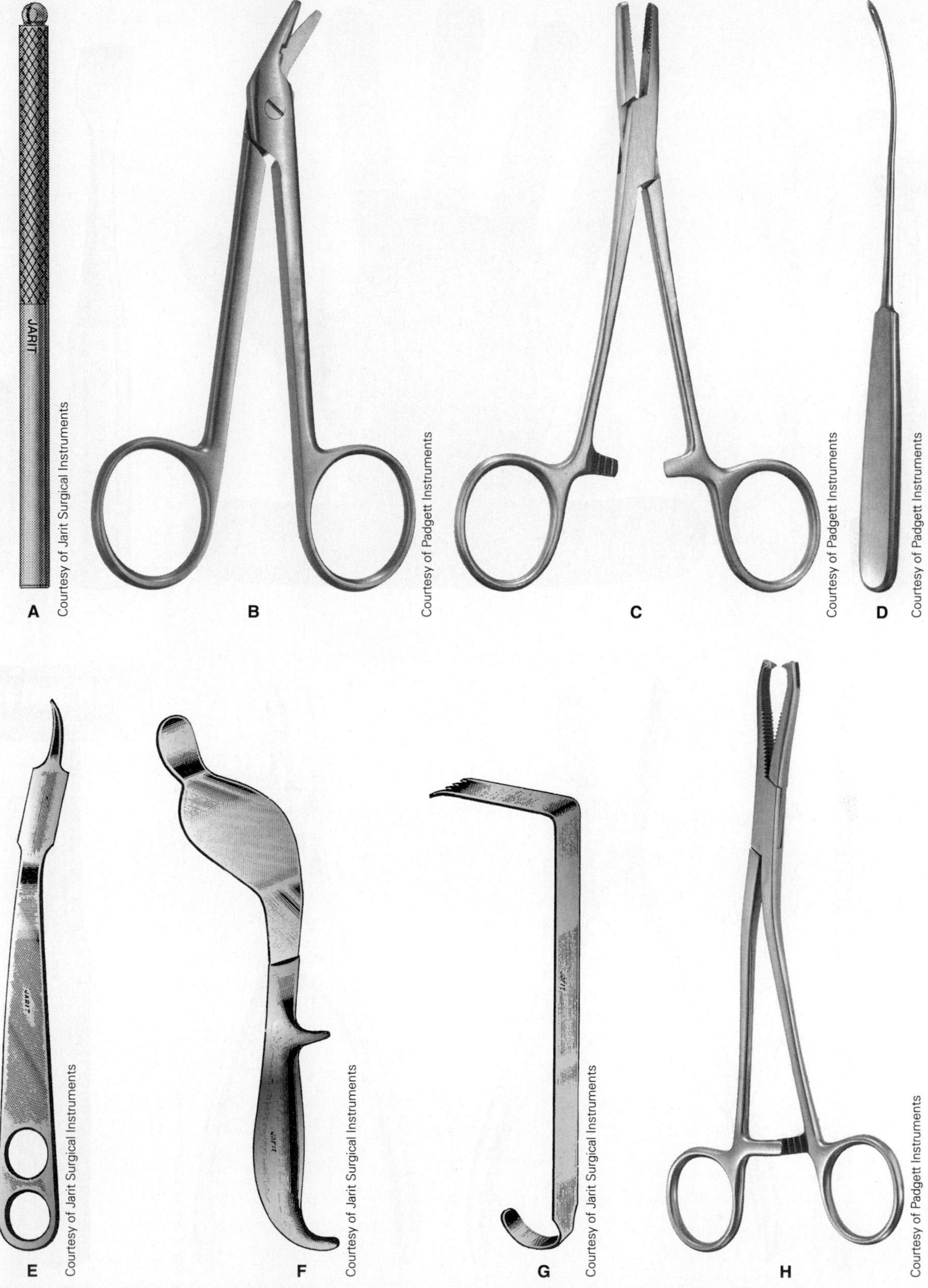

Figure 21-9 Orthopedic instrumentation: (A) Beaver knife handle, (B) wire suture scissors, (C) wire twisting forceps, (D) malleable suture passer, (E) Hohmann retractor, (F) Bennett tibia retractor, (G) Hibbs retractor, (H) Dingman bone-holding clamp

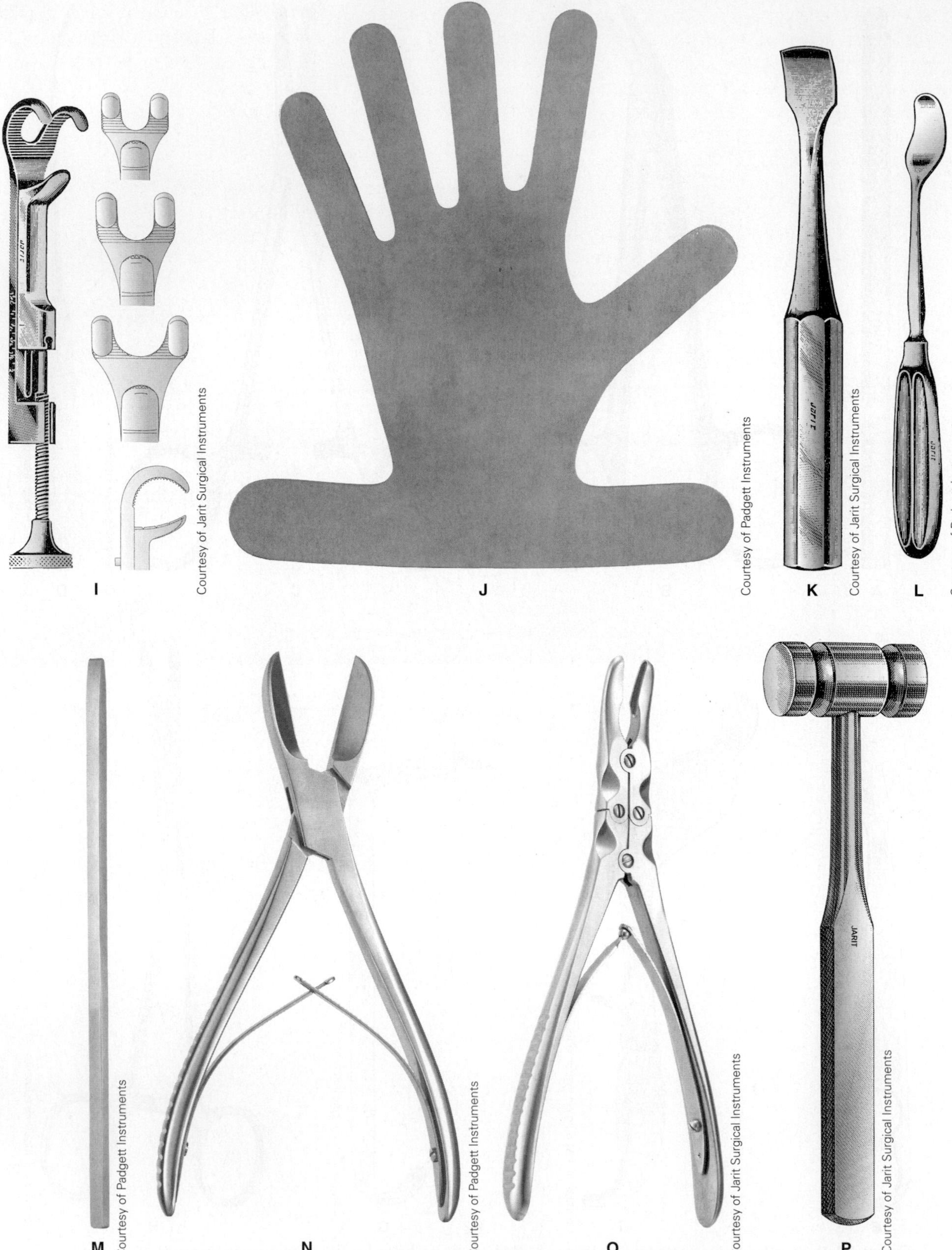

Figure 21-9 Orthopedic instrumentation: (I) Lowman bone-holding clamp, (J) lead hand, (K) Key elevator, (L) Chandler elevator, (M) Lambotte osteotome, (N) Liston's bone-cutting forceps, (O) Ruskin bone rongeur, (P) bone mallet

includes instruments unique to orthopedic surgery and adding to your knowledge as you first scrub advanced procedures. Also remember that during advanced procedures such as a total arthroplasty, not all of the instruments from the multiple trays will be used for the procedure; there are specific instruments used for the procedure on a routine basis and the other instruments are for unique circumstances that you will become familiar with over time.

Orthopedic procedures require a general orthopedic set with soft tissue and basic bone instrumentation. They also require specific sets with instruments for exposure, reduction, and internal fixation of a bone, for replacement of a joint, or for the placement of an intramedullary rod. Procedures for the hand or foot typically require a minor orthopedic, or hand, set. Table 21-5 presents a basic orthopedic instrument set. See Figure 21-9A–P for illustrations of commonly used instruments.

Routine Equipment

Orthopedic surgery is known for its special requirements in terms of equipment and instrumentation. The following is a brief introduction to the complex and continuously progressing world of orthopedic equipment.

Table 21-5 Basic Orthopedic Instrument Set

Qty	Instrument
3	knife handles: #3 × 2, #7
1	Beaver knife handle (Figure 21-9A)
1	Mayo scissor, straight
1	Mayo scissor, curved
2	Metzenbaum scissors, curved: regular and long
1	Bandage scissor
1	Wire cutting/suture scissors (Figure 21-9B)
4	Mosquito clamps, curved
8	Crile clamps, straight × 4; curved × 4
4	Kelly clamps, curved
2	Pean clamps, curved
4	Kocher clamps
1	Wire twisting clamp (Figure 21-9C)
8	Towel clips, blunt × 4, sharp × 4
2	Sponge-holding forceps
4	Adson forceps, smooth × 2; with teeth × 2
2	Tissue forceps with teeth
2	Crile-Wood needle holders
4	Mayo-Hegar needle holders
1	Malleable suture passer (Figure 21-9D)
4	Senn retractors, blunt × 2; sharp × 2
2	U.S. Army retractors
4	Rake retractors, blunt × 2; sharp × 2
2	Weitlaner self-retaining retractors
2	Gelpi self-retaining retractors
4	Hohmann retractors, small to large (Figure 21-9E)
3	Bennett retractors, small to large (Figure 21-9F)
3	Hibbs retractors, small to large (Figure 21-9G)
2	Israel retractors
2	Meyerding retractors
2	Dingman bone-holding clamps (Figure 21-9H)
2	Lowman bone-holding clamps (Figure 21-9I) (slang term for this retractor that surgeons will use is "turkey foot")
1	Lead hand (Figure 21-9J)
2	Rasps, small and large
2	Langenbeck elevators
2	Joker elevators
5–7	Key elevators (Figure 21-9K)
2	Chandler elevators (Figure 21-9L)
2	Freer dissectors
6	Bone curettes, #0 -#5
3–4	Gouges, small to large
5–7	Lambotte osteotomes, small to large (Figure 21-9M)
3	Bone cutters, small to large (Figure 21-9N)
1	Pituitary rongeur
1	Duckbill rongeur
2	Ruskin double-action rongeurs, straight and curved (Figure 21-9O)
1	Stille-Luer rongeur
1	Liston rongeur
1	Nerve hook, blunt
1	Ruler
2	Pliers, needlenose; regular
1	Mallet (Figure 21-9P)

Note: Surgeons will use the term "cobra retractor" interchangeably for the Hohmann and Bennett retractors.

Positioning Devices

The positioning of the orthopedic surgical patient can be quite involved, particularly when the patient has sustained a severe fracture. The selected position should provide adequate exposure of the operative site while maintaining body alignment and possibly alignment of the fractured bones, prevent pressure on the muscles and nerves, and prevent compression of blood vessels.

The choice of position is based on the type of procedure, location of the injury, and the surgeon's preference. Often, the OR table safety strap is not sufficient to stabilize the patient and other positioning devices are required to secure the patient. When positioning the patient, the OR team must know the meaning of common orthopedic directional terms such as **flexion**, extension, lateral, medial, **abduction**, and **adduction**.

Many positioning devices are commercially available to hold an extremity in place during surgery. Some of the positioning devices can be sterilized in order to be utilized intraoperatively at the sterile field. Two popular types of devices are the foot holder utilized during total knee arthroplasty procedures and the shoulder positioner, which allows for distraction of the joint to aid in visualization. The advantage of using sterile positioning devices is the ability to reposition the extremity during the surgical procedure.

The lateral position is frequently used for operations on the hip and shoulder. The vacuum beanbag is often used to stabilize the patient in the lateral position, eliminating the need for roll towels and tape over the hips. The beanbag can be contoured to the body shape of the patient by adjusting the beanbag while the air is suctioned out.

The prone position is used for procedures on the back, posterior portion of the shoulder, and Achilles tendon. The prone position is often facilitated with the use of the Wilson frame, Andrews frame, and OR table. The Andrews frame maintains the patient in a modified knee-chest position. The Wilson and Andrews frames are placed on top of the OR table and the patient is rolled onto the frame after being anesthetized on the stretcher.

A fracture table is commonly used for surgery on a hip fracture and for femoral nailing. The fracture table must be well understood by the personnel using it in order for it to be properly set up. Fracture tables have several moving parts and can cause injury to the patient and OR personnel if not correctly handled. The patient can be placed in the supine or lateral position using a fracture table. The following description is for placing the patient in the supine position on the fracture table.

The pelvis is stabilized against a perineal post that must be well padded, usually with Webril, to prevent damage to the external genital structures and perineal nerve. The foot of the injured extremity is placed in a "boot" that is also well padded. The boot is attached to a traction bar that can rotate the leg or apply traction to it. The foot can be secured in the boot with the use of Velcro straps or by wrapping an Ace or Coban bandage around the foot. The unaffected leg is placed in a boot that is abducted to allow for the C-arm fluoroscope to be positioned over the injured site.

Pneumatic Tourniquets

Pneumatic tourniquets are frequently used for surgical procedures on extremities. The use of the tourniquet provides a bloodless surgical site, which aids visualization. The surgeon will exsanguinate the extremity by elevating it and wrapping, distally to proximally, with an Ace or Esmarch bandage. After exsanguination is accomplished, the tourniquet is inflated. A popular tourniquet is the double-cuffed pneumatic tourniquet. If one cuff fails to inflate, the second cuff provides the needed pressure. In addition, the cuffs can be inflated alternately to reduce constant pressure on one site of the extremity. To avoid a pressure-induced injury to the nerves and blood vessels, continuous tourniquet pressure should not be applied for more than 1 hour on an upper extremity or for more than 1½ hours on the thigh. After 1 hour of pressure, the surgeon should be notified, and again every 15 minutes thereafter. During a lengthy procedure the surgeon may request the tourniquet to be temporarily deflated and then reinflated.

Traction

Traction alignment can be used preoperatively, intraoperatively, and postoperatively. Traction is used to immobilize a joint, reduce a fracture, and align a body part. The three types of traction are manual, skin, and skeletal. Skeletal traction is frequently applied in the OR.

Application of skeletal traction is a sterile procedure. The sterile instruments used for the insertion of skeletal traction include knife handle with #15 knife blade, hand or power drill, Steinmann pins, traction bow, and pin cutter. Traction frames are placed on the patient's postoperative bed and weights are used to apply the traction.

Lasers

The use of lasers in orthopedic surgery has been slowly increasing. With the development of new techniques and improved instrumentation, the laser may become even more attractive in the future.

The CO_2 and contact Nd:YAG lasers have seen use during knee arthroscopy. The same two lasers have been successfully used on the soft tissues during a total joint arthroplasty and lumbar laminectomy. CO_2 is used to aid in the removal of methyl methacrylate (MMA) during a revision arthroplasty. The laser changes the consistency of the MMA, allowing for its easy removal.

Air Flow

The prevention of infection is critical during orthopedic procedures, especially those involving open bone from a fracture or during a total joint arthroplasty. The invasion of the interior of bone by microorganisms can have devastating effects for the patient. Body exhaust suits are frequently worn by the members of the sterile surgical team during repair of severe fractures and total joint replacement. Laminar air-flow systems provide highly filtered air, one-direction flow of air, and continuous air exchanges that reduce the microbial count.

Continuous Passive Range-of-Motion Machines

Surgeons frequently order the use of a continuous passive range-of-motion machine (CPM) for the patient after major knee, elbow, shoulder, and femoral surgical procedures. The CPM provides the following advantages:

1. Aids in decreasing pain and swelling at the operative site
2. Reduces joint stiffness resulting from the patient being bedridden
3. Inhibits the formation of adhesions
4. Provides early mobility
5. Decreases the effects of immobilization, such as muscle wasting

Transcutaneous Electric Nerve Stimulation

The transcutaneous electric nerve stimulation (TENS) unit can be used to suppress postoperative pain by stimulating large sensory nerve fibers. It is a portable, battery-operated unit with electrodes that are placed on the skin near the source of the pain. Because the overstimulation of the large-diameter sensory neurons blocks the perception of pain sensations carried by unmyelinated fibers, TENS is effective after total joint replacements and repair of severe fractures.

Electrical Stimulation of Bone

Osteogenesis is influenced by artificially applied electrical stimulation. Due to the low level of current generated by the device, electrical stimulation can be used in the presence of implants, both internal and external. The types of stimulators available include implantable, percutaneous, and external. The disadvantage of using electrical stimulation is that it requires immobilization of the extremity for a long period of time, which can slow the rehabilitation.

The electrical stimulator is used in the treatment of nonunion or delayed union of bone fractures to speed the healing process. Infected nonunions that have undergone debridement also benefit from electrical stimulation that inhibits bacterial growth.

Saws, Drills, and Reamers

Instruments powered by air, nitrogen, or electricity have virtually eliminated the need for hand-operated saws and drills. The use of power instruments reduces operative time and improves both surgical technique and postoperative results. The manufacturer's instructions must be followed for cleaning, sterilizing, and lubricating power instruments.

The surgical technologist must be familiar with the assembly of the power instruments, including safety factors. The majority of power instruments include a safety device that prevents the inadvertent activation of the instrument. Power instruments can be heavy and should not be placed on the patient when not in use.

Two directional terms must be understood in relation to the use of power saws. An oscillating saw is one in which the saw blade moves from side to side, or oscillates. In a reciprocating saw, the saw blade moves back and forth, or reciprocates. Various bone cuts can be achieved using the two types of motion. The operative procedure or particular step in the procedure will dictate which will be needed.

Arthroscopic Equipment

Arthroscopic surgery is frequently performed for diagnostic purposes, for repair of tissues within a joint, and as an adjunct to surgical procedures such as anterior cruciate ligament repair. Arthroscopy is usually performed on the shoulder, elbow, wrist, knee and ankle joints. To perform the arthroscopy the surgeon requires well-functioning equipment that allows clear visualization of the interior of the joint.

The required equipment includes:

1. Video monitor
2. Light source box
3. Arthroscopy pump and tubing for fluids
4. Powered shaving system
5. Camera system
6. Video recording system
7. Photograph system

Other Routine Equipment

- ESU
- Tourniquet machine
- Nitrogen tank for power instruments
- Suction device

Routine Supplies

The field of orthopedics requires a large number of supplies. Casting materials were discussed earlier. Other commonly used supplies are discussed in this section.

Implants

Implants are a routine part of many orthopedic surgical procedures. Implants include screws, plates, wires, pins, intramedullary nails and rods, and total joint components. An adequate inventory of implants is required in order to meet the needs of surgery. The inventory can be based on surgeon's preference, number of procedures performed per year requiring the use of implants, and cost.

The U.S. Food and Drug Administration requires proper documentation and tracking of implants. The majority of implants, particularly total joint implants, nails, and rods, include a manufacturer's label with the required information that can be attached to the patient's operative record and filed in the patient's permanent record. The surgical technologist assists the circulator by supplying the information if a label is not available. The information should include:

1. Number of implants used
2. Type of implant(s)
3. Size of implant(s)
4. Manufacturer's serial number(s)

TABLE 21-6 Suture Used in Orthopedic Surgery

Suture Material	*Description*	*Use*
FiberWire™	Polyethylene-based, braided suture material promoted as providing increased strength to provide the potential for stronger repairs	Tendon and meniscal repairs
Surgical steel	Most inert and strongest of all suture material; lacks elasticity	Tendons; bone to bone, such as sternum closure
Polyester (Ethibond)	Braided suture that is superior to any other braided suture in decreasing drag through tissue	Tendon to bone
Polypropylene (Prolene)	Monofilament strand almost as inert as stainless steel; acceptable substitute for steel, but easier to handle	Tendon to bone
Nylon (Nurolon)	Multifilament with minimal tissue reaction	Tendon to bone
Chromic	Moderate tissue reaction; chemically treated to slow absorption	Periosteum
Polyglactin (Vicryl)	Coated multifilament; slow absorption	Periosteum

Various alloys are used to manufacture implants. The most frequently used alloys include titanium, stainless steel, and cobalt-chromium. It is very important that implants of the same alloy are used when surgery is performed. If implants composed of different alloys are placed in the patient, they will corrode, causing a breakdown of the implant. This will delay healing and may possibly cause an infection.

Implants should never be reused. Scratches that can occur on the surface of an implant can cause complications if the implant is reused. These complications may include corrosion of the implant, irritation, and infection of the bone due to the imperfection's "digging" into the bone. If an implant, particularly a total joint implant, is dropped, it should not be used because it may have become marred or scratched.

Suture

Orthopedic surgeons use a wide range of sutures (Table 21-6). Ligaments and tendons are made of tough collagen tissue that has a poor vascular supply and, compared to vascular tissues, they heal more slowly. Generally, nonabsorbable suture is used to repair ligaments, tendons, muscles, and bone. Absorbable suture is preferred to close the periosteum.

Polymethyl Methacrylate

Polymethyl methacrylate (PMMA), also referred to as bone cement, is routinely used during total joint arthroplasty. Bone cement stabilizes and keeps the implants in the correct anatomical position. The cement fills the cavity and spaces of the bone to form a bond between the implant and bone. The surgical technologist is responsible for mixing the sterile powder and liquid to create the cement. The majority of ORs have incorporated the use of a closed mixing system that is attached to suction to exhaust the fumes created during the process of mixing the cement. The fumes are irritating to the mucous membranes and possibly toxic to the liver.

Other Routine Supplies

- Ortho back table pack
- Arthroscopic back table pack (specific for arthroscopic procedures)
- Drapes according to surgical procedure, may include
  - Three-quarter sheets
  - Hip drape
  - Extremity drape
  - Split sheet drape
  - Arthroscopic drape
  - Impervious stockinette
- Knife blades: #10 × 3; #15 × 2
- Gloves
- Basin set
- Marking pen
- Dressing materials, may include:
  - ABD
  - Ace bandage
  - Webril or Kerlix
  - 4 × 4 nonradiopaque sponges

ORTHOPEDIC SURGICAL PROCEDURES

There are many orthopedic procedures and most have several variations. The procedures in this chapter illustrate common types of procedures with their unique characteristics and techniques. The procedures are presented in the following order: shoulder, radius, hip; femur, knee, ankle, and foot.

Shoulder Procedures

PROCEDURE 21-1 Shoulder Arthroscopy

Surgical Anatomy and Pathology

- The clavicle, referred to as the collarbone, is a long, slender, doubly curved bone that acts as a brace for the scapula and aids in keeping the shoulder in place.
  - It articulates medially with the manubrium and laterally with the acromion process of the scapula.
  - It is attached to the underlying coracoid process of the scapula by the coracoclavicular ligaments.
- The scapula or shoulder blade is a broad, flat, triangle-shaped bone located on either side of the upper back forming the posterior portion of the shoulder girdle.
  - The posterior surface of each scapula is divided into unequal portions by a spine. This spine, or ridge of bone, leads to the acromion process and the coracoid process.
  - The acromion process articulates with the clavicle and provides attachments for muscles of the arm and chest.
  - Between the processes on the lateral side of the scapula is a fossa called the glenoid cavity that serves as the socket for the head of the humerus. This forms the ball-and-socket **shoulder joint**.
- The pectoral or shoulder girdle consists of the glenohumeral, sternoclavicular, and acromioclavicular (AC) joints.
  - Of the three joints, the glenohumeral has the widest ROM.
  - The **AC joint**, located at the top of the shoulder, is an articulation between the lateral end of the clavicle and the flattened, small process located on the border of the acromion (Figure 21-10).
  - Surrounding the shoulder joint are four muscles collectively referred to as the rotator cuff. The four muscles are the infraspinatus, teres minor, subscapularis, and supraspinatus. The tendons of the four muscles insert onto the

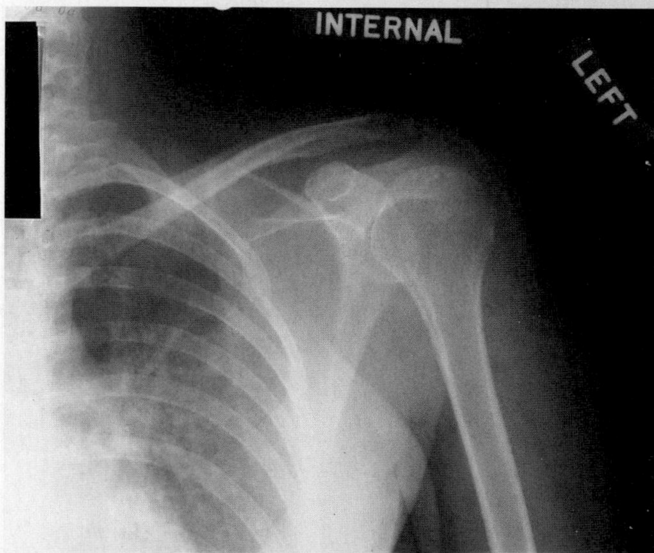

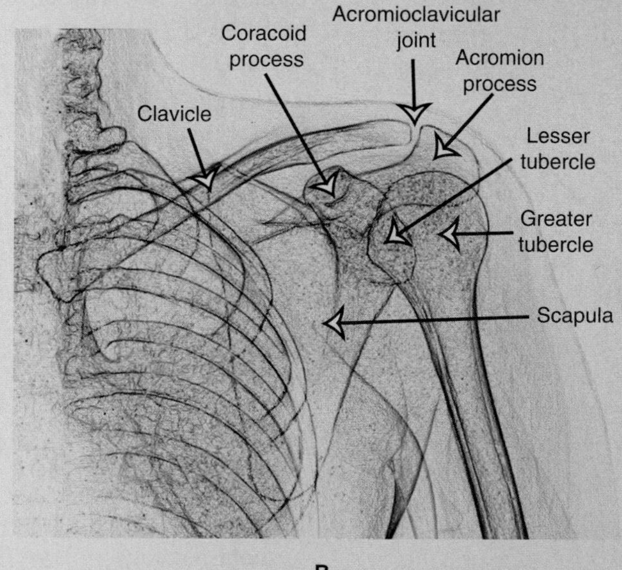

Figure 21-10 Shoulder: (A) X-ray, (B) schematic

(*continues*)

PROCEDURE 21-1 (continued)

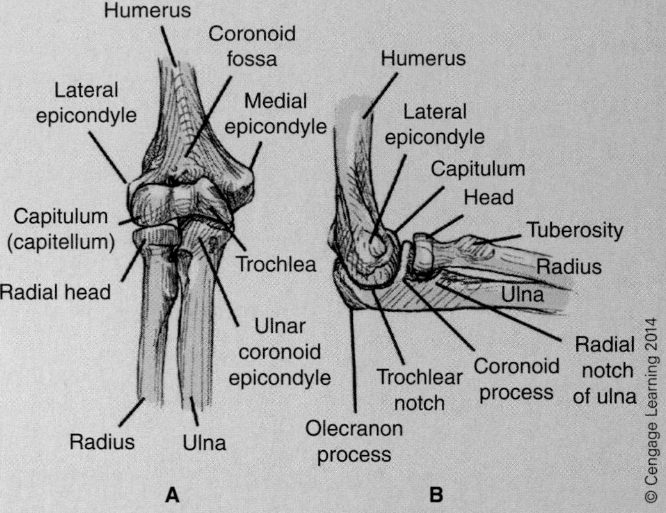

Figure 21-11 Elbow: (A) Anterior, (B) lateral

capsule of the humeral head, allowing the muscles to provide a variety of movements of the shoulder joint. The main function of the rotator cuff is to provide stability and strength to the shoulder joint.

- The humerus is the longest and largest bone of the upper extremity. It extends from the scapula to the elbow (Figure 21-11).
  - Its upper end is the smooth and rounded ball that fits into the glenoid fossa of the scapula.
  - Just below the head of the humerus are two processes called the greater and lesser tuberosities. The greater tubercle is located on the lateral side of the humeral head. The supraspinatus, infraspinatus, and teres minor tendons insert on the greater tubercle. The lesser tubercle is located on the anterior side and serves as the site of insertion of the subscapular tendon.
  - Lying in a deep groove between the tuberosities called the bicipital groove is the tendon of the biceps muscle.
  - Just below the tubercles is a region called the surgical neck, so named because it is a common site for fractures.
  - A narrow circumferential depression along the lower margin of the articular surface of the humerus separating the head from the tubercles is called the anatomical neck.
  - Near the middle of the humeral shaft is the deltoid tuberosity. It provides an attachment for the deltoid muscle that raises the arm horizontally and laterally.
  - At the distal end of the humerus there are two condyles. The lateral condyle is called the capitulum; it articulates with the head of the radius. The articular surface of the medial condyle, called the trochlea, articulates with the ulna.
- Shoulder arthroscopy is highly beneficial as a diagnostic tool for evaluating patients with chronic shoulder problems and for repairing some types of defects.
  - Procedures that can be performed include the removal of loose bodies, bursectomy, rotator cuff repairs, labral tear repair and repair of impingement syndrome. The following describes an arthroscopy for diagnostic reasons.

PROCEDURE 21-1 (continued)

Preoperative Diagnostic Tests and Procedures	• See Table 21-4.
Equipment, Instruments, and Supplies Unique to Procedure	• See previous list of arthroscopic equipment. • Arthroscopy instrument set *Note:* Instruments and equipment that are used for a shoulder arthroscopy. Disposable A-scope sheaths and trocars may be used according to surgeon's preference. • Arthroscopic ESU • Nitrogen tank for arthroscopic powered shaver • 4-mm, 30° arthroscope • 70° arthroscope (have available) • 3000-mL bags of lactated Ringer's solution • Arthroscopic back table pack • Marking pen • #11 knife blade • 18-gauge spinal needle • 20-mL LuerLok syringe • Distraction supplies and weights for patients in lateral position

Preoperative Preparation	• Position: Lateral or semi-Fowler's, surgeon's preference. If the patient is placed in lateral position, a vaccum beanbag is used to maintain the position. The operative arm is placed in suspension with 5–15 pounds of weight placed on the pulley system to achieve distraction of the glenohumeral joint. Once the procedure begins, the surgeon may ask for additional weight to be added.
	• Anesthesia: General or regional; usually general anesthesia is used for the patient in the lateral position; general or regional when semi-Fowler's position is used.
	• Skin prep: Base of neck, shoulder, scapula, chest to midline, and circumference of the arm up to the level of the elbow
	• Draping: Draping can widely vary according to the surgeon's preference. Split sheets may be used with three-quarter sheets or a shoulder arthroscopy drape. The draping procedure for a patient in the lateral position may include the following:
	  • Four towels to widely square off the shoulder joint; towel clamps are used to keep the towels in place.
	  • Plastic adhesive incise drape
	  • Split sheet × 2: One up and one down
	  • Three-quarter sheet × 2: One above to isolate patient's head and upper torso; second to cover lower torso
	  • Impervious stockinette, Coban or Ace bandage for arm; stockinette is applied prior to placing the arm in traction.

Practical Considerations	• Prior to skin prep, the surgeon will perform an examination under anesthesia (EUA). • Radiographs should be in the OR. • Test arthroscopic equipment prior to patient entering the OR. • To help in controlling bleeding, the surgeon may request 1 mL of epinephrine added to each 3000-mL bag of lactated Ringer's solution; the surgeon will confirm with the anesthesia provider if this can be done. Arthroscopic ESU will also be used to control bleeding. • The surgical technologist may be responsible for manipulating the arm to rotate the shoulder to allow the surgeon to better visualize specific anatomical structures. The surgical technologist should know the directional terms and how to manipulate the arm and shoulder in the correct directions.

(continues)

PROCEDURE 21-1 (continued)

Surgical Procedure

1. Using the marking pen, the surgeon marks the incisions/portal sites. The surgeon will begin by establishing the posterior portal, which is the primary entry portal for visualization of the shoulder joint and used to visualize the sites for establishing the other portals. The surgeon positions his or her index finger at the point of the coracoid process and inserts an 18-gauge spinal needle just lateral to the process. The surgical technologist hands the surgeon a 20-mL Luer-Lok syringe filled with normal saline for injection through the spinal needle into the shoulder joint to distend the joint and facilitate placement of the trocar and arthroscope. If epinephrine has not been injected into the bags of lactated Ringer's solution, the surgeon may inject the shoulder joint with up to 5 mL of Marcaine with epinephrine to aid in controlling bleeding.

2. The spinal needle is removed and the surgeon uses a #11 knife blade to make the stab incision at the point of the spinal needle insertion. The sharp trocar with sleeve is inserted through the joint capsule. The sharp trocar is removed and replaced with the blunt trocar, which is used to enter the shoulder capsule.

3. The blunt trocar is removed and the arthroscope is placed. The camera and light source are attached to the arthroscope as are the inflow and outflow tubing to facilitate the distention of the joint.

   Procedural Consideration: The surgical technologist must be familiar with the arthroscopic equipment in order to assist the surgeon with placement of the camera and hooking up the light source cord and tubings.

4. The anterior portal is now established in the same manner. The surgeon uses the posteriorly placed arthroscope to visualize and assist in the placement of the anterior portal.

   Procedural Consideration: Other portals will be established as the procedure progresses to allow the surgeon to view specific anatomical structures.

5. Upon entering the shoulder joint, the surgeon first examines the biceps tendon, which is used as a landmark throughout the procedure. The initial examination continues with the superior portion of the shoulder joint, biceps tendon, articular cartilages of the glenoid, and humeral head.

   Procedural Consideration: The surgeon will frequently use the arthroscopic probe (also called a switching stick) placed through the anterior port to examine the stability of structures as well as to determine if an injury, such as a tear, has occurred to the structure. When not being used, the surgical technologist should keep hold of the probe as much as possible rather than placing on the back table in order to quickly hand to the surgeon. The surgical technologist may be requested by the surgeon to slowly internally and externally rotate the shoulder to view the articular cartilages; the surgical technologist must manipulate the arm slowly to prevent damage to the shoulder joint structures and allow the surgeon to follow along with the arthroscope.

6. The surgeon advances the arthroscope anteriorly to view the superior and inferior surfaces of the biceps tendon to examine for injury at its attachment to the shoulder joint.

   Procedural Consideration: The biceps tendon at its attachment can be injured from a fall on the shoulder joint or repeated hard throwing such as by a baseball pitcher.

PROCEDURE 21-1 (continued)

7. The surgeon now moves the arthroscope to the inferior area of the shoulder joint to view the inferior and middle glenohumeral ligaments, posterior humeral articular surface, and back to the biceps tendon to complete the circular examination.

8. The superior and inferior surfaces of the biceps tendon are now evaluated. The surgeon will place the probe through the anterior portal to examine for labral or SLAP (superior labrum anterior and posterior) tears or synovitis.

9. The rotator cuff is now thoroughly examined. The surgeon initially withdraws the scope to view the posterior portion of the cuff.

   Procedural Consideration: The surgical technologist may be requested by the surgeon to gently manipulate the arm from the extended, externally rotated position to an internally rotated, slightly flexed position.

10. The surgeon moves the scope to the anterior portal and places the probe through the posterior probe. The posterior of the rotator cuff is viewed and evaluated for tears, synovitis, fraying from instability, or inflammation.

11. The surgeon moves the scope back to the posterior portal to examine the subacromial bursa for impingement syndrome and inflammation. The surgeon may use the shaver to perform a bursectomy.

    Procedural Consideration: The surgical technologist may be requested by the surgeon to internally and externally rotate the shoulder.

12. One of the last structures to be examined is the AC joint through the anterior and posterior portals. If an AC joint bone spur is discovered, arthroscopic ESU and the shaver will be used to remove the spur.

13. At the conclusion of the procedure, the surgeon allows plenty of fluid to flow through the joint for irrigation purposes and removal of any loose bodies. Additional Marcaine may be injected into the joint to minimize postoperative pain. Skin closure tapes and 4 × 4 dressing sponges are placed on the stab wounds and the arm is placed in a sling.

Postoperative Considerations

Immediate Postoperative Care

- Patient is transported to the PACU.
- Patient is observed for hemorrhage.

Prognosis

- No complications: Patient usually discharged the same day of surgery; length of time taken to return to full normal activities depends on if additional procedures were performed and if the patient has to undergo physical therapy; however, anticipation is that the patient will have a full recovery.
- Complications: Postoperative SSI; hemorrhage; return of pathology such as impingement.

Wound Classification

- Wound Class I: Clean

PROCEDURE 21-2 Bankart Procedure, Open

Surgical Anatomy and Pathology	• The shoulder joint has a cuff of cartilage called the labrum that lines the cup of the joint that the ball of the humerus rests within. The labrum provides additional cushion to the joint as well as additional stability. • A Bankart lesion is an avulsion (tear) injury of the anterior capsule and labrum of the glenoid rim; it is usually caused by subluxation or luxation of the joint. The tear affects that portion of the labrum called the inferior glenohumeral ligament; when the ligament is torn is called a Bankart lesion. • The lesion can cause the patient to have recurrent shoulder joint dislocations, chronic soreness and pain, and catching sensations.
Preoperative Diagnostic Tests and Procedures	• See Table 21-4.
Equipment, Instruments, and Supplies Unique to Procedure	• Bankart instruments • Shoulder immobilizer • Power drill • 3.2-mm drill bit • #15 knife blades × 3–4 • Nitrogen tank
Preoperative Preparation	• Position: Supine; an arm board is placed on the operative side for the surgeon to lay the arm as well as an arm board for the nonoperative arm. • Anesthesia: General • Skin prep: Begin at incision site on anterior of the shoulder joint; extend from lower border of mandible to the level of the umbilicus; medially using the middle of the chin and sternum as the border; laterally as far as possible; entire axillary region and arm • Draping: Arm is draped free in order to manipulate during the surgical procedure; impervious stockinette is rolled over arm up to axillary region and held in place with Coban; three-quarter sheet is tucked under posterior of patient's shoulder and used to cover arm board; split sheet × 2—one up and one down; three-quarters sheets to cover upper and lower torso or extremity drape (Figure 21-12).
Practical Considerations	• There are several types of procedures for the repair of recurrent anterior dislocation of the shoulder joint, including Putti-Platt and Bristow, as well as variations of the Bankart. However, the instrumentation, equipment, and supplies are similar for all the procedures; • Radiographs should be in the OR. • Confirm with the surgeon if postoperative X-rays will be take in the OR or PACU. • Have C-arm ready for use.
Surgical Procedure	1. Using a #10 knife blade, the surgeon makes the incision from the coracoid process to the axillary fold.
	2. The pectoralis major and deltoid muscles are retracted laterally away from each other, making sure to include the cephalic vein with the deltoid muscle in order to prevent injury to the vein.
	3. The coracobrachialis muscle and conjoined tendon are retracted superiorly. **Procedural Consideration:** The second scrub surgical technologist must gently retract the conjoined tendon to avoid injury to the musculocutaneous nerve.

PROCEDURE 21-2 (continued)

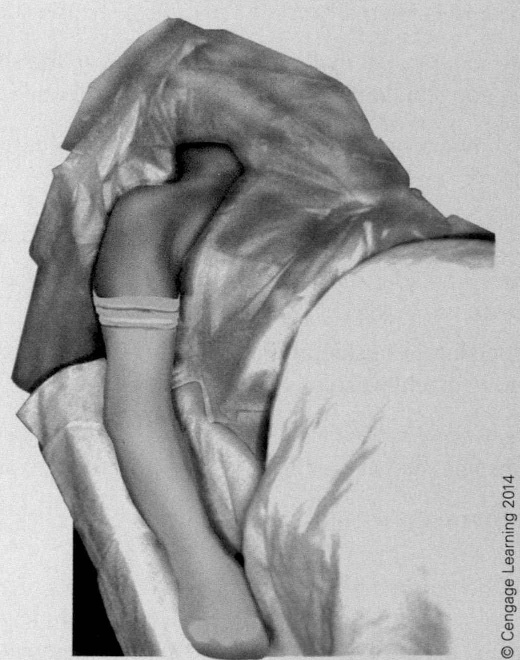

Figure 21-12 Position and draping

4. The coracoid is now osteotomized from the scapula. Beginning at the tip of the coracoid, a hole is dilled using the 3.2-mm drill bit. Using a ¼-in. osteotome, the surgeon divides the coracoid and it is retracted medially and inferiorly.

   Procedural Consideration: The drill hole makes it easier for the surgeon to divide the coracoid from the scapula.

5. Using the #15 knife blade and Metzenbaum scissors, the subscapularis muscle and tendon are dissected off the anterior capsule of the shoulder. The inferior portion of the muscle and tendon is left in place to prevent injury to the axillary nerve.

6. The surgeon places the shoulder in external rotation before incising the capsule. Using the #15 knife blade, the surgeon makes a vertical incision in the capsule lateral to the rim of the glenoid.

7. The Bankart humeral head retractor is placed to retract the humeral head laterally; the Bankart single-spiked retractor is placed along the anterior glenoid neck to retract the medial capsule and glenoid labrum.

8. The capsule is now reattached to the glenoid rim:
   A. The glenoid rim is curetted to promote the capsule attaching to the bone and healing.
   B. Using the drill, three holes are made on the anterior of the glenoid rim. The holes are completed with a Bankart curved spike.
   C. A #1 nonabsorbable suture is placed through the holes to connect the lateral section of the capsule directly to the glenoid rim. The sutures are not yet tied.

9. The medial flap/margin of the capsule that laps over the lateral part is sutured into place with #1 nonabsorbable suture to reinforce the capsular repair.

(continues)

PROCEDURE 21-2 (continued)

10. The arm is internally rotated in order to tie the suture knots to the glenoid rim.
11. The surgeon externally rotates the arm with the shoulder in the neutral position; the surgeon should be able to attain 30° of external rotation.
12. Any other openings in the anterior capsule are sutured with #1 nonabsorbable suture.
13. The subscapularis tendon is sutured back into place.
14. The coracoid is reattached by placing two #1 nonabsorbable sutures through the previously made drill hole in the base and tip of the coracoid process and tied.

    Procedural Consideration: Some surgeons may use a screw to reattach the coracoid and reattach the soft tissue with suture.

14. The wound is closed in layers; the subcutaneous layer is closed with suture and skin closure tapes are placed. The 4 × 4 dressing sponges are placed; the surgeon may use ABD.
15. The arm is placed in a shoulder immobilizer.

Postoperative Considerations

Immediate Postoperative Care

- Patient is transported to the PACU.
- Patient is discharged on day 3 or 4 of hospitalization.

Prognosis

- No complications: Shoulder immobilizer is removed on the second or third postoperative day. Passive exercises begin on the third postoperative day; an arm sling is used for comfort by the patient as needed. At 3 weeks postoperatively, isometric exercises are begun. By 6 months full motion should be achieved. At 3 months resistive exercises such as swimming are started, and by 6 months full function of the shoulder should be regained.
- Complications: Postoperative SSI; hemorrhage; reinjury; stiff joint.

Wound Classification

- Class I: Clean

PROCEDURE 21-3 Bankart Procedure, Arthroscopic with Suture Anchors

Note: Surgical anatomy and pathology, preoperative diagnostic tests and procedures, preoperative preparation, and practical considerations are the same as for shoulder arthroscopy and open Bankart procedure.

Equipment, Instruments, and Supplies Unique to Procedure

- Equipment and instruments are the same as for a shoulder arthroscopy with the addition of absorbable MITEK suture anchors and insertion instrumentation, use of threaded cannulas, full-radius cutter and burr for shaver, drill guide, #1 or 0 PDS and 0 DEXON suture.
- Free needles

Surgical Procedure

1. Surgeon performs an EUA to confirm the degree of shoulder instability.
2. The posterior, anterosuperior, and anteroinferior portals are established in the same manner as for a shoulder arthroscopy using the 18-gauge spinal needle, #11 knife blade, and placement of the cannulas with the use of trocars.

   Procedural Consideration: Blunt, not sharp, trocars are used. Threaded cannulas should be used to prevent their dislodgement during the surgical procedure.

PROCEDURE 21-3 (continued)

3. The outflow cannula is placed in the posterosuperior portal and the arthroscope is placed in the anterosuperior port in order to view the glenohumeral ligament. The anteroinferior portal is the port through which the majority of the repair is performed.

4. The anterior glenoid rim and scapular neck are prepared as follows:
   A. The surgeon places the shaver with abrader tip through the anteroinferior portal and abrades the anterior glenoid rim to begin creating a trough.
   B. Next the surgeon switches to a full-radius cutter on the shaver to smooth out the trough. Suction is attached to the shaver.
   C. The surgeon uses a periosteal evlevator to mobilize the inferior glenohumeral ligament along the glenoid rim and scapular neck. This step is performed because often the ligament has healed.
   D. The surgeon now uses a burr on the shaver to remove the cortical tissue from the glenoid rim and scapular neck. The cortical tissue is removed down to the bone.

   Procedural Consideration: The surgical technologist must be familiar with the equipment and be able to quickly change out tips on the shaver. The circulator should be told to lower the power on the suction device in order to help the surgeon in preventing sucking into the full-radius cutter viable tissue from the inferior glenohumeral ligament that may be needed for the repair.

5. The surgeon is now ready to drill the holes in preparation for the suture and anchors.
   A. The cannula in the anteroinferior portal is removed and replaced with an 8.5-mm threaded cannula; the drill guide, drill bits, and suture hooks are more easily inserted through the 8.5-mm sized cannula.
   B. The surgeon is given the drill guide and power drill with drill bit to be inserted through the cannula. The first hole is drilled inferiorly on the anterior of the glenoid rim, the second hole is placed superoanteriorly, and the third is placed between the two holes.

6. Placement of suture and anchors for repair of the lesion:
   A. A suture hook is placed through the inferior section of the detached glenoid ligament. Using the suture hook, a #1 or 0 PDS suture is placed into the joint; the suture hook is withdrawn, which leaves the suture through the detached ligament.
   B. A suture grasper is used to pull out the inside strand of suture, which creates a loop of suture that is through the cannula, through the ligament, and back out through the cannula.
   C. The surgical technologist hands an anchor and inserter to the surgeon. The surgeon loads the anchor onto the inserter and ties a 0 DEXON tie over the handle of the inserter to prevent losing the anchor within the joint.
   D. The suture anchor is inserted over and slid down the strand of suture that was brought out through the cannula; the anchor is inserted into the first drill hole (inferior drill hole) and the suture is cut.
   E. The inserter and suture are pulled out, which leaves a loop of suture down the cannula, through the detached ligament, into the anchor, and back out through the cannula.

(*continues*)

PROCEDURE 21-3 (continued)

F. The suture loop is tied outside of the cannula. The surgical technologist gives the surgeon the knot pusher to slide the knot down the cannula and tighten the knot to approximate the inferior portion of the inferior glenohumeral ligament.

G. Steps 6A–F are performed two additional times.

7. The wound is thoroughly irrigated. Then 15–20 mL of 0.25 Marcaine with epinephrine is injected into the joint. Arthroscopic cannulas are removed and the incisions closed with 3-0 or 4-0 nylon suture. Then 4 × 4 dressing sponges are applied; the surgeon may want an ABD placed; the patient is placed in a shoulder immobilizer.

Postoperative Considerations

Immediate Postoperative Care

- Patient is transported to the PACU.
- Patient is hospitalized for 3–4 days.
- Dressing is removed after 24 hours.

Prognosis

- No complications: Sutures are removed after 5 days. Patient must wear shoulder immobilizer for 3 weeks. After 3 weeks immobilizer must only be worn at night for 6 weeks. Passive exercises are begun at 3 weeks. At 6 weeks active and resistive full ROM exercises are begun. At 12 weeks the majority of patients have full motion.
- Complications: Postoperative SSI; hemorrhage; impingement syndrome; reinjury.

Wound Classification

- Class I: Clean

PROCEDURE 21-4 Acromioplasty, Open

Pathology

- Candidates for an acromioplasty are afflicted by impingement syndrome, which limits the ROM of the shoulder. Often the patient will have completed a rehabilitation program for up to 6 months to attempt to relieve the symptoms and if no improvement is noted, the patient is a candidate for acromioplasty surgery.
- The cause of the syndrome is the impingement of the rotator cuff and humeral head under the coracoacromial arch during forward flexion of the shoulder joint.

Preoperative Diagnostic Tests and Procedures

- X-rays, CT scan, MRI
- Impingement sign during physical examination: Pain that is produced in the shoulder joint by forceful abduction of the internally rotated arm against the acromion
- Impingement injection test: A temporary relief of pain occurs when 10 mL of lidocaine is injected into the subacromial space.

Equipment, Instruments, and Supplies Unique to Procedure

- Same as for an open Bankart procedure
- Oscillating saw

PROCEDURE 21-4 (continued)

Preoperative Preparation	• Position: semi-Fowler's • Anesthesia: General	• Skin prep: Same as for open Bankart procedure	• Draping: Same as for open Bankart procedure
Practical Considerations	• Same as for Bankart procedure		

Surgical Procedure

1. Using the marking pen, the surgeon marks the incision along the skin lines across the anterior corner of the acromion.
2. The surgeon injects 10 mL of Marcaine with epinephrine into the shoulder joint.
3. The surgeon makes an incision with the #10 knife blade in an anteroposterior direction between the tip of the acromion and the AC joint. The incision is carried down to the fascia and two Gelpi retractors are placed for exposure.
4. The fascia is freed from its attachments to the deltoid, but left in place for closure at the end of the procedure.
5. Surgeons have two options concerning the deltoid muscle:
   A. Dissect through the muscle fibers, or
   B. Detach for later reattachment; the description of this procedure involves detaching the deltoid muscle. The division between the anterior and middle deltoid is identified and split by blunt and sharp dissection with the use of electrosurgery using a needle tip on the Bovie handle. The deltoid is dissected from the anterior acromion. Blunt retractors are placed for exposure.

   Procedural Consideration: The surgeon uses the Bovie needle tip to preserve as thick of a flap of deltoid muscle as possible for later reattachment. If the deltoid is not securely reattached it will diminish the desired results of the acromioplasty due to decreased deltoid function.
6. Using electrocautery, the coracoacromial ligament is resected. The resection exposes the subacromial space.

   Procedural Consideration: Electrocautery is used in order to also cauterize the acromial branch of the coracoacromial artery that is within the ligament.

8. The bursa and adhesions, if present, are dissected from the undersurface of the acromion.
9. Using an oscillating saw or rongeur, the section of acromion that projects anterior to the anterior border of the clavicle is removed. The acromioplasty is completed with the oscillating saw or osteotome.

   Procedural Consideration: Every few seconds the surgical technologist should place a few drops of irrigating fluid into the area being resected to keep the saw blade and bone from overheating. An Hohmann or malleable retractor is used to protect the rotator cuff and humeral head during resection.
10. A rongeur and bone rasp are used to smooth the bone surface and remove any sharp edges.
11. The surgical wound is thoroughly irrigated to remove any debris and check for bleeding.

(*continues*)

PROCEDURE 21-4 (continued)

12. The deltoid muscle is sutured from side-to-side. The rest of the wound is closed in layers. Then 4 × 4 dressing sponges are placed; ABD may be placed and the arm may be placed in a sling.

Postoperative Considerations

Immediate Postoperative Care

- Patient is transported to the PACU.
- Patient can discontinue the use of the sling as soon as he or she is comfortable.

Prognosis

- No complications: Passive exercises are begun the day after surgery. At 3 weeks postoperatively, active and resistive exercises are begun. At 6 weeks the patient should be at full activity.
- Complications: Complication that the surgeon wants to most avoid is loss of anterior deltoid function caused by axillary nerve injury or detachment of the deltoid from the acromion; loss of function produces a poor surgical outcome and the surgeon cannot do much to restore the function. Other complications include postoperative SSI; hematoma; biceps rupture; acromial fracture; and continued pain and joint stiffness due to noncompliance or poor compliance by patient during rehabilitation.

Wound Classification

- Class I: Clean

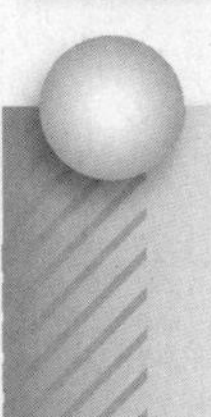

PEARL OF WISDOM

Small amounts of irrigation fluid are dropped onto the bits of power drives that are used to create the trough. The water prevents overheating and damage to the bone. Be sure all team members are wearing appropriate PPE. Fluid will splatter.

PROCEDURE 21-5 Acromioplasty, Arthroscopic

Notes: Surgical anatomy, pathology, and preoperative diagnostic tests and procedures are the same as for an open acromioplasty. Equipment, instruments, supplies, preoperative preparation, and practical considerations are the same as for arthroscopic Bankart repair.

Surgical Procedure—Described with Patient in Lateral Position

1. The surgeon performs an EUA to evaluate the shoulder joint for instability and/or stiffness before the skin prep is performed.
2. Using the marking pen, the surgeon marks the bony landmarks—acromion, acromioclavicular joint, distal clavicle, and coracoid process.
3. Using a 6.0- or 6.2-mm cannula with blunt trocar, the posterior portal is established for the insertion of the arthroscope. The surgeon moves the blunt trocar back and forth medially and laterally to break up adhesions in the subacromial space. The arthroscope with inflow tubing connected is inserted through the posterior portal.

Procedure 21-5 (continued)

4. The arthroscope is used to assist in establishing the lateral (also called the mid-lateral) portal, which will be used for instrumentation. An 18-gauge spinal needle is inserted through the lateral area 3 cm distal to the acromion and along a line with the posterior of the AC joint. The cannula and blunt trocar are inserted, and the blunt trocar is removed.
5. The shaver with a full-radius resector is inserted through the lateral portal and a bursectomy is performed in order to view the rotator cuff and undersurface of the AC joint.
6. The surgeon places a spinal needle through the AC joint and another at the anterolateral aspect of the acromion to help identify these anatomical landmarks throughout the procedure.
7. Using a surgical thermal probe, the surgeon dissects the periosteum and acromial undersurface to release the coracoacromial ligament.

   Practical Consideration: Throughout the procedure, hemostasis is maintained by electrocautery and injection of 1 mL of epinephrine in each 3000-L bag of irrigating fluid.
8. A 5.5-mm full-radius resector is placed through the lateral portal and the soft tissues on the undersurface of the acromion are removed.

   Practical Consideration: It should be communicated to the circulating person to keep the suction unit at half power to prevent the shaver from sucking up viable tissue.
9. The full-radius resector is replaced with a 5.5-mm burr and the lateral edge of the acromion is resected. The resection is continued to the AC joint. The surgeon uses even strokes from anterior to posterior resecting a small portion of bone, each time tapering it down. The AC joint is located by the previously placed spinal needle and is resected last due to the vascularity of this area.
10. Once the acromioplasty is completed, the surgeon uses a full-radius resector or arthroscopic rasp to smooth the undersurface of the acromion.
11. Using the thermal probe, the soft tissue on the undersurface of the clavicle is removed.
12. If radiographic studies showed the presence of bony spurs on the undersurface of the clavicle, they are removed with a burr.
13. The surgeon views the acromioplasty to evaluate the cut of the acromion and to confirm the undersurface of the AC joint is smooth.
14. The joint is thoroughly irrigated and arthroscopic equipment removed. The small incisions are closed with nonabsorbable suture; skin closure tapes are placed; 4 × 4 dressing sponges are applied and the arm is placed in a sling.

Postoperative Considerations

Immediate Postoperative Care

- Patient is transported to the PACU.
- Passive exercises are started on the first postoperative day.

Prognosis

- No complications: Sling is removed as soon as the patient is comfortable; ROM and isometric exercises are begun during the first week postoperative; in the second postoperative week resistive exercises are begun; patients usually have full ROM by the third week postoperative.
- Complications: Postoperative SSI; hematoma; loss of anterior deltoid function; continued pain and joint stiffness due to noncompliance or poor compliance by patient during rehabilitation.

Wound Classification

- Class I: Clean

PROCEDURE 21-6 Total Shoulder Arthroplasty

Pathology	• The primary pathology for performing a total shoulder arthroplasty is chronic pain from glenohumeral arthritis with significant loss of ROM and joint function the condition has not been resolved by conservative medical therapy. Complications include narrowing of the joint space, osteophyte formation, and cysts. • Rheumatoid arthritis that causes destruction of the cartilage (labrum) of the joint is another cause. • Shoulder arthroplasty may be performed for arthritis that is secondary to traumatic injuries to the joint such as dislocations and/or fractures of the glenohumeral joint or chronic displaced fractures. • Osteonecrosis of the humeral head is another reason for performing an arthroplasty. Osteonecrosis is usually caused by sickle cell disease, alcoholism, or corticosteroid use and occasionally by systemic lupus erythematosus.
Preoperative Diagnostic Tests and Procedures	• Standard X-rays including anteroposterior, scapular, and axillary lateral. Anteroposterior X-rays are taken with the arm in neutral position as well as externally and internally rotated. The condition of the AC joint is evaluated with the use of X-rays; an arthritic AC joint can compromise the surgical outcome of an arthroplasty and must be first resolved. • CT scan is useful in determining if there will be a need for glenoid bone grafting. • MRI is used to evaluate the rotator cuff as well as rule out other pathologies such as osteonecrosis. • Electromyography is performed for patients who are suspected to have nerve conduction disorder. • Aspiration and nuclear medical studies are performed on patients who have had previous shoulder surgery to rule out an infection.
Equipment, Instruments, and Supplies Unique to Procedure	• Basic orthopedic instrument set • Total shoulder instrumentation and trial prostheses: Specialty instruments and trial prostheses for performing the shoulder arthroplasty. It can be several instrument trays that are shipped to or brought to the health care facility by a sales representative. • Permanent shoulder implants: Also usually either shipped or brought to the health care facility. • Nitrogen tank • Batteries if cordless power drill and saw are used • Power drill and saw • Drill bits: Usually available in a set called the drill bit box • Oscillating and reciprocating saw blades • #10 knife blades × 5 • GelFoam and thrombin (available in the OR) • PMMA kit (purchased commercially) • Self-contained unit for mixing the PMMA • Jackson-Pratt drain • Full-coverage sterile attire (space suits) • Multiple pairs of gloves for each team member

PROCEDURE 21-6 (continued)

Preoperative Preparation	• Position: Semi-Fowler's; patient must be positioned as close to the edge of the OR table as possible to facilitate the surgeon's access to the shoulder region and allow for hyperextending the arm and shoulder joint in order to be able to dislocate the humerus and resurface the glenoid. The torso is flexed 45° and the knees are flexed 30°. • Anesthesia: General; regional is rarely used. • Skin prep: Same as for an open Bankart procedure • Draping: The arm is draped free such as for a Bankart procedure and rested on a padded armboard with the shoulder slightly hanging off the OR table to allow extension, rotation, and some adduction. A folded towel is placed under the scapula for stabilization.
Practical Considerations	• All radiographic studies should be in the OR. • Surgical technologist should confirm the day before surgery that the specialty instrument trays and trial prostheses arrived and are being sterilized. The first thing on the morning of surgery, the surgical technologist should confirm everything has been sterilized. • There are several types of shoulder arthroplasty systems. The surgical technologist must find out prior to the day of surgery the prosthesis and specialty instrumentation that will be used; the surgical technologist must be familiar with the instrumentation and the order in which it is used. The manufacturer can be contacted for procedural information to study and the sales representative can be consulted. • Some surgeons may have the team remove the outer gloves of the double-gloving and replace after draping. Studies have shown that the highest risk for breaks in sterile technique during orthopedic procedures is during draping, due to the complicated draping procedures. • Some surgeons may have the team remove the outer gloves and replace just prior to the permanent implants being opened and implanted. • Confirm on the day of surgery that the blood bank received the blood order and it is ready for use. • Check the nitrogen level in the nitrogen tank or make sure the batteries are charging the day before surgery for the cordless power instruments. The batteries must be sterilized the morning of surgery by immediate-use steam sterilization. • Test the power equipment prior to the patient entering the OR. • Ask surgeon if he or she will want X-rays taken in the OR before transporting the patient to the PACU or the X-rays taken in the PACU. • The day before surgery, make sure the batteries for air flow for the space suits are charging. • Health care facility policy must be followed for recording the prostheses that are implanted.

(*continues*)

PROCEDURE 21-6 (continued)

Surgical Procedure

1. The skin incision is made from the mid-acromion distally and follows the deltopectoral groove. The cephalic vein is identified and gently retracted away from the incision site to avoid injury. The groove is opened and retracted.
2. The long head of the biceps is visualized as the surgical anatomical landmark located between the tuberosities and rotator interval.
3. A Hohmann retractor is placed above the coracoid to provide superior traction. A Charnley retractor is placed in the subpectoral space.
4. The subscapularis is elevated and fully mobilized off the anterior glenoid, and divided approximately 2 cm medial to the bicipital groove.
5. An Hohmann retractor is then placed on the anterior glenoid to provide anterior retraction. The subscapularis is retracted medially along with the lesser tuberosity to expose the joint. An elevator is placed beneath the capsule to protect the axillary nerve from injury. Deep exposure of the shoulder joint is completed when the shoulder can be easily externally rotated without placing torque on the humerus.
6. The humeral head is dislocated from the shoulder socket. A blunt Hohmann retractor is placed behind the humeral head to maintain the dislocation. The arm is extended, adducted, and rotated to maximize the exposure of the humeral head.
7. Peripheral osteophytes are trimmed away from the humeral head using an osteotome and rongeur.
8. The arm is externally rotated 30–40° and, using the reciprocating saw, the humeral head is excised. A humeral cutting guide may be used to fine-tune the cut.
9. The glenoid is inspected and the size of prosthesis is selected.
10. A blunt Hohmann is placed in front of the proximal humerus and behind the posterior glenoid in order to provide full exposure of the glenoid. Using a high-speed power burr and curette, a centralized fossa is created in the glenoid for the prosthesis to fit.
11. The opening into the intramedullary canal of the humerus is now made. The stem diameter and length are determined. The largest stem diameter possible is used.
12. The humeral shaft is elevated upward using a blunt Hohmann. The intramedullary canal is identified with the use of a curette. Next a drill bit is selected that corresponds to the diameter of the canal and the canal is drilled 5–7 in. down. The first power intramedullary reamer is inserted into the canal adjacent to the greater tuberosity. The canal is reamed with subsequent larger sizes of reamers until the opening in the canal corresponds to the diameter of the shaft of the prosthesis.
13. Suture drill holes are placed through the bicipital tuberosity on either side. Two holes are made anteromedially, two holes anteriorly, and two holes anterolaterally in the proximal humerus. A heavy-gauge nonabsorbable suture is passed through the holes.
14. Trial prostheses are inserted into the glenoid and humeral shaft, and trial reduction is performed. Neck length and the stability of the joint are confirmed.

PROCEDURE 21-6 (continued)

15. The trial prostheses are removed. In younger patients, press-fit prostheses are used; in the older patient PMMA will most likely be used. If PMMA is going to be used, as soon as the trial prostheses are removed and the size of the permanent prostheses confirmed, the PMMA should be mixed. While the cement is being mixed the surgeon will thoroughly irrigate the humeral canal, glenoid, and shoulder joint. The surgeon may use a brush that has been slipped onto the outside of the suction tip to clean the humeral canal of any debris.
16. The glenoid prosthesis is placed. The humeral implant is seated with the use of the calcar and mallet. Just before the humeral implant is fully seated, high spots on the humerus may need to be removed with an osteotome or power high-speed burr.
17. The sutures previously placed through the suture holes of the tuberosities are passed through holes in the neck of the prosthesis, thereby reducing the tuberosities beneath the neck, and they are tied.
18. The shoulder is reduced and ROM is confirmed. The rotator cuff subscapularis tendon is sutured. The subscapularis tendon can be sutured to the coracohumeral ligament with a large-gauge suture. The biceps tendon is reattached.
19. The joint is thoroughly irrigated and closed in layers.
20. The drainage tube to the Jackson-Pratt closed drain is inserted between the cuff and deltoid; the tube must be placed in such a manner as to avoid contact with the axillary artery.

Postoperative Considerations

Immediate Postoperative Care

- Patient is transported to the PACU.
- Patient is discharged 3–4 days postoperatively.

Prognosis

- No complications: Patient undergoes shoulder rehabilitation for up to 16 weeks, at which time the patient should have close to full ROM.
- Complications: Postoperative SSI; axillary nerve injury; glenoid loosening; tuberosity malunion or nonunion; rotator cuff tear; fracture of the bone around the prosthesis; deltoid rupture; impingement syndrome; glenohumeral instability; loss of ROM.

Wound Classification

- Class I: Clean

Procedures of the Radius

PROCEDURE 21-7 External Fixation of a Colles' Fracture

Surgical Anatomy and Pathology

- The radius extends from the elbow to the wrist and rotates around the ulna (Figures 21-11 and 21-13).
- An easy way to remember on which side of the arm the radius lies is to recall that it is on the "thumb" side of the arm and hand.
- The proximal end articulates with the capitulum of the

(*continues*)

PROCEDURE 21-7 (continued)

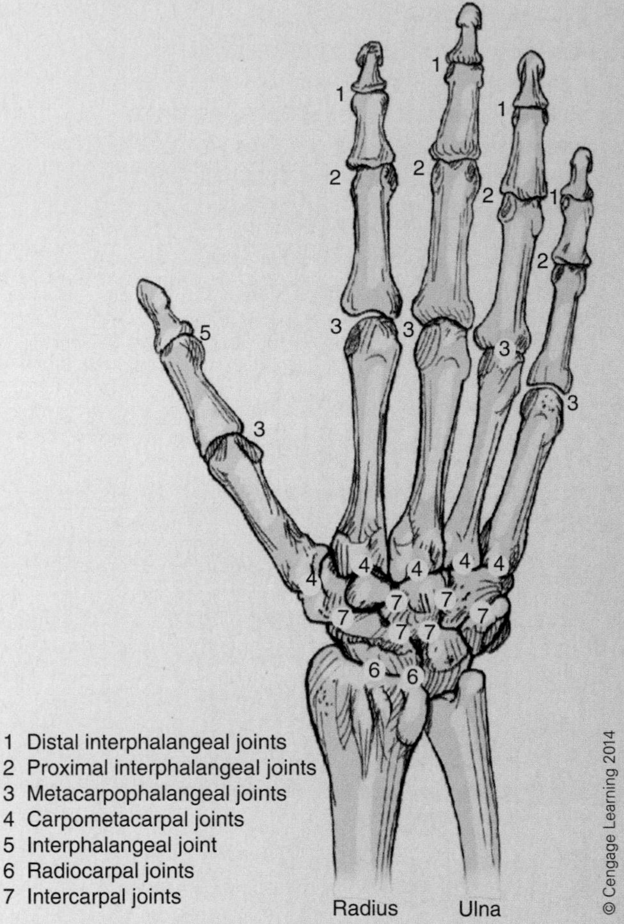

Figure 21-13 Hand and wrist joints

humerus and the radial notch of the ulna. This allows the radius to rotate around the ulna during movement.

- Just below the head of the radius is a process called the radial tuberosity, which serves as an attachment for the tendon of the biceps muscle.
- The distal end is divided into two articular surfaces. The lateral surface articulates with the carpal bones of the wrist. Located on the lateral surface is the styloid process, which provides attachments for the ligaments of the wrist. The medial surface articulates with the distal end of the ulna.
- The proximal portion of the ulna, the trochlea, articulates with the humerus. Two processes, called the olecranon and coronoid processes, are located on each side of this articulation. Both processes provide attachments for muscles.
- The somewhat rounded head on the distal end of the ulna articulates with

PROCEDURE 21-7 (continued)

	a notch of the radius called the ulnar notch. The ulna also has a styloid process that provides attachments for	ligaments of the wrist. • Colles' fracture is an angulated fracture of the distal radius at the epiphysis	approximately 1 in. from the wrist joint. The fracture causes the hand to assume a dorsal and lateral position until treated.
Preoperative Diagnostic Tests and Procedures	• Standard anteroposterior and lateral X-rays • CT scan	• MRI **Note:** Radiographic studies help the surgeon decide the procedure to	perform, e.g., ORIF, external fixation.
Equipment, Instruments, and Supplies Unique to Procedure	• C-arm • Basic orthopedic instrument set • Power drill • Nitrogen tank • Drill bit box • Pin cutter	• Tourniquet and insufflator • Webril—placed around upper arm for cushion under tourniquet • Kirschner wires (K-wires) or Steinmann pins	• External fixation device and specialty instrumentation • Drill guide • Hand table • Xeroform dressing
Preoperative Preparation	• Position: Supine with operative arm on hand table • Anesthesia: Bier block; general • Skin prep: Starting at incision area on wrist	extending from fingertips to middle of upper arm up to lower border of tourniquet • Draping: Three-quarter sheet laid underneath arm to cover hand	table or Mayo stand cover inserted over the table; extremity draping technique
Practical Considerations	• Radiographic studies are in the OR. • Level of nitrogen tank is checked prior to the patient entering the OR. • Power equipment is tested prior to the patient entering the OR. • Have C-arm in the OR. • Notify radiology department to be on stand-by for possible intraoperative X-rays. • Many types of external fixators are commercially available, varying in design depending on	the area of the body for which they are intended. • The advantages of using an external fixating device include decreased interference with the joint, early mobilization for the patient, and elimination of the need for casting. • The external fixator is usually available from the manufacturer in its own sterile package and does not require any type of processing by the	central sterile supply department. • The surgical technologist must be familiar with the external fixator and its components, including the specialty instrumentation. The manufacturer can be contacted to provide information to study or consult with the sales representative who can provide information, including a hands-on in-service.

(continues)

Procedure 21-7 (continued)

- Common features of external fixation devices include:
- Clamps and rings to connect and hold the device together
- Long smooth rods that serve as the supporting device for the clamps and rings

Surgical Procedure

1. The fracture is reduced under fluoroscopy. An external frame may be placed to stabilize the fracture.

   Procedural Consideration: Assist with positioning and stabilizing the extremity as needed.

2. A small longitudinal incision is made from the base of the second metacarpal to the middle of the shaft. The soft tissue is bluntly dissected down to the bone. Small Hohmann retractors may be used.

   Procedural Consideration: A #15 knife blade is used. The metacarpal incision is performed first to ensure proper length of the fixator.

3. A drill guide is used as a directional aid and to protect the surrounding soft tissues from the drill bit.

   Procedural Consideration: Be sure that the size of the drill guide coordinates with the selected drill bit. The size is usually imprinted on the guide.

4. Pins are inserted with the use of a power drill.

   Procedural Consideration: Pins will be placed above and below the fracture site.

5. The distal (metacarpal) pins are inserted at a 45–60° angle with the tips imbedded in, but not penetrating, the far cortex.

   Procedural Consideration: A marking pen may be used to mark the sites of insertion.

6. A longitudinal incision is made in the forearm and tissues are bluntly dissected down to the bone. The sensory branch of the radial nerve must be preserved.

   Procedural Consideration: Blunt rakes are used to provide gentle retraction.

7. Fluoroscopy is used throughout the procedure to confirm the placement of the pins and that the reduction of the fracture is maintained.

   Procedural Consideration: Wear lead gloves if necessary.

8. Proximal (radial) pins are inserted in the fashion described for the distal pins.

   Procedural Consideration: The surgeon may place pins so that a slight protrusion is achieved through the far cortex for osteopenic bone.

9. Clamps and/or joints are slipped over the pins and the longitudinal supportive rod is put in place.

   Procedural Consideration: Be sure the securing screws on the frame are facing laterally to facilitate tightening.

10. A frame is placed over the pins and the clamps are secured. Tightening the clamps holds the fracture in reduction.

    Procedural Consideration: Wrenches are used to tighten the frame (Figure 21-14).

Procedure 21-7 (continued)

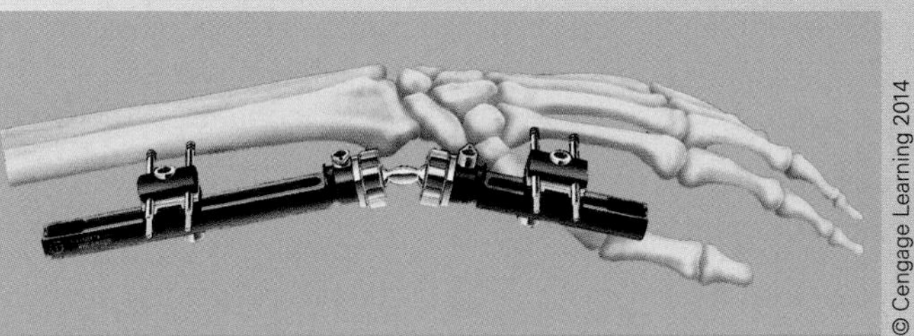

© Cengage Learning 2014

Figure 21-14 External fixation—Colles' fracture

11. Any flexion/extension, radial/ulnar, length, and supination/pronation deviations are corrected by adjusting the frame.

    Procedural Consideration: More than one wrench may be useful.

12. A final X-ray is taken to confirm pin placement and fracture reduction.

    Procedural Consideration: Be sure patient and all team members are protected from radiation.

13. Dressing is applied.

    Procedural Consideration: Sutures are generally not needed. The surgeon may loosely wrap strips of Xeroform around the base of each pin at the insertion site.

Postoperative Considerations

Immediate Postoperative Care

- Patient is transported to the PACU.
- Patient is observe for local hemorrhage.
- Provide pain management.
- Patient is usually discharged the same day.

Prognosis

- No complications: Active finger motion started immediately; at 8–10 weeks, bone should be healed and external fixator removed in the surgeon's office.
- Complications: Postoperative wound infection including local pin site infection; hemorrhage; nerve damage

Wound Classification

- Class I: Clean

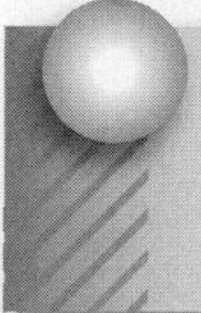

Pearl of Wisdom

Anticipate the use of fluoroscopy and X-ray machines. Follow all radiation safety procedures.

Procedure 21-8 ORIF Radius

Pathology	• See Table 21-2 for types of fractures.
Preoperative Diagnostic Tests and Procedures	• Standard X-rays

(*continues*)

PROCEDURE 21-8 (continued)

Equipment, Instruments, and Supplies Unique to Procedure	• Hand table • Tourniquet and insufflator • Webril • Nitrogen tank • Batteries if cordless poswer drill is being used • Basic orthopedic instrument set • Internal fixation small fragment instrument tray; contains screws, plates, malleable plate templates, drill guide, countersink, drill bits, depth gauge, tap and tap handle with tap holding sleeve, hexagonal screwdriver, screw holding sleeve, bone-holding forceps, compression device, plate benders, K-wires, quick coupling device for power drill • Large plate bender available in OR. • Additional K-wires available in OR. • Power drill
Preoperative Preparation	• Position: Supine with operative arm on hand table • Anesthesia: Bier block; general • Skin prep: Starting at incision site, middle of forearm, extend from fingers to lower border of tourniquet • Draping: Three-quarter sheet laid underneath arm to cover hand table or Mayo stand cover inserted over the table; extremity draping technique
Practical Considerations	• Radiographic studies are in the OR. • Level of nitrogen tank is checked prior to the patient entering the OR. • Make sure batteries for cordless power instruments are charging the day before surgery. The morning of surgery the batteries will need to be sterilized by immediate-use steam sterilization. • Power equipment is tested prior to the patient entering the OR. • Have C-arm in the OR. • Notify radiology department to be on stand-by for possible intraoperative X-rays. • The surgical technologist must know the internal fixation instrumentation and the order of the use of instruments for inserting a screw to decrease the operative time; the surgeon should not have to ask for each instrument when placing the screws. • The surgical technologist must remember the plate that is used and types, sizes, and number of screws and communicate the information to the circulating person, who must document the implants that were placed in the patient in order to be compliant with FDA device laws.
Surgical Procedure	1. The incision depends on the location of the fracture. A. If the fracture is located in the distal half of the radius, the forearm is supinated and a longitudinal incision is made over the interval between the brachioradialis and flexor carpi radialis muscles. When making this incision, the radial nerve, which is posterior to the brachioradialis muscle, must be identified and preserved. B. If the fracture is located in the proximal half, the forearm is pronated and the incision made over the proximal radius along a line from the center of the dorsum of the wrist up to the humeral epicondyle. C. For fractures located in the middle of the radius, either incision can be used.

PROCEDURE 21-8 (continued)

2. The incision is carried through the subcutaneous and muscle layer, and the bone is exposed.
3. Using a ¼-in. Key periosteal elevator, the periosteum is stripped from the area of bone where the plate will be applied.
4. Using a small curette, the clotted blood is removed from the fractured ends of the bone.
5. The fracture is reduced using the self-retaining bone clamps to hold the reduction in place. Reduction may include fitting bone fragments back into anatomical position. Large bone fragments may require fixation with a screw.
6. Next the surgeon places a malleable plate template against the bone and contours it to the radius. The surgeon requests a 3.5-mm AO dynamic compression plate of sufficient length, a 5- or 6-holed plate and rarely a 4-holed. The malleable template is placed against the plate and, using plate benders, the plate is contoured in order to fit securely to the bone.

   Procedural Consideration: The plate must be contoured to fit the radius in order for it to heal with its normal anatomical bow and restore normal function.
7. The plate is placed on the bone and held in place with two to three self-retaining bone-holding forceps. Using the drill and drill guide, the first hole is drilled; the hole nearest one end of the bone is drilled first, tapped (if self-tapping screws used, not necessary to tap the drill hole), and the depth gauge and screws are is placed. The surgeon will place one screw at a time.

   Procedural Consideration: As previously mentioned, the placement of screws follows the same sequence, which the surgical technologist must remember: (a) The quick-coupling device should have been loaded onto the power drill while setting up for the procedure; the correct-size drill bit is loaded onto the quick-coupling device; gently pull on the drill bit to make sure it is seated; the drill guide is placed over the bit and the drill handed to the surgeon; (b) be prepared to hand the depth gauge to the surgeon; (c) while the surgeon is using the depth gauge, load the correct-size tap onto the handle using the tap-holding sleeve and pass to the surgeon holding your hand under the tap in case it is knocked loose from the holding sleeve when passing (if using self-tapping screws, this step is not performed); (d) the surgeon will communicate the size of screw that is needed after using the depth gauge; the surgical technologist places the screw onto the hexagonal screwdriver using the screw-holding sleeve to keep it in place; when passing the screwdriver to the surgeon verbally confirm the size of the screw and hold your hand under the screw in case it is knocked loose during passing; and (e) steps are repeated for all screws.
8. The bone-holding forceps are removed after the last screw is placed.
9. The surgeon may thoroughly irrigate the surgical wound. The muscles are allowed to go back into normal anatomical position and do not require suturing. The tourniquet is released in order to identify bleeders. The subcutaneous layer and skin are closed. Xeroform dressing and 4 × 4 dressing sponges are placed.

(continues)

PROCEDURE 21-8 (continued)

Postoperative Considerations

Immediate Postoperative Care

- Patient is transported to the PACU.
- Patient is usually discharged the same day.

Prognosis

- No complications: In 10–12 days patient usually has good motion of the wrist, forearm, and elbow. Strenuous activity is restricted until full healing has occurred. The plate and screws are not removed before 2 years.
- Complications: Postoperative SSI; hemorrhage; wound infection; malunion; nonunion.

Wound Classification

- Class I: Clean

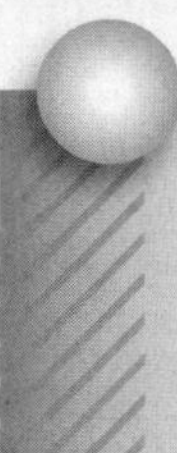

PEARL OF WISDOM

Two of the main categories of screws available are self-tapping and nontapping (other types of screws available include cannulated, locking and non-locking): You must be able to identify them on sight. Nontapping screws require that the drill hole be tapped with a tapping device prior to placement of the screw. Screws that are self-tapping can be identified by an angled notch near the tip of the screw.

Hip Procedures

PROCEDURE 21-9 ORIF Hip Fracture

Surgical Anatomy and Pathology

- The sacrum, coccyx, and pelvic girdle form the circular pelvis. (Refer to Chapter 15 for more details on the pelvis.)
  - The pelvis provides support for the trunk and attachments for the femur.
  - The pelvis is created from the fusion of three bones called the ilium, ischium, and pubis. Together they are referred to as the ox coxae or innominate bone.
- The ilium forms the superior portion of the pelvis and is the largest of the three bones. The ilium flares outward in a ridge called the iliac crest. This crest serves as a primary site for obtaining bone for bone grafts.
- The ischium forms the inferior portion of the pelvis and is the strongest of the three pelvic bones. Located on the lower portion of the ischium is the ischial tuberosity, which provides attachments for the ligaments and leg muscles.
- The pubis is the anterior portion of the pelvis. The two pubic bones join at the midline to form the symphysis pubis. The symphysis pubis is actually a disk of fibrous cartilage that serves to connect the two pubic bones.

(continues)

PROCEDURE 21-9 (continued)

- The hip is a ball-and-socket joint formed by the deep, round fossa, called the acetabulum, located in the innominate bone and the head of the femur (Figure 21-15).
- A capsule, ligaments, and muscles stabilize the hip. The iliofemoral ligament connects the ilium with the femur anteriorly and superiorly, and the ischiofemoral and pubofemoral

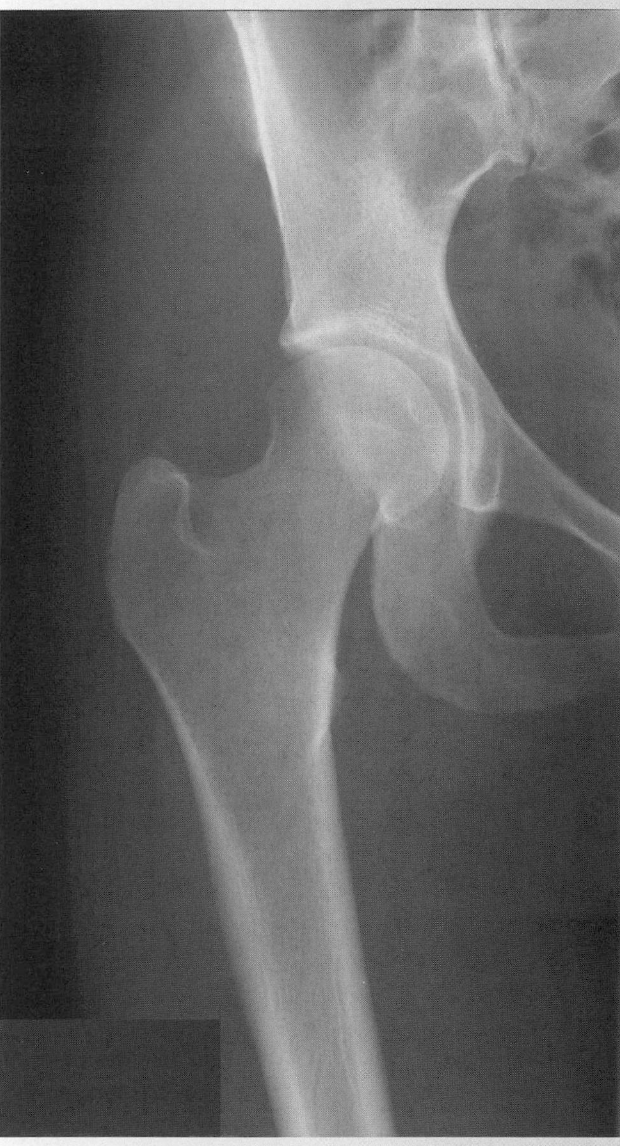

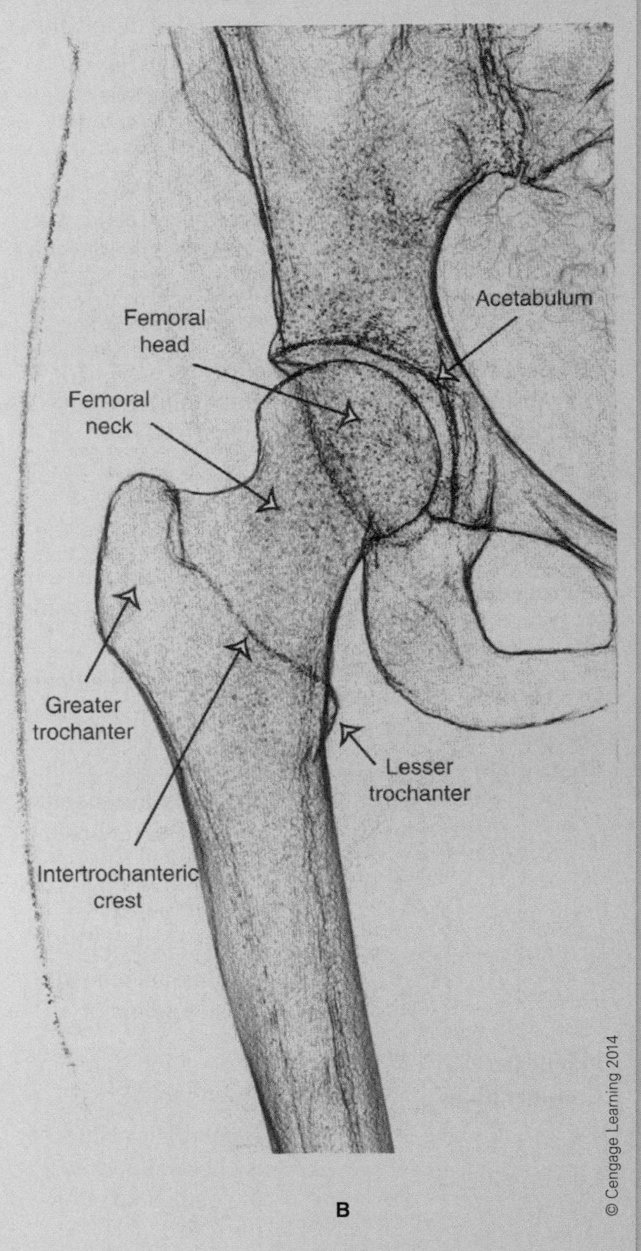

Figure 21-15 Hip: (A) AP X-ray, (B) schematic

(*continues*)

PROCEDURE 21-9 (continued)

	ligaments join the ischium and pubis to the femur. • There are several categories of hip fractures and hip fractures with an associated dislocation. The type of fracture determines the treatment, including whether the treatment is nonoperative or operative. The operative fractures that require ORIF are intertrochanteric,	subtrochanteric, femoral neck, and basilar neck fractures. • Fractures are common in the elderly and in females who have osteoporosis. The fracture can disrupt the blood supply to the femoral head, resulting in bone necrosis; consequently, fractures should be treated as soon as possible.	• The following discussion is for repair of intertrochanteric fractures with the use of the AO Dynamic Hip Screw/Dynamic Condylar Screw (DHS/DCS) system. Intertrochanteric fractures most often reduce without complications; however, ORIF is indicated to prevent malunion due to the rotation of the lower extremity.
Preoperative Diagnostic Tests and Procedures	• Standard anteroposterior and lateral X-rays	• MRI to evaluate soft tissues • CT scan	
Equipment, Instruments, and Supplies Unique to Procedure	• Fracture table • Nitrogen tank • Batteries if cordless power drill and reamer are used • Power drill and reamer	• C-arm • Basic orthopedic instrument set • Dynamic hip screw (DHS) specialty instruments	• DHS implants • Bone reduction clamps • Barrier drape
Preoperative Preparation	• Position: A fracture table is used with the patient in the supine position to reduce the fracture. • Anesthesia: General • Skin prep: Beginning at hip joint, extend down midline of	abdomen on operative side up to mid-chest and laterally as far as possible, and entire operative leg to the ankle • Draping: Four towels to square off; plastic adhesive incise drape;	laparotomy sheet; or four towels to square off and large barrier drape that has adhesive to stick to hip and is draped over three IV poles and extends close to the floor.
Practical Considerations	• Radiographic studies are in the OR. • Level of nitrogen tank is checked prior to the patient entering the OR. • Power equipment is tested prior to the patient entering the OR.	• Have C-arm in the OR; it will be used throughout the procedure. If the barrier drape is not used the C-arm must have a C-arm drape placed; if barrier drape is used, the C-arm can be brought in over the	hip joint of the patient on the opposite side of the surgical team. • Notify radiology department to be on stand-by for possible intraoperative X-rays. • The surgical technologist must know the DHS

PROCEDURE 21-9 (continued)

instrumentation and the order of the use of instruments for inserting the lag screws and plate/barrel assembly to decrease the operative time; the surgeon should not have to ask for each instrument when placing the implants.

- Fluoroscopy is used throughout the procedure to confirm the reduction and placement of the implants.
- The surgical technologist must remember the types and sizes and how many implants were used and communicate the information to the circulating person, who must document the implants that were placed in the patient in order to be compliant with FDA device laws.
- The surgeon may want everyone to change the outer glove when double-gloved after the draping procedure.
- Make sure the batteries for the cordless power instruments are charging the day before surgery. The morning of surgery the batteries will need to be sterilized by immediate-use steam sterilization.

Surgical Procedure

1. The surgeon makes an incision distally from the greater trochanter downward the approximate length of the implant. The dissection is carried downward with the #10 knife blade through the fascia lata and vastus lateralis to expose the fracture site.

   Procedural Consideration: Initially small to medium retractors will be needed; as the wound is deepened deeper retractors will be placed.

2. The DHS/DCS guide pin is handed to the surgeon for placement in the femoral head.

   Procedural Consideration: The guide pin that comes with the DHS/DCS instrument set is designed for use with the set, so no other guide pin should be substituted.

3. The appropriate angle guide is placed along the axis of the femoral shaft and the guide pin is inserted with the power drill into the center of the femoral head.

   Procedural Consideration: The guide pin remains in place for the rest of the procedure and care must be taken to prevent its removal. However, if the guide pin is accidentally removed it must be immediately reinserted. The guide pin often comes out when the triple reamer is removed. To reinsert, a lag screw is inserted backward into the short centering sleeve. This is placed partway into the femoral head for use as a guide to reinsert the guide pin. The surgeon uses a mallet to reseat the guide pin.

4. The surgeon now determines the reaming and tapping depth and screw length. The direct measuring device is slid over the guide pin to measure the depth of the guide pin insertion. The measurement is a direct reading. The surgeon communicates the reading to the surgical technologist, who then subtracts 10 mm from the reading. For example, if the direct reading is 100 mm, the reamer setting, tapping depth, and screw length will be 90 mm. For the rest of this description, 90 mm will be used.

5. The appropriate triple reamer is assembled. To assemble, select the reaming head that goes with the DHS plate and barrel length. The standard 38-mm barrel length for the plate and 135° barrel angle is most commonly used. The set screw on the reaming head is aligned with the flat side of the drill bit. Slide the cutting end of the reaming head over the coupling end of the drill bit and continue sliding the reaming head until the noncutting end of the reaming head is level with the calculated depth, which in this instance is 90 mm. The reaming head is secured into the notch and locked into place with the locking nut.

   Procedural Consideration: Extra care must be taken while assembling the triple reamer because it is very sharp. The triple reamer can be assembled by the surgical technologist during setup and the depth established intraoperatively.

(*continues*)

Procedure 21-9 (continued)

6. The triple reamer assembly is placed on the power drill using the large quick-coupling device.
7. The reamer is placed over the guide pin and drilled into the femoral head.

   Procedural Consideration: This accomplishes three things: (1) drills for the lag screw, (2) countersinks for the plate/barrel junction, and (3) reams in preparation for the plate barrel. While the surgeon is drilling, the surgical technologist should frequently irrigate the area with small amounts of normal saline to prevent thermal necrosis of the bone.
8. If necessary the surgeon will use the calibrated tap. The tap is assembled by sliding the short centering sleeve over the tap and the tap is inserted into the T-handle quick-coupling device. Release the collar of the T-handle and tug on the tap to make sure it is fully seated in the T-handle quick-coupler. The surgeon now inserts the tap over the guide pin and taps to the correct 90-mm depth.
9. At this point the surgical technologist puts the lag screw insertion assembly together with the correct-size lag screw. To assemble, the coupling screw is inserted into the guide shaft. The coupling screw is screwed into place on the end of the lag screw. The tabs on the guide shaft should fit into the slots located on the lag screw. The long centering sleeve is placed over the wrench. Last, the guide shaft/lag screw assembly is inserted into the wrench until it stops.
10. The assembly is placed over the guide pin and the lag screw is inserted. The wrench, long centering sleeve, coupling screw, guide shaft, and guide pin are removed. Removal of the guide pin requires the use of the power drill in reverse.
11. The surgeon uses the impactor and mallet to seat the plate.
12. The last step of the procedure involves placing 4.5-mm cortex screws using the standard AO screw insertion technique to fix the plate against the femur.
13. The surgeon thoroughly irrigates the wound, traction on the fracture table is slowly released, one or two Jackson-Pratt drains are placed, and the wound is closed in layers. Xeroform dressing, 4×4 dressing sponges, and ABD are placed.

Postoperative Considerations

Immediate Postoperative Care

- Patient is transported to the PACU.
- Patient is observed for local hemorrhage.
- Pain control is provided.

Prognosis

- No complications: Patient is hospitalized for 3–5 days. The patient should begin partial weight bearing as soon as possible, often the first postoperative day. Full weight bearing should be occurring by 6–8 weeks postoperative.
- Complications: Postoperative SSI; hemorrhage; failure of implant; disruption of blood supply to hip joint; nerve damage.

Wound Classification

- Class I: Clean

PROCEDURE 21-10 Total Hip Arthroplasty

Pathology	• The primary indication for total hip arthroplasty (THA) is decreasing the incapacitating pain in patients who are older than 65 years of age and for whom the pain has not been resolved by conservative medical therapy. • Other indications for a THA include rheumatoid arthritis, ankylosing spondylitis, degenerative joint disease (DJD), avascular necrosis of the hip joint due to previous fracture or dislocation, alcoholism, systemic lupus erythematosus, nonunion of femoral neck and/or trochanteric fractures, tuberculosis, congenital luxation or subluxation, and bone tumor of the acetabulum or proximal femur.
Preoperative Diagnostic Tests and Procedures	• Physical examination is very important to determine if the pain is at a level of debilitation that justifies performing a THA. It is also of importance to rule out an alternate diagnosis and avoid performing a THA that would not relieve the symptoms of the primary condition. • Nuclear scans and aspiration of fluid from the hip joint for culture in the lab to rule out any presence of infection • Standard anteroposterior and lateral X-rays of the hip joint • Surgeon will create plastic overlay templates using the standard X-ray marking measurements that show the size of implants that will be needed.
Equipment, Instruments, and Supplies Unique to Procedure	• Nitrogen tank • Batteries if cordless power drill and saw are used • Vacuum suction beanbag • Extra gloves for surgical team • Space suits • Basic orthopedic instrument set or basic THA instrument set (the instruments listed may be included in the basic THA instrument set) • Meyerding retractors • Curettes • Serrated rongeur • Hohmann retractors • Self-retaining hip retractor (Charnley retractor is one example that is often used) • Cobb elevators • Lambotte osteotomes • Gouges • Hip skid • Rasps • Mallet • Long Bovie tip • Pulse lavage • PMMA kit • Closed cement mixing system with suction tubing • Brush tip for placement over regular suction tip for lavage • 4 × 4 radiopaque sponges soaked in thrombin • Cement gun • Power drill and saw • Oscillating and reciprocating saw blades • Drill bits ¼ and ½ in. • #10 knife blades × 3 • Gelfoam available in OR. • THA instrument trays that include trial prostheses and specialty instrumentation such as femoral head extractor, acetabular reamers, T-handle intramedullary canal reamer, femoral reamers, cookie cutter, and femoral rasps

(continues)

Procedure 21-10 (continued)

General List of Instruments for the Mayo Stand	**Note:** Due to the extensive nature of a THA procedure, the following is presented as a suggested list of instruments for the instrument Mayo stand. • #3 knife handles with #10 knife blades • Curved Mayo scissors • Two long tissue forceps	• Suture scissors • Two curved Crile clamps • Sharp and blunt Hohmann retractors • Small and medium Meyerding retractors • Medium curved and straight Lambotte osteotomes • Two Kocher clamps • Medium curette	• Freer elevator • Large Key periosteal elevator • Medium Cobb elevator • Bone hook • Serrated rongeur • Pliers • Mallet • Self-retaining hip retractor available on back table
Preoperative Preparation	• Position: Lateral most often used; supine may be used • Anesthesia: Continuous epidural block, spinal or general • Skin prep: Starting at the hip region extending down the midline of the abdomen to the level of the umbilicus and laterally as far as possible, and the entire leg and foot on the operative side	• Draping: (1) Four towels to square off the operative site and kept in place with four perforating towel clamps; (2) with the leg held up, a plastic U-drape is placed under the leg; one tail is placed using the lateral edge of the buttock and iliac crest a as guide and the other tail placed along the midline of the abdomen covering the genitals;	(3) impervious stockinette placed on leg and rolled up to mid-thigh; Coban is wrapped around the stockinette; (4) two three-quarter sheets: First is laid transversely at the level of the umbilicus; the other is placed transversely at the mid-thigh; (5) impervious U-drape is placed with the tails toward the feet.
Practical Considerations	• All radiographic studies including X-ray templates should be in the OR. • The surgical technologist should confirm the day before surgery that the specialty instrument trays and trial prostheses arrived and are being sterilized. The first thing on the morning of surgery the surgical technologist should	confirm everything has been sterilized. • There are several types of hip arthroplasty systems offered by various orthopedic medical companies. The surgical technologist must find out prior to surgery the system that will be used; the surgical technologist must be familiar with the instrumentation and the order in which it is	used. The manufacturer can be contacted for procedural information to study the sales representative can be consulted. • The surgeon's preference usually dictates which company's system will be used. Because each system requires specific instrumentation, there is no

PROCEDURE 21-10 (continued)

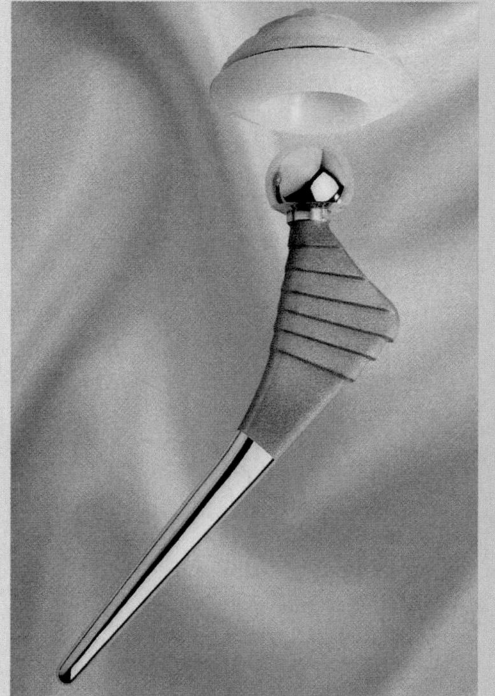

© Alila Sao Mai/www.Shutterstock.com

Figure 21-16 Hi-Nek total hip prosthesis: (A) Acetabular component, (B) femoral component

"universal" set of hip instruments.

- The femoral prosthesis is available in different sizes, types, and length of neck to accommodate the size of the patient. The stem of the prosthesis is either collarless or has a collar that rests on the rim of the resected femur.
- The development of modular components has greatly increased the efficiency of the acetabular component and decreased the amount of surgery required in the event of a total hip revision. Metal acetabular cups that are used when cementing is indicated have a slightly rough, textured posterior surface and a polyethylene cup that snaps into the metal shell. Cups not requiring cement have a porous surface on the posterior side (Figure 21-16).
- Active individuals with healthy bones and no previous bone diseases or complications are ideal candidates for a noncemented total hip replacement. Conversely, a cemented prosthesis is usually best for patients with osteoporosis, particularly older individuals.
- Some surgeons may have the team remove the outer gloves of the double-gloving and replace after draping. Studies have shown that the highest risk for breaks in sterile technique during orthopedic procedures is during draping due to the complicated draping procedures.
- Some surgeons may have the team remove the outer gloves and replace just prior to the permanent

(continues)

PROCEDURE 21-10 (continued)

implants being opened and implanted.

- Confirm on the day of surgery that the blood bank received the blood order and it is ready for use. The average blood loss during a THA is 1000 to 1500 mL, so the possibility of blood transfusion is high. The surgical technologist must keep careful track of the irrigation that is used in order to help in determining the amount of blood loss.
- Check the nitrogen level in the nitrogen tank or make sure the batteries are charging the day before surgery for the cordless power instruments. The batteries must be sterilized the morning of surgery by immediate-use steam sterilization.
- Test the power equipment prior to the patient entering the OR.
- Ask the surgeon if he or she will want X-rays taken in the OR before transporting the patient to the PACU or the X-rays taken in the PACU.
- The day before surgery, make sure the batteries for air flow for the space suits are charging.
- Health care facility policy must be followed for recording the prostheses that are implanted.
- The permanent implants must not be opened until the surgeon requests the prostheses and communicates the types and sizes.
- It is suggested that the surgical technologist use two Mayo stands, one for instrumentation and the other for power equipment and specialty hip instrumentation.
- It is also suggested that new saw blades and drill bits be used for each THA procedure. Often the medical company whose THA system is being used will provide new saw blades and drill bits.

Surgical Procedure

1. A posterolateral approach is the most common approach to the hip joint. Once the patient is placed in lateral position, prepped, and draped, a slightly curved incision centered over the greater trochanter is made.

   Procedural Consideration: The incision is long and large. Electrocautery and appropriate retractors will be needed.

2. The incision is extended following the femoral shaft to approximately 10 cm distal of the greater trochanter.

   Procedural Consideration: The assistant will need laparotomy sponges for soaking up blood and as an aid in manually retracting tissues.

3. Continuing to use the #10 blade and electrosurgery, the subcutaneous tissues are incised in a single plane down to the fascia lata and fascia of the gluteus maximus.
4. The subcutaneous tissue is dissected free from the fascial plane anteriorly and posteriorly to facilitate wound closure at the end of the procedure.
5. The fascia is divided with the scissors over the center of the greater trochanter.
6. The surgeon divides the gluteus maximus in blunt fashion proximally in the direction of its fibers.
7. The fascial incision is extended to expose the insertion of the gluteus maximus on the posterior femur. The Charnley hip retractor is positioned.

(continues)

PROCEDURE 21-10 (continued)

Procedural Consideration: The surgical technologist should have the self-retaining Charnley hip retractor with blades readily available at this point in the procedure. At this point, the surgical technologist should change the Bovie blade from a short blade to a long blade.

8. The surgeon divides the trochanteric bursa in order to visualize the edge of the gluteus medius. Once this posterior dissection is complete, the knee is flexed and the hip joint is internally rotated.
9. The external rotators and quadratus femoris are now divided at their insertion on the femur.
10. Hemostasis is attained with electrocautery and a long Bovie tip throughout the dissection. In particular, the surgeon identifies the branches of the medial circumflex artery that are located within the quadratus femoris and coagulates the vessels.
11. The interval between the gluteus medius and superior hip joint capsule is located and blunt dissection is performed between the two structures. Two Hohmann retractors are placed to expose the entire joint capsule.
12. The capsule is incised. A Steinmann pin is placed in the ilium superior to the acetabulum. Using electrocautery, the surgeon makes a mark on the greater trochanter; these anatomical landmarks are later used to determine if the leg length is correct after insertion of the trial prosthetic components.

    Procedural Consideration: The surgeon will most likely need a #7 or long #3 knife handle with a #10 blade to incise the capsule.
13. The hip joint is now dislocated; it is flexed, adducted, and gently rotated. A bone hook is used as an aid in lifting the femoral head out from the acetabulum.

    Procedural Consideration: When the surgeon and/or assistant is dislocating the hip joint, the surgical technologist may be asked to provide manual traction if necessary.
14. The femoral osteotomy guide is placed over the lateral femur and neck and, using electrocautery, the point is marked where the oscillating saw will be used to remove the head of the femur.

    Procedural Consideration: Hand the femoral osteotomy guide to the surgeon. While the marks are being made for the femoral neck cut, the oscillating saw should be prepared for use. Blunt Hohmann retractors are placed around the femoral neck; one large Hohmann is placed under the neck and one sharp Hohmann is placed distal to the lesser trochanter to deliver the femur into the wound.
15. The oscillating saw is used to cut and remove the femoral head. The femoral head can be removed with a corkscrew or bone clamp.

    Procedural Consideration: The surgical technologist should not immediately pass off the femoral head in case bone can be used for grafting purposes. However, the femoral head is considered a tissue specimen.
16. The femur is retracted anteriorly to expose the acetabulum and allow the use of the acetabular reamers. The rim of the acetabulum is inspected for osteophytes. If present, they are removed with the rongeur to create a smooth acetabular rim.

(continues)

Procedure 21-10 (continued)

Procedural Consideration: The surgical technologist should have a laparotomy sponge ready to remove and clean dissected bits of osteophytes from the jaws of the rongeur.

17. Acetabular reamers (informally referred to as cheese graters) are used to ream the acetabular cup to remove the articular cartilage. Reaming is complete when all cartilage has been removed and osteochondral bone is exposed.

    Procedural Consideration: The acetabular reamers are hemispheric in shape with several small, sharp blades on their surface for cutting the cartilage. The smallest size of reamer is used first and progression to larger reamers is 2 mm at a time. The surgical technologist should verbalize the size of the reamer when handing it to the surgeon. Additionally, the surgical technologist should save some of the cartilaginous shavings for later use as grafting material; place the shavings on a saline-soaked lap sponge on the back table.

18. The surgeon checks the reamed acetabulum to verify if any subchondral cysts are present. If necessary, a curette is used to remove the cysts.

    Procedural Consideration: The surgical technologist should have a small-size curette available for use in removal of the subchondral cysts.

19. The trial acetabular shell is attached to the acetabular positioning device and inserted; the mallet is used to tap on the end of the positioning device to seat the trial component. The edges of the trial component should match the angle of the acetabular rim. If the fit is not correct, the trial is removed and the next size trial is inserted until the correct size is attained. The trial plastic insert is now positioned inside the trial acetabular shell.

    Procedural Consideration: The surgeon will inform the surgical technologist of the size of the trial acetabular shell to be inserted. The surgical technologist should know how to attach the trial to the acetabular positioning device.

20. The foot is lowered toward the floor and is internally rotated to expose the proximal end of the femur. Hohmann retractors are placed and the femoral end is visualized to determine if bone and soft tissue needs to be removed with the use of a rongeur. Usually bone must be removed from the medial aspect of the trochanter in order to facilitate placement of the femoral reamer.

    Procedural Consideration: Again, the surgical technologist should have a laparotomy sponge ready to remove and clean dissected bits of bone and tissue from the jaws of the rongeur.

21. The T-handle intramedullary canal reamer is used to start the opening and expose the femoral canal opening.

    Procedural Consideration: While the surgeon is using the T-handle reamer, the surgical technologist should be preparing the first power reamer to be used. Unless communicated otherwise by the surgeon, the smallest reamer should be prepared. Each additional reamer that is used will be the next size up. The surgical technologist should verbalize the size of the reamer when handing it to the surgeon.

Procedure 21-10 (continued)

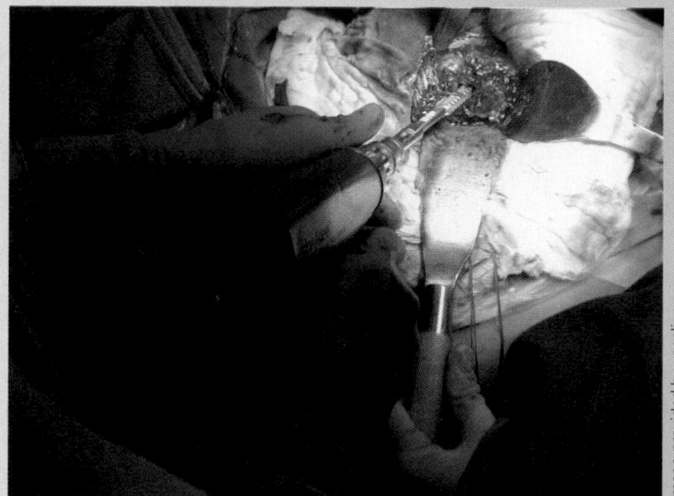

Image provided by vesalius.com

Figure 21-17 Femoral reamer

22. The surgeon now begins using the reamers attached to the power reamer to further open up the canal (Figure 21-17). Reaming is continued until cortical bone is reached. Some total hip arthroplasty systems provide reamers that ream both proximally and distally.

23. Additional bone may need to be removed at the end of the femur using a box chisel (also called a box osteotome) or a cookie cutter before the rasps are used.

24. The femoral rasps are used next. Care is taken not to penetrate the femur, which could cause a femoral fracture. The rasp is attached to the rasp handle, aligned with the axis of the femoral neck, and inserted into the reamed femoral canal. Using a back-and-forth motion, the surgeon rasps the canal to enlarge it, facilitating placement of the femoral component.

    Procedural Consideration: While the surgeon is using the box chisel or cookie cutter, the surgical technologist should obtain the rasp handle and attach the first rasp to be used. The surgeon is given the smallest rasp, also called a broach, and utilizes a back-and-forth motion to remove the cancellous bone. The surgeon uses the rasp manually and/or with a mallet. Larger rasps are successively used until cortical bone is exposed. The surgical technologist should verbalize the size of the rasp when handing it to the surgeon

25. The final rasp is left seated and serves as the femoral trial component. Next, the femoral neck is prepared with a round calcar plane; the calcar plane removes any excess bone around the trial femoral implant and creates a smooth surface.

    Procedural Consideration: Once the last rasp is used, the surgical technologist should prepare the calcar plane on the power drill.

26. A trial head and neck is placed on the trial femoral implant. The hip is reduced and put through an ROM. The leg length is checked.

(continues)

PROCEDURE 21-10 (continued)

Procedural Consideration: The surgeon communicates the size of the trial head and neck to be placed on the femoral implant. While the hip is reduced and put through an ROM and then redislocated, the surgical technologist should prepare the pulse lavage with the brush tip. Clean, dry laparotomy sponges should be kept up on the field at all times, in particular during the pulse lavage.

27. When it has been confirmed that the components are the correct size, the hip is redislocated and the acetabular and femoral trials are removed. Pulse lavage with regular and brush tips is used to clean out the femoral canal.

28. If cement will be used, a cement restrictor is placed in the distal portion of the femoral canal to prevent cement from entering the nonreamed portion of the medullary canal.

    Procedural Consideration: The surgical technologist should prepare the cement restrictor on the end of the insertion device.

29. Most often the acetabular prosthesis is placed first. If cement is being used, it is injected into the acetabulum first. The metal shell is placed and the acetabular impactor with mallet is used to gently seat the component. Excess cement is removed from around the cup both manually and with a small curette. Next, the plastic liner is snapped into place inside the shell.

    Procedural Consideration: If the components will be cemented, the surgical technologist should prepare the first batch of cement. The surgical technologist should keep track of the time to help the surgeon estimate when the bone cement will be sufficiently hardened after injection into the acetabulum and the acetabular prosthesis is seated. Hint: Save a small piece of cement; roll it into a ball and place on the back table. The surgical technologist and surgeon can check this cement piece for hardness.

30. Cement is injected down the femoral canal.

    Procedural Consideration: While the cement is hardening around the acetabular component, the surgical technologist prepares the second batch of cement for injection into the femoral canal.

31. The femoral prosthesis is placed in the canal with the use of the femoral impactor. Great care is taken to introduce the prosthesis in such a way as to obtain valgus position.

    Procedural Consideration: After the femoral prosthesis is seated, the surgical technologist should again keep track of the time from when the cement is injected down the femoral canal.

32. Once the cement hardens, the femoral head and neck is positioned onto the stem. The femoral head impactor and mallet are used to seat the head on the stem.

33. The hip is reduced and moved through a ROM to check for stability and positioning (Figure 21-18).

    Procedural Consideration: The femoral head prosthesis is small, round, and smooth. Be careful not to drop it when passing it to the surgeon.

34. One or two HemoVac drains will be placed. The first is placed deep in the hip joint and the second is placed in the subcutaneous area.

35. The fascia is closed with interrupted sutures and the skin is closed with staples. Xeroform dressing, 4 × 4 dressing sponges, and ABDs are placed.

    Procedural Consideration: Prepare drains for insertion. Anticipate closure.

PROCEDURE 21-10 (continued)

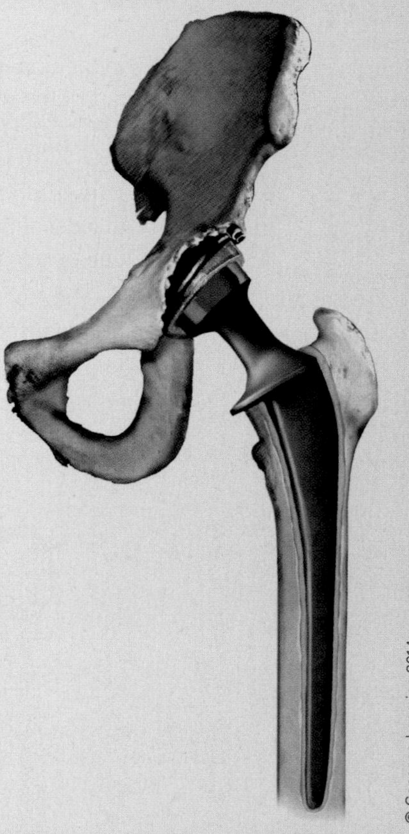

Figure 21-18 Total hip arthroplasty (prosthesis in place)

Postoperative Considerations

Immediate Postoperative Care

- An abduction triangular splint is placed between patient's legs to immobilize the joint.
- Patient is transported to the PACU.
- Observe for local hemorrhage.

Prognosis

- No complications: Drains are removed 24–48 hours after surgery; discharge from hospital after 3–6 days; patient will undergo a lengthy recovery period with progressive rehabilitation from passive non-weight-bearing exercises to full ROM.
- Complications: Postoperative SSI that can be localized to joint; hemorrhage; intraoperative femoral fracture.

Wound Classification

- Class I: Clean

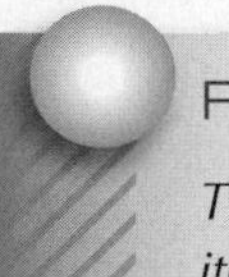

PEARL OF WISDOM

The surgical technologist should verbalize the size of the rasp when handing it to the surgeon. In fact, all items that are sized should be verbally identified when used.

Femoral Procedures

Procedure 21-11 Repair of Femoral Shaft Fracture with AO Titanium Femoral Nail System

Surgical Anatomy and Pathology

- The femur is the largest bone in the body, extending from hip to the knee.
  - The proximal end of the femur consists of the femoral head and neck, and the greater and lesser trochanters (Figure 21-19).
    - The greater trochanter is located on the upper, lateral part of the upper shaft of the femur. It serves as the point of insertion for the gluteus medius and gluteus minimus.
    - The iliopsoas muscle inserts onto the lesser trochanter.
- Located at the distal end of the femur are the lateral and medial condyles that articulate with the condyles of the tibia to form the knee joint. The femoral condyles are separated by a depression called the patellar surface (groove), forming the articulating surface for the patella.
- See Table 21-2 for the various types of fractures.

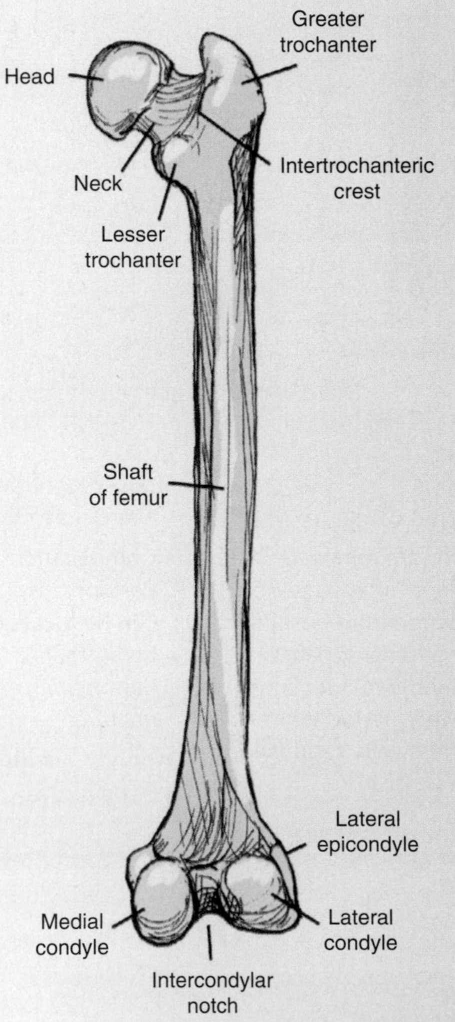

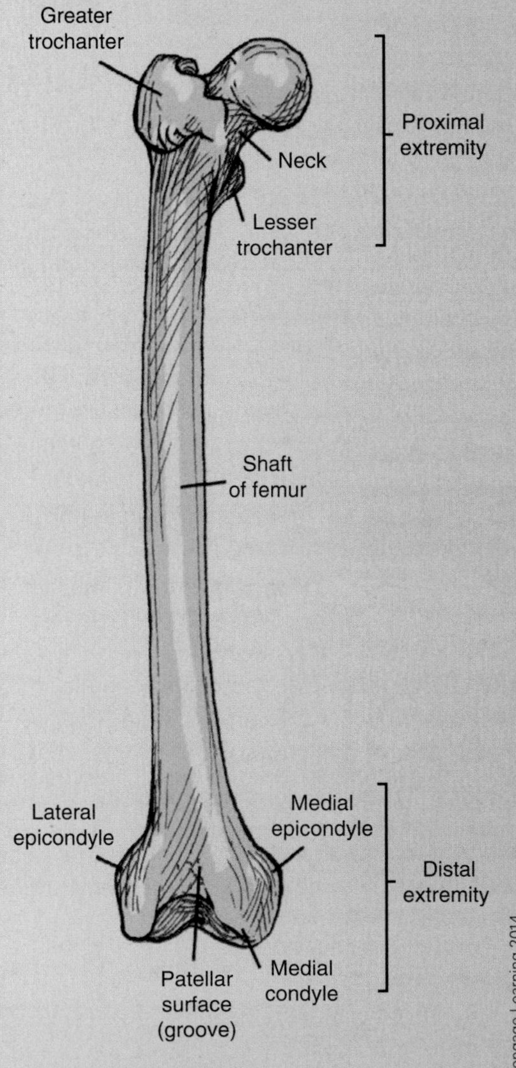

Figure 21-19 Femur: (A) Posterior, (B) anterior

PROCEDURE 21-11 (continued)

	Fractures of the femoral shaft are due to either trauma or pathological disease. The common femoral shaft fractures are comminuted, transverse, oblique, and spiral. • Ipsilateral trochanteric or condylar fractures often occur in conjunction with a femoral shaft fracture. • Femoral fractures require attention and repair as soon as possible after the injury occurs. A delay of 12 hours or more can lead to difficulties in reducing the fracture. If surgery must be delayed, it is recommended that the leg be put in traction. • The choices for treatment of a femoral fracture include closed reduction, skeletal traction, and surgical repair. • Surgical repairs that have been used in the past but have fallen out of favor include external fixation and plates and screws. The complications associated with plates and screws include infections and broken or bent screws and plates, which have contributed to femoral refracture. • The standard method of treatment is the use of intramedullary fixation nails, which in this instance are referred to as femoral intramedullary nails. • The type of nail to be used depends on the type and location of the fracture, whether ipsilateral trochanteric or condylar fractures are present, and whether bone fragments are present. Types of nails include flexible nails such as the Rush and Ender; interlocking nails such as the Trigen; retrograde interlocking intramedullary nails; and standard nails such as the AO (surgical procedure description is for AO titanium femoral nail system).
Preoperative Diagnostic Tests and Procedures	• Standard anteroposterior and lateral X-rays • The surgeon determines the correct length of the nail preoperatively using the X-rays. A nail is placed on the lateral side of the nonoperative leg of the patient. Two anteroposterior X-rays are taken; the surgeon performs the measurements on the X-rays to determine the length to nail that will be needed.

Equipment, Instruments, and Supplies Unique to Procedure	• Fracture table
	• Nitrogen tank
	• Batteries if cordless power drill and reamer are used
	• Power drill
	• C-arm
	• Basic orthopedic instrument set
	• Drill bit box
	• AO system and nails, system includes:
	  • Calibrated guide pin
	  • 13-mm cannulated drill bit
	  • Large reverse awl
	  • Tissue protector
	  • Radiographic ruler
	  • Guide rod—required if using cannulated nails
	  • Medullary and trochanteric reamers, drivers, and extractors
	  • Centering device for the guide pin
	  • Nails of various lengths and diameters
	• The special instruments, in particular the guide pin and reamers that

(continues)

PROCEDURE 21-11 (continued)

	are provided with the AO instrument set, must be used and not substituted with other instrumentation. The	instruments, guide pin, and reamers are specially designed for the insertion of AO nails and only those	types of nails. The diameters of nails and reamers vary from one manufacturer to another.
Preoperative Preparation	• Position: A fracture table is used with the patient in the supine position to reduce the fracture. • Anesthesia: General • Skin prep: Beginning at hip joint extend down midline of abdomen on operative side up to mid-chest and laterally as far as possible, and entire operative leg to the ankle	• Draping: (1) Three-quarter sheets x 2; one placed over upper body; second placed with upper edge at knee joint; (2) Barrier drape placed; (3) two plastic U-drapes placed—one up and one down; (4) impervious stockinette placed on leg and rolled up to just above the knee; Coban is wrapped	around the stockinette; (5) two three-quarter sheets: First is laid transversely at the level of the umbilicus; the other is placed transversely at the mid-thigh; (6) impervious U-drape is placed with the tails toward the feet.
Practical Considerations	• Radiographic studies are in the OR including X-rays with nail measurements. • Level of nitrogen tank is checked prior to the patient entering the OR. • Make sure the batteries for the cordless power instruments are charging the day before surgery. The morning of surgery the batteries will need to be sterilized by immediate-use steam sterilization. • Power equipment is tested prior to the patient entering the OR. • Have C-arm in the OR; it will be used throughout the	procedure. The C-arm must be draped with a C-arm drape. • Notify radiology department to be on stand-by for possible intraoperative X-rays. • The day before the surgical procedure, the surgical technologist must confirm the AO instruments have been received and are being sterilized. Also confirm that the nails, which come in separate sterile packages, have been received. • The surgical technologist must know the AO intramedullary nail instrumentation and the order of the use of instruments for	inserting the nail to decrease the operative time; the surgeon should not have to ask for each instrument when placing the implants. • The surgical technologist must remember the types, sizes, and how many implants were used and communicate the information to the circulating person, who must document the implants that were placed in the patient in order to be compliant with FDA device laws. • The surgeon may want everyone to change the outer glove when double-gloved after the draping procedure.

PROCEDURE 21-11 (continued)

Surgical Procedure

1. The surgeon will confirm the nail length with the use of fluoroscopy and compare the measurement with the preoperative measurement. An anteroposterior view of the proximal femur is taken. The radiographic ruler is held along the lateral side of the thigh and placed until the top is level with the tip of the greater trochanter. The skin is marked at this level. An anteroposterior view of the distal femur is taken. The proximal end of the radiographic ruler is placed at the skin mark and the nail length is read from the ruler.
2. The surgeon makes a longitudinal incision proximal to the greater trochanter through the gluteus medius and maximus.
3. Using the power drill, the 3.2-mm calibrated guide pin is placed in the medullary canal to a depth of 100 mm at the entry point where the nail will be placed.
4. The 13-mm cannulated drill bit with tissue protector is placed over the guidewire and drilled to a depth of 100 mm. The opening that is created will allow the insertion of 9- to 12-mm nail. For a 13- to 15-mm nail, the broach is used instead to enlarge the opening. The drill bit is removed after the opening has been created.
5. The surgical technologist now assembles the insertion instruments. The use of cannulated nails is described.
   A. The correct connecting screw is placed into the insertion handle and secured to the nail with the hexagonal screwdriver.
   B. The driving cap is screwed onto the insertion handle. This serves as the striking point when the mallet is used.
6. The surgical technologist hands the assembly to the surgeon, who manually inserts the nail into the femoral opening as far as possible. For cannulated nails, the nail is inserted over the guide pin, which passes through an opening in the side of the insertion handle. The surgeon now uses the mallet to drive the nail into the distal metaphysis and the guidewire is removed.
7. The proximal locking bolts are placed next.
   A. The standard aiming arm is attached to the insertion handle.
   B. The surgical technologist assembles the triple trocar assembly: 11.0/8.0-mm protection sleeve, 8.0/4.0-mm drill sleeve, and 4.00-mm trocar. The assembly is inserted into the handle through the stab incision to the bone and the 4.0-mm trocar is removed.
   C. The surgical technologist loads the 4.0-mm calibrated drill bit onto the power drill and hands it to the surgeon, who drills through both cortices until the drill sleeve presses against the cortex.
   D. The locking bolt length is read from the calibrated drill and communicated by the surgeon to the surgical technologist.
   E. The locking bolt, protection sleeve, and screwdriver are handed to the surgeon for insertion of the locking bolt.
   F. The procedure is repeated for the second proximal locking bolt.
8. The distal locking bolt is now placed with the use of fluoroscopy.
   A. The C-arm is placed to show the most distal hole in the femoral nail.
   B. Using the #10 knife blade, a stab incision is made over the site of the distal hole.

(continues)

Procedure 21-11 (continued)

C. The surgical technologist loads the 4.0-mm drill bit and hands the drill to the surgeon. The drill bit is placed through the distal hole and a hole drilled through both cortices.

D. Using the depth gauge, the length of the locking bolt is obtained. The surgical technologist hands the surgeon the correct-size bolt, holding sleeve, and screwdriver for insertion of the bolt.

Procedural Consideration: The surgical technologist should help the surgeon remember to add 2–4 mm to the reading of the depth gauge to make sure the thread of the bolt engages the far cortex.

9. The insertion instruments are removed.

10. The surgical technologist hands the surgeon the hexagonal screwdriver and end cap to be threaded onto the proximal end of the nail.

    Procedural Consideration: The surgical technologist should be prepared to hand the surgeon the ratchet wrench to tighten the end cap.

11. The surgeon closes the stab incisions, and 4 × 4 dressing sponges are placed. The leg may be splinted.

Postoperative Considerations

Immediate Postoperative Care
- Patient is transported to the PACU.
- Patient is observed for local hemorrhage.
- Pain control is provided.

Prognosis
- No complications: Splint remains in place for 5–7 days; crutch ambulation begins within 7–10 days; nail is not removed until fracture is completely healed, which requires 12 months to 2 years.
- Complications: Postoperative SSI; delayed union; malunion; nonunion; bone marrow fat embolization; malrotation of femur; shortening of femur; failure of implant—breaks.

Wound Classification
- Class I: Clean

Knee Procedures

Procedure 21-12 Arthroscopy of the Knee Joint with Repair of Torn Meniscus

Surgical Anatomy and Pathology

- The patella is a sesamoid bone
  - The proximal quadriceps femoris tendon passes down bilaterally to the patella and inserts on the upper tibia; the patellar tendon originates on the distal portion of the patella and inserts on the tibial tuberosity and its fibers are continuous over the patella with the fibers of the quadriceps femoris tendon.
  - The posterior surface of the patella articulates with the femur.
- The capsule of the knee joint is attached as follows (Figure 21-20A):
  - Proximally to the lateral and medial condyles of the femur
  - Distally to the lateral and medial condyles of the tibia
  - Superior end of the fibula
- The capsule is stabilized as follows:
  - Anteriorly by the patellar and quadriceps tendons

PROCEDURE 21-12 (continued)

- Laterally and medially by the medial and lateral collateral ligaments
- Posteriorly by the popliteus and gastrocnemius muscles

- Two large **ligaments** located in the knee joint help stabilize the movement of the joint (Figure 21-20B, C). The ligaments are called the anterior and posterior cruciate ligaments and are located in the intercondylar region of the knee joint.
    - The posterior cruciate ligament (PCL) is attached to the posterior midline surface of the tibia and passes anteriorly, attaching to the medial condyle of the femur. The PCL prevents the femur from sliding anteriorly on the tibia, especially when the knee is bent.
    - The anterior cruciate ligament (ACL) is attached to the posterior lateral condyle of the femur and to a notch in the midline of the tibia between the tibial condyles. The ACL prevents the femur from sliding posteriorly on the tibia, prevents hyperextension of the knee, and limits the medial rotation of the femur when the leg is in a fixed position with the foot planted. A common injury of the knee is

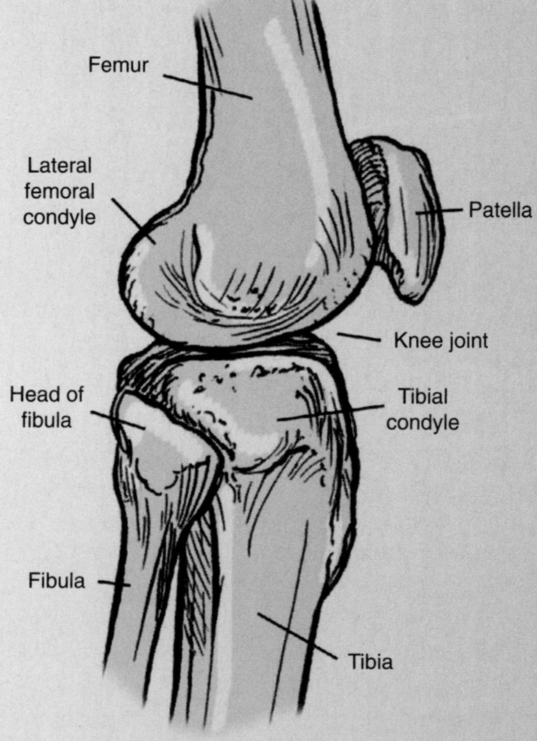

Figure 21-20 Knee: (A) Lateral,

(continues)

Procedure 21-12 (continued)

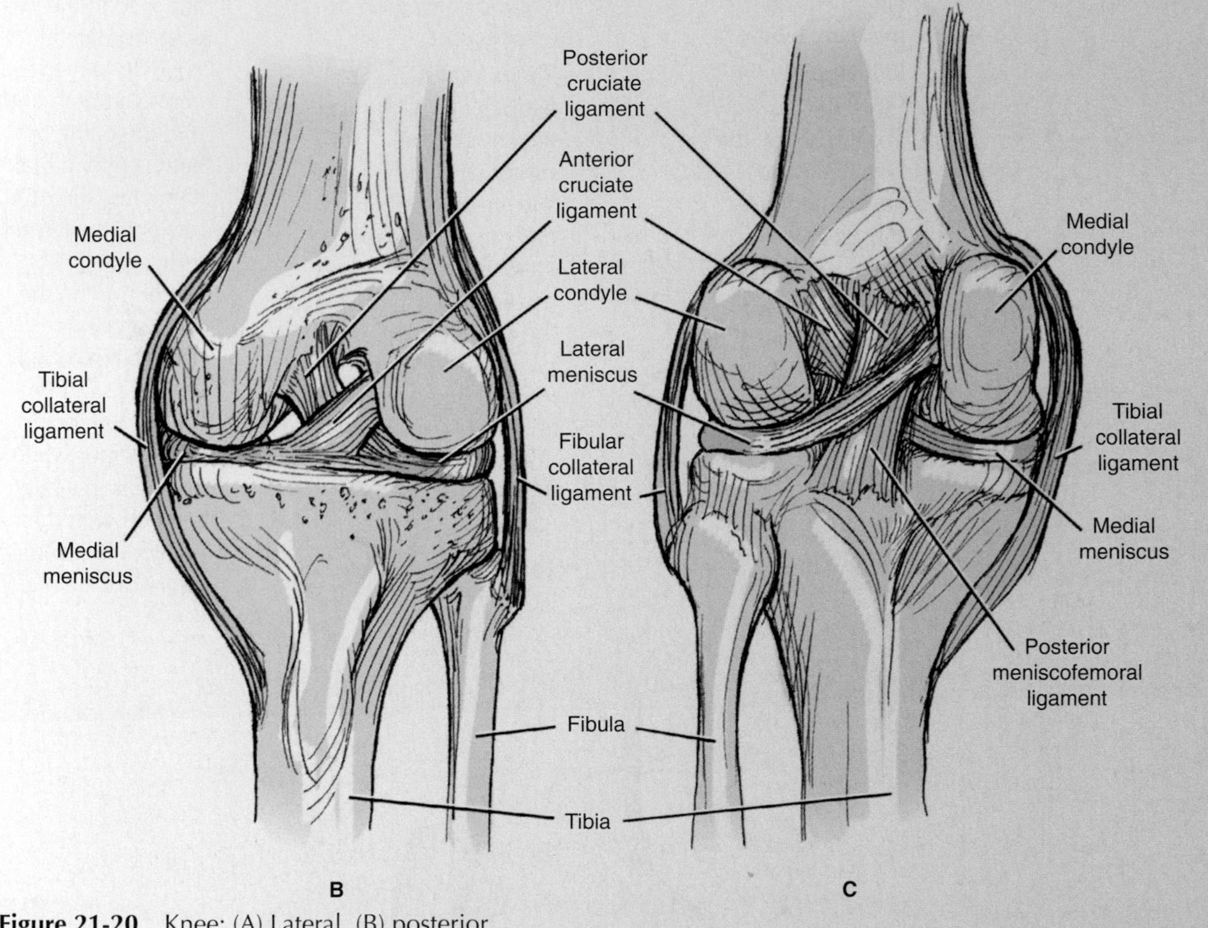

Figure 21-20 Knee: (A) Lateral, (B) posterior

a torn ACL, which requires surgery to either repair or replace the ACL.

- The knee joint is cushioned to withstand activities such as walking, jumping, and running by a pair of menisci called the lateral and medial meniscus.
    - The menisci are thick, crescent-shaped pads of cartilage that rest on the upper articular surface of the tibia. Injuries to the menisci, particularly athletic injuries, are common and result in various types of tears in the cartilage.
- The tibia, or shinbone, is the larger, thus stronger bone of the lower leg. It is located on the medial side.
    - Located at the proximal end of the tibia are the medial and lateral condyles that articulate with the condyles of the femur to form the knee joint.
    - Distally, the tibia articulates with the talus bone, forming part of the ankle joint.
    - Laterally, it articulates with the fibula.
    - The medial prominence at the ankle joint is called the medial malleolus.
- The fibula is located on the lateral side of the lower leg. It is a non-weight-bearing bone that serves as a site for attachment of ligaments and muscles of the lower leg.
    - A prominence called the lateral malleolus articulates with the talus bone to form the other

PROCEDURE 21-12 (continued)

portion of the ankle joint.

- Knee pathology is usually diagnosed by physical examination, with radiography (Figure 21-21A) and with MRI (Figure 21-21B).
- Knee arthroscopy is performed for diagnostic purposes, for removal of loose bodies that can cause the knee joint to lock in place, for shaving the patella and torn meniscus, and for insertion of instruments to perform a meniscectomy or repair.
- Injury to the menisci is one of the most common knee injuries (Figure 21-22).
  - Various types of tears can occur in the meniscus, the most common being what is called the *bucket handle* (see Table 21-2). The bucket handle consists of an incomplete longitudinal tear with displacement of the inner portion of the meniscus. When a tear of this type is encountered, an arthroscopic partial meniscectomy or repair can be completed.
- The goals of meniscal surgery are to preserve as much of the cartilage as

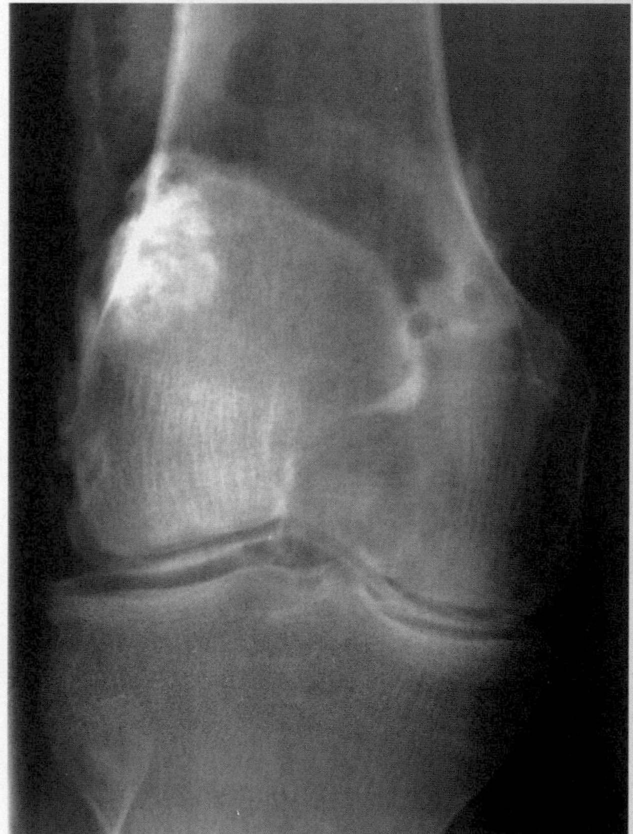

A

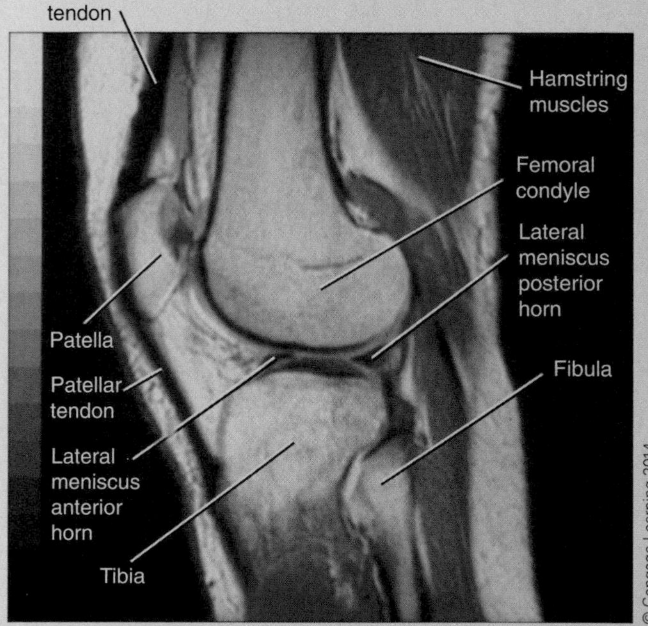

B

Figure 21-21 Knee diagnostics: (A) X-ray, (B) MRI

(*continues*)

PROCEDURE 21-12 (continued)

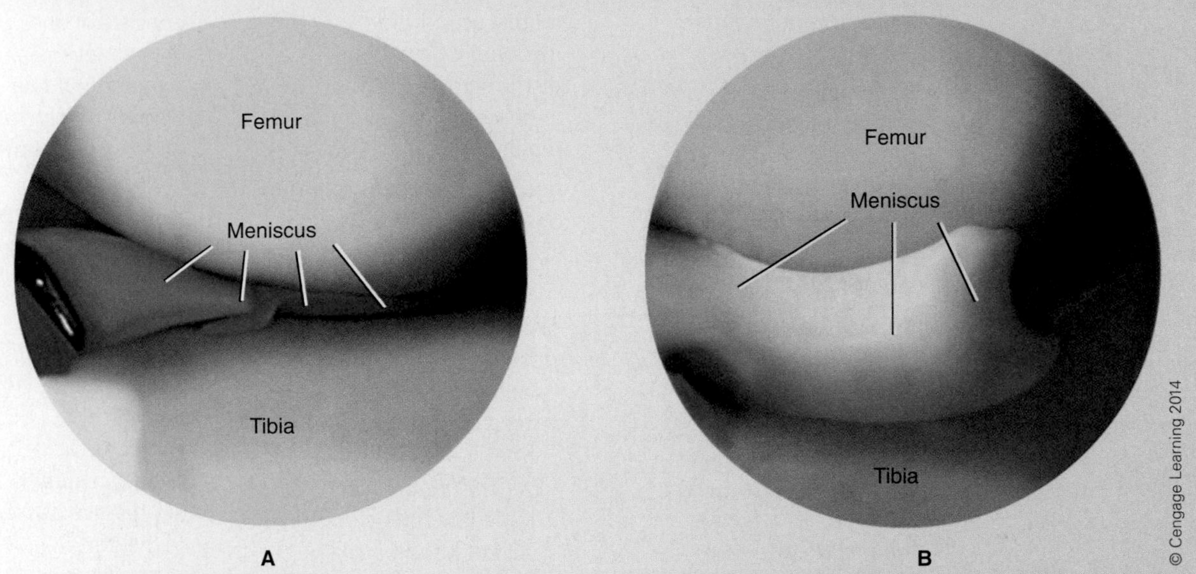

Figure 21-22 Torn meniscus: (A) Medial meniscus tear with fragment, (B) fragment dislocated into knee joint

	possible and to leave the rim of meniscus intact to aid in cushioning	and stabilizing the knee joint. • Extensive tears require a total	meniscectomy, but this leaves the knee somewhat unstable.
Preoperative Diagnostic Tests and Procedures	• See Table 21-4.		
Equipment, Instruments, and Supplies Unique to Procedure	• A-scope tower: Video monitor, light source, shaver power unit, recording device • Tourniquet and insufflators • Webril • Fluid pump • Minor orthopedic instrument set • Long Beaver knife handle with #64 blade • Arthroscopy instrument set: Includes nerve hooks,	probe (switching stick), scissors, punches, and arthroscopic "biters" including up-biter, down-biter, right-biter, left-biter, down-biter • 30° and 70° arthroscopes • Shaver with the following cutting tips: abraders, full-radius resector, side cutter • Meniscal repair instrument set • Meniscal suture	• #11 knife blade • 18-gauge spinal needle • 3000-mL bags of lactated Ringer's solution—need 6–7 bags available • 0.25% Marcaine with epinephrine • Arthroscopic back table pack • Dressing: 4 × 4 sponges, Kerlix, Ace bandage • Leg holding device/ stand for skin prep.

PROCEDURE 21-12 (continued)

Preoperative Preparation

- Position:
  - Supine
  - End of OR table may be lowered according to surgeon's preference.
  - A padded lateral post is attached to the side of the OR table approximately at the level of the mid-thigh of the operative leg to facilitate placing countertraction on the knee joint to open the medial side.
  - Webril and tourniquet are placed prior to the prep.
- Anesthesia: Continuous epidural block, spinal or general
- Skin prep: Starting at the knee joint, the entire leg circumferentially from the groin fold to the toes; a leg holding device/stand may be used for performing the prep.
- Draping: Extremity draping technique

Practical Considerations

- Prior to skin prep the surgeon will perform an EUA to confirm diagnostic findings.
- Have radiographic studies in the OR.
- Notify radiology department of possible intraoperative X-rays.
- Have C-arm near OR.
- Check arthroscopic equipment prior to the patient entering the OR.
- Arthroscopy pump tubing must be primed prior to use.
- The surgical technologist must be familiar with all of the arthroscopic equipment and supplies to ensure correct setup and assist the surgeon with connections such as camera placement on the arthroscope, light source cord connection on the arthroscope, and inflow tubing connected to inflow cannula. The surgical technologist must also be familiar with which ends of the cords to hand off to the circulating person.
- The surgical technologist must know the specialty meniscal repair instrumentation, including order in which it is used and how to load the suture, in order to prevent delay of the surgical procedure.
- The surgical technologist must know how to manipulate the leg and understand the directional terms the surgeon communicates in order for the surgeon to view the various compartments and structures of the knee joint.

Surgical Procedure

1. A #11 knife blade is used to make an incision that is lateral to the patellar tendon and just above the joint line.

   Procedural Consideration: Observe findings of diagnostic procedure; the location of the tear determines where the scope and instruments will be inserted. For a medial tear, the scope is inserted into the medial portal and the cannula is inserted into the lateral portal. The reverse is true for a lateral tear.

2. The irrigation/inflow cannula is inserted using the sharp trocar and/or blunt trocar according to the surgeon's preference.

   Procedural Consideration: Tubing leading from a bag of lactated Ringer's or saline solution is connected to the opening on the side of the cannula.

3. The joint is distended either by fluids entering the joint by gravity or with the use of the arthroscopy pump.

   Procedural Consideration: Finish passing equipment to the circulator to connect.

(continues)

PROCEDURE 21-12 (continued)

4. A second stab incision is made anterolaterally, allowing for insertion of the sharp trocar and sheath just inside the capsule of the knee.

   Procedural Consideration: Employ necessary sharps precautions for #11 blade and trocars.

5. The sharp trocar is removed and replaced with the blunt. The sheath is now advanced into the knee joint. The blunt trocar is removed and the 30-degree scope is inserted.

   Procedural Consideration: The camera is attached to the top of the scope and the light source to the side. Tubing attached to the inflow trocar is usually switched to the inlet valve/port on the side of the arthroscope sheath. The inflow trocar is now the outflow trocar.

6. For additional incisions, the surgeon inserts the spinal needle under direct vision as a guide to make an anteromedial stab incision.

   Procedural Consideration: This incision serves at the entry for inserting probes and instruments.

7. Beginning in the suprapatellar pouch, the patellofemoral joint is visualized. Next the medial and lateral aspects of the knee are viewed to examine the menisci and ACL.

   Procedural Consideration: Assist with leg stabilization as needed. Remote control may be used to document procedure with still photos.

8. The probe or nerve hook is inserted. It is used to determine if the menisci and ACL are intact or have suffered a tear.

   Procedural Consideration: The shaver may be used to shave the posterior surface of the patella that displays a frayed appearance due to osteoarthritis. Gently pressing down on the patella will aid the surgeon in shaving the movable patella.

9. The scope is inserted in the opposite portal (medial side of knee joint) to complete the examination by looking at the medial femoral condyle, medial meniscus, and posterior cruciate ligament.

   Procedural Consideration: A common tear of meniscus is the "bucket handle" tear.

10. The rest of the steps describe the repair of a meniscal tear. A probe is inserted to identify and free the torn section of the meniscus.

    Procedural Consideration: An 18-gauge spinal needle may be used to identify a fourth incision site.

11. A clamp is inserted to grasp the torn meniscus. A cutting instrument such as the Beaver knife or arthroscopic scissors is used to resect the meniscus (Figure 21-23).

    Procedural Consideration: The surgical options are to resect or repair. Adjust instrumentation according to the surgeon's decision.

12. An arthroscopic biter or arthroscopic shaver with side cutting blade can be used to smooth the edge of the torn area and create an even line of tissue.

    Procedural Consideration: If the meniscal tear is going to be repaired, the instrumentation from the meniscal repair set will be used. The instrument set will contain various cannulas that are straight or curved; the type of cannula required is determined by the location of the tear.

Procedure 21-12 (continued)

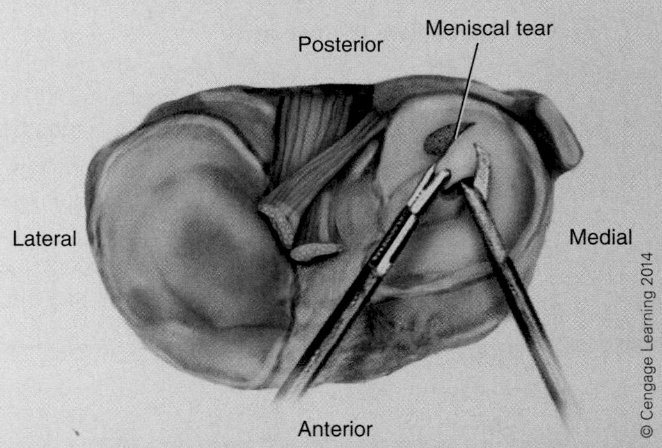

Figure 21-23 Arthroscopic meniscal resection

13. The cannula is positioned and each needle with suture is inserted into the cannula, through the meniscus, and across the tear, forming a loop of suture over the tear.

    Procedural Consideration: Meniscal repair kits are commercially available that contain two Keith needles attached by suture. The suture of preference is usually 0 or 2-0 Vicryl, PDS, or Prolene.

14. The needle is passed through the anterolateral portal so the sutures pass through the medial meniscus.

    Procedural Consideration: The surgical technologist may be asked to operate the camera while the surgeon performs the repair.

15. The needle tips are palpated under the skin and the surgeon, using a #15 knife blade, makes a small incision in order to pull the suture out of the knee joint.

    Procedural Consideration: After the sutures are placed, the knee is flexed and extended to ensure that the range of movement is not constricted. Watch sterile field carefully during manipulation. A needle holder may be used to initially grasp and deliver the needle from the wound.

16. The needles are cut off and the suture is tied to bring the torn edges of the meniscus together.

    Procedural Consideration: The sutures are usually tied with the knee extended. Prepare for closing while the sutures are tied.

17. At the end of the procedure, the fluid is allowed to freely flow through the knee joint, thoroughly irrigating the site.

    Procedural Consideration: Small pieces of tissue that are not irrigated out can get wedged in the joint, causing the knee to lock into place.

18. The sheaths are removed. The wounds are closed.

    Procedural Consideration: Adson tissue forceps and needle holder with suture are used to close the portals; ½-in. Steri-Strips are applied over the incision sites. It is a routine practice for the surgeon to inject a local anesthetic, usually 0.25% Marcaine, within the joint to aid in postoperative pain management.

(*continues*)

PROCEDURE 21-12 (continued)

Postoperative Considerations	**Immediate Postoperative Care** • Patient is transported to the PACU. • Patient is usually discharged the same day. **Prognosis** • No complications: No weight bearing with use of crutches for 5–7 days; passive exercises leading to full ROM in 3–4 months. • Complications: Postoperative SSI including local joint infection; hemorrhage; reinjury due to noncompliance with rehabilitation. **Wound Classification** • Class I: Clean

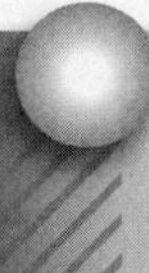

PEARL OF WISDOM

Be sure all videoscopic equipment is in working order prior to use.

- Prime fluid pump.
- Balance camera color field.
- Be sure cable/electrical connections are secure.
- Be sure camera remote has charged batteries.

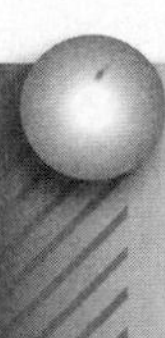

PEARL OF WISDOM

If the surgical technologist is required to operate the camera or stabilize the extremity during the repair, be sure all necessary items are within the surgeon's reach.

PROCEDURE 21-13 ACL Repair

Surgical Anatomy and Pathology	• The ACL averages a length of 38 mm and width of 10 mm and is made up of collagen fibers.
	  • The blood supply to the ACL is from the middle genicular artery, and innervation is from the tibial nerve.
	  • The femoral attachment is the medial aspect of the lateral femoral condyle in the intercondylar notch.
	  • The ACL inserts into the interspinous area of the tibia.
	  • It is an important stabilizing structure and the most frequently injured ligament of the knee.
	• ACL tears often occur in younger athletic patients who play basketball and football; in older patients, the tears are most often from skiing injuries.
	  • The tear is usually due to noncontact deceleration that produces a **valgus** twisting injury. An example is an athlete who places the foot and pivots in a quick manner in the opposite direction.

Preoperative Diagnostic Tests and Procedures	• See Table 21-4. • MRI is used as an aid to diagnose and confirm an ACL tear. • Several clinical diagnostic tests can

PROCEDURE 21-13 (continued)

	also be used as aids in diagnosing a tear. • A popular test is the Lachman test, and the following is a description for a tear of the right knee. The knee is placed in 15° of flexion and slight external rotation to relax the iliotibial band. The surgeon will place the right hand on the medial side of the calf while the left hand grabs the	lateral aspect of the thigh. The right hand pulls the lower leg slightly in an anterior direction, while the left hand pushes the upper part of the leg slightly posteriorly. In this way, the surgeon can determine if a tear has occurred and the millimeters of displacement. • If the patient does not respond to	rehabilitation, exercises, and other nonoperative treatment, arthroscopic repair has become the standard for surgical treatment. ACL repair involves replacement of the ligament with autograft, synthetic ligament, or allograft. Autografts are most often used and include patellar tendon graft (the most frequently used), iliotibial band, or semitendinosus tendon.
Equipment, Instruments, and Supplies Unique to Procedure	• Basic orthopedic instrument set • Knee arthroscopic instrument set • A-scope tower • ACL guide system • Bone tunnel plugs • Fixation device: bone screws, staples or spiked washers—surgeon's preference • Power drill • Microsagittal saw • Drill bit box	• Sagittal saw blade • Tourniquet and insufflator • Webril • Fluid pump • Long Beaver knife handle with #64 blade • 30° and 70° arthroscopes • Shaver with the following cutting tips: abraders, full-radius resector, side cutter	• #11 and #15 knife blades • 18-gauge spinal needle • 3000-mL bags of lactated Ringer's solution—need 6–7 bags available • 0.25% Marcaine with epinephrine • Arthroscopic back table pack • Dressing: 4 × 4 sponges, Kerlix, Ace bandage
Preoperative Preparation	• Position: • Supine • End of OR table may be lowered according to the surgeon's preference. • A padded lateral post is attached to the side of the OR table approximately at the level of the mid-thigh	of the operative leg to facilitate placing countertraction on the knee joint to open the medial side. • Webril and tourniquet are placed prior to the prep. • Anesthesia: Continuous epidural block, spinal or general	• Skin prep: Starting at the knee joint, the entire leg circumferentially from the groin fold to the toes; a leg-holding device/stand may be used for performing the prep. • Draping: Extremity draping technique

(continues)

PROCEDURE 21-13 (continued)

Practical Considerations	• Prior to skin prep the surgeon will perform an EUA to confirm diagnostic findings. • Have radiographic studies in the OR. • Notify radiology department of possible intraoperative X-rays.	• Have C-arm near OR. • Check arthroscopic equipment prior to the patient entering the OR. • Arthroscopy pump tubing must be primed prior to use.	• The surgical technologist must be familiar with all of the arthroscopic ACL specialty instrumentation in order to be able to correctly set it up and assist the surgeon.

Surgical Procedure

1. A diagnostic A-scope will be carried out to confirm the diagnosis and perform any preliminary procedures such as repairing a meniscal tear. Refer to Procedure 21-12, Knee Arthroscopy. The rest of this discussion concentrates on the ACL repair.

2. Notchplasty

   A. The portion of the ACL that remains is debrided using a full-radius resector attached to the A-scope shaver.

   B. A notchplasty can be performed using a 4.5-mm arthroplasty burr, osteotome, and rasp.

   C. Notchplasty widens the anterior portion of the intercondylar notch by removing 3–5 mm of bone and recessing the roof of the intercondylar notch to prevent impingement on the ACL graft.

3. ACL graft choice: Graft selection is based on the surgeon's preference, graft availability, and the patient's choice. There are two types of grafts: autograft, which is a graft taken from the patient's own tissue, and allograft, which is tissue taken form another person (cadaver). Steps 4–7 describe if the surgeon decides to use the patellar tendon, hamstring, quadriceps tendon, or allograft.

   A. The surgeon continues the procedure by making a small incision on the distal lateral portion of the femur downward to the lateral aspect of the femoral condyle.

   B. The femoral aiming device is positioned and the guide pin is inserted at the femoral site into the posterior and superior area of the intercondylar notch.

   C. A second anterior incision is made that is medial to the tibial tubercle below the knee.

   D. The tibial aiming device is positioned and the guide pin is inserted on the anterior tibial incision into the intercondylar notch, just medial to the site of ACL attachment to the tibia.

   E. The pins are now replaced with #1 or #2 suture that is passed through the pin sites. The surgeon then moves the knee through a series of motions to confirm that the measurements of the aiming devices are correct.

4. Patellar tendon harvest and preparation

   A. A longitudinal incision is made near the patellar tendon. Small self-retaining retractors are placed to expose the tendon.

   B. The surgeon inserts a Cushing periosteal elevator (also referred to as a Joker) underneath the tendon and moves it proximally and distally to loosen the tendon from its attachments.

(continues)

PROCEDURE 21-13 (continued)

C. The surgeon uses either a marking pen or the cautery to outline a 1-in. long patellar and tibial bone plugs. Two 2-mm holes are drilled in the patellar and tibial bone plugs.

D. Using the microsagittal saw, the surgeon begins the removal of the central one-third portion of the patellar tendon with the 2.5-cm tibial and patellar bone plugs. The bone saw is initially used for the harvest, but the task is completed with a ¼-in. curved osteotome.

E. The surgical technologist should clear a small area on the back table where the surgeon may prepare any type of graft that will be used for insertion (Figure 21-24). A green towel should be laid down to reinforce the area and prevent a tear in the sterile back table cover. The surgeon uses a tendon-sizing device to stretch the tendon to full length to aid in preparation.

F. The surgeon then uses curved Mayo scissors to debride the graft and size it to the appropriate width, usually 10–12 mm.

G. The sharp edges of the bone plugs may be gently crushed and formed with pliers. Additionally, the surgeon will mark the bone plugs with a marking pen or methylene blue stain to aid in visualization later in the procedure.

H. The surgeon will place heavy nonabsorbable synthetic sutures (usually #2 or #5 Ethibond) through the drill holes for the tibial and femoral tunnels.

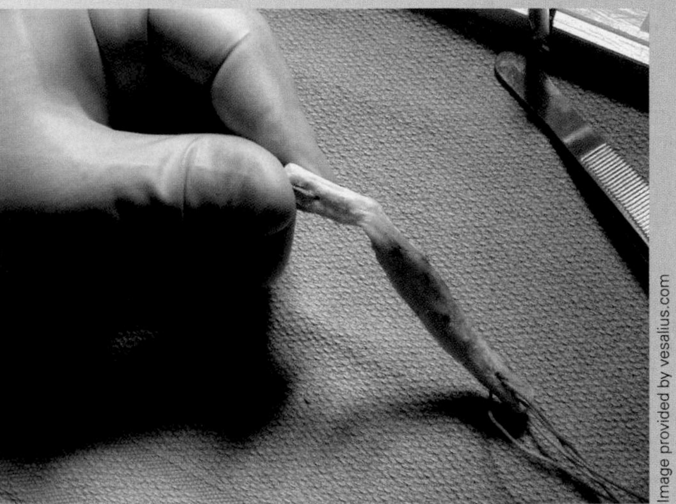
Image provided by vesalius.com

Figure 21-24 Preparing ACL graft on back table

5. Hamstring harvest and preparation

A. The incision for hamstring autograft is much smaller than for a patella tendon autograft. The 2- to 3-cm vertical incision is made approximately 4 cm inferior to the medial port.

B. The semitendinosis and gracilis are identified. A portion of the gracilis is dissected from the tibial insertion. A #2 polyester suture is placed in the distal end of the gracilis.

C. The tendon stripper is placed over the partially dissected gracilis. The surgeon carefully strips the gracilis from the patient's leg. The surgeon follows the same procedure to remove the semitendinosis.

(continues)

Procedure 21-13 (continued)

D. The surgeon dissects the muscle from the two pieces of graft. The hamstrings are folded in half to form a four-stranded graft. Sutures are placed in the folded ends of the graft. A #5 polyester suture is placed through the folded portion of the graft.

6. Quadriceps tendon harvest
   A. A vertical or horizontal incision is made just above the kneecap.
   B. The graft consists of harvesting the end of the tendon and a bone block from the anterior surface of the patella; therefore, the graft will have a bone block on one end and soft tissue on the other.
7. Allograft
   A. To reduce patient morbidity and recovery time, the use of allograft tissue can be a good alternative for an ACL reconstruction. The types of allografts include patella tendon, Achilles tendon, and anterior tibialis tendon. The grafts are removed and prepared the same as for autografts.
8. Femoral and tibial tunnels
   A. The two-incision approach is the established standard for A-scope ACL reconstruction as opposed to the one-incision technique that presents obstacles to proper placement of the graft.
   B. The lateral condyle is exposed in the second incision and Hohmann retractors are placed to protect the soft tissues and the vastus lateralis.
   C. An angled curette is used to create the starting point for the femoral tunnel.
   D. The guide pin is reinserted and overdrilled with the cannula to create a 10-mm tunnel. The tibial tunnel is created in the same fashion.
   E. The tunnels are smoothed using a curette or egg-shaped abrader placed on the A-scope shaver.
9. Graft insertion and fixation
   A. Prior to placing the graft each end of the graft is marked with a skin marker.
   B. The inflow should be turned off because the saline will cause the graft to expand.
   C. As one last step prior to graft insertion, the surgeon may use a pituitary rongeur to remove soft tissue that surrounds the outer portion of the femoral tunnel to facilitate passage of the graft.
   D. The smaller of the bone plugs is placed into the tunnel first, ensuring that the cortical side of the proximal bone plug is facing posteriorly.
   E. Under arthroscopic visualization, a Schnidt clamp is passed up the tibial tunnel to grab the stay sutures to pull them out of the tibial tunnel and help in passing the graft. The surgeon also confirms that the bone plugs are in place by viewing the blue marks that were made on the edge of each bone plug.
   F. Both ends of the graft are fixed with either staples, bone screws with spiked washers, interference screws, or bioabsorbable screws. The graft is fixed with the knee in 20–30° of flexion to maintain the physiological tension. Under A-scope exam the surgeon will confirm there is no impingement of the graft with the knee in full extension.

PROCEDURE 21-13 (continued)

10. Wound closure and postoperative rehabilitation
    A. Prior to wound closure, the joint is thoroughly irrigated.
    B. During the procedure the surgical technologist should have collected as many bone chips as possible that were created during the reaming of the femoral and tibial tunnels. The surgeon may place the chips in the defect caused by the harvesting of the patellar tendon as an aid in healing. A bone tamp may be used to keep the chips in place.
    C. Other options from which surgeons can choose are either not repairing the tendon at all or repairing the tendon with a 0 Vicryl, simple or horizontal mattress suture technique. Regardless of the choice, the paratenon, the synovial material between a tendon and its sheath, must be repaired. The rest of the wound closure is accomplished in the usual fashion for knee surgery procedures.
11. Dressing is placed: Xeroform dressing, 4 × 4 dressing sponges or Fluffs, Kerlix, and Ace bandage. A hinged knee brace may be placed–surgeon's preference.

Postoperative Considerations

Immediate Postoperative Care

- Patient is transported to the PACU.
- Pain management is provided.

Prognosis

- No complications: During the postoperative period up to the eighth week the patient will use crutches or a cane for assisted ambulation in combination with rehabilitation that includes ROM exercises, straight leg raises, TENS unit, toe raises, and minisquats. By 2 weeks postoperative, the patient should be able to obtain 0° of extension and 90° of flexion by 4 weeks.
- Complications: Postoperative SSI; postoperative prolonged immobilization or poor compliance with rehabilitation can lead to loss of achieving full ROM; anterior knee pain is the most common chronic complication; surgical failure of the graft due to poor surgical technique; chronic effusion; of allograft is used complications include risk of acquiring hepatitis or HIV and graft rejection.

Wound Classification

- Class I: Clean

PROCEDURE 21-14 Above-the-Knee Amputation (AKA)

Pathology

- Amputations are most often performed because of trauma or disease that inhibits a good vascular supply to the extremity.
  - Diabetic patients, who are prone to nonhealing ulcers and poor vascularity to the extremities, are at risk for amputation, in particular of the foot and leg.
- Nonischemic limbs are amputated due to bone or bone marrow tumor, trauma, infection, or congenital defect.
- The goal of the surgery is to preserve as much of the movement of the proximal leg as possible and to allow the patient to eventually ambulate with a prosthesis. However, the health of the patient often determines if he or she will be a good candidate for a prosthesis.

(continues)

PROCEDURE 21-14 (continued)

Preoperative Diagnostic Tests and Procedures	• History and physical • Standard X-rays		
Equipment, Instruments, and Supplies Unique to Procedure	• Basic orthopedic instrument set • Power saw • Oscillating saw blade • Nitrogen tank • Batteries if cordless power saw is being used	• Liston amputating knife (Figure 21-25A) • Gigli saw (Figure 21-25B) • Satterlee bone saw (Figure 21-25C) • Large bone hook	• Tourniquet and insufflator • Culture tubes, aerobic and anaerobic • Closed wound drainage unit, usually HemoVac

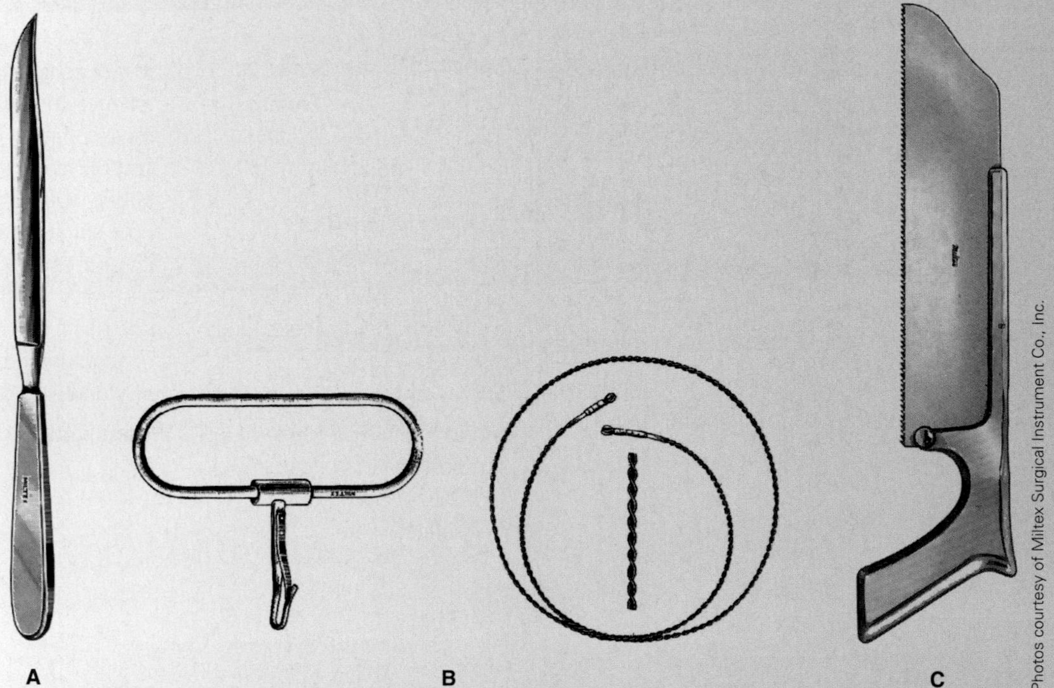

Figure 21-25 Amputation instruments: (A) Liston amputating knife, (B) Gigli-Strully saw handle and Gigli 12-in. saw, (C) Satterlee bone saw

Preoperative Preparation	• Position: Supine • Anesthesia: Continuous epidural block, spinal, general • Skin prep: The skin prep may not be performed on the part of the leg to be amputated due to sepsis; the section that will be removed can be isolated by covering and wrapping it with a Mayo stand cover and taping in place, or using a sterile plastic adhesive drape. The rest of the leg is prepped from the incision site up to the groin fold. If the entire leg is to be prepped and sepsis is present, follow the aseptic rule of clean to dirty; begin at the cleanest non-infected area and work towards the dirtiest (infected/gangrenous)

PROCEDURE 21-14 (continued)

	part of the leg. Perform a circumferential prep extending from the groin fold to the toes. The person responsible for holding the leg must be careful due to the condition of the gangrenous section of the leg; do not hold the leg by the toes as they may be in such	bad condition they could easily detach/amputate. Hold the leg underneath the heel. • Draping: Leave the Mayo stand cover or plastic adhesive drape in place. Perform a standard extremity draping technique using the impervious	stockinette, three-quarters sheets or split sheet, and extremity drape. Another Mayo stand cover may be placed around the section of leg to be amputated and used for handing off to the circulating person and transport to pathology.
Practical Considerations	• Have X-rays in OR. • Webril and tourniquet are applied prior to skin prep • Check to make sure batteries are placed in the charger the day before surgery if using cordless saw. The batteries must be sterilized the morning of surgery using immediate-use steam sterilization. • Check power equipment prior to the	patient brought into the OR. • Amputations are performed quickly in order to control hemorrhaging; consequently, the surgical technologist must be prepared to keep up with the surgeon during the procedure. The surgical technologist should have a large number of lap sponges ready for use on the sterile back table. The	surgical technologist may be required to help the surgeon in using the sponges to soak up blood and aid in exposure. • It should be confirmed with pathology department if amputated leg should be given to the family. Some religions require that the amputated portion be buried with the individual upon death.
Surgical Procedure	1. The level of the bone resection is approximately 4–6 inches proximal to the knee joint line. The surgeon will use a #10 knife blade to make an incision that is in the shape of the mouth of a fish. **Procedural Consideration:** The surgical technologist must be prepared to quickly hand Crile clamps to the surgeon for controlling bleeding as well as the electrocautery and DeBakay forceps.		
	2. Using sharp and blunt dissection, the surgeon creates two skin flaps: an anterior flap so the scar will be in the posterior, and a long adductor muscle flap that will be used to suture across the end of the resected femur.		
	3. The anterior muscles are transected with a #10 knife blade or Liston amputating knife.		
	4. The femur is now transected. The femoral periosteum is elevated with a Key elevator or #10 knife blade. The surgeon may use either a power saw, Gigli saw, or Satterlee bone saw. The posterior muscles are identified and transected.		

(*continues*)

Procedure 21-14 (continued)

Procedural Consideration: The surgical technologist must be prepared with several clamps and nonabsorbable suture ties for the surgeon to doubly clamp, ligate, and cut the major blood vessels.

5. The end of the sciatic nerve is clamped with a Schnidt clamp and ligated with cautery.
6. The posterior muscles are freed from their attachments to the femur with a Key elevator and the periosteum is cut circumferentially with the knife blade at the level of the femoral bone transection.
7. The surgeon uses a $^{7}/_{64}$ drill bit to drill holes into the cortex of the transected end of the femur.
8. The adductor flap is sutured across the femoral end, utilizing the drill holes, while the surgical technologist keeps the femur in adduction as the surgeon ties down the adductors.
9. A HemoVac drain may be place according to the, surgeon's preference. The surgeon will suture the quadriceps to either the posterior femur or adductor flap. While the surgeon is suturing the quadriceps in place, the surgical technologist will keep the femur in extension position to avoid hip flexion contracture.
10. A bulky dressing is placed.

Postoperative Considerations

Immediate Postoperative Care

- Patient is transported to the ICU for an overnight stay and then moved to the ward; hospitalization is 4–5 days.
- Patient may experience "phantom limb syndrome" (patient experiences discomfort or pain in the missing limb) and must be reassured.

Prognosis

- No complications: Stump is protected from weight bearing until the tissues have healed. Drain is removed 1–3 days after surgery. The dressing is changed in 7- to 10-day day intervals. The stump is usually well healed 3–4 weeks after surgery.
- Complications: Postoperative SSI; phantom limb syndrome causing a perceived severe pain; chronic effusion; necrosis of tissue.

Wound Classification

- Class I: Clean for nonischemic limb or,
- Class III or IV: Contaminated or Dirty-infected, respectively, due to presence of gangrene

Procedure 21-15 Below-the-Knee Amputation (BKA)

Note: Pathology, preoperative diagnostic tests and procedures, equipment, instruments, and supplies, preoperative preparation, practical considerations, and Postoperative Considerations are the same as for AKA.

Surgical Procedure

1. The surgeon makes an incision in the shape of the mouth of a fish approximately at the halfway mark of the lower leg. When the incision is extended across the tibial crest the surgeon deepens the incision to make a mark on the periosteum to serve as a landmark.

PROCEDURE 21-15 (continued)

2. The incision is carried through the deep fascia, but the surgeon is careful not to separate the skin and deep fascia from the underlying muscle.
3. Using sharp and blunt dissection, two flaps of the deep fascia and periosteum are formed, distal and proximal flaps, and reflected back over the tibia.
4. Using the landmark made with the knife in the periosteum, the surgeon determines the section of bone where the amputation cut will be made; the surgeon marks this point with the power saw.
5. Using a curved Kelly clamp, the surgeon identifies and places the clamp under the superficial peroneal nerve. Using the electrosurgery or knife blade, the nerve is divided.
6. Using electrosurgery and knife blade, the anterior compartment muscles are divided distal to where the bones will be cut in order to allow the muscles to retract and be flush with the end of the bone. As the muscles are being divided, the surgeon identifies and divides the anterior tibial vessels and deep peroneal nerve.
7. Before the surgeon resects the tibia and fibula, he or she uses a saw to bevel the tibial crest.
8. Using the saw, the tibia and fibula are transversely resected.
9. The distal segments of each bone are grasped with large bone-holding clamps and pulled anteriorly and distally to expose the posterior muscles. The muscles are divided to the level of the bone resection in order that they retract to the cut end of the bones. This also exposes the posterior tibial and peroneal vessels as well as the tibial nerve; the vessels are doubly ligated and divided.
10. Using the Liston amputation knife, the surgeon cuts the gastrocsoleus muscle in a bevel fashion so it forms a flap that is long enough to go across the end of the tibia.

    Procedural Consideration: The lower section of the leg is now completely amputated and is handed off to the circulating person; the surgical technologist should verbally confirm right or left leg with the circulator.
11. The ends of the tibia are smoothed in round fashion with a rasp.
12. The area is thoroughly irrigated to remove all bone debris and dust.
13. The tourniquet is released and bleeders are clamped and ligated or cauterized.

    Procedural Consideration: The control of bleeding is important prior to suturing the flaps over the ends of the bone. The surgical technologist must have several ties and clamps on hand for use. The surgical technologist may be responsible for using the cautery on a clamp and removing it while the surgeon is placing clamps on the other bleeders.
14. The gastrocsoleus muscle flap is brought over the ends of the bones and sutured to the deep fascia and the periosteum anteriorly.
15. The HemoVac drain is placed deep in the muscle flap and fascia and brought out laterally in the skin approximately 10–12 cm proximal to the end of the stump.
16. The skin flaps are trimmed with the knife blade and Metzenbaum scissors in preparation for suturing. The skin flaps are brought over the muscle flap and sutured together with interrupted nonabsorbable sutures.

Procedure 21-16 Total Knee Arthroplasty (TKA)

Pathology	• TKA is indicated for patients who demonstrate radiographic intra-articular disease and severe knee pain or other symptoms that cannot be controlled by nonsurgical methods (Plate 21-1). • The normal surfaces may have become damaged due to disease, such as degenerative joint disease, or through years of wear and tear, such as in athletes who are involved in impact sports. • When pain, limping, and joint dysfunction become so severe that the individual's daily living is affected and nonsurgical therapy is not providing adequate relief, surgery is the next option. • The knee is one of the more difficult, challenging joints for which an implant system has been developed. The reason is because the knee motion occurs in three planes: (1) abduction and adduction, (2) extension and flexion, and (3) rotation. In addition, the knee prosthetic system should preserve the normal ligaments while replacing the worn bone surfaces. The goal of the procedure is to restore normal function of the joint and relieve chronic pain.
Preoperative Diagnostic Tests and Procedures	• Physical examination is very important to determine if the pain is at a level of debilitation that justifies performing a TKA. It is also of importance to rule out an alternate diagnosis and avoid performing a TKA that would not relieve the symptoms of the primary condition. • Nuclear scans and aspiration of fluid from the knee joint for culture in the lab to rule out any presence of infection • Standard anteroposterior and lateral X-rays of the hip joint • Surgeon will create plastic overlay templates using the standard X-ray marking measurements that show the size of implants that will be needed.
Equipment, Instruments, and Supplies Unique to Procedure	• Nitrogen tank • Batteries if cordless power drill and saw are used • Extra gloves for surgical team • Space suits • Basic orthopedic instrument set or basic TKA instrument set (the following instruments listed may be included in the basic TKA instrument set) • Rake retractors • Richardson retractors • Curettes • Serrated rongeur • Lambotte osteotomes • Gouges • Rasps • Mallet • Pulse lavage • PMMA kit • Closed cement mixing system with suction tubing • Brush tip for placement over regular suction tip for lavage • 4 × 4 radiopaque sponges soaked in thrombin • Cement gun • Power drill and saw • Oscillating and reciprocating saw blades • Tourniquet and insufflator • Drill bits • #10 knife blades × 3 • GelFoam available in OR. • TKA instrument trays that include trial prostheses and specialty instrumentation

PROCEDURE 21-16 (continued)

Preoperative Preparation	• Position: Supine with sandbag taped in position on the OR table in order for the surgeon to flex the leg and place the heel on the bag to keep the leg in position • Anesthesia: Continuous epidural block, spinal, or general • Skin prep: Starting at the knee joint region extending upward to the lower border of the tourniquet and the entire leg and foot. A foot-holding stand may be used for performing the prep. • Draping: (1) Operative leg is elevated by the circulator; (2) three-quarter sheet is placed under the leg on the OR table; (3) sterile towel is wrapped around lower edge of tourniquet and held in place with penetrating towel clip; (4) toes of foot are grasped within the impervious stockinette. The circulator steps away and the stockinette is unrolled down the leg, covering the sterile towel; (5) split sheet is placed along lower border of thigh tourniquet with the split ends going toward the head of the patient. The split ends are brought around and placed together by the adhesive; (6) extremity drape is placed.
Practical Considerations	• All radiographic studies including X-ray templates should be in the OR. • The surgical technologist should confirm the day before surgery that the specialty instrument trays and trial prostheses arrived and are being sterilized. The first thing on the morning of surgery the surgical technologist should confirm everything has been sterilized. • There are several types of knee arthroplasty systems offered by various orthopedic medical companies. The surgical technologist must find out prior to surgery the system that will be used; the surgical technologist must be familiar with the instrumentation and the order in which it is used. The manufacturer can be contacted for procedural information to study and the sales representative can be consulted. • The surgeon's preference usually dictates which company's system will be used. Because each system requires specific instrumentation, there is no "universal" set of knee instruments. • Knee implants are divided into three different categories based on the section of the knee to be replaced: unicompartmental, bicompartmental, and tricompartmental. Unicompartmental implants are used to replace either the medial or lateral side of the corresponding articular surface of the femur and tibia. Bicompartmental implants replace the medial and lateral surfaces of the femur and tibia. Tricompartmental implants replace the medial and lateral surfaces of the femur and tibia, including the patella. • Tricompartmental implants are further subdivided into categories: (1) Unconstrained implant: Requires minimal resurfacing of the tibia and femur, and good collateral and posterior cruciate ligaments; (2) semiconstrained implant: Used when there is a difficulty with ligament balance; (3) fully constrained implant: Implant is jointed

(continues)

PROCEDURE 21-16 (continued)

together by hinges and only allows motion in a sagittal plane. Used when there is a severe deformity with the ligaments or for TKA revisions.

- Some surgeons may have the team remove the outer gloves of the double-gloving and replace after draping. Studies have shown that the highest risk for breaks in sterile technique during orthopedic procedures is during draping due to the complicated draping procedures.
- Some surgeons may have the team remove the outer gloves and replace just prior to the permanent implants being opened and implanted.
- Confirm on the day of surgery that the blood bank received the blood order and it is ready for use. The surgical technologist must keep careful track of the irrigation that is used in order to help in determining the amount of blood loss.
- Check the nitrogen level in the nitrogen tank or make sure the batteries are charging the day before surgery for the cordless power instruments. The batteries must be sterilized the morning of surgery by immediate-use steam sterilization.
- Test the power equipment prior to the patient entering the OR.
- Ask surgeon if he or she will want X-rays taken in the OR before transporting the patient to the PACU or the X-rays taken in the PACU.
- The day before surgery make sure the batteries for air flow for the space suits are charging.
- Health care facility policy must be followed for recording the prostheses that are implanted.
- The permanent implants must not be opened until the surgeon requests the prostheses and communicates the types and sizes.
- It is suggested that the surgical technologist use two Mayo stands, one for instrumentation and the other for power equipment and specialty knee instrumentation.
- It is suggested that new saw blades and drill bits be used for each TKA procedure. Often the medical company whose TKA system is being used will provide new saw blades and drill bits.

Surgical Procedure

1. Incisions
   A. An anterior midline skin incision is made with the knee in flexion (Plate 21-3).
   B. The standard retinacular incision is a medial parapatellar approach. It is extended proximally the length of the quadriceps tendon around the medial aspect of the patella, and extends 3–4 cm onto the anteromedial surface of the tibia, along the border of the patellar tendon.

   Procedural Consideration: When preparing the instruments and equipment the surgical technologist should confirm that the saw blade and drill bits are of the correct size, and fit in the cutting slot or drill holes of the cutting guides.

2. The medial side of the knee is exposed by stripping the anteromedial knee capsule and medial collateral ligaments off the tibia with a curved osteotome.

   Procedural Consideration: The surgical technologist may be asked at times to stabilize the leg/ foot while it is flexed and the foot is positioned against the bump.

PROCEDURE 21-16 (continued)

3. The leg is extended and the patella everted. The lateral patellofemoral plicae and adhesions are released with the Mayo scissors.

   Procedural Consideration: The surgeon will frequently use electrocautery for hemostasis and electrosurgery for soft tissue dissection. The surgical technologist should make sure to keep the Bovie pencil blade clean.

4. The knee is again flexed and the remaining meniscus and ACL are excised with Mayo scissors and a rongeur. Osteophytes on the rim of the femur and tibia are removed with a rongeur.

   Procedural Consideration: The surgical technologist should be prepared to remove bone and tissue bits from the rongeur when the surgeon is removing the osteophytes.

5. Femoral preparation
   a. An opening is created in the femoral canal with a 3/8-in. drill bit.
   b. The intramedullary (IM) reamer (also referred to as the T-handle reamer) is inserted into the femoral canal while irrigation and aspiration with the pulse lavage is repeated several times to reduce the risk of fat embolism (Plate 21-4).

   Procedural Consideration: The surgical technologist should keep clean laparotomy sponges on the sterile field throughout the procedure.

6. Femoral alignment
   a. The valgus angle is set on the valgus angle alignment guide. The guide is attached to the IM reamer, rests against the distal femoral condyle, and is secured.
   b. The guide is locked in place by tightening a large screw (Plate 21-5).
   c. The distal resection crosshead is locked onto the valgus alignment guide by tightening the locking screw with a hexagonal screwdriver (Plate 21-6).

   Procedural Consideration: During the femoral resection retractors are kept in place to protect the patellar tendon, MCL, LCL, and all other soft tissues such as muscle.

7. Femoral resection
   a. The distal femoral resection is performed.
   b. The valgus angle alignment guide and IM reamer rod with T-handle are removed.
   c. The distal femur is resected using the appropriate-size saw blade. The surgeon will place the saw blade through the standard resection guide (Plate 21-7).
   d. The pins or drill bits are removed and the crosshead is removed.

   Procedural Consideration: The surgical technologist should load the appropriate-size saw blade in anticipation of its use by the surgeon. Test the saw prior to handing it to the surgeon; the team members should be told that the saw is being tested so as not to startle them with the noise. The safety locking device should then be kept in place until the surgeon is ready to use the saw.

8. Femoral sizing
   a. The anterioposterior (AP) femoral sizer is placed flush against the resected distal femur and adjusted so that the feet rest against the posterior condyles, and the point of the stylus barely touches the most prominent aspect of the anterior cortex just proximal to the anterior condyles. The AP femoral sizer is a template for indicating the placement of the pins for the AP cutting guide (Plate 21-8).

(continues)

Procedure 21-16 (continued)

b. The holes that were previously created in the distal femur are redrilled to accept the fixation pegs of the femoral resection block.

Procedural Consideration: The surgical technologist should always have extra pins available to stabilize the cutting blocks and sizers.

9. Anterior and posterior resections

c. The calipers are used to measure the size of the femoral resection block. The fixation pegs and pins are used to hold the cutting block flush against the distal femur (Plate 21-9).

d. The anterior, posterior, and chamfer cuts are made with the appropriate size saw blade.

e. The cutting block is removed.

Procedural Consideration: The surgeon will communicate to the surgical technologist the correct size of femoral resection block that is needed for the anterior and posterior resections. When the surgeon is cutting bone, the surgical technologist should irrigate the bone with the Asepto syringe to prevent the bone from being overheated by the cutting action of the saw, thus causing charring and thermal necrosis of the bone.

10. Trochlear groove resection

f. The final femoral resection is performed. The trochlear groove resection guide is secured to the femur with pins (Plate 21-10).

g. The appropriate size saw blade is used for the resection.

h. The cutting guide is removed.

Procedural Consideration: The surgical technologist should be aware that the saw blade could become dull. An extra sterile saw blade should be available.

11. Tibial preparation

a. The ankle yoke is positioned and secured against the lower portion of the leg, proximal to the malleolus.

b. The tibial resection guide is positioned and centered on the proximal tibia and secured with pins (Plate 21-11).

12. Extramedullary tibial resection

a. The medial/lateral adjustment screw at the ankle is used to align the resection guide parallel to the tibia.

b. The stylus is attached to the crosshead and the crosshead adjustment knob is turned to raise or lower the crosshead until the level of the resection is indicated by the stylus.

c. Pins are used to fix the crosshead to the proximal tibia.

d. An alignment rod is used to check alignment to the ankle.

e. The appropriate-size saw blade is used for the tibial resection (Figure 21-26; Plates 21-12 and 21-13).

13. Tibial sizing

a. The tibial trial handle is attached to the trial base and placed against the proximal tibial surface (Plate 21-14).

(continues)

Procedure 21-16 (continued)

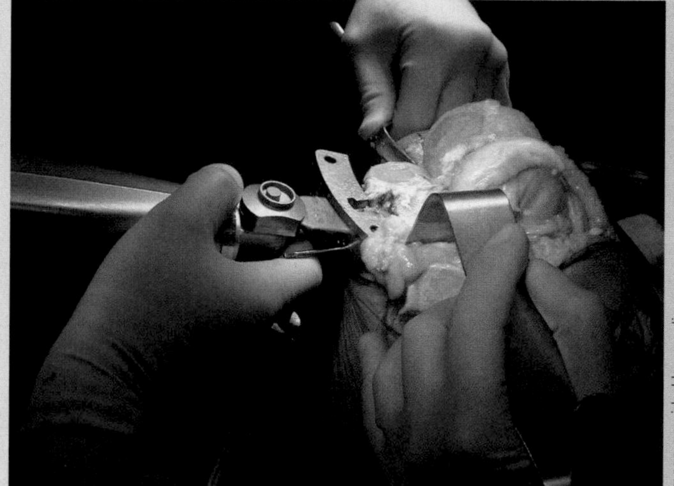

Figure 21-26 Tibial resection

b. Alignment is confirmed by inserting the alignment rod through the handle to check the alignment to the ankle (Plate 21-14).

c. The entry hole for the tibial stem is prepared using the appropriate-size drill guide and reamer (Plates 21-15 and 21-16).

d. The keel punch guide is attached to the keel punch handle and secured to the trial base.

e. Using the mallet, the keel punch on the keel punch handle is hammered into place through the guide until the punch is fully seated (Plate 21-17).

f. Once the punch is seated, the keel punch handle is removed, leaving the tibial trial base and stem in place for trial reduction.

14. Patellar preparation

a. For patellar preparation, the patella is laterally retracted with the articular surface facing upward.

b. The calipers are used to determine the size of the patella and amount of bone that will need to be resected (Plate 21-18).

c. Once the size of the patella is determined, the patella cutting guide is placed. The purpose of the cutting guide is to ensure the proper cut of the patellar apex is made.

d. Using the appropriate-size saw blade, the patellar cut is made (Plate 21-19).

e. The patellar peg holding guide is placed flush onto the resected patella and the peg holes are drilled using the appropriate-size drill bit (Plate 21-20).

15. Trial reduction

a. Keeping the knee flexed, the appropriate-size femoral trial is placed on the distal femur using the femoral impactor and mallet.

b. The appropriate tibial trial insert is snapped into place on the trial base.

c. The surgeon puts the knee through a series of motions to confirm normal joint movement and alignment.

(*continues*)

PROCEDURE 21-16 (continued)

d. Once the correct fit and alignment of the trials are confirmed, the trial components are removed. The joint is copiously irrigated with the pulse lavage.

e. The surgeon injects the cement on the cut bone surfaces and the prostheses are placed.

Procedural Consideration: Once the trial reduction has been completed, the surgeon will communicate the size of the prostheses that are needed. Before opening the implant containers, the surgical technologist should confirm the correct sizes with the surgeon. The surgical technologist will receive the prostheses from the circulator.

While the surgeon is irrigating the bone surface in preparation for placement of the implants, the surgical technologist should ask the surgeon when the bone cement should be mixed.

When the surgeon has finished irrigating the cut bone surfaces with the pulse lavage and is ready for the cement, the surgical technologist should replace the laparotomy sponges on the field with clean ones.

16. Implant insertion (Plate 21-21)
    a. The femoral implant is inserted with the femoral impactor and mallet.
    b. The metal tibial base is inserted with the tibial base impactor and mallet.
    c. The patellar implant is secured with bone cement and held in place with the parallel patellar recessing clamp.
    d. The tibial polyethylene insert is seated and locked into place on the metal tibial base.
    e. The leg is placed in 35° of flexion and the cement is allowed to harden.

Procedural Consideration: The surgeon will use a Freer elevator, smooth forceps, and/or knife blade to trim excess cement from around the prostheses. The surgical technologist should keep a small piece of cement on the back table and let the surgeon know when it has hardened.

17. Wound closure and dressing (Plates 21-22–21-24)
    a. The surgeon will thoroughly irrigate the wound.
    b. The tourniquet is released and hemostasis is achieved with electrocautery.
    c. The surgeon's preference will determine if a closed-suction drainage device will be placed.
    d. The wound is closed in layers.
    e. A bulky compressive dressing is placed.

Postoperative Considerations

Immediate Postoperative Care

- Patient is transported to the PACU.
- Patient is observed for hemorrhage.
- Pain management is implemented if necessary.

Prognosis

- No complications: Patient is discharged 3–4 days postoperatively. A rigorous physical therapy program may be ordered to assist the patient in gaining strength and maintaining balance. Assistive devices, such as a walker or cane, may be needed initially.
- Complications: Postoperative SSI; hemorrhage; deep vein thrombosis; restricted ROM; neurovascular complications related to tourniquet use; uneven leg length.

Wound Classification

- Class I: Clean

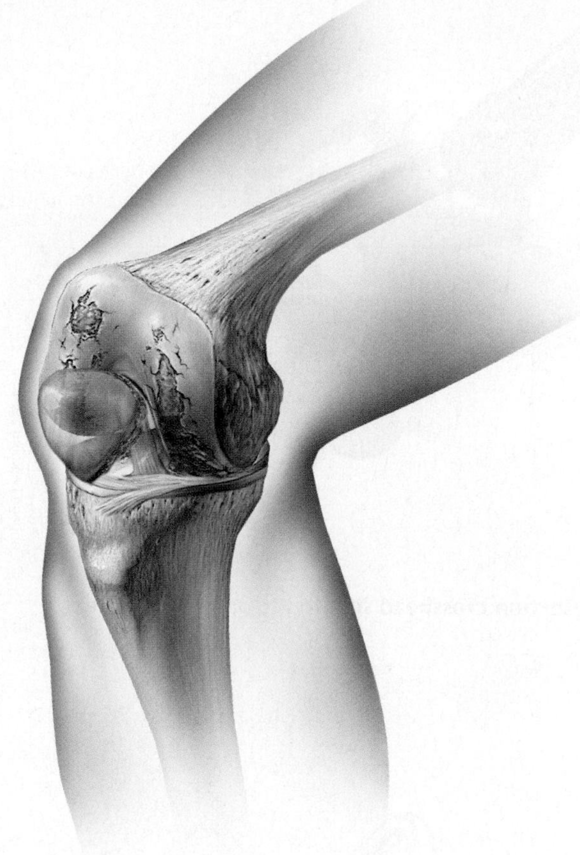

Intraarticular pathology of the knee joint

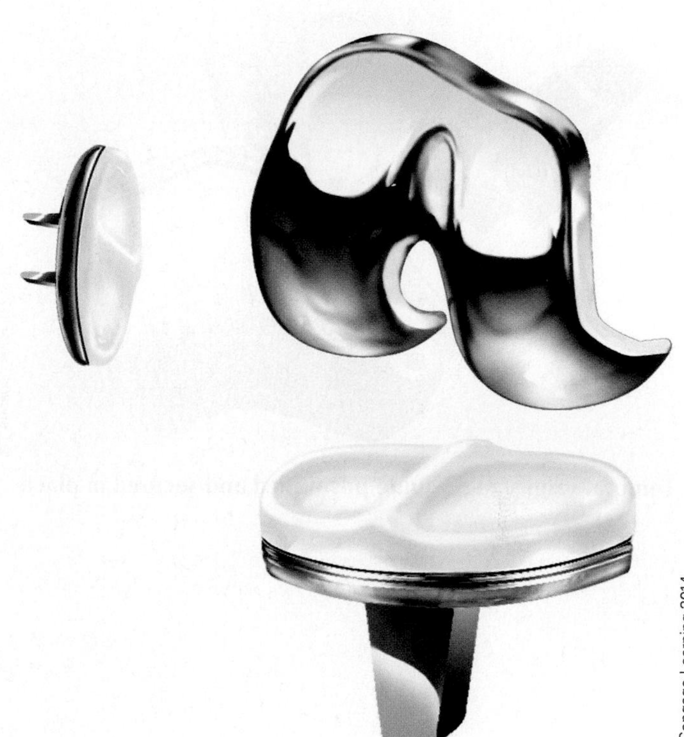

Prosthetic components

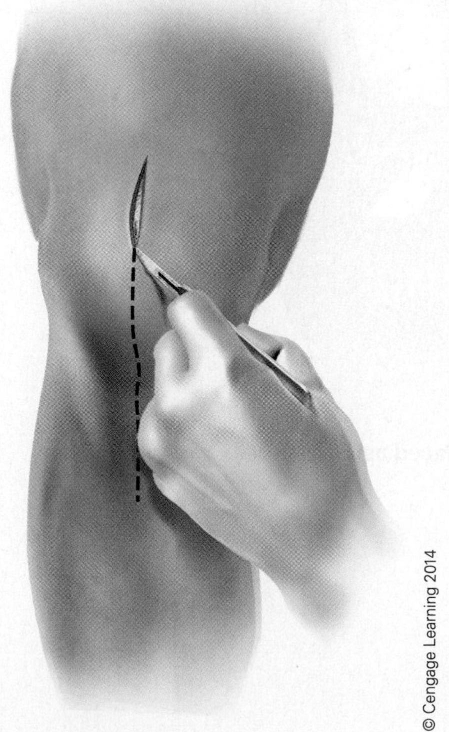

Anterior midline skin incision

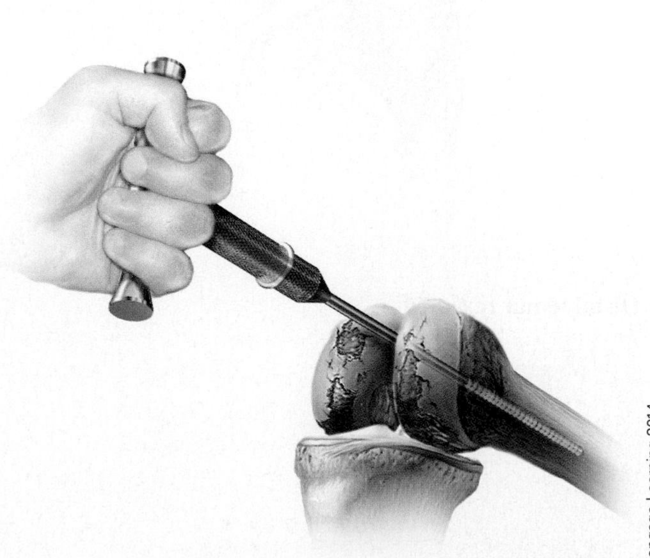

IM reamer placed into femoral canal

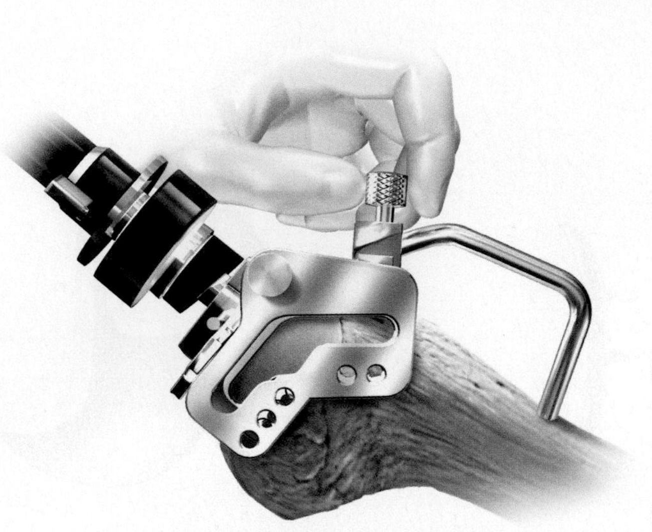

Femoral valgus angle guide positioned and secured in place

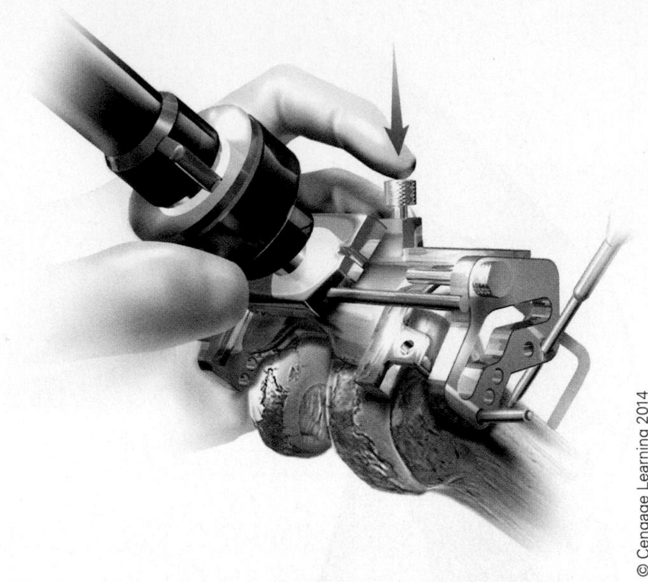

Distal resection crosshead secured to valgus alignment guide

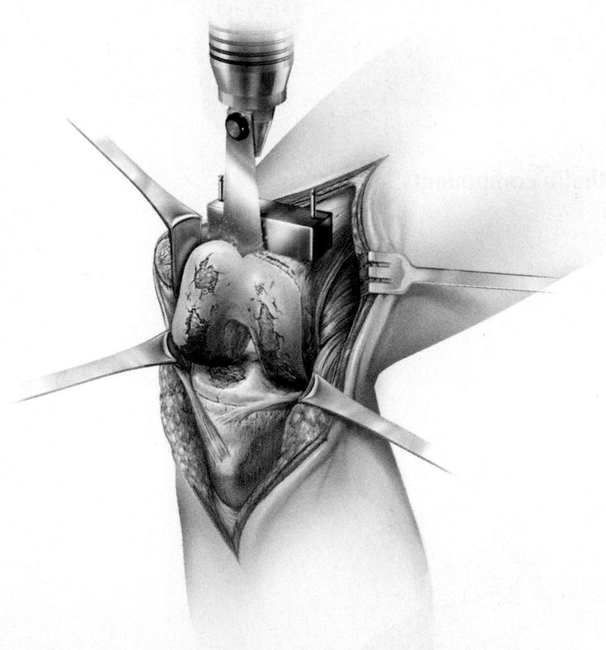

Distal femur resected

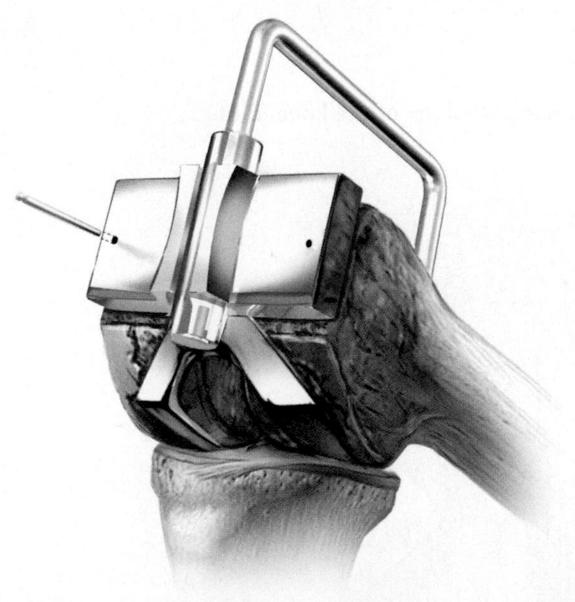

A-P femoral sizer placed against resected femur

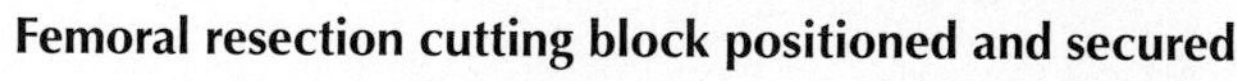

Femoral resection cutting block positioned and secured

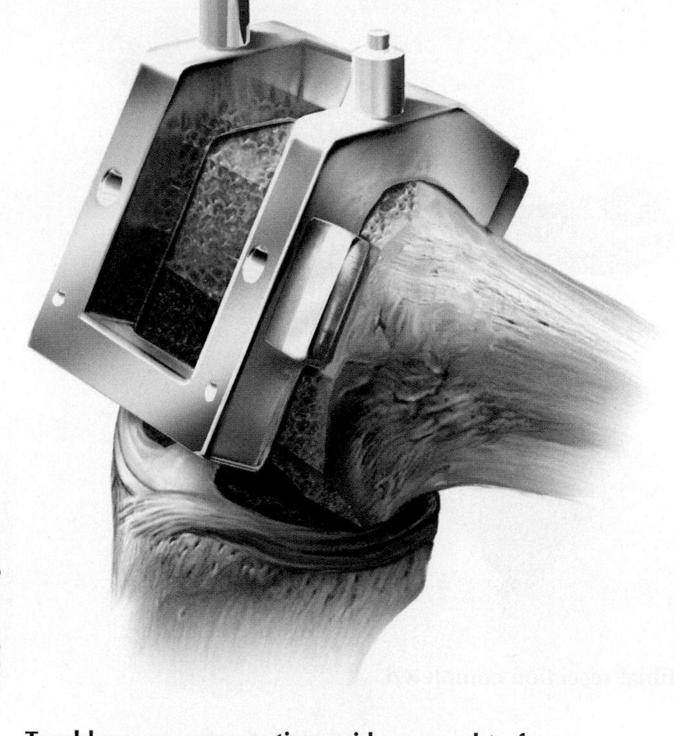

Trochlear groove resection guide secured to femur

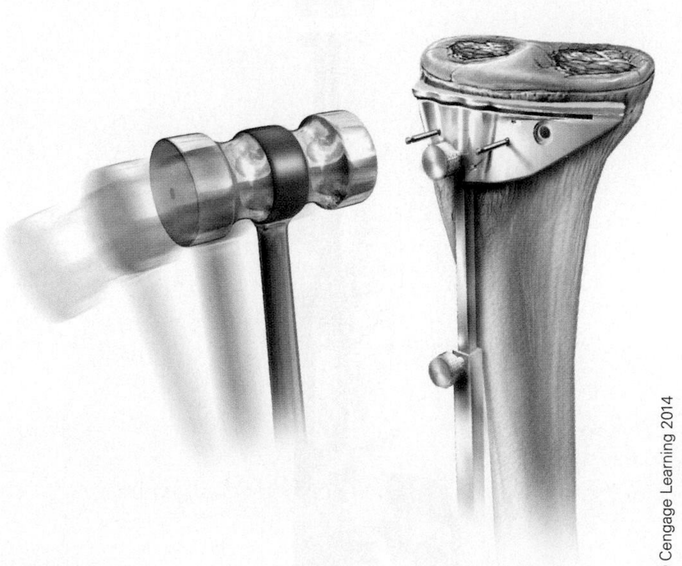

Tibial resection guide positioned and secured on tibia

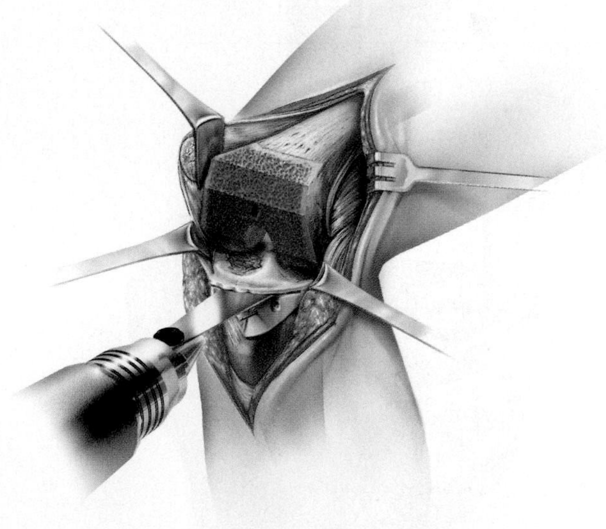

Tibial resection

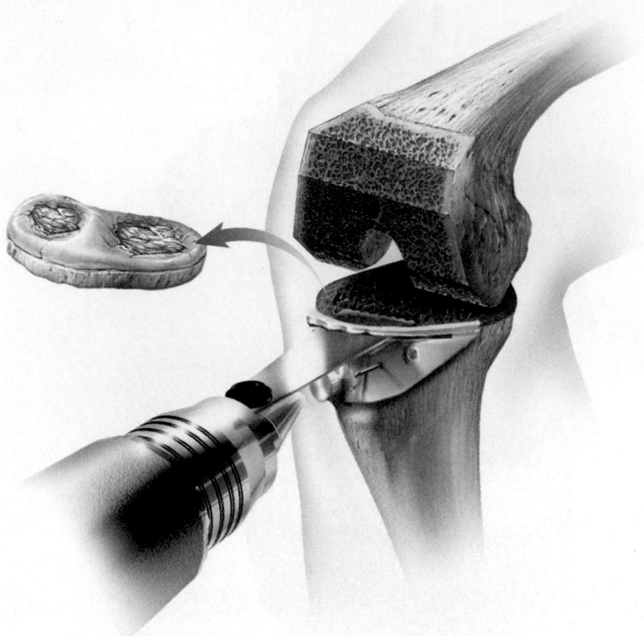

Tibial resection completed

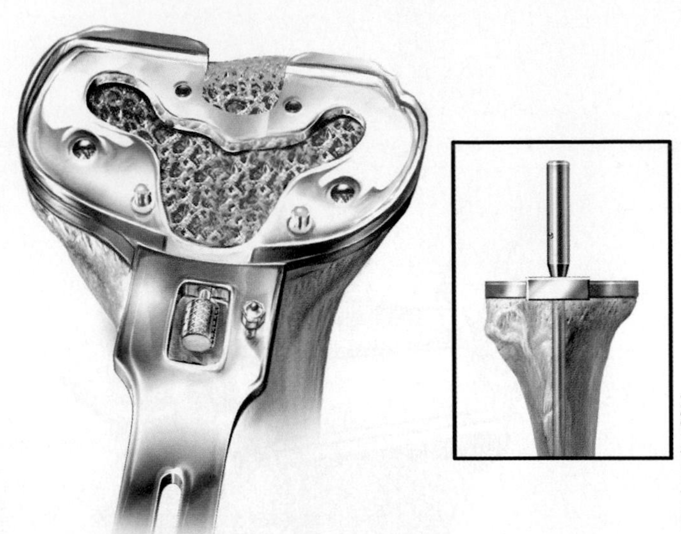

Tibial trial handle and trial base placed on tibial surface alignment confirmed with alignment rod

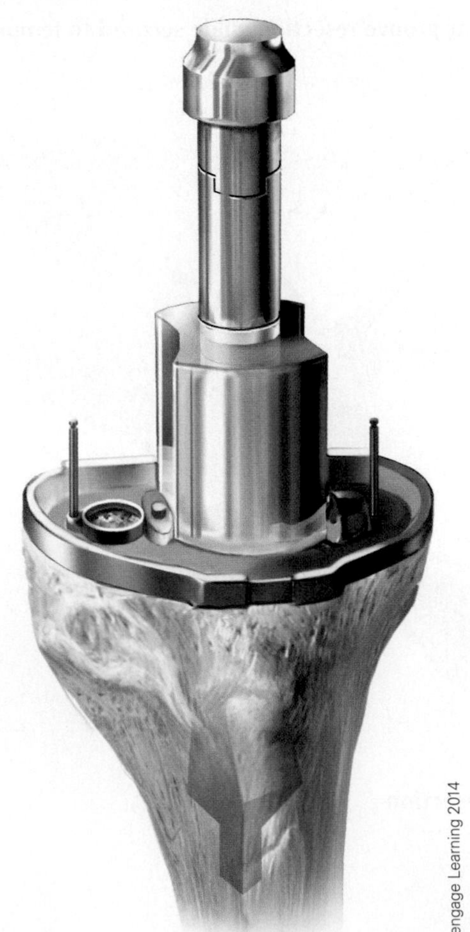

Entry hole for tibial stem prepared

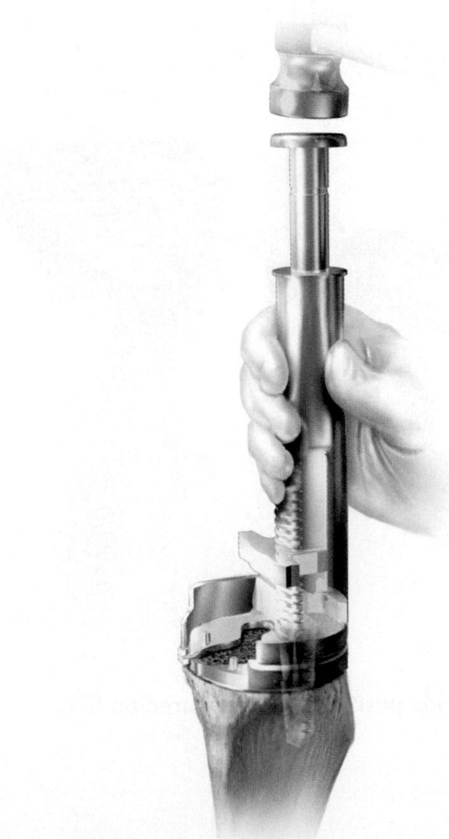

Entry hole for tibial stem completed

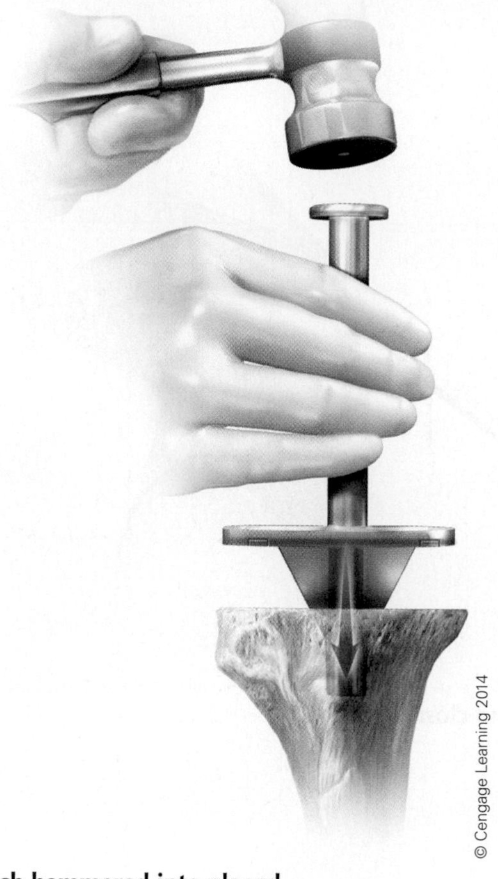

Keel punch hammered into placed

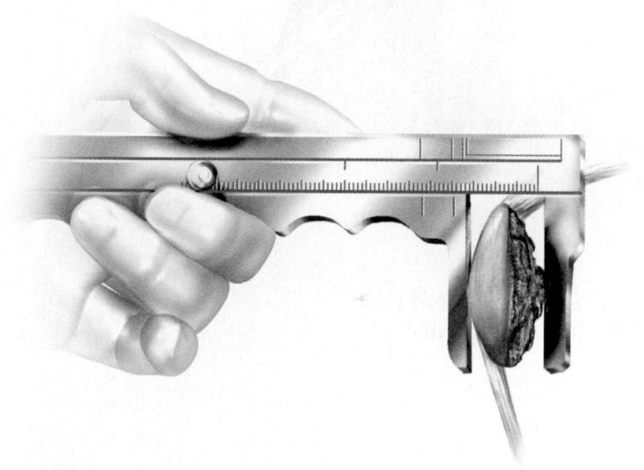

Calipers used to determine amount of bone to be resected

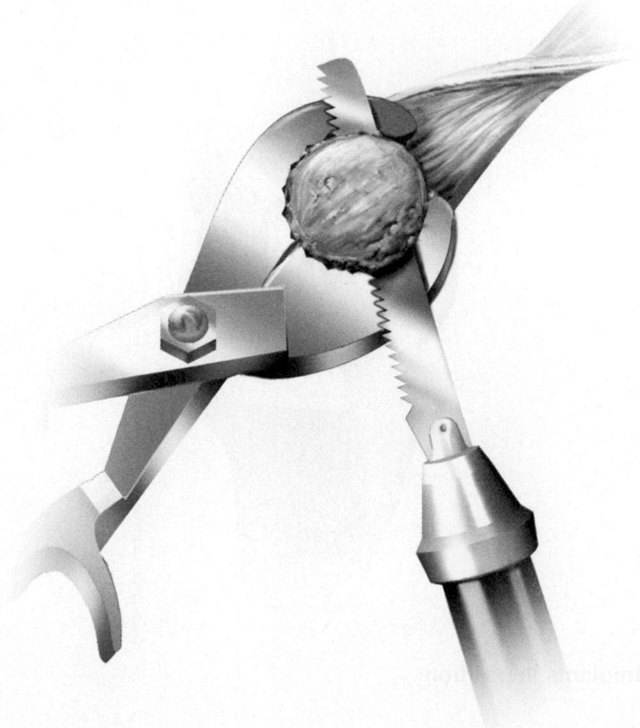

Patellar cut made

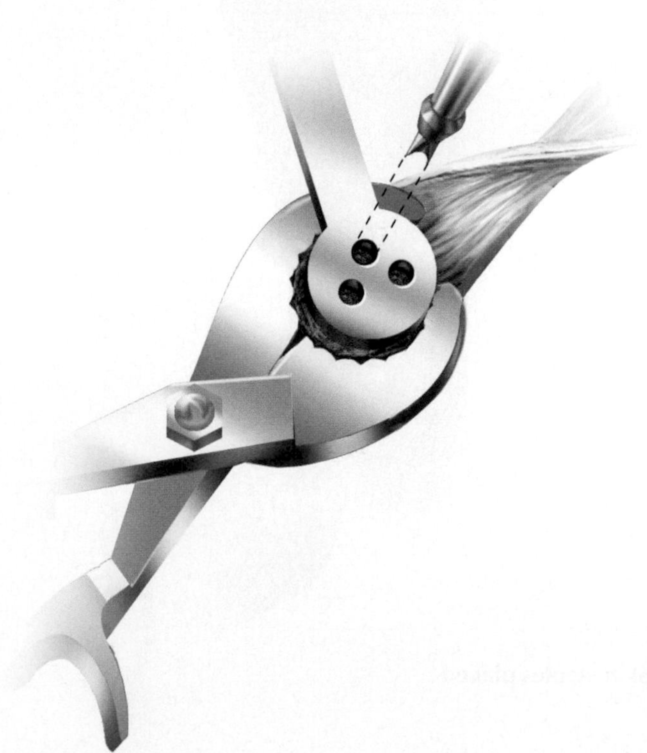

Peg holes drilled in resected patella

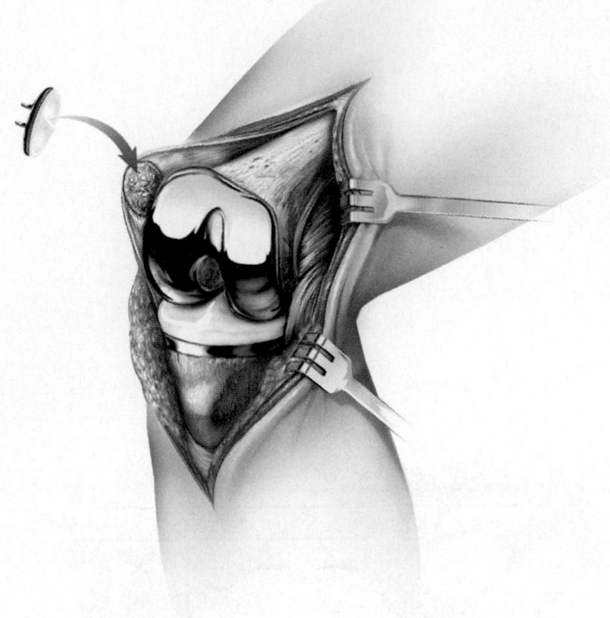

Insertion of implants

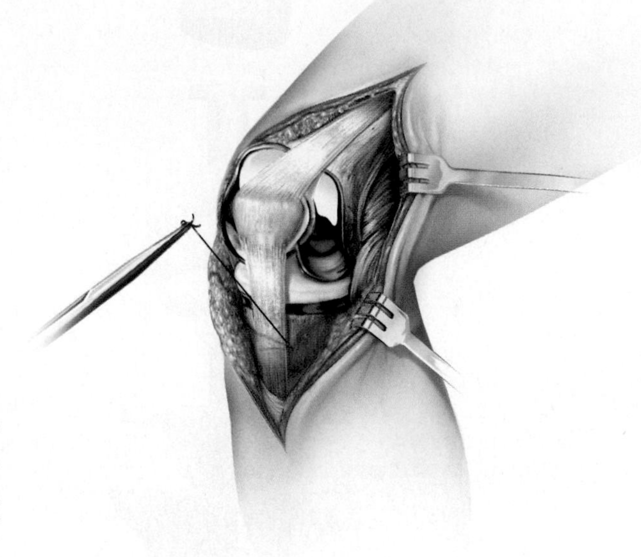

Wound closure

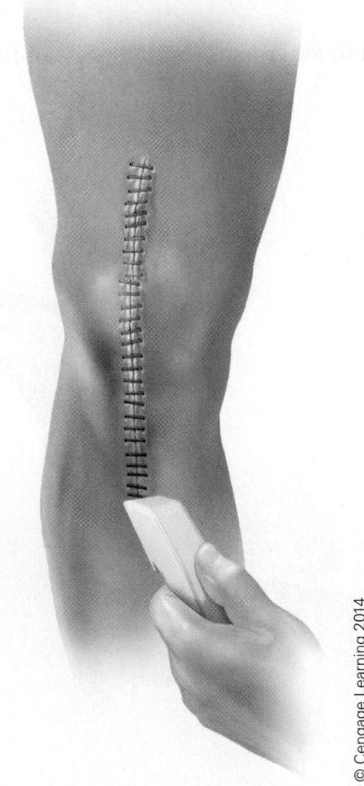

Skin staples placed

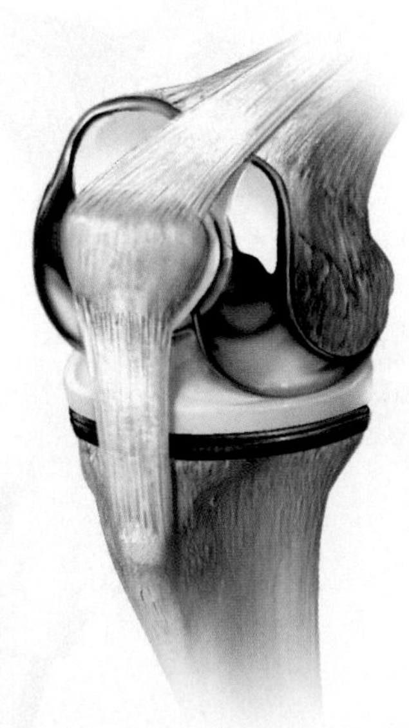

Implants in position

Ankle and Foot

Procedure 21-17 Triple Arthrodesis

Surgical Anatomy and Pathology

- The ankle joint consists of seven tarsal bones named as follows: calcaneus, navicular, cuboid, medial cuneiform, middle cuneiform, and lateral cuneiform (Figure 21-27).
- The largest of the ankle bones is the calcaneus, which is located inferiorly to the talus

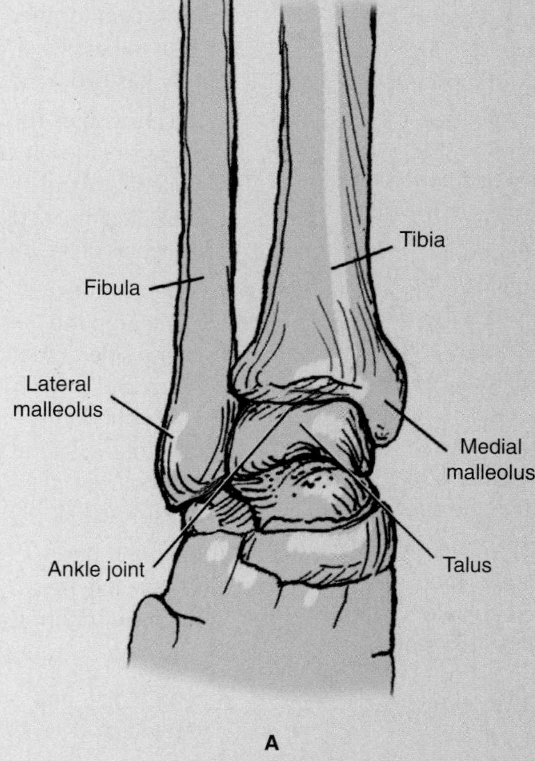

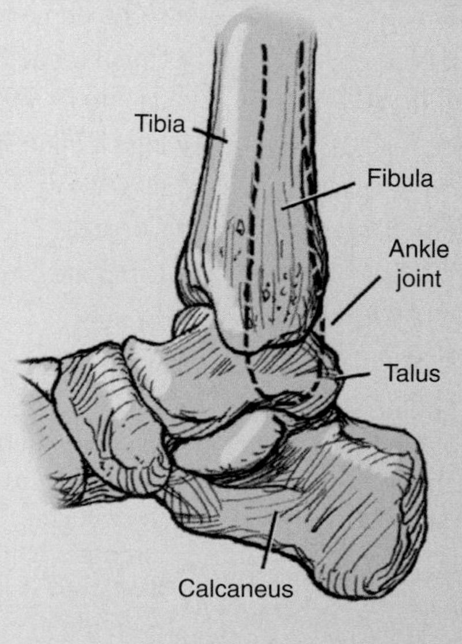

Figure 21-27 Ankle: (A) Anterior, (B) lateral

(*continues*)

Procedure 21-17 (continued)

	and forms the heel. A process located on the medial side of the calcaneous is called the sustentaculum tali, which serves to support part of the talus. The calcaneus aids in supporting the weight of the body and provides an attachment for the muscles of the foot. • The talus is a small bone that lies between the calcaneus and tibia and fibula. Where the talus meets the calcaneous and navicular bones is called the subtalar joint. • The five metatarsals are equivalent to the metacarpals of the hand (Figure 21-28). The distal ends of the metatarsals articulate with the first phalanges of the toes. The phalanges consist of three per toe except for the great toe, which only has two. • The ankle joint also consists of the lateral malleolus of the fibula and the medial malleolus of the tibia. • A depression located on the lateral side of the tarsus and distal to and at the same level of the lateral malleolus is called the sinus tarsi. • Triple arthrodesis is most effective for individuals suffering from a forefoot or hind foot deformity. • Such deformities are the result of clubfoot, rheumatoid arthritis, or poliomyelitis. • The procedure is contraindicated in children younger than 10–12 years of age because the procedure limits foot growth and has a high failure rate. • Postoperatively the procedure only allows plantar flexion and dorsiflexion. • The result of triple arthrodesis is the fusion of the subtalar, calcaneocuboid, and talonavicular joints.
Preoperative Diagnostic Tests and Procedures	• History and physical • Standard anteroposterior, anteromedial, and anterolateral X-rays
Equipment, Instruments, and Supplies Unique to Procedure	• Nitrogen tank • Batteries if cordless power drill is used • Extra gloves for surgical team • Basic orthopedic instrument set • AO compression plates and screws • Hohmann retractors • Crego retractors (Figure 21-29) • Inge lamina spreader (Figure 21-30) • Curettes • Lambotte osteotomes • Gouges • Rasps • Bone graft instruments • K-wires • Mallet • Power drill and saw • Tourniquet and insufflator
Preoperative Preparation	• Position: Supine with sandbag bump placed under the hip on the operative side • Anesthesia: Spinal or general • Skin prep: Starting at the ankle joint region extending upward to the midcalf circumferentially. The iliac crest is also prepped in case bone is needed for the bone grafting portion of the procedure. • Draping: Extremity draping technique except ensure the iliac crest is exposed.

PROCEDURE 21-17 (continued)

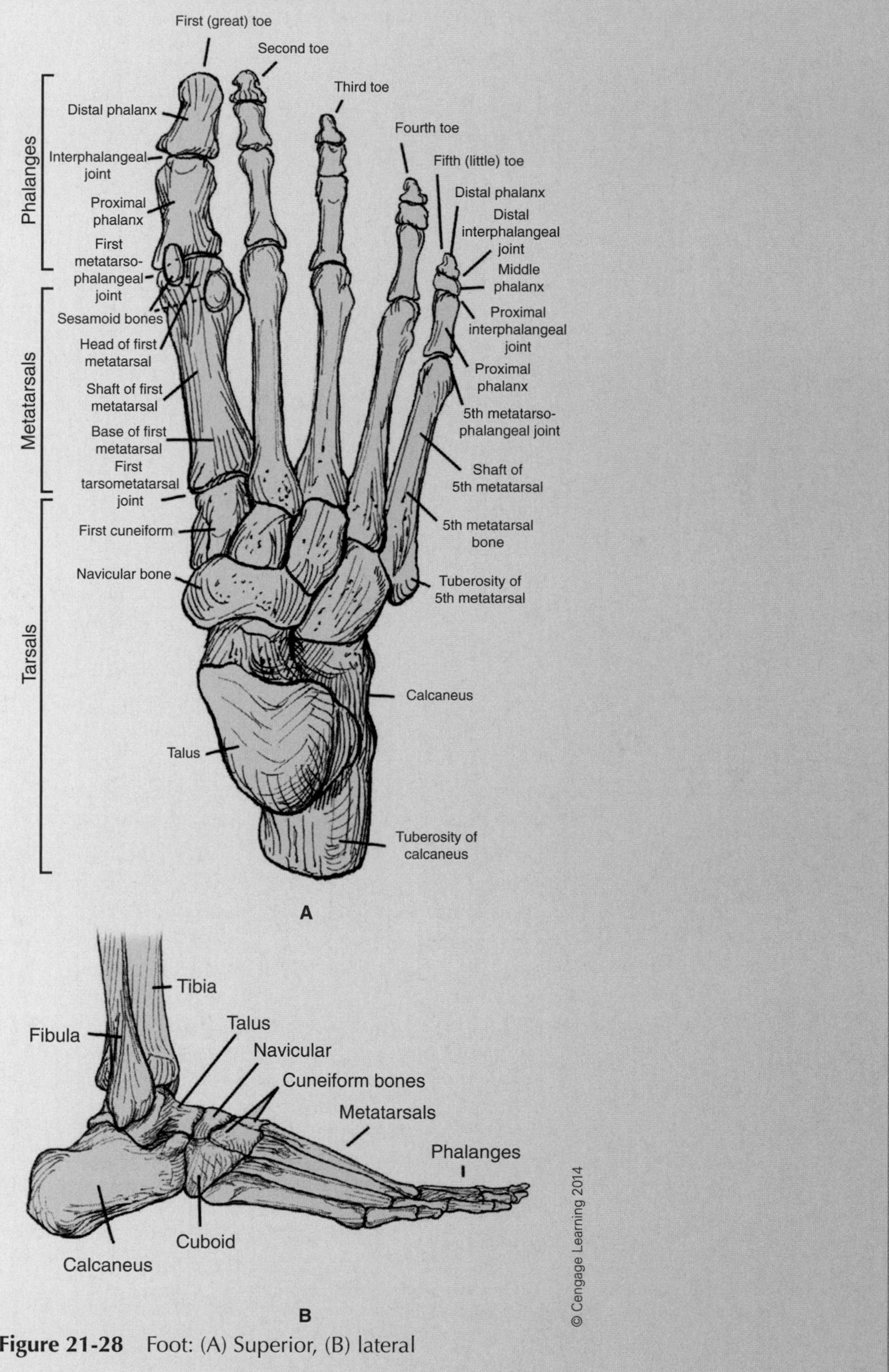

Figure 21-28 Foot: (A) Superior, (B) lateral

(continues)

PROCEDURE 21-17 (continued)

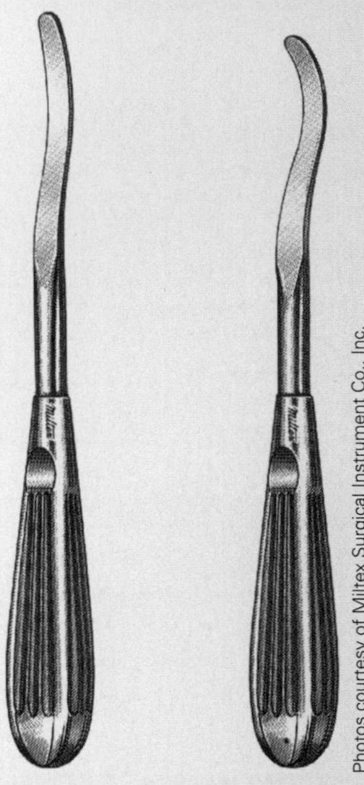

Figure 21-29 Crego periosteal elevators

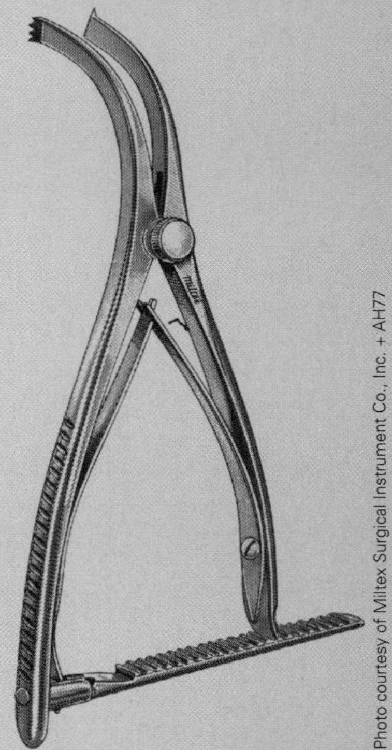

Figure 21-30 Inge lamina spreader, 6 in.

Practical Considerations

- Have radiographic studies in the OR.
- Some surgeons may have the team remove the outer gloves of the double-gloving and replace after draping. Studies have shown that the highest risk for breaks in sterile technique during orthopedic procedures is during draping due to the complicated draping procedures.
- Check the nitrogen level in the nitrogen tank or make sure the batteries are charging the day before surgery for the cordless power instruments. The batteries must be sterilized the morning of surgery by immediate-use steam sterilization.
- Test the power equipment prior to the patient entering the OR.
- Ask surgeon if he or she will want X-rays taken in the OR before transporting the patient to the PACU or the X-rays taken in the PACU.

Surgical Procedure

1. Depending on the surgeon's preference, the incision will be oblique, which parallels the subtalar joint, or anterolateral, which is a longitudinal incision between the tip of the lateral malleolus and the base of the fourth metatarsal.
2. The extensor digitorum brevis is resected from its point of insertion, and soft tissue dissection is continued with a #15 knife blade and rongeur.
3. The first resection is the subtalar joint. A Crego elevator is placed around the calcaneus at the level of the joint. The joint capsule is incised and the lamina spreader placed. The articular surface of the subtalar joint is removed and smoothed using the power saw, osteotome, curette, and rasp.
4. Next the articular surface of the calcaneocuboid joint is removed by the same method.

PROCEDURE 21-17 (continued)

5. Last, the articular surface of the talonavicular joint is removed. The head of the joint is manually brought into the wound to facilitate the resection. If the head of the joint cannot be exposed well enough, the surgeon will use a #15 knife blade to release the joint to attain as much mobility as possible.

   Procedural Consideration: The surgical technologist must ensure that as much of the resected bone as possible is saved for the bone graft, which might enable the surgeon to avoid having to obtain bone from the iliac crest.

6. The correction of the hind foot valgus is achieved by fixation of the subtalar joint. The surgeon places a screw, the usual length being 65 mm, anterior to posterior or posterior to anterior.

7. The forefoot rotation is corrected with fixation of the talonavicular joint. A smooth Steinman pin is inserted toward the center of the head of the talus.

8. Third fixation involves the calcaneocuboid joint, which corrects the forefoot abduction and adduction. Two 4.5-mm cannulated screws will be crossed placed from the anterior process of the calcaneus to the cuboid.

9. After fixation is achieved, the bone graft is placed. A rongeur is used to cut the bone into small pieces. The bone is placed around the talonavicular joint, in the gap at the calcaneocuboid joint, and in the sinus tarsi. Bone tamps with a mallet may be used to tap the bone graft into place.

10. The surgeon will thoroughly irrigate the surgical wound site, check the foot and heel for alignment, place a Jackson-Pratt suction drain, and close the wound in layers. A short leg cast or splint will be applied.

Postoperative Considerations

Immediate Postoperative Care

- Patient is transported to the PACU.
- A good amount of bleeding should be expected during the first 6–8 hours from the wound itself and through the drain. The dressings need to be frequently checked and changed as needed.

Prognosis

- No complications: Patient remains hospitalized for 3–4 days. The foot should be elevated to reduce swelling. The drain is removed 24–48 hours postoperative. The pins are removed 6–8 weeks postoperatively and a short walking cast is applied and worn until healing is complete after approximately 4 more weeks. The patient may begin weight bearing 10–12 weeks postoperative.
- Complications: SSI; mobility in one plane not be attained; malunion; nonunion.

Wound Classification

- Class I: Clean

PROCEDURE 21-18 Achilles Tendon Repair

Surgical Anatomy and Pathology

- The Achilles tendon (medical terms are tendo Achillis or tendo calcaneus) serves the purpose of connecting the gastrocnemius, soleus, and plantaris muscles to the calcaneus; the

(continues)

PROCEDURE 21-18 (continued)

	aponeuroses of those muscles form the beginning of the tendon. • It is the thickest and strongest tendon in the body and is approximately 6 in. long. • It begins with a width of 3–4 in. and narrows down to its insertion on the posterior tuberosity of the calcaneous. • Externally it is covered by paratenon, fascia, and the skin. In comparison to the flexor tendons in the hand, which have an outside synovial sheath covering the tendon, the Achilles tendon has no such sheath and is covered by the paratenon. It is separated from the	deep muscles and vessels by areolar and adipose tissue. • The primary blood supply to the tendon is through its mesotendon, with the most supply through the anterior mesentery. • The Achilles tendon is most often ruptured, either partially or totally, by a traumatic incident. • Middle-aged athletes are a common group of individuals at risk for an Achilles tendon rupture, in particular, "weekend athletes." • The common mechanisms of rupture include pushing off with the weight-bearing forefoot while	extending the knee, extreme dorsiflexion of the plantar-flexed foot such as when falling from a considerable height, direct hard contact with the tendon, traumatic laceration, and sudden and unexpected dorsiflexion of the ankle. • As a person ages the anterior mesenteric blood supply decreases, contributing to the loss of viscoelasticity in the tendon and predisposing to rupture. • The treatment is surgical repair of the rupture, which must be performed as soon as possible before the tendon atrophies.
Preoperative Diagnostic Tests and Procedures	• History and physical • Palpable tendon defect • Inability to perform a toe-raise	• Thompson "squeeze test"—calf is squeezed just distal to its maximal diameter while the patient is in prone position to cause	plantar flexion of the ankle joint. The test is positive for tendon rupture when no flexion occurs. • MRI
Equipment, Instruments, and Supplies Unique to Procedure	• Basic orthopedic instrument set • Flexible or rigid tendon-pulling forceps (Figure 21-31)	• Tendon stripper • Tourniquet and insufflator	
Preoperative Preparation	• Position: Prone • Anesthesia: Spinal or general • Skin prep: Beginning at the ankle joint	extending up to the lower border of the tourniquet and to the toes, circumferential	• Draping: Extremity draping technique

PROCEDURE 21-18 (continued)

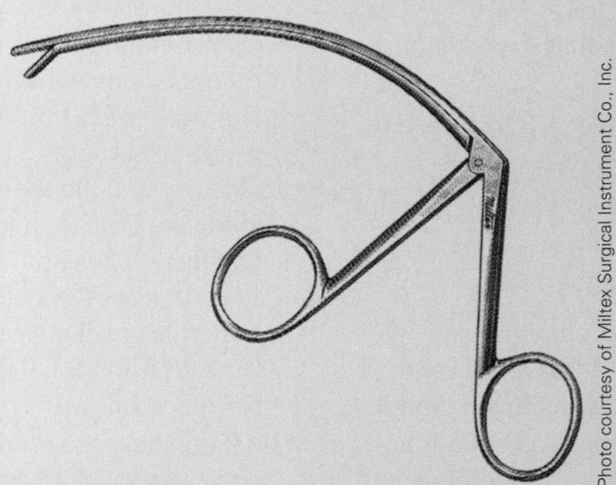

Figure 21-31 Miltex tendon-pulling forceps

Practical Considerations

- Place the tourniquet while the patient is in the supine position, before turning him or her to the prone position; it is difficult to apply the tourniquet in the prone position.
- The surgical technologist must be familiar with the suture the surgeon prefers to use for repairing the rupture of the tendon as well as the suturing technique used by the surgeon.

Surgical Procedure

1. A posteromedial longitudinal incision 10–12 cm long is made with the #10 knife blade. The incision is approximately 1 cm medial to the tendon. The incision is carried down to the paratenon.

   Procedural Consideration: If an assistant is not present, the surgeon will have the surgical technologist maintain the foot in equinus position during surgery.

2. The ruptured ends of the Achilles tendon are identified. Exploration of the proximal end may occur. The Achilles tendon is always under some degree of tension, even when an individual is at rest. Consequently, on rupture, the proximal end may retract upward along the gastrocnemius muscle and require retrieval with the tendon-pulling forceps or other atraumatic clamp. Another atraumatic clamp is placed on the other ruptured end of the tendon and the ends are brought together to achieve the original tendon length.

3. Several suture techniques can be utilized by the surgeon. One popular type is called the Krachow whip stitch, in which suture is placed 2.5 cm from the edge of the rupture to accomplish the approximation. The suture used to repair the rupture is the surgeon's preference; it can range from 2-0 nonabsorbable to #5 Ticron or Ethibond, but always on a noncutting needle.

   Procedural Consideration: The surgeon will have the surgical technologist place the foot in plantar flexion up to 5° and flex the leg at 15° when approximating the ends of the tendon.

4. The surgeon next closes the paratenon and subcutaneous layer over the site of the tendon repair to aid in healing and preventing adhesions from forming; a 4-0 nonabsorbable suture is used. The rest of the wound is closed in layers. Then 4 × 4 dressing sponges or Fluffs are placed. A posterior splint or short leg cast is applied with the foot maintained in gravity equinus position.

(*continues*)

PROCEDURE 21-18 (continued)

Postoperative Considerations	**Immediate Postoperative Care** • Patient is transported to the PACU. • Patient stay in hospital is usually 1–2 days. **Prognosis** • No complications: After 10–14 days the splint or cast is removed, and the staples and sutures are removed. Another short leg cast with the foot in gravity equinus position is applied and worn for another 2 weeks. At 4 weeks the cast is changed and the foot is gradually brought into plantigrade position. At 6–8 weeks postoperative a short leg walking cast is applied and full weight bearing is allowed with rehabilitative exercises. At 12 weeks an ankle brace is worn until full ROM is achieved, which usually occurs within 6 months. • Complications: Deep postoperative SSI; fistula; skin necrosis; rerupture; failure of repair; less plantar flexion strength as compared to pre-rupture injury. **Wound Classification** • Class I: Clean

PROCEDURE 21-19 Bunionectomy

Pathology	• A bunion, medically referred to as *hallux valgus,* is a bony exostosis located on the medial side of the first metatarsal head of the great toe causing a lateral deviation of the toe.
	  • Bunions are common in females due to the common shoe styles worn by women, including pointed toes and high heels.
	  • Other dispositions to developing a bunion include flat feet, imbalance due to muscle difficulties, and foot pronation.
	  • The patient experiences pain and swelling of the great toe as well as difficulty walking.
	• Various types of surgical procedures are used to treat the condition, such as the Aken, Chevron, McKeever, Keller, and McBride techniques.
	  • All of these procedures have the same outcome of removing the exostosis and realigning the great toe. The goals of surgery are to correct the deformity by removing the exostosis, restore the normal ROM, and remove the abnormal bony portions to prevent reoccurrence. The modified McBride technique is described here.

Preoperative Diagnostic Tests and Procedures	• History and physical • The type of surgical technique to be used is not determined by the surgeon until the entire foot is thoroughly examined with the patient standing, sitting, and lying supine and prone. • Standard X-rays: standing dorsoplantar and lateral; sitting oblique and axial • Vascularity and nerve supply to area must be examined to determine that no irregularities or conditions exist.
Equipment, Instruments, and Supplies Unique to Procedure	• Basic orthopedic instrument set • Small Inge lamina spreader • Lambotte osteotomes • Small rongeur • Microsagittal saw • 9-mm microsagittal saw blade • Bovie needle tip • Nitrogen tank • Several #15 knife blades • Tourniquet and insufflator • Bone wax

Procedure 21-19 (continued)

Preoperative Preparation

- Position: Supine
- Anesthesia: Spinal or general
- Skin prep: Starting a medial side of foot extend to lower border of tourniquet on thigh and toes, circumferentially
- Draping: Extremity draping technique; foot drapes are commercially available with either a single fenestration or double fenestration if both feet will be operated on.

Practical Considerations

- It is important to confirm which foot will be operated on because patients often have bunions on both feet and the foot with the worse deformity will usually be operated on first, unless both feet are being operated on.
- The surgical technologist must understand the directional terms such as dorsal, plantar flexion, lateral, and medial in order to assist the surgeon in positioning the foot during surgery and understanding the location of anatomical structures.
- Confirm X-rays are in the OR, including those in which the surgeon has marked measurements on the foot.
- Check the level of the nitrogen tank.
- Test the power equipment prior to the patient's entry into the OR.
- The surgeon will use several #15 knife blades; the surgical technologist must make sure to frequently change them out to prevent a dull blade from being used.

Surgical Procedure

Steps 1–5 are considered the first stage of the procedure.

1. Using a #15 knife blade, the surgeon makes a straight, midline medial incision from the middle of the proximal phalanx to where the bony exostosis meet with the metatarsal shaft.
2. Small skin flaps are made anteriorly and posteriorly. The blade sides of two Senn retractors are placed to expose the surgical site.

   Procedural Consideration: Electrocautery with needle tip is used to control bleeding in order to prevent postoperative hemorrhaging. The surgical technologist should have fine-toothed Adson tissue forceps for the surgeon to use when cauterizing.
3. Using the #15 knife blade, the surgeon makes a longitudinal incision over the capsule of the exostosis and continues by dissecting the periosteum away from the capsule. The capsule is gently retracted anteriorly and posteriorly with small blunt rake retractors to expose the metatarsal head and exostosis.

   Procedural Consideration: The surgical technologist must avoid placing too much tension on holding the capsule retractors; the attachment of the capsule to the metatarsal neck must be preserved.
4. The exostosis is now removed. Using a ¼-in. straight osteotome, the surgeon scores (marks) the proximal edge of the exostosis where it meets the metatarsal shaft.
5. The exostectomy is completed with the use of the microsagittal saw. A small rongeur is used to round off the edges of the metatarsal head.

(continues)

PROCEDURE 21-19 (continued)

Steps 6–8 are considered the second stage of the procedure.

6. Using the #15 knife blade, the surgeon makes a dorsal longitudinal incision beginning 2 cm proximal to the first web space and extends it between the first and second metatarsal heads.

   Procedural Consideration: Gentle retraction is provided with the dull-blade side of the Senn retractors to avoid damage to nerves.

7. The Senn retraction exposes the dorsal digital branches of veins that are cauterized.

8. Using a curved Mosquito clamp, the surgeon identifies the adductor hallucis tendon in order to free it up. A small Inge lamina spreader is placed to spread the first and second metatarsal heads to expose the lateral head of the flexor hallucis brevis muscle. The insertion of the adductor hallucis tendon to the flexor hallucis brevis muscle is severed with the #15 knife blade and an incision is made in the deep transverse intermetatarsal ligament as well as a lateral capsule release (incision), thus allowing free and independent movement of the tendon.

   Procedural Consideration: A neurovascular bundle is located right underneath the transverse intermetatarsal ligament that must be preserved. To protect the bundle a Freer elevator is inserted underneath the ligament and then the incision is made.

Steps 9A–D are considered the third stage of the procedure.

9. If the release of the adductor hallucis tendon and lateral capsule does not fully correct the valgus deformity, a fibular sesamoidectomy is needed.

   A. Using the Inge lamina spreader, the first and second metatarsal heads are exposed.

   B. The surgeon will have the surgical technologist plantar flex the metatarsophalangeal joint to reduce the tension on the fibular sesamoid.

   C. Using a small Kocher clamp, the fibular sesamoid is grasped and pulled laterally into the metatarsal space.

   D. Using the #15 knife blade, the intersesamoid ligament is released and the fibular sesamoid removed.

   Procedural Consideration: When the ligament is incised, the surgeon must avoid cutting the flexor hallucis longus tendon that rests next to the ligament.

Steps 10A–B are considered the fourth stage of the procedure.

10. The medial capsule is imbricated (closing the capsule with layers of tissue) and the wound closed.

    A. 3-0 absorbable suture is placed through the dorsal flap and then the plantar flap; when the sutured is tightened and tied it brings the plantar flap over the dorsal flap to close the capsule. It also pulls the adductor hallucis tendon back into normal pre–hallux valgus anatomical position. This step is not performed if the fibular sesamoid was removed.

    B. The remaining part of the capsule is closed with 2-0 absorbable sutures and the skin is closed with interrupted sutures. Fluffs are placed as the dressing.

PROCEDURE 21-19 (continued)

Postoperative Considerations	**Immediate Postoperative Care** • Patient is transported to the PACU. • Patient is usually released the day of surgery, but with strict instructions to elevate the foot as high as comfortable for 48–72 hours and can only get up from bed rest during that time period to go to the bathroom and must wear a wood-soled shoe when doing so.	**Prognosis** • No complications: Increased ambulation occurs using a wood-soled shoe over the 72 hours postoperative. After 3 weeks the sutures are removed. A toe spacer/immobilizer must be used for 6 weeks postoperatively and wood-soled shoes for 3–4 weeks postoperatively. After 3–4 weeks the patient can switch to a	wide shoe and after 12–14 weeks regular shoes with a normal, but not constricted toe box can be worn. • Complications: Postoperative SSI; local hemorrhage; nerve injury; tendon or ligament injury; reoccurrence of hallux valgus. **Wound Classification** • Class I: Clean

CASE STUDY Cheryl is a downhill skier. She fell while cutting through deep powder. She said that she heard a "pop" while she was twisting and falling. Cheryl was diagnosed with a tear of the anterior cruciate ligament. She is in the OR for an arthroscopic repair.

1. What equipment is necessary for all arthroscopic procedures?
2. Can ligaments be repaired? How? Provide examples

QUESTIONS FOR FURTHER STUDY

1. What safety steps should be followed when using cement in orthopedic procedures?
2. What is the difference between a Steinmann pin and a K-wire?
3. What is the difference in structure between a self-tapping and a nontapping screw?
4. What is the purpose of placing a cement restrictor within the femur during a total hip arthroplasty?
5. Place the following in their order of use during a knee arthroscopy: blunt trocar, irrigation/inflow cannula, sharp trocar, #11 knife blade.

BIBLIOGRAPHY

Agur, A. M., & Dalley, A. F. (2008). *Grant's atlas of anatomy* (12th ed.). Philadelphia: Lippincott Williams & Wilkins.

Butler, J. L., Lewis, R., & Shier, D. N. (2005). *Hole's essentials of human anatomy & physiology* (10th ed.). New York: McGraw-Hill.

Canale, S. T., & Beatty, J. H. (Eds.). (2007). *Campbell's operative orthopaedics* (11th ed.). Maryland Heights, MO: Mosby.

Ethicon, Inc. (2007). *Ethicon wound closure manual.* Somerville, NJ: Ethicon, Inc.

Goldman, M. A. (2007). *Pocket guide to the operating room* (3rd ed.). Philadelphia: F. A. Davis Company.

Hitner, H., & Nagle, B. T. (2004). *Pharmacology: An introduction* (5th ed.). New York: McGraw-Hill.

Junge, T. (1999, Summer). Bone healing: Normal and disrupted. *The Surgical First Assistants, 4*(2).

Marks, S. C., Jr., & Hermey, D. C. (1996). The structure and development of bone. In J. P. Bilezikian, L. G. Raisz, & G. A. Rodan (Eds.), *Principles of bone biology.* San Diego: Academic Press.

Salerno, E. (2000). *Pharmacology for health professionals.* St. Louis, MO: Mosby.

Sanders, T., & Scanlon, V. C. (2006). *Essentials of anatomy and physiology* (5th ed.). Philadelphia: F. A. Davis.

Standring, S. (Ed.). (2008). *Gray's anatomy: The anatomical basis of clinical practice* (40th ed.). Philadelphia: Churchill Livingstone.

Synthes. (1995). DHS®/DCS® dynamic hip and condylar screw system: Technique guide [Brochure]. Paoli, PA: Author.

Vile, J. (1981, July/August). Scoliosis and spinal fusion. *The Surgical Technologist, 11,* pp. 9–13.

Welling, K. R. (n.d.). Rotator cuff surgery. *The Surgical Technologist, 31,* 11–18.

Wheeless' Textbook of Orthopaedics. (n.d.). [Online]. Retrieved from http://www.wheelessonline.com

CHAPTER

22

Cardiothoracic Surgery

CASE STUDY

Robert, a 54-year-old mechanic, arrives in the emergency department complaining of severe chest pain that radiates to his back and difficulty taking a deep breath. He has smoked two packs of cigarettes a day for 20 years and is grossly overweight. His father and brother both died of heart disease.

1. What does the physician suspect is wrong?
2. What tests should the physician order?
3. Will surgical intervention be necessary, and if so, what kind?
4. What procedure is typically attempted before surgery, and where is this procedure performed? What specialist performs this procedure?

OBJECTIVES

After studying this chapter, the reader should be able to:

A 1. Recognize the relevant anatomy of the cardiovascular and respiratory systems.

P 2. Summarize the pathology that prompts cardiac or thoracic surgical intervention and the related terminology.

3. Determine any special preoperative diagnostic procedures/tests for the patient undergoing cardiac or thoracic surgery.
4. Determine any preoperative preparation procedures.
5. Indicate the names and uses of cardiovascular and thoracic equipment, instruments, and supplies.

O 6. Summarize the surgical steps of the cardiac and thoracic procedures.

7. Interpret the purpose and expected outcomes of the cardiac and thoracic procedures.
8. Recognize the immediate postoperative care and possible complications of the cardiac and thoracic procedures.

S 9. Assess any specific variations related to the preoperative, intraoperative, and postoperative care of the patient undergoing a cardiac or thoracic procedure.

SELECT KEY TERMS

alveoli	hyaline cartilage	oxygenated	stent
aneurysm	infarction	pericardium	systole
arrhythmia	infiltrate	pleura	tachycardia
atria	mediastinum	prolapse	tamponade
cardiac cycle	myocardium	regurgitation	ventricles
ductus arteriosus			

PART I: Thoracic Surgical Procedures

INTRODUCTION

Although the lungs are the primary focus of thoracic surgical procedures, surgical treatment of chest wall deformities and identification of lesions within the **mediastinum** are also included. The surgical procedures that will be discussed in this section are bronchoscopy, mediastinoscopy, thoracoscopy, pectus excavatum repair, and lung procedures.

DIAGNOSTIC PROCEDURES AND TESTS

Imaging studies that are used most frequently in the diagnosis of thoracic diseases and disorders include standard X-rays, CT scanning, MRI, and pulmonary angiography. Anteroposterior (AP) and lateral standard X-rays of the chest can determine the size of the heart and great vessel configuration, as well as any valvular or intracoronary calcification. Asymptomatic pericardial cysts and cardiac tumors may also be detected.

CT scan and MRI are useful for the evaluation of pericardial and intracardiac masses. CT scan is especially useful for the detection and evaluation of thoracic aorta dissection. MRI can detect abnormal positioning of intracardiac structures.

Pulmonary angiography is primarily used to detect pulmonary embolism and other blockages of the arterial circulation in the lungs. It is also used to help diagnose congenital narrowing of pulmonary vessels, pulmonary artery **aneurysms**, and changes to the arteries due to pulmonary hypertension (Figure 22-1).

Electrocardiography, echocardiography, and cardiac catheterization are also useful diagnostic procedures for the evaluation of cardiac disease. For a detailed description of these procedures, refer to Chapter 13.

However, the three definitive diagnostic procedures for the diagnosis of suspected lesions are bronchoscopy, mediastinoscopy, and thoracoscopy with the excision of tissue and fluid specimens. The three procedures are described later in detail.

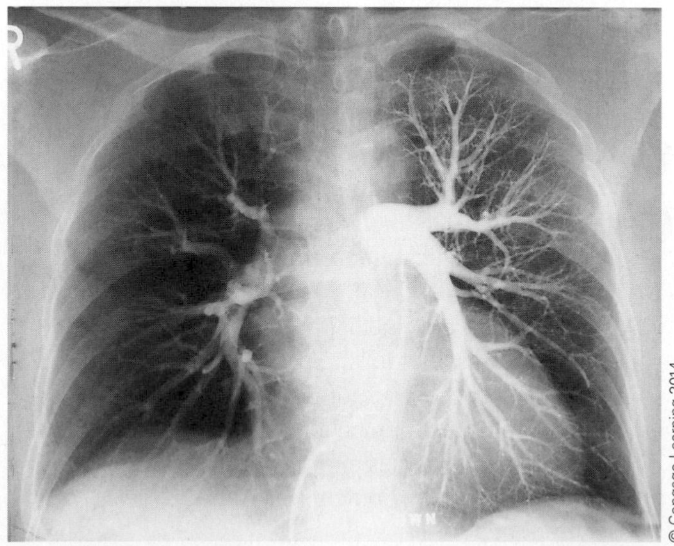

Figure 22-1 Pulmonary arteriogram

INSTRUMENTATION, ROUTINE EQUIPMENT, AND SUPPLIES

The instrumentation, equipment, and supplies for the three endoscopic procedures will be presented within the procedural descriptions. The following lists are the routine items that are needed for lung procedures.

Instrumentation

Instrumentation for thoracotomy includes vascular and thoracotomy instrument sets. The thoracotomy set will include instruments to remove a rib (e.g., Bethune rib shears and Matson rib stripper/elevator) and expose and repair the organs of the thorax.

If exposure requires median sternotomy, a sternal saw and retractor are opened separately. Thoracic procedures may also require a laparotomy or general vascular instrument set with additional cardiovascular instruments. Hemoclip appliers of various sizes are often in a separate instrument set. Table 22-1 presents a list of the instruments that are included in a routine vascular instrument set. Table 22-2 provide the thoracotomy instrument set.

Equipment

The following is a list of the routine equipment that is required for thoracic surgery:

- ESU
- Cell Saver
- Suction system
- Fiberoptic headlight
- Fiberoptic light source
- Defibrillation unit available

Anesthesia Monitoring Equipment

Anesthesia personnel prepare and apply or insert monitoring equipment that may include a Swan-Ganz catheter for pulmonary wedge pressure and central venous pressure (CVP) readings, an arterial catheter for the monitoring of arterial blood pressure and blood gases (ABGs), and electrocardiography, oxygen saturation, temperature, and blood pressure equipment. For intrathoracic procedures, the anesthesia provider may prefer to use a double-lumen endotracheal tube so that the affected lung can be collapsed during the surgical procedure without interfering with the unaffected lung's ventilation. The use of the double-lumen endotracheal tube requires careful monitoring of ABGs and O_2 saturation because of the increased possibility of right-to-left shunt through the nonventilated lung (Figure 22-3).

TABLE 22-1 Vascular Instrument Set

2	45° Potts-Smith Scissors
2	Potts-Smith Forceps (Figure 22-2A)
4	DeBakey Forceps (2 regular and 2 long)
2	Curved Cooley clamps
2	Straight Cooley multipurpose clamps
2	Curved Cooley multipurpose clamps
2	DeBakey angled clamps
4	DeBakey aorta clamps
4	DeBakey tangential occlusion clamps
2	DeBakey multipurpose clamps
2	Straight Glover clamps
2	Curved Glover clamps
2	Straight Glover coarctation clamps
2	Curved Glover coarctation clamps
2	Straight Glover patent ductus clamps
2	Angled Glover patent ductus clamps
2	Sarot bronchus clamps (Figure 22-2B)
2	Satinsky vena cava clamps (Figure 22-2C)
1	Davidson scapula retractor (Figure 22-2D)
1	Bailey rib contractor (Figure 22-2E)
2	Allison lung retractors (Figure 22-2F)
2	Lovelace lung-grasping forceps (Figure 22-2G)
4	Ryder needle holders (Figure 22-2H)
1	Bethune rib shears (Figure 22-2I)
2	Castroviejo needle holders, straight and curved tip

Supplies

The following is the list of routine supplies needed for thoracic surgery:

- Cardiothoracic back table pack
- Double basin set
- Gloves
- Knife blades: #11, #10, and #15
- Transverse laparotomy drape
- Plastic adhesive incise drape (surgeon's preference)
- Hemoclips of various sizes
- Magnetic instrument pad
- ESU pencil
- ESU tips, regular and long
- Suction tubing × 2
- Suction tips × 2, Yankauer
- Cell Saver suction tubing

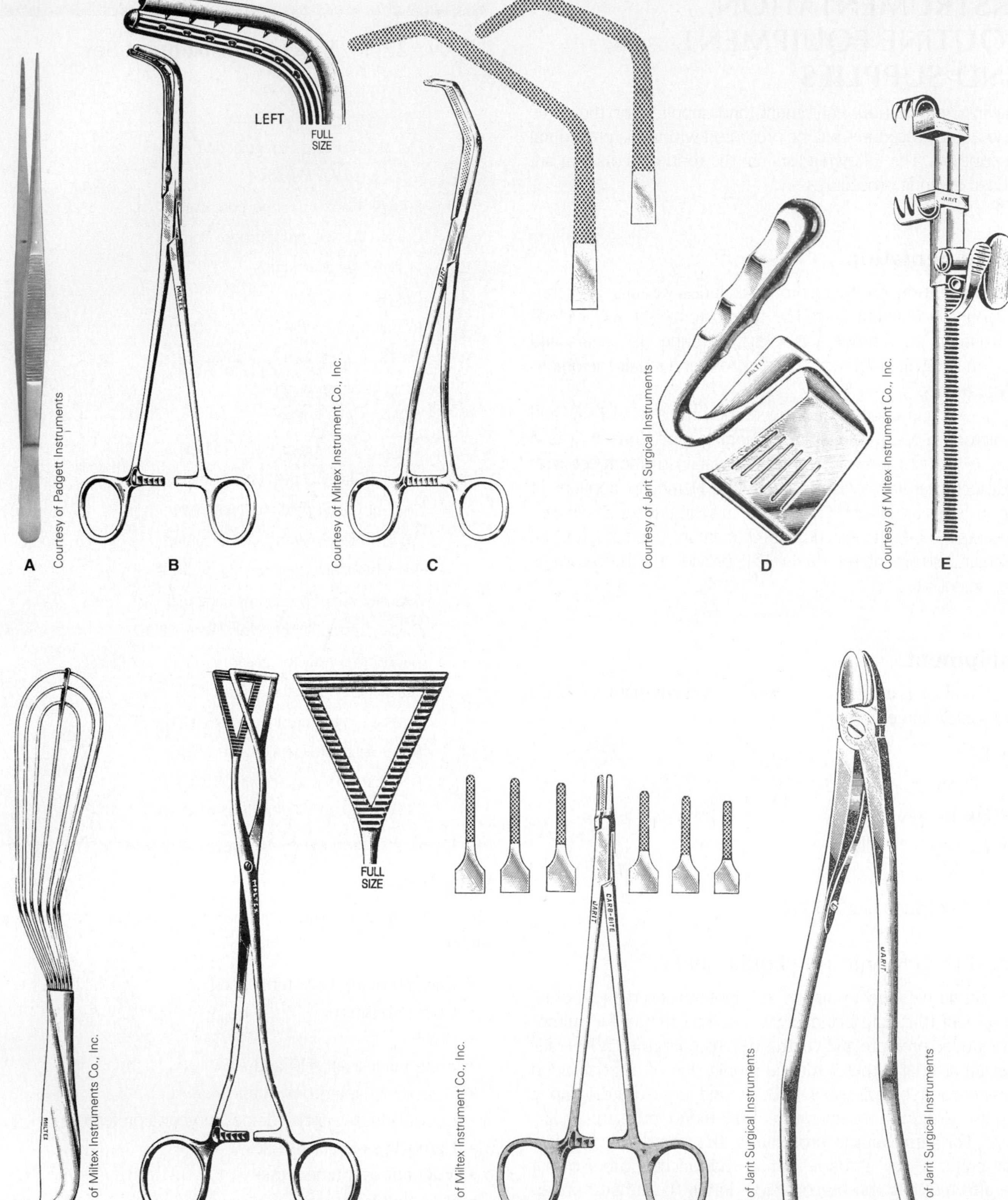

Figure 22-2 Thoracic instrumentation: (A) Potts-Smith forceps, (B) Sarot bronchus clamp, (C) Satinsky vena cava clamp, (D) Davidson scapula retractor, (E) Bailey rib contractor, (F) Allison lung retractor, (G) Lovelace lung-grasping forceps, (H) Ryder needle holder, (I) Bethune rib shears

TABLE 22-2 Thoracotomy Instrument Set

2	Curved Metzenbaum scissors, regular and long
2	Curved Mayo scissors, regular and long
2	Tissue forceps with teeth, regular and long
2	DeBakey forceps, regular and long
4	Babcock clamps
4	Mixter clamps
4	Right angle clamps
2	Lovelace or Duval lung-grasping forceps
1	Bethune rib shear
1	Stille rongeur
1	Duckbill rongeur
2	Bailey rib contractors
2	Finochietto rib retractors, adult and pediatric
2	Alexander periosteotomes
2	Alexander rib rasps
2	Doyen elevator and rasp
2	Langenbeck periosteal elevators

- Asepto syringes × 2
- Kitner sponges
- 4 × 4 sponges loaded onto sponge sticks
- Laparotomy sponges, adult or pediatric
- Argyle chest tubes of various adult or pediatric sizes
- Pleur-evac closed seal drainage system
- Straight or Y-type connector if more than one chest tube is inserted
- Vessel loops
- Vascular stapling devices
- 2-0 and 3-0 silk suture ties loaded on tonsil or right-angle clamps
- Polypropylene vascular suture
- Pledgeted double-armed polypropylene sutures
- Antibiotic irrigating solution
- 1% xylocaine without epinephrine for postoperative pain control
- Three-layer dressing: nonadherent contact layer; 4 × 4s; ABD; tape

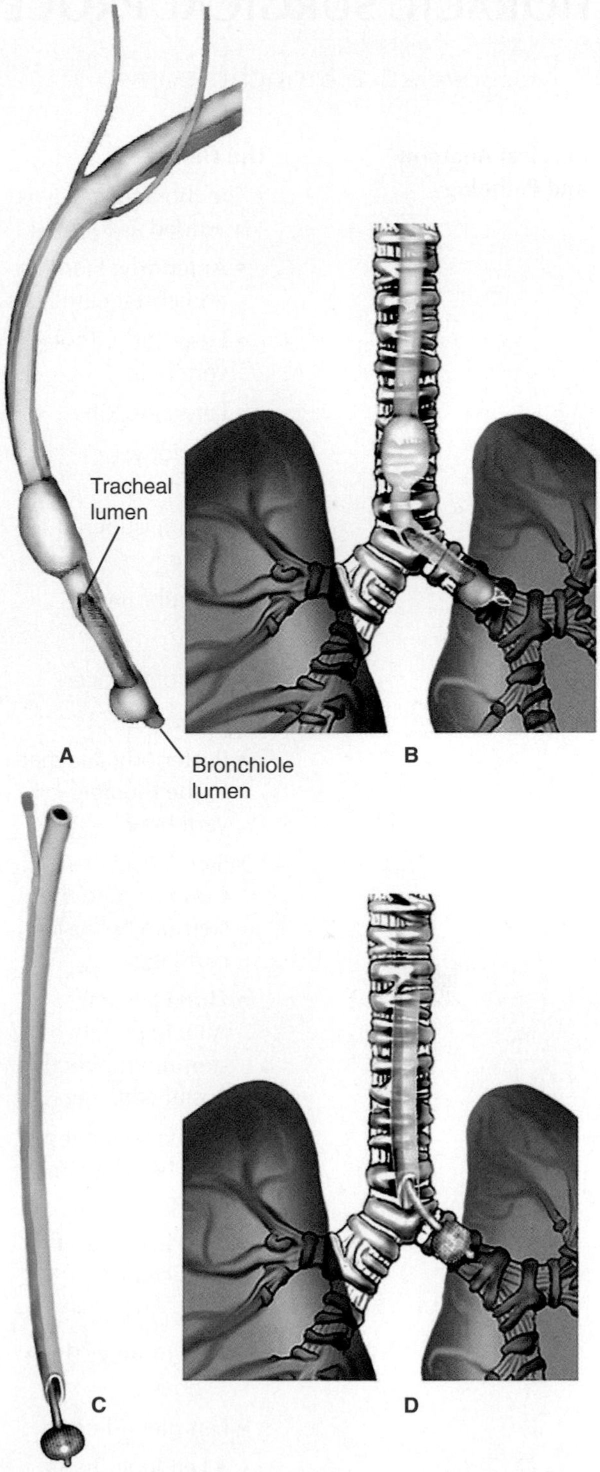

Figure 22-3 Specialized endotracheal tubes: (A) Double-lumen endotracheal tube with separate bronchial and tracheal balloons; (B) tubes are most often placed with the tip (bronchial lumen) in the left mainstem bronchus; (C) single-lumen endotracheal tube with an endobronchial balloon; (D) balloon positioned to occlude the left mainstem bronchus

THORACIC SURGICAL PROCEDURES

PROCEDURE 22-1 Bronchoscopy

Surgical Anatomy and Pathology

The Thorax

- The thoracic cavity is bounded as follows.
  - Anteriorly: Sternum and costal cartilages
  - Posteriorly: Thoracic vertebrae
  - Laterally: Ribs
  - Inferiorly: Diaphragm
- Sternum (superior to inferior)
  - Manubrium
  - Body
  - Xiphoid process
- Twelve ribs
  - Posteriorly attached to the thoracic vertebrae
  - Seven true ribs: Connected to the sternum by costal cartilage
  - Three false ribs: Attached to the sternum indirectly by costal cartilage
  - Two false (floating) ribs: No attachment to the sternum
- Three divisions of thoracic cavity
  - Right pleural cavity
    - Right lung: Three lobes
  - Left pleural cavity
    - Left lung: Two lobes
- Mediastinum
  - Esophagus
  - Trachea
  - Thymus
  - Lymph nodes
  - Heart with great vessels
- **Pleura**
  - Parietal pleura: Lines inner surface of ribs, **pericardium** of the heart, and superior surface of the diaphragm
  - Visceral pleura: Covers outer surface of each lung
  - Pleural space: Small space between parietal pleura and visceral pleura; contains serous fluid that prevents friction between the lungs and pleura during respiration
- Respiration (Figure 22-4)
  - Principal muscles associated with inspiration are the diaphragm and external intercostals.
  - Accessory muscles of inspiration are the sternocleidomastoid and scalenes (Figure 22-5).
  - Principal muscles associated with expiration are the internal intercostals, external oblique, internal oblique, transversus abdominis, and rectus abdominis.
  - Act of respiration
    - Diaphragm and external intercostals muscles contract.
    - Ribs and sternum elevate.
    - Size of thoracic cavity increases.
    - Pulmonary pressure decreases, thus forcing air into the lungs.

The Trachea

- Trachea (Figure 22-6)
  - Extends from larynx to bronchi
  - Formed by
    - Smooth muscle
    - **Hyaline cartilage**: C-shaped rings; prevent trachea from collapsing
    - Inner wall lined with ciliated mucosa
    - Functions as passageway for air to and from the lungs
- Bronchial tree
  - Bronchi
    - Trachea divides at carina into right and left bronchi.
    - Bronchi are composed of smooth muscle and cartilaginous rings.
    - Inner wall is lined with ciliated mucosa. Mucosa is composed of goblet cells.
    - Goblet cell secretions trap foreign particles; cilia pass the particles forward into the throat to be expelled as an aid in preventing respiratory tract infection.
  - Bronchial divisions
    - Bronchus enters lung and divides into secondary lobar branches (Figure 22-7).

PROCEDURE 22-1 (continued)

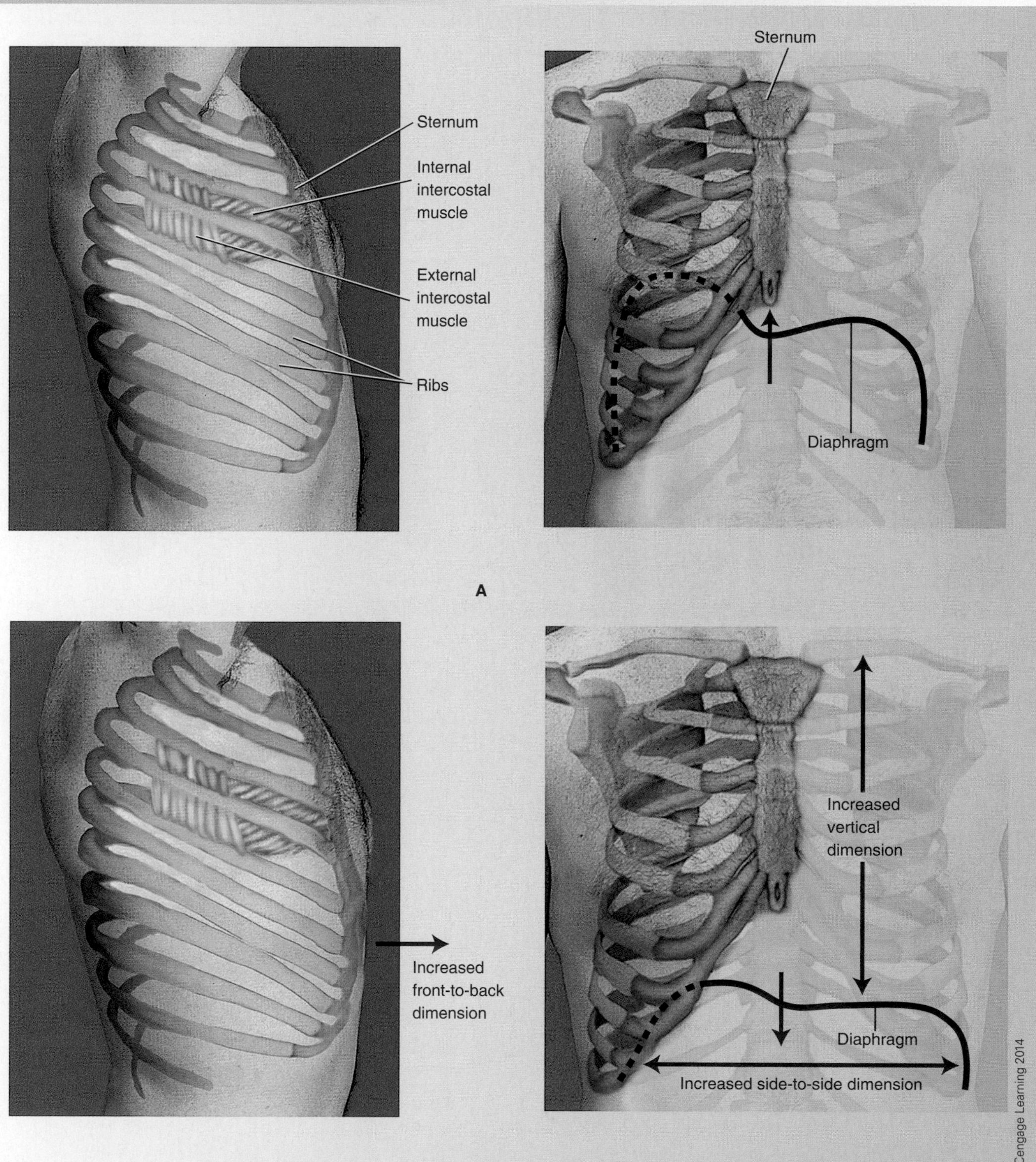

Figure 22-4 Thoracic changes during respiration: (A) Expiration, (B) inspiration

(continues)

PROCEDURE 22-1 (continued)

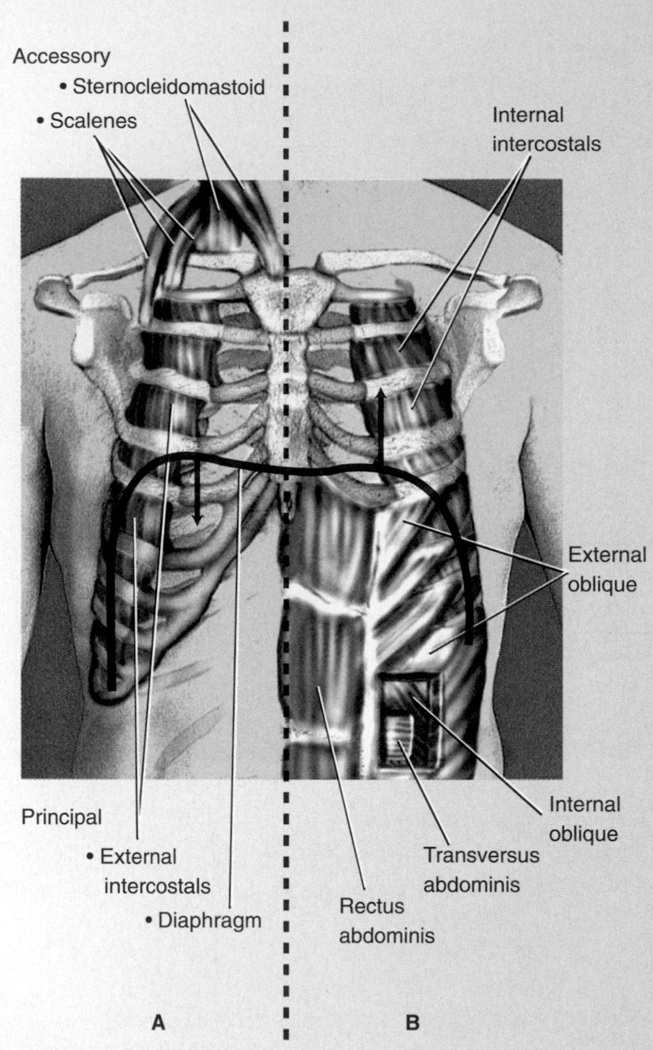

Figure 22-5 Muscles of respiration: (A) Inspiration, (B) expiration

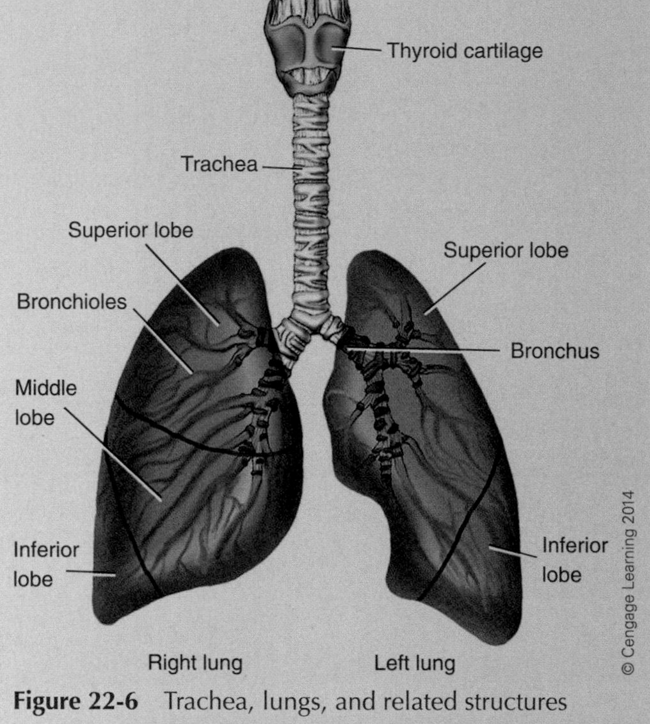

Figure 22-6 Trachea, lungs, and related structures

- Lobar branches divide into segmental bronchi.
- Segmental bronchi divide into bronchioles.
- Bronchioles end in alveolar ducts and **alveoli**.
- Alveoli (Figure 22-8)
  - Composed of simple squamous epithelium
  - Exchange oxygen and carbon dioxide

The Lungs

- Lungs
  - Extend from just slightly below the clavicle to the diaphragm
  - Ancillary structures: Bronchus, pulmonary artery, superior pulmonary vein, inferior pulmonary vein, lymphatic vessels
  - Hilum: Slight concave portion on medial side of each lung where the bronchus and other structures enter
  - Left lung lobes: Superior and inferior lobes separated by fissure
  - Right lung lobes: Superior, middle, inferior; each lobe is separated by a fissure.
  - Blood flow

PROCEDURE 22-1 (continued)

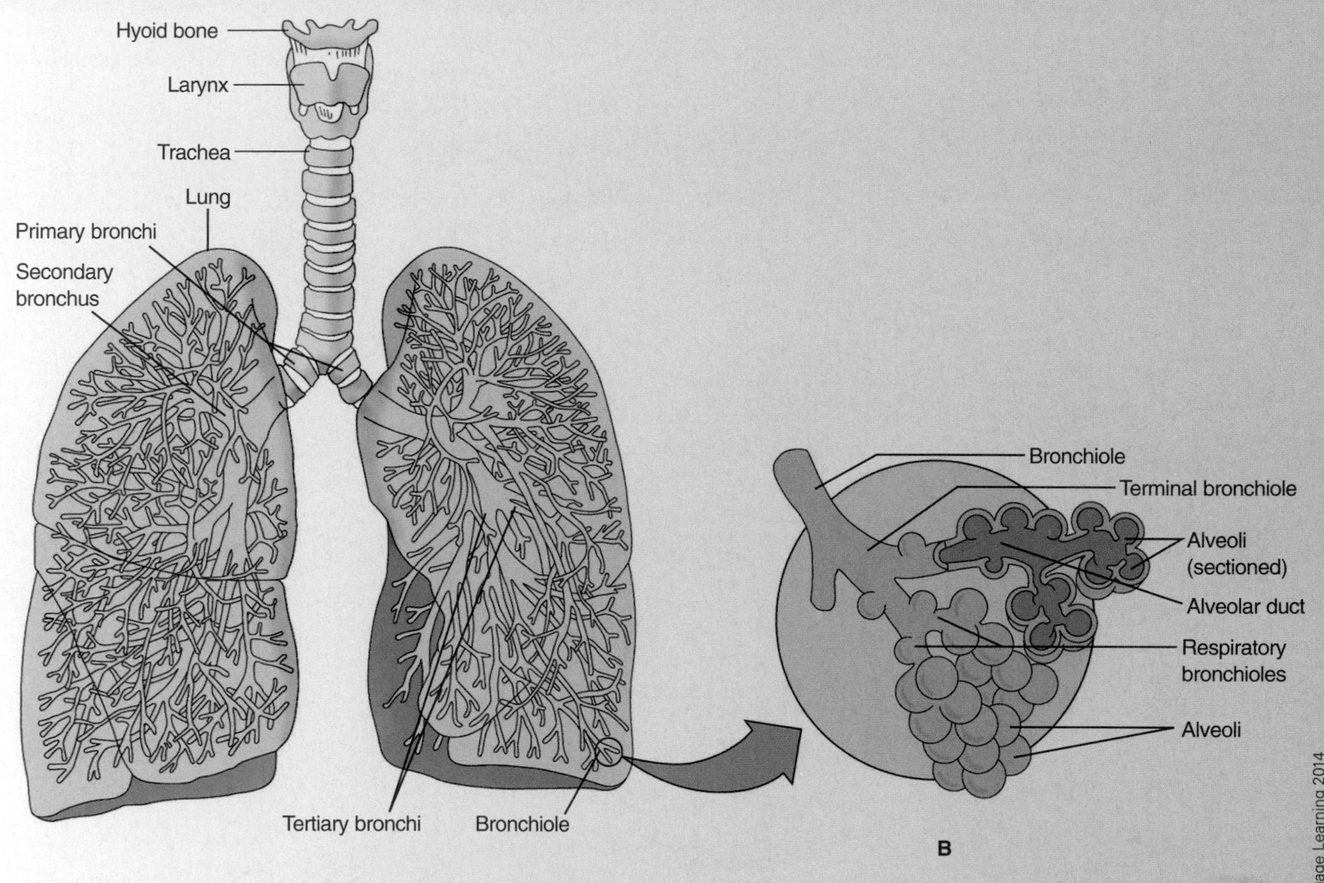

Figure 22-7 Bronchial tree: (A) Bronchial divisions, (B) bronchioles

- Blood low in oxygen travels from the right ventricle of the heart through the left branch of the pulmonary artery to the left lung to be oxygenated.
- Blood travels in the same way to the right lung, except it travels through the right branch of the pulmonary artery.
- **Oxygenated** blood leaves the lungs through the pulmonary veins and enters the left atrium of the heart (Figure 22-9).
- Bronchial arteries that arise from the aorta supply the bronchi, bronchioles, and tissue of the lungs.
- Bronchoscopy is an invasive diagnostic and/or therapeutic procedure for the evaluation of hemoptysis, infection, carcinoma of the lung, and damage to the lungs due to smoke inhalation. It is useful for retrieving foreign objects lodged in an airway and for laser treatment of endobronchial tumors. Brochoscopy is also useful for postoperative evaluation of the transplanted lung.
- Carcinoma of the lung is the leading cause of death due to cancer in the United States.
- In most cases, lung cancer is the result of cigarette smoking. Cigarette smoke contains a number of known carcinogens,

(*continues*)

PROCEDURE 22-1 (continued)

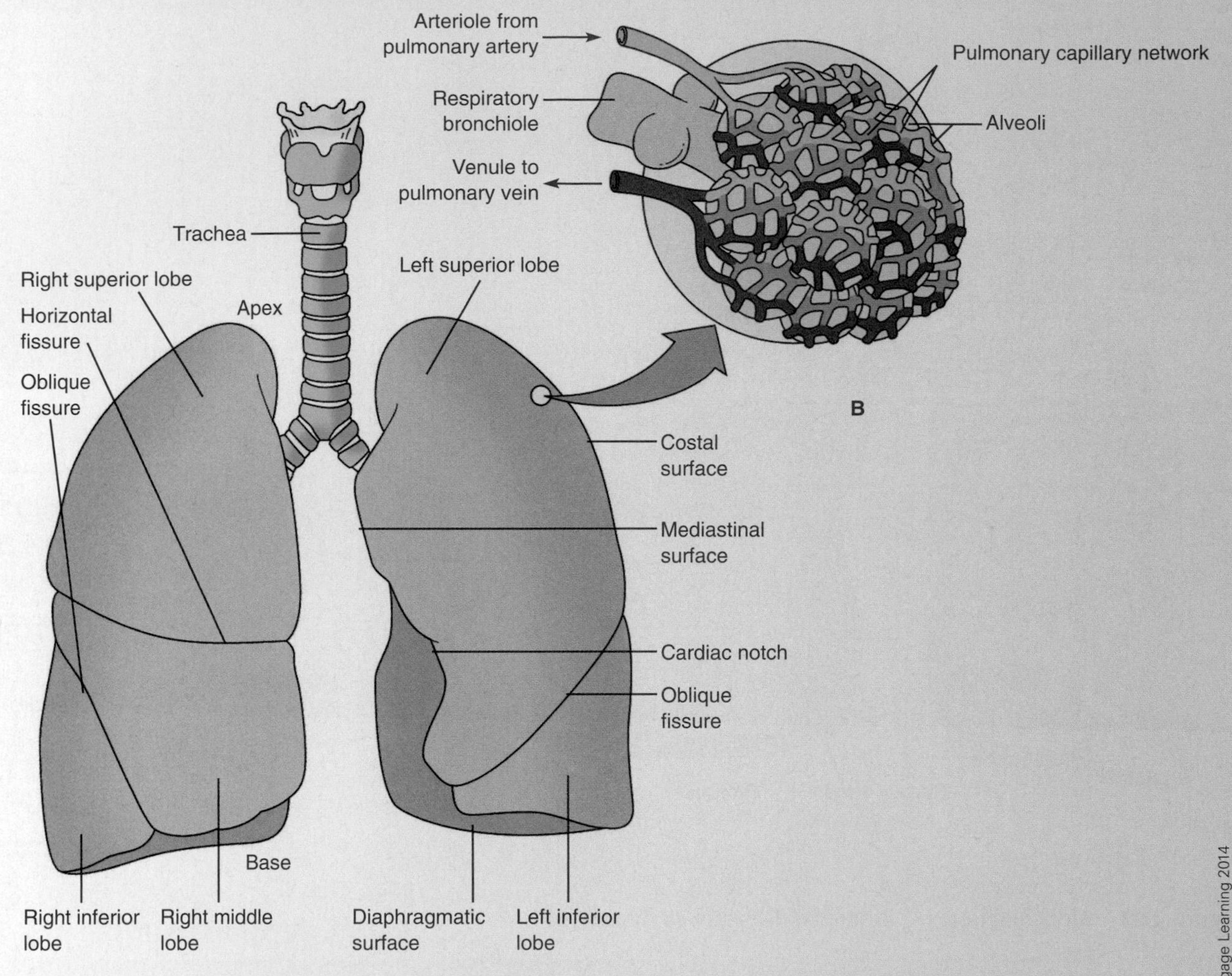

Figure 22-8 Lung structure: (A) Lobes and fissures, (B) alveoli and exchange of gases

the worst of which are the polycyclic hydrocarbons. These substances promote malignant transformation of bronchial cells through the activation of oncogenes and tumor suppression gene inhibition. Cigarette smoke also contains irritants that, in combination with the carcinogens, create lesions that eventually become cancerous.

- Lung tumors are divided into four subgroups: small cell carcinoma; squamous cell carcinoma; adenocarcinoma; and large cell carcinoma. Tumors may also be of a mixed type. Tumors of the lung are usually metastases from other sites, most commonly the kidney or the colon, although primary lung tumors are not uncommon. Primary lung tumors are highly invasive, and may metastasize locally to the thoracic lymph nodes,

Procedure 22-1 (continued)

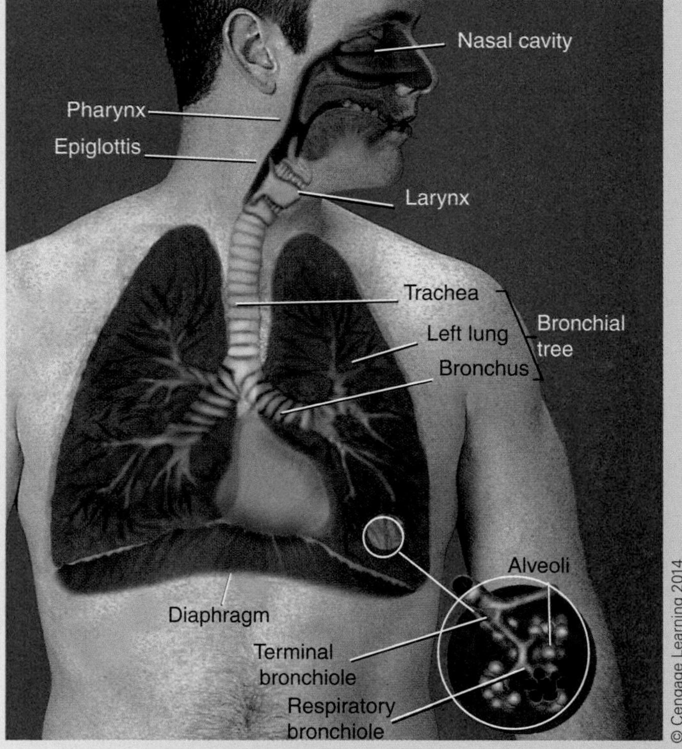

Figure 22-9 Pathway of respiration

	esophagus, and pericardium. Distant metastatic sites include the brain, adrenal glands, liver, or skeleton. • Patients usually present with a persistent cough, hemoptysis, and shortness of breath. Other signs and symptoms include pleural effusion, pain on inspiration, and/or clubbing of fingers if the cancer has invaded the pleural space.
Preoperative Diagnostic Tests and Procedures	• Initial diagnosis is made by chest X-rays and sputum cytology test, but definitive diagnosis is made with a tissue and cytology biopsy from bronchoscopy. Early detection of bronchial tumors cannot be made with X-rays, only with bronchoscopy.
Equipment, Instruments, and Supplies Unique to Procedure	Typically, a bronchoscopy cart with all the necessary supplies and equipment is available for the surgical technologist and need only be checked for completeness.
Equipment, Instruments, and Supplies Common to Rigid and Flexible Bronchoscopy	• Fiberoptic light source • Fiberoptic light cord • Endotracheal adaptor for anesthesia • Two-piece metal sponge carrier • Suction tubing • Straight and curved aspirating tubes • Biopsy forceps • Lukens tubes • Lubricant • Telfa for tissue specimens • Several specimen containers • Antifog solution

(continues)

Procedure 22-1 (continued)

	• Wire-cutting scissors • Topical anesthesia supplies set up on a separate small sterile table or Mayo stand: • Local anesthetic spray or poured into a medicine cup	• Local anesthetic drugs often used include lidocaine, tetracaine, and procaine with or without epinephrine, depending on surgeon's preference. • Emesis basin	• Laryngeal mirror • Lingual retractor/spatula • Laryngeal syringe with straight and curved metal cannulae • 10-mL Luer-Loc syringe • 22-gauge needle • Medicine cups
Equipment, Instruments, and Supplies Common to Rigid Bronchoscopy	• Rigid bronchoscope of surgeon's diameter preference	• Fiberoptic telescope • Plastic teeth guard	• Small basin with sterile saline and 10-mL syringe to take cytology specimens
Equipment, Instruments, and Supplies Common to Flexible Bronchoscopy	• Flexible bronchoscope • Biopsy brush • Microscopic slides	• Container for microscope slides • 95% ethanol alcohol	
Preoperative Preparation	• Position: Supine with scapular roll to hyperextend neck or the head is slightly lowered by lowering the head piece of the OR table. The anesthesia provider will be seated at the patient's side while the	surgeon is at the head of the table. • Anesthesia: Flexible brochoscopy is generally performed under a local anesthetic in the endoscopy department, but for the evaluation of intrabronchial tumors	before thoracotomy, the procedure is performed in the OR under general anesthesia. • Skin prep: No skin prep is performed. • Draping: Three-quarter sheet placed over upper body of patient.

Practical Considerations	• Bronchoscopes are either rigid or flexible.
	  • The rigid scope is equipped with a fiberoptic light carrier for illumination of the trachea and primary bronchi and side channels for anesthetic gas and oxygen administration. Rigid bronchoscopy is typically performed for the removal of foreign objects in children, although it may occasionally be used for biopsy of a large
		central mass or for evaluating hemoptysis.
		  • The smaller-diameter flexible fiberoptic bronchoscope allows for visualization of the upper, middle, and lower lobe bronchi and may have a video camera attached for viewing on a monitor. Transbronchial lung biopsy for examination of pulmonary **infiltrate** is also performed through the flexible bronchoscope.
			• Because the scope is inserted through the mouth and into the bronchial tubes, the procedure is not treated as a sterile one. The scope should either be sterilized or undergo high-level disinfection.
			• The bronchoscope and light source should be tested prior to the entry of the patient into the OR.
			• Prior to the start of the procedure, loose teeth may have to be removed.

PROCEDURE 22-1 (continued)

- Prior to the start of the procedure, confirm that the anesthesia provider has an endotracheal adaptor.
- The surgical technologist should apply the antifog solution to the lens of the scope just prior to insertion.
- The surgeon may sit for the procedure; have a sitting stool positioned at the head of the OR table.
- The overhead OR lights may be turned off according to surgeon's preference; the circulator will turn on the X-ray viewing box to provide some light.
- The surgical technologist may be responsible for assisting the surgeon inserting a brush or biopsy forceps into the channel of the scope and advancing the forceps. The forceps are flexible; therefore, the surgical technologist should assist the surgeon in maintaining control of the forceps and prevent contamination. The surgical technologist should make sure the forceps are in the closed position prior to inserting into the channel.
- The 10-mL syringe should be filled with 5 mL of saline prior to the start of the procedure in preparation for taking cytologic specimens.
- The surgical technologist must be familiar with the procedure for taking fluid washings when performing a flexible bronchoscopy in order to prevent the specimen from being lost through the suction.
- Cytologic specimens from bronchial washings delivered through the flexible bronchoscope are essential for the diagnosis of lung disease. Bronchial brushings and needle aspirations may also be performed through the flexible bronchoscope, and specimens taken with a flexible biting tip forceps may be sent to the laboratory for tissue identification.
- Lung tissue specimens are friable; the surgical technologist should take care removing the specimen from the jaw of the biopsy forcep using a 22-gauge needle or let the surgeon "tap" the specimen onto the Telfa pad.
- The circulator should prepare four or five specimen containers prior to the start of the procedure.

Surgical Procedure

1. One of two methods is used for applying the topical anesthetic. In the first method, the anesthesia provider or surgeon sprays the local anesthetic to numb the tongue, palate, pharynx, larynx, and trachea. The second method involves the surgeon or anesthesia provider using a straight or curved metal cannula that is attached to a laryngeal syringe. The topical anesthetic is squirted onto the surface of the vocal cords and then through the glottis and onto the surface of the trachea.
2. *Flexible:* The surgeon inserts the flexible bronchoscope through the endotracheal adaptor and endotracheal tube.

   Rigid: If not using a scapular roll, the head of the OR table is slightly lowered after the patient has been administered general anesthesia. A plastic tooth guard is placed over the upper teeth for protection. The surgeon inserts the rigid bronchoscope into the mouth and over the anterior surface of the tongue. The surgical technologist may be asked to retract the upper lip slightly upward or the surgeon will do it himself or herself. The surgeon identifies the epiglottis and moves it upward using the tip of the bronchoscope.

   Procedural Consideration: When setting up for the procedure, the circulator should squirt lubricant onto a 4 × 4 sponge on the back table or Mayo stand.

(*continues*)

PROCEDURE 22-1 (continued)

The surgical technologist should lubricate 2–3 inches of the end of either type of scope just prior to insertion.

When positioning the patient for a rigid bronchoscopy, the head is slightly tilted to the left when the surgeon wants to view the right bronchi and slightly tilted to the right to view the left bronchi.

3. *Flexible:* The surgeon advances the scope through the vocal cord and into the trachea to view the tracheal rings and tissues. Next, the surgeon advances the scope into the right or left bronchi. Using the tissue biting forceps, the surgeon may take tissue specimens as well as take fluid specimens and use the biopsy brush.

Procedural Consideration: The surgical technologist will be responsible for assisting the surgeon in taking fluid specimens. The suction tube with specimen container is positioned for collecting bronchial washings; the specimen container must be held upright and not tipped to prevent the specimen from going through the suction. When the surgeon gives the order, the surgical technologist connects the suction tubing to the bronchoscope. The suction tubing is disconnected and the surgical technologist injects 5 mL of saline solution into the channel of the scope and quickly reconnects the suction to take additional fluid specimen; the surgical technologist must be familiar with the brand/type of bronchoscope being used and know the correct channel in which to inject the saline solution. The surgeon may have the procedure repeated several times.

When a brush biopsy is taken, the surgical technologist must complete two actions along with the circulator. First, the surgical technologist will take the brush and rub it on a microscope slide that the circulator is holding. The circulator will then "fix" the specimen to the slide by spraying it with 95% ethanol alcohol. Next, the surgical technologist will use the wire-cutting scissors to cut the brush off the end of the forceps while holding it over the specimen container the circulator is holding.

Rigid: The surgeon advances the scope through the vocal cords and into the trachea to view the tracheal tissues. The patient's head is moved slightly to the left and the scope advanced to view the right bronchi. The right-angle telescope is inserted into the bronchoscope to view the right bronchial branches and upper lobe. The surgeon may take fluid and tissue specimens at this time (Figure 22-10).

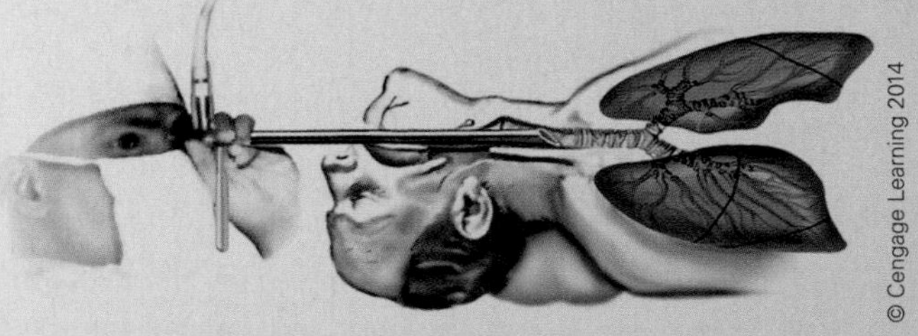

Figure 22-10 Rigid bronchoscopy

Practical Considerations

The straight aspirating tube is used to take cytology specimens from the pharynx, larynx, and esophagus. The curved aspirating tubes are used to remove cytology specimens from the upper portions of the bronchi. The surgical technologist must communicate where the specimen was obtained to the circulator so he or she can correctly label the specimen container.

Procedure 22-1 (continued)

4. *Flexible:* The surgeon withdraws the flexible bronchoscope and reinserts in the opposite bronchi to view and remove tissue and fluid-washing specimens.

   Rigid: The surgeon withdraws the bronchoscope and telescope into the trachea, the patient's head is straightened and the scope advanced to view the middle lobes.

5. *Rigid:* The scope is withdrawn again, the patient's head is slightly turned to the right, and the left bronchi and upper lobe are inspected. Additional fluid and tissue specimens may be taken.

6. *Flexible and Rigid:* The bronchoscope is removed.

Postoperative Considerations

Immediate Postoperative Care

- Patient is transported to the PACU.
- Patient is discharged the same day of surgery.

Prognosis

- No complications: Patient returns to normal activities once the sedation and local anesthetic has worn off. Patient may have to undergo additional follow-up procedures depending on analysis of specimens.
- Complications: Postoperative SSI; hemoptysis

Wound Classification

- Class V: Unclassified

Procedure 22-2 Mediastinoscopy

Pathology

- Mediastinoscopy is performed for the evaluation of nodal involvement or mediastinal masses in patients with lung carcinoma. Typical of the lesions found within the mediastinum are thymomas, lymphomas, and germ cell tumors.
- Mass lesions tend to be enterogenous cysts, lymphomas, neurogenic tumors, and pleuropericardial cysts.
- The most common tumors found within the mediastinum of children are neurogenic tumors; in adults, thymomas and lymphomas appear most frequently.
- Complaints typically include cough, dyspnea, and chest pain. Symptomatic lesions are malignant in 60% of all patients.

Preoperative Diagnostic Tests and Procedures

- CT scan that shows hilar or paratracheal adenopathy.

Equipment, Instruments, and Supplies Unique to Procedure

- Mediastinoscope
- Fiberoptic light source
- Fiberoptic light cord
- Suction tips
- Suction tubing
- Aspiration tubes
- Biopsy forceps
- Minor instrument set
- Single basin
- ESU
- Electrocautery pencil
- Basic back table pack
- Gowns

(*continues*)

PROCEDURE 22-2 (continued)

	• Gloves • 4 × 4 radiopaque sponges	• Telfa • 20- or 22-gauge needle	• Towels • Thyroid or transverse drape
Preoperative Preparation	• Position: Supine with scapular roll to hyperextend neck • Anesthesia: General. The anesthesia provider will be seated at the patient's side while the surgeon	is at the head of the table. • Skin prep: Beginning at suprasternal notch where incision will be made, extend from the lower border of the mandible to mid-	chest, including entire neck and bilaterally as far as possible. • Draping: Four towels to square off incision site; thyroid or transverse drape
Practical Considerations	• Mediastinoscopy is a sterile procedure. It is preferable that the mediastinoscope be sterilized for use rather than use high-level disinfection. • Sponge counts are completed because the incision involves entering the neck region down to the trachea. • The tissue specimens are friable; the surgical technologist should take care removing the specimen from the jaw of the biopsy forcep using a 22-gauge needle or let the surgeon "tap" the specimen onto the Telfa pad. • The circulator should prepare	4–5 specimen containers prior to the start of the procedure. • The mediastinoscope and light source should be tested prior to the entry of the patient into the OR. • The surgical technologist should apply the antifog solution to the lens of the scope just prior to insertion. • The overhead OR lights may be turned off according to surgeon's preference; the circulator will turn on the X-ray viewing box to provide some light. • The surgical technologist may be responsible for	assisting the surgeon in inserting the biopsy forceps into the channel of the scope and advancing the forceps. When using flexible forceps, the surgical technologist should assist the surgeon in maintaining control of the forceps and prevent contamination. The surgical technologist should make sure the forceps are in the closed position prior to insertion into the channel. • The 10-mL syringe should be filled with 5 mL of saline prior to the start of the procedure in preparation for taking cytologic specimens.

Procedure 22-2 (continued)

Surgical Procedure

1. Using a #15 knife blade, the surgeon makes a 1- to 2-cm transverse incision just above the suprasternal notch and carried down to the platysma muscle.
2. Dissection is continued through the pretracheal fascia until the trachea is exposed.
3. Using blunt dissection, the surgeon creates a tunnel along the trachea into the mediastinal space.
4. The mediastinoscope is inserted and advanced through the tunnel into the space.
5. The surgeon visualizes the lymph nodes, tracheal bifurcation, and bronchi (Figure 22-11).

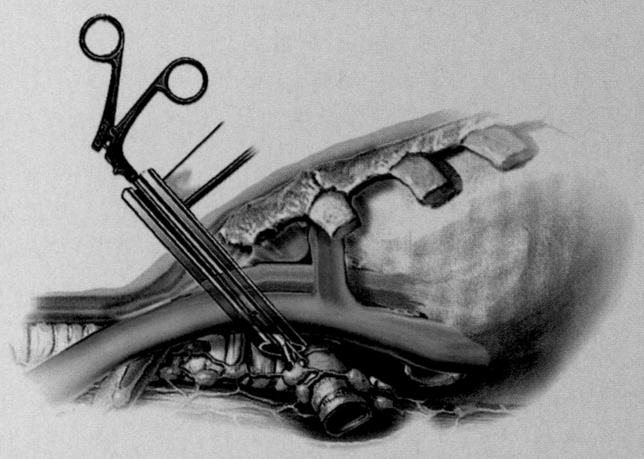

Figure 22-11 Mediastinoscopy

6. Using the tissue biopsy forcep, the surgeon excises lymph node tissue specimens.
7. The mediastinoscope is removed. The platysma muscle is closed with interrupted absorbable sutures. The skin is closed with interrupted nonabsorbable sutures or skin staples. A small dressing is applied.

Postoperative Considerations

Immediate Postoperative Care

- Patient is transported to the PACU.
- Patient is discharged the same day of surgery.

Prognosis

- No complications: Patient expected to return to normal activities in 2–3 days. Patient may have to undergo additional follow-up procedures depending on analysis of specimens.
- Complications: Postoperative SSI; hemorrhage

Wound Classification

- Class I: Clean

Procedure 22-3 Video-Assisted Thoracic Surgery (VATS)

Pathology

- VATS evolved from thoracoscopy as well as the advances made in minimally invasive surgical techniques and instrumentation. VATS is used for the diagnosis and treatment of several

(continues)

PROCEDURE 22-3 (continued)

	thoracic diseases and disorders of the esophagus, lungs, mediastinum, pericardium, and pleura. • Pleural disorders that can be treated include blebs (irregular bulge) and cysts as well as tissue	biopsy of mediastinal masses. • Procedures that have been performed through VATS include lung wedge resection, lobectomy, lung volume reduction, creation of a pericardial window,	pericardiectomy, and thymectomy. • VATS is also indicated when the patient has impaired pulmonary functions and the risk of performing open surgery is outweighed by the pathology.
Preoperative Diagnostic Tests and Procedures	• As previously listed for thoracic procedures		
Equipment, Instruments, and Supplies Unique to Procedure	• 5- and 10-mm endoscopes, 0° and 30° lenses • Fiberoptic light cord • Camera • Fiberoptic light source • Videocassette recorder • Printer • Insufflator • ESU • #11 and #15 knife blades • Endoscopic scissors: Straight, curved, hooked, micro • Endoscopic graspers: Toothed, serrated with no teeth, smooth • Endoscopic Allis clamps • Endoscopic Babcock clamps	• Endoscopic Pennington clamps • Endoscopic probes • Endoscopic fan lung retractor • Trocars: 10/11 mm × 2; 10/12 mm × 2 • Endoscopic hemoclip appliers of various sizes • Hemoclips of various sizes • Endoscopic linear stapler • Tissue specimen bag • Minor instrument set–instruments needed for incision and closure, including long Pean clamps and Cushing vein retractors • Endoscopic suture ligators and carriers	• Endoscopic tissue and lung endostaplers • Major cardiovascular instrument set available in OR • Laparoscopy back table pack • Transverse or laparoscopy drape • Plastic adhesive incise drape • Kitners • Vessel loops • Lens defogger • 28 Fr chest tube • Pleur-evac closed water-seal drainage system • Marcaine 0.25% or lidocaine 1% with epinephrine
Preoperative Preparation	• Position: Usually lateral, but may vary according to the planned procedure • Anesthesia: General with a double-lumen	endotracheal intubation tube • Skin prep: Extends from the shoulder and axilla to the iliac crest and bilaterally as far as possible	• Draping: Four towels to square off incision site; plastic adhesive incise drape (surgeon's preference); transverse or laparoscopy drape

PROCEDURE 22-3 (continued)

Practical Considerations	• Patient's X-rays are in the OR. • Verify if surgeon wants a Foley catheter inserted. • The surgical technologist should be prepared for conversion to an open thoracotomy. • The surgical technologist should be prepared to assist the surgeon with intraoperative complications of VATS, including air embolism, injury to the diaphragm, and hemorrhage, all of which can be reason to convert to an open procedure. • The surgical technologist should use the lens defogger on the endoscope just before it is inserted. • Contact the blood bank to confirm that blood has been ordered and is available. • This is a sterile procedure; therefore, the camera, scopes, light cord, insufflator cord, etc. must be sterile. • The ESU may be connected to endoscopic instruments such as the scissors and probe.
Surgical Procedure	The following is a description of a VATS wedge resection. 1. Lidocaine or Marcaine is injected into incision site. Using the #15 knife blade, the surgeon makes a 1.5- to 3-cm incision between the fourth and seventh intercostal space at the posterior axillary line. A digital examination is completed to verify the entrance into the pleural cavity. The anesthesia provider deflates the lung. 2. The first 10/12-mm trocar is inserted and removed, leaving the sheath in place. The 0° 10-mm endoscope is inserted and camera and light cords are attached (Figure 22-12A). 3. Under endoscopic visualization, the second incision is made between the fourth and seventh intercostal space at the anterior axillary line. The 10/11-mm trocar is inserted and removed, leaving the sheath in place. 4. The third incision is made at the upper posterior axillary line and the second 10/11-mm trocar is inserted. The surgeon may replace the 0° scope with the 30° scope. **Procedural Considerations:** The second and third ports are for the insertion of endoscopic instruments (Figure 22-12B). 5. A fourth incision is made; it is a 6-cm submammary incision that will be used for removing the tissue specimen. 6. An atraumatic endoscopic grasper is inserted; the lung is grabbed and retracted downward and anterior. 7. The surgeon identifies the blood vessels that will need to be divided (Figure 22-12D). An endoscopic vascular clamp is placed on the vessel proximal to where the endoscopic staples will be placed. The endoscopic stapler is inserted and fired to divide the vessel. This process will be repeated several times until all major vessels have been divided. **Procedural Consideration:** The surgical technologist will need to quickly refill the stapler when it is empty in order to avoid delays. The surgical technologist should have at least two endoscopic staplers available; when one is empty, the full stapler can be handed to the surgeon to allow the surgical technologist time to fill the first stapler.

(continues)

Procedure 22-3 (continued)

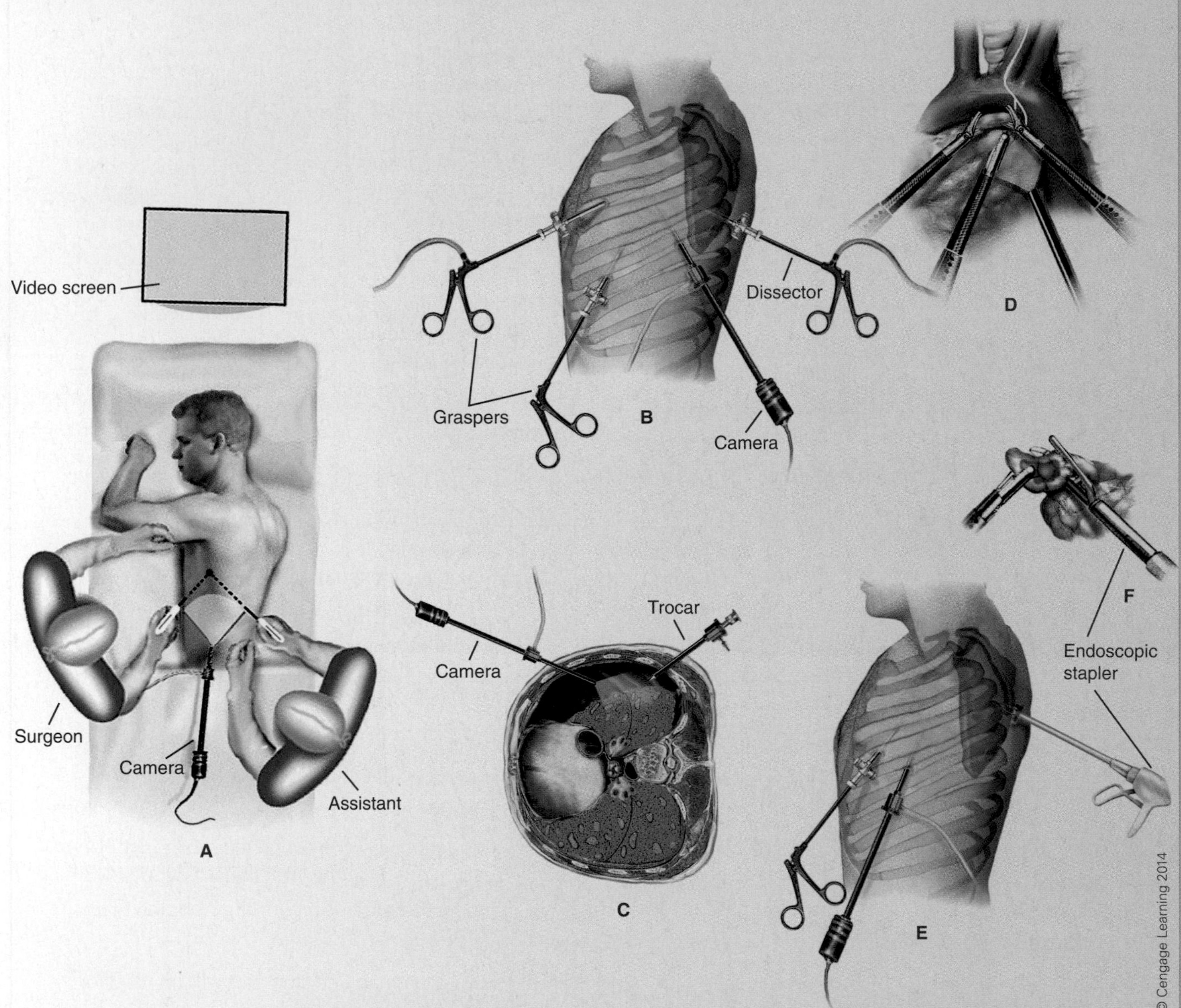

Figure 22-12 Video-assisted thoracoscopic surgery (VATS): (A) Trocar placement, (B) trocar and instrument placement, (C) intrathoracic view, (D) exposure and dissection of lung lesion, (E) introduction of endoscopic stapler, (F) stapling of lung lesion

8. Using graspers and scissors, the lymph nodes that are situated around the bronchus are removed.

   Procedural Consideration: The lymph nodes are considered tissue specimens; the surgical technologist should ask the surgeon if they are to be sent to pathology together or as separate specimens. If to be sent as separate specimens, the surgical technologist should communicate the location from where each one is excised in order for the specimen container label to have the correct information.

Procedure 22-3 (continued)

9. The wedge of lung tissue to be removed is identified by the surgeon. A grasper is placed on the lower part of the wedge. An endoscopic stapler is placed across the lung and fired (Figure 22-12E, F).
10. A tissue specimen bag is rolled up and inserted. The wedge is placed inside the bag and brought out through the submammary incision.

    Procedural Consideration: If the specimen is infected or has a malignant tumor, the bag prevents the spread of infectious fluid or seeding of malignant cells. Routine, non-endoscopic instrumentation may be inserted through the submammary incision to grasp the specimen bag and remove.
11. The surgical site is inspected for hemorrhage and the staple line is viewed to verify closure.
12. The surgeon places a chest tube though the lower posterior incision site and it is connected to the Pleur-evac.
13. The sheaths are removed and the incisions closed. The chest tube is secured to the skin with a suture. Small dressings are placed over the incisions.

Postoperative Considerations

Immediate Postoperative Care

- Patient is transported to the PACU, ICU, or CCU.
- Patient will remain hospitalized for 4–7 days.

Prognosis

- No complications: Patient is expected to make a full recovery and return to normal activities in 4–6 weeks. Patient may have to undergo additional follow-up procedures depending on analysis of specimens.
- Complications: Postoperative SSI; atelectasis; acute pulmonary edema; hemorrhage; mediastinal shift; pneumonia; pneumothorax; pulmonary embolus; respiratory insufficiency; subcutaneous emphysema

Wound Classification

- Class I: Clean

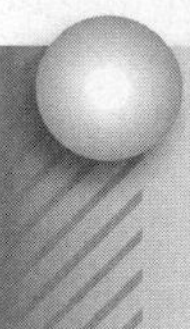

Pearl of Wisdom

As with any endoscopic procedure, proper camera positioning is essential. But unlike with laparoscopic procedures, the thorax cannot be insufflated for expansion; therefore, double-lumen endotracheal tubes that allow single-lung ventilation and collapse of the lung on the affected side are essential.

Procedure 22-4 Nuss Pectus Excavatum Repair by VATS

Pathology

- The most common congenital deformity of the chest is a funnel-shaped, asymmetrical depression due to a posterior displacement of the sternal body, referred to as pectus excavatum (funnel chest). The deformity usually affects 4–5 ribs on each side of the sternum. In extreme cases, the sternum may even reach the vertebral column.

(continues)

Procedure 22-4 (continued)

	• The cause of the abnormal growth of the costal cartilage and sternum is not known, but its occurrence along with Marfan's syndrome and/or kyphosis is common.	• Symptoms include bronchospasm, exercise intolerance, dysrhythmias, chest pain, and dyspnea. Surgical repair before the age of 5 years produces the best results.	• Treatment is for aesthetic and psychological reasons as well as restoration of normal respiratory functions in extreme cases.
Preoperative Diagnostic Tests and Procedures	• History and physical • Standard X-rays of the chest, lateral and posteroanterior	• CT scan of chest • Comprehensive cardiologic	examination with electrocardiography • Spirometry

Equipment, Instruments, and Supplies Unique to Procedure	• Thoracoscopy equipment and instrumentation
	• Minor orthopedic instrument set
	• Vascular instrument set
		• Pectus bar instruments:
		  • Metal bar lock
		  • Pectus bar clamp
		  • Pectus bar bender
		  • Pectus bar introducer
		  • Pectus bar plate flipper
			• Pectus bar stabilizer plates × 2
			• Templates, various lengths that range from 7 to 17 in.
			• Insufflator and tubing
			• Umbilical tape

Preoperative Preparation	• Position: Supine; chest may be slightly elevated with use of a roll sheet, surgeon's preference • Anesthesia: General with double-lumen ET tube. An epidural	catheter is inserted preoperatively in order to provide postoperative pain control. • Skin prep: Lower border of the mandible to the level of the	umbilicus; bilaterally as far as possible • Draping: Four towels to square off chest region—do not cover the marks made for the bilateral incisions; transverse drape.
Practical Considerations	• Test all the video equipment prior to the patient entering the OR. • X-rays are in the OR. • Using a permanent marker, the surgeon will mark the bilateral incisions in the mid-axillary line, as well as indicate the deepest point of the pectus excavatum and mark the top of the rectus ridge bilaterally. These	serve as anatomical landmarks for the insertion of the pectus bar. • Preoperatively, the surgeon will measure the chest using the anatomical marks that were marked as indicated in the previous bullet. The length of the pectus bar is determined by the distance from the	right to the left incision marks minus 1–2 cm. The surgeon will communicate the needed length of the pectus bar to the surgical technologist. • The surgical technologist should set up a small separate sterile table for the surgeon to use the plate bender to bend the pectus bar.

PROCEDURE 22-4 (continued)

Surgical Procedure

1. After draping the patient, the surgeon will place a template on the chest of the patient and bend it to the desired shape. The pectus bar is placed on the template, and in the pectus bar bender to bend the pectus bar to match the shape of the template.

   Procedural Consideration: The surgical technologist should place the bended pectus bar in a safe place on the back table until needed. If the pectus bar were to fall on the floor, the surgeon will most likely want a new bar to bend because the bar that fell on the floor could have scratches.

2. Using a #15 knife blade, two bilateral 2.5-cm incisions are made at the previous skin marks (Figure 22-13A).

3. A tunnel is made just below the skin from both incisions toward the marks that were made on each rectus ridge.

4. The anesthesia provider collapses the right lung and the thoracoscope is inserted two intercostal spaces below the right lateral incision. The thoracoscope is advanced subcutaneously to the pectus ridge.

5. The pectus bar introducer is inserted through the right-side incision and advanced across the mediastinum until the tip appears through the left-side incision.

6. The umbilical tape is tied to the introducer and it is slowly pulled back, out left to right.

   Procedural Consideration: The umbilical tape will be used to guide the pectus bar through the tunnel.

7. The umbilical tape is untied from the introducer and tied to the pectus bar on the right side. The pectus bar is advanced through the tunnel right to left under the sternum.

   Procedural Consideration: The pectus bar is inserted with the convexity facing posteriorly.

8. The umbilical tape is untied from the pectus bar. The pectus bar plate flipper is used to turn the pectus bar into position, which raises the sternum and anterior chest wall into the desired anatomic position. The distal ends of the pectus bar lie along the lateral sides of the chest wall (Figure 22-13B).

9. Stabilizer plates are placed to secure the pectus bar to the chest and prevent migration. The plates are either sutured together with a large-diameter nonabsorbable suture, #2 or #3 steel wire, or with the use of a metal bar lock that is placed in a distal hole of the plates.

10. The stabilizer is further secured to the lateral chest wall muscles with several sutures placed through the holes. The pectus bar stabilization is further achieved by the surgeon placing a suture around the bar and ribs.

11. The surgeon performs a final examination of the thorax with the thoracoscope to verify no injury to the pericardium, lungs, and mediastinal structures, as well as no bleeding.

12. Two chest tubes are inserted and the right lung is reexpanded. The thoracoscope is removed. Lateral incisions are closed in layers, including a subcuticular closure. Small dressings are placed.

(*continues*)

PROCEDURE 22-4 (continued)

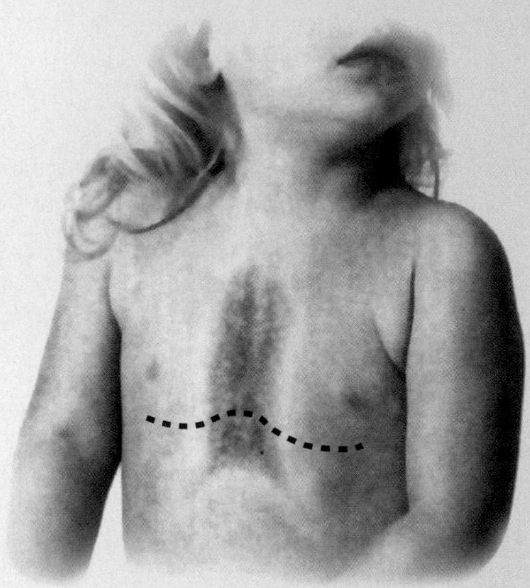

A

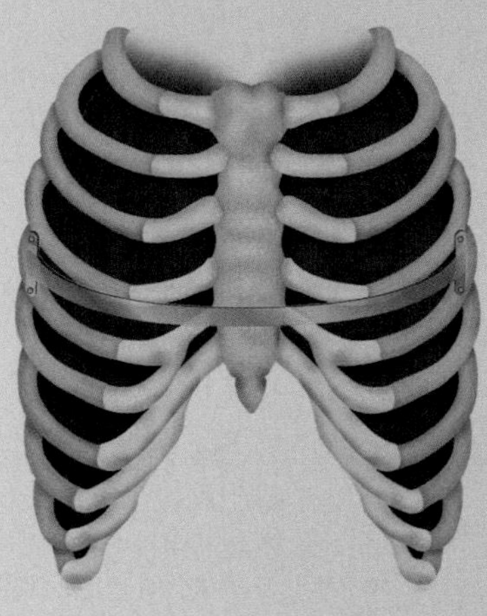

B

Figure 22-13 Pectus excavatum repair: (A) Defect and incision outline, (B) chest wall stabilized with pectus bar following repair

Postoperative Considerations

Immediate Postoperative Care

- Patient is transported to the PACU, ICU, CCU, or PCCU.
- Chest tubes are usually removed the day after chest X-ray confirms complete bilateral lung reexpansion and no air leaks.

Prognosis

- No complications: Patient is expected to have a full recovery with return to normal activities in 5–7 weeks. The pectus bar will not be removed for at least 3 years.
- Complications: Postoperative SSI; migration of the bar; pneumothorax; pleural and cardial effusion; pectus bar adhesions

Wound Classification

- Class I: Clean

PROCEDURE 22-5 Pulmonary Thromboendarterectomy

Pathology

- Pulmonary embolism obstructs the pulmonary artery, resulting in life-threatening chronic pulmonary hypertension and its associated complications.
- Patients are often asymptomatic until the disease has progressed and right heart failure is occurring. The earliest sign is severe pulmonary hypertension when exercising; however, the patient may not consider the symptoms abnormal and not report to the physician.
- Other signs and symptoms include enlarged pulmonary

PROCEDURE 22-5 (continued)

	arteries, septal hypertrophy, tricuspid regurgitation,	chronic cough, syncope, palpitations, and hemoptysis.	• The disease is always bilateral.
Preoperative Diagnostic Tests and Procedures	• History and physical: Pulmonary flow murmurs when listening to heart activity through the stethoscope. • Echocardiography: Used to visualize septal hypertrophy, tricuspid regurgitation, right atrial enlargement.	• CT angiography: Used to visualize and assess the pulmonary artery tree. • Lung perfusion scan: Reveals the patches of occlusion within the pulmonary artery. • Pulmonary arteriogram: Definitive	test for diagnosing pulmonary embolism; the arteriogram will clearly show the lack of blood flow to the periphery of the thoracic cavity from branches of the pulmonary artery.
Equipment, Instruments, and Supplies Unique to Procedure	• Refer to the coronary artery bypass with grafting (CABG) procedure.		
Preoperative Preparation	• Position: Supine • Anesthesia: General • Skin prep: Lower border of mandible to	mid-thigh; bilaterally as far as possible • Draping: Four towels to square off thoracic	region; plastic adhesive incise drape (surgeon's preference); cardiac/chest drape
Practical Considerations	• X-ray studies are in the OR. • Confirm with the blood bank that blood has been ordered and is available. • The surgical technologist should be particularly meticulous in keeping the instruments free of dried blood and tissue, and plaque.	• 4 to 5 liters of iced slush saline solution may be used when placing the patient on the cardiopulmonary bypass pump (CPB). • Warm saline solution will be needed when the patient is being taken off the CPB. • CBP is essential to the procedure. When the pulmonary arteries are	obstructed, the lung tissue is kept viable by a greater-than-normal bronchial blood flow. If circulatory arrest is not used, the pulmonary arteries and branches will not be able to be visualized due to the bronchial blood flow.

Surgical Procedure

1. The surgeon may insert an inferior vena cava filter prior to the start of the primary procedure.

   Procedural Consideration: Based on the surgeon's preference, the filter may be inserted preoperatively in a separately scheduled procedure, before the median sternotomy incision is made, or within 24 hours postoperatively.

2. The surgeon performs a median sternotomy with the powered sternal saw.

3. The pericardial sac is opened (called a pericardiotomy) and CPB is established by venous cannulation and ascending aortic cannulation.

(continues)

Procedure 22-5 (continued)

Procedural Consideration: Refer to the CABG procedure for details concerning cannulation.

4. The body of the patient is cooled 18°–20°C followed by circulatory arrest. While the body is cooling the surgeon will dissect free and mobilize the superior vena cava in order to gain access to the right pulmonary artery.

   Procedural Consideration: The surgeon will identify and preserve the phrenic nerves during this step of the procedure.

5. Beginning with the right pulmonary artery, the surgeon makes an arteriotomy using the #11 knife blade and extends the incision with the 45° Potts-Smith scissors.

   Procedural Consideration: The following is the surgeon's preference: (a) Due to the increased bronchial blood flow, the surgeon may call for intermittent periods of circulatory arrest and reperfusion in order to obtain exposure of the surgical site; or, (b) The surgeon will work on the right pulmonary artery, reperfuse, and repeat the procedure on the left pulmonary artery.

6. Using smooth vascular forceps, Freer elevator, and Jamieson dissector, the plaque is raised and excised from the right pulmonary artery. Dissection begins on the posterior wall of the artery and continues in a circumferential manner.

7. The surgeon continues the removal of the plaque from the segmental and subsegmental arterial branches using a combination of suction and dissection.

   Procedural Consideration: The surgeon may use a choledochoscope to first identify the location of the plaque in the arterial branches.

8. The surgeon closes the right pulmonary artery arteriotomy and performs the procedure on the left pulmonary artery.

9. Upon completion of the endarterectomy, CPB is resumed and the patient is re-warmed.

   Procedural Consideration: This is when the surgical technologist will need to request warm saline to be poured into a basin by the circulator for use by the surgeon.

10. The median sternotomy is closed and the dressings are applied.

Postoperative Considerations

Immediate Postoperative Care

- Postoperative care of the patient is similar to that provided for any patient who has undergone a thoracic/heart procedure. The patient is transported to the CCU.
- Patients usually remain ventilated for up to 48 hours.

Prognosis

- No complications: Pulmonary thromboendarterectomy is a curative procedure. A decrease in the pulmonary pressures and vascular resistance as well as improvement in the pulmonary blood flow are immediate. The enlarged right ventricle will decrease and return to normal size over a short period of time, which eliminates the tricuspid regurgitation. The average hospitalization is 10 days.
- Complications: Postoperative SSI; reperfusion response, also called reperfusion pulmonary edema that occurs in a small percentage of patients; however, it is the most significant complication associated with the procedure in which edema occurs in the area of the artery where the endarterectomy was performed; it is treated with conservative medical therapy.

Wound Classification

- Class I: Clean

Procedure 22-6 Decortication of the Lung

Pathology	• If blood or pus from a chest injury is not properly drained from the pleural cavity, it coagulates and forms a fibrin layer over the visceral and parietal pleura that interferes with the proper expansion of the lung. The condition is called empyema. • The main goal of decortication is to restore the normal lung function. Two other goals include controlling infection, such as in the case of empyema, and prevention of deformity. If not treated, deformity can occur in the chest and spine of adolescents.
Preoperative Diagnostic Tests and Procedures	• Standard chest X-ray • CT scan of chest • Bronchoscopy • Bronchospirometry
Equipment, Instruments, and Supplies Unique to Procedure	• As previously listed at beginning of chapter for thoracic procedures
Preoperative Preparation	• Position: Posterolateral • Anesthesia: General • Skin prep: Shoulder extending to iliac crest; arm up to the elbow; bilaterally as far as possible • Draping: Four towels to square off incision site; plastic adhesive incise drape; transverse drape
Practical Considerations	• X-rays are in the OR. • Confirm with the blood bank that blood has been ordered and is available. The procedure is associated with blood loss that will most likely need to be replaced.
Surgical Procedure	1. A posterolateral incision is made in the fifth or sixth intercostal space. The incision is carried through the subcutaneous and muscle layers using the #15 knife blade and ESU.
	2. The fifth or sixth rib may or may not be stripped and removed depending on the extent of the disease process.
	3. The rib retractor is placed and opened.
	4. The lung is inflated to visualize the extent of the entrapment. Using the #15 knife blade, the fibrin layer is incised.
	5. The dissection is performed with long Metzenbaum scissors and vascular forceps, blunt dissection with the finger, and Kitner sponge. The dissection is completed in the following manner: superior to inferior; medially to the superior vena cava, esophagus, and aorta; inferiorly and medially to the diaphragm and phrenic nerve (Figure 22-14). **Procedural Consideration:** During the dissection, extra care is taken to avoid injuring the subclavian vessels and phrenic nerve. It is important that the diaphragm be included in the dissection; if it is not included, it defeats the purpose of the decortication procedure in allowing the lung to fully expand. Additionally, injury to the phrenic nerve is avoided in order to prevent the paralysis of the diaphragm. The dissection can be a tedious process, and the surgical technologist must remain alert and vigilant throughout the procedure.

(continues)

PROCEDURE 22-6 (continued)

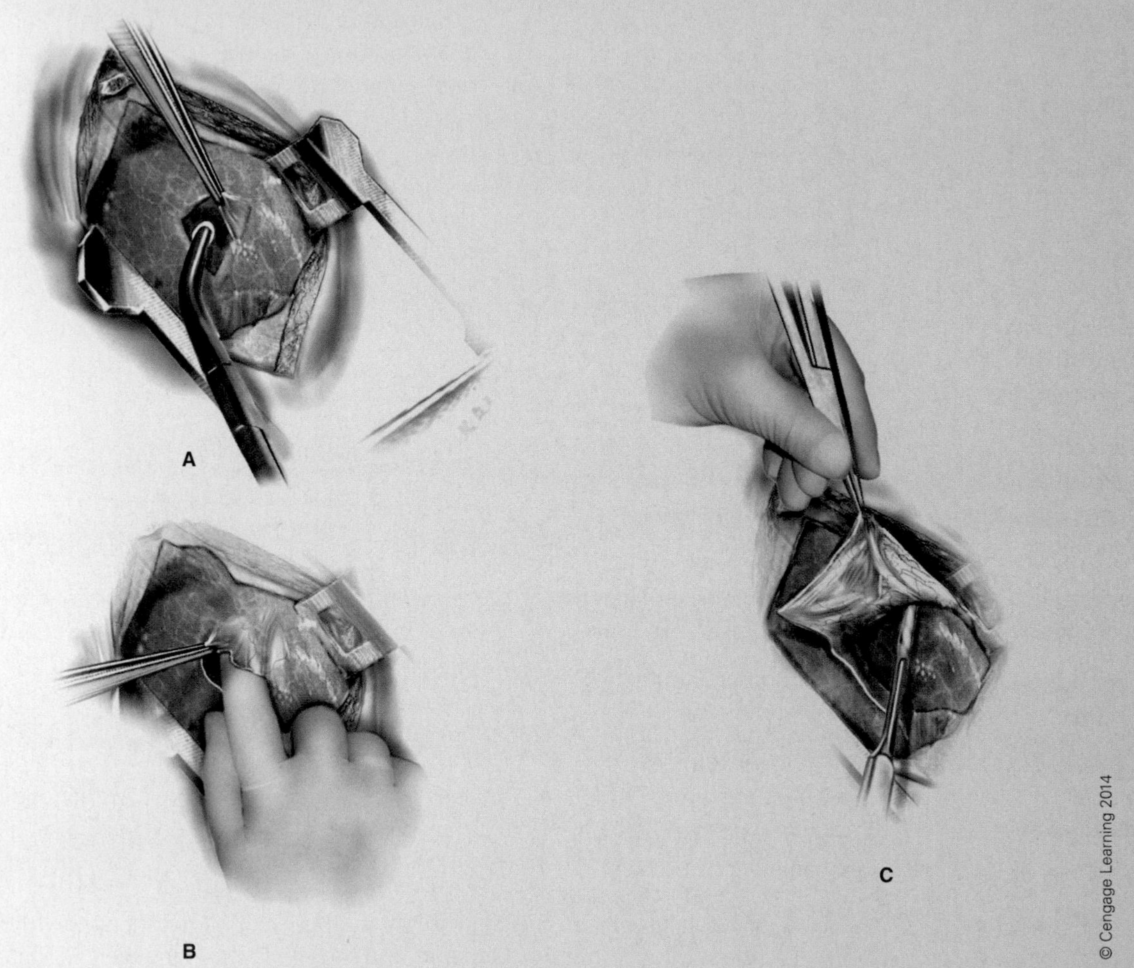

Figure 22-14 Decortication of the lung: (A) An incision is made in the fibrous membrane, (B) begins with blunt dissection, (C) sharp dissection may be required if membrane is adhered to visceral pleura

6. Upon completion of the dissection, the anesthesia provider will inflate the lung again in order for the surgeon to check for air leaks and hemorrhage from the lung.
7. The rib retractor is removed, two chest tubes are placed, and the posterolateral incision is closed in layers.

Postoperative Considerations

Immediate Postoperative Care

- Patient is transported to the PACU.

Prognosis

- No complications: Patient will be hospitalized for 7–10 days. Patient immediately begins physical therapy and continues for several months to achieve restoration of full lung expansion and avoid postural deformities, especially in adolescent patients. Patient is expected to make a full recovery as long as physical therapy regimen is completed.
- Complications: Postoperative SSI; hemorrhage; dissection not thorough and patient still experiences difficulty with breathing; diaphragm paralysis due to phrenic nerve damage

Wound Classification

- Class I: Clean

Procedure 22-7 Upper Lobectomy

Pathology	• If a neoplasm is confined to a particular lobe of the lung and hilar nodes are not involved, a lobe of the lung can be removed without disturbing other portions of the lung.
Preoperative Diagnostic Tests and Procedures	• Routine X-rays and tests for thoracic surgery
Equipment, Instruments, and Supplies Unique to Procedure	• As previously listed at beginning of chapter for thoracic procedures
Preoperative Preparation	• Position: Posterolateral • Anesthesia: General • Skin prep: Routine posterolateral skin prep • Draping: Routine draping procedure for posterolateral incision
Practical Considerations	• X-rays are in the OR. • Confirm with the blood bank that blood has been ordered and is available. • The surgical technologist should set up two suction tubes with tips on the sterile field. • The surgical technologist should have extensive knowledge of anatomy and physiology of the thorax. Procedures of the chest should be studied extensively. • Thoracic surgery can be challenging for even the most experienced surgical technologist, especially during emergency procedures. Proximity to major vessels should alert the surgical technologist to be prepared for vessel injury at any moment. Pledgeted double-armed polypropylene sutures should be always at the ready, as should silk or polypropylene suture ligatures; 2-0 or 3-0 silk ties of 24–32 in. length loaded onto carriers should be available at all times.
Surgical Procedure	1. After the patient has been prepped and draped, an incision is made into the fourth intercostal space (fifth or sixth interspace incision is made for the right middle lobe and lower lobe dissections). **Procedural Consideration:** Incision is made with a #10 blade on a No. 3 handle.
	2. A rib spreader is placed, and the pleura is incised. The anterosuperior portion of the hilar pleura is incised and separated. **Procedural Consideration:** Once the thorax is opened, it is unlikely that the rib instruments will be reused. Remove them from the Mayo stand.
	3. The fissure between the upper and lower lobes is opened, and dissection of the pulmonary artery is begun. **Procedural Consideration:** During the thoracic procedure, the surgical technologist should keep a calculation of the amount of irrigation used because of the potential for blood replacement. If sponges are to be weighed, throw off sponges only after they are completely soaked with blood.
	4. Pulmonary artery and pulmonary vein lobar branches are identified, isolated, doubly ligated, and divided.

(continues)

PROCEDURE 22-7 (continued)

Procedural Consideration: Thoracic procedures require the surgical technologist to always think a few steps ahead of the surgeon so that the surgeon never has to wait for a loaded suture or instrument. Time is of the essence during an injury to a major vessel of the thorax, and it requires the surgical technologist to move quickly and think clearly.

5. The upper lobe bronchus is freed by blunt dissection, and a bronchus clamp or staple gun is placed at least 1.5–2 cm from the main bronchial trunk.

   Procedural Consideration: Have stapler loaded and sutures prepared. The bronchus is divided quickly. Entry of the bronchial tree will change the wound classification and may result in contaminated instruments. Be prepared to isolate any contaminated instruments or supplies.

6. The bronchus is divided and closed with nonabsorbable sutures or staples fired from the autosuture device.

   Procedural Consideration: Be aware of the surgeon's and surgical assistant's moves at all times. Closely listening and watching during the procedure allows for anticipation. During an emergency, this is vital because the procedure may quickly deviate from normal.

7. A pleural flap is placed over the bronchial stump and secured with sutures. The remaining lobes are checked for air leaks, and the wound is closed after placement of chest tubes. The surgeon may inject 0.25% Marcaine during skin closure for postoperative pain control.

   Procedural Consideration: Body-temperature irrigation will be needed to fill the thorax to check for leaks. The anesthesia provider will perform the Valsalva maneuver (forcible exhalation or induced cough). Prepare for chest tube placement, wound closure, and appropriate counts. The lines from the chest tubes must be hooked up to the closed suction drainage unit and suction immediately turned on to prevent clotting within the chest tubes. The surgical technologist should not break scrub and keep the Mayo stand and back table sterile until the patient has left the OR.

Postoperative Considerations

Immediate Postoperative Care

- After the thoracic procedure, the patient may be transferred to the CCU with the endotracheal tube in place to ensure adequate postoperative ventilation and air exchange, the two most important factors for postoperative consideration in thoracic procedures.

Prognosis

- No complications: Patient will be hospitalized for 7–10 days. Patient is expected to make a full recovery; however, additional treatments such as chemotherapy and radiation can determine extent of return to normal activities.
- Complications: Postoperative SSI; hemorrhage; atelectasis; pneumonia; respiratory insufficiency; pneumothorax; pulmonary embolus; subcutaneous emphysema; mediastinal shift; acute pulmonary edema

Wound Classification

- Class I: Clean

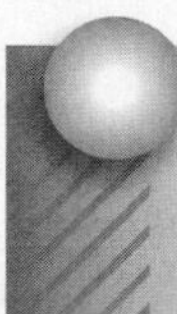

Pearl of Wisdom

Emergency chest procedures allow little time for a proper setup. Find out what approach the surgeon will be taking (usually posterolateral or median sternotomy) and prepare the items first that will allow you access to the injury. If approach is through median sternotomy, a scalpel followed by an electrosurgical pencil will be the first items the surgeon will want.

While the surgeon is making the incision, prepare the sternal saw and pass off the Cell Saver suction line. After the sternotomy, a sternal retractor will be required. At this point, laparotomy sponges and the suction from the Cell Saver will be necessary. Once hemorrhage is controlled, the surgical technologist can properly set up for the remainder of the procedure.

Procedure 22-8 Pneumonectomy

Pathology	• The chief indication for pneumonectomy is bronchogenic carcinoma. Less common indications include multiple lung abscesses, bronchiectasis, and extensive unilateral tuberculosis.
Preoperative Diagnostic Tests and Procedures	• Routine X-rays and tests for thoracic surgery
Equipment, Instruments, and Supplies Unique to Procedure	• As previously listed at beginning of chapter for thoracic procedures
Preoperative Preparation	• Position: Posterolateral • Anesthesia: General • Skin prep: Routine posterolateral skin prep • Draping: Routine draping procedure for posterolateral incision
Practical Considerations	• X-rays are in the OR. • Confirm with the blood bank that blood has been ordered and is available. • The surgical technologist should set up two suction tubes with tips on the sterile field. • The surgical technologist should have extensive knowledge of anatomy and physiology of the thorax. Procedures of the chest should be studied extensively.
Surgical Procedure	1. Using the #10 knife blade, the surgeon makes a posterolateral incision in the skin and carries it through the subcutaneous and muscle layer with the knife and ESU.
	2. If necessary, a rib is stripped and resected.
	3. The rib retractor is placed and opened to expose the lung in the thoracic cavity. The surgeon explores the cavity to determine if metastasis is present. If extensive metastasis is confirmed, the surgeon will terminate the procedure; two chest tubes will be inserted and the wound closed.
	4. Using long Metzenbaum scissors, vascular forceps, and blunt dissection, the surgeon dissects cavity adhesions and the mediastinal pleura to completely free up the lung. In the process of dissection the pulmonary ligament is doubly clamped, cut, and tied (CCCT).

(*continues*)

PROCEDURE 22-8 (continued)

5. Using a vessel loop, the superior pulmonary vein is retracted laterally to expose the pulmonary artery. The artery is CCCT.

   Procedural Consideration: When dividing the arteries and veins, the surgeon takes care to identify and preserve the vagus nerve. The surgeon may use a vessel loop to gently and slightly retract the nerve from the area of dissection; the vessel loop may be moved several times according to where the dissection is taking place.

6. The superior pulmonary vein is CCCT.

7. Branches of the superior pulmonary vein and pulmonary artery are isolated and CCCT.

   Procedural Consideration: The division of branches can be tedious and time consuming, but it is necessary to prevent postoperative hemorrhage in the thoracic cavity. The surgical technologist must remain focused and anticipate each time the surgeon needs clamps by keeping one or two clamps in the hand ready to be passed. Additionally, the surgeon will use a large number of ties; the surgical technologist must make sure not to run out of ties to pass to the surgeon.

8. The lung is retracted anteriorly using an Allison lung retractor. Using the Metzenbaum scissors and vascular forceps, the surgeon incises the hilar pleura to expose the inferior pulmonary vein. The vein is CCCT.

9. The bronchus clamp is placed on the bronchus near the bifurcation of the trachea. The bronchus is divided and the stump closed with nonabsorbable sutures using a mattress suture technique, or with the clamp still in place the bronchus is divided with the bronchial stapler. If staples are used, the surgeon will use a #15 knife blade on a long knife handle to divide the bronchus. The lung is removed and given to the surgical technologist.

   Procedural Consideration: The surgical technologist may need an extra-large basin to place the lung and hand off to the circulator. Confirm with the circulator whether it is right or left lung.

10. The thoracic cavity is thoroughly irrigated with warm normal saline solution. The cavity is inspected for hemorrhage and the bronchial stump is checked for air leakages. The empty pleural space must be thoroughly suctioned to prevent the irrigation solution and blood, if present, from entering the opposite lung.

    Procedural Consideration: The surgical technologist should anticipate when the surgeon will want the saline irrigation and ask the circulator to pour it just before it is needed in order to prevent it from becoming cold.

11. The surgeon excises the peripheral lymph nodes within the thoracic cavity, including the mediastinal space.

12. Using the pleura, the surgeon creates a flap that is sutured over the bronchial stump using nonabsorbable suture.

13. Two chest tubes are placed and the pleural space is closed. After the space is closed the chest tubes are connected to the closed water-seal drainage unit.

14. The rib retractor is removed and the Bailey rib contractor is placed. The thoracic cavity is closed with nonabsorable suture using interrupted suture technique.

15. The muscle and subcutaneous layers are closed. The skin is closed with skin staples or subcuticular closure and skin closure tapes.

Procedure 22-8 (continued)

16. The dressing is applied. Chest tubes are sutured to the skin with large-diameter nonabsorbable suture.

Postoperative Considerations	**Immediate Postoperative Care** • After the thoracic procedure, the patient may be transferred to the CCU with the endotracheal tube in place to ensure adequate postoperative ventilation and air exchange, the two most important factors for postoperative consideration in thoracic procedures.	**Prognosis** • No complications: Patient will be hospitalized for 10–14 days. Patient is expected to make a full recovery; however, additional treatments such as chemotherapy and radiation can determine extent of return to normal activities.	• Complications: Postoperative SSI; hemorrhage; atelectasis; pneumonia; respiratory insufficiency; pneumothorax; pulmonary embolus; subcutaneous emphysema; mediastinal shift; acute pulmonary edema **Wound Classification** • Class I: Clean

Procedure 22-9 Double Lung Transplant

Pathology	• A lung transplant is performed for a variety of reasons, including emphysema, COPD, idiopathic pulmonary fibrosis, cystic fibrosis, and primary pulmonary hypertension. • The procedure is not performed for patients	who have a history of cancer or currently have cancer, who have a history of chronic liver and kidney disease, who currently have an infection such as HIV or hepatitis, who had tobacco use in the last 6 months, or who have a history of	alcohol and drug abuse. • The patient must be psychologically stable in order to cope with the life-long challenges that a lung transplant presents, including ability to remember medication regimen.
Preoperative Diagnostic Tests and Procedures	• Routine X-rays and tests for thoracic surgery • Blood tests and skin tests to check for infections • Echocardiogram	• Possibly cardiac catheterization • Tests to look for cancer, e.g. Pap smear, mammogram, colonoscopy • Tissue typing	• The patient will have been undergoing preoperative immunosuppressive and antibiotic drug therapy.
Equipment, Instruments, and Supplies Unique to Procedure	• As previously listed at beginning of chapter for thoracic procedures	• Bronchoscopy instrumentation and equipment	
Preoperative Preparation	• Position: Supine with arms placed on armboards. Patients with emphysema may	have the arms positioned alongside the body. • Anesthesia: General	• Skin prep: Lower border of mandible to mid-thigh

(continues)

PROCEDURE 22-9 (continued)

	• Draping: Four towels to square off entire thoracic region; plastic adhesive incise drape (surgeon's preference); chest or transverse drape. The groin region is prepped and draped separately because an arterial femoral line may have to be inserted for monitoring or if cannulation for cardiopulmonary bypass (CPB) becomes necessary.
Practical Considerations	• X-rays are in the OR. • Confirm with the blood bank that blood has been ordered and is available. • The surgical technologist should set up two suction tubes with tips on the sterile field. • The surgical technologist should have extensive knowledge of anatomy and physiology of the thorax, as well as of the lung transplant procedure. The procedure is challenging and the surgical technologist is required to efficiently manage a large number of instruments and supplies. The surgical technologist should undergo training with an experienced Certified Surgical Technologist (CST) before attempting to perform the first scrub role on a solo basis. • The surgical technologist must be prepared for the use of CPB. • The donor will be a cadaver or individual who has been declared brain dead. • The surgical technologist should not break scrub and should preserve the sterility of the Mayo stand and back table until the patient has left the OR.
Surgical Procedure	*Steps 1–5: Removal of Lungs from Recipient* 1. A clamshell incision is made in the mammary fold. The incision extends mid-axillary region from right to left with the gentle curve at the sternum. A small skin flap is created with ESU and forceps to the level of the fourth intercostal space and the pectoralis muscle is divided at that level. 2. The fourth intercostal space is entered laterally and the rib spreader is placed to aid in the dissection of the mammary vessels as close to the sternum as possible. The mammary vessels are divided; the vessels are doubly clamped and divided with hemoclips or CCCT with 2-0 silk ties. 3. The tissue posterior to the sternum is dissected and the sternum cut with the sternal saw. The self-retaining sternal retractors are placed bilaterally and slowly opened while the retrosternal mediastinal tissue is incised to provide exposure of the aorta and the right atrium in case CPB becomes necessary. **Procedural Consideration:** The surgical team must be ready for the surgeon to indicate that CPB must be used. Hypoxia and/or chronic low pH combined with hemodynamic instability are two intraoperative complications that demand the use of CPB. **Note:** The following steps of the procedure are for transplantation of the right lung. However, the first lung to be transplanted is the one identified as having the lesser perfusion of the two lungs. 4. The anesthesia provider collapses the right lung. The pleura lying over the pulmonary hilum and the inferior pulmonary ligament are incised. The superior

PROCEDURE 22-9 (continued)

pulmonary vein, pulmonary artery, and inferior pulmonary vein are dissected free and divided. The superior division of the right pulmonary artery is CCCT; next, two vascular staplers are used to divide the superior pulmonary vein as close to the lung to be removed as possible in order to preserve the length for anastomosis. The inferior division of the right pulmonary artery and inferior pulmonary vein are also divided with vascular staples as close to the lung as possible.

Procedural Consideration: The surgeon is careful to identify and prevent injury to the phrenic nerve during the dissection of the hilum. The nerve supplies the diaphragm, and injury can result in diaphragmatic paralysis.

5. The bronchus is the last structure to be divided and the lung is then removed.

   Procedural Consideration: The surgeon will exercise great care in achieving hemostasis at this point in the procedure, in particular for patients who have bronchiectasis or cystic fibrosis, as they tend to have enlarged bronchial arteries.

6. Before the donor lung can be implanted the bronchus, pulmonary veins and the pulmonary artery must be prepared for anastomosis. Allis clamps are placed on the corners of the bronchus and held in place by the surgeon. Using a sponge for blunt dissection and the Metzenbaum scissors, the surgeon dissects away the tissue that surrounds the bronchus (called peribronchial tissue) toward the mediastinum. Next, the cartilaginous wall is cut from around the end of the bronchus, but left attached on the posterior side. The surgeon will place 3-0 PDS or Vicryl at the corners of the cartilaginous wall, but the needles are not cut off. Now the membranous wall located behind the cartilaginous wall is cut with valve scissors.

7. Two Judd-Allis clamps are placed on the stumps of the pulmonary vein. The pericardium is incised around the veins in order to obtain as much length as possible of the left atrium in order to apply the atrial clamp when the atrial anastomosis is performed.

8. Two Judd-Allis clamps are placed on the pulmonary artery and the tissue around the artery is removed. Hemostasis is confirmed in the hilar region and a cooling jacket is placed in the pleural cavity. The donor lung will lie on the jacket during the anastomoses.

9. *Donor Lung Preparation:* The donor lungs are separated and prepared on a separate sterile back table. The bronchus, pulmonary artery, and atrial cuff are prepared.

   A. To separate the lungs, the atrial cuff is divided at the midline.

   B. The right and left pulmonary arteries are divided at their attachment to the primary pulmonary artery.

   C. The bronchus is divided with a GIA linear stapler and left stapled until implantation to keep the lung inflated.

   D. The right pulmonary artery is cut to a short length to avoid kinking at the site of anastomosis. The first branch of the artery is identified and preserved to serve as an anatomical landmark to avoid kinking or twisting at the site of the anastomosis.

   E. The left atrium is dissected free from its pericardial attachments. The surgeon will hold the atrial cuff upward with vascular forceps, and a Kelly clamp is applied to the pericardial tissue flap. The surgeon performs the dissection with the Metzenbaum scissors and preserves the flap, which to will be used to help cover the bronchial anastomosis; 5 mm or slightly more of the atrium is left around the pulmonary veins.

(*continues*)

PROCEDURE 22-9 (continued)

Steps 10–11: Implantation of the Donor Lung

10. Right before the donor lung is placed in the pleural space on top of the cooling jacket, the surgeon opens the bronchus using a #15 knife blade.

11. The order of the anastomosis is bronchus, pulmonary artery, atrial cuff.
   A. *Bronchus:* The previously placed sutures in the cartilaginous wall of the recipient bronchus are placed at the corners of the donor bronchus, but not tied; Crile clamps are placed on the sutures to provide traction. The membranous wall is anastomosed first with a continuous 4-0 Maxon or PDS suture. When the membranous portion anastomosis is completed, the surgeon gently pulls on the two traction sutures to tighten the membranous wall sutures. Next the cartilaginous wall is sutured with 3-0 or 4-0 polypropylene. When the diameters of the lumens match up, an end-to-end anastomosis is performed using interrupted suture technique. If the diameters do not match up, a telescoping anastomosis is used; the donor bronchus will be telescoped outside the recipient bronchus. The mediastinal tissue posterior to the pulmonary artery and donor peribronchial tissue is used to cover the bronchus at the site of the anastomosis.
   B. *Pulmonary artery:* The surgical assistant gently pulls on the mediastinum to reveal the pulmonary artery. Two Judd-Allis clamps are placed on the end of the artery stump. A vascular clamp is placed further down the artery to aid in providing as much length as possible for the anastomosis. A 5-0 polypropylene suture is placed in the bottom corner of the artery, but not tied. A suture is placed in the top corner and tied. The back wall of the artery is anastomosed first using a continuous suture. The front wall is then anastomosed; the first continuous suture is from the bottom corner to the middle and the second continuous suture is from the top corner to the middle. Before the surgeon ties the front wall suture, the pulmonary artery is filled with warm normal saline to remove the air; the surgeon will use a 14-gauge angiocatheter attached to a 20-mL syringe filled with the saline solution.
   C. *Atrial cuff:* The pulmonary veins are cut open just below the staple lines. The atrial tissue between the two veins is cut in order to create a single atrial cuff for anastomosis. Two Judd-Allis clamps are placed on the superior and inferior vein stumps. An atrial clamp is placed on the recipient's left atrium to aid in providing as lengthy of an atrial cuff as possible. The posterior wall of the atrium is sutured first; an everting mattress suture technique is used to create an end-to-end anastomosis. The anterior wall is sutured using the same suture technique. The sutures are not immediately tied; a curved Kelly clamp is placed between the suture line into the inferior pulmonary vein to keep the suture line open. While the anesthesia provider inflates the lung, the pulmonary artery clamp is slowly released; the surgeon will take 8–10 minutes to remove the clamp in order to provide a controlled reperfusion of the lung. While the clamp is being removed and the lung inflated, blood flow through the suture line is allowed and air is also allowed to escape. Once this is complete, the Kelly clamp is removed and the suture is tied.

12. The surgeon explores the pleural space to confirm there is no air leakage from the anastomoses and to confirm hemostasis.

13. The procedure is performed for the left lung.

PROCEDURE 22-9 (continued)

14. After the left lung is in place, two 28 Fr chest tubes are inserted in each pleural cavity, one straight tube and the other curved.

15. Four #2 Vicryl sutures are used to close each hemithorax. Three or four #5 steel wires are used to close the sternum. The muscle and subcutaneous layers are sutured with absorbable suture. The skin is closed with suture or staples.

16. The anesthesia provider changes the double-lumen ET tube to a single-lumen ET tube. The surgeon performs a bronchoscopy to aspirate secretions and internally recheck the anastomoses.

Postoperative Considerations

Immediate Postoperative Care

- Patient is transported to the CCU with the endotracheal tube in place to ensure adequate postoperative ventilation and air exchange, the two most important factors for postoperative consideration in thoracic procedures.
- If possible, attempt to have patient walk the same day as surgery.
- TED stockings should be worn to prevent DVT.
- Patient will be instructed to perform deep breathing exercises to prevent infection and pneumonia, and inflate the transplanted lung as fully as possible.
- Numerous chest X-rays will be taken during the hospital stay.

Prognosis

- No complications: Patient will be hospitalized for 14–21 days. Full recovery takes 6–8 months. Patient is expected to make a full recovery. However, the patient's lifestyle will not be the same as it was prior to lung disease and transplantation. Patient will undergo physical therapy with the goal of being able to function independently and lead as active of a lifestyle as possible with limitations. The patient will undergo numerous chest X-rays and blood tests during his or her lifetime. The patient will be required to be on medication to prevent the rejection of the lungs. One in five patients develops cancer or heart disorders within 5 years after the lung transplant.
- Complications: Postoperative SSI; hemorrhage; atelectasis; pneumonia; respiratory insufficiency; pneumothorax; pulmonary embolus; mediastinal shift; acute pulmonary edema; rejection of lung(s)

Wound Classification

- Class I: Clean

PART II: Adult Cardiac Surgical Procedures

INTRODUCTION

The surgical procedures of the adult heart described in this section include CABG, intra-aortic balloon pump (IABP), ventricular assist device (VAD) insertion, aortic valve replacement, ventricular aneurysm, and heart transplant.

Cardiac surgery is typically performed in the largest room of the OR suite to accommodate a larger number of OR personnel and the equipment, which can be large, such as the CPB pump machine.

The cardiac patient may come from the cardiac care unit on an ICU bed with monitoring lines in place. Occasionally, the patient will be brought over from the cardiac catheterization lab, usually for an emergency procedure. Percutaneous transluminal coronary angioplasty (PTCA) procedures are performed in the "cath lab," and the OR's cardiac team is typically asked to stand by in case the patient requires an emergency open-heart procedure. Coronary angioplasty balloons can dissect a coronary artery during inflation, and this will require immediate surgical repair. These emergencies require the team to open sterile supplies and to set up for the procedure very quickly, often as the patient is being moved to the OR table. The patient brought over from the cardiac catheterization lab will generally have a sheath still inserted into the femoral artery (sheath is used to facilitate insertion of cardiac catheter in the lab); the surgical team should be careful not to dislodge the catheter until surgeon is ready for it to be removed and insertion site closed with suture.

DIAGNOSTIC PROCEDURES AND TESTS

Electrocardiography, echocardiography, and cardiac catheterization are also useful diagnostic procedures for the evaluation of cardiac disease. For a detailed description of these procedures, refer to Chapter 13. The following preoperative diagnostic studies are routinely performed for the patient scheduled to undergo a cardiac procedure:

- Chest X-ray
  - AP and lateral X-rays of the chest can determine the overall size of the heart and great vessel configuration, as well as any valvular or intracoronary calcification. Asymptomatic pericardial cysts and cardiac tumors may also be detected on plain films.
- CT scan and MRI
  - CT scan and MRI are useful for the evaluation of pericardial and intracardiac and extracardiac masses. CT scan is especially useful for the detection and evaluation of thoracic aorta dissection. MRI can detect abnormal positioning of intracardiac structures.
- Resting electrocardiography
- Stress test electrocardiography
- Echocardiography
- Radionuclide imaging
- Electrophysiology studies
- Cardiac catheterization studies that include ventricular, atrial, and pulmonary pressures, and cardiac output with ejection fraction recordings
- Digital subtraction cine-arteriograms of the left ventricle and coronary arteries; often a drawing is made by the cardiologist of the coronary arteries and coronary artery stenoses.
- Thoracic aorta arteriograms if the patient is to have a ventricular aneurysm repaired

In addition to diagnostic findings, the anesthesia provider should examine preoperative pulmonary function, coagulation studies, and arterial blood gas studies.

ROUTINE INSTRUMENTATION, EQUIPMENT, AND SUPPLIES

Most cardiac procedures require the same instrumentation, equipment, and supplies, with specialty items added that are unique to the procedure.

Instrumentation

Coronary bypass procedures typically require one set of instruments for exposure of the heart and great vessels and cannulization for CPB, and another set with instruments for saphenous vein harvesting or inferior mammary artery (IMA) dissection and coronary anastomosis. Delicate coronary artery anastomosis instruments (e.g., Dietrich instrument set) are generally kept in a separate smaller set. A sternal saw, sternal retractor, and IMA retractor are usually opened separately. Valve retractors and sizers for aortic or mitral valve replacement are also opened separately. Table 22-3 is a list of instruments that are typically included in a cardiac instrument set.

Equipment

The following is a list of the routine equipment needed when performing cardiac procedures:

- CPB machine
- Hypothermia/hyperthermia unit
- Hypothermia mattress
- Cell Saver
- External pacemaker
- Defibrillator unit
- ESU
- Suction system
- Ice slush machine
- Endoscopic equipment for saphenous vein removal

Supplies

The following is a list of the routine supplies needed when performing cardiac procedures:

- Cardiac back table pack
- Double basin set
- Gloves
- Knife blades: #10 × 4; #11 × 2; #15 × 4
- Beaver knife handles × 2
- Beaver blades #64 and #69
- Three-quarter sheets × 5
- Plastic adhesive incise drape
- Split sheet
- Suture:
  - Cannulation sutures of the surgeon's choice (e.g., polypropylene or polyester)

Table 22-3 Cardiac and Diethrich Instrument Sets

Basic Cardiac Instrument Set

4	Knife handles: #3 × 2; #3L; #7
1	Lebsche sternal knife
2	Mayo scissors, straight, regular and long
2	Mayo scissors, curved, regular and long
4	Metzenbaum scissors, regular × 2; long × 2
4	Potts-Smith scissors, 25°, 45° × 2, 60°
2	Wire-cutting scissors
4	Tissue forceps with teeth, regular × 2, long × 2
2	Adson tissue forceps with teeth
2	Adson tissue forceps, smooth
4	DeBakey forceps, regular × 2, long × 2
6	Mosquito clamps, curved
6	Crile clamps, straight
20	Crile clamps, curved
6	Kelly clamps, curved
6	Pean clamps, curved
4	Kocher clamps
4	Right angle clamps
4	Schnidt (tonsil) clamps
2	Crawford aortic aneurysm clamps
8	DeBakey bulldog clamps, straight × 4, curved × 4
2	DeBakey coarctation clamps
2	DeBakey patent ductus clamps, straight and angled
2	DeBakey tangential occlusion clamps
2	Herrick kidney clamps
2	Satinsky clamps
6	Hemoclip appliers, small, medium, large
3	Richardson retractors, small, medium, large
2	U.S. Army retractors
2	Cushing vein retractors
4	Senn retractors, blunt × 2, sharp × 2
4	Rake retractors, blunt × 2, sharp × 2
2	Adson self-retaining retractors
2	Weitlaner self-retaining retractors
2	Self-retaining sternal retractors (surgeon's preference)
6	Needle holders, regular × 3, long × 3
8	Ryder vascular needle holders
2	Sternal needle holders
6	Sponge forceps
10	Towel clamps, blunt tip
20	Towel clamps, sharp tip
2	Yankauer suction tips
1	Aortic punch
1	Awl
1	Pituitary rongeur
1	Needlenose pliers
1	Mallet
1	Ruler

Endoscopic instrumentation for saphenous vein removal

Diethrich Instrument Set

4	Diethrich coronary scissors
2	Aortic dilators
10	Vessel dilators
6	Heparin needles
6	Vascular forceps
4	Castroviejo needle holders, straight × 2; curved × 2

- 5-0, 6-0 polypropylene; 0, 2-0, 3-0, 4-0 silk for pericardial stays
- Chest tube suture: 0 silk
- Silk and Vicryl ties, 0, 2-0, and 3-0
- Stainless steel sternal wires
- Absorbable suture for wound closure

- Drains: chest tubes (Argyle), various sizes
- Dressings: 4 × 4 sponges; ABD; tape
- Drugs:
    - Heparinized saline for intra-arterial irrigation and for soaking the saphenous vein before anastomosis
    - Topical papaverine for the prevention of vasospasm, especially involving the internal mammary artery
    - Antibiotic solution of surgeon's choice mixed with saline for irrigation
    - Various topical coagulants
- Internal defibrillator paddles and cord
- Venous and arterial cannulas
- Cardioplegia needle and administration set
- Cell Saver suction tubing
- Asepto syringe × 2

- Alligator pacing cables
- IV tubing and needles for intrachamber pressure readings
- Bone wax
- Gelfoam
- Surgicel
- Electrosurgical pencil × 3 (one for saphenous vein retrieval and two for the chest: two spatula tips and one needle tip)
- Hemoclips, various sizes
- Teflon felt pledgets
- Left ventricular sump catheter
- Coronary artery direct perfusion cannula
- Pacemaker wires
- Closed seal drainage unit (e.g., Pleur-evac)
- Hemoclips of various sizes
- Teflon or Dacron patch material
- Red rubber catheters for tourniquets and rubber shods
- Vessel loops
- Y-connector for chest tubes
- Fogarty inserts for aortic cross-clamp
- Saphenous vein cannula
- Various sizes of syringes and needles

ANATOMY AND PHYSIOLOGY OF THE HEART

The role of the heart within the cardiovascular system is essential for the circulation of blood, which carries waste substances away from cells to excretory organs for elimination, and vital nutrients and oxygen from the respiratory and digestive organs to cells throughout the body. Due to the extensive anatomy and physiology of the heart, it is presented in the next section rather than within the cardiac surgical procedures.

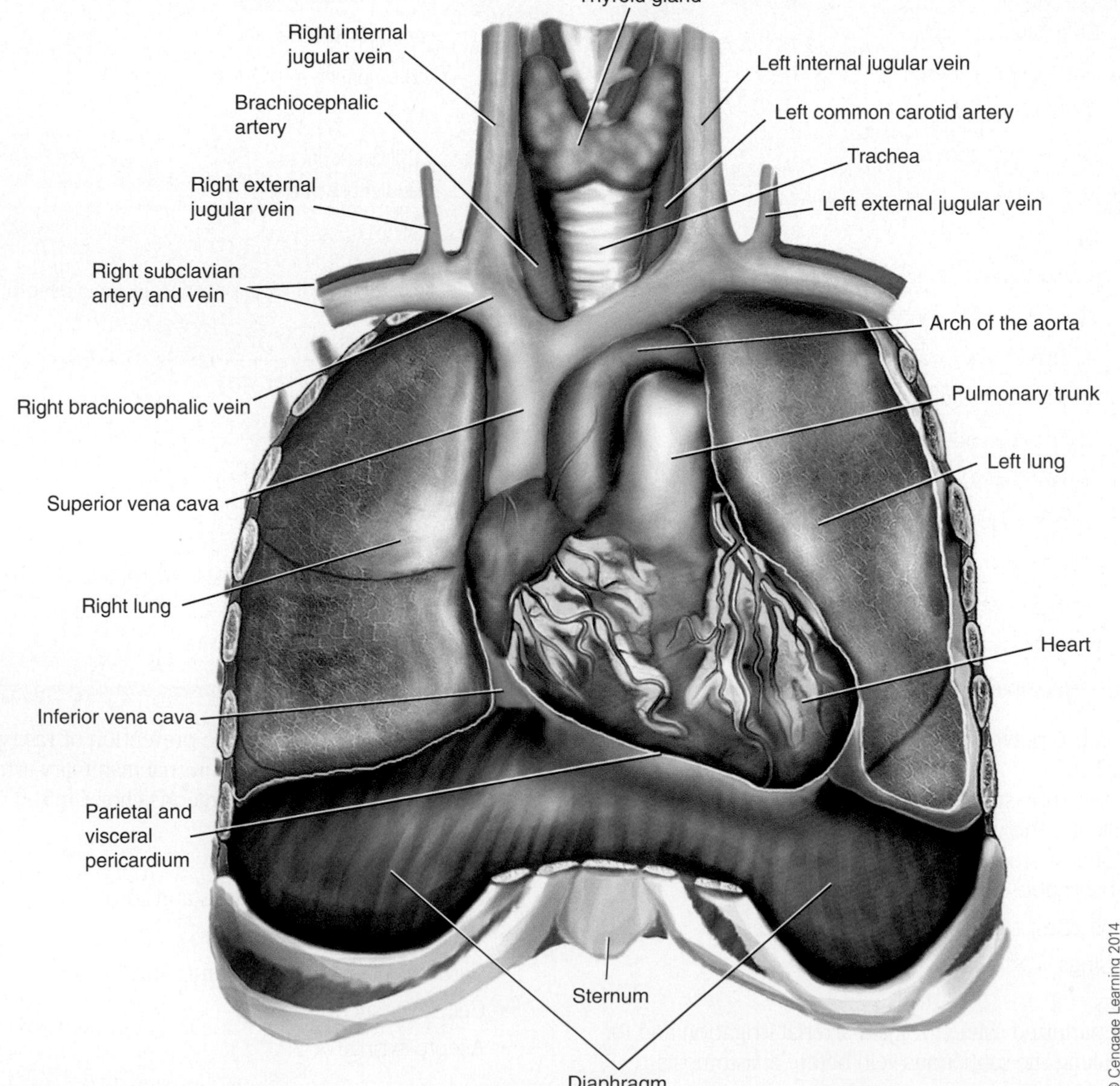

Figure 22-15 Structures within the thorax

Location of the Heart

- Hollow, muscular organ
- Size of a man's fist
- Located within mediastinum, with two-thirds of the organ on the left side (Figure 22-15)
- Rests behind the body of the sternum and on the diaphragm
- Lies diagonally, with distal apex tapering to the left

Coverings of the Heart

The pericardium (Figure 22-16) protects the heart and prevents it from rubbing against the thoracic cavity wall. It consists of two parts:

- Fibrous pericardium
  - Outer layer of pericardium
  - Consists of white fibrous connective tissue
  - Fits loosely around the heart and attaches to large blood vessels, but does not attach to the heart itself
  - Inelastic
  - Protects the heart
- Serous pericardium
  - Parietal layer: Lines the inside of the fibrous pericardium
  - Visceral layer: Attached to the surface of the heart
  - Pericardial space: Space between the two layers that contains pericardial fluid, which acts as a lubricant on the surfaces of the two layers, reducing friction and allowing the heart to easily contract

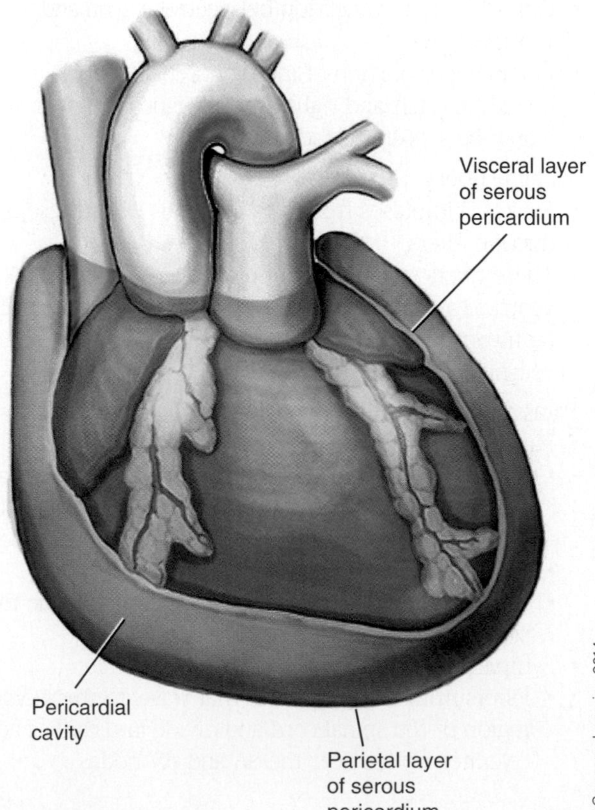

Figure 22-16 Pericardium

The Heart Wall

The wall of the heart is composed of three layers:

- The epicardium, which is the outer layer of the heart, provides protection and is composed of the visceral pericardium.
- The **myocardium**, which makes up the bulk of the heart wall, is composed of specially constructed cardiac muscle cells that contract and force blood from the heart's chambers.
- The endocardium, which is the inner lining of the heart wall, lines all of the heart's chambers and valves. The endocardium is composed of endothelial tissue, which consists of a single layer of flattened cells.

The Heart Chambers

The heart has four chambers: two **atria** and two **ventricles**. The atria are the upper chambers and the ventricles are the lower chambers.

- Atria (sing., atrium)
  - Receive blood from the veins of the body
  - Have walls thinner than those of the ventricles
  - Are divided by the interatrial septum
- Ventricles
  - Pump blood into the arteries leading away from heart
  - Have a thicker myocardium than do atria
  - The right ventricle pumps blood to the lungs.
  - The left ventricle pumps blood into arteries that transport blood to all other regions of the body.
  - Are divided by the interventricular septum

The Heart Valves

- Atrioventricular valve (AV valve): Located between each atrium and ventricle
  - Tricuspid valve
    - The tricuspid valve is located between the right atrium and the right ventricle. It is named for its three leaf-like cusps.
    - When blood pressure increases in the right atrium, the cusps of the tricuspid valve open, allowing the blood to flow into the right ventricle.
    - When the pressure in the right ventricle is greater than the pressure in the right atrium, the cusps close.
  - Pulmonary semilunar valve
    - Formed by three half-moon-shaped cusps.
    - The blood exits the right ventricle through the semilunar valve into the pulmonary artery to be transported to the lungs for oxygenation.
  - Mitral valve
    - Is also called bicuspid valve because it has two cusps.
    - Blood returns from the lungs and enters the left atrium.
    - The mitral valve opens, allowing blood to flow from the left atrium to the left ventricle.

- When the left ventricle contracts, the mitral valve closes.
- A pathological condition that can occur is mitral valve **regurgitation**. The valve does not close, allowing blood to backflow into the atrium.
- Aortic semilunar valve
  - Located at the base of the aorta
  - When the left ventricle contracts, the valve opens, allowing blood to flow into the aorta.
- Chordae tendineae
  - These fibrous cords are attached to the cusps of valves on the ventricle side.
  - They originate from papillary muscles that project outward from the walls of the myocardium.
  - The chordae tendineae prevent the cusps of the valve from folding back into the atrium, which would cause incomplete closure of the valve and lead to regurgitation of the blood back into the atrium.

Blood Flow Through the Heart

- The right atrium receives deoxygenated blood from the superior vena cava (drains upper portion of body), inferior vena cava (drains lower portion of body), and coronary sinus (drains blood from wall of the heart).
- The tricuspid valve opens, allowing blood to flow into the right ventricle; then the valve closes.
- The pulmonary semilunar valve opens and blood enters the pulmonary artery and travels to the lungs for oxygenation. When the right ventricle relaxes, the blood in the pulmonary artery pushes against the valve, causing it to close.
- Blood travels from the branches of the pulmonary artery to eventually enter the capillaries that surround the alveoli. Oxygen and carbon dioxide are exchanged between the blood in the capillaries and the air in the alveoli.
- The oxygenated blood returns to the heart through four pulmonary veins and enters the left atrium.
- The atrial wall contracts, the mitral valve opens, and blood enters the left ventricle.
- The left ventricle contracts, the mitral valve closes, the aortic semilunar valve opens, and blood enters the aorta for transport to the rest of the body.

Blood Supply for the Heart

- Two coronary arteries originate from the ascending aorta.
  - Right coronary artery
    - Posterior descending artery: branches to both ventricles
    - Marginal artery: branches to right ventricle and right atrium
  - Left coronary artery
    - Anterior descending artery: supplies blood to both ventricles
    - Circumflex artery: supplies blood to left ventricle and left atrium
- Deoxygenated blood is returned to the right atrium through coronary veins into the coronary sinus. The path of the coronary veins parallels the path of the coronary arteries.

Cardiac Conduction

The cardiac conduction system coordinates the events of the **cardiac cycle**. Located throughout the heart are specialized areas of tissue that transmit electrical impulses throughout the myocardium for the rhythmical activity of the heart.

- Sinoatrial node (SA node)
  - Located in the right atrial wall inferior to opening of the superior vena cava
  - Referred to as the "pacemaker" of the heart
  - Fires an electrical impulse that travels through the myocardium and stimulates it to contract in a rhythmic manner
- AV node
  - Located in the interatrial septum
  - Impulses from the SA node travel to the AV node.
  - Provides conduction pathway between atrium and ventricles
  - Pulse stimulates fibers. Fibers are interconnected, forming a branching network that contracts as a unit.
  - The action potential slows at the AV node because the fibers are smaller, thus allowing time for the atria to empty the blood into the ventricles.
- Bundle of His (AV bundle)
  - Only electrical connection between the atria and ventricles
  - Enters upper portion of interventricular septum and divides into left and right bundle branches that travel along the septum to the apex
- Purkinje fibers
  - Electrical impulses from bundle of His enter these conduction fibers.
  - These fibers spread the impulse to the apex of the left ventricle and upward to the remainder of the ventricular myocardium, resulting in contraction of the ventricle.
- Parasympathetic and sympathetic nerve fibers
  - Parasympathetic division
    - Fibers that originate within the medulla oblongata of the brain stem, become a part of the right and left vagus nerve, and terminate in the SA and AV nodes
    - Responsible for slowing the heart rate
    - Utilize the neurotransmitter called acetylcholine to slow down SA and AV node activity.
  - Sympathetic division
    - Fibers from the brain stem that travel to the thoracic region of the spinal cord and divide into cardiac accelerator nerves near the SA and AV nodes

  - The nerves secrete the neurotransmitter norepinephrine, which accelerates heart rate and myocardial contraction.
- Homeostasis of the parasympathetic and sympathetic divisions
  - Adult normal resting heart rate averages 72 beats/minute; parasympathetic division is in control through the secretion of acetylcholine, which decreases SA and AV nodal activity

Techniques of Cardiopulmonary Bypass

The invention of CPB was a significant step forward in the specialty of cardiac surgery that allows surgeons to perform procedures that previously they were not able to perform. Due to its complexity and because it is routinely used during cardiac procedures, the techniques are presented as a separate section.

The pump oxygenator, or "heart-lung machine," is the apparatus used in cardiac surgery to remove unoxygenated blood from the venous system, oxygenate and filter it, and return it to the arterial system. By assuming the roles of the heart and lungs, the pump oxygenator (Figure 22-17) allows the heart to be stopped so that delicate cardiac procedures may be performed. It also allows the lungs to be deflated for better exposure of the heart and major vessels.

The name "heart-lung machine" indicates what is required to produce extracorporeal circulation: the oxygenation of blood (replacing the function of the lungs) and the pumping of blood (replacing the function of the heart).

The pump oxygenator is relatively simple in design. Venous blood is removed from the body by way of a sterile plastic tube (cannula) that is placed into the right atrium or venae cavae and shunted through an oxygenator. The oxygenator may be a bubble or microporous-membrane type, and it is equipped with a reservoir and heat exchanger that allows the temperature of the blood to be manipulated as needed. After blood has been oxygenated, a roller pump moves the blood from the reservoir back to the arterial system. Additional pumps are used for removing blood from the operative site (using "cardiotomy suckers" on the operative field) and vented blood from the left ventricle (Figure 22-18). This blood is added to a reservoir for oxygenation and sent back into the arterial system, preventing blood loss.

The placement of cannulae into the right atrium or venae cavae for draining venous blood to the pump oxygenator and the ascending aorta for the return of arterial blood from the pump oxygenator is referred to as *cannulation* (Figure 22-19). Before cannulation, heparin (300 U/kg) must be administered to prevent clotting.

Note: If the right atrium is to be opened (for tricuspid valve replacement or repair of ASD), a venous cannula is placed into the superior vena cava and another in the inferior vena cava. For most cardiac procedures, however, a two-stage venous cannula is sufficient.

After venous and arterial cannulation, saline-filled polyvinyl chloride tubing from the pump oxygenator is attached to each cannula and secured. As the connections between the

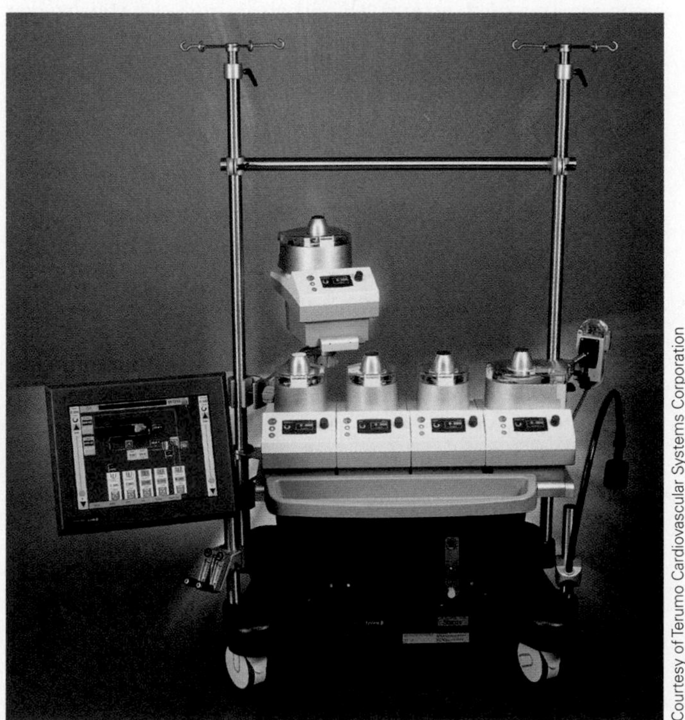

Figure 22-17 Terumo® Advanced Perfusion System 1

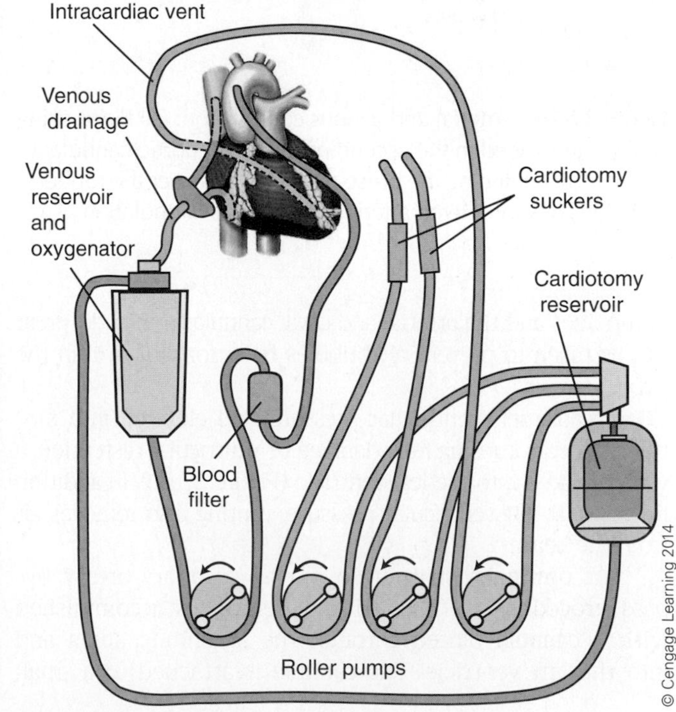

Figure 22-18 Cardiopulmonary bypass

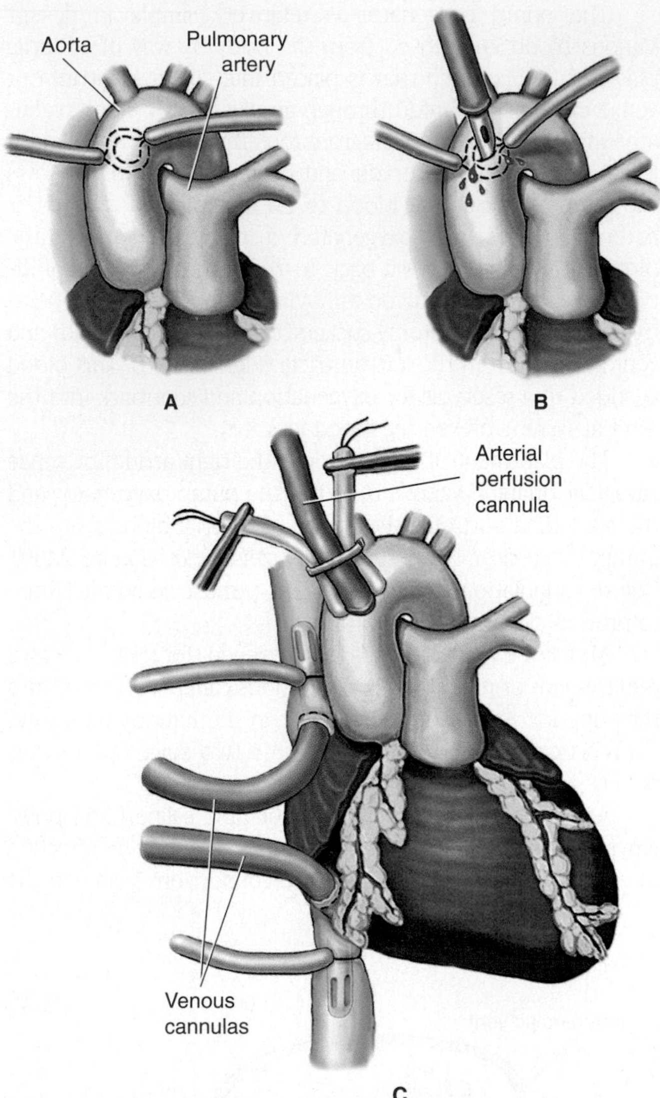

Figure 22-19 Arterial and venous cannulation: (A) Purse-string sutures are placed in the ascending aorta; (B) aortic cannula is secured by tightening the purse-string sutures over the rubber catheters; (C) completed arterial and venous cannulation

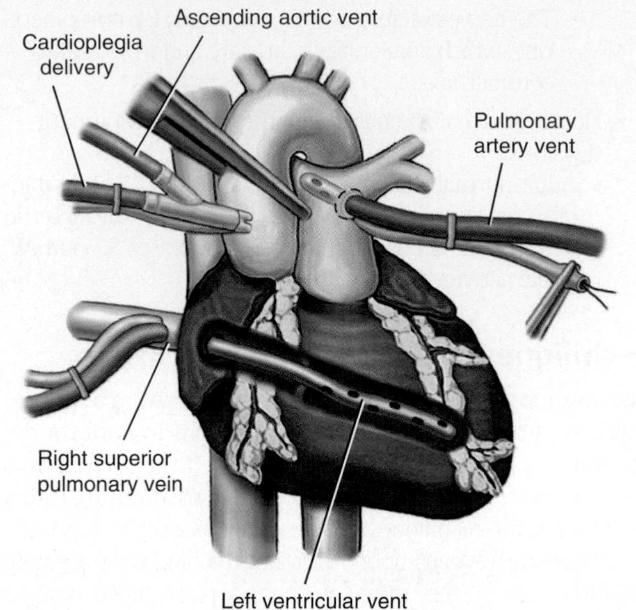

Figure 22-20 Left ventricular venting

pump lines and the arterial and caval cannulas are made, great care is taken to prevent air bubbles from forming within the bypass circuit.

Because left ventricular pressures are elevated in a motionless heart, causing lung damage or ventricular distention, a vent is placed into the left ventricle (Figure 22-20). In addition to lowering left ventricular pressure, venting also removes air from the heart.

For optimal visualization during coronary artery bypass procedures, left ventricular venting is accomplished with a cannula placed through the ascending aorta and into the left ventricle. The cannula is attached to a small needle-vented suction line from the pump oxygenator. Utilizing a Y-shaped cannula, the cardioplegia solution can be administered through the same aortic puncture site as the venting line.

Myocardial protection during CPB is accomplished with systemic hypothermia, topical myocardial hypothermia, and the administration of cold potassium cardioplegia solution into the coronary arteries via the aortic root and/or the coronary sinus via the right atrium. Hypothermia reduces the oxygen demands of the myocardium, and so is the technique utilized most often for cardiac procedures.

After cannulation and the initiation of CPB, a Fogarty cross-clamp is placed across the ascending aorta. A needle/cannula assembly for the administration of cold (4°C) potassium cardioplegia solution that inhibits myocardial contraction is inserted into the aortic root, and the paralyzing solution is infused into the coronary arteries at frequent intervals. Retrograde administration of cardioplegia is useful for second operations for coronary artery stenosis and valvular procedures and can be accomplished via a catheter placed into the coronary sinus via the right atrium that is held in place with a purse-string/tourniquet combination.

After cardioplegia infusion, ice slush, or ice-cold saline (4°C) is placed around the heart. A myocardial insulating pad may also be placed behind the heart. After hypothermic techniques have been employed, the systemic temperature of the patient often falls to 32°C. Utilizing the heat exchanger on the pump oxygenator, the temperature can be taken down even further. A moderate temperature of approximately 28°C reduces oxygen demand on the myocardium by half.

Continuous warm-blood cardioplegia is an alternative to hypothermic techniques for myocardial preservation, but is not widely used because of visualization problems during the coronary artery anastomoses.

If the patient has an inadequate ascending aorta due to short length, or if scarring from a previous procedure prevents quick access through a sternotomy, then cannulae for CPB may be inserted into the common femoral or external iliac artery.

TECHNIQUE

Aortic Cannulation

1. After median sternotomy, a self-retaining retractor is placed and an incision is made into the pericardium. Traction sutures are placed into the pericardium and secured to the retractor or chest wall.
2. The aorta is exposed, and two purse-string sutures are placed high on the ascending aorta to allow room for proximal vein grafts and the cardioplegia/venting cannula.
3. Large red rubber catheters that have been cut into 4-in. pieces are placed over each purse-string suture and the needles are cut off of the suture ends. A Rochester-Pean or Crile hemostat clamp is placed on the ends of each purse-string. A Satinsky partial-occlusion clamp may be placed onto the aorta if the aorta is not calcified.
4. An incision is made into the aorta between the purse-string sutures with a #11 knife blade, and the metal, bevel-ended tip of the aortic cannula is placed into the arteriotomy. The cannula is allowed to fill with arterial blood that is held in check by a stopper on the proximal end.
5. The cannula is held in place by rubber catheter tourniquets (keepers) that are cinched tightly over the purse-string sutures and clamped with a hemostat. A heavy silk suture is tied around the cannula and rubber keepers.

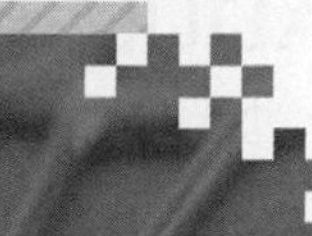

TECHNIQUE

Venous Cannulation

1. A single purse-string suture is placed into the right atrial appendage, and a red rubber catheter is placed over the purse-string suture. The needles are removed from the suture and either a Rochester-Pean hemostat clamp or a Crile hemostat clamp is placed on the suture ends.
2. A Satinsky partial-occlusion clamp is secured over the incision site.
3. The incision is made into the right atrial appendage with a #15 blade or Metzenbaum scissors.
4. A two-stage venous cannula that drains blood from the right atrium, inferior vena cava, and coronary sinus is inserted, and the red rubber catheter is cinched tightly over the purse-string suture, securing the cannula. The hemostat is clamped to the rubber catheter tourniquet.
5. A heavy silk suture is placed around the cannula and the rubber keepers.

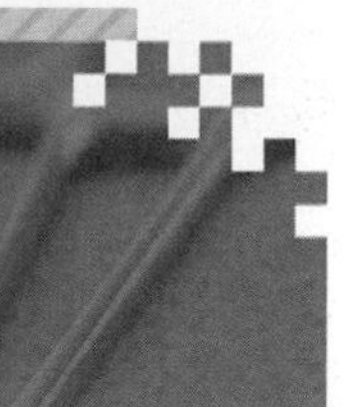

TECHNIQUE

Left Ventricular Vent Placement Via the Left Atrium

1. A single purse-string suture is placed into the anterior surface of the right superior pulmonary vein.
2. A small incision is made in the pulmonary vein and dilated.
3. A 20 Fr left heart venting catheter is inserted and guided into the left ventricle.
4. The venting catheter is attached to a suction line from the pump oxygenator.

ADULT CARDIAC SURGICAL PROCEDURES

PROCEDURE 22-10 Coronary Artery Bypass with Grafting (CABG)

Pathology

Due to the amount of information about coronary artery disease, it is presented in paragraph format.

Coronary atherosclerotic heart disease is the most common type of coronary artery disease and is recognized as the leading cause of death in the industrialized Western world. Each year approximately 1 million Americans die from the disease, and the annual economic costs are staggering, averaging in the tens of billions of dollars.

Risk factors for coronary atherosclerosis include

- *Age:* Older people are far more likely to be affected.
- *Gender:* The disease affects more males than females. Female sex hormones are thought to play a role, and estrogen therapy for postmenopausal women is currently being studied.
- *Race:* There is a higher mortality rate among nonwhites.
- *Genetics:* A familial disposition is thought to have both genetic and environmental origins.
- *Hypertension:* High blood pressure will accelerate the development of atherosclerosis, particularly if it develops at an early age.
- *Cigarette smoking:* This is one of the most important risk factors associated with the disease. The negative effects on the cardiovascular system are partially related to nicotine, tar, carbon monoxide, and other harmful components of cigarette smoke.
- *Diet:* A diet rich in saturated fats, especially animal fats contributes to the development of the disease.
- *Obesity:* Overall, obese people develop atherosclerosis at an earlier age and have more significant lesions than do those who weigh less. Elevated serum levels of lipids, such as cholesterol, lipoproteins, and triglycerides, directly correlate with the extent and severity of the atherosclerosis. Obese individuals are also more prone to hypertension, diabetes, and glucose intolerance; it is these associated factors that may be the link between obesity and atherosclerosis.
- *Clotting factors:* Soluble clotting factors, such as thrombin, fibrin, and platelets, play a role in the formation of atherosclerotic lesions.
- *Psychosocial influences:* Individuals in lower socioeconomic positions are more likely to smoke, are more obese, and have higher rates of hypertension than those in positions of higher economic status. Individuals who are under constant pressure to perform, or who can be labeled "overachievers," are more likely to develop atherosclerosis.

The term atherosclerosis describes a condition that involves the formation of an atheroma in the intima of medium and large arteries. The first step in the formation of the atheroma (Figure 22-21) is believed to be an injury to the endothelial lining of the arterial wall. Blood platelets and lipoproteins are deposited into the injury as a repair mechanism, and growth factors released from the platelets stimulate the growth of new smooth muscle tissue in the arterial wall. Changes in the metabolism of the smooth muscle cells promote the accumulation of cholesterol

Procedure 22-10 (continued)

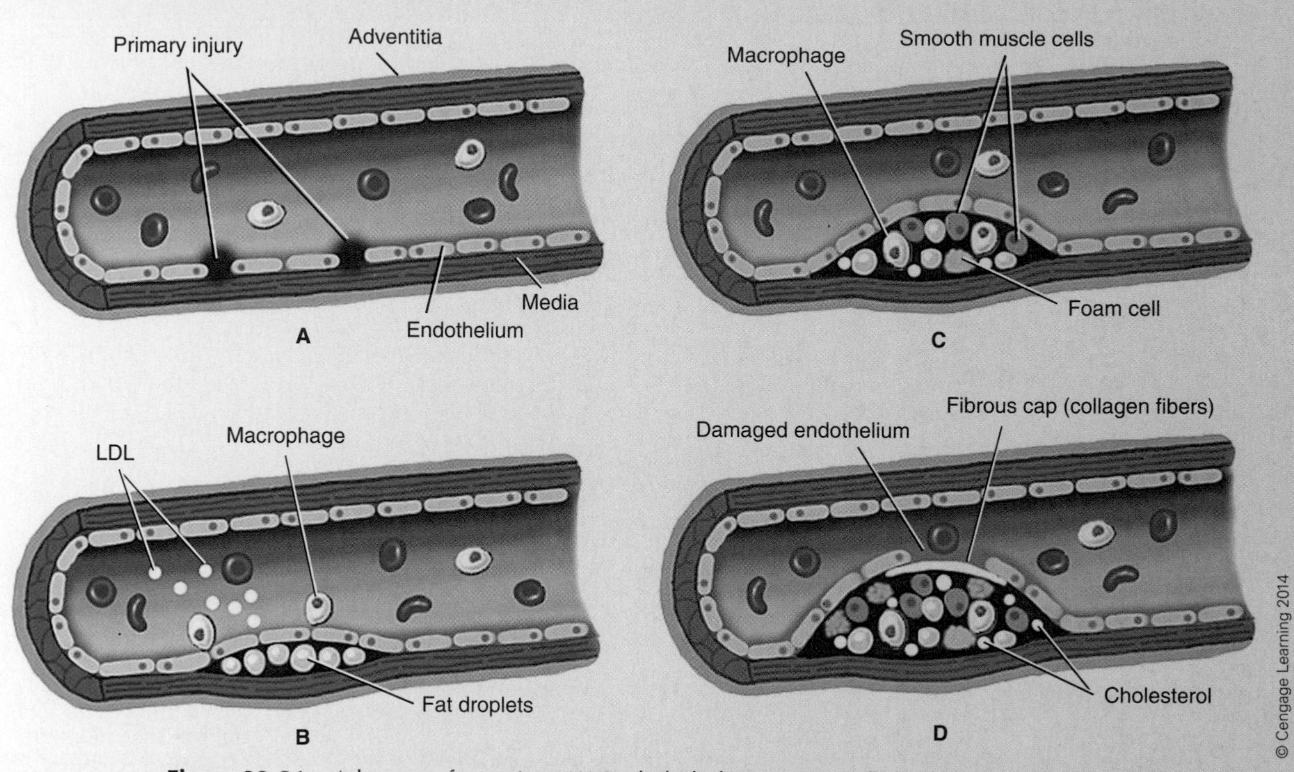

Figure 22-21 Atheroma formation: (A) Endothelial injury, (B) influx of lipids, (C) accumulation of lipids, proliferation of smooth muscle cells and accumulation of macrophages, (D) atheroma

and other lipids within the cells' cytoplasm, which, when leaked across the cell membrane into the interstitial spaces, attract scavenger macrophages. The macrophages secrete biologically active substances that cause further damage to the arterial wall. Eventually, collagen is deposited into the lesion and scar tissue begins to form, narrowing the lumen of the artery.

Progressive, chronic myocardial ischemia, the underlying pathogenic mechanism of coronary atherosclerosis, develops as a result of the progression of narrowing of the lumen of the coronary artery due to atheroma formation. It is ischemia that is responsible for the clinical manifestations of coronary atherosclerosis: angina pectoris, which occurs when myocardial oxygen demand exceeds supply, and is characterized by substernal or retrosternal "crushing" pain that often radiates to the throat, back, or left arm; acute myocardial **infarction**, which results in the death of heart muscle tissue; and sudden cardiac death.

Sudden occlusion of the vessel results in acute myocardial infarction (MI) and treatment must be immediate. The area of damage by MI depends on the coronary artery affected and the amount of myocardial tissue served by the artery. For example, an occlusion of the proximal right coronary artery will result in infarction of the right ventricle and posterior wall of the left ventricle; an occlusion of the proximal circumflex branch of the left coronary system will result in infarction of the lateral wall of the left ventricle; and an anterior ventricular wall infarction is

(*continues*)

Procedure 22-10 (continued)

typically caused by occlusion of the proximal left anterior descending artery. Smaller areas of damage occur in the myocardium when occlusion occurs in one or more distal branches of the coronary arteries.

Coronary artery lesions usually occur near the origin and bifurcation of the main coronary vessels, but diffuse involvement throughout the branches is seen in advanced cases. Most lesions occur in the left anterior descending artery, or LAD. The LAD accounts for 50% of all atherosclerotic lesions of the coronary system, the right coronary artery accounts for 30%–40%, and the circumflex branch of the left coronary system accounts for 15%–20% of the lesions.

- Within 24 hours of an MI, temperature is elevated and white cell count is increased due to myocardial necrosis. Death of the myocardial cells also brings about the release of enzymes that enter the bloodstream.

Sudden death from MI occurs usually as a result of ventricular fibrillation, heart block, and asystole (cardiac arrest).

Diagnosis of MI is based on the presenting symptoms and evidence of impaired heart function that is found by physical examination, electrocardiography, and abnormal serum enzyme levels.

Complications of MI include:

- Myocardial rupture, which may occur as a result of a softening of the necrotic ventricular myocardium and an increased ventricular pressure. As blood escapes from the ventricle into the pericardial sac, the heart is compressed, interrupting normal rhythm. This potentially lethal condition is known as cardiac **tamponade** and is usually treated by pericardiocentesis.
- Cardiac aneurysm, or a ballooning of the ventricular wall, can be a result of increased ventricular pressure and scar tissue in the ventricular wall formed by massive MIs.
- Heart failure and cardiogenic shock. As a result of inadequate perfusion of tissues by a failing heart, multisystem organ failure may develop. The most dangerous of these is cerebral ischemia, which may lead to irreversible brain damage. But it is the kidneys that are most often damaged. Typical signs of renal failure, such as oliguria and anuria, are common.

Preoperative Diagnostic Tests and Procedures

- See list at beginning of Part II.

Equipment, Instruments, and Supplies Unique to Procedure

- See list at beginning of Part II.

PROCEDURE 22-10 (continued)

Preoperative Preparation	• Position: Supine with legs externally rotated
	• Anesthesia: General
	  • Intraoperative invasive monitoring includes the following:
	    • An arterial line within the radial or femoral artery for measurement of direct arterial blood pressures and arterial blood gas studies
	    • A Swan-Ganz pulmonary artery catheter that indirectly measures left atrial and left ventricular pressures by assessing right atrial, right ventricular, and pulmonary artery wedge pressures. The Swan-Ganz may also be used to monitor central venous pressures.
	  • Urinary drainage catheter with temperature sensor for the measurement of urinary output and core temperature
	  • Transesophageal echocardiography
	• Noninvasive intraoperative monitoring includes:
	  • Blood pressure cuff for the indirect measurement of arterial blood pressure
	  • Pulse oximeter for the measurement of oxygen saturation of hemoglobin
	  • Electrocardiogram
	• Skin prep: Lower mandible to toes of both legs; bilaterally as far as possible for the chest and abdomen and circumferentially for both legs
	• Draping: *Thorax:* Folded towel is placed over the genitals; 4 towels to square off chest region; plastic adhesive incise drape; heart drape. *Legs:* Three-quarter sheet underneath both legs; impervious stockinette placed on both legs; legs laid on sheet and slightly externally rotated for access to the saphenous veins.

Practical Considerations	• Surgical technologists who desire to be on the heart team must build their skills in other surgical specialties and eventually may be eligible to be a member of the team. However, the surgical technologist must begin learning the first scrub role on simpler procedures, such as harvesting the saphenous vein, and eventually complete training to first scrub solo on difficult procedures such as a CABG. • The surgical technologist must have excellent anticipatory skills, and should thoroughly understand cardiovascular anatomy and physiology, as well as cardiac procedural sequence. • The surgical technologist should be thinking five steps ahead of the surgeon throughout the procedure, and should pay attention at all times. • It is important that the surgical technologist understand cardiac dysrhythmias and their relationship to the cardiac procedure, and be able to understand all pressure readings. • For repeat cardiac procedures, be prepared to cannulate femorally. The oscillating saw may be used for sternotomy to prevent cutting into ventricular adhesions to the sternal wall. • Pass off defibrillation cables at the same time as electrosurgical cords. The surgeon will

(*continues*)

Procedure 22-10 (continued)

not want to wait for the defibrillation paddles if they are suddenly needed.

- Wet the surgeon's hands with saline when tying polypropylene sutures to prevent breaking them.
- Remind the circulator to turn on the suction to the closed-seal drainage unit as soon as the chest tubes are connected to it. This prevents clots from forming in the chest tubes.
- Do not confuse the terms "atrial" and "arterial" when passing cannulation stitches. One is for the right atrium, and the other is for the aorta. Typically, the arterial cannulation stitch is placed first, but if aortic pressure is high, the right atrium will be cannulated first.
- Typically, three Mayo stands are utilized for CPB procedures. CPB procedures that will utilize a saphenous vein graft will require a third Mayo stand for saphenous vein harvesting.
- In usual fashion, the surgical technologist should not break scrub and keep the back table and Mayo stand sterile until the patient has safely left the OR. Wire cutters, sternal retractor, cannulation stitches loaded on needle holders, and cannulas should be available in case the patient must be placed back on CPB.

Surgical Procedure

1. An incision is made extending from the sternal notch to the xiphoid process and vessels are coagulated (Plate 22-1).

   Procedural Consideration: Prepare the sternal saw and the sternal retractor. For repeat sternotomies, an oscillating saw is used so that a ventricle that may be adhered to the chest wall is not cut.

2. The sternum is opened with a sternal saw, and a self-retaining sternal retractor is inserted (Plate 22-2).

   Procedural Consideration: If the IMA is dissected for coronary artery anastomosis, a mammary retractor is placed instead of the sternal retractor.

3. The pericardium is incised and retracted with sutures (Plate 22-3).

   Procedural Consideration: Retraction sutures are prepared in advance as their use is anticipated.

4. If the left IMA is to be used for left anterior descending artery anastomosis, the IMA is dissected as a pedicle graft proximally from the level of the subclavian artery and distally to the costal margin. Side branches are occluded with small clips (Plate 22-4).

   Procedural Consideration: The pedicle graft is soaked in a papaverine solution to prevent vasospasm. A papaverine-soaked 4 × 4 gauze is usually wrapped around the graft.

5. The saphenous vein is harvested from one or both legs by a separate team at the same time that the chest is opened. Tributaries are ligated during dissection with small hemoclips and 4-0 silk ties (Plate 22-5; Figure 22-22).

   Procedural Consideration: If the saphenous vein is not taken endoscopically, then dissection is carried out with a #10 blade on a No. 3 handle, Metzenbaum scissors, and DeBakey forceps. Hemoclip appliers must be reloaded for immediate reuse.

PROCEDURE 22-10 (continued)

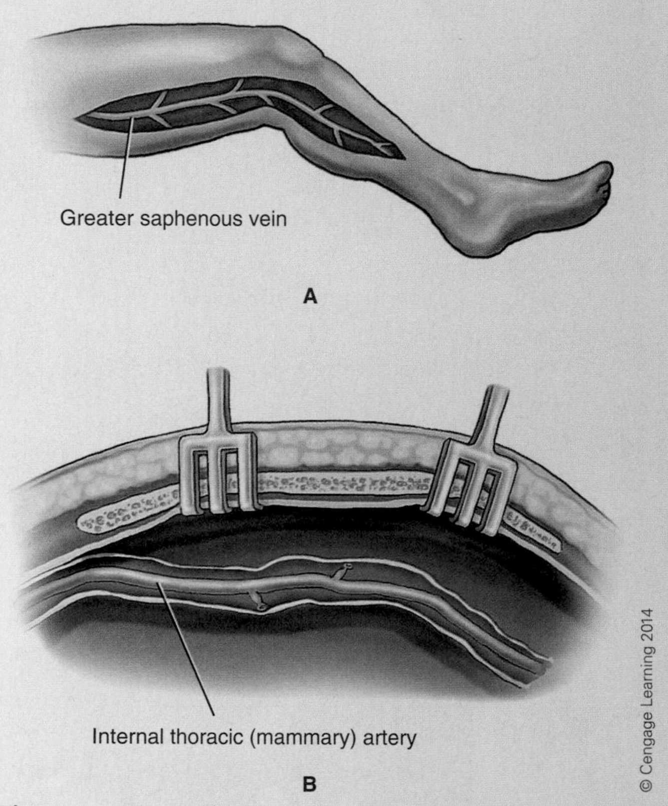

Figure 22-22 Graft options for CABG: (A) Saphenous vein dissection, (B) internal mammary artery dissection

6. The vein is flushed with heparinized saline to identify any branches that may have been missed, and the vein is stored in a heparin/saline solution until needed.

   Procedural Consideration: Flushing is facilitated by a saphenous vein cannula inserted into the vein and secured with a silk tie. Tributaries are tied off with a 4-0 silk tie.

7. CPB is initiated utilizing techniques discussed previously (Plate 22-6).

   Procedural Consideration: The pump lines should be easily accessible and ready to hook up to the cannulas. An Asepto filled with warm saline should be ready to displace air bubbles during hookup.

8. Coronary artery stenoses are identified, and an arteriotomy is made just distal to the stenosis (Plate 22-7)

   Procedural Consideration: A #64 Beaver blade and handle are useful for the arteriotomy. Tenotomy scissors and Diethrich angled coronary scissors should be available.

9. The internal mammary artery or saphenous vein is anastomosed to the affected coronary artery with 6-0- or 7-0-gauge polypropylene sutures (Plate 22-8; Figure 22-23).

   Procedural Consideration: A disposable bulldog vascular clamp is used to occlude the distal end of the IMA.

(continues)

PROCEDURE 22-10 (continued)

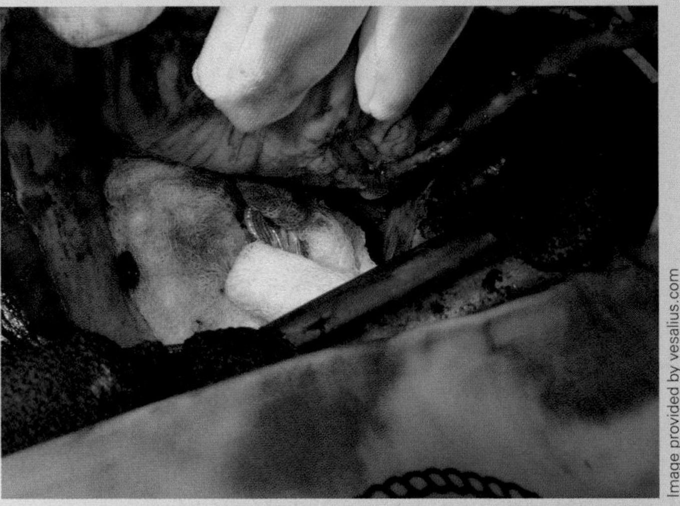

Figure 22-23 Internal mammary artery or saphenous vein is anastomosed to affected coronary artery

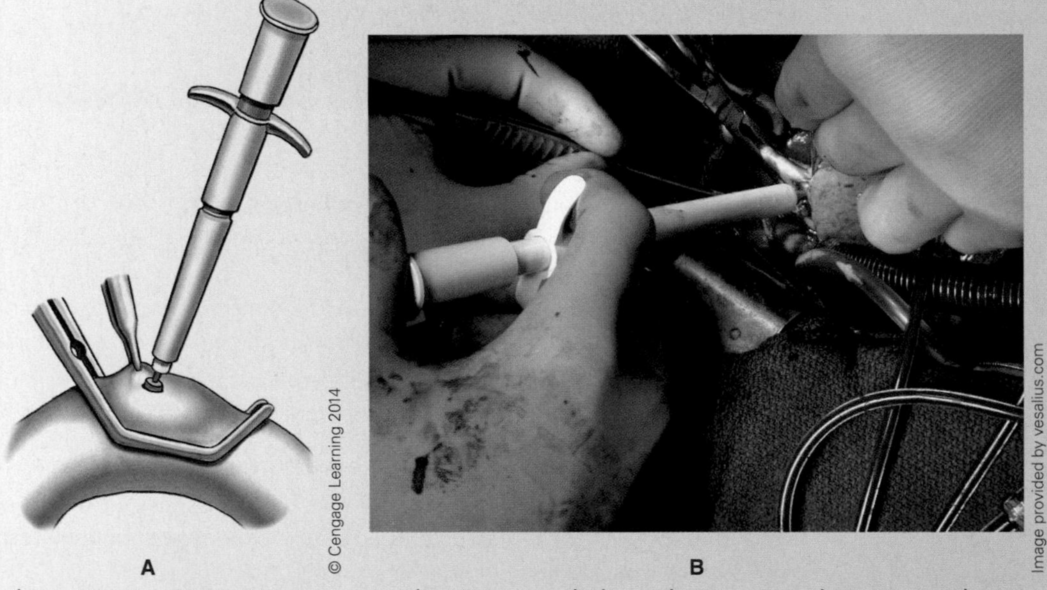

Figure 22-24 CABG: (A) Aortic punch, (B) 4.5-mm hole made in aorta with aortic punch

10. A Satinsky partial-occlusion clamp is applied to the ascending aorta, and a 4.5-mm hole is made in the isolated section of the aorta with an aortic punch (Figure 22-24).

    Procedural Consideration: Pass vascular clamp of appropriate size as needed. Prepare aortic punch and sutures if saphenous vein graft is used.

11. The proximal saphenous vein is anastomosed to the aorta in an end-to-side fashion with size 6-0 polypropylene sutures (Plates 22-9 and 22-10; Figure 22-25).

    Procedural Consideration: No proximal anastomosis is necessary for the IMA because only the distal end of the artery is transected. The proximal portion remains intact at its origin of the subclavian artery.

PROCEDURE 22-10 (continued)

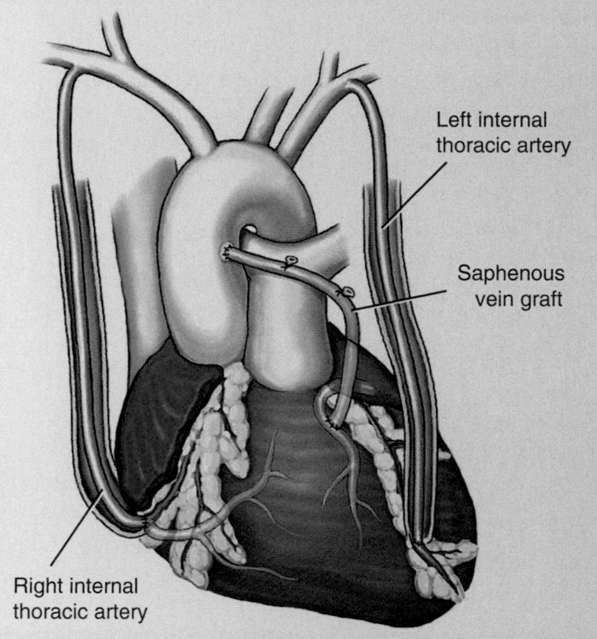

Figure 22-25 Internal mammary (thoracic) artery and saphenous vein anastomosed to coronary arteries

12. The Satinsky partial-occlusion clamp is removed and needle aspiration of the graft is performed to remove air.

    Procedural Consideration: Needle aspiration is carried out with a 25-gauge, 5/8-in. needle on a 10-mL syringe.

13. CPB is discontinued, chest tubes are placed for the evacuation of fluid and air, and the sternum is closed with heavy-gauge stainless steel wire. The chest is closed in the usual manner.

    Procedural Consideration: Use caution when passing wire to avoid puncture of gloves. Have wire twisters, cutters, and closing suture ready. Count as necessary. Chest tubes are secured to the skin with 0 silk on a cutting needle.

Postoperative Considerations

Immediate Postoperative Care

- Care must be taken when transferring the patient from the OR table to the CCU bed. The patient will have monitoring lines, an ET tube, and urinary and chest drainage tubes in place. These can be easily disturbed if tension is placed on them during the move. Patient is transported to the CCU.

Prognosis

- No complications: Recovery depends on the condition of the myocardium, especially the left ventricle, and the degree of atherosclerosis. Time spent on CPB is also a factor. The patient's life-style will be altered to a certain degree. However, if the patient experiences none to minimal complications,

(continues)

Procedure 22-10 (continued)

he or she will be hospitalized for 15–21 days. Recovery time is 6–8 months.

Complications

- Postoperative SSI: Thoracic cavity and/or leg from which saphenous vein was harvested
- Clotting problems related to systemic heparinization and CPB, which can damage platelets as they pass through the machine.
- Electrolyte imbalances, hypervolemia, pulmonary edema, atelectasis, and metabolic acidosis may occur if CPB time is extended.
- Transient cerebral ischemia and cerebral edema may also result from prolonged CPB.
- Postoperative bleeding is monitored through the chest tube drainage. Excessive hemorrhage may be caused by clotting mechanism deficiencies related to CPB, and can lead to cardiac tamponade. If hemorrhage is excessive, the patient is returned to the OR (referred to as a "bring-back heart") and the chest reopened for hemorrhage control.

Wound Classification

- Class I: Clean (CABG and saphenous vein harvesting)

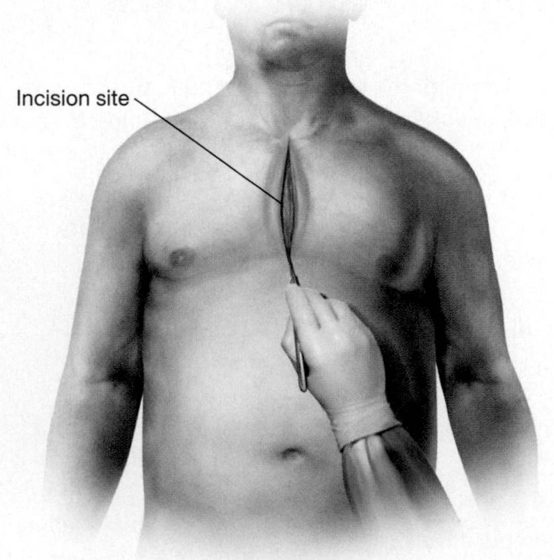

Plate 22-1 Incision from sternal notch to xiphoid

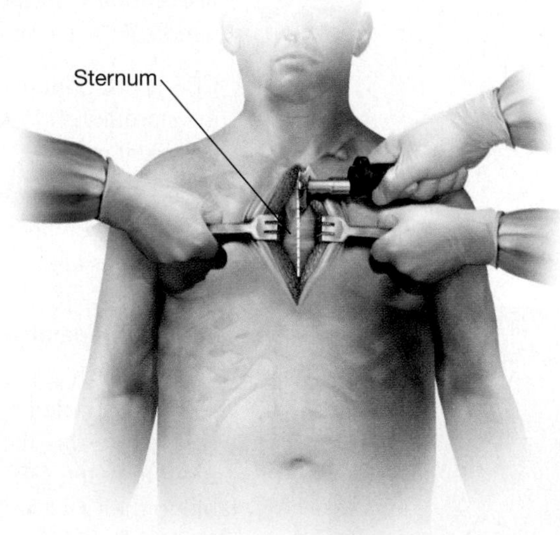

Plate 22-2 Sternum opened with sternal saw

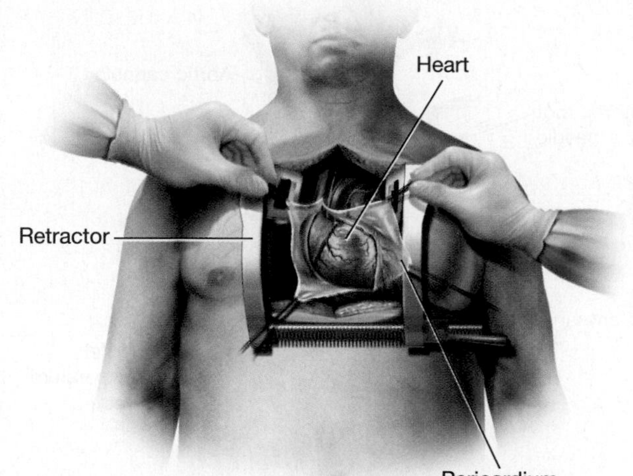

Plate 22-3 Pericardium is incised and retracted with sutures

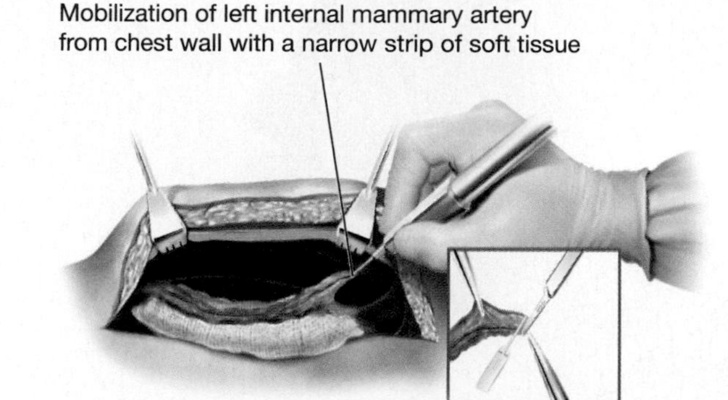

Plate 22-4 Harvesting the left IMA

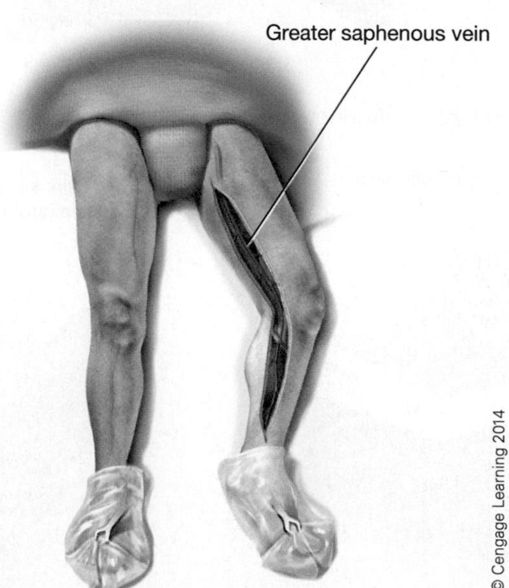

Plate 22-5 Exposure of saphenous vein and branches

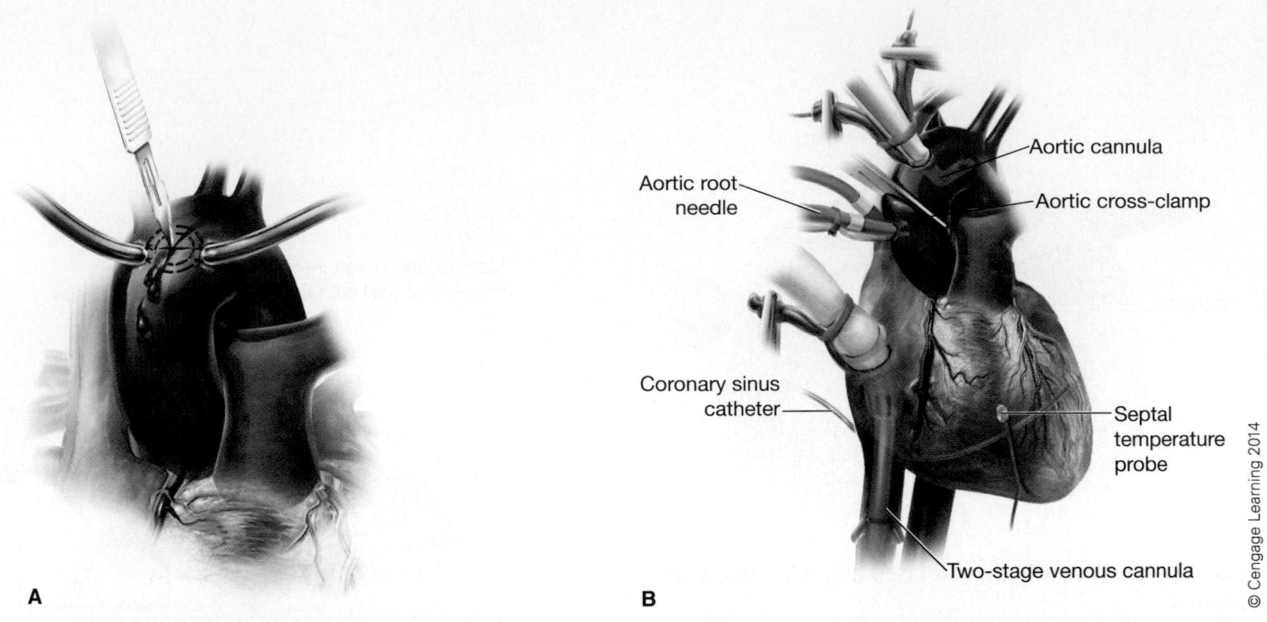

Plate 22-6 (A) Arterial cannulation: Purse-string sutures placed in ascending aorta and incision to facilitate placement of aortic cannula; (B) completed arterial and venous cannulation

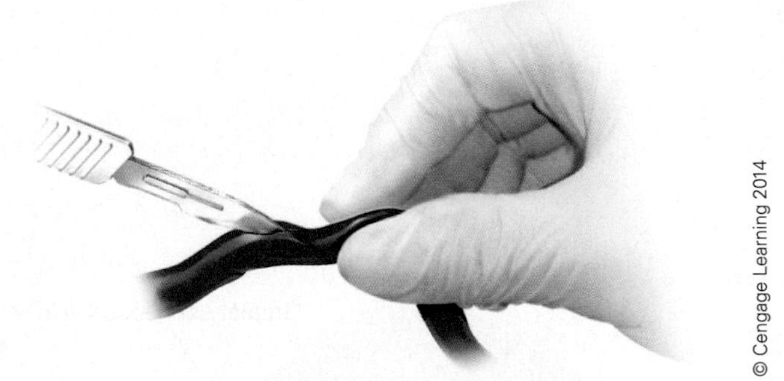

Plate 22-7 Arteriotomy made in coronary artery

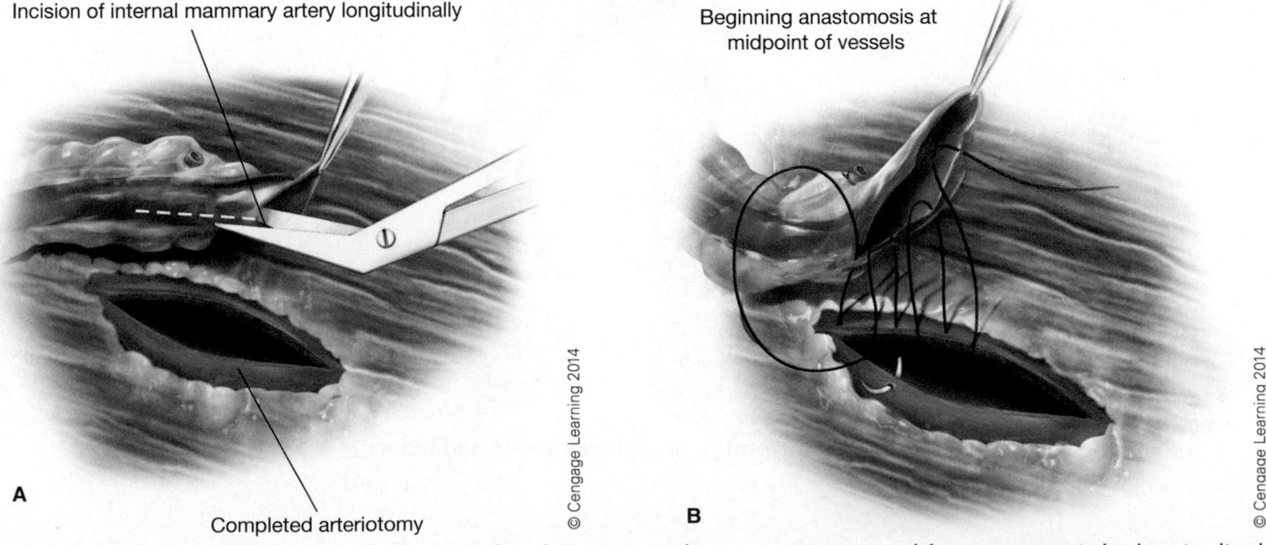

Plate 22-8 (A) Coronary artery arteriotomy completed; IMA or saphenous vein prepared for anastomosis by longitudinal cut with Potts-Smith scissors to match length of arteriotomy; (B) polypropylene suture is used to anastomose the IMA or saphenous vein to the coronary artery

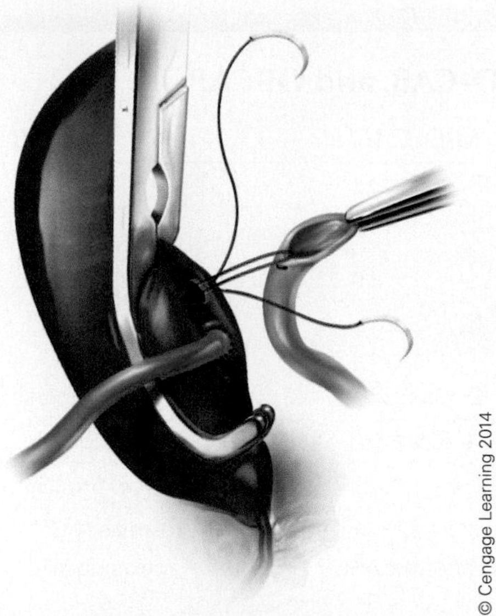

Plate 22-9 End-to-side anastomosis of proximal end of IMA or saphenous vein to aorta with polypropylene suture

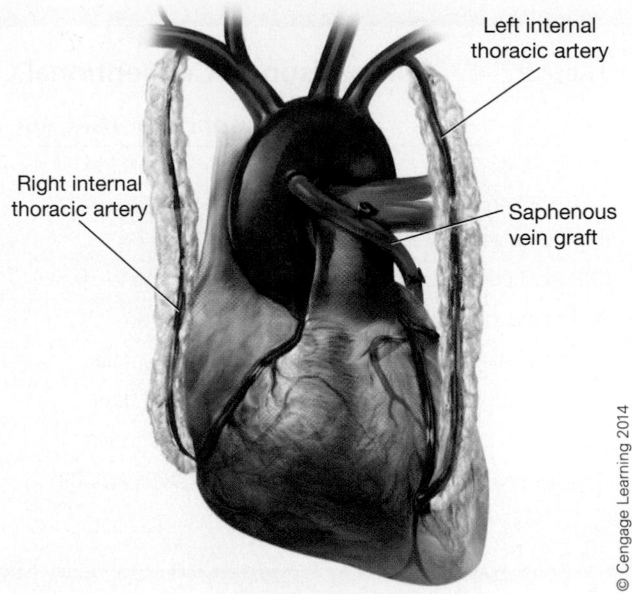

Plate 22-10 Completed anastomosis

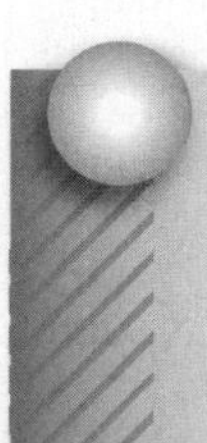

PEARL OF WISDOM

In emergencies, think about what you will be doing first, and prepare the items necessary to do those things. Think about what you need to get into the chest and cannulate (scalpel, electrosurgical pencil, sternal saw, sternal retractor, Cell Saver suction, pump lines, cannulation stitches). Anything else can wait, including counts.

The next two procedures, minimally invasive direct coronary artery bypass with graft (MID-CABG) and off-pump CABG (OPCAB), were developed as part of the minimally invasive surgery trend that has been occurring over the course of the last few years. Before describing the procedures, information that is important to being able to understand the procedures will be first presented. The procedural descriptions will be brief because the procedures are fairly similar to those of the conventional CABG procedure.

The most significant difference between a conventional CABG and the minimally invasive surgery (MIS) is that MID-CAB and OPCAB do not require the use of the CPB machine. Therefore, surgery is performed on a beating heart; hence the term that is also used to describe these two procedures, beating heart surgery. The other major difference is the size of incisions. The conventional CABG incision is a median sternotomy that is approximately 30 cm long, whereas the length of the incision for the MID-CAB is 10 cm and for OPCAB, 20–30 cm.

There are several advantages to the MIS procedures:

- The procedural time is significantly shortened.
- The recovery time is also considerably decreased from months to days or weeks.
- Complications of the heart-lung machine are avoided.
- The need for a blood transfusion is reduced; usually a transfusion is not required.
- Patients are moved out of the CCU sooner.
- Patients experience less pain as compared to those patients who underwent a conventional CABG.
- Estimates are up to 40% decrease in the cost of MIS procedures as compared to conventional CABG.

However, as with any type of surgical procedure, there are disadvantages:

- MID-CAB is only conducive to being able to graft a maximum of two arteries and OPCAB four arteries because the incisions are smaller, the heart is beating, and the suturing of the graft(s) must be completed under direct vision.
- The anastomosis is technically more difficult because the heart is beating. The surgeon must develop technically excellent skills in order to perform the surgery.
- Ischemia is a complication that can occur that may lead to hemodynamic compromise of the patient. Therefore, the surgical

Table 22-4 Comparison of Conventional CABG, MID-CAB, and OBCAP

	Conventional CABG	*MID-CAB*	*OPCAB*
Length of incision	30 cm (12 in.)	10 cm (4 in.)	20–30 cm (8–12 in.)
Maximum number of arteries that can be grafted	5	2	4
CPB machine required	Yes	No	No
Beating heart surgery	No	Yes	Yes
Length of surgery	3–6 hours	2–3 hours	2–5 hours
Hospitalization	7–10 days	4–6 days	6–10 days
Length of full recovery	6–10 weeks	2–4 weeks	4–6 weeks
Cost of surgery	$35,000–$40,000	Approximately 40% less than conventional CABG	Approximately 25% less than conventional CABG

team must be prepared for a quick conversion to conventional CABG and placing the patient on the CPB machine.

- Bleeding can obscure the surgical field of vision, causing the conversion to a conventional CABG.

Table 22-4 summarizes the differences between the three procedures.

To overcome some of the challenges of performing beating heart surgery, special loop suture and instrumentation has been developed to aid the surgeon in visualization and slowing down the heart. The description of the use of the loop suture will be provided in the MID-CAB procedure.

Specially designed stabilizers have been developed that can be attached to the chest wall and have two prongs at the end of a long handle. The prongs place gentle pressure on the area of the heart between the prongs to restrict movement. This slows the heart movement to 1 millimeter of motion, allowing the surgeon to perform the procedure. Three types of stabilizers that are frequently used are:

- Medtronic OCTOPUS® 2+ Tissue Stabilization System: The system has multiple small suction cups that are placed on the surface of the heart. When suction is turned on the cups affix to the surface to reduce the heart movement; the movement of the heart is less than 1 mm for each heart beat. This device is reusable.
- Guidant Ultima OPCAB® system: The system consists of a rigid arm with two prongs (called stabilizer feet) on the end that is attached to a quick mount; the quick mount is attached to one of two side pieces, which can be spread apart or brought closer together. This device is reusable.
- Heartport's OPTrac STILLSITE Stabilizer®: The stabilizer consists of a locking device to hold the arm in place. This is a disposable device.

A device called the site blower is used to remove blood from the surgical site. It consists of a handpiece with an on/off switch and a long malleable shaft that delivers an irrigation mist that clears the blood while not drying out the tissues. Several medical manufacturers have designed a site blower, which is usually disposable.

Two drugs that are used to slow the heart beat are adenosine, a metabolite used in treating **arrhythmias**, and esmolol, a beta-receptor antagonist. They have been found to also temporarily stop the heartbeat for a few seconds.

Procedure 22-11 MID-CABG

1. The surgeon makes a 10-cm posterolateral incision. The incision is carried through the subcutaneous layer down to the pectoralis muscle, which is divided with the ESU.

   Procedural Consideration: The coronary artery to be bypassed must lie directly beneath the incision due to the small size of the incision.

Procedure 22-11 (continued)

2. A small section of the rib is stripped and removed. The minimally invasive chest retractor of the surgeon's preference is placed and the IMA is harvested.
3. The frame for the MID-CAB stabilizer system is fitted into the incision and the rigid arm with stabilizer foot is positioned. Three other items positioned are the site blower, site light for illumination, and a site manipulator to move the heart.
4. The surgeon continues in much the same fashion as when performing a conventional CABG. An incision is made in the pericardium to expose the LAD.

   Procedural Consideration: The surgical team must be prepared to quickly switch to a conventional CABG and placing the patient on the CPB due to complications such as bleeding.
5. One end of the IMA is sutured to the LAD above the blockage and the other end is sutured below the blockage.
6. The site is checked for control of hemorrhage, the MID-CAB instrumentation is removed, and the layers are closed in routine fashion.

Procedure 22-12 OPCAB

1. The surgeon makes a median sternotomy that will vary in length depending on the physiology of the patient. However, the incision is usually smaller than that made for a conventional CABG. The self-retaining sternal retractor is placed.

   Procedural Consideration: While the surgeon is opening the chest, the saphenous vein or IMA is harvested. Once the surgeon has entered the chest and the retractor is placed, either adenosine or esmolol is used to slow the heart rate.
2. To permit access to the entire heart muscle, cardiac displacement must be accomplished. Special instruments are placed that move the heart into position to allow the surgeon access to blocked arteries.
3. The pericardium is incised. Sponges are used to soak up blood; they also serve to aid in further displacing.

   Procedural Consideration: Displacement of the heart is important because it is a challenge for the surgeon to perform a bypass on the lateral and posterior of a beating heart.
4. The Octopus® stabilizer with suction cups is positioned.
5. The surgeon may prepare the heart and vessels for attachment of the CPB in case it becomes necessary; not all surgeons will do so.
6. The rest of the procedure is performed similar to a CABG, including closure, with the exception that a **stent** is used because the heart is still beating. After the arteriotomy is made in the artery that is blocked, the stent is placed to allow blood to flow through while the bypass is performed. The ends of the graft are placed above and below the blockage.

Procedure 22-13 Intra-aortic Balloon Pump (IABP)

Pathology	• For patients who need cardiac support because they are waiting for cardiac transplantation or cannot be weaned from CPB, mechanical devices designed to assist in circulatory functions may be utilized. • The mechanical device designed for circulatory support after cardiac procedures is called an IABP. Insertion of the balloon pump may increase cardiac output to a level that would permit separation from the pump oxygenator and allow time for the heart to recover. • To be completely effective, the IABP must lower left ventricular pressure during **systole** (when the balloon is deflated) and increase coronary artery circulation during diastole (when the balloon is inflated).
Preoperative Diagnostic Tests and Procedures	• Routine for cardiac procedures
Equipment, Instruments, and Supplies Unique to Procedure	• IABP catheter set that includes needle/cannula assembly, dilators, balloon sheath/dilator assembly, IABP catheter and balloon • Peripheral vascular instrument set • Cardiac instrumentation available
Preoperative Preparation	• Position: Supine with leg slightly flexed • Anesthesia: General • Skin prep: Leg from groin region to toes • Draping: Four towels to square off insertion site; three-quarter sheet × 2 to cover bottom part of leg and upper part of leg, including groin region
Practical Considerations	• The surgical technologist should be familiar with the IABP tray, including the order in which supplies are used and how they are connected.
Surgical Procedure	1. After percutaneous needle/cannula assembly placement into the femoral artery, a guidewire is threaded through the arterial cannula and the cannula is removed (Figure 22-26A). 2. The artery is dilated to a 12 Fr diameter with plastic, graduated dilators threaded over the guidewire (Figure 22-26B). 3. A balloon sheath/dilator assembly is inserted over the guidewire, and the dilator is removed (Figure 22-26C). 4. The IABP catheter with a large balloon wound tightly around the distal end is inserted through the sheath and advanced slowly to a position just distal to the left subclavian artery (Figure 22-26D). 5. The balloon is unwound and the catheter is attached to the pump. The pump is then activated (Figure 22-27).

PROCEDURE 22-13 (continued)

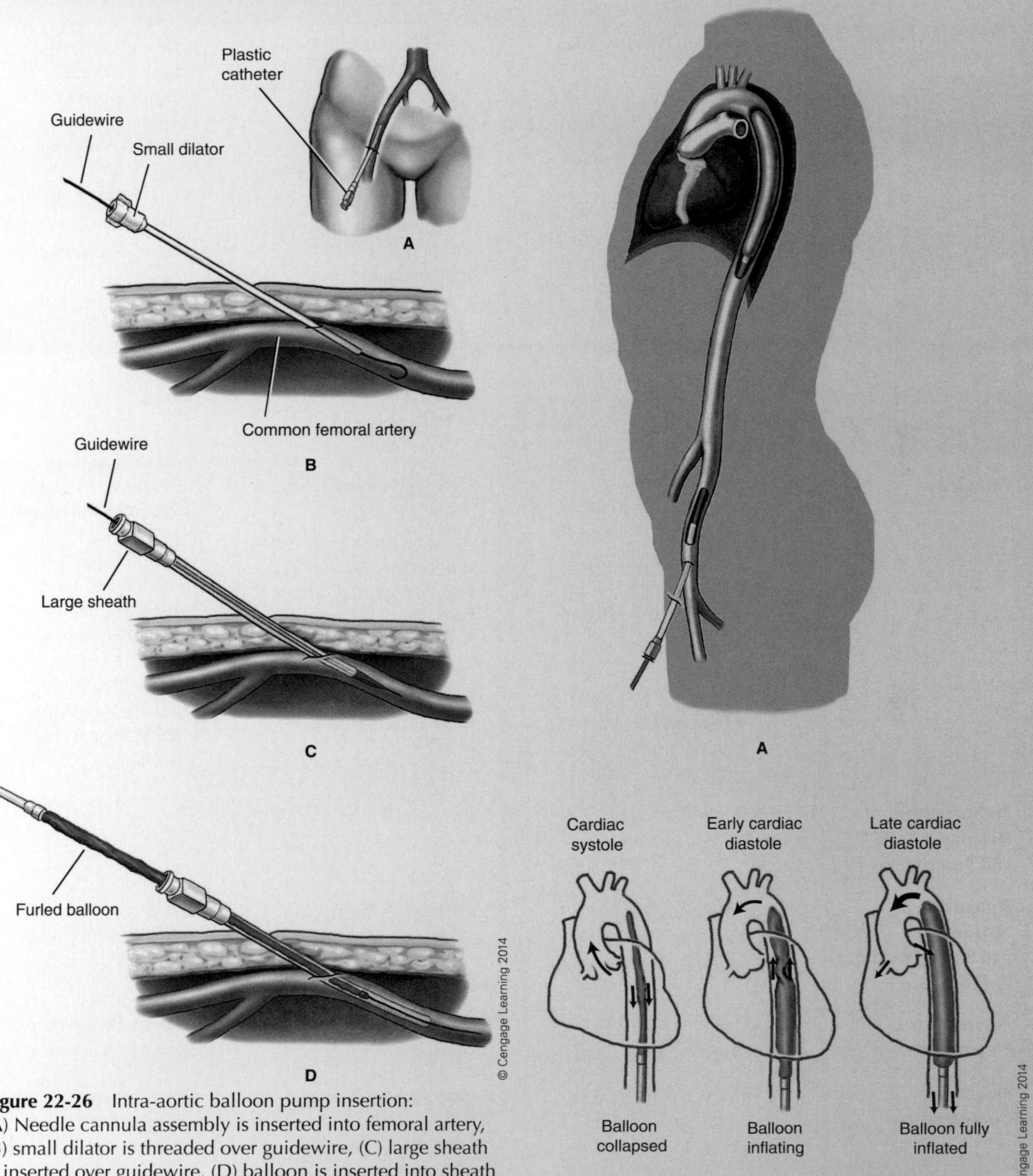

Figure 22-26 Intra-aortic balloon pump insertion: (A) Needle cannula assembly is inserted into femoral artery, (B) small dilator is threaded over guidewire, (C) large sheath is inserted over guidewire, (D) balloon is inserted into sheath

Figure 22-27 IABP mechanics: (A) Balloon is situated in the descending aorta, (B) balloon is deflated during cardiac systole and inflated during diastole

(*continues*)

PROCEDURE 22-13 (continued)

Postoperative Considerations	**Immediate Postoperative Care** • Patient is transported to the CCU. **Prognosis** • No complications: Patient is expected to make a full recovery. When counterpulsation to increase the coronary blood flow and decrease the afterload (resistance the ventricle must override in order for the aortic valve to open) is no longer necessary, the IABP is removed. • Complications: Postoperative SSI; ischemia and compartment syndrome in the leg; cerebral embolism during insertion; dissection of the aorta or iliac artery; hemorrhage in the mediastinum; mechanical failure of the balloon **Wound Classification** • Class I: Clean

PROCEDURE 22-14 Ventricular Assist Device (VAD) Insertion

Pathology	• Insertion of a VAD is performed for two reasons:
	  • Serve as a temporary device that maintains circulation in patients who need a heart transplant
	  • Temporarily support an open-heart patient who cannot yet be removed from the CPB.
	• A VAD is used to support the circulation from the left, right, or both ventricles. For patients who require a heart transplant, a left ventricular assist device (LVAD) is placed. The device decreases the workload of the heart by diverting the blood from the ventricle to a pump that pushes the blood into the systemic circulation. The VAD helps to keep the patient ambulatory and to lead as normal of a life as possible while waiting for a donor heart.

Preoperative Diagnostic Tests and Procedures	• Routine tests for cardiac patient
Equipment, Instruments, and Supplies Unique to Procedure	• VAD device • There are several types of VADs on the market. One type is a whole device in which the VAD is implanted and connected to an external power source/box.
Preoperative Preparation	• Position: Supine • Anesthesia: General • Skin prep: Routine for cardiac procedures • Draping: Routine for cardiac procedures
Practical Considerations	• The surgical technologist should find out well in advance of the procedure the type of VAD that will be used and study the literature that is provided by the manufacturer as well as the surgical procedure. The manufacturer's sales reps are also often very knowledgeable about their product and can answer questions as well as provide guidance and suggestions. Additionally, the surgeon is, obviously, an excellent resource to discuss the device and procedure.

PROCEDURE 22-14 (continued)

Surgical Procedure

1. The surgeon makes a median sternotomy with the sternal saw and extends the incision to the umbilicus with the #10 knife blade.
2. Using blunt and sharp dissection (Metzenbaum scissors, ESU), the surgeon creates a round preperitoneal pouch. The top of the pouch is just below the mammary line and the bottom at the level of the umbilicus, extending laterally to the line with the axilla and medially in line with the umbilicus. The VAD is inserted into the pouch.
3. CPB is established and the aorta is cross-clamped.
4. A Dacron graft is anastomosed to the aorta in end-to-side fashion.
5. Using a device that is part of the VAD instrumentation called a core-cutting device, the surgeon makes a round opening in the apex of the left ventricle.
6. The surgeon inserts the apex connector into the opening of the left ventricle. The connector has a flange with small holes for suture. Pledgets are used; suture is placed through the holes in the flange and sutured to the myocardium of the left ventricle in interrupted fashion.
7. The inflow conduit is connected to the apex connector.
8. A round opening is made in the diaphragm that is just large enough to accommodate inserting the inflow conduit through the opening and attaching it to the VAD.
9. The Dacron graft that was anastomosed to the aorta is attached to the outflow conduit, which is then attached to the VAD.
10. The driveline (or what we would refer to in layperson's terms as the electrical or power cord) is subcutaneously tunneled from the VAD and exteriorized through a small incision in the groin to be connected to the battery pack.

    Procedural Consideration: The flow of blood is from the left ventricular apex to the VAD through the aortic conduit and into the circulatory system.
11. The surgeon confirms that hemostasis has been achieved, CPB is discontinued, and the surgical site is closed in routine fashion.

Postoperative Considerations

Immediate Postoperative Care

- The patient is transported to the CCU.
- The VAD should be kept running and checked to make sure battery pack is kept fully charged.

Prognosis

- Patient is expected to make a full recovery and adjust to the use of the VAD. Hospitalization is for 7–10 days. Patient should have improved circulation and ability to be more ambulatory while waiting for donor heart.
- Complications: Postoperative SSI; hemorrhage; VAD device failure; thromboembolism

Wound Classification

- Class I: Clean

PROCEDURE 22-15 Orthotopic Heart Transplant

Pathology	• Cardiomyopathy is a general term designating primary disease of the myocardium, often of obscure and unknown etiology. In response to injury, the heart often enlarges, restricting its normal function. Cardiomyopathy can appear in many forms, including alcoholic, congestive, hypertrophic, infiltrative, and restrictive cardiomyopathies.
	  • Alcoholic cardiomyopathy may occur in the individual who consumes large amounts of ethanol over a long period. Ethanol has a toxic effect on cardiac tissue, and eventually results in cardiac enlargement and low cardiac output. The onset of alcoholic cardiomyopathy is gradual with fatigue and dyspnea on exertion as the first symptoms. Physical examination usually reveals a cardiac murmur, edema, hypertension, and an increasing central venous pressure.
	  • Congestive cardiomyopathy is characterized by cardiac enlargement, especially of the left ventricle, myocardial dysfunction, and congestive heart failure.
	  • Hypertrophic cardiomyopathy is characterized by an extensive thickening of the left ventricular myocardium and septum. Blood flow from the atria to the ventricles may be affected as well. Young males are most often affected, but the disease can also occur in a familial form that affects males and females equally.
	  • Infiltrative cardiomyopathy results in the deposition of abnormal substances in the myocardium, as may occur in amyloidosis. The foreign material results in restrictive cardiomyopathy because the heart cannot expand adequately to receive the inflowing blood. The ventricular walls become excessively rigid, impeding ventricular filling. Restrictive cardiomyopathy is marked by normal systolic function of the heart but abnormal diastolic function.
	  • Cardiomyopathies are incurable. Currently, the best treatment is heart transplantation.
	• Heart transplants are also indicated for patients with severe myocardial damage caused by coronary artery disease, heart valve disease with congestive heart failure, and severe congenital heart disease.

Preoperative Diagnostic Tests and Procedures; Equipment, Instruments, and Supplies; Preoperative Preparation; Practical Considerations	• Same as for a CABG, except the skin prep is to mid-thigh because a graft does not have to be taken. • The primary principles when removing the donor heart are rapid arrest and cooling of the donor organ to preserve the myocardium.

PROCEDURE 22-15 (continued)

Surgical Procedure

Harvest of Donor Heart

1. The surgeon exposes the donor heart through a median sternotomy.
2. The aorta and pulmonary artery are mobilized superiorly to the level of the aortic arch and bifurcation to provide as long of a length as possible for the anastomosis.
3. The superior vena cava is mobilized superiorly to the level of the azygos vein. Two ties are placed around the vena cava, but left in place and the strands left uncut.
4. The inferior vena cava is mobilized from the pericardium. The patient is now systemically heparinized. A cardioplegia cannula is inserted in the ascending aorta.
5. The superior vena cava is now divided between the two ties which is followed by CCCT of the inferior vena cava at the level of the diaphragm.
6. Using an aortic clamp, the aorta is cross-clamped at the level of the innominate artery and cold cardioplegia is administered (Figure 22-28A).
7. An incision is made in the right superior pulmonary vein to vent the left atrium. Cold cardioplegia is administered to this area.

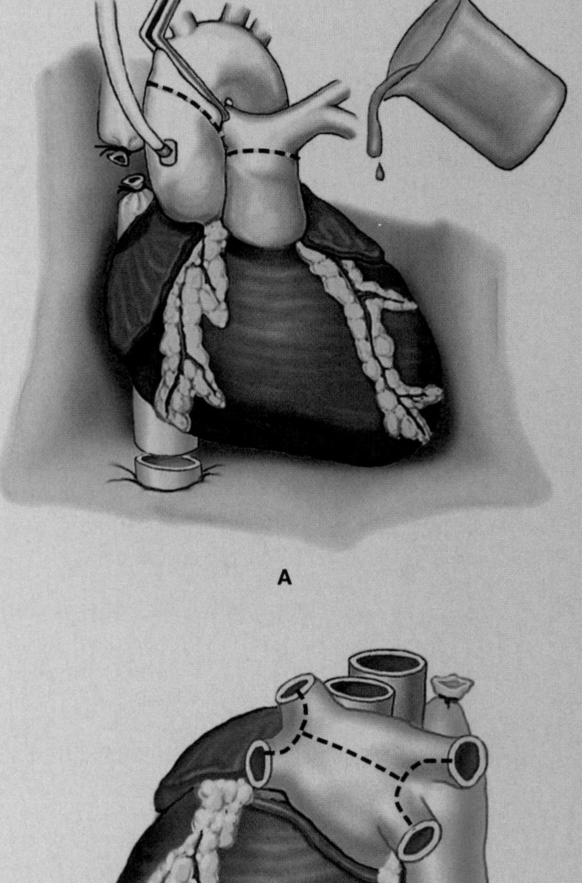

Figure 22-28 Donor heart: (A) Procurement (anterior view), (B) great vessel anastomosis sites (posterior view)

8. The heart is slightly lifted out of the pericardium to allow the surgeon to CCCT the pulmonary veins.
9. The pulmonary artery is CCCT at the bifurcation and the aorta CCCT at the origin of the innominate artery.
10. The heart is removed and placed in a basin of cold slush saline solution and transported to the recipient OR (Figure 22-28B).

(*continues*)

PROCEDURE 22-15 (continued)

Orthotopic Heart Transplantation

1. The surgeon exposes the recipient's heart through a median sternotomy and CPB is begun by inserting a superior vena cava cannula and a cannula in the right atrium.
2. Using an aortic clamp, the aorta is cross-clamped above the aortic valve and proximal to the innominate artery. The heart is removed by incising the atria next to the AV groove and cutting the great arteries distal to the aortic and pulmonary valves.
3. The donor heart is brought up onto the surgical field. The first anastomosis is the left atrium of the donor heart to the left atrium of the recipient heart. The surgeon uses a 3-0 double-armed polypropylene suture to accomplish the anastomosis (Figure 22-29A).
4. A curved left heart catheter (also called a vent) is inserted through the left atrial appendage and advanced into the left ventricle of the donor heart. The catheter aids in air removal at the end of the procedure when the aortic cross-clamp is removed.
5. The right atrium is incised; the incision extends superiorly from the inferior vena cava and is angled away from the junction of the superior vena cava and right atrium of the donor heart. This incision protects and preserves the SA node.
6. The right atrial anastomosis is accomplished using a double-armed 3-0 polypropylene suture in continuous fashion.
7. The lateral and inferior edges of the donor right atrium are anastomosed with the placement of sutures through the atrial septal region of the previous left atrial anastomosis.
8. The pulmonary anastomosis is completed using 4-0 double armed polypropylene in continuous fashion. The posterior wall is sutured first and then the anterior wall.
9. The last anastomosis is the aortic anastomosis, which is completed in the same manner as the pulmonary artery. During this step the patient's body temperature is slowly increased (Figure 22-29B).
10. The patient is placed in slight Trendelenburg position and air is removed from the heart and aorta by lowering the bypass flow, and the air bubbles are released through the ventricular and ascending aortic vents. While the venting continues, the aortic cross-clamp is slowly removed over a 5- to 10-minute period.
11. When the air has been removed the heart is defibrillated and after adequate reperfusion of the new heart has been achieved, the CPB is stopped.
12. The cavity and heart are checked one last time for bleeding and the anastomosis for leaks.
13. The surgical site is closed in layers in routine fashion.

Procedure 22-15 (continued)

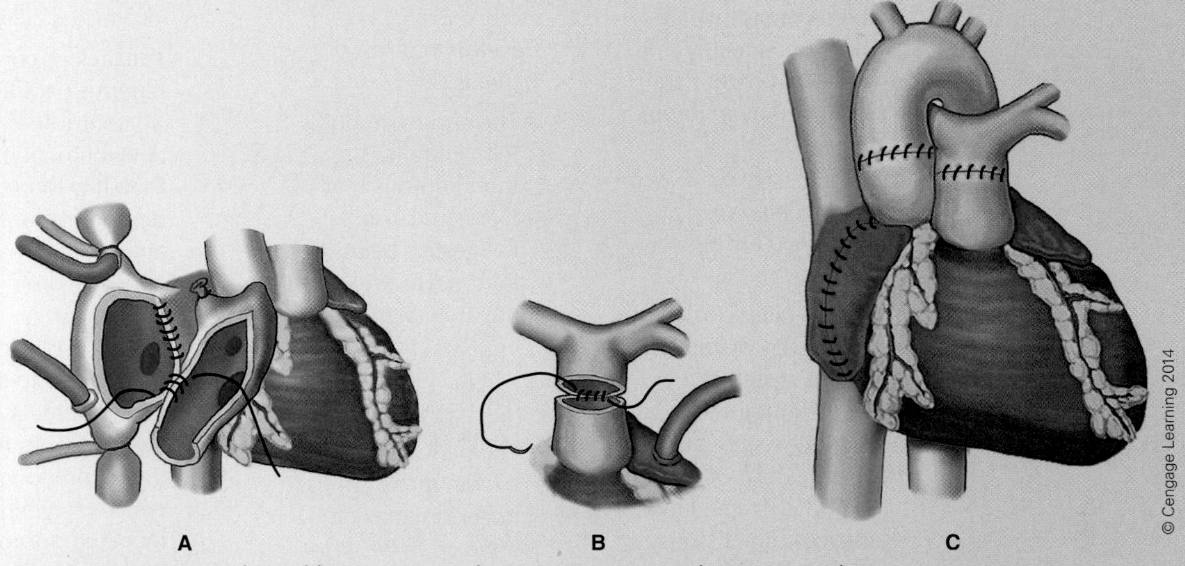

Figure 22-29 Transplanted heart: (A) Atrial anastomosis, (B) pulmonary trunk anastomosis, (C) completed anastomoses

Postoperative Considerations

Immediate Postoperative Care

- Patient is transported to the CCU.
- Short-term drug therapy is initiated to maintain the heart rate at 90–110 beats per minute in order to compensate for the denervated heart. The drug therapy includes vasodilators and inotropics to control the central venous pressure and edema.

Prognosis

- No complications: The 5-year survival rate for heart transplant patients has increased and the risks and complications significantly decrease for patients who survive past the first year. The patient will be closely monitored for the rest of his or her life as well as be on a drug therapy regimen. However, the patient will be able to be ambulatory and lead a much more normal life as compared to the previous state of health.
- Complications: Rejection of heart; postoperative SSI; coronary artery disease; most common causes of early mortality include poor donor selection, poor donor preservation, recipient has prohibitive pulmonary hypertension

Wound Classification

- Class I: Clean

Procedure 22-16 Ventricular Aneurysm Repair

Pathology

- An aneurysm is a sac formed by localized dilatation of the walls of an artery due to structural weakening. The strength of an arterial wall is in the elastic tissue of the tunica media. Destruction of this layer by any disease diminishes the strength of the vessel wall.
- Arterial aneurysms may be classified according to cause, shape, location, or structure.
- There are two types of aneurysm: true aneurysm, in which the wall of the sac consists of one or more of the layers that make up the wall of the blood vessel; and false, or pseudoaneurysms,

(continues)

PROCEDURE 22-16 (continued)

	which are pulsatile hematomas that are not contained by the vessel layers but are confined by a fibrous capsule. Atherosclerotic aneurysms are classified as true aneurysms. • False aneurysms are caused by disruption of the vessel wall or of the anastomotic site between graft and vessel, with blood contained by surrounding tissue (Figure 22-30).	• Left ventricular aneurysms (LVAs) develop in post-MI patients. • The aneurysm of the left ventricle is a mural fibrous scar that can cause congestive heart failure. The wall of the aneurysm is thin. • The mural thrombus can be a large size and calcify over time. The pericardium overlying the aneurysm may be adhered to the epicardial surface of	the aneurysm and also may calcify. • The lack of coronary reperfusion after an MI contributes to the development of an LVA. It is thought that reperfusion of the affected coronary artery by drug therapy or angioplasty contributes to a lower incidence of LVA by improving the blood flow, and hence oxygen, to the infarcted portion of the myocardium.
Preoperative Diagnostic Tests and Procedures	• Routine tests for cardiac surgery • Positron-emission tomography • Left ventriculography is the gold standard for diagnosis of LVA.	• Preoperative assessment of the ventricular function as well as degree of mitral regurgitation, ventricular septal defect (VSD), and	coronary artery disease is important to achieving satisfactory surgical results.
Equipment, Instruments, and Supplies Unique to Procedure	• Routine for cardiac surgery	• Dacron fabric patch	
Preoperative Preparation	• Position: Supine; slight Trendelenburg after sternotomy and exposure of the heart	• Anesthesia, skin prep, draping: Routine for cardiac surgery	
Practical Considerations	• Routine for cardiac surgery		
Surgical Procedure	1. The surgeon makes a median sternotomy. The anesthesia provider heparinizes the patient. The ascending aorta and right atrium are cannulated and CPB is begun, including administration of cardioplegia. The aorta is now cross-clamped. **Procedural Consideration:** Cardioplegia and aortic cross-clamping are first performed to prevent the dislodging of the mural thrombus when the aneurysm is dissected from the pericardial sac.		
	2. The left ventricle is vented by placing a vent through the junction of the right superior pulmonary vein and left atrium.		

PROCEDURE 22-16 (continued)

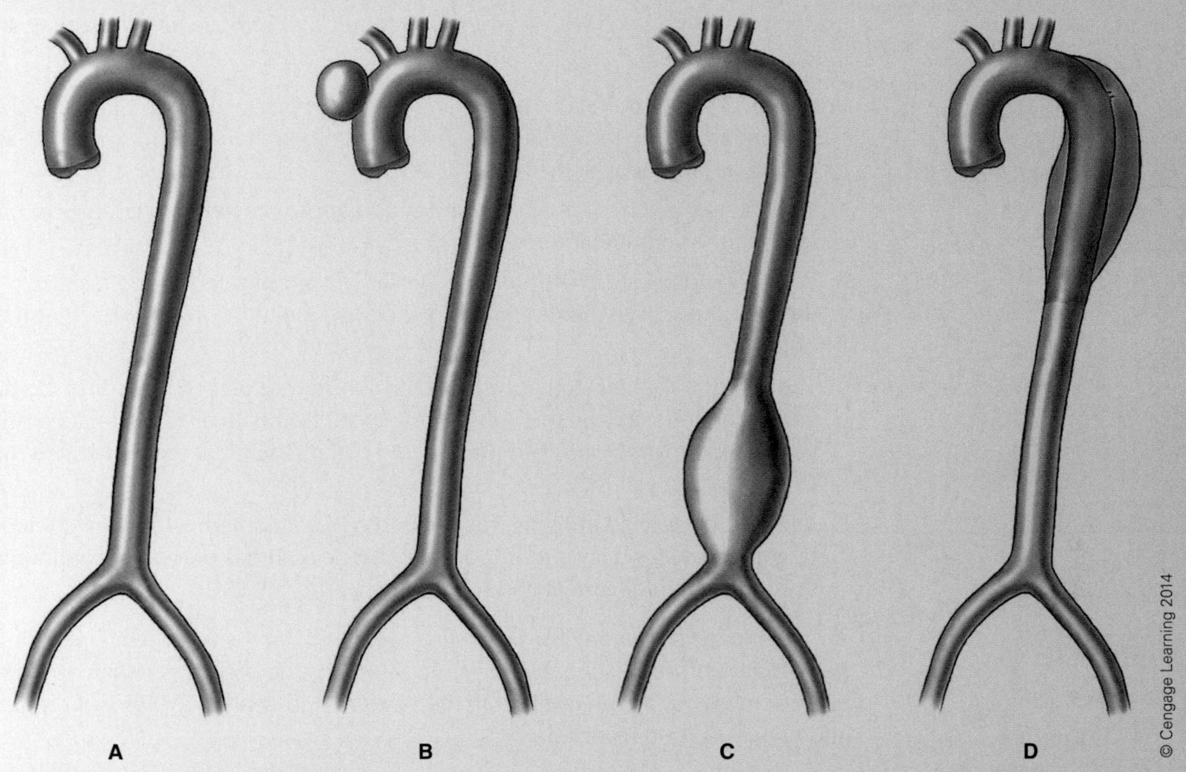

Figure 22-30 Various forms of aneurysms: (A) Normal aorta, (B) saccular aneurysm, (C) fusiform aneurysm, (D) dissecting aneurysm

3. The pericardial adhesions that overly the aneurysm are divided by blunt and sharp dissection, freeing the aneurysm from the pericardial sac.

4. The surgeon inspects the left ventricle and confirms the location of the aneurysm. Using the #15 knife blade and Potts-Smith scissors, a ventriculotomy is made on the anterior aneurysm wall 3–4 cm from the left anterior descending (LAD) coronary artery. The heart is slightly elevated from the pericardial sac and the center of the incised wall of the aneurysm is identified.

5. With the left ventricle open, the mural thrombus is carefully dissected from the ventricle. The margins of viable myocardium are identified and the scar tissue is excised. Loose thrombi are removed. Care is taken to preserve the papillary muscles from injury.

   Procedural Consideration: A wet lap sponge may be placed inside the ventricle to cover the aortic and mitral valves to prevent debris from entering the aorta or left atrium.

6. The remaining portion of the aneurysm is excised, but a 2- to 3-cm rim of scar tissue is left in place for the placement of sutures when the Dacron patch is placed rather than placing the sutures through viable myocardium. The ventricle is

(*continues*)

Procedure 22-16 (continued)

inspected and irrigated with warm saline solution to remove any remaining small pieces of thrombus.

7. Inferior and posterior located aneurysms require repair with a circular Dacron patch, but anteriorly located aneurysms can also be repaired with the patch. The following are the steps of the repair.
   A. The Dacron patch is cut in circular fashion approximately 2 cm larger in diameter than the ventricular opening.
   B. Polypropylene suture with felt pledgets is placed in purse-string fashion through the scar tissue rim and tightened to reduce the size of the ventricular opening.
   C. The 2-0 or 3-0 pledgeted polypropylene sutures are placed in interrupted horizontal mattress fashion through the aneurysm fibrous scar tissue located on the ventriculotomy rim and then through the patch. The pledgets are located on the exterior of the ventricle.
   D. The sutures are tied bringing the patch into place and covering the ventricular opening. A second layer of 2-0 polypropylene suture is placed in continuous fashion for reinforcement and hemostasis.
8. Air is removed by venting the ascending aorta and left ventricle while allowing the heart to fill and ventilating the lungs. Additionally, the patient is rewarmed. Temporary pacing wires are placed on the right atrium and ventricle. CPB is discontinued and heparinization reversed.
9. The surgical site and median sternotomy are closed in routine fashion.

Postoperative Considerations

Immediate Postoperative Care

- Patient is transported to the CCU.
- Patient is closely monitored for low cardiac output and ventricular arrhythmias.

Prognosis

- No complications: The short- and long-term results of LVA have significantly improved over the last 10–15 years due to improvements in surgical technique, instrumentation, equipment, and preoperative diagnostic testing. The patient is expected to make a full recovery with a few limitations in activity. The hospitalization is 14–21 days.
- Complications: Left ventricular failure is the most common cause of hospital mortality; low cardiac output; ventricular arrhythmias; respiratory failure.

Wound Classification

- Class I: Clean

PROCEDURE 22-17 Aortic Valve Replacement

Pathology

- Disease of the semilunar or AV valves of the heart can lead to stenosis of the valves, a condition that can obstruct the normal flow of blood from one region of the heart to another, or to valvular insufficiency, which can cause a reflux of blood into the area from which the blood was ejected during systole. This reverse flow, usually involving the mitral and tricuspid valves, is known as regurgitation. As the valvular disease progresses, the myocardium enlarges to compensate for insufficient flow, and, unless treated surgically with prosthetic valve replacements, congestive heart failure is bound to ensue. Aortic valve dysfunction may result from rheumatic disease, acute infection, atherosclerotic heart disease, or congenital defects. Stenotic valves are often due to the aging process.
- Rheumatic fever may cause calcium deposition and fibrous tissue formation on the leaflets of the mitral valve. This results in an immobile valve, and the AV orifice between the left atrium and left ventricle becomes progressively narrower. Half of the patients with the disease will develop atrial fibrillation and blood flow from the atria to the ventricles is not ejected normally because the contraction is eliminated. Blood stagnated in the atria may form thromboses that could result in arterial embolization.
- Aortic valve stenosis is less common than mitral valve disease and usually affects males. It can be caused by rheumatic fever, but atherosclerosis can be responsible for the condition in the elderly. Congenital valvular malformation is the predominant factor in aortic stenosis, causing the patient to become more susceptible to endocarditis or rheumatic fever.
    - Aortic stenosis impedes the flow from the left ventricle into the aorta, resulting in hypertrophy of the left ventricle as the ventricle struggles to overcome the increased resistance of its outflow tract. As the hypertrophied ventricle becomes dysfunctional, cardiac output is decreased; backflow to the left atrium and pulmonary circulation results in left atrial and pulmonary hypertension. The enlarged ventricle may also compress the coronary arteries at a pressure exceeding coronary perfusion pressure, resulting in myocardial ischemia and angina, exacerbated by the increased oxygen demands of the hypertrophied ventricle's myocardium. Eventually, heart failure will ensue.
- Aortic regurgitation, like aortic stenosis, is frequently caused by rheumatic fever, which damages the leaflets of the valve and results in an incomplete closure. Marfan syndrome is another etiologic factor. This disease, which affects connective tissue systemically, results in necrosis and aneurysm formation of the ascending aorta. The dilation of the aortic annulus pulls the leaflets apart, resulting in valvular insufficiency. Congenital malformation of the valve results in

(*continues*)

PROCEDURE 22-17 (continued)

	susceptibility to bacterial endocarditis and rheumatic fever; aortic regurgitation is therefore imminent. • When the leaflets of the aortic valve close improperly, the outlet between the	left ventricle and the aorta remains open to a degree, and blood that has been expelled into the aorta across the aortic valve flows back into the left ventricle during	diastole. The ventricle hypertrophies and must contract more forcefully to expel this increased volume of blood.
Preoperative Diagnostic Tests and Procedures	• The true extent of aortic stenosis and cor pulmonale (overload of the right ventricle due to pulmonary hypertension) can be attained with cardiac catheterization. Echocardiography will show a thickened	aortic valve and ventricular wall with abnormal movement of the aortic leaflets. • Diagnosis of aortic regurgitation is made on auscultation with a blowing diastolic murmur over the	ascending aorta. Cardiac catheterization reveals the extent of the valvular insufficiency, the degree of ventricular overload, the stroke volume, and the ejection fraction.
Equipment, Instruments, and Supplies Unique to Procedure	• Routine for cardiac procedures • Add the following for valve procedures: • Valve prosthesis • 6 Allis clamps, 3 regular, 3 long	• 6 Babcock clamps, 3 regular, 3 long • Valve retractors to retract leaflets and annulus • Atrial retractor • Valve dilator	• Valve sizers, handle and rings to size the annulus • Valve scissors to excise diseased valve • Valve suture, typically polyester
Preoperative Preparation	• As previously described for cardiac procedures		
Practical Considerations	• Aortic valves are the most frequently replaced valves in cardiac surgery. There are basically two types of valves used for replacement: biologic (tissue) and mechanical. A valve that combines	synthetic material with animal tissue is also frequently used. The tissue valves may be harvested from a pig or a human cadaver, and may also be constructed from the pericardium of a cow. Unlike mechanical	valves that have a tendency to form blood clots, placement of a tissue valve does not require anticoagulant therapy for the recipient. Porcine (pig) and human donor valves usually wear out

PROCEDURE 22-17 (continued)

after a period of 10–15 years, and so are not suitable for implantation in younger patients.

- Mechanical valves are constructed from modern ceramics, and are usually implanted into patients under the age of 65 because of their longer life span. These valves require the use of anticoagulant therapy because of their tendency to form blood clots. Other risks associated with the use of the mechanical valves are hemorrhage and endocarditis.
- A valve that combines bovine pericardium with polyester and plastic, such as the Carpentier-Edwards bioprosthesis valve, lasts approximately 14 years and is another option for patients over the age of 65. The leaflets of the valve are constructed from pericardial tissue, while the supporting structure is made from polyester and plastic.
- In certain instances, a diseased aortic valve can be replaced with the patient's own healthy pulmonary semilunar valve. The pulmonary valve is then replaced with a human donor valve. The benefit to this type of valve replacement is that no foreign synthetic substance or animal tissue is introduced into the body, so there is little risk of rejection or clot formation.
- Room-temperature saline should be used up to the point of aortic cross-clamping; thereafter, cold saline is to be used until the rewarming period. Warm saline should be used after rewarming begins.
- There should never be water on the back table. It would be too easy to accidentally use water instead of saline when filling the cannulas. Water will cause lysing of RBCs.
- Be ready to go back on the pump at a moment's notice. Do not discard cannulas after removal and keep cannulation sutures ready after the patient is removed from CPB. Keep wire cutters and the sternal retractor sterile until the patient is safely out of the OR.
- Pass off defibrillation cables at the same time as the ESU cords. The surgeon will not want to wait for the defibrillation paddles if suddenly needed.
- Keep the field clear of instruments, blood-soaked sponges, etc. Wring out blood from laparotomy sponges into a bowl specifically labeled for blood from the sponges and suction with the pump sucker.
- The surgical technologist should ensure the valve sizers are for the valve being replaced. Do not use aortic valve sizers for mitral valves and vice versa.
- Do not open the valve prosthesis until you have confirmed with the surgeon that is the one he or she needs.
- The surgical technologist should not break scrub and should maintain the sterility of the Mayo stand and

(continues)

PROCEDURE 22-17 (continued)

back table until the patient has safely left the OR. Wire cutters, sternal retractor, cannulation stitches loaded on needle holders, and cannulas should be available in case the patient must be placed back on CPB.

Surgical Procedure

1. A median sternotomy is performed and CPB is initiated.

   Procedural Consideration: Bone wax is used to seal off bleeders from the sternal walls. The 2-0 silk pericardial stays retract the pericardium and are often secured to the sternal retractor.

2. For the maintenance of a bloodless field, a left ventricular vent is placed through the right superior pulmonary vein and into the left ventricle.

   Procedural Consideration: Follow sequence for cannulation previously outlined. Cardioplegia solution is prepared in advance of need.

3. The aorta is cross-clamped and cardioplegia is infused in a retrograde fashion through the coronary sinus. If the aortic valve is incompetent, cardioplegia may be infused through the ascending aorta.

   Procedural Consideration: A large Fogarty aortic cross-clamp with plastic, atraumatic inserts is frequently used to occlude the aorta.

4. An incision is made into the aorta, the edges are retracted with sutures, and the exposed aortic valve is inspected.

   Procedural Consideration: Retraction sutures are ready. Prepare valve retractors and scissors for use.

5. Leaflets are resected and calcium deposits are carefully removed from the annulus for eventual placement of sutures.

   Procedural Consideration: The surgical technologist should ready the valve sizers at this point and the circulator should be ready to open the proper valve. Be sure the prosthesis holder is readily available.

6. The annulus is sized and the prosthesis is selected. The prosthesis is delivered to the annulus on a prosthesis holder.

   Procedural Consideration: Tissue prosthetics must be rinsed in saline according to protocol. Follow the manufacturer's instructions for rinsing porcine valves, typically, 2–3 minutes in three different bowls.

7. Interrupted, nonabsorbable, multifilament sutures of alternating colors are placed into the annulus and through the skirt of the valve, and the valve is carefully pushed down into place (Figure 22-31A).

   Procedural Consideration: The surgical technologist should keep close track of the sutures to be loaded and of the needles that are returned by the surgeon. Wet valve and sutures with saline when placing valve into annulus.

8. The sutures are tied and the motion of the prosthetic leaflets is tested (Figure 22-31B).

   Procedural Consideration: The surgical technologist should have a French-eyed needle available in case the surgeon needs to place another suture through the annulus after the needles have been cut off.

PROCEDURE 22-17 (continued)

9. The aortic incision is closed with nonabsorbable sutures and the cross-clamp is removed (Figure 22-31C).

   Procedural Consideration: Polyester is the suture of choice for aortic incision closure.

10. Air is removed from the left ventricle, the cross-clamp is removed, and CPB is discontinued. Chest tubes are placed for the evacuation of fluid and air, and the chest is closed in the usual manner.

    Procedural Consideration: Patient is warmed, the heart is restarted, and the cannulas are removed. Prepare chest tubes and closing suture. Count as needed.

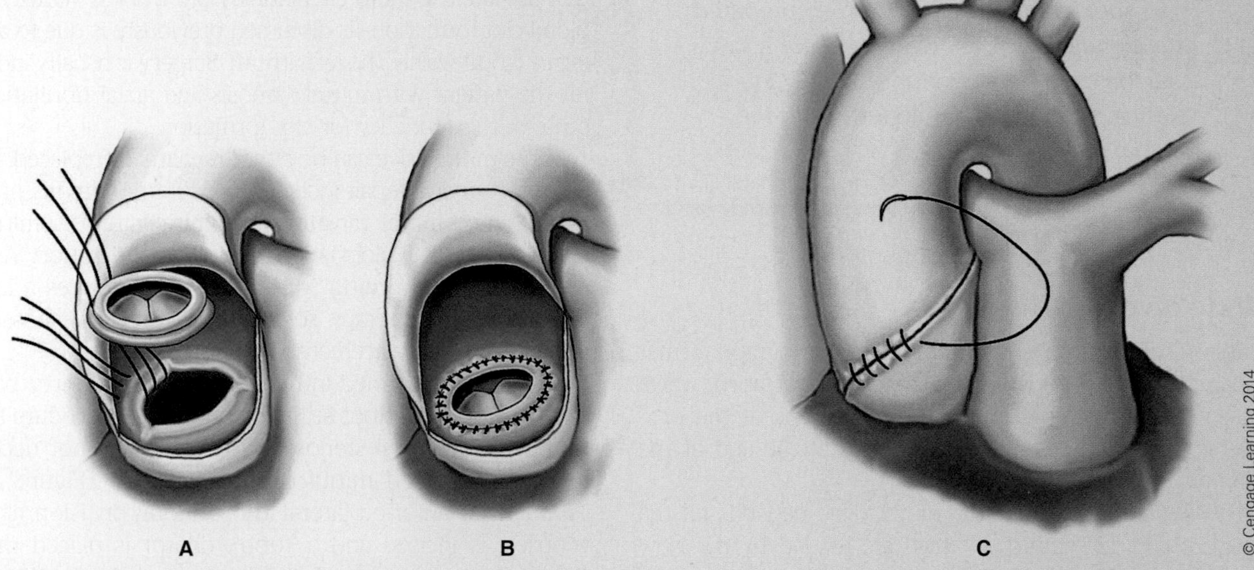

Figure 22-31 Aortic prosthetic valve placement: (A) Sutures are placed through the annulus and the skirt of the valve prosthesis, (B) valve is positioned and sutures are tied, (C) aortic incision is closed

Postoperative Considerations

Immediate Postoperative Care

- Care must be taken when transferring the patient from the OR table to the CCU bed. The patient will have monitoring lines, IV line, ET tube, and urinary and chest drainage tubes in place. These can be easily disturbed if tension is placed on them during the move.
- Patient is transported to the CCU.

Prognosis

- No complications: Patient is expected to make a full recovery and return to normal activities. Hospitalization is 14–21 days.

(continues)

PROCEDURE 22-17 (continued)

- Complications: Postoperative SSIs can be potentially fatal. Implanted cardiac prosthetics increase the risk for infection and should be handled with strict attention to sterile technique. An infection of a valve prosthetic can cause embolism, endocarditis, or mechanical failure, any of which is potentially fatal. Infections of the sternum generally require debridement. Other complications include failure of implanted valve, pneumonia, and complications due to CPB.

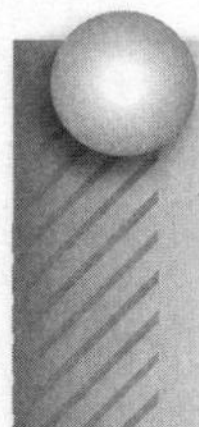

PEARL OF WISDOM

For repeat cardiac procedures, be prepared to cannulate femorally. The oscillating saw may be used for sternotomy to prevent cutting into ventricular adhesions to the sternal wall.

Mitral Valve Replacement

Discussion of mitral valve replacement is in paragraph format because the procedure is so similar to that for aortic valve replacement. A brief presentation of the steps of the procedure is presented in the Technique box at the end of the discussion.

The decision to replace the mitral valve depends on the severity of clinical symptoms which are graded by the New York Heart Association (NYHA) method. Dyspnea on exertion as a result of pulmonary hypertension is graded as 3 or 4 on the NYHA scale, and generally indicates a need for surgery. Other clinical symptoms for the diagnosis of mitral valve stenosis include: dysphagia or bronchitis as a result of left atrial hypertrophy; and excessive fatigue and weakness due to decreased cardiac output. Auscultation helps to confirm the stenosis; an opening snap may be heard which is the result of a forceful opening of the valve, followed by a diastolic rumbling (murmur). Stenosis can also be diagnosed by cardiac catheterization that provides information on cardiac output from the left ventricle as well as pulmonary artery pressures. A comparison of pressures within the atrium and ventricle provides a pressure gradient across the valve. Noninvasive diagnosis is achieved with ECG that outlines the left atrial enlargement, fusion of the mitral leaflets, and obstruction of flow from the left atrium to the left ventricle.

Mitral stenosis and atrial fibrillation may cause systemic embolization from blood clots formed within the left atrium that are launched into circulation from the left ventricle. This blood clot formation, as discussed previously, is due to a pooling of blood within the left atrium. Surgery is usually indicated for the patient with mitral stenosis and atrial fibrillation because of this tendency for clot formation.

The mitral valve can be either repaired or replaced. Procedures for surgical repair include closed mitral commissurotomy (CMC), open mitral valvotomy for mitral stenosis, mitral annuloplasty, or valvuloplasty for mitral regurgitation. As with the aortic valve, a mitral valve prosthesis requires a lifetime of anticoagulant therapy, so mitral valve repair, if possible, is preferable over replacement.

CMC is performed infrequently in this country, but certain developing nations still depend on the procedure for the treatment of mitral stenosis because CPB is not necessary to perform closed mitral commissurotomy (Figure 22-32). Through an anterior lateral thoracotomy incision, the left ventricle is incised and a Tubb's dilator is placed through the wall of the ventricle and across the left AV orifice (a finger in the left atrium serves as a guide for the dilator). The blades of the dilator are spread, and the stenotic mitral valve is widened.

Open mitral commissurotomy for mitral stenosis requires a median sternotomy and CPB. An incision is made into the left atrium and the mitral valve is visualized. If the valve leaflets are fused together at the line of closure (commissure), an incision is made into the leaflets and they are separated. Areas of calcification are removed, and the atrium is closed.

Mitral valve annuloplasty (Figure 22-33) is performed to correct an annular dilatation of the posterior leaflet of the mitral valve due to a contraction of the papillary muscle that shortens the chordae tendineae. The leaflet edges of the valve do not come together properly, and mitral regurgitation results. A prosthetic ring is selected and interrupted sutures are placed through the annulus and into

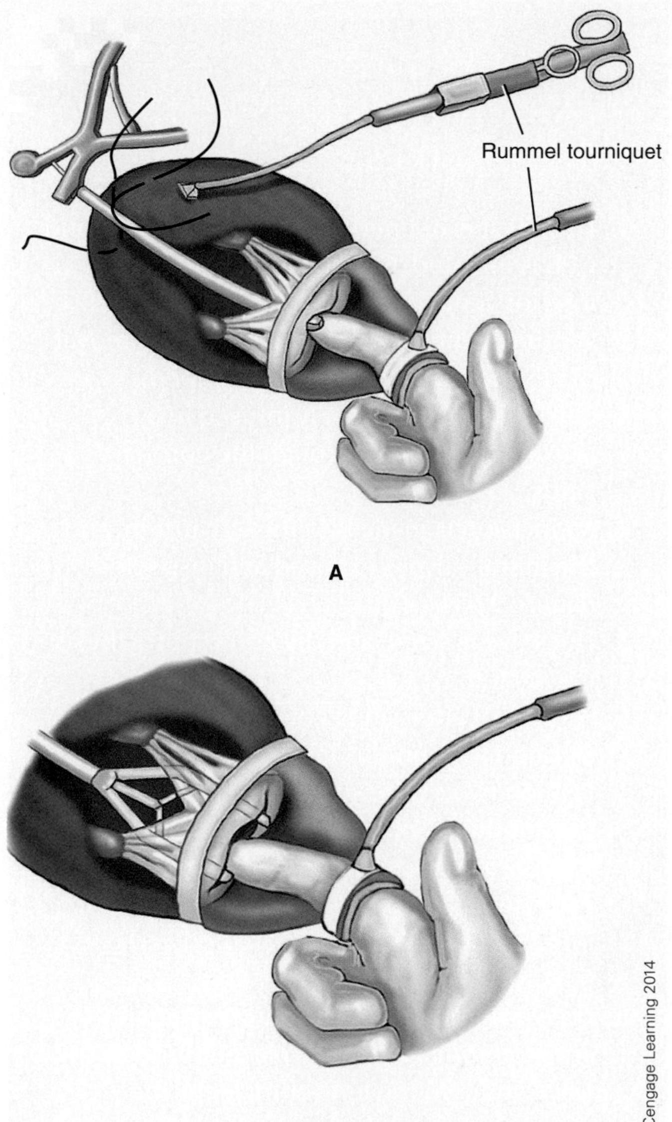

Figure 22-32 Closed mitral commissurotomy: (A) A mitral valve dilator is inserted through the left ventricle and into the mitral valve after the valve is explored with the index finger, (B) dilator is opened

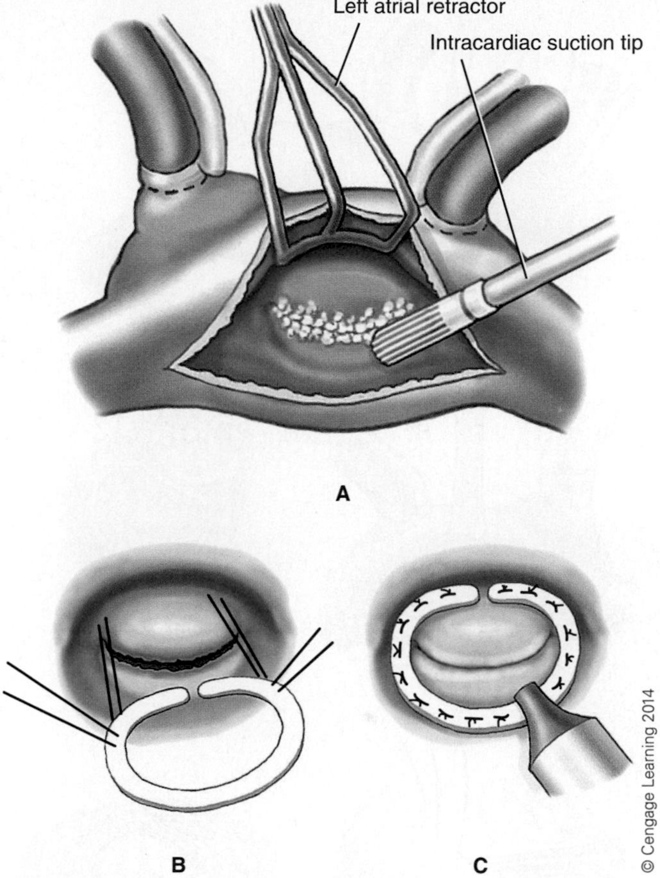

Figure 22-33 Mitral valve annuloplasty: (A) The left atrium is opened and retracted to expose the mitral valve; (B) sutures are placed through the annulus and the ring; (C) the ring is positioned, the sutures are tied, and an Asepto syringe filled with saline is used to check valve competency

the prosthetic ring. The sutures are tied and the annulus is drawn snugly against the ring, thus creating a competent valve.

Mitral valvuloplasty for mitral regurgitation is done to repair the valve's leaflets or to shorten or repair the chordae tendineae associated with the leaflets. Mitral regurgitation can also be caused by mitral valve **prolapse** (MVP). This form of mitral insufficiency is a condition in which some portion of the mitral valve is pushed back too far during ventricular contraction, usually due to redundant tissue on one or both leaflets or papillary muscle dysfunction. The valve leaflets are pushed in the direction of the left atrium during systole, and blood flows backward. MVP, in the vast majority of patients, is a benign condition requiring no treatment.

Mitral valve replacement is performed when damage is too extensive for repair. Many types of prosthetic valves are available for this procedure (bovine pericardial, porcine, bileaflet, or disk). The surgeon chooses the prosthesis after assessing factors associated with each patient. As with the aortic valve prosthesis, risks include thromoembolism, hemorrhage, and endocarditis. Patients with a mitral valve prosthesis must receive anticoagulant medication for the remainder of their lives.

Preservation of as much valve tissue as possible is preferable, especially the posterior leaflet and its supporting structures.

Occasionally, the tricuspid valve will become leaky, resulting in tricuspid regurgitation. If the condition is severe, a De Vega annuloplasty may be performed. This type of repair

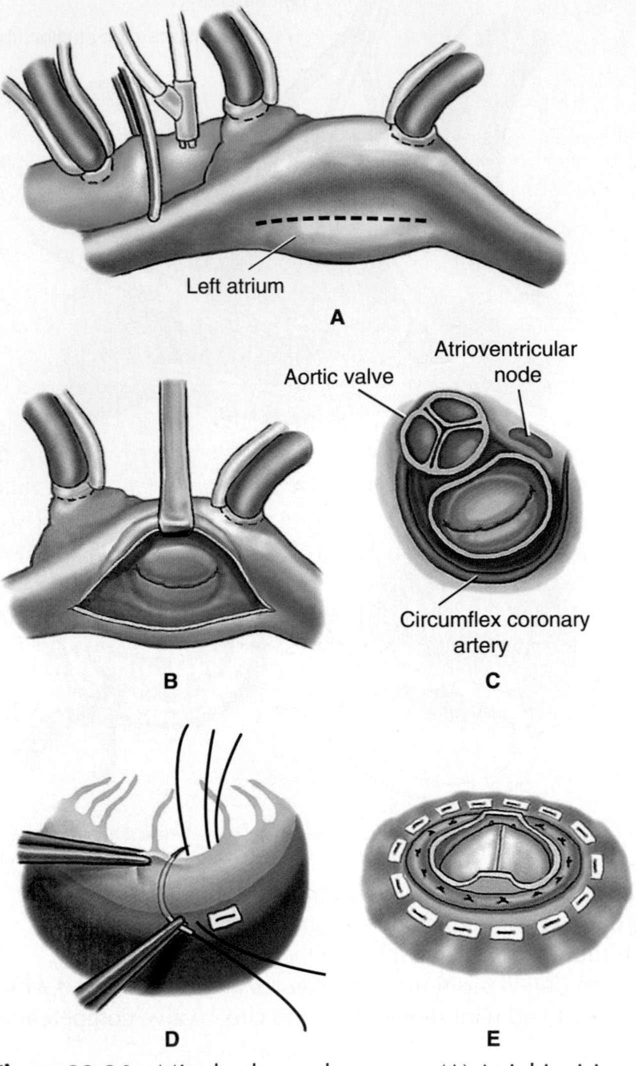

Figure 22-34 Mitral valve replacement: (A) Atrial incision site, (B) mitral valve exposed, (C) cross-section showing related anatomical structures, (D) sutures are placed in the annulus, (E) prosthesis in place

involves the placement of a purse-string suture around the circumference of the annulus. The purse-string is drawn tightly enough to reduce the backflow of blood from the right ventricle into the right atrium.

TECHNIQUE

Replacement of the Mitral Valve with a Prosthesis

1. The chest is opened in the usual manner, and CPB is initiated. Generally, superior and inferior vena cavae cannulation is utilized.
2. Venting catheters are placed for the removal of air, and the aorta is cross-clamped.
3. Cardioplegia is generally infused in a retrograde fashion through the coronary sinus.
4. An incision is made into the left atrium, and the mitral valve is exposed and inspected (Figure 22-34A–C).
5. The valve is sized, and the correct prosthesis is selected.
6. Sutures of alternating colors are placed through the annulus in an interrupted fashion (*Note:* The sutures are pledgeted if the annulus is not stable; Figure 22-34D).
7. Sutures are placed through the ring of the prosthesis, and the prosthetic is lowered into position. The sutures are tied and cut (Figure 22-34E).
8. The valve is inspected for proper function, and a venting catheter is placed through the valve and into the left ventricle for the removal of air while the left atrium is closed.
9. Air removal techniques are employed, the cross-clamp is removed, and CPB is discontinued. Chest tubes are placed for the evacuation of fluid and air, and the chest is closed in the usual manner.

PART III: Pediatric Cardiac Procedures

INTRODUCTION

Surgical procedures for repair of congenital heart defects include repair of atrial septal defect (ASD) and VSD, closure of patent ductus arteriosus (PDA), repair of coarctation of the aorta, and repair of tetralogy of Fallot (TOF).

Preoperative Preparation

The information that has been typically introduced at the beginning of each part of this chapter is not presented here because it would be a repeat of what is listed for adult cardiac procedures. The primary difference is that pediatric cardiac instruments are smaller and more delicate than adult cardiac instruments, but they basically are the same in type. A sternal saw is not necessary for infants. The sternum is typically cut with Mayo scissors.

Prosthetic patch materials or pericardial pieces are frequently used in pediatric cardiac procedures for repair of congenital defects. Small-gauged polypropylene sutures with and without pledgets are also frequently used.

Most adult cardiac procedures are coronary bypasses or valve replacements. Pediatric heart procedures are typically congenital heart defect repairs of acyanotic or cyanotic classification.

The pediatric patient is at greater risk of hypothermia than the adult patient, so the OR temperature is generally raised well before the patient arrives. Warming blankets are utilized during the procedure, and the patient's temperature is closely monitored with temperature probes.

Blood loss should be closely monitored by the surgical team because of the pediatric patient's low blood volume. Sponges should be weighed by circulating personnel, and irrigation amounts should be measured accurately by the surgical technologist.

Ventricular Septal Defect

The VSD repair is similar to the ASD repair; therefore the following is a brief overview of the procedure. A VSD is an abnormal opening in the wall between the right and left ventricle. The size of the defect may vary from the size of a pinhole to a complete absence of the septum, resulting in a common ventricle. This opening allows a certain amount of oxygenated blood from the left ventricle to be shunted through the defect to the right ventricle. From the right ventricle, the blood is pumped back to the lungs, even though it has already been refreshed with oxygen. This inefficient shunting of oxygenated blood displaces blood that needs oxygenation. The heart must pump an increased amount of blood, resulting in an enlargement of the heart.

Symptoms associated with VSD may not occur until several weeks after birth. An infant with a large VSD will not grow normally and may appear undernourished. Pulmonary hypertension is often present because of the increased amount of blood within the pulmonary artery and its branches. If the defect is small, the only clinical finding is a heart murmur. These smaller defects often close spontaneously, but if the defect is large, surgical repair with either a synthetic prosthetic patch or a pericardial patch is recommended to prevent serious problems.

A VSD is repaired in a fashion similar to the ASD, that is, with a small Dacron patch sewn over the defect (primary closure is rare for the VSD). Smaller VSDs are generally left alone, especially if the patient is asymptomatic. Asymptomatic patients should undergo cardiac catheterization at the age of 1, and if pulmonary pressures are elevated, the VSD should be repaired at that time to prevent irreversible pulmonary vascular disease later in life. Large VSDs should be repaired surgically, especially if the patient has a significant left-to-right shunt or an elevated right ventricular pressure.

Septal defects of the ventricle may occur as conoventricular septal defects (the most common of the VSDs), with an outer rim composed of membranous tissue; as muscular VSDs, with an outer rim composed of muscle only and occurring anywhere in the trabecular portion of the septum; as AV-canal-type VSDs that lie beneath the tricuspid valve with all or part of the septum of the AV canal missing; and as conal septal defects that result from a defect within the infundibular septum.

Our discussion will concern the conoventricular septal defect. The challenge for this procedure is to close the VSD completely without damaging the conduction system of the heart.

1. The heart is approached through median sternotomy, and the patient is placed on CPB and cooled. (*Note*: For patients weighing less than 8 kg, deep hypothermia to a temperature of 18°C with total circulatory arrest is also an option.)
2. If a patent **ductus arteriosus** is present, it is ligated and divided before the right atrium is opened to prevent air from entering the systemic circulation.
3. After antegrade cardioplegia delivery, the defect is repaired. The surgeon makes the incision according to the anatomical location of the VSD.
    A. Canal VSD: The surgeon will make an incision in the right atrium, retract the atrium, and insert a suction pump through the tricuspid valve into the right ventricle to verify the location of the VSD.
    B. Muscular VSD: Repair performed through a short transverse ventriculotomy.
    C. Supracristal VSD: Incision is made in the pulmonary artery and extended into the right ventricle.
    D. Pledgeted, interrupted, nonabsorbable sutures of 6-0 gauge are utilized to hold a Dacron patch in place over the VSD. The VSD is rarely repaired by primary closure.
4. The atrium is closed, and CPB is discontinued.

Procedure 22-18 Repair of Atrial Septal Defect (ASD)

Pathology

- An ASD is an abnormal opening in the wall between the two atria. There are three types of ASD: ostium secundum, sinus venosus, and ostium primum.
  - The ostium secundum type is in the midatrial septum and is the most common.
  - The sinus venosus type of defect occurs high in the septum near the entrance of the superior vena cava in the right atrium. This type of defect is usually associated with anomalous pulmonary venous drainage, in which one or more pulmonary veins drain into the right atrium rather than the left.
  - The ostium primum is located low in the anterior portion of the septum and is associated with other defects in the AV canal, usually with a cleft of the mitral valve.
- The ASD results in a shunting of oxygenated blood from the left atrium across the defect into the right atrium. If the defect is large or of the ostium primum type with marked shunting of flow, the workload of the right side of the heart is increased. Pulmonary hypertension, enlargement of the pulmonary artery and its branches, and enlargement of the heart's right side may be a result of this increased workload. In later stages, right-sided heart failure and a reversal of the shunt with subsequent cyanosis may ensue.
- The primary indication for surgical repair of the ASD is the presence of symptoms. Surgery may also be indicated in the infant who is asymptomatic but has clear echocardiographic evidence of right ventricular volume overload.
  - The child who is asymptomatic for the defect should undergo surgical repair around the age of 4–5.
  - If symptoms are present, intervention should come at any age without hesitation.

Preoperative Diagnostic Tests and Procedures

- Electrocardiography
- Standard chest X-ray
- Cardiac catheterization
- Two-dimensional echocardiography

Equipment, Instruments, and Supplies Unique to Procedure

- Same as described for other open-heart procedures
- Dacron patch

Preoperative Preparation

- Position: Supine; rarely right anterior oblique
- Anesthesia: General
- Skin prep: Lower mandible to mid-thigh; bilaterally as far as possible
- Draping: Four towels to square off chest region; pediatric chest drape

Practical Considerations

- Same as described for other open-heart procedures

Surgical Procedure

1. The surgeon makes a median sternotomy and CPB is begun. The patient's core body temperature is established at 32°C. The aorta is cross-clamped and the heart is stopped with cardioplegia solution injected into the aortic root.

PROCEDURE 22-18 (continued)

Procedural Consideration: There are two methods of CPB that the surgeon will choose to use. When bicaval cannulation is used, the pediatric patient remains on CPB during the procedure and the blood flow bypasses the right atrium by traveling through the superior and inferior venae cavae cannulas. However, this method of cannulation can block the view of the surgical site. Therefore, single cannulation may be used by placing the cannula into the right atrium.

2. Using a finger inserted into the right atrium through a stab wound, the defect is inspected and a decision is made as to whether primary closure or patch closure is to be performed. If significant tension will be the result of a primary closure, then the patch will be used.

   Procedural Consideration: If single venous cannulation is used, the venous line is clamped just before the incision is made in the right atrium. Palpation before making the atrial incision eliminates the need to explore the atrium, which decreases the hazards of the formation of an air embolism.

3. Using a #15 knife blade, the right atrium is incised.

4. Small ASDs may be closed directly with polypropylene suture with continuous suture technique.

5. Large defects are closed with a Dacron patch or autologous pericardium.

   A. The patch is sutured to the defect with a double-armed 4-0 or 5-0 polypropylene. The suture is begun at the inferior margin of the defect; each end is placed around the sides in continuous fashion to meet at the superior margin and tied.

   B. The right atrium is closed with a 4-0 or 5-0 polypropylene suture.

   Procedural Consideration: Before the atrium is completely closed the right atrium and pulmonary artery are deaired by allowing blood to fill the atrium. Autologous pericardium patches are an excellent choice for the repair because they are resistant to postoperative SSI.

6. The clamp is removed from the aorta in order to allow blood to flow from the left atrium to the right atrium to prevent air embolism. The lungs are ventilated to deair the pulmonary veins and left atrium. CPB is discontinued; suction is applied to the vent in the ascending aorta for a few minutes after the heart is beating. The chest is closed as described for open-heart procedures.

Postoperative Considerations

Immediate Postoperative Care

- Patient is transported to the NICU.
- Patient is closely monitored for arrhythmias.

Prognosis

- No complications: Patient is expected to make a full recovery; due to the improvement in surgical technique, instrumentation, and equipment, most pediatric patient recovery is uneventful. Hospitalization is 14–21 days.
- Complications: Postoperative SSI; failure of synthetic patch; hemorrhage; heart block (rare); mitral insufficiency remains–if the insufficiency progresses, the patient may have to undergo a reoperation.

Wound Classification

- Class I: Clean

Procedure 22-19 Closure of Patent Ductus Arteriosus (PDA)

Pathology	• PDA is a failure of that fetal structure to completely close after birth. • In fetal life, the ductus arteriosus connects the pulmonary artery to the aorta in order to shunt oxygenated blood directly into the systemic circulation by bypassing the lungs. It usually extends from the origin of the left pulmonary artery to just distal to the origin of the left subclavian artery. • PDA may coexist with other anomalies, such as VSD, coarctation of the aorta, and pulmonary stenosis. • Once the diagnosis of PDA is established, surgical intervention should be planned because it is highly unlikely that spontaneous closure will occur in the few weeks after birth, especially if the PDA is large. If symptoms are present surgery should be performed immediately. The ductus should be divided after 1 year of age or earlier if there is congestive heart failure. • If the patient is asymptomatic, an elective procedure should be performed within 3 months of diagnosis. • If a ductus is found late in life and there is a small shunt, surgery is usually not recommended. Surgery in the adult can present problems because the ductus is usually calcified, brittle, and aneurysmal. • Because the defect is outside the heart chamber, CPB is not required.
Preoperative Diagnostic Tests and Procedures; Equipment, Instruments, and Supplies; Practical Considerations	• Same as described for open-heart procedures
Preoperative Preparation	• Position: Right lateral position (majority of PDAs are located on the left) • Anesthesia: General • Skin prep: Lower border of mandible to mid-thigh; bilaterally as far as possible, including axillary region • Draping: Four towels to square off lateral thoracotomy incision; pediatric transverse drape
Surgical Procedure	1. Infants: Surgeon makes incision through the third intercostal space. Children: Incision is through the fourth intercostal space. The incision through either space is short and spares the serratus anterior muscle (Figure 22-35A). 2. The apex of the lung is retracted downward and anteriorly. The mediastinal pleura is opened over the aorta and retracted with retention sutures; mosquito clamps are placed on the ends of the sutures. The incision is extended upward along the proximal side of the left subclavian artery. The left superior intercostal vein is identified and CCCT. 3. The dissection continues over the anterior surface of the aorta up to and across the PDA toward the pulmonary artery. The direction of the dissection prevents injury to the recurrent laryngeal nerve.

Procedure 22-19 (continued)

4. The aorta, main pulmonary artery, vagus and recurrent laryngeal nerves, and thoracic duct are identified. Intraoperative injury to these structures must be prevented.
5. The parietal pleura and pericardium are incised over the anterior surface of the PDA, dissected free, and retracted medially with retention sutures. The PDA is now exposed (Figure 22-35B).
6. Dissection of the posterior wall of the PDA is critical.
   A. First, the aorta must be prepared for possible occlusion in the event of hemorrhage. Two umbilical tapes are placed around the aorta above and below the PDA, and two tapes are placed around the left subclavian artery; the tapes are loosely clamped.
   B. The aorta is retracted superiorly and anteriorly to expose the posterior wall of the PDA.
7. The PDA clamps are placed as close to the aorta and pulmonary artery as possible (Figure 22-35C).
8. There are three methods of closing the PDA:
   A. Any additional tissue surrounding the ductus is dissected to allow a small right-angle clamp to be passed underneath the lower margin of the ductus. A silk tie is placed in the tip of the right-angle clamp and the tie brought around the ductus and tied.
   B. The PDA is divided as close to each clamp as possible and a continuous suture is placed to close the lumen of each stump (Figure 22-35D).
   C. Four or five metal clips are placed to close the PDA.

   Procedural Consideration: The placement of metal clips avoids having to place the right-angle clamp behind the thin, friable ductus and possibly tearing it, causing life-threatening hemorrhage. Second, the placement of metal clips shortens the surgical time. Last, using metal clips decreases the amount of time the left lung must be retracted, thus decreasing the intraoperative complications with ventilation that can arise.

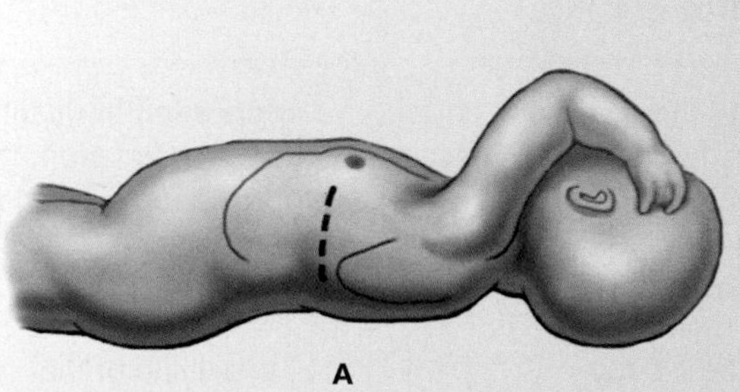

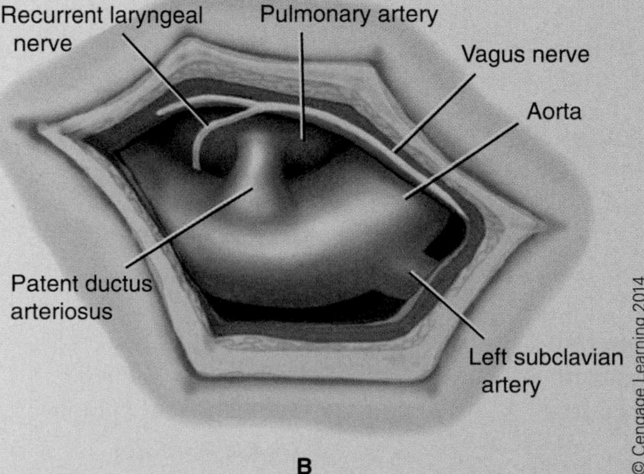

Figure 22-35 Repair of patent ductus arteriosus: (A) Planned incision site, (B) exposure of the patent ductus arteriosus

(*continues*)

Procedure 22-19 (continued)

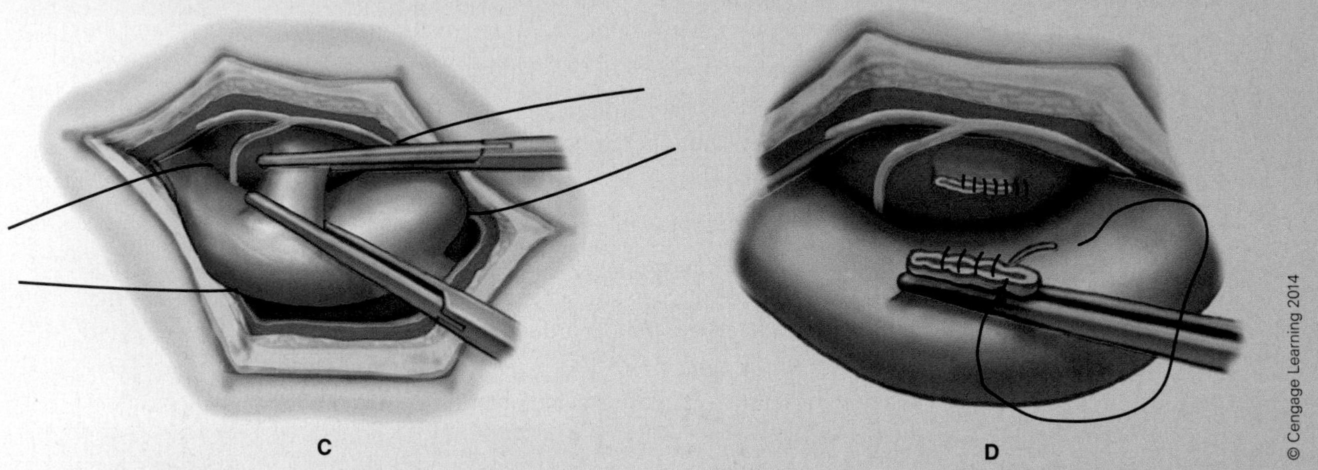

Figure 22-35 Repair of patent ductus arteriosus: (C) clamp application, (D) suturing of free edges

9. After ligation or division, the pleura is left open, and a small drainage catheter is placed into the left pleural space for the drainage of fluid and air for 24 hours. The ribs are approximated and the wound is closed in two layers with running sutures.

Postoperative Considerations

Immediate Postoperative Care

- Patient is transported to the NICU.
- Drain is removed after 24 hours.

Prognosis

- No complications: The patient is hospitalized an average of 3–5 days. Full recovery and return to normal activities takes 6–8 weeks. The prognosis is good when PDA is the only pathology that is present. If additional pathologies or disorders are present, the complications increase.
- Complications: Postoperative SSI; hemorrhage; injury to the recurrent laryngeal nerve; vocal cord paralysis; injury to the vagus nerve; damage to the thoracic duct; incomplete surgical closure of the PDA

Wound Classification

- Class I: Clean

Procedure 22-20 Repair of Coarctation of the Aorta

Pathology

- Coarctation of the aorta is a localized narrowing of the aorta in an otherwise normal vessel. In the adult form, the narrowing is usually distal to the left subclavian artery or just distal to the ligamentum arteriosum. In infantile aortic coarctation, the obstruction is proximal to the ductus arteriosus.

Preoperative Diagnostic Tests and Procedures

- Neonatal: Diagnosis is accurately obtained with echocardiography.
- Adolescents and adults:
  - Electrocardiography
  - Chest X-ray
  - Echocardiography
  - Heart catheterization and aortography should be performed to demonstrate the exact site of the narrowing, extent of the narrowing, and to evaluate or detect any associated lesions.

PROCEDURE 22-20 (continued)

Equipment, Instruments, and Supplies Unique to Procedure	• Same as previously described for open-heart procedures • Adult patients: Dacron tubular prosthesis
Preoperative Preparation	• Position: Posterolateral • Anesthesia: General • Skin prep: Lower border of mandible to mid-thigh; bilaterally as far as possible, including axillary region • Draping: Four towels to square off posterolateral incision site; pediatric transverse drape
Practical Considerations	• Elective surgery is often recommended at 3–6 months of age because, if performed earlier, obstruction may recur. However, some surgeons prefer to wait until the third or fourth year. • Surgery is necessary because of the high incidence of complications, including stroke, hypertension, ruptured aorta, and congestive heart failure. • Because the defect is outside the heart chambers, only the thoracic cavity is entered. • Coarctation of the aorta is often seen in conjunction with other congenital cardiac abnormalities, and it is often surgically repaired at the same time that the other defects are addressed. • The neonate or infant with coarctation of the aorta usually has a PDA and presents with dramatic symptoms after the ductus closes and the coarctation remodels. Collapse of the cardiovascular system ensues rapidly, with hypotension, **tachycardia**, and tachypnea as the initial symptoms, followed within hours by anuria and metabolic acidosis. Prompt resuscitation and stabilization of the cardiovascular system is necessary before surgical correction can be attempted.
Surgical Procedure	1. A posterolateral incision is made in the fourth intercostal space. In adult patients, the fourth rib will be stripped and resected. **Procedural Consideration:** The collateral circulation that formed may have contributed to the enlargement of the arteries in the muscle layer and intercostal space. Controlling bleeding is essential to maintaining normal hemodynamic stability in the patient. The surgical technologist should be prepared for the surgeon to frequently use the ESU and have a large number of ties.
	2. The lung is retracted anteriorly and inferiorly, and the coarctation is exposed by incising the mediastinal pleura over the aortic isthmus. Using a vessel loop, the vagus nerve will be retracted medially (Figure 22-36A). **Procedural Consideration:** The aortic isthmus is a small area of the aortic arch just distal to the left subclavian artery and right before the aorta that is termed the descending aorta. To keep bleeding at a minimum, the surgeon is meticulous in the dissection of tissue surrounding the aorta and intercostals vessels. The dissection will be carried out in blunt fashion; the surgical technologist should provide the surgeon with an unfolded 4 × 4 radiopaque sponge that he or she will place around the fingers to facilitate the blunt dissection.

(continues)

Procedure 22-20 (continued)

3. The supreme intercostal vein (most superior vein in the line of intercostal veins) crosses over the aortic isthmus; it is CCCT to expose the coarctation.

   Procedural Consideration: The intercostal vessels have thin walls and therefore must be carefully handled throughout the procedure.

4. The intercostal arteries distal to the supreme intercostals vein are ligated; however, it is not necessary to cut the arteries. They are retracted inferiorly and medially with vessel loops.

5. In the event heavy bleeding occurs, the surgeon places large-gauge silk sutures or vessel loops around the subclavian artery and aorta; Crile clamps are placed on the ends of the sutures or vessel loops.

6. The aorta is mobilized almost up to the diaphragm.

7. The surgeon now determines the length of aorta to be excised above and below the coarctation. Usually, the aortic lumen proximal to the coarctation is narrower than the lumen distal to the coarctation, demanding the excision of a long segment in order to achieve lumens that are matching in size (Figure 22-36B).

   Procedural Consideration: In adults, usually primary anastomosis cannot be performed even with extensive mobilization of the aorta due to excessive tension placed on the anastomosis. In this case, a Dacron tubular graft will be placed.

8. Arterial clamps are placed on the aorta above and below the area of dissection, and a clamp is placed on the left subclavian artery.

9. Using the #15 knife blade, an incision is made either above or below the area of constriction and, with the Potts-Smith scissors, is carried circumferentially. The procedure is performed on the opposite end. The aortic specimen with constriction is removed.

10. The end-to-end anastomosis is begun by suturing the posterior wall of the aorta with 5-0 or 6-0 absorbable monofilament suture placed in continuous fashion (Figure 22-36C, D).

11. The anterior wall is anastomosed with either the continuous suture or with simple interrupted sutures (Figure 22-36E).

    Procedural Consideration: When using a Dacron tubular graft after the coarctation has been excised, the synthetic graft is positioned between the two aortic segments and sutured into place with a 4-0 continuous polypropylene suture.

12. The lower arterial clamp is removed first and the upper clamp is removed slowly. The surgical technologist should be ready to quickly hand the clamps back to the surgeon if bleeding occurs and quickly provide sutures to be placed to control the bleeding.

13. The pleura is closed with a continuous absorbable suture.

14. Before the chest is closed in layers, the surgeon ensures that hemostasis has been achieved.

Procedure 22-20 (continued)

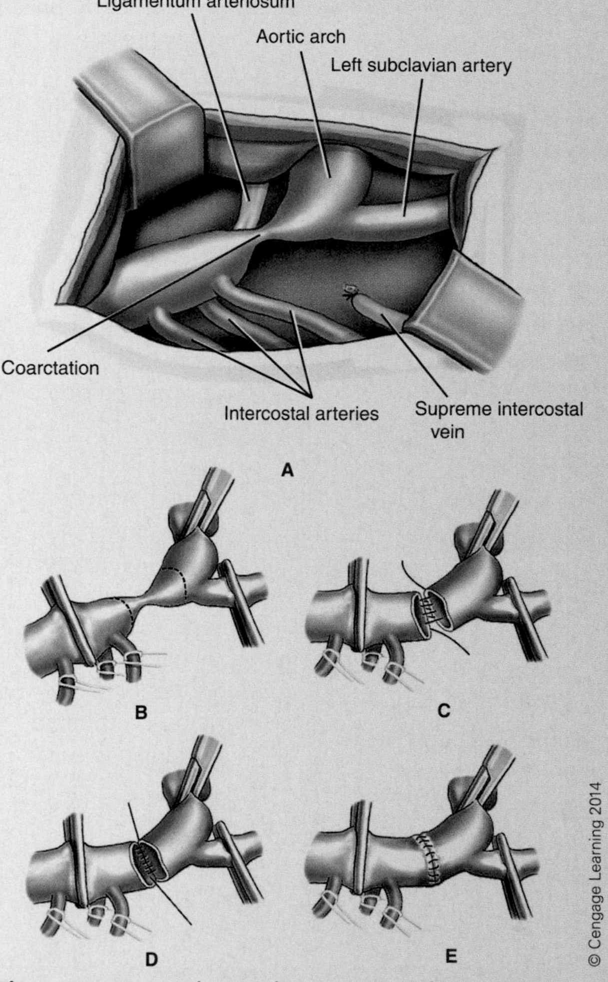

Figure 22-36 End-to-end anastomosis for repair of aortic coarctation: (A) Exposure of coarctation, (B) incision sites, (C) anastomosis of free edges, (D) advance of closure, (E) anastomosis complete

Postoperative Considerations

Immediate Postoperative Care

- Patient is transported to the NICU (adults to the CCU).
- Patient is closely monitored for arrhythmias and signs of hemorrhage.
- Antibiotics are administered for 1–3 days.

Prognosis

- No complications: Patient is expected to make a full recovery; due to the improvement in surgical technique, instrumentation, and equipment most pediatric patients recovery is uneventful. Hospitalization is 7–8 days.
- Complications: Postoperative SSI; failure of Dacron prosthesis; hemorrhage; paraplegia—most devastating complication due to ischemia of the spinal cord during cross-clamping of the aorta; hypertension, usually affects the adult patient during the first 48–72 postoperative hours and is controlled with hypertensive medications.

Wound Classification

- Class I: Clean

PROCEDURE 22-21 Repair of Tetralogy of Fallot (TOF)

Pathology	• TOF is the most common cyanotic heart defect in children. The classic form of which there are several variations, includes the following four defects: 1. VSD 2. Infundibular or pulmonary valve stenosis 3. An aorta that overrides the VSD 4. Right ventricular hypertrophy • The first three defects are congenital and the fourth is acquired as a result of the increased pressure within the right ventricle. • Older children with this disease often give a history of squatting after exercise and are subject to hypoxic spells. Squatting relieves the symptoms of dyspnea and faintness that can occur after exertion by causing a rise in the common ventricular pressure. Pulmonary artery flow is enhanced as a result of the increased ventricular pressure, and more oxygenated blood enters the left side of the heart. • TOF results in cyanosis, which may appear soon after birth, in infancy, or later in childhood. These "blue babies" may have sudden episodes of severe cyanosis with rapid breathing and may even lose consciousness. • Other complications of the disease include infective endocarditis, blood clotting problems, cerebral infarction or embolism, cerebral abscess, and, rarely, right ventricular failure. Therefore, early total surgical correction should be done for all cases to avoid these complications. • Infants with severe TOF may require a shunt between the aorta or subclavian artery and the pulmonary artery to increase blood flow to the lungs. This shunt allows for more blood flow to the lungs for increased oxygen saturation, which reduces cyanosis and allows the child to grow and develop until a total repair can be done when the child is older.
Preoperative Diagnostic Tests and Procedures	• As previously described for open-heart procedures
Equipment, Instruments, and Supplies Unique to Procedure	• Same as for open-heart surgery with the addition of the following items: • 2 × 2 in. intracardiac patch • 2 × 2 in. outflow cardiac patch • 4 × 4 in. Gore-Tex patch
Preoperative Preparation	• Position: Supine • Anesthesia: General • Skin prep: Lower border of mandible to mid-thigh; bilaterally as far as possible • Draping: Four towels to square off chest region; pediatric chest drape
Practical Considerations	• Most children with TOF have the defects repaired before school age. • Due to symptoms of hypoxemia and hypoxia, the majority of patients with TOF and pulmonary stenosis will require surgical correction during the first year of life. • Early repair minimizes secondary damage to the brain, heart, and lungs.

Procedure 22-21 (continued)

Surgical Procedure

1. A median sternotomy is performed. At this time a small pericardial patch is excised for later use in reconstruction of the right ventricular outflow tract. If the surgeon uses a synthetic graft this step will not be performed.
2. CPB and cooling are initiated in the usual manner.
3. The pulmonary trunk is dissected away from the right and left pulmonary branches and the ascending aorta, and the aorta is cross-clamped for cardioplegia infusion. Circulation is stopped and the right atrial cannula is removed for exposure.
4. Using a #15 blade and Metzenbaum scissors, the surgeon makes a right vertical ventriculotomy over the infundibular area.
5. Self-retaining retractors are positioned and a small portion of the hypertrophied infundibular muscle is excised from the right ventricular outflow tract using smooth forceps and Metzenbaum scissors.
6. The VSD is identified and incised. Hypertrophied septal and parietal bands on each side of the defect are excised. In the majority of cases the closure of the VSD requires the use of an intracardiac patch; the patch is either synthetic (Dacron) or a piece of excised pericardium. Interrupted horizontal mattress sutures reinforced with Teflon patches are used for placement of the patch.
7. If the pulmonary annulus is determined to be small, it is also enlarged with use of a Gore-Tex patch or other synthetic material of the surgeon's preference.
8. If the pulmonary valve leaflets are fused, a pulmonary valvulotomy is performed by blunt and sharp dissection. Using two clamps or smooth forceps, the edges of the valve are grasped and inverted. Using a #15 blade, the surgeon incises the fused leaflets to release them and also inserts a finger gently through the valve opening to ensure patency.
9. The right ventricular outflow patch is placed to enlarge the right ventricular outflow tract located inferior to the pulmonary valve. The patch will be either synthetic (Dacron or Teflon) or pericardial homograft.
    i. The right side of the heart is filled with saline.
    ii. CPB is reinstated with a single cannula placed into the right atrium, just below the opening of the superior vena cava.
    iii. While the patient is warming, the patch is sewn to the right ventricular outflow tract with a continuous 5-0 Prolene suture.
    iv. A 19-gauge catheter is pushed through a purse-string suture into the epicardium of the right ventricle for postoperative monitoring.
10. Air is withdrawn from the left ventricle by inserting a needle into the ascending aorta.
11. Air is removed from the pulmonary veins by inflating the lungs.
12. The pressures of the pulmonary artery and right ventricle are taken to ensure success of the procedure. If the pressures are not normal, the procedure may continue to achieve the desired results.
13. CPB is discontinued; chest tubes are inserted; the chest is closed in the usual manner and dressings are applied. The patient is transported to the pediatric ICU.

(*continues*)

Procedure 22-21 (continued)

Postoperative Considerations

Immediate Postoperative Care

- Patient is transported to the NICU.
- Close monitoring of intrathoracic bleeding is required during the first 24 hours postoperatively; patients have an increased chance of hemorrhage due to the long-term polycythemia. Close observation is required to detect intrathoracic collection of blood with cardiac tamponade.
- Cardiac output must be closely monitored for 24 hours postoperatively.

Prognosis

- No complications: Postoperative prognosis varies a great deal. Usually it is good, but it depends largely on the severity of the defects, especially the severity of pulmonary stenosis. However, the majority of patients experience immediate improvements such as the absence of cyanosis. Full recovery takes a few months, but the patient builds up to performing normal activities including ability to fully exercise.
- Complications: Postoperative SSI; hemorrhage; reduced cardiac output; heart block (rare)

Wound Classification

- Class I: Clean

Case Study Jim, a 50-year-old with diabetes, is taken to the cardiac cath unit for a coronary angiogram and left ventriculogram after arriving in the emergency department with severe chest pain. The cardiologist discovers a lesion in the left main coronary branch and immediately orders an emergency CABG.

1. Why is a lesion in this location more dangerous than any other coronary lesion?
2. Could an angioplasty be performed to repair the lesion?

Questions for Further Study

1. What is the proximal saphenous vein sutured to during CABG?
2. What is the purpose of the left ventricular vent?
3. What is the purpose of the IABP, and where is it positioned?
4. During cannulation, where are the cannulas of the pump oxygenator machine placed for CPB surgery?
5. Describe what occurs when a patient experiences a mediastinal shift.

BIBLIOGRAPHY

Beauchamp, D. R., Courtney, M., Evers, M. B., Mattox, K. L., Sabiston, D. C., & Townsend, M. D. (Eds.). (2007). *Sabiston textbook of surgery: The biological basis of modern surgical practice* (18th ed.). Philadelphia: W. B. Saunders.

Boasquevisque, C. H. R., Yildirim, E., Waddel, T. K., & Keshavjee, S. (2009). Lung transplant and lung volume reduction. *Proceedings of the American Thoracic Society, 6*, 66–78. doi:10.1513/pats.200808-083GO

Butler, J. L., Lewis, R., & Shier, D. N. (2009). *Hole's human anatomy and physiology* (12th ed.). New York: McGraw-Hill.

Cleveland Clinic Foundation. (2002–2006). *TMR (transmyocardial laser revascularization): A surgical procedure for inoperable coronary artery disease patients with angina (chest pain)* [Online]. Retrived from http://www.clevelandclinic.org/

Dauphine, C., & Omari, B. (2005). Pulmonary embolectomy for acute massive pulmonary embolism. *Annals of Thoracic Surgery, 79*, 1240–1244. doi:10.1016/j.athoracsur.2004.08.081

Derrickson, B. H., & Tortora, G. J (2008). *Principles of anatomy and physiology* (12th ed.). Hoboken, NJ: John Wiley & Sons.

Gazes, P. C. (1997). *Clinical cardiology* (4th ed.). New York: Hodder Arnold Publication.

Glower, D. D., & Lowe, J. E (2003). Left ventricular aneurysm. In L. H. Cohn & L. H. Edmunds Jr. (Eds.), *Cardiac surgery in the adult* (pp. 771–788). Retrieved from http://cardiacsurgery.ctsnetbooks.org/cgi/content/full/2/2003/771 ?ck=nck

Jamieson, S. W. (2004). Pulmonary thromboendarterectomy. *US Cardiology*, 1–3. Retrieved from http://www.touchcardiology.com/files/article_pdfs/5228.pdf

Luckraz, H., & Dunning, J. (2001). Pulmonary thromboendarterectomy. *Annals of the Royal College of Surgeons of England, 83*, 427–430.

Mickleborough, L. (2005). Ventricular reconstruction or aneurysm repair using a modified linear repair technique with septal patch when indicated. *European Association for Cardio-thoracic Surgery*, 1–10. doi:10.1510/mmcts.2004.000588

Minimally invasive direct coronary artery bypass, MIDCAB. (n.d.). Retrieved from http://biomed.brown.edu/Courses/BI108/BI108_2000_Groups/Heart_Surgery/MIDCAB.html

Molins, L., Fibla, J. J., Perez, J., & Vidal, G. (2007). Chest wall surgery: Nuss technique for repair of pectus excavatum in adults. *European Association for Cardio-thoracic Surgery*, 1–9. doi:10.1510/mmcts.2004.000315

Mancini, M. C. (2011). Patent ductus arteriosus surgery. Medscape Reference. Retrieved from http://emedicine.medscape.com/article/904895-overview

Off pump coronary artery bypass,opcab (n.d.). Retrieved from http://biomed.brown.edu/Courses/BI108/BI108_2000_Groups/Heart_Surgery/OPCAB.html

O'Toole, M. T. (2005). *Miller-Keane encyclopedia & dictionary of medicine, nursing and allied health* (7th ed.). Philadelphia: W. B. Saunders.

Sanders, T., & Scanlon, V. C. (2006). *Essentials of anatomy and physiology* (5th ed.). Philadelphia: F. A. Davis.

Techniques and instrumentation used to operate on a beating heart. (n.d.). Retrieved from http://biomed.brown.edu/Courses/BI108/BI108_2000_Groups/Heart_Surgery/Instrumentation.html

Thibodeau, G. A. (2009). *Anthony's textbook of anatomy and physiology* (19th ed.). St. Louis: Mosby.

Chapter

23

Peripheral Vascular Surgery

Case Study Gregory is a 67-year-old man who has come to the emergency department complaining of bouts of weakness in his right leg that have been progressively getting worse. His wife has noted that he appears confused during these bouts and often has trouble speaking. The speech difficulties and confusion last only about a day, and then he is back to normal. The right extremity weakness, however, improves only slightly after each bout, leaving Gregory a bit weaker each time. Gregory put off seeing a doctor because of the transient nature of his attacks. His wife, however, is worried that he is having a stroke. Gregory has been a pack-a-day smoker for 40 years.

1. What tests may be ordered?
2. What is the possible diagnosis?
3. What surgical procedure will be scheduled?

Objectives

After studying this chapter, the reader should be able to:

A 1. Recognize the relevant anatomy of the peripheral vascular system.

P 2. Summarize the pathology that prompts surgical intervention of the peripheral vascular system and the related terminology.

3. Determine any special preoperative peripheral vascular diagnostic procedures.
4. Determine any special preoperative preparation procedures.

O 5. Indicate the names and uses of peripheral vascular instruments and supplies.

6. Indicate the names and uses of special equipment.
7. Determine the intraoperative preparations of the patient undergoing peripheral vascular procedures.
8. Summarize the surgical steps of peripheral vascular procedures.
9. Interpret the purpose and expected outcomes of peripheral vascular procedures.
10. Recognize the immediate postoperative care and possible complications of peripheral vascular procedures.

S 11. Assess any specific variations related to the preoperative, intraoperative, and postoperative care of the patient undergoing peripheral vascular surgery.

Select Key Terms

adventitia
bifurcation
capillaries
claudication
contralateral
embolus
Fogarty embolectomy catheter
in situ
innominate
intima
ischemia
morbidity
mortality
occlusion
patency
phrenic
pledget
plethysmography
sinuses
thrombus
valve

PERIPHERAL VASCULAR SURGICAL ANATOMY

The peripheral vascular system refers to a closed system of blood vessels that transports blood away from the heart to the body's tissues, and then back again to the heart. The anatomy is discussed at the beginning of this chapter rather than addressed within the context of surgical procedures due to the complexity of the peripheral vascular system.

Blood Vessels

Arterial blood is pumped by the heart through a large system of blood vessels called arteries; therefore, arterial blood refers to blood that is transported away from the heart to the tissues of the body. The arteries are large in size as they leave the heart, but begin subdividing into progressively smaller arteries as they move into various regions of the body. These arteries grow progressively smaller until they become arterioles, which in turn become **capillaries**. Capillaries are microscopic vessels designed to exchange nutrients and wastes between the blood and tissue fluid around the cells in specialized areas called capillary beds. After this exchange, capillaries unite to form venules, the smallest of veins (Figure 23-1). These venules, in turn, unite to form progressively larger blood vessels called veins, which eventually become the superior and inferior vena cava, the largest of veins. Veins, then, are designed to transport blood back to the heart.

Arterial blood pumped away from the left ventricle of the heart enters the aorta, the largest of the arteries, and begins its trip through the progressively smaller arteries toward the arterioles, which become capillaries (Figure 23-2). Wastes, nutrients, oxygen, and carbon dioxide are exchanged, and then venous blood begins its trip back to the heart in the venules, which grow progressively larger to become veins. Venous blood is then emptied into the inferior and superior vena cava, and deposited into the right atrium of the heart.

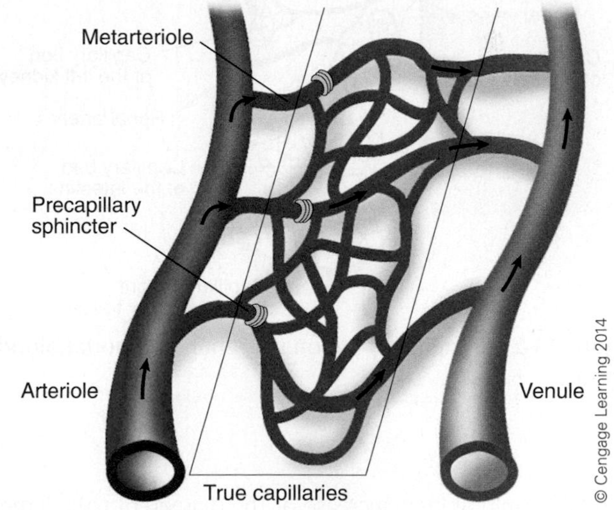

Figure 23-1 Capillary bed connecting an arteriole to a venule

Structure of the Artery and the Vein

The wall of an artery consists of three layers called tunics. The outer layer is called the tunica **adventitia** and consists of connective tissue. This layer attaches the artery to the surrounding tissues and also contains tiny vessels called vasa vasorum that nourish the cells of the arterial wall.

The middle tunic is called the tunica media and is the thickest of the three layers of the arterial wall. This layer includes elastic fibers and smooth muscle fibers that completely encircle the artery. The smooth muscles in this layer are innervated by sympathetic branches of the autonomic nervous system. Impulses from these nerves can cause the smooth muscles to contract, resulting in a narrowing of the lumen, which is the channel for blood flow within the vessel. This process is referred to as vasoconstriction. The inhibition of the impulses from the autonomic nervous system allows the smooth muscles

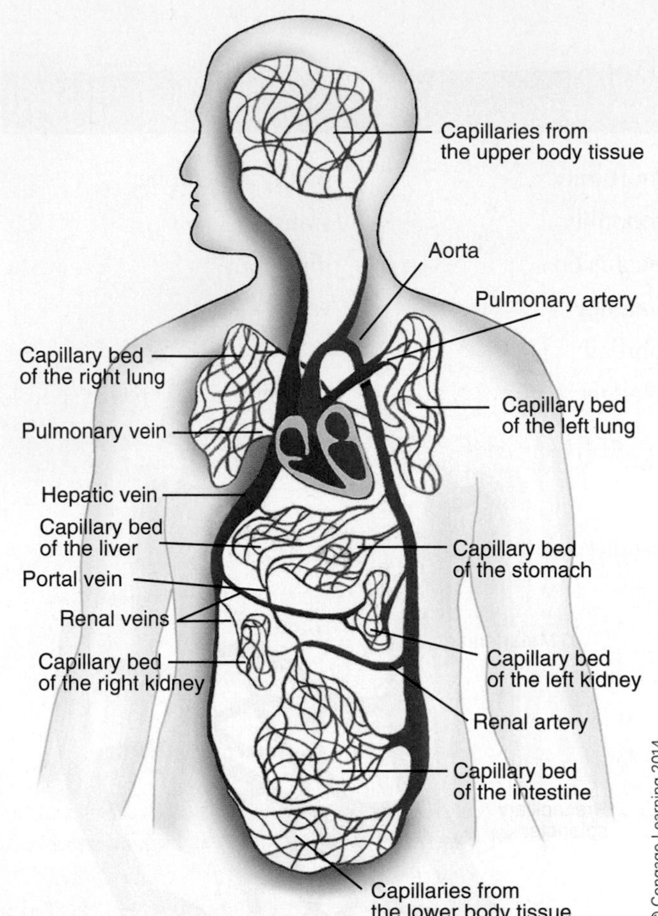

Figure 23-2 Systemic, pulmonary, renal, and portal blood circuits

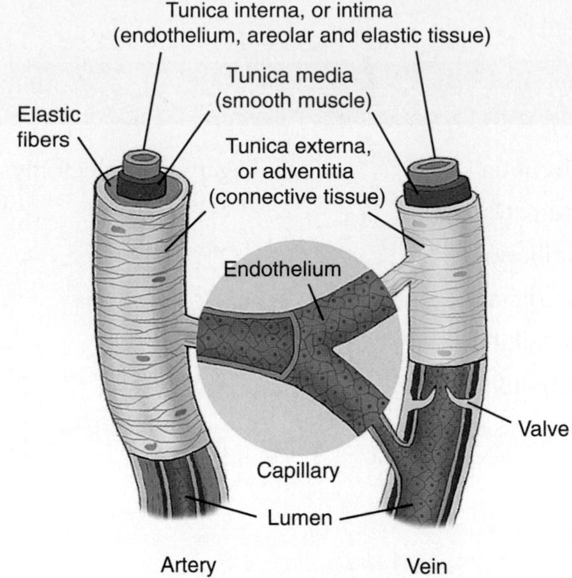

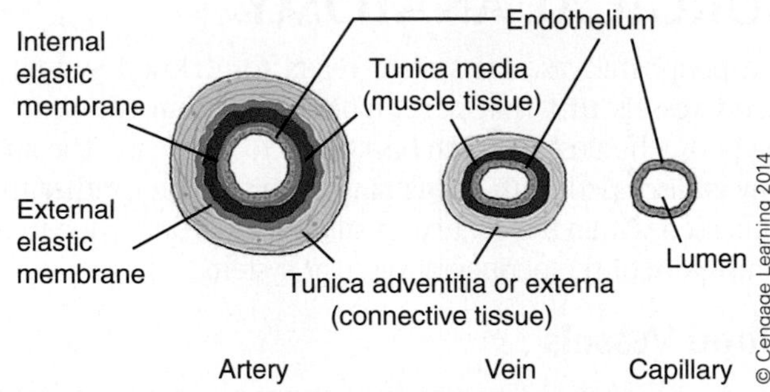

Figure 23-3 Blood vessel types and structure

to relax, resulting in an increase of the diameter of the lumen. This is referred to as vasodilation. Vasoconstriction results in a rise in blood pressure, while vasodilation results in decrease in blood pressure.

The inner tunic is called the tunica **intima** and is composed of a lining of endothelium. This layer is in contact with the blood; the lining of this layer must be smooth so that platelets can flow without being damaged and clotting will be prevented.

The walls of arterioles are very thin, and consist of only a layer of simple squamous epithelium surrounded by a small amount of smooth muscle and connective tissue.

The epithelial layer of the capillaries is also very thin, and contains openings or pores where two adjacent epithelial cells overlap. These pores vary in size, depending on their location. Within the endocrine and digestive systems, the pores are very large, with increased permeability due to their larger diameter. The pores of the capillaries of the muscular system, however, are very small. Within the nervous system, the brain has capillaries with tightly packed endothelial cells, comprising a system of protection for delicate neurons called the blood–brain barrier.

Veins are composed of the same three layers as arteries, but there are differences in their relative thickness. The middle layer of the venous wall is poorly developed, with far less smooth muscle tissue. The tunica adventitia is the thickest layer of the vessel, consisting of collagen and elastic fibers, while the tunica intima is much thinner than that of the artery. The lumen of a vein, however, is larger than that of an artery (Figure 23-3).

Blood pressure within a vein is low and venous blood must work against gravity in most regions of the body on its trip back to the heart. Therefore, the veins are equipped with flaplike **valves** made of thin layers of tunica intima that close if blood begins to back up in a vein. Veins pass between groups of skeletal muscles, and when these muscles contract, blood is pushed upward in the vein toward the heart (Figure 23-4). When the skeletal muscles relax, the vein's valves prevent the blood from moving back away from the heart (Figure 23-5).

The Arterial System

The aorta, which is the largest artery in the body, begins as the ascending aorta, ascending from the left ventricle of the heart. Just beyond the aortic semilunar valve are the left and right

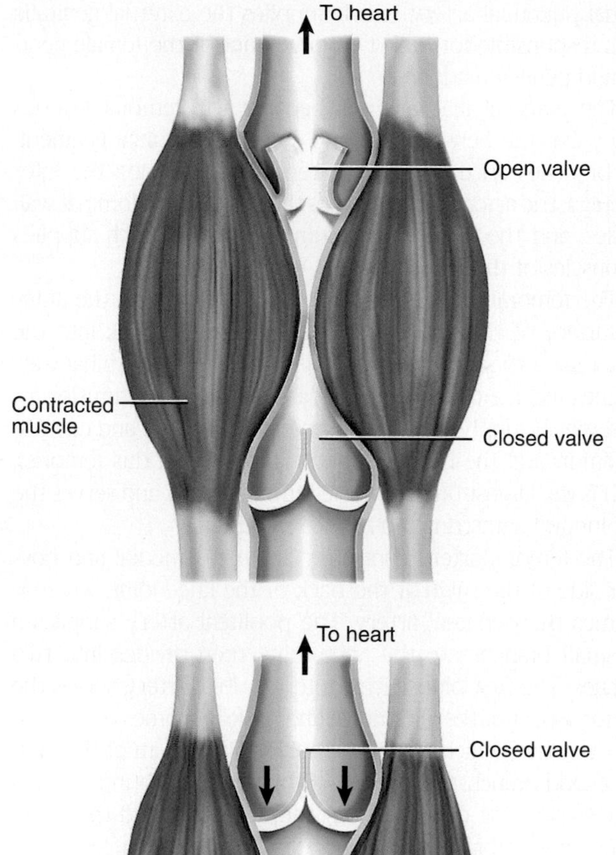

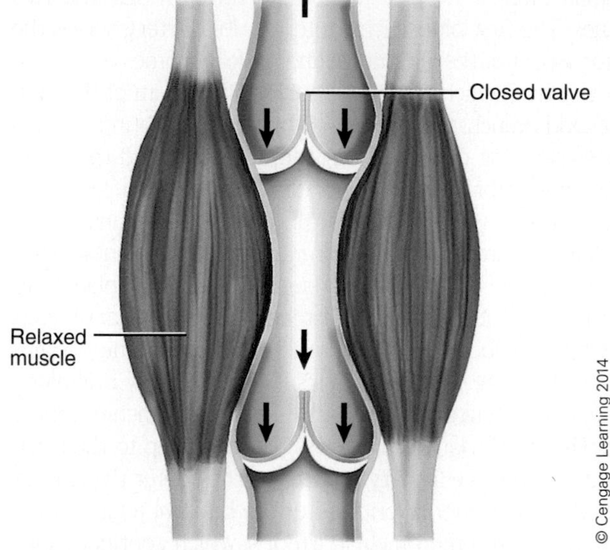

Figure 23-4 Skeletal muscle moves venous blood

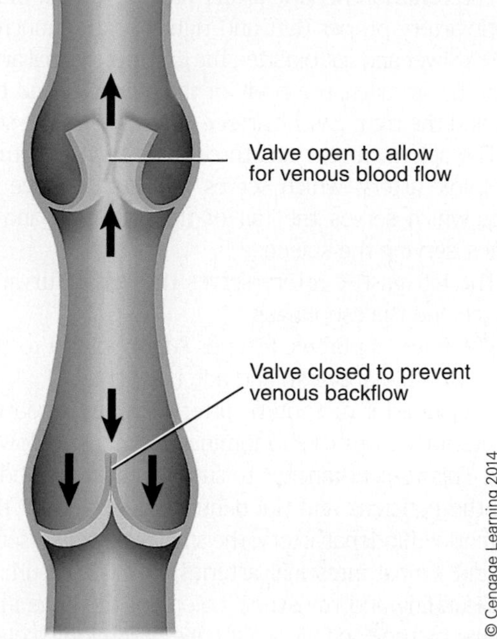

Figure 23-5 Venous valves

aortic **sinuses**, which are small dilatations of the aorta that precede the only branches of the ascending aorta, the left and right coronary arteries. The aortic sinuses contain the aortic bodies, which are specialized receptors within the epithelial lining that function to control blood pressure and oxygen and carbon dioxide concentrations.

The coronary arteries directly supply the myocardium with oxygenated blood. They lie within a groove that encircles the heart called the atrioventricular sulcus. Branches of the left coronary artery are the anterior interventricular artery (also known as the anterior descending artery), which supplies both ventricles, and the circumflex artery, which serves the left atrium and the left ventricle. Branches of the right coronary artery are the posterior interventricular artery (also known as the posterior descending artery), which supplies both ventricles, and the marginal artery, which serves the right atrium and right ventricle.

Three major arteries emerge from the aortic arch: the brachiocephalic artery (also known as the **innominate** artery), the left common carotid artery, and the left subclavian artery.

The brachiocephalic artery supplies the blood to the tissues of the arm and head, and is the first branch of the aortic arch, veering to the right. Near the junction of the sternum and the right clavicle, the brachiocephalic artery bifurcates into the right subclavian artery, which leads into the right arm, and the right common carotid artery, which serves the brain and the right side of the neck and head.

The left common carotid and the left subclavian arteries are the second and third branches of the aortic arch, and serve the same function as their counterparts on the right side. Just beyond the left subclavian artery, the aorta becomes the descending aorta. The portion of the descending aorta that lies above the diaphragm is known as the thoracic aorta, which passes downward from the 4th through 12th thoracic vertebrae; that portion below the diaphragm is known as the abdominal aorta.

Branches of the descending aorta supplying the thoracic wall are the superior **phrenic** arteries and the posterior intercostal arteries. Branches supplying the viscera of the thorax are the bronchial, pericardial, mediastinal, and esophageal arteries.

In the abdominal aorta, branches serve the abdominal wall and the abdominal viscera. The visceral branches include the celiac artery, which is a thick, short artery that immediately divides into three arteries: the left gastric, splenic, and common hepatic arteries.

The common hepatic artery has three main branches: the hepatic artery proper (left and right hepatic branches), which serve the liver and gallbladder; the gastroduodenal artery, which serves the stomach, the body of the pancreas, and the duodenum; and the right gastric artery, which serves the stomach.

The splenic artery has three main branches: the left gastroepiploic artery, which serves the stomach; the pancreatic artery, which serves the tail of the pancreas; and the polar arteries, serving the spleen.

The left gastric artery serves the lesser curvature of the stomach and the esophagus.

The inferior phrenic arteries supply blood to the inferior surface of the diaphragm and adrenal glands.

The superior mesenteric artery is an unpaired vessel arising anteriorly from the abdominal aorta, just below the celiac trunk. This vessel branches to supply numerous abdominal organs: the pancreas and duodenum are served by the inferior pancreaticoduodenal artery; the small intestine is served by the ileal and jejunal intestinal arteries; and the cecum, appendix, and ascending and transverse colons of the large intestine are supplied by the ileocolic, right colic, and middle colic arteries.

The suprarenal artery is a paired artery that serves the adrenal glands, which are also well supplied by branches of the renal and inferior phrenic arteries.

The renal arteries pass laterally from the aorta to each kidney and also serve a small portion of the adrenal glands.

In the male, the right and left gonadal arteries are referred to as the testicular arteries; they arise from the aorta and pass through the body wall by way of the inguinal canal to serve the testes. In the female, the arteries are referred to as the ovarian arteries; they arise from the aorta and pass into the pelvis to supply the ovaries.

The inferior mesenteric artery is an unpaired vessel arising anteriorly from the abdominal aorta, just above the **bifurcation** of the aorta. This vessel supplies the lower abdominal organs, including the descending and sigmoid colons of the large intestine (left colic and sigmoid arteries) and the rectum (superior rectal artery).

The lumbar arteries arise from the posterior surface of the aorta and serve the spinal cord and its meninges, as well as various muscles and skin of the lumbar region of the back.

The middle sacral artery is a small, unpaired vessel that supplies the sacrum, coccyx, and rectum.

The abdominal aorta bifurcates into the left and right common iliac arteries at the level of the fourth lumbar vertebra. These arteries divide inferiorly into two main branches: the right and left external iliac arteries, and the right and left internal iliac arteries.

The internal iliac arteries are the principal blood supply for the pelvis and perineum. Their branches include the iliolumbar and lateral sacral arteries, which serve the pelvic wall and muscles; the middle rectal artery, which serves the internal pelvic organs; the vesicular arteries (superior, inferior, and middle), which serve the urinary bladder; the superior and inferior gluteal arteries, which supply the buttocks; the obturator artery, which supplies the upper medial thigh muscles; and the internal pudendal artery, which supplies the external genitalia and is responsible for blood engorgement of the female genitalia and penile erections in men.

The external iliac arteries become the femoral arteries as they exit the pelvic cavity and cross the inguinal ligament. Two branches arise from the external iliac arteries: the inferior epigastric artery, which serves the skin and abdominal wall muscles; and the deep iliac circumflex artery, which supplies the muscles of the iliac fossa.

The femoral arteries, which pass fairly close to the anterior surface of the upper thigh, send branches back into the pelvic region to supply the genitals and lower abdominal wall. Branches include the medial and lateral femoral circumflex arteries, which supply muscles in the proximal thigh and encircle the femur; and the deep femoral artery (profundus femoris), which is the largest branch of the femoral artery and serves the hip joint and hamstring muscles of the thigh.

The femoral artery continues down the medial and posterior side of the thigh at the back of the knee joint, where it becomes the popliteal artery. The popliteal artery supplies a few small branches to the knee joint, then divides into two branches. The first branch, the anterior tibial artery, serves the anterior aspect of the leg, and, at the ankle, becomes the dorsalis pedis artery, which serves the ankle and dorsum of the foot. The second branch, the posterior tibial artery, continues down the posterior side of the leg between the knee and the ankle. The posterior tibial artery sends off a large branch called the peroneal artery, which supplies the peroneal leg muscles. At the ankle, it bifurcates into the lateral and medial plantar arteries, which supply the bottom of the foot. The lateral plantar artery joins with the dorsal pedis artery to form the plantar arch.

Arterial blood supply for the left upper extremity begins at the aortic arch, where the left subclavian artery originates. The right subclavian artery branches from the brachiocephalic artery. The subclavian arteries pass laterally deep to the clavicle, and become the axillary arteries as they enter the axillary region. As the axillary arteries enter the brachial region of the arm, they become the brachial arteries, which continue along the medial side of the humerus. The major branch of the brachial artery is the deep brachial artery, which serves the triceps muscle. At the end of the elbow, the brachial artery divides into the medial ulnar and lateral radial arteries. The largest branch of the radial artery is the radial recurrent artery, which supplies the elbow. The branches of the ulnar artery are the anterior and posterior ulnar recurrent arteries. The ulnar and radial arteries pass inferiorly to the palm, where branches fuse to form palmar arches. From these arise palmar digital arteries, which supply the fingers and thumb.

Blood for the head and neck originates from the two common carotid arteries that pass along either side of the trachea in the neck. The right common carotid originates from the brachiocephalic artery, and the left common carotid arises directly from the aortic arch. Small branches of the common carotid artery supply the larynx, thyroid gland, anterior neck muscles, and lymph glands.

The common carotid artery bifurcates into the internal and external carotid arteries at the superior border of the larynx. The external carotid artery supplies structures in the neck and head area external to the skull. The main branches include the superior thyroid artery, which serves the hyoid muscles, larynx, vocal cords, and the thyroid gland; the ascending pharyngeal artery; the lingual artery, which supplies the tongue and sublingual salivary gland; the facial artery, which supplies the palate, chin, lips, and nose; the occipital artery, which serves the posterior scalp, the meninges of the brain, and the posterior neck muscles; and the posterior auricular artery, which supplies the ear.

Near the mandibular condyle, the external carotid divides into the superficial temporal artery, which serves the parotid salivary gland; and the maxillary artery, which supplies the teeth and gums, muscles of mastication, nasal cavity, eyelids, and meninges of the brain.

The internal carotid and the vertebral arteries supply blood to the brain. The internal carotid artery enters the base of the skull through the carotid canal of the temporal bone. After arising from the subclavian arteries, the paired vertebral arteries enter the skull through the foramen magnum. Once inside the skull these two arteries unite to form the single basilar artery. The two internal carotid arteries and the basilar artery unite in a circular arrangement at the base of the brain near the sella turcica called the circle of Willis. This circle is formed by the union of the anterior cerebral arteries, which branch from the internal carotid arteries, and the posterior cerebral arteries, which branch from the basilar artery. The posterior communicating arteries connect the posterior cerebral arteries and the internal carotid arteries. The anterior cerebral arteries are connected by the anterior communicating artery (refer to Plate 15A in Appendix A).

The Venous System

The dural sinuses are blood channels that receive blood from the cerebral, ophthalmic, cerebellar, and meningeal veins of the brain. These include the superior sagittal sinus, inferior sagittal sinus, straight sinus, and basilar plexus, which are all unpaired sinuses of the brain. The paired sinuses include the cavernous, superior petrosal, inferior petrosal, occipital, transverse/lateral, and sigmoid sinuses.

The veins of the brain include the superior cerebral vein, inferior and medial veins, the great cerebral vein of Galen, and the superior and inferior ophthalmic veins. The veins that receive blood from these numerous sinuses and veins within the brain are the right and left internal jugular veins. The internal jugular veins drain the brain and the meninges, as well as the deep regions of the face and neck. These veins course downward, beneath the sternocleidomastoid muscle and alongside the common carotid artery in the neck, and eventually empty into the right and left subclavian veins. The union of the internal jugular and the subclavian veins creates the brachiocephalic, or innominate, veins. The brachiocephalic veins then merge into a single superior vena cava, which enters into the right atrium of the heart.

The right and left external jugular veins course downward laterally alongside the internal jugular vein and superficial to the sternocleidomastoid muscle. These veins drain the parotid glands and superficial structures of the face and scalp, eventually emptying into the right and left subclavian veins.

The right and left vertebral veins descend through the transverse foramina of the cervical vertebra alongside the vertebral arteries. These veins drain deep structures of the neck, including the vertebrae, and eventually empty into the subclavian veins.

The superficial tissues of the upper extremities are drained by the cephalic and basilic veins. The cephalic vein courses along the lateral side of the arm from the hand to the shoulder, eventually emptying into the axillary vein. Just beyond the axilla, the axillary vein becomes the subclavian vein.

The basilic vein passes upward along the medial side of the arm and merges with the brachial vein just below the head of the humerus to form the axillary vein. The deep tissues of the upper extremity are drained by the radial, ulnar, and brachial veins, which course upward within the same regions as their counterpart arteries. The radial veins receive blood from the dorsal metacarpal veins; the ulnar veins receive blood from the palmar venous arch; and the brachial veins join into the axillary veins.

The abdominal and thoracic walls are drained by tributaries of the brachiocephalic and azygos veins. The right and left brachiocephalic, as mentioned earlier, are formed by the union of the subclavian and internal jugular veins. The brachiocephalic vein drains the head, neck, arms, and upper thorax. The left brachiocephalic vein is the entry point for the thoracic duct of the lymphatic system. The thoracic duct enters the right brachiocephalic vein at the junction of the right internal jugular and subclavian veins. The azygos vein receives the ascending lumbar, hemiazygos, accessory azygos, and bronchial veins in the thorax, as well as certain intercostal and subcostal veins that drain the muscles of the thoracic wall. The azygos originates in the dorsal abdominal wall and courses superiorly to the right side of the vertebral column to join the superior vena cava. Blood from the abdomen and pelvis enters the inferior vena cava for return to the right atrium of the heart. The inferior vena cava, however, does not drain the veins of the spleen, pancreas, gastrointestinal tract, or gallbladder. The blood from these organs is drained into the hepatic portal vein, which is formed by the union of the superior mesenteric vein and the splenic vein. The superior mesenteric vein drains blood from the small intestine and the splenic vein drains blood from the spleen. The hepatic portal vein transports the blood to the liver. In the liver, the blood, which contains absorbed nutrients of digestion, enters capillaries called hepatic sinusoids, which filter the blood through the hepatic liver cells. This venous pathway is called the hepatic portal system.

Bacteria that are present in the portal vein are filtered by the phagocytic action of the Kupffer cells within the hepatic sinusoids. After passing through the hepatic sinusoids, blood is carried through a series of merging vessels into the hepatic veins, and eventually makes its way back to the inferior vena cava.

As the inferior vena cava ascends through the abdomen, it picks up other tributaries from the abdomen. These include the left and right renal veins from the kidney, the suprarenal veins from the adrenal glands, the inferior phrenic veins, and the gonadal veins from the ovaries or testicles.

The veins of the lower extremities are divided into two groups: the superficial group and the deep group. The deep veins of the lower extremities have the names of their corresponding arteries. The anterior and posterior tibial veins drain blood from the deep veins of the foot. At the knee, these veins unite to form the popliteal vein, which continues upward into the thigh and becomes the femoral vein, which drains blood from the deep femoral vein and lateral-medial circumflex veins in the upper thigh. As the femoral vein approaches the inguinal ligament, it receives blood from the great saphenous vein, the longest vein in the body. Near its junction with the femoral vein, the great saphenous vein receives blood from the upper thigh, groin, and lower abdominal wall.

At the level of the sacroiliac joint, the external iliac vein merges with the internal iliac vein, which carries blood away from the reproductive, urinary, and digestive organs, and becomes the common iliac vein. The left and right common iliac veins merge at the level of the fifth lumbar vertebra to form the inferior vena cava (refer to Plate 15B in Appendix A).

PERIPHERAL VASCULAR SURGERY

Peripheral vessel procedures are often performed on patients with advanced atherosclerosis that affects the extremities, abdominal and thoracic viscera, and the brain. The surgical technologist should be aware of this, and should take proper precautions during patient preparation. The surgical technologist should have a good understanding of the pathology and the anatomy and physiology involved in peripheral vascular procedures. Knowledge of any preoperative procedures that may have been used for diagnosis is essential. The outcome of each peripheral vascular procedure performed depends on the ability of OR personnel to function as a team, trusting that each member will perform with utmost skill and professionalism.

DIAGNOSTIC PROCEDURES AND TESTS

Diagnostic procedures and tests for the evaluation of peripheral vascular disease are listed below. Preoperative diagnostic tests and procedures will not be listed again within the description of surgical procedures because they are listed here and discussed in detail in Chapter 13.

- **Plethysmography** for patients with diffuse small vessel arterial disease
- Doppler probe for the measurement of blood flow to a particular artery
- Phleborheography for diagnosis of deep vein thrombosis
- Computed axial tomography, magnetic resonance imaging, and ultrasonography for the detection and evaluation of carotid artery atherosclerosis or thoracic or abdominal aortic aneurysm
- Angiography, the gold standard for the diagnosis and evaluation of vascular disease

INSTRUMENTATION, SUPPLIES, AND EQUIPMENT

The structure of blood vessels and the surgical treatment of pathological conditions are relatively similar throughout the body. Many of the features of peripheral vascular surgery are, therefore, common to most of the procedures, including instrumentation, supplies, and equipment, which are presented in the next section. The lists of instruments, supplies, and equipment will not be repeated within the description of surgical procedures, with the exception of any specialty items that are unique to a procedure.

Instrumentation

Peripheral vascular procedures require a vascular set with instruments that are the proper size and fit for the exposure and repair of the vessel to be repaired. Many ORs have vascular sets related to the size of the artery to be worked on. For example, small arteries would require a minor set for soft tissue dissection and exposure instruments, and an AV fistula set with delicate vascular forceps, clamps, and scissors. Arteries of medium size, such as the femoral or carotid arteries, may require a minor set and a carotid set. Large arteries, such as the aorta, will require a major laparotomy set and a general vascular set with larger and longer vascular instruments. Here are some examples of instrument sets used for particular procedures:

- Abdominal aortic aneurysmectomy or aortofemoral bypass: Major laparotomy set with large abdominal retractors and soft tissue instruments; vascular set with medium and large vascular instruments.
- Carotid endarterectomy: Carotid set (some health care facilities have sets specific to peripheral vascular procedures). The carotid set could also be used for procedures on medium-sized arteries, such as a femoral thrombectomy.

Table 23-1 provides a generalized list for a peripheral vascular instrument set.

Supplies

General supplies used for most vascular procedures include:

- Laparotomy back table pack
- Extremity drape
- #10, #11, #12, #15 knife blades
- Closed-wound drainage system, surgeon's preference
- Kitners
- 4 × 4 sponges

TABLE 23-1 Typical Peripheral Vascular Instrument Set

Qty	Instrument
2	#3 Knife handles
1	#3L Knife handle
1	#7 Knife handle
2	Beaver knife handles
1	Curved Mayo scissors
1	Curved long Mayo scissors
1	Straight Mayo scissors
1	Curved Metzenbaum scissors
1	Curved long Metzenbaum scissors
3–4	Potts-Smith scissors of various angles
1	Curved Stevens tenotomy scissors
4	Straight mosquito hemostats
4	Curved mosquito hemostats
6	Straight Crile hemostats
6	Curved Crile hemostats
4	Curved Pean or Kelly clamps
4	Schnidt clamps
4	Right-angle clamps
4	Long right-angle clamps
6	Towel clamps
4	Sponge forceps
4–6	Bulldog clamps of various sizes, straight and curved (Clamps may be included in a separate instrument set called the Diethrich Coronary Artery Set; Figure 23-7F)
2	DeBakey multipurpose clamps (Figure 23-6A)
2	DeBakey tangential occlusion clamps (Figure 23-7A)
2	DeBakey aortic clamps (Figure 23-7B)
2	DeBakey peripheral vascular clamps (Figure 23-7D)
2	DeBakey patent ductus clamps (Figure 23-7G)
2	Straight Cooley multipurpose clamps (Figure 23-6B)
2	Angled Cooley multipurpose/peripheral vascular clamps (Figure 23-7E)
2	Curved Cooley and/or Satinsky multipurpose clamps
2	Straight Glover clamps
2	Curved Glover clamps
2	Straight Glover coarctation clamps
2	Angled Glover coarctation clamps
2	Straight Glover patent ductus clamps
2	Angled Glover patent ductus clamps
2	Angled Lambert-Kay vascular clamp (Figure 23-7C)
2	Straight Fogarty Hydragrip Clamps
2	Angled Fogarty Hydragrip Clamps
2	Adson tissue forceps with teeth
2	Smooth Adson tissue forceps
1	Tissue forceps with teeth
1	Long tissue forceps with teeth
2	DeBakey forceps
2	Long DeBakey forceps
2	Senn retractors, sharp and blunt
2	Rake retractors, sharp and blunt
2	Cushing vein retractors
2	U.S. Army retractors
4	Richardson retractors, various sizes
4	Deaver retractors, various sizes
1	Weitlaner, sharp and blunt
4	Ryder needle holders, various lengths
2	Castroviejo needle holders, curved and straight tips
1	Malleable probe
1	Grooved director
6–10	Vascular dilators
6–10	Rubber shods of various sizes
2	Frazier suction tips
Instruments not included in instrument tray	
1	Self-retaining abdominal retractor, e.g., Balfour or surgeon's preference
4	Harrington retractors, various sizes
4–6	Hemoclip appliers, various sizes

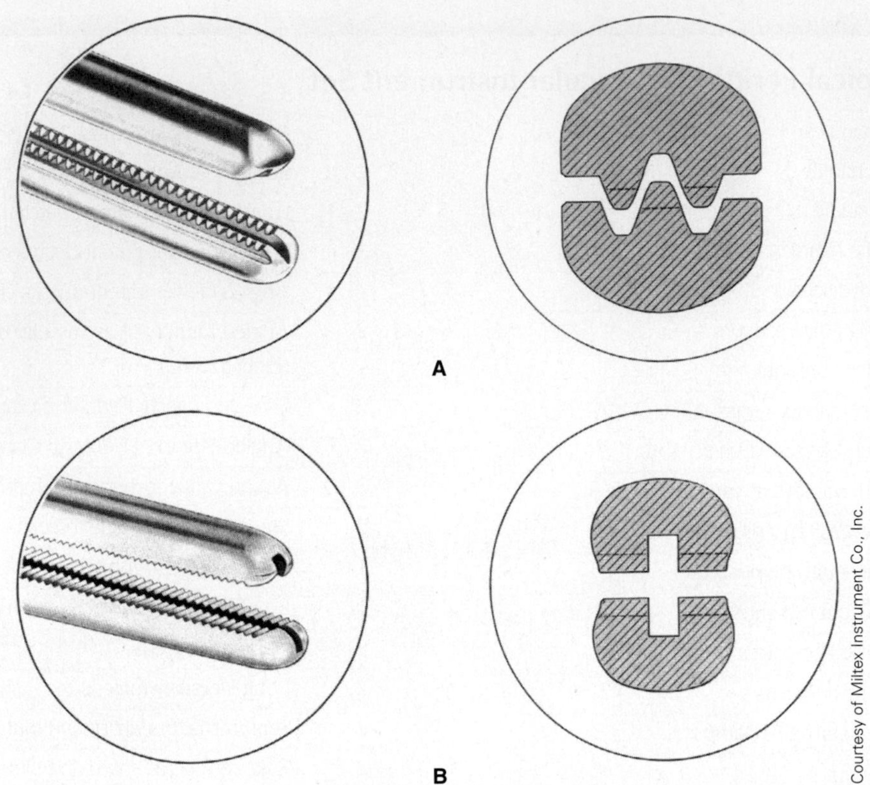

Figure 23-6 Atraumatic serrations for cardiovascular instruments: (A) DeBakey-type serration, (B) Cooley-type serration

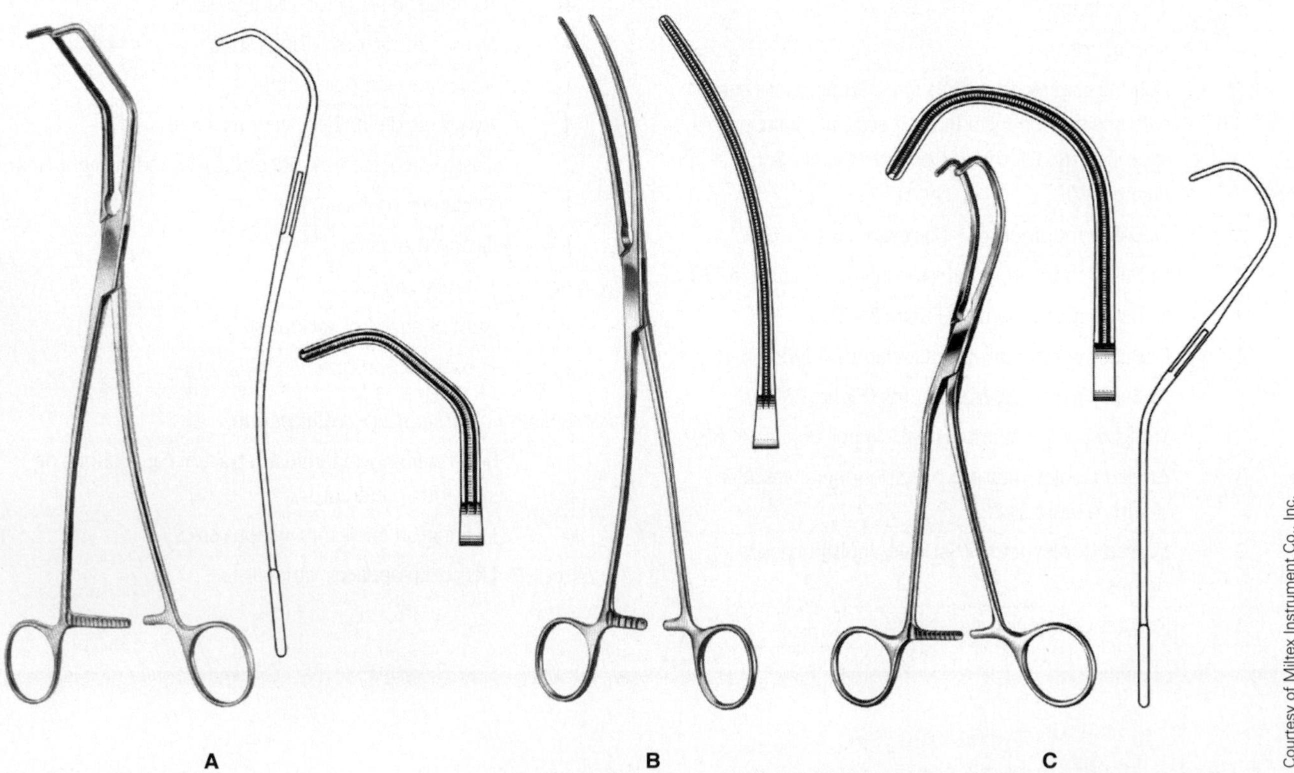

Figure 23-7 Selected peripheral vascular instruments: (A) DeBakey tangential occlusion clamp, (B) DeBakey vascular clamp for aortic aneurysm, (C) Lambert-Kay vascular clamp for aortic anastomosis

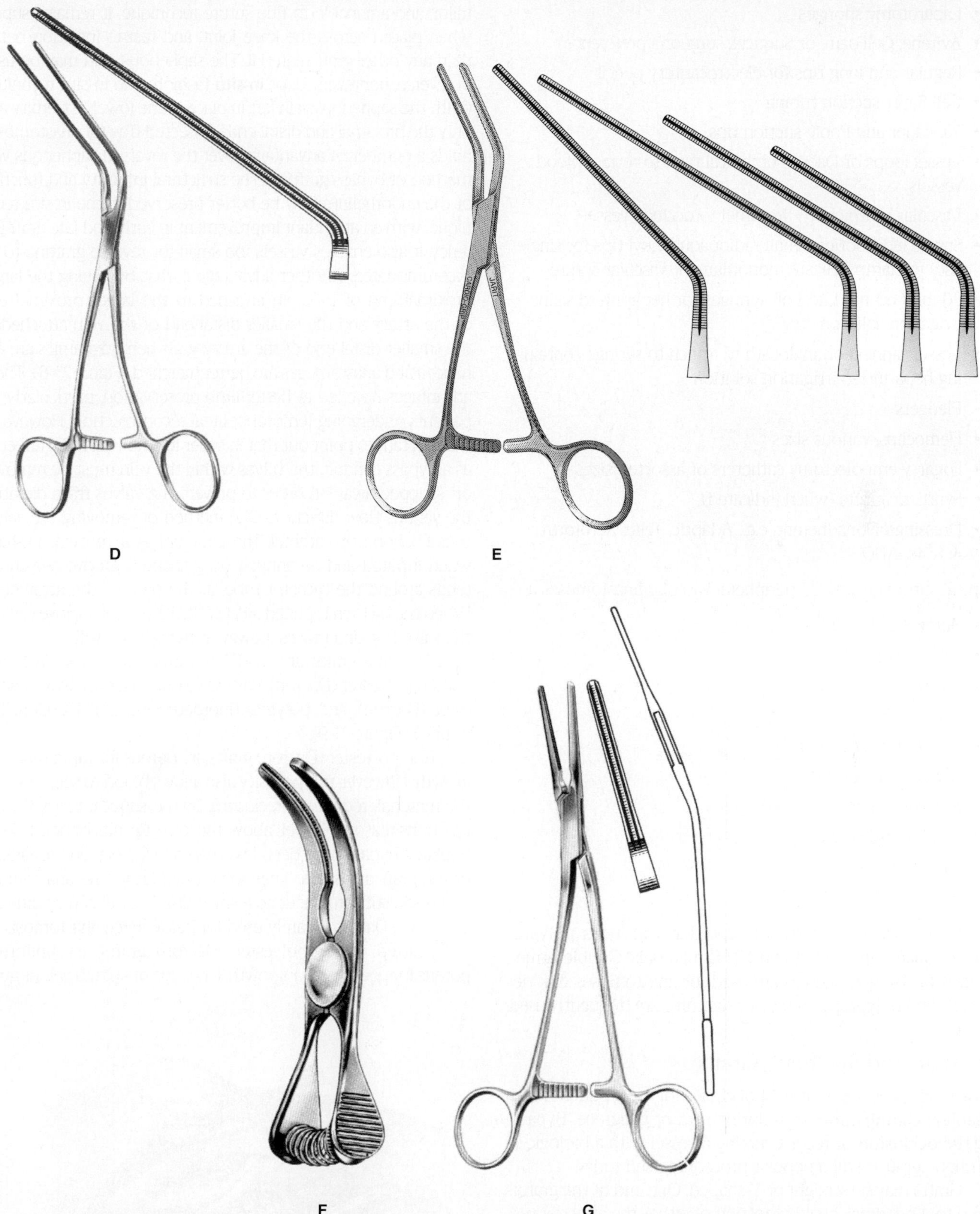

Figure 23-7 Selected peripheral vascular instruments: (D) DeBakey peripheral vascular clamp, (E) Cooley peripheral vascular clamp, (F) Glover bulldog peripheral vascular clamp, (G) DeBakey patent ductus and peripheral vascular clamp

- Laparotomy sponges
- Avitene, GelFoam, or Surgicel, surgeon's preference
- Regular and long tips for electrocautery pencil
- Cell Saver suction tubing
- Yankauer and Poole suction tips
- Vessel loops or Dacron umbilical tape to retract blood vessels
- Vascular tourniquet – Rommel to occlude vessel
- Suture aid booties (small radiopaque vinyl tips for single use) to clamp delicate monofilament vascular suture
- 30- and 60-mL LuerLok syringes for heparinized saline irrigation solution
- Vessel cannula or angiocath to attach to syringe containing heparinized irrigation solution
- Pledgets
- Hemoclips, various sizes
- Fogarty embolectomy catheters of assorted sizes
- Synthetic grafts (when indicated)
- Dressings: Nonadherent, e.g., Adaptic, Telfa, Xeroform, 4 × 4s, ABD

Typical suture gauges for peripheral vascular anastomoses are:

- *Aorta*: 3-0 or 4-0
- *Iliac*: 4-0 or 5-0
- *Femoral*: 5-0 or 6-0
- *Popliteal*: 5-0 or 6-0
- *Posterior tibial*: 6-0 or 7-0
- *Common carotid*: 6-0
- *Internal carotid*: 6-0 or 7-0
- *Brachial*: 6-0 or 7-0
- *Subclavian*: 6-0
- *Radial or ulnar*: 6-0 or 7-0

Suture for peripheral vascular procedures includes polypropylene, Dacron, polyester, and PTFE materials. Double-armed sutures on swaged needles are used for anastomoses. Silk ties and silk and polypropylene suture ligatures are frequently used.

Biologic and Synthetic Grafts

Surgery remains the treatment of choice for most patients with disabling **claudication**, pain during rest, or gangrene. Bypassing the **occlusion** or reconstructing a vessel with a biologic or synthetic graft is still a popular procedure used today.

Grafts may be straight or Y-shaped. One end of the graft is sewn to a proximal, healthy portion of either the affected vessel or another vessel altogether. The other end of the graft is sewn to the distal portion of the affected vessel, bypassing the obstruction and serving as a substitute conduit for blood flow.

Autogenous saphenous vein remains the material of choice for distal bypasses of the lower extremity. It is pliable, easy to tailor, and amenable to fine suture technique. It remains supple when placed across the knee joint, and resists infection better than any other graft material. The saphenous vein may be used in reverse, nonreversed, or **in situ** fashion. The in situ technique (with the saphenous vein left in place in the lower extremity and only the proximal and distal ends dissected free for anastomosis) holds a number of advantages over the reversed saphenous vein method of bypass grafting. The structural integrity and function of the endothelium may be better preserved in the in situ technique, with an attendant improvement in early and late graft patency. It also enables vessels too small for reverse grafting to be accommodated. Another advantage is that by having the larger proximal end of the vein attached to the larger proximal end of the artery and the smaller distal end of the vein attached to the smaller distal end of the artery, graft hemodynamics are enhanced and anastomoses are better matched (Figure 23-8). These advantages have led to better limb preservation, particularly for patients undergoing femoropopliteal reconstruction. However, it is important to point out that in order for the vein to be effective as a bypass conduit, the valves within the vein must be removed or "stripped away" in order to prevent the valves from dictating the venous flow direction. One method of removing the valves uses a balloon-tip catheter. The catheter has an arrowhead shape when inflated and an annular (ring-shaped) groove, which extends around the catheter tube, at the base of the arrowhead. When the balloon is pulled against the valves, the groove catches the valve flap and moves it away from the vein wall.

Synthetic grafts are made of various materials, including knitted polyester (Dacron), knitted velour (Dacron), woven polyester (Dacron), and polytetrafluoroethylene (PTFE) (Gore-Tex®, Impra®) (Figure 23-9).

Knit polyester (Dacron) grafts are porous for rapid tissue ingrowth. However, this porosity also allows blood to seep through the material, requiring preclotting by the surgical team. Dacron functions reasonably well above the knee. Results of below-knee popliteal bypass have been less than satisfactory due to kinking of the graft across the knee joint. In addition, the anastomosis of a thick, stiff prosthetic to a small distal vessel is very difficult. Therefore, Dacron is rarely used for below-knee anastomosis.

Knitted velour polyester (Dacron) grafts are uniformly porous for good tissue ingrowth. One type of knitted velour graft,

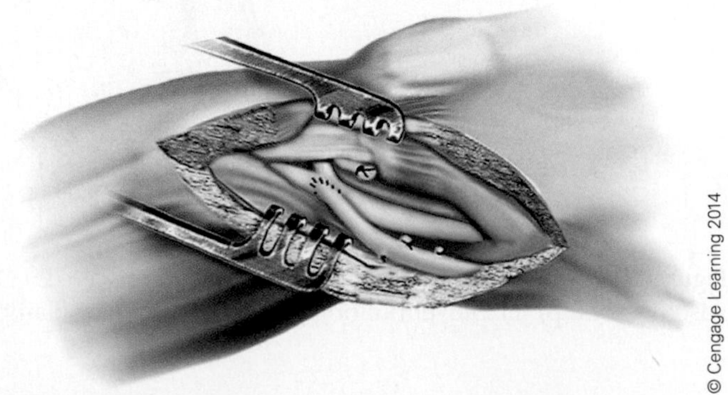

Figure 23-8 In situ saphenous vein anastomosis

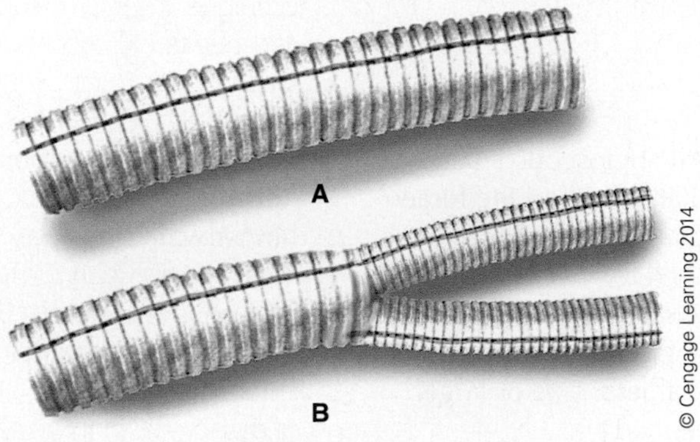

Figure 23-9 Vascular grafts: (A) Tubular, (B) bifurcated

the exoskeleton (EXS) prosthesis, has a spiral polypropylene support within the graft, and was specially designed for use across the knee joint. Another type has the antibiotic amikacin impregnated into the prosthetic wall, making the graft impervious to leaks and obviating the need for preclotting.

Woven polyester construction of the Dacron graft is leak proof and does not need to be preclotted. Because of their inflexibility, however, these grafts are relegated to larger arterial bypass grafting.

Expanded polytetrafluoroethylene can be taken across the knee joint without risk of kinking. Although effective at the popliteal level, PTFE may be less satisfactory for more distal bypasses. The microporous wall of PTFE serves as a lattice framework for tissue ingrowth, creating an ultra-thin layer for contact with blood and obviating the need for preclotting. The PTFE graft may have rigid rings built into the prosthetic wall for support.

A composite of synthetic and autogenous vein may substitute for an insufficient length of saphenous vein. These grafts retain the advantage of a distal vein–artery anastomosis, which is particularly important at the infrapopliteal level. Dacron-vein composites have been used in the past, but are liable to stenosis and false aneurysm at the intermediate anastomosis. PTFE-vein grafts appear to be less prone to this problem, and results have been superior to PTFE alone for infrapopliteal bypass.

Equipment

- ESU
- Suction system
- Doppler ultrasound unit and sterile probe
- Cell Saver
- Hypo/hyperthermia unit
- Headlamp

PERIPHERAL VASCULAR SURGICAL PROCEDURES

Peripheral vascular surgery ranges from uncomplicated endoscopic and minor procedures such as angioscopy and vein ligation to treating life-threatening conditions including abdominal aortic aneurysm. The following section will describe the commonly performed procedures that the entry-level surgical technologist should be familiar with in order to competently assist the surgeon.

Procedure 23-1 Angioscopy

Equipment, Instruments, and Supplies Unique to Procedure	• Flexible angioscope, 0.5–3.0 mm, surgeon's preference • Video camera • Light cord	• Endoscopic equipment (monitor, light source) • Vein catheter • 1000-mL bag of Ringer's saline solution	• Pneumatic pressure cuff or irrigation pump, surgeon's preference
Preoperative Preparation	• Position: Supine • Anesthesia: General • Skin prep: Depends on site of insertion of	angioscope, but the prep should still be extended in a wide margin regardless that	it is an endoscopic procedure.
Practical Considerations	• The primary challenge of performing an angioscopy is clearing the visual field of blood; if this cannot be accomplished the	surgeon will not be able to perform the procedure. Even a small volume of blood causes blurring of the visual field. Methods	of blood displacement include saline irrigation, transparent balloon inflation, and intra-arterial injection of CO_2,

(continues)

PROCEDURE 23-1 (continued)

the most commonly used being saline irrigation.

- The surgical technologist should confirm the size of the angioscope to be used with the surgeon.

An angioscope smaller in diameter than the lumen of the vessel should be used to avoid inducing vasospasm. An angioscope the same diameter size or larger than the vessel lumen pushes against the inner wall as well as irritates the wall as the scope is advanced, causing vasospasm.

Surgical Procedure

1. The vessel to be visualized is exposed through a cut-down incision.
2. The segment of vessel to be viewed is isolated by the placement of two vascular clamps, one distal and the other proximal.
3. A small arteriotomy or venotomy is made with the #11 or #15 knife blade.
4. The blood is flushed from the segment with saline irrigation.
5. The vein irrigating catheter is inserted and the Ringer's solution allowed to flow into the vessel.

   Procedural Consideration: A pneumatic pressure cuff is placed around the bag of Ringer's solution and inflated to a pressure between 200 and 300 mm Hg. However, some surgeons may use an irrigation pump that, when turned on, can provide a constant pressure of 200 mm Hg. Additionally, some angioscopes have an irrigation port to attach the irrigating tubing.
6. The angioscope is positioned centrally and inserted into the vessel. The distal vascular clamp is removed. The vein irrigating catheter is advanced parallel with the angioscope.

   Procedural Consideration: The surgical technologist may be responsible for helping the surgeon to advance the vein-irrigating catheter. When internally viewing a vein the force of the irrigation fluid helps to open the valves to facilitate advancing the angioscope.
7. Upon completion of the procedure, the angioscope is carefully withdrawn along with the irrigating catheter. The vessel incision is closed and the proximal vascular clamp removed.

   Procedural Consideration: The surgeon may use the Doppler ultrasound to confirm the reestablishment of normal blood flow within the vessel.

Postoperative Considerations

Immediate Postoperative Care

- Transport to PACU
- Depending on extent of procedure, patient may be discharged same day of surgery or kept overnight.

Prognosis

- No complications: Depending on extent of procedure, patient is expected to resume normal activities in 5–7 days. Additional procedures may be scheduled depending on the results of the angioscopy.
- Complications: Postoperative SSI; vasospasm; intimal damage from the angioscope and/or force of irrigation; dislodging of atheroma causing an embolism or thrombus

Wound Classification

- Class I: clean

PROCEDURE 23-2 Peripheral Vessel Angioplasty

Pathology	• Arteriosclerosis obliterans is a common disorder of the arteries characterized by thickening and loss of elasticity of the arterial walls. This results in a decreased blood flow to the organs that the arteries supply. A type of arteriosclerosis is atherosclerosis. • Atherosclerosis usually occurs with age and is associated with tobacco use, hypertension, obesity, diabetes mellitus, and high levels of low-density lipoprotein cholesterol. • Atherosclerosis is characterized by the formation of yellow-colored plaques of cholesterol and lipids called atheromas on the inner layers of the walls of medium-sized and large arteries. The formation of the atheroma is usually segmental. • The vessel walls become fibrotic and calcified and the lumen narrows, causing reduced blood flow to the organs the artery supplies. • The two main areas of early peripheral involvement are the aortic bifurcation and the distal superficial femoral artery. The disorder may then progress to involve other arteries. • The plaque places the patient at risk for thrombosis, coronary heart disease (CHD), angina pectoris, and myocardial infarction.
Preoperative Diagnostic Tests and Procedures	**History and physical** • Physical examination of patients reveals severely thickened, deformed nails; shiny skin; and decreased hair growth. Significant pallor of the skin during examination and, when the extremity is exercised, is an important sign.

Equipment, Instruments, and Supplies Unique to Procedure	• Angioplasty balloon catheter tray: Commercially purchased, includes the needed supplies:
	  • Arterial introducer needle
	  • Sheath introducer
	  • Guiding catheter
	  • Coronary guidewire
	  • Angioplasty balloon catheter (Figure 23-10)
	Stent
	• Stents are made out of stainless steel mesh, titanium, or polypropylene.
	• Heparin
	• Contrast dye
	• Fluoroscopy (C-arm)
	• C-arm drape

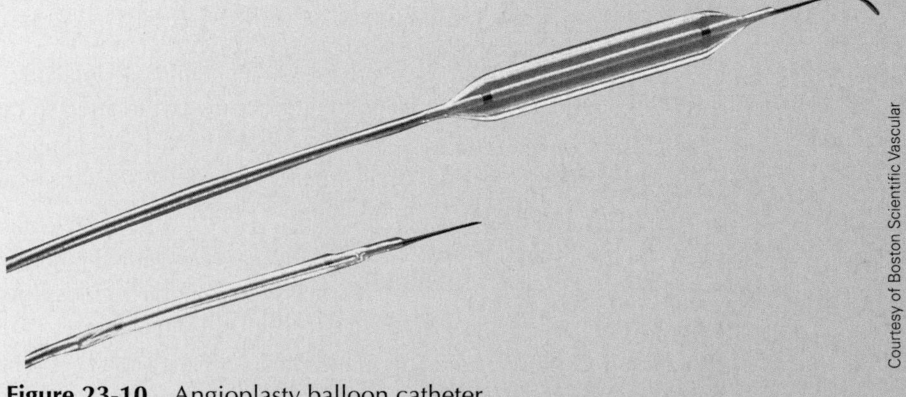

Courtesy of Boston Scientific Vascular

Figure 23-10 Angioplasty balloon catheter

(continues)

Procedure 23-2 (continued)

Preoperative Preparation

Position
- Supine

Anesthesia
- Local with MAC

Skin prep
- Inguinal groin to knee joint above and below site of catheter insertion

Draping
- Four towels to square off; three-quarters sheet

Practical Considerations

- Balloon dilation of the peripheral artery (percutaneous transluminal angioplasty) is an option for patients with symptomatic atherosclerosis.
- Initial theories of the mechanism of angioplasty advocated compression of plaque against the arterial wall as the most significant factor in reducing the narrowness of the lumen, but more recent evaluation has demonstrated that a "cracking" of the plaque with subsequent healing and growth of a new intima layer is what underlies the physiological process.
- Balloon sizing and selection are crucial elements in successful peripheral artery angioplasty.
- Selection of a balloon that is too small may result in underdilation and early stenosis. A balloon that is too large may result in dissection of the vessel. Most physicians base their balloon selection on measurements from angiographic studies that allow for magnification. Balloon length should be sufficient to extend 1–2 cm beyond the lesion (Figure 23-9).
- Angiographic studies should be in the OR for the surgeon to view. Detailed angiographic mapping is necessary before performing an angioplasty in order to locate and define the lesion.

Surgical Procedure

The following procedure describes percutaneous transluminal coronary angioplasty for treating blockage of the coronary artery.

1. Under fluoroscopic guidance, an arterial introducer needle is inserted into the femoral artery.

   Procedural Consideration: Antegrade percutaneous puncture of the femoral artery is the best approach for most peripheral stenoses. The most common approach is through the ipsilateral femoral artery, but the **contralateral** approach is occasionally used.

2. A sheath introducer is placed over the needle into the artery to keep it open and control bleeding. The needle is removed.

3. A long, flexible plastic tube called the guiding catheter is placed through the sheath introducer and the tip inserted up to the opening of the affected coronary artery.

   Procedural Consideration: The placement of the guiding catheter allows for the injection of contrast dye into the coronary artery to allow the surgeon to visualize the location and extent of the lesion under fluoroscopy.

4. With the use of fluoroscopy, the surgeon is able to estimate the diameter of the coronary artery and communicates the size of coronary guidewire and balloon catheter that will be needed to the surgical technologist.

   Procedural Consideration: The surgical technologist should also be ready to provide heparin to the surgeon for injection through the guiding catheter to prevent the formation of blood clots.

Procedure 23-2 (continued)

5. The coronary guidewire is inserted through the guiding catheter, advanced into the coronary artery and through the site of stenosis or blockage and past the lesion.

   Procedural Consideration: Passage of the guidewire through a lesion is the most crucial part of the procedure. Steps to prevent and reverse vessel spasm should be taken during the procedure; the surgical technologist should always have nitroglycerine ready for intra-arterial injection.

6. A balloon-tipped angioplasty catheter is threaded over the guidewire, carefully advanced, and positioned across the coronary artery lesion.

7. The balloon is slowly inflated to compress the atheromatous plaque against the wall of the coronary artery.

   Procedural Consideration: The surgeon will use fluoroscopy throughout the procedure.

8. An intraluminal expandable wire mesh stent may be placed within the vessel after balloon angioplasty to maintain **patency** of the vessel lumen. The Palmaz stent is delivered to the site of the lesion with the balloon angioplasty catheter. Once in position, the balloon is inflated and the stent is expanded against the arterial wall and left in place as the balloon is deflated and removed.

9. Fluoroscopy is used to confirm the repair and images are permanently recorded.

Postoperative Considerations

Immediate Postoperative Care

- Transport to PACU or CCU
- Patient closely monitored for dysrhythmias

Prognosis

- Patient is discharged same day or hospitalized overnight. Patient is expected to make a full recovery and return to normal activities in 1–2 days.
- Complications: Postoperative SSI; hematoma at the insertion point into the femoral artery, which may delay hospital discharge because the blood flow may continue into the hematoma requiring surgical repair; allergic reaction to the contrast dye; myocardial infarction; angioplasty performed soon after a myocardial infarction places the patient at an increased risk for suffering a stroke.

Wound Classification

- Class I: clean

Procedure 23-3 Insertion of Double-Lumen Groshong Venous Catheter

Pathology

- Groshong catheters are a type of central indwelling catheter that is placed to facilitate the long-term intravenous administration of chemotherapy, antibiotic therapy, intravenous (IV) fluids, and pain medications. The catheter allows for the patient to infuse IV fluids and pain medications at home.

Preoperative Diagnostic Tests and Procedures

- History and physical

(continues)

PROCEDURE 23-3 (continued)

Equipment, Instruments, and Supplies Unique to Procedure	• Groshong catheter kit, commercially purchased	• 12F Groshong catheter frequently used • Minor instrument set	• Contrast dye • Fluoroscopy (C-arm) • C-arm drape
Preoperative Preparation	• Position: Supine with slight Trendelenburg to increase the diameter of the sublcavian vein; head slightly turned to the left, away from the operative site	• Anesthesia: Local with MAC • Skin prep: Right side of neck down to mid-chest and laterally as far as possible	• Draping: Small fenestrated drape that usually comes with the catheter tray
Practical Considerations	• The primary duties of the surgical technologist during the procedure are providing the surgeon the instrumentation and	supplies in the correct order, and anticipating the next needed item. Entry has been made into the subclavian vein,	a major vein, and the surgeon wants to avoid delays in placement of the catheter.

Surgical Procedure

1. Under fluoroscopy, the surgeon selects the insertion site 1–2 cm lateral to the insection of the clavicle and first rib.

   Procedural Consideration: The right subclavian vein is used unless it has been affected by infection or thrombosis due to a previously placed catheter. In that instance, the left subclavian vein will be used. Fluoroscopy will be used throughout the procedure.

2. Using the micropuncture device, a 21-gauge introducer needle is inserted at the site into the subclavian vein. Contrast dye is injected through the needle to confirm correct insertion. Modified Seldinger Technique is a technique to obtain safe access to blood vessels using a needle, guidewire, dilator and sheath.

   Procedural Consideration: A micropuncture device allows for the placement of a 0.035-in.-diameter guidewire into a vessel later in the procedure. It also allows the use of the 21-gauge introducer needle for the initial venous puncture instead of the larger 18-gauge needle that is provided in the Groshong catheter kit. The use of the 21-gauge needle decreases the risk for pneumothorax and bleeding from an accidental puncture of the subclavian vein.

3. A 0.018-in. guidewire is inserted through the needle and advanced into the superior vena cava.

   Procedural Consideration: A challenge with inserting the guidewire is to prevent it from travelling cephalad into the jugular vein. If this occurs, the guidewire will curve upward, looking like a "J," meaning it has entered the jugular vein. The surgeon will carefully withdraw the guidewire from the jugular vein and reposition into the superior vena cava.

4. The micropuncture device is used to change from the 0.018-in. guidewire to the larger-diameter 0.035-in. guidewire. The guidewire is advanced into the right atrium or inferior vena cava.

   Procedural Consideration: The surgeon avoids placing the guidewire into the right ventricle to avoid causing dysrhythmias.

5. The peel-away sheath is inserted over the guidewire into the subclavian vein.

Procedure 23-3 (continued)

6. The Groshong catheter is advanced through the sheath, over the guidewire to the junction of the superior vena cava and right atrium. The position is confirmed with the injection of 1 mL of contrast solution and a permanent image recorded.

   Procedural Consideration: Hand the Groshong catheter to the surgeon coiled and tip first. The surgeon may need the assistance of the surgical technologist in controlling the catheter until a good length of it has been inserted.

7. The small Dacron cuff that is attached around the catheter is subcutaneously tunneled along with the catheter end and tubing. The cuff is left in the subcutaneous layer at the exit site and the rest of the tubing exteriorized.

   Procedural Consideration: The cuff helps to prevent the catheter from migrating inward or being pulled out.

8. The catheter is secured to the skin with 3-0 or 4-0 silk suture for approximately 2 weeks to allow the cuff to become imbedded in the subcutaneous tissue layer.

9. A standard chest X-ray may be taken in the OR to exclude a pneumothorax.

Postoperative Considerations

Immediate Postoperative Care

- Transport to PACU
- Discharge same day unless unexpected procedural complications have occurred

Prognosis

- No complications: Patient returns to normal activities in 2–3 days; however, due to chemotherapy and other treatments such as radiation, activities may be limited.
- Complications: Subclavian artery puncture; pneumothorax; cephalic placement of the catheter that is not observed at the time of insertion

Wound Classification

- Class I: clean

Procedure 23-4 Embolectomy or Thrombectomy

Pathology

- A sudden loss of circulation to an extremity is usually an indication of arterial embolism.
- An **embolus** can be a blood clot, fat, air, or even a small portion of a tumor that circulates through the cardiovascular system until it eventually becomes lodged in smaller vessels, at which point it is now called a **thrombus**, blocking the blood flow to an extremity or organ.
- **Morbidity** associated with embolism remains high; however, not necessarily because of the ischemic limb, but because of the underlying disease that led to the formation of the embolus.
- Emboli lodge at bifurcations or the origin of large vessel branches, at sites of anatomical narrowing, and at sites of pathological narrowing, such as an atherosclerotic

(continues)

PROCEDURE 23-4 (continued)

	superficial femoral artery. Approximately 80% of peripheral emboli affect the lower limb, with the common femoral bifurcation accounting	for approximately 50% of cases. • Emboli may originate from the left atrium in patients with atrial fibrillation or from the	left ventricle when the endocardium is damaged and the ventricle contracts poorly. Emboli may also originate from the aorta to the extremities.
Preoperative Diagnostic Tests and Procedures	• As previously listed		
Equipment, Instruments, and Supplies Unique to Procedure	• Fogarty embolectomy catheters, various sizes	• Irrigation catheters • Vessel loops	• Heparinized saline solution
Preoperative Preparation	**Position** • Supine **Anesthesia** • General	**Skin prep** • Depends on site of procedure—extremity prep is the most common	**Draping** • Depends on site of procedure—extremity drape is the most common
Practical Considerations	• The underlying source for arterial embolism must be established for proper treatment and to prevent recurrence. The first practical decision in the treatment of the patient with arterial embolism is whether the patient can tolerate angiography and general anesthesia. Treatment of recent myocardial infarction or ventricular dysrhythmia assumes priority. However, simultaneous attempts should be made to restore peripheral circulation.	• For the unstable patient, nonoperative therapy is the best option. High dosages of anticoagulants such as heparin allow the patient's own fibrinolytic system to lyse the occluding clot. More recently, enzymatic lysis of the embolus has been advocated. The enzyme (urokinase or streptokinase) is delivered through an intra-arterial catheter placed at the proximal extent of the clot. If enzyme therapy is not successful, surgery for the direct removal	of the embolus or thrombus is the next option. • For the patient with no acute complicating cardiovascular condition, evaluation should be thorough but delay in treatment should be avoided. Electrocardiogram and echocardiogram should be obtained, and enzymatic therapy during angiography should be attempted. If unsuccessful, surgery is the next option.
Surgical Procedure	1. Using a #10 knife blade, the surgeon makes an incision in the groin and cuts down to expose the femoral artery.		
	2. Vessel loops are placed around the common, deep, and superficial femoral arteries.		
	3. Vascular clamps are placed proximally on the common and deep femoral arteries. The backflow of blood within the superficial femoral artery is confirmed.		
	4. Vascular clamps are placed distally on the common and superficial femoral arteries. The clamp is removed from the deep femoral artery and backflow is confirmed.		

Procedure 23-4 (continued)

5. Using the #11 knife blade, an arteriotomy is made into the common femoral artery and extended with the 45° Potts-Smith scissors.

6. The surgeon inserts the **Fogarty embolectomy catheter** into the superficial femoral artery, advances it slightly past the thrombus, and inflates the balloon (Figure 23-11).

   Procedural Consideration: A variety of sizes of catheters should be available in the OR. The surgeon will communicate the size to the surgical technologist, who will request the circulator to open the catheter onto the sterile back table.

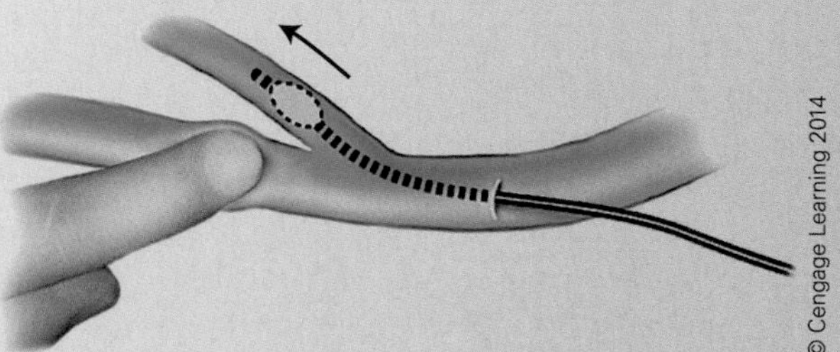

Figure 23-11 Insertion of Fogarty catheter

7. The surgeon slowly pulls the catheter backwards with the balloon inflated in order to dislodge the thrombus, and it is removed as the catheter is taken out of the artery.

8. A vascular clamp is placed on the artery because backflow is now reestablished.

   Procedural Consideration: The surgical technologist must have the vascular clamp ready to quickly hand to the surgeon when the catheter with the thrombus is removed from the artery.

9. The vascular clamp is removed from the common femoral artery and a small-diameter irrigating catheter is inserted. The heparinized saline solution is injected to irrigate the common femoral artery.

10. The surgeon may perform an angioscopy or take an arteriogram.

11. The artery is closed in continuous fashion. The wound is closed, and dressings are placed.

Postoperative Considerations

Immediate Postoperative Care

- Transport to PACU, ICU, or CCU
- Patient remains hospitalized 1–2 days

Prognosis

- No complications: Patient is expected to make a full recovery and return to normal activities in 14–21 days with blood flow to the affected extremity restored.
- Complications: Postoperative SSI; vasospasm; puncture of the artery causing hemorrhage; blood flow not completely restored, requiring additional surgery

Wound Classification

- Class I: clean

Procedure 23-5 Carotid Endarterectomy

Pathology	• The primary indication is carotid stenosis which may cause endarterectomy is transient cerebral **ischemia**. • Small pieces of plaque break away from the common carotid or internal carotid artery and are flushed upstream to lodge in small cerebral vessels, temporarily blocking blood flow to that particular area of the brain. • The warning sign of a stroke is referred to as transient ischemic attacks (TIAs). Patients suffering from TIAs often demonstrate a weakness on the opposite side of the body (plaque is located on right side of body, patient experiences the weakness on the left side of the body) that worsens over a series of TIAs. The patient may exhibit confusion and/or slurred speech that resolves within 1–2 days after a TIA.
Preoperative Diagnostic Tests and Procedures	• Transfemoral arteriography; Carotic arteriography: Performed to outline the specific location of the lesion; view intracerebral vasculature for possible occlusions. • CT scan or MRI: Performed to rule out cerebral infarction
Equipment, Instruments, and Supplies Unique to Procedure	• Shunt clamps • 20-mL syringe and heparin needle or angiocath cannula for intra-arterial irrigation • Javid or Argyle shunts, surgeon's preference
Preoperative Preparation	**Position** • Supine with arms placed at the sides; head placed on donut headrest and slightly turned toward unaffected side; scapular roll to slightly hyperextend neck. If a saphenous vein patch graft is to be taken, the affected leg should be slightly bent and externally rotated. **Anesthesia** • General • Local anesthesia/MAC **Skin prep** • Beginning at incision site on neck, extend midline of neck from lower border of ear to the level of the axilla and laterally as far as possible. If saphenous vein is to be taken, the leg is prepped starting at the incision site extending from the toes to the groin crease. **Draping** • Neck: four towels to square off incision; thyroid or transverse drape. Leg: three-quarters sheet placed under affected leg and over unaffected leg; impervious stockinette rolled over the foot and up to the groin crease; extremity drape positioned above incision; bandage scissors to cut stockinette to expose incision site.
Practical Considerations	• Have patient's imaging studies in the OR. • It is important to minimize the anesthesia time and time that the carotid artery is clamped to avoid cerebral ischemia and stroke (primary complication of carotid endarterectomy). The surgical technologist must be highly organized, including efficiency of movements, as well as know the surgeon's routine in detail in order to avoid any unnecessary intraoperative delays. • Dull Senn's and rakes should be used to avoid injury to the vessels in the neck.

PROCEDURE 23-5 (continued)

- When setting up the back table, the surgical technologist should load the vessel loops onto the tonsil clamps and place them in small basin of saline to keep them moist.
- Confirm with the blood bank on the morning of surgery that blood has been ordered and is immediately available.
- Some surgeons prefer to divert cerebral blood flow with a Javid or Argyle shunt during the procedure, whereas other surgeons believe that the shunt is unnecessary and obstructs the view of the surgery site, especially if the surgeon works quickly and cerebral functions are closely monitored. If a shunt is not used, electroencephalogram should be used to monitor the patient for signs of cerebral hypoxia.
- Confirm with the surgeon whether a shunt will be used and the size prior to opening.
- If a graft will be used, a small portion of the saphenous vein will be taken and trimmed to size.

Surgical Procedure

1. An incision is made in the anterior line of the sternocleidomastoid, over the carotid bifurcation.

   Procedural Consideration: Incision is made with a #10 blade on a #3 knife handle. Two folded sponges should be placed on opposite sides of the operative site. A magnetic mat placed over the chest is useful for procedures of the neck.

2. The common, internal, and external carotid arteries are dissected free and isolated with vessel loops.

   Procedural Consideration: Dissection is accomplished with small or medium Metzenbaum scissors and small or medium DeBakey forceps.

3. Heparin is administered systemically, and clamps are applied first to the internal carotid, then to the external carotid, and finally to the common carotid artery (Figure 23-12).

   Procedural Consideration: Angled vascular and bulldog vascular clamps are used for occlusion. The internal and external carotid arteries may be occluded with vessel loops. The anesthesia provider and circulator will record the time heparin was administered and the clamps placed on the carotid arteries.

4. An arteriotomy is made along the lateral portion of the distal common carotid artery and, with the use of Potts-Smith scissors, is extended into the internal carotid artery.

   Procedural Consideration: Arteriotomy is begun with a #11 or #12 knife blade on a #7 knife handle. Surgeon's preference determines the choice of knife blade.

5. A Javid or Argyle shunt is placed into the common carotid and internal carotid artery. The Javid shunt is held in place with Javid shunt clamps. The Argyle shunt is held in place with clamped vessel loops or tapes (Figure 23-13).

   Procedural Consideration: If the surgeon prefers to proceed without shunting, the surgical technologist should be prepared for a faster-paced procedure. The surgeon will not delay with blood flow shutoff to one side of the brain.

(*continues*)

PROCEDURE 23-5 (continued)

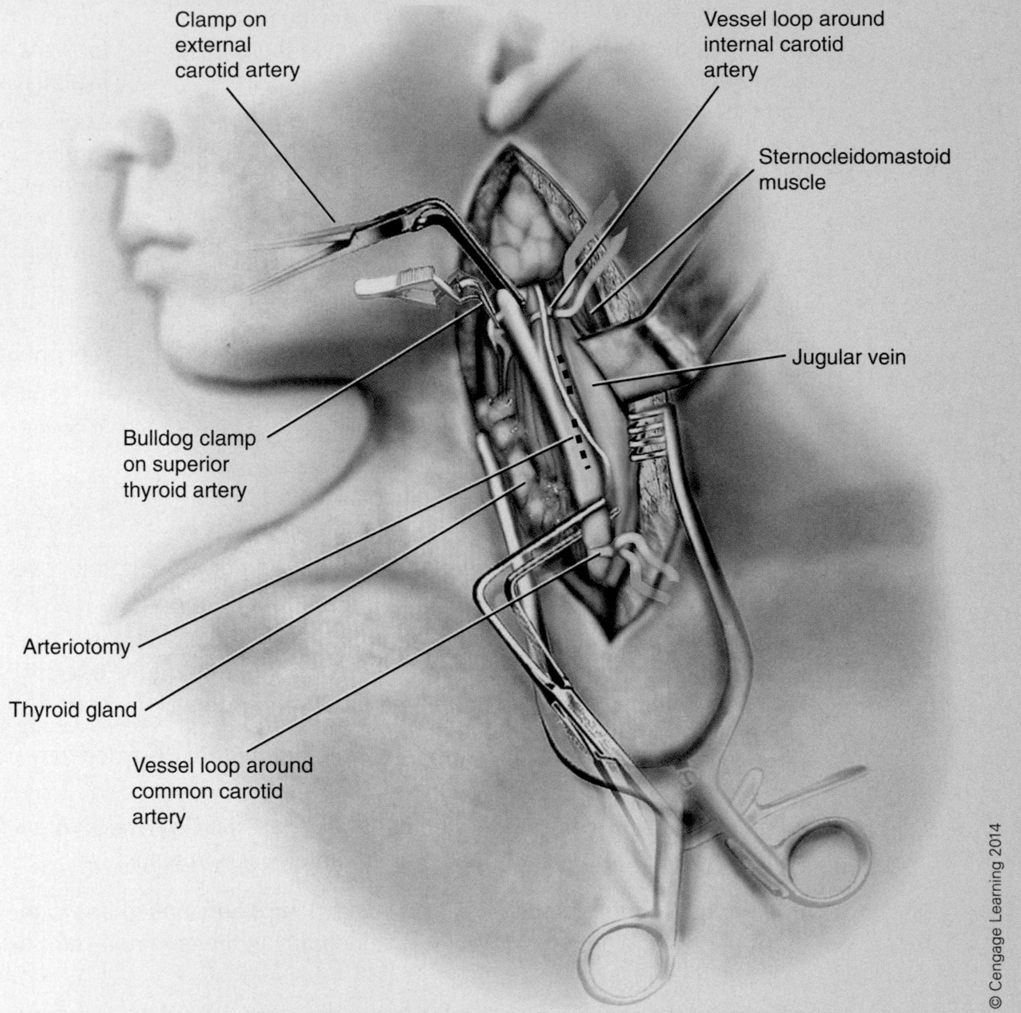

Figure 23-12 Carotid endarterectomy

6. The atheromatous core is carefully lifted from the arterial wall with a blunt dissector, beginning in the distal common carotid artery and moving into the external and internal carotid arteries.

   Procedural Consideration: The plaque is elevated with a Freer elevator or Penfield #4 dissector. Remaining pieces are removed with DeBakey forceps and mosquito clamp. Tenotomy scissors may also be used.

7. An end point is established for the plaque in the distal internal carotid artery, and the arteries are irrigated with heparinized saline to wash away any stray media or fibrin strands.

   Procedural Consideration: If a heparin needle is not available, the plastic cannula of an Angiocath needle works nicely.

PROCEDURE 23-5 (continued)

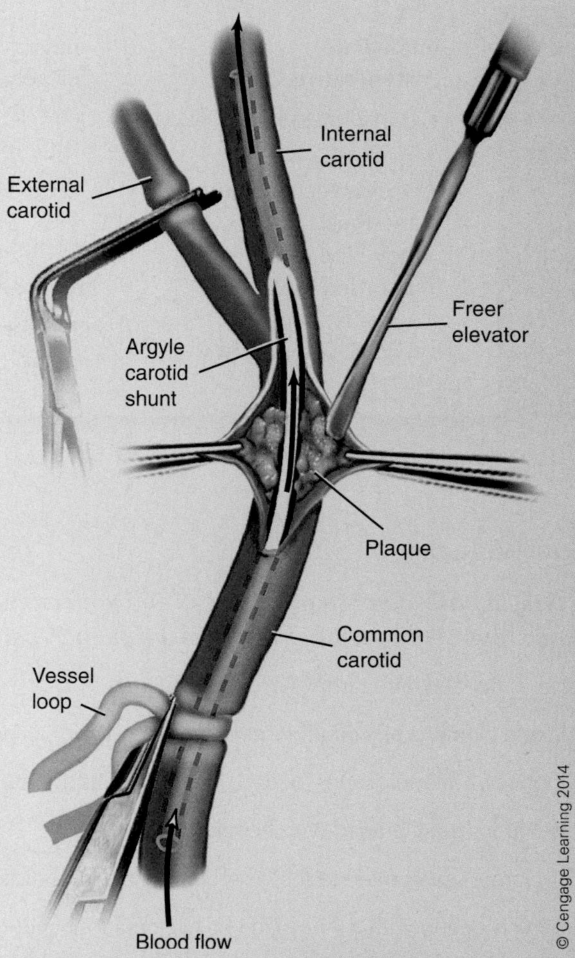

Figure 23-13 Carotid endarterectomy—clamps and shunt in place

8. The arteriotomy is closed directly with 6-0 and 7-0 Prolene sutures. (Note: An autogenous vein or synthetic patch may be utilized for closure of the arteriotomy.)

   Procedural Consideration: Note time blood flow is restored. Vein patch may be procured at this time, but it is likely that it has been secured prior to neck incision if its use is anticipated.

9. The vascular clamps are removed from the common, external, and internal carotid arteries (in that order), a drain is placed and secured, and the wound is closed.

   Procedural Consideration: The ½-in. Penrose drain is frequently used for procedures of the neck. The surgical technologist should ensure the Penrose drain is secured to prevent migration back into the wound. 4 × 4 dressings are applied; a Penrose drain requires additional 4 × 4s for fluid absorption.

(continues)

Procedure 23-5 (continued)

Postoperative Considerations

Immediate Postoperative Care

- Transport to PACU, ICU, or CCU
- During recovery from anesthesia, ability to move the extremities is recorded in the postoperative patient's record. The patient's neurological signs are closely monitored for postoperative changes.
- Patient will be hospitalized for 3–5 days, possibly more if complications occur.

Prognosis

- No complications: If neurological signs are intact, the prognosis is good. Patient will return to normal activities in several weeks.
- Complications: Postoperative SSI; stroke; hemorrhage

Wound Classification

- Class I: clean

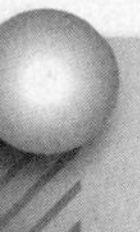

Pearl of Wisdom

There is a typical procedural sequence to all endarterectomies after vessel exposure is achieved. The sequence represents a pattern that appears often in peripheral vascular surgery. It is as follows:

1. The vessel is dissected free from surrounding tissues.
2. A right-angle clamp is placed underneath the vessel and opened.
3. Vessel loops or umbilical tapes loaded onto hemostats are fed into the right-angle clamp proximally and distally.
4. The vessel loops are clamped with hemostats.
5. Vascular clamps are applied to the vessel proximally and distally.
6. Arteriotomy is begun with a #11 blade or #12 on a #7 handle and extended with Potts-Smith scissors.

Procedure 23-6 Abdominal Aortic Aneurysm with Graft

Pathology

- The majority of patients with abdominal aortic aneurysm (AAA) are diagnosed while the patient is still asymptomatic.
- AAAs are generally fusiform.
- The majority occur below the origin of the renal arteries and terminate at the bifurcation of the aorta or common iliac arteries. Rarely one or both renal arteries may arise from an AAA without involving the superior mesenteric artery or extend beyond the bifurcation of the common iliac arteries into the external or internal iliac arteries (Figure 23-7).
- Aneurysms may also occur in the smaller peripheral arteries. Atherosclerotic aneurysms of the femoral and popliteal arteries are likely to shed emboli and finally thrombose rather than rupture. The patient typically complains of foot or calf pain. Examination reveals a pulsating mass in the groin or behind the knee and irregular red-blue patches of skin on the foot. Continued embolization and loss

PROCEDURE 23-6 (continued)

	of the extremity are inevitable in the untreated patient. • Iliac artery aneurysm rupture is more likely than aneurysms of the popliteal and femoral arteries. These aneurysms are generally not detected on physical examination or routine X-rays, and so they progress until they rupture. • Severe abdominal and back pain with a	pulsatile abdominal mass signifies aneurysm rupture. The aneurysm may rupture into the peritoneal cavity with rapid exsanguination, but it more commonly ruptures into the retroperitoneal space, where it is briefly contained before fatal hemorrhage occurs. • Hypertension increases the likelihood of rupture	for any given size of aneurysm. Operative **mortality** is very low (2%–3%) for the elective procedure, but once rupture has occurred, operative mortality rises steeply and may exceed 80% for the patient in shock. Therefore, elective surgical correction is highly advisable.
Preoperative Diagnostic Tests and Procedures	• CT scan is useful in the diagnosis of abdominal aortic aneurysm. It can provide information about the extent of the aneurysm, the location of thromboembolytic material, and whether leakage has occurred. • Ultrasound is also useful for initial detection but cannot provide much more information. Once the aneurysm is detected, the patient should	undergo aortic angiography so that surgery may be planned in detail. • An aortogram can reveal important factors such as renal artery involvement, renal artery stenosis, visceral arterial disease, and additional occlusive or aneurysmal disease in the internal iliac and runoff vessels. Intimal degeneration in the juxtarenal aorta that	would preclude safe infrarenal clamping may also be revealed by aortogram. • The patient with an abdominal aortic aneurysm should be assessed for coronary artery disease before undergoing aneurysmal repair because atherosclerosis of the coronary arteries is a major determinant of mortality after arterial reconstruction.
Equipment, Instruments, and Supplies Unique to Procedure	• Peripheral vascular instrument set (see Table 23-1) • Aortic compressor (have available) • Suction system × 2 • Antibiotic irrigation • Heparinized saline solution	• Protamine sulfate (neutralize heparin) • Contrast medium • Fogarty embolectomy catheters, various sizes • PTFE or Dacron polyester tube grafts • Butterfly needle with extension tubing	• Angiocath cannula for intra-arterial irrigation • Headlight • ½- and 1-in. Penrose drains
Preoperative Preparation	**Position** • Supine **Anesthesia** • General	**Skin prep** • Mid-chest to mid-thigh; bilaterally as far as possible **Draping** • Folded towel over genitalia; four towels	to square off incision—towels are placed wide—lateral towels in line with nipples, folded edge of superior towel placed

(continues)

Procedure 23-6 (continued)

	right below nipple line, folded edge of posterior towel placed along line of	symphysis pubis; adhesive incise drape (emergency procedure may not have time to	place); laparotomy drape (bandage scissors used to extend fenestration)
Practical Considerations	• For grafting, the Y-shaped, bifurcated Dacron material is used if the common iliac arteries are involved; if not, a straight Dacron graft is used. • If the patient is asymptomatic for aneurysmal disease but has symptomatic coronary artery disease, coronary artery bypass grafting or percutaneous transluminal coronary angioplasty should be attempted before the aneurysm repair. If the patient is symptomatic for both diseases, simultaneous repair for both the aneurysm and the coronary stenoses is advisable. • Patient's imaging studies should be in the OR.	• Confirm with the surgeon the type and size of graft. The surgical technologist should prepare the graft according to the manufacturer's and surgeon's instructions. • Pedal pulses should be marked using a marking pen prior to performing the skin prep to aid the circulator in quickly finding the pulses intraoperatively. • Confirm with blood bank on the morning of surgery that blood has been ordered and is immediately available. • The surgical technologist must be highly organized, including efficiency of movements, as well as know the surgeon's routine in detail in order to avoid any	unnecessary intraoperative delays, in particular during an emergency AAA. • When setting up the sterile back table, the surgical technologist should preload several vessel loops on long tonsil clamps and place them in a small basin of saline to keep them moistened. • The surgical technologist should keep the Mayo stand and back table setup sterile until the patient has left the OR. • If the aneurysm has ruptured, control of hemorrhage is the first consideration. The surgical technologist should set up two suction tubes and Yankauer tips and have several laparotomy sponges.
Surgical Procedure	1. An incision is made from the xiphoid to the pubis, and the aorta is exposed. **Procedural Consideration:** The surgical technologist should prepare a large self-retaining retractor (Balfour or Bookwalter) for the abdominal wall and large Deaver and Harrington retractors for the bowel.		
	2. The inferior mesenteric artery is isolated at the left border of the aneurysm with a vessel loop. The peritoneal incision is extended to the area over the common iliac arteries.		
	3. The external and internal iliac arteries are cleared for eventual vascular clamp placement. However, if the common iliac artery is aneurysmal, only the external iliac artery is mobilized. Often only one vascular clamp is applied to the distal portion of the common iliac artery bilaterally. **Procedural Consideration:** Atraumatic Potts vascular or angled DeBakey clamps are frequently used to occlude the iliac artery.		

PROCEDURE 23-6 (continued)

4. The aorta is mobilized proximal to the aneurysm up to the level of the renal arteries and cleared for eventual placement of a vascular clamp.

   Procedural Consideration: A large right angle may be useful to mobilize the aorta.

5. A bifurcated knitted Dacron graft is selected after sizing, and blood is drawn from the vena cava for preclotting. (If a PTFE or woven polyester is used as graft material, preclotting is not necessary.)

   Procedural Consideration: A 20-mL plastic syringe with a 20- to 23-gauge hypodermic needle is used to draw venous blood for preclotting. The surgical technologist should have the graft in a metal bowl for saturation with blood.

6. The patient is given intravenous heparin, and vascular clamps are applied to the external and internal iliac arteries bilaterally (or to the common iliac arteries).

   Procedural Consideration: Note the time that the heparin is administered and the time of placement of proximal and distal vascular clamps.

7. An aortic vascular clamp is carefully applied to the aorta above the aneurysm (Figure 23-14).

   Procedural Consideration: The surgical technologist should ensure that all anastomosis sutures are loaded and ready.

8. The aneurysm is opened longitudinally along the anterolateral wall and stopped just short of the aortic bifurcation. Thrombus material is removed from the interior of the aorta, and lumbar vessels are oversewn with non-absorbable synthetic suture of surgeon's preference from within the aneurysm sac (Figure 23-15).

   Procedural Consideration: The aneurysm is opened with #11 blade on #7 knife handle and completed with Mayo scissors. Thrombus material should be saved for specimen.

9. A T-shaped extension is cut into the proximal border of the aneurysm, and the anterior aneurysm wall is opened for copious irrigation with heparinized saline.

   Procedural Consideration: The jet action of the 20-mL syringe/heparin needle combination with heparinized saline forces small pieces of thrombus from the aortic wall.

10. The proximal anastomosis is begun with a continuous, double-armed 4-0 Prolene suture and taper-cut needle.

    Procedural Consideration: The 4-0 Prolene should be loaded onto a long, vascular needle holder with a narrow diamond jaw.

11. A Fogarty clamp is placed across the graft immediately distal to the anastomosis, the aortic vascular clamp is released, and the two ends of the Prolene suture are tied together, completing the anastomosis.

    Procedural Consideration: Any leaks in the proximal anastomosis are patched with interrupted, pledgeted Prolene sutures. Most patch sutures are single-armed, so the surgeon may ask the surgical technologist to cut a double-armed Prolene suture in half.

12. The right limb of the graft is aspirated, brought down to the common iliac bifurcation, and cut to the correct length.

    Procedural Consideration: Prepare to cut the graft to the appropriate size. An additional vascular clamp may be placed on the distal graft.

13. An arteriotomy is performed on the right common iliac vessel, and the graft limb is anastomosed in an end-to-side fashion with a double-armed 5-0 or 6-0 Prolene.

    Procedural Consideration: Do not try to remove knots from Prolene sutures. If a knot is found while loading the suture, simply discard the knotted Prolene and load another.

(continues)

PROCEDURE 23-6 (continued)

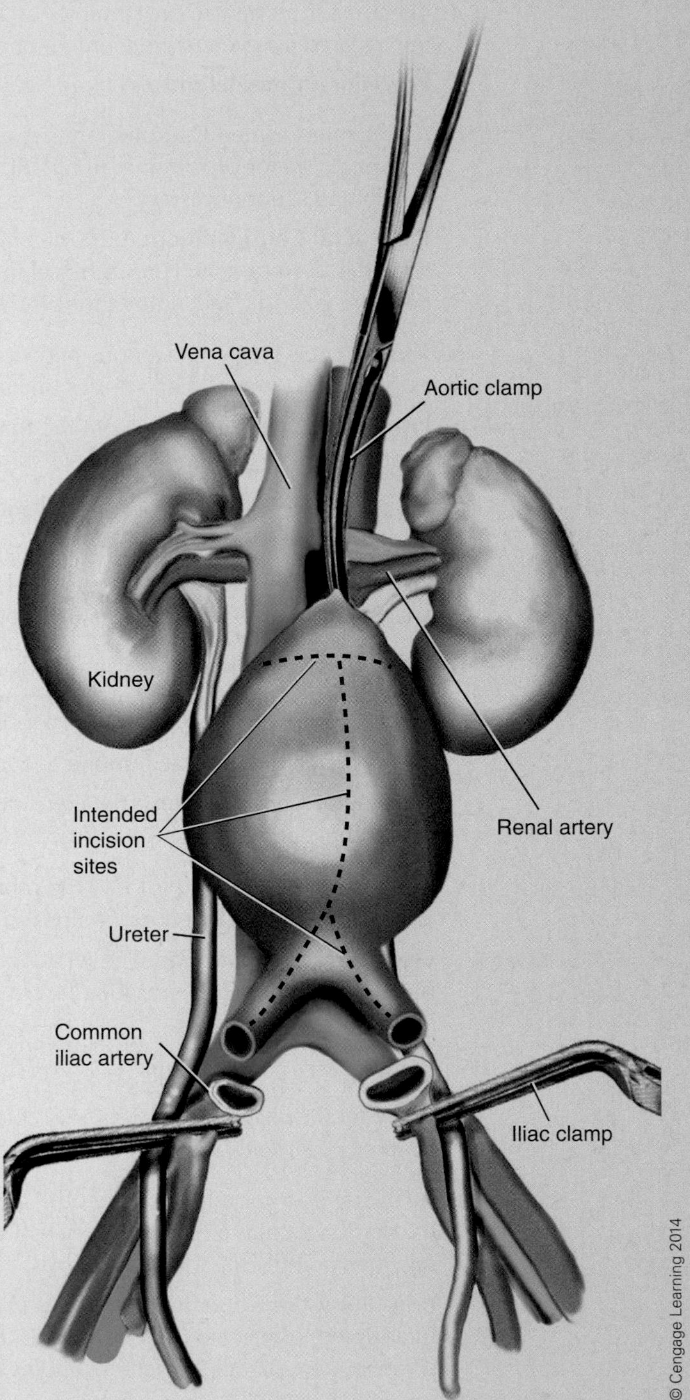

Figure 23-14 Abdominal aortic aneurysm

14. Before completion of the iliac anastomosis, the distal and proximal clamps are opened for flushing. The suture ends are tied, and circulation is opened (Figure 23-16).

    Procedural Consideration: Wet the hands of the surgeon with saline before the tying of polypropylene sutures. Note time blood flow is restored to limb. Patch sutures may be needed.

PROCEDURE 23-6 (continued)

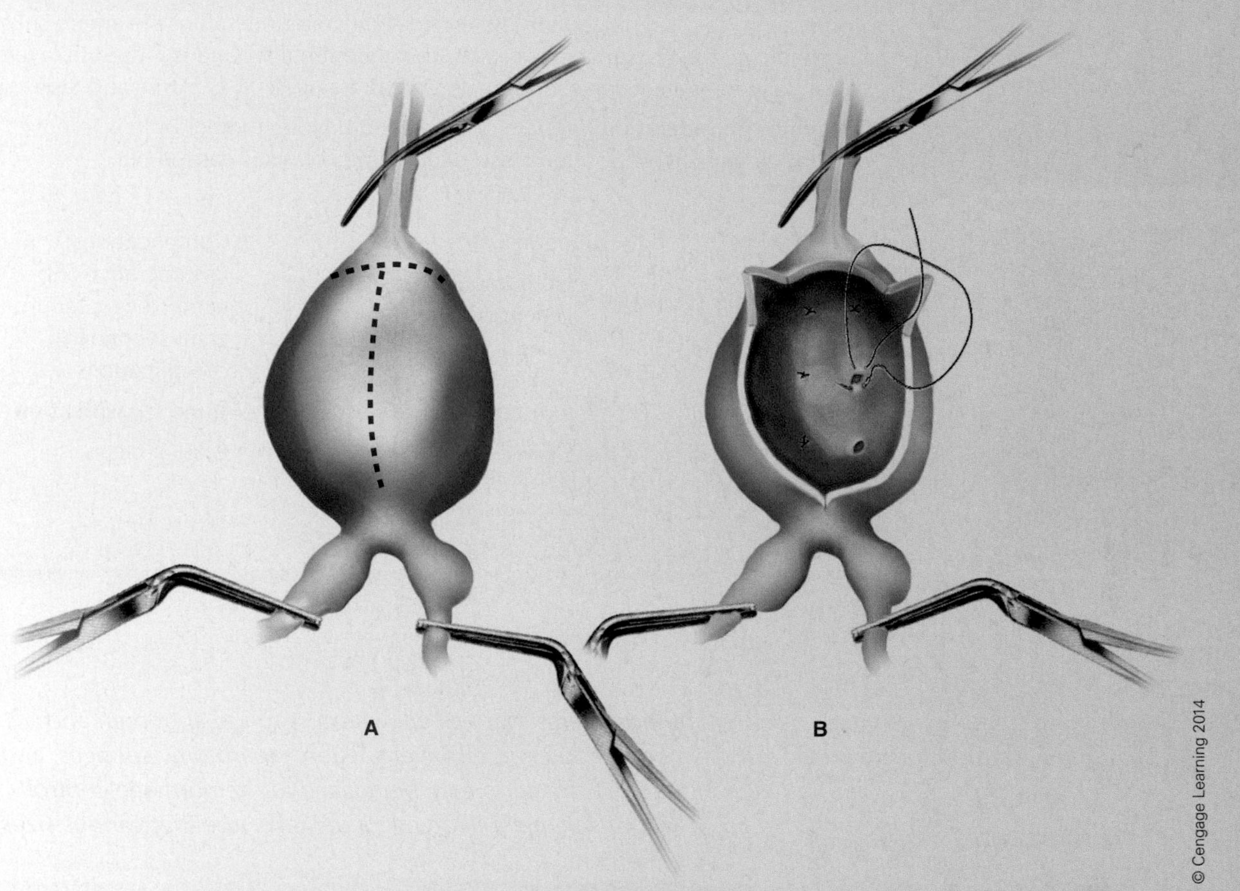

Figure 23-15 Aortic aneurysm: (A) Planned incision sites, (B) lumbar vessels oversewn

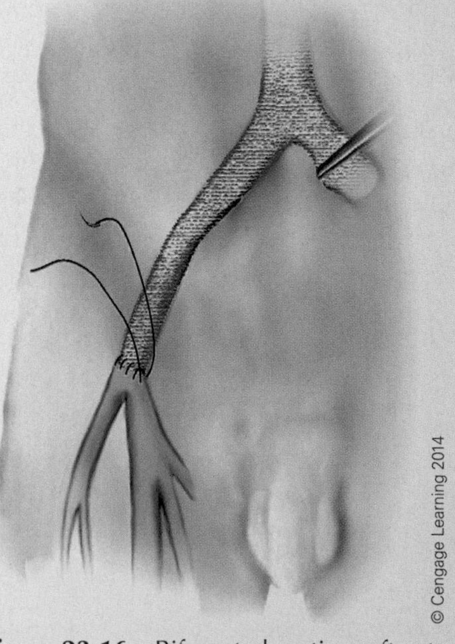

Figure 23-16 Bifurcated aortic graft sutured in place

(*continues*)

Procedure 23-6 (continued)

15. The same process is repeated for the left side. The anterior wall of the aneurysm sac is sutured over the proximal aortic graft. The abdominal wound is closed in layers. A three-layer dressing is placed: nonadherent dressing, 4 × 4s, ABD, and tape.

    Procedural Consideration: Prepare closure suture. Note number of laps removed from abdominal cavity. Routine closure including counts is carried out.

Postoperative Considerations

Immediate Postoperative Care

- Transport to PACU, ICU, or CCU
- Patient will remain hospitalized for several days until stable and able to walk without assistance.

Prognosis

- No complications: Patient is expected to make a full recovery with adjustments made to normal activities. Long-term prognosis may vary depending on secondary effects.
- Complications: Postoperative SSI; hemorrhage; failure of graft; secondary complications

Wound Classification

- Class I: clean

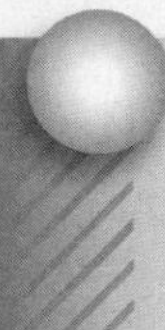

Pearl of Wisdom

For ruptured abdominal aneurysms, prepare those items that will allow access to the abdomen and exposure of the ruptured vessel first. Have a knife, cautery, Cell Saver suction, laparotomy sponges, and retractors ready to go. A Foley catheter with a 30-mL balloon may be utilized for hemorrhage control. A large aortic cross-clamp, such as a Fogarty aortic clamp, will be needed. Make sure that various sizes of grafts are available for inspection.

Procedure 23-7 Aortofemoral Bypass

Pathology

- Arterial obstructions due to atherosclerosis occur most frequently in the aortoiliac segment of the arterial system causing claudication. Results of arterial bypass in this region are good because of its high flow rate and large-diameter vessels.

Preoperative diagnostic tests; equipment, instruments, and supplies the same as for AAA plus add tunneling device of surgeon's preference, e.g., Sarot clamp, uterine dressing forceps, or specialty CV tunneler.

PROCEDURE 23-7 (continued)

Preoperative Preparation	**Position** • Supine **Anesthesia** • General **Skin prep** • Mid-chest to toes on both legs; bilaterally as far as possible and entire legs **Draping** • Genitalia are covered with a folded towel; four towels to square off abdomen and inguinal region; adhesive incise drape placed; laparotomy drape–bandage scissors used to extend fenestration over the femoral arteries
Practical Considerations	• Imaging studies should be in the OR. • Confirm with surgeon the type and size of graft. • Confirm if the surgeon wants to perform an intraoperative angiography and notify the radiology department. Verify the type of catheters, syringes, and contrast medium the surgeon prefers. • Contact the blood bank to confirm blood has been ordered and is immediately available. • The surgical technologist should keep the Mayo stand and back table setup sterile until the patient has left the OR.
Surgical Procedure	1. With the patient in the supine position, incisions are made in each groin lateral to the vascular axis with dissection of the profunda femoris down to the first perforating branch or beyond. **Procedural Consideration:** Dissection is accomplished using medium Metzenbaum scissors and tissue forceps. The surgical technologist should have Weitlaner retractors ready for placement.
	2. The inguinal ligament is partially excised at the upper limit of the incision for unlimited passage of the Dacron graft from the abdomen. The deep circumflex iliac vein is divided to make way for eventual tunneling. **Procedural Consideration:** Dissection will continue with the electrocautery and sharp and blunt techniques. Suction may be used intermittently.
	3. The abdomen is opened from the xiphoid to the pubis, and the transverse colon and omentum are reflected superiorly. The small bowel is displaced over the right-hand wound margin and covered with warm moist packs. **Procedural Consideration:** Incision is made with #10 knife blade. The surgical technologist should have bowel bag or warm moist packs completely wrung and ready for coverage of small bowel.
	4. The posterior peritoneum is incised and extended toward the aortic bifurcation. **Procedural Consideration:** The surgical technologist should be prepared for sudden hemorrhage.
	5. The portion of the aorta just below the renal arteries is isolated and cleared, and the left renal vein is mobilized. **Procedural Consideration:** The 18-in. silk ties of 3-0 or 4-0 gauge are good for ligating small superficial vessels. For ligation of larger, deeper vessels, 2-0 or 3-0 silk ties of 30-in. length on carriers are necessary. Typical carriers are Schnidt tonsil clamps or Sarot clamps for deeper ligation.

(*continues*)

Procedure 23-7 (continued)

6. A retroperitoneal tunnel is developed with a tunneling device or long clamp lateral to the vascular axis and behind the ureter.

   Procedural Consideration: A device for tunneling may be a Sarot clamp, uterine dressing forceps, or a specialty CV tunneler with a bullet tip that the graft end can be tied onto with heavy silk ties and pulled through the tunnel. If a clamp is used to create the tunnel, it can also be used to grasp the graft end and pull it through.

7. Blood is drawn from the vena cava, and a knitted Dacron graft is selected and preclotted.

   Procedural Consideration: Have various graft sizes available (but unopened) for the surgeon to choose. (Note: PTFE grafts do not require preclotting.)

8. The patient is heparinized systemically, and a large vascular clamp is applied to the aorta just below the left renal vein. A 2–3-cm section of aorta is excised and the distal aortic stump is oversewn.

   Procedural Consideration: Make sure the vascular clamps chosen are the proper size and angle for the vessel being repaired or bypassed. The aorta is typically occluded with a large Fogarty or DeBakey aortic clamp.

9. The proximal stump of the aorta is prepared for anastomosis, and the Dacron graft is sewn to the aorta in an end-to-end fashion with a continuous 4-0 Prolene suture.

   Procedural Consideration: If the aorta is friable, Teflon-coated **pledgets** may be used with the suture to reinforce the anastomosis, preventing the suture from tearing the tissue. The pledget is loaded by carefully folding the pledget in half with one hand, and placing the needle (loaded on a needle holder) through the top half of the fold (Figure 23-17).

10. A vascular clamp is applied to the common femoral artery. (*Note:* If the anastomosis site is further distal, clamps are applied to the superficial and deep femoral vessels.)

    Procedural Consideration: Angled vascular or Potts vascular clamps are frequently used for femoral artery occlusion. The superficial and deep femoral vessels are frequently occluded with bulldog vascular clamps.

11. An incision is made into the common femoral artery, and the graft is cut to the correct length and its end beveled.

    Procedural Consideration: Arteriotomy is begun with a #11 blade on a #7 knife handle. It is completed with 45° Potts-Smith scissors. The Dacron graft is cut with straight Mayo scissors. A PTFE should be cut with a fresh #15 knife blade.

12. The graft limb is anastomosed to the femoral artery using a continuous, double-armed 5-0 or 6-0 Prolene suture. Just before the completion of anastomosis, the proximal and distal clamps are released to flush the graft, and the femoral suture line is flushed with heparinized saline.

    Procedural Consideration: The surgical technologist should be familiar with the art of "running" polypropylene suture. A small basin may be useful to contain blood when the graft is flushed to remove clotted blood and air. Heparin solution is prepared in advance of need.

Procedure 23-7 (continued)

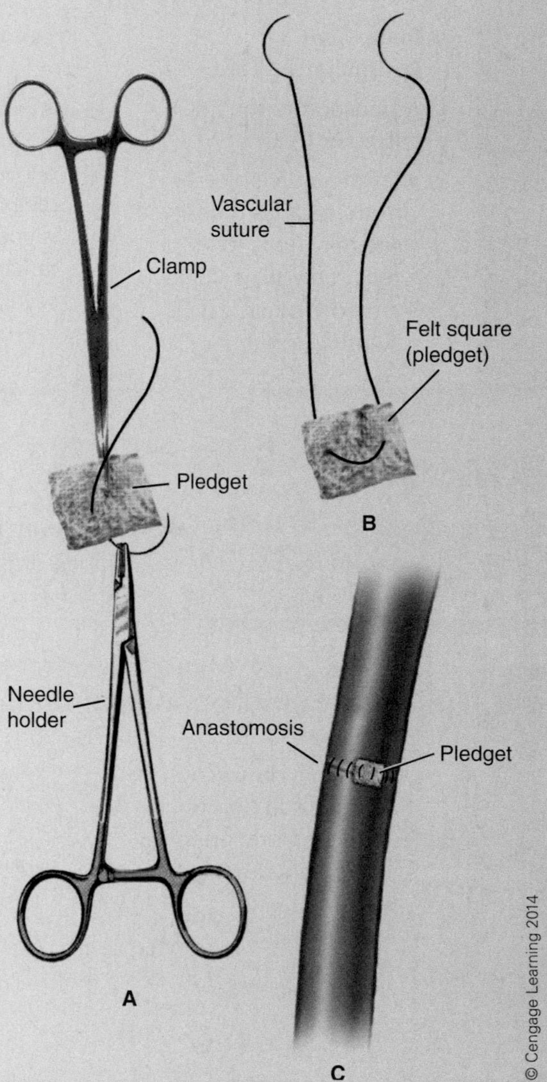

Figure 23-17 Pledget preparation and use: (A) Loading the pledget, (B) pledget ready for use, (C) pledgeted suture incorporated in the anastomosis

13. The suture line is completed for the right side, and the same process is repeated for the left. The posterior peritoneum and preaortic fascia are closed over the graft, and the abdomen and groins are closed in layers. A three-layer dressing is placed for each incision: nonadherent dressing, 4 × 4s, ABD, and tape.

    Procedural Consideration: Be prepared for an intraoperative arteriogram. Supplies needed are arterial needle (or butterfly needle), 20-mL syringe, X-ray cassette or C-arm drape, injecttable saline, and contrast solution. Make sure that bubbles are completely removed from the syringe and tubing. Glass syringes are preferred over plastic for intra-arterial injection because they do not retain air bubbles as much as plastic. Three incisions are used. Doppler ultrasound may be used to assess the blood flow. Be sure the appropriate number of counts is completed.

(*continues*)

Procedure 23-7 (continued)

Postoperative Considerations	**Immediate Postoperative Care** • Transport to the PACU, ICU, or CCU • Postoperative bleeding from the anastomosis site may need to be repaired with a single-armed Prolene patch suture.	**Prognosis** • No complications: If arterial flow is reinstated before tissue damage has become too severe, then the prognosis for recovery is good. The patient will remain hospitalized for several days until stable and walking without	assistance. Anticoagulants are necessary to prevent clot formation postoperatively. • Complications: Postoperative SSI; failure of graft; rejection of graft material **Wound Classification** • Class I: Clean

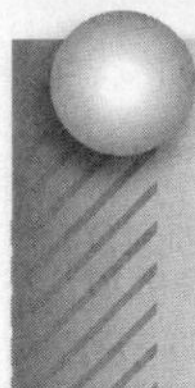

Pearl of Wisdom

The surgical technologist should have a variety of atraumatic vascular clamps available for aortofemoral bypass. Anatomical variables require different shapes, angles, and curves for the vascular clamp.

Procedure 23-8 Unilateral Femoropopliteal Bypass

Pathology	• Although obstruction in the distal portion of the femoral artery can be adequately bypassed with synthetic graft	material, the material of choice remains the autogenous saphenous vein, particularly for more distal obstructions. For in	situ bypass, the valves of the vein must stripped for unimpeded flow of arterial blood.
Preoperative diagnostic tests same as for other peripheral vascular procedures			
Equipment, Instruments, and Supplies Unique to Procedure	• Peripheral vascular instrument set (see Table 23-1) • Valvulotome • Heparinized saline solution • Protamine sulfate	• Antibiotic irrigation • Contrast medium • Fogarty embolectomy catheter, various sizes • Butterfly needle with extension tubing	• Angiocath cannula for intra-arterial irrigation • Tunneling device of surgeon's preference, e.g., Sarot clamp, uterine dressing forceps, or specialty CV tunneler
Preoperative Preparation	**Position** • Supine • Affected leg externally rotated & abducted **Anesthesia** • General	**Skin prep** • Midabdomen to toes; leg circumferentially **Draping** • Three-quarter sheet under leg; folded towel over genitalia	• 6-in stockinette placed over foot • Femoral area square-draped with 4 towels • Split sheets may be placed around leg or laparotomy sheet used

PROCEDURE 23-8 (continued)

Practical Considerations	• Imaging studies should be in the OR. • Confirm if the surgeon wants to perform an intraoperative angiography and notify the radiology department. Verify the type of catheters, syringes, and contrast medium the surgeon prefers. • Contact the blood bank to confirm that blood has been ordered and is immediately available. • The surgical technologist should keep the Mayo stand and back table setup sterile until the patient has left the OR. • The procedure for femorotibial bypass is essentially the same as the one described here, except that the tibial artery is used as the distal anastomosis site rather than the popliteal artery.
Surgical Procedure	1. The first incision is made over the distal portion of the popliteal artery, extending from the posterior border of the medial femoral condyle to just below the tibial tuberosity. **Procedural Consideration:** The surgical technologist should keep contact with the exposed leg to a minimum. Weitlaner retractor will likely be used.
	2. The saphenous vein is identified and inspected for size and quality and is dissected free with its branches ligated and divided with 4-0 or 5-0 silk ties. **Procedural Consideration:** The surgical technologist should have synthetic graft material available in case the saphenous vein is inadequate for grafting.
	3. The distal popliteal artery is exposed by retracting the tendons of sartorius, gracilis, and semitendinosus superiorly. The gastrocnemius is retracted posteriorly. **Procedural Consideration:** Retractors for this phase may be U.S. Army, Richardson (small double-ended), Cushing, or vein.
	4. The dissection continues distally and the anterior tibial vein is identified, ligated, and divided. **Procedural Consideration:** The anterior tibial vein is ligated with 4-0 silk ties, 18 in. in length, and/or small or medium-sized hemoclips
	5. A longitudinal incision is made into the groin over the saphenofemoral junction and the proximal portion of the saphenous vein is located, inspected, and dissected free. **Procedural Consideration:** Dissection is made with medium Metzenbaum scissors and medium DeBakey forceps. Handheld and/or self-retaining retractors will be necessary.
	6. The tributaries of the saphenous vein are ligated with 4-0 or 5-0 silk ties and small clips. **Procedural Consideration:** Small, short hemoclip applicators are used with clips from the small (blue) carrier.
	7. The common femoral vein is cleared in the area of its junction with the saphenous vein, and a small Satinsky partial-occlusion clamp is applied. **Procedural Consideration:** The partial-occlusion clamp allows blood flow to continue through the vessel because the clamp is applied to only the top portion of the vessel.
	8. The saphenous vein and a small cuff of the common femoral vein are cut free from the saphenofemoral junction. The junction is closed with 6-0 Prolene suture. **Procedural Consideration:** The 6-0 Prolene is frequently loaded onto a Castroviejo needle holder.

(*continues*)

Procedure 23-8 (continued)

9. The patient is administered systemic heparin. The common femoral artery is exposed and clamped with a DeBakey angled vascular clamp.

   Procedural Consideration: The femoral artery will be isolated with vessel loops placed proximally and distally.

10. An arteriotomy is performed on the anterolateral portion of the common femoral artery, and the saphenous vein is anastomosed in an end-to-side fashion with a continuous 6-0 Prolene suture. If the valvulotome is used, the vein is reversed prior to anastomosis.

    Procedural Consideration: Arteriotomy is performed with #11 blade on #7 knife handle and Potts-Smith scissors.

11. The clamp is removed, and blood is allowed to flow up to the first valve.

    Procedural Consideration: Clamp will be replaced several times as procedure progresses.

12. The distal end of the saphenous vein is transected at the anastomosis site, and a Cartier valvulotome is introduced and passed through the full length of the vein.

    Procedural Consideration: The valvulotome will remove any valves that may prevent the flow of arterial blood to target tissues.

13. The arterialized saphenous vein is ligated at its distal end, and its medial side is marked to prevent torsion.

    Procedural Consideration: Marking of the vein is done with a purple marking pen so that the vein is anastomosed without a twist.

14. The knee is flexed and the popliteal artery is occluded with small vascular clamps.

    Procedural Consideration: Popliteal artery occlusion is usually accomplished with small bulldog vascular clamps or vessel loops tightened around the artery.

15. An incision is made into the popliteal artery and the spatulated saphenous vein is anastomosed with a continuous 6-0 or 7-0 Prolene suture. Before completion of the suture line, clamps are released to flush and the lumen is irrigated with heparinized saline (Figure 23-18).

    Procedural Consideration: Rubber shods (Prolene clamps) should be available for all vascular anastomoses. Heparin solution is prepared in advance.

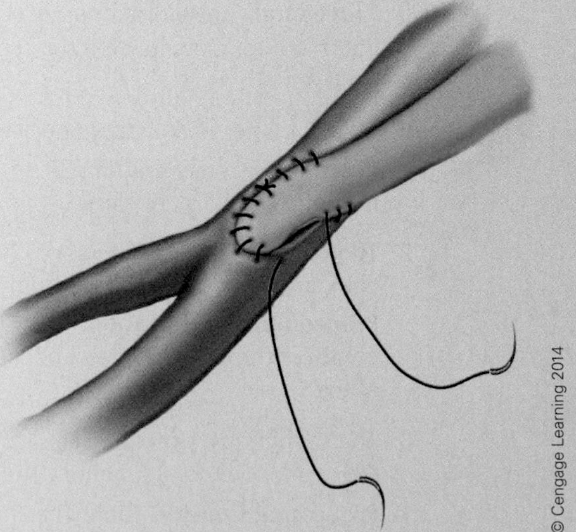

Figure 23-18 Popliteal artery—saphenous vein anastomosis

PROCEDURE 23-8 (continued)

16. The suture ends are tied, and the anastomosis is completed. The wounds are closed in layers.

    Procedural Consideration: Have the Doppler probe and unit available for postanastomosis vessel evaluation.

Postoperative Considerations

Immediate Postoperative Care

- Transport to the PACU, ICU, or CCU.
- Postoperative bleeding from the anastomosis site may need to be repaired with a single-armed Prolene patch suture.

Prognosis

- No complications: If arterial flow is reinstated before tissue damage has become too severe, then the prognosis for recovery is good. The patient will remain hospitalized for several days until stable and walking without assistance. Anticoagulants are necessary to prevent clot formation postoperatively.
- Complications: Postoperative SSI; failure of graft; rejection of graft material

Wound Classification

- Class I: Clean

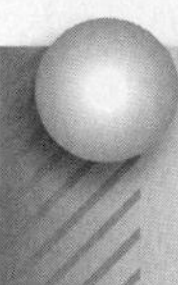

PEARL OF WISDOM

The surgical technologist should be adept at handling small polypropylene sutures and small, delicate needles. A white paper towel laid between the Mayo and the operative site, or on the Mayo tray itself, helps to visualize the blue suture. Needles should be returned from the surgeon directly to the surgical technologist, because the needles are small and easily lost.

PROCEDURE 23-9 Arteriovenous Fistula and Shunt

Pathology

- Arteriovenous fistula and shunt is established for vascular access for patients who require long-term renal dialysis.

Preoperative Diagnostic Tests and Procedures

- Patients with renal disease must have their creatinine level regularly monitored by the lab through the creatinine clearance test; it measures the rate at which creatinine is cleared from the blood by the kidney. When the creatinine level is determined to be abnormal, the patient will be scheduled to undergo an arteriovenous fistula and shunt procedure in preparation to start long-term dialysis treatment.

(*continues*)

Procedure 23-9 (continued)

Equipment, Instruments, and Supplies Unique to Procedure	• Peripheral vascular instrument set (see Table 23-1) • Loupes, surgeon's preference • Coronary artery dilators • Shunt clamps • Silastic cannulas, various sizes • Teflon tips • Shunt connector • Heparinized saline solution
Preoperative Preparation	• Position: Supine with nondominant arm extended on hand table • Anesthesia: Local with MAC • Skin prep: Beginning at site of incision on forearm extending from fingertips to 3 in. above elbow • Draping: Arm is help up and a three-quarters sheet is placed on hand table or Mayo stand cover draped over the table; impervious stockinette is placed over the arm; a split sheet is placed under the arm with tails in cephalad direction and the tails are crossed; a three-quarters sheet is used to cover the shoulder.
Practical Considerations	• The procedure involves using the patient's own vessels and subcutaneously anastomosing an artery and vein, which is called an arteriovenous shunt. • The four types of anastomoses are artery side–to–vein side, artery end–to–vein side, artery end–to–vein end, and vein end–to–artery side. • One of the most common and popular procedures to be performed is the Cimino fistula and shunt, which forms a shunt between the radial artery and cephalic vein in the wrist region.
Surgical Procedure	1. Using a #15 knife blade, the surgeon makes the incision over the radial artery and cephalic vein in the forearm.
	2. The incision is carried down to the vessels, which are identified. The vessels are mobilized for the length of the anastomosis and vessel loops are placed.
	3. Small vascular clamps or bulldog clamps are placed proximally and distally on each vessel.
	4. Branches that are near the site of anastomosis in both vessels are identified, doubly clamped, cut, and tied.
	5. Using the #11 knife blade, the surgeon makes an arteriotomy in the radial artery, which is slightly extended with the 45° Potts-Smith scissors.
	6. The radial artery is dilated with the DeBakey or Garrett vascular dilators. **Procedural Consideration:** The surgical technologist should have the dilators lined up in order of size (smallest to largest diameter) and communicate the size of the dilator to the surgeon when handing to him or her.
	7. The cephalic vein is doubly clamped, cut, and tied distally.
	8. Using the #11 knife blade, a venotomy is made in the cephalic vein.
	9. Using continuous suture technique, the radial artery is anastomosed to the cephalic vein (Figure 23-19). **Procedural Consideration:** Just before the last 2–3 stitches are placed, the surgeon will inject a small amount of heparin into the area of the anastomosis.

PROCEDURE 23-9 (continued)

10. The area is thoroughly irrigated with antibiotic irrigation solution and the anastomosis checked for bleeding.
11. The wound is closed in layers and dressing placed. The area of the anastomosis is gently palpated to confirm blood flow.

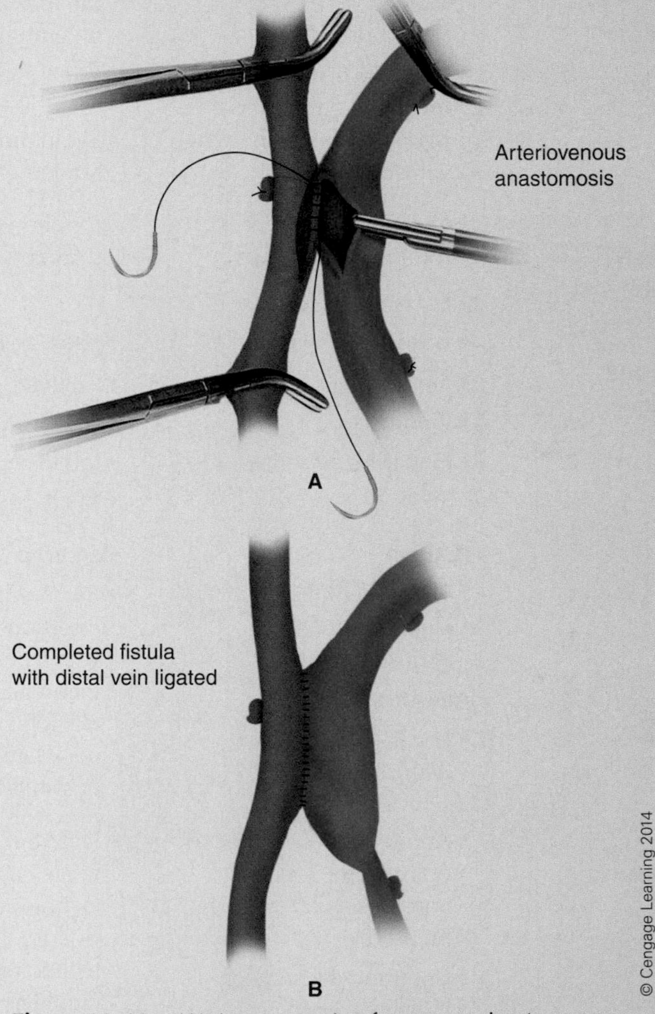

Figure 23-19 (A) Anastomosis of artery and vein, (B) completed anastomosis

Postoperative Considerations

Immediate Postoperative Care

- Transport to PACU
- Patient will be hospitalized overnight for observation of postoperative complications.

Prognosis

- No complications: Patient expected to recover from surgery; other factors such as renal disease are responsible for patient not being able to return to full normal activities.
- Complications: Risk factors for complications include being elderly, female, or black or having diabetes. The most common complication is stenosis, which can lead to thrombosis and must be surgically treated. Additional complications include postoperative SSI; hemorrhage at site of anastomosis; aneurysm forms at site of anastomosis

Wound Classification

- Class I: clean

PROCEDURE 23-10 Inferior Vena Cava Filter Placement–Jugular Vein Access

Pathology	• Placing an inferior vena cava (IVC) filter is indicated for preventing pulmonary embolism (PE) due to deep vein thrombosis (DVT). • DVT is a disorder involving a thrombus in one of the deep veins of the body. The deep veins most commonly affected are the iliac and femoral veins. It is a life-threatening disorder; if the thrombus becomes an embolus, it is likely it will enter the lungs, causing a PE. • Symptoms include tenderness, claudication, swelling, and discoloration of the skin. • IVC filter placement is performed when medical therapy, including bed rest and anticoagulant drugs, does not resolve the disorder.
Preoperative Diagnostic Tests and Procedure	• Diagnostic tests are routinely performed for peripheral vascular disorders.
Equipment, Instruments, and Supplies Unique to Procedure	• Ultrasound with probe • Sterile cover for probe • Fluoroscopy • Heparinized saline solution • Basic angiography set • Catheter • 0.035-in. guidewire • 0.038-in. guidewire • Micropuncture device • Cook Gunther Tulip or Celect filter kit • Contrast medium
Preoperative Preparation	**Position** • Supine with head slightly turned to expose operative site **Anesthesia** • Local—1% lidocaine with sedation **Skin prep** • Beginning at site of insertion over jugular vein extending from inframandible to clavicle, midline of neck laterally as far as possible **Draping** • Four towels to square off and three-quarters sheets × two or four towels to square off and transverse drape
Practical Considerations	• Approximately 5 mL of lidocaine local anesthesia will be used. • Confirm with surgeon if the micropuncture device will be used to anticipate if a 0.035-in. guidewire will be needed. • Different types of filters have different techniques for insertion. The surgical technologist should be familiar with the type of filter the surgeon prefers and study the manufacturer's instructions that come with the filter kit prior to the procedure. • The surgical technologist must be careful to prevent bumping the OR bed and fluoroscopy machine because the surgeon has carefully positioned the fluoroscopy.
Surgical Procedure	1. The surgeon palpates for the jugular vein and injects 3–5 mL of lidocaine 1%.
	2. Using the #15 knife blade, the surgeon makes a small horizontal skin incision.
	3. Depending on surgeon's preference, an 18-gauge needle or ultrasound-guided micropuncture device is used to enter the jugular vein. The surgeon may use a Modified Seldinger technique to obtain entry into the vessel. Venous blood is aspirated to verify entry into the vein.
	4. The course for inserting the guidewire is viewed on fluoroscopy. If the surgeon is using the micropuncture device, the 0.035-in. wire will be used.

PROCEDURE 23-10 (continued)

5. The 0.035- or 0.038-in. guidewire is advanced into the IVC. The sheath is placed over the guidewire and then the catheter is inserted through the sheath and over the guidewire.
6. The guidewire is removed and a small amount of contrast medium is injected to verify location of the catheter.

   Procedural Consideration: The surgeon will perform a cavogram. The cavogram is performed to measure the diameter of the IVC, verify the anatomical location of the renal veins, rule out that an IVC does not exist on the left side of the body, and make sure the IVC is patent.
7. The catheter is removed and replaced with the introducer sheath.

   Procedural Consideration: When placing the IVC filter through the jugular vein, a 7F introducer sheath will be used; femoral vein is entered and an 8.5F sheath is used.
8. The sheath is advanced to the spot where the IVC filter will be placed.
9. The inner dilator is removed, and the deployment catheter with the pre-attached filter is inserted.

   Procedural Consideration: The surgeon is careful not to push the filter all the way out of the sheath, but just to the end so it is ready for deployment.
10. The sheath and filter are advanced to the position of deployment distal to the lowest renal vein.
11. The sheath is drawn back and the filter is uncovered and opens, but it is still attached to the sheath. If the filter is not in the correct position or incorrectly angled, it can be resheathed and fluoroscopy continued so the surgeon can reposition the sheath and filter. When the correct position is achieved, the filter hook is released and the filter is positioned.
12. The surgeon will perform another cavogram to verify IVC filter position.
13. The sheath is removed and the incision closed with interrupted sutures, and small dressing is placed.

Postoperative Considerations

Immediate Postoperative Care

- Transport to PACU
- Patient usually has an overnight stay unless other predisposing conditions require a longer stay.

Prognosis

- No complications: Patient is expected to have a full recovery from surgery.
- Complications: Pneumothorax; persistent hemorrhage from insertion site; PE; filter migration; filter infection; caval thrombosis; penetration of the IVC wall by the filter that can lead to retroperitoneal hematoma

Wound Classification

- Class I: clean

PROCEDURE 23-11 Vein Ligation and Stripping (Unilateral)

Pathology	• Varicose veins are veins that have become elongated, dilated, and tortuous. • Varicose veins are characteristic of a disorder that is progressive and there is no cure. • They are categorized as primary and secondary. Primary varicose veins are the result of dilated, visible protrusions of superficial veins. • Secondary varicose veins are the result of deep venous disorders such as DVT. • Veins in the legs are more frequently affected, in particular, the saphenous vein and its branches. • Risk factors include heredity, female gender, hormones (particularly progesterone), constricted clothing, long periods of standing, obesity, incompetent venous valves, pregnancy, physical inactivity, smoking, and hypertension. • Varicose veins can result in venous stasis, which can lead to stasis ulcers. • Symptoms include aching and heaviness of the lower extremity that worsens during the day, nighttime leg cramping, edema, fatigue, visible protrusions of the veins, skin pigmentation, ulceration, eczema, tenderness, and internal and external bleeding. • Indications for therapy and/or surgery include pain, easy fatigability, recurrent thrombophlebitis, external bleeding, external appearance of the leg(s), and complications of varicose veins such as dermal atrophy, hemorrhage, ulceration, and cellulitis. • Contraindications to treatment include pregnancy during the first and second trimesters, significant leg edema, arterial occlusive disease, and immobility.
Preoperative Diagnostic Tests and Procedures	• History and physical
Equipment, Instruments, and Supplies Unique to Procedure	• Vein stripper with various sizes of acorns or PIN stripper • #0 or #1 silk ties
Preoperative Preparation	**Position** • Supine with affected leg externally rotated and abducted to expose saphenous vein; once the skin prep and draping are completed, the surgeon may request to have the patient placed in slight Trendelenburg's position to aid in decreasing the venous congestion. **Anesthesia** • General, spinal, or epidural **Skin prep** • Circumference of leg, upper thigh to toes • During prep be careful to not remove marks on skin made by surgeon **Draping** • Holding leg up, three-quarters sheet is placed under leg and over unaffected leg; genitalia is covered by folded towel; impervious stockinette is placed over the leg; a split sheet is placed under the leg with tails cephalad and the upper body is covered by three-quarters sheet or extremity drape placed.

PROCEDURE 23-11 (continued)

Practical Considerations

- Surgical technologist should confirm with surgeon the size of acorn that will be used.
- The vein stripper is prepared by screwing the selected size of acorn onto the end. The surgical technologist must be careful to prevent the stripper from becoming contaminated because it is long and highly flexible. It should be kept coiled up on the back table or Mayo stand until ready for use.
- The surgical technologist will be responsible for removing the inverted vein from the vein stripper as the tissue specimen. The surgical technologist will need to use a #15 knife blade to incise down the midline of the vein and, using tissue forceps with no teeth and fingers, remove the vein from the stripper.
- Before the patient is transported to the OR, the surgeon will have the patient stand and, using a nonerasable marker, indicate the location of the varicose veins.

Surgical Procedure

1. Using the #15 knife blade, the surgeon makes a small transverse incision in the upper thigh above the location of the proximal portion of the saphenous vein.
2. The incision is carried down to the saphenous vein. Bleeders are cauterized or clamped and tied with silk ties. A Weitlaner self-retaining retractor is placed.
3. The proximal end of the vein is mobilized with sharp and blunt dissection. It is mobilized up to where it connects to the femoral artery. While dissecting upward, the surgeon ligates vein branches by double clamping, cutting, and tying with silk ties.
4. At the junction with the femoral artery, the saphenous vein end is double clamped and cut, but not tied. One clamp is removed.
5. The surgeon moves to the distal saphenous vein in the ankle region and makes a transverse incision over the saphenous vein.

   Procedural Consideration: A new #15 knife blade should be loaded on the knife handle for the surgeon to use. Another Weitlaner retractor is placed to expose the surgical site.
6. The incision is carried down to the saphenous vein, which is double clamped and cut but not tied.
7. The clamps are removed and the vein stripper is inserted into distal opening of the saphenous vein at the ankle and advanced to the proximal end. Just before the stripper comes through the opening at the proximal end, the clamp that was left in place is removed (Figure 23-20).
8. The surgeon or surgical technologist screws the acorn onto the exteriorized end of the stripper. The surgeon tightly ties a large-diameter silk tie around the vein and stripper just below the acorn.
9. The surgeon pulls the stripper back toward the ankle, which inverts and strips the ankle from the leg.

   Procedural Consideration: As the surgeon is pulling the stripper, he or she may have the surgical technologist follow along and apply external pressure to keep the stripper and vein from excessive movement within the leg.
10. The surgeon pulls the stripper back toward the ankle, which inverts and strips the vein from the leg.

(continues)

Procedure 23-11 (continued)

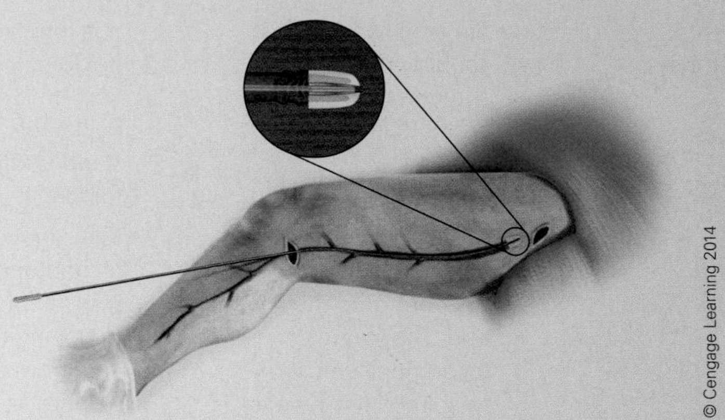

Figure 23-20 Insertion of the vein stripper through the saphenous vein

Postoperative Considerations

Immediate Postoperative Care

- Transport to PACU
- Patient discharged same day

Prognosis

- No complications: Patient expected to have full recovery and good results both clinically and cosmetically. Return to full normal activities in 6–10 days.
- Complications: Postoperative SSI; hemorrhage; recurrence of varicose veins; hematoma

Wound Classification

- Class I: clean

Case Study Hugo is a 65-year-old with diabetes. He is scheduled for a femoropopliteal bypass. The OR team knows him from past visits to the OR. His overall health appears to them to be worsening.

1. What is the relationship between diabetes and the condition leading to this procedure?
2. What is Hugo's prognosis?
3. What are the complications related to the procedure and for which of these is Hugo at high risk?

Questions for Further Study

1. What is meant by collateral flow?
2. What is the difference between ischemia and infarction?
3. Why aren't the neurological deficits associated with transient ischemia attacks permanent?
4. Describe the method for loading a pledget with a double-armed needle for use during an aortofemoral bypass.
5. Why is preclotting a PTFE or woven polyester graft not necessary?
6. What two surgical instruments are used to create the arteriotomy in the common carotid artery during an endarterectomy?

BIBLIOGRAPHY

Association of Surgical Technologists. (2011). *Core curriculum for surgical technology* (6th ed.). Littleton, CO: Association of Surgical Technologists.

Burnett, A. F., Lossef, S. V., Barth, K. H., Grendys, E. C., Johnson, J. C., Barter, J. F., & Barnes, W. A. (1994). Insertion of Groshong central venous catheters utilizing fluoroscopic techniques. *Gynecologic Oncology, 52*, 69–73.

Cameron, J. L. (2007). *Current surgical therapy* (9th ed.). St. Louis: Mosby.

Casserly, I. P., Sachar, R., & Yadav, J. S. (2011). *Practical peripheral vascular intervention* (2nd ed.). Philadelphia: Lippincott Williams & Wilkins.

Davies, A. H. (2006). *Vascular surgery*. New York: Springer.

Haimovici, H. (2003). *Haimovici's vascular surgery*. Hoboken, NJ: Wiley-Blackwell.

Lau, K. Y. (2002). Percutaneous insertion of Hickman central venous catheter: Jugular approach. *Journal of the Hong Kong College of Radiologists, 5*, 69–72.

Puppala, S. (2011). *Inferior vena cava vascular filter placement.* Retrieved from http://emedicine.medscape.com/article/1377859-overview

Rutherford, R. B. (2005). *Vascular surgery* (6th ed.). Philadelphia: W. B. Saunders.

Sanders, T., & Scanlon, V. C. (2006). *Essentials of anatomy and physiology* (5th ed.). Philadelphia: F. A. Davis.

Salenius, J. (1995). Experience of peripheral angioscopy in Scandinavia. *International Journal of Angiology, 4*, 65–68.

Shier, D. N., Butler, J. L., & Lewis, R. (2009). *Hole's human anatomy & physiology* (12th ed.). New York: McGraw-Hill.

Tortora, G. J., & Derrickson, B. H. (2008). *Principles of anatomy and physiology* (12th ed.). Hoboken, NJ: John Wiley & Sons.

Townsend, C. M., Beauchamp, R. D., Evers, B. M., & Mattox, K. L. (Eds.). (2007). *Sabiston's textbook of surgery: The biological basis of modern surgical practice* (18th ed.). Philadelphia: Elsevier.

Uflacker, R. (2006). *Atlas of vascular anatomy: An angiographic approach* (2nd ed.). Philadelphia: Lippincott Williams & Wilkins.

CHAPTER

24

Neurosurgery

CASE STUDY Katy is a 10-year-old girl who was admitted to the emergency department after falling from a schoolyard slide and sustaining an injury to her head. Katy initially lost consciousness, but awoke soon afterward complaining of nausea and a severe left-sided headache. She developed right-sided hemiparesis within minutes of the injury. On arrival at the emergency department, she was conscious and responding to verbal commands.

A neurosurgeon called to the emergency room examined Katy. During the examination, Katy's condition began to deteriorate rapidly. As she lost consciousness, her blood pressure rose rapidly and her pulse rate fell. Her left pupil became fixed and dilated. The neurosurgeon informed the OR that an emergency procedure should be scheduled and appropriate personnel summoned.

1. **What is the suspected diagnosis?**
2. **Why did the neurosurgeon schedule an emergency procedure?**
3. **What procedure did the neurosurgeon schedule?**

OBJECTIVES

After studying this chapter, the reader should be able to:

A 1. Recognize the relevant anatomy and physiology of the neurological system.

P 2. Summarize the pathology that prompts surgical intervention of the neurological system and the related terminology.

O 3. Determine any special preoperative neurological diagnostic procedures/tests.

S 4. Indicate the names and uses of neurosurgical instruments, supplies, and drugs.

5. Indicate the names and uses of special equipment related to neurosurgery.
6. Determine the intraoperative preparation of the patient undergoing a neurosurgical procedure.
7. Summarize the surgical steps of the neurosurgical procedures.
8. Interpret the purpose and expected outcomes of the neurosurgical procedures.

9. Recognize the immediate postoperative care and possible complications of the neurosurgical procedures.
10. Assess any specific variations related to the preoperative, intraoperative, and postoperative care of the neurosurgical patient.

SELECT KEY TERMS

abscess
acute
cerebellum
cerebrum
Craniosynostosis
circle of Willis
CNS
decompress
epidural
extruded
glioma
hematoma
intracranial pressure
meninges
osteophyte
PNS
transphenoidal

INTRODUCTION TO NEUROLOGICAL SURGERY

The field of neurological surgery is one of the most sophisticated surgical specialties and encompasses advanced surgical and imaging technology. Surgery on the nervous system involves the brain, spinal cord, peripheral nerves, and the protective structures that surround them. common indications include congenital defects, traumatic injury, degeneration, and cancer. This chapter will familiarize the student with neurological procedures commonly performed as preparation for surgical rotation.

INSTRUMENTS, ROUTINE EQUIPMENT, AND SUPPLIES

Instruments

Cranial

Instrument sets for craniotomy include a minor set with basic instrumentation and a basic craniotomy or neurological set. A basic neurological set is equipped with the following basic instruments:

- Hudson brace with bits and attachments (Figure 24-1)
- Gigli saw, handles, and guide for bone flaps (Figure 24-2)
- Various bone rongeurs (Love-Kerrison, Leksell, Stille-Leur, Adson, Ferris-Smith) (Figure 24-3)
- Various pituitary rongeurs (straight, up-biting, down-biting)
- Penfield dissectors (Figure 24-4)
- Self-retaining retractors (Gelpi—shallow and deep, Weitlaner, Adson-Beckman, Adson cerebellar)
    - Leyla-Yasargil or Greenberg self-retaining retractor (may be separate)
- Manual retractors (Cushing, Meyerding, U.S. Army, Taylor, Love, Scoville) (Figure 24-5A–C)
- Malleable brain spoons (Silastic, Scoville) (Figure 24-6)
    - Pituitary spoons
    - Nerve hooks
    - Dura hooks
    - Dural separators and elevators
- Bayonet, Cushing, Adson, and Gerald forceps, with and without teeth (Figure 24-7)
- Periosteal elevators (Adson, Langenbeck, Freer, Cushing)
    - Bone curettes, gouges, and osteotomes (may be separate)
- Suction tips of various sizes (Frazier or Adson)
- Scalp clip applicators or scalp gun (may be separate) (Figure 24-8)
- Dandy clamps
- Aneurysm clips (Figure 24-9)
- Hemoclip applicators (short)
- Bipolar forceps

Power instrumentation includes Midas Rex or Anspach pneumatic drill with attachments, burrs, and bits; air-, battery-, or electric-powered cranial perforator and craniotome with dura guard; and wire-pass air drill with burrs and bits.

Microsurgical instruments include arachnoid knife, microforceps (bayonet-type), curettes, scissors, needle holders, dissectors, and bipolar forceps (Figure 24-10).

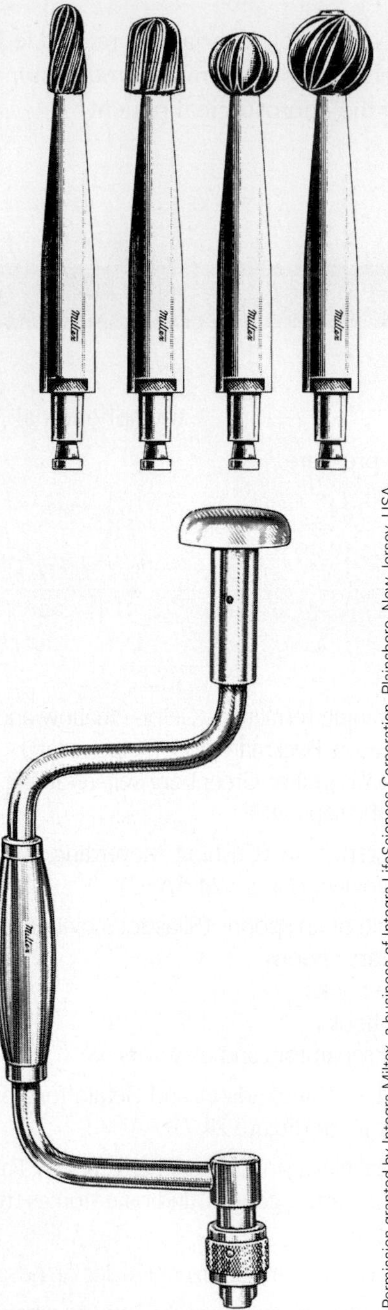

Figure 24-1 Hudson brace with attachments

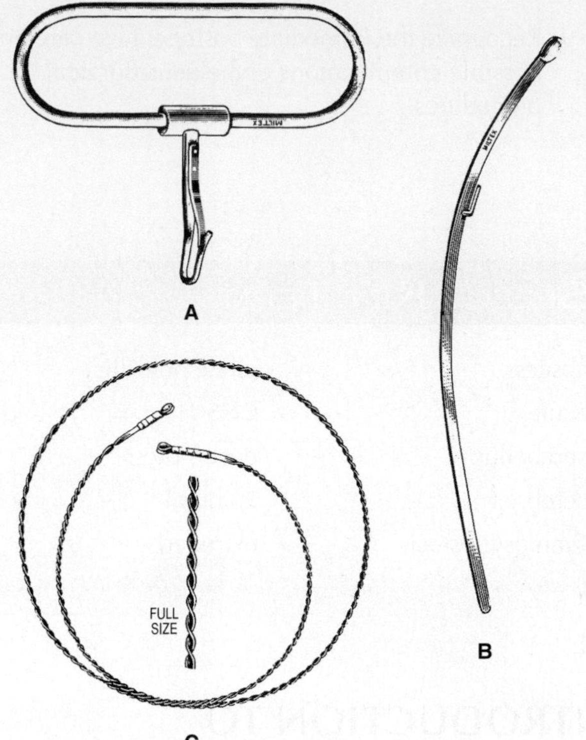

Figure 24-2 Gigli saw: (A) Handle, (B) guide, (C) blade

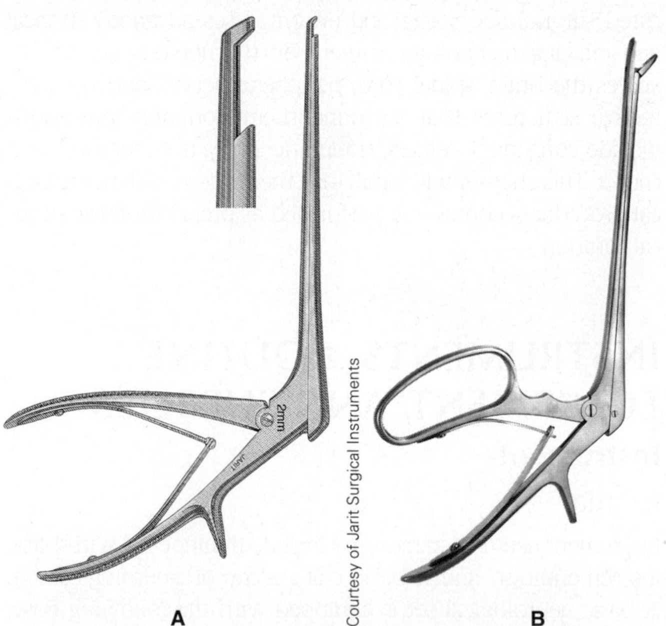

Figure 24-3 Bone rongeurs: (A) Love-Kerrison rongeur, 40° forward biting angle, (B) Ferris-Smith spurling rongeur

Spinal

Instrument sets for spinal procedures include a basic laminectomy or neurological set for posterior approaches and an anterior cervical discectomy set that includes the instruments necessary for the exposure and removal of the anterior cervical disk and the excision and placement of a bone graft.

Fusion of the posterior spine typically requires the following specialty instrumentation for the removal of cancellous and cortical bone from the iliac crest:

- Bone curettes of variable sizes, curved and straight
- Osteotomes of various sizes, curved and straight
- Gouges of various sizes, curved and straight
- Large mallet
- Oscillating saw (optional)
- Gelpi self-retaining retractors
- U.S. Army and/or Hibbs retractors
- Periosteal elevator (Cobb, Key, Langenbeck)

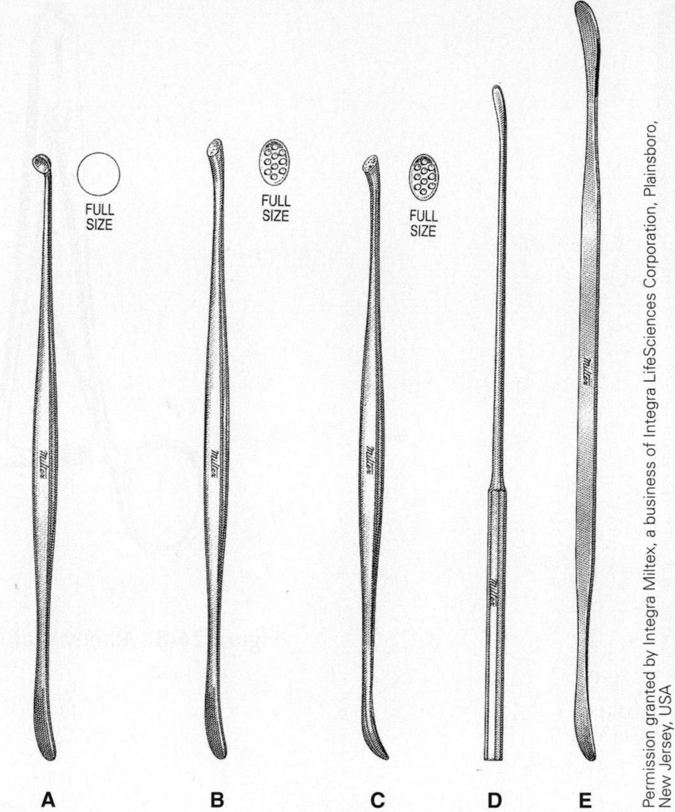

Figure 24-4 Penfield dissectors: (A) Style #1, (B) style #2, (C) style #3, (D) style #4, (E) style #5

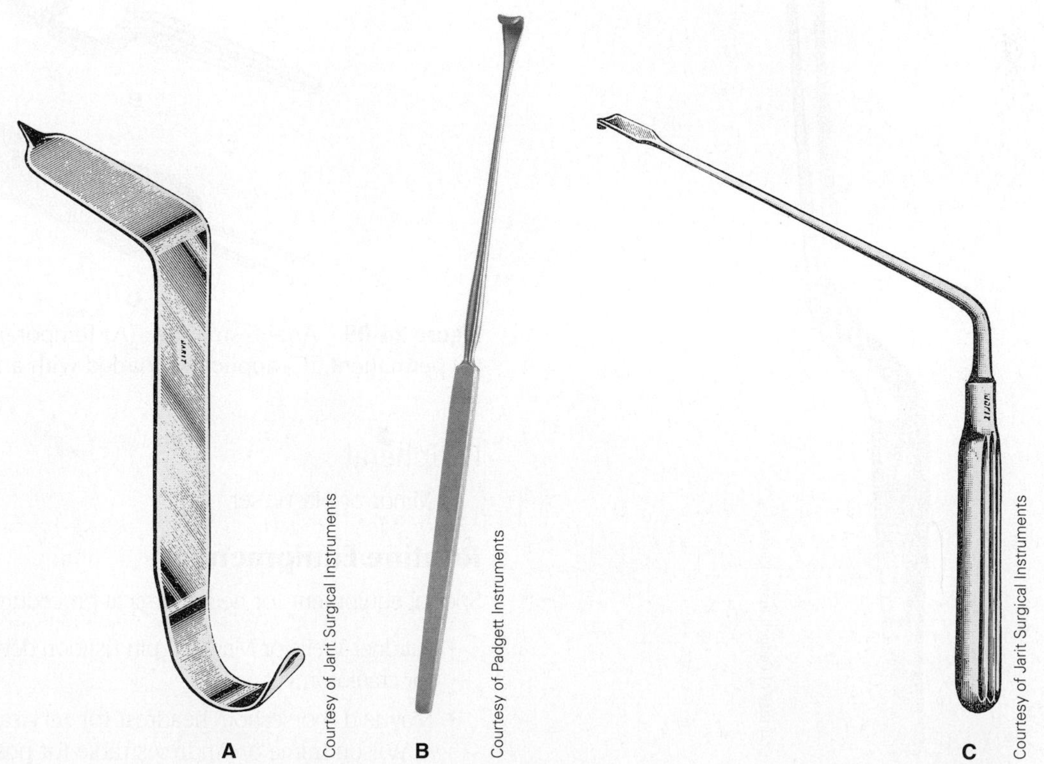

Figure 24-5 Manual retractors: (A) Taylor spinal retractor, (B) Love nerve retractor, (C) Scoville nerve root retractor

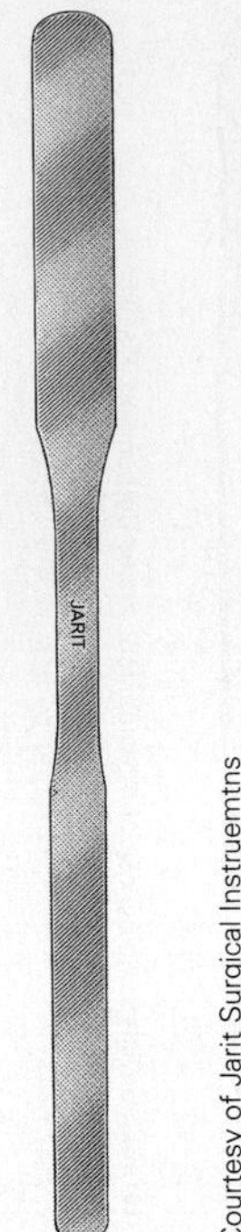

Courtesy of Jarit Surgical Instruemtns

Figure 24-6 Scoville brain spatula

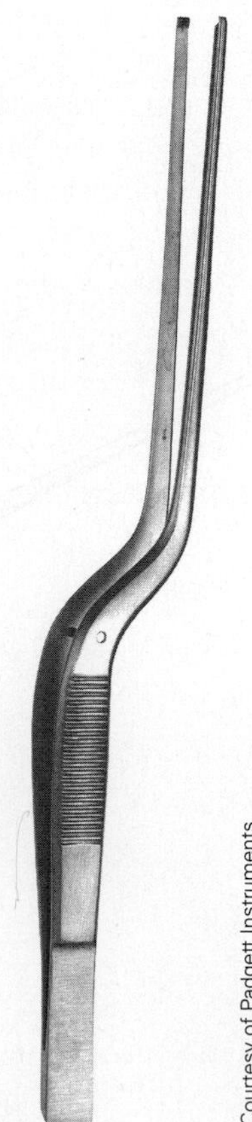

Courtesy of Padgett Instruments

Figure 24-7 Cushing bayonet forceps

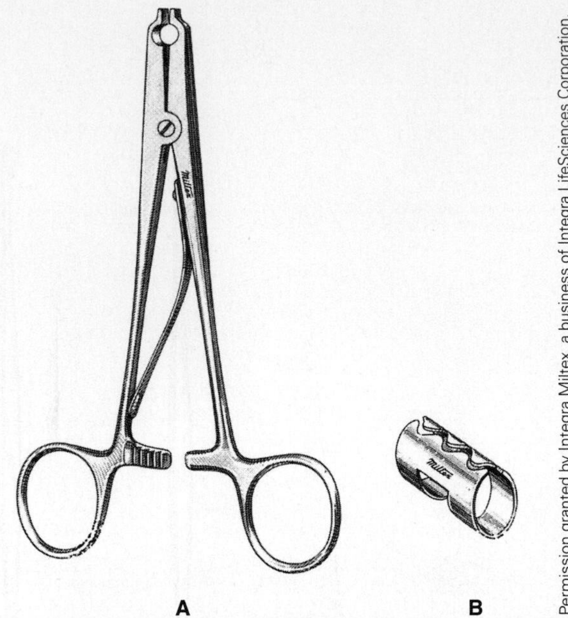

Permission granted by Integra Miltex, a business of Integra LifeSciences Corporation, Plainsboro, New Jersey, USA

Figure 24-8 Raney scalp system: (A) Applicator, (B) clip

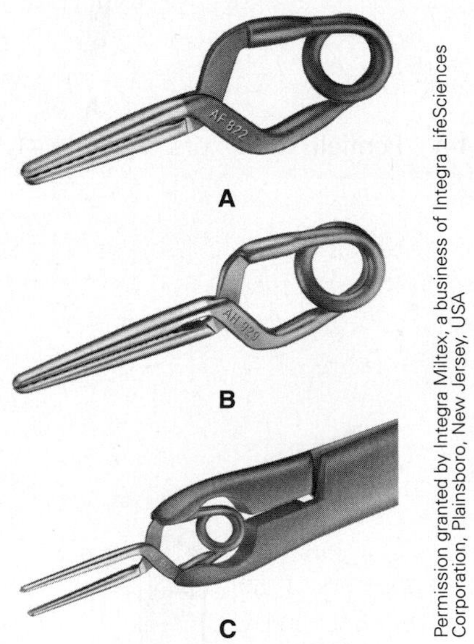

Permission granted by Integra Miltex, a business of Integra LifeSciences Corporation, Plainsboro, New Jersey, USA

Figure 24-09 Aneurysm clips: (A) Temporary, (B) permanent, (C) applicator loaded with aneurysm clip

Peripheral

- Minor or plastic set

Routine Equipment

Special equipment for neurosurgical procedures includes:

- Gardner-Wells or Mayfield pin fixation device (Figure 24-11) for craniotomy
- Mayfield "horseshoe" headrest for cervical spine
  - Wilson frame or Andrews table for posterior thoracic or lumbar spine

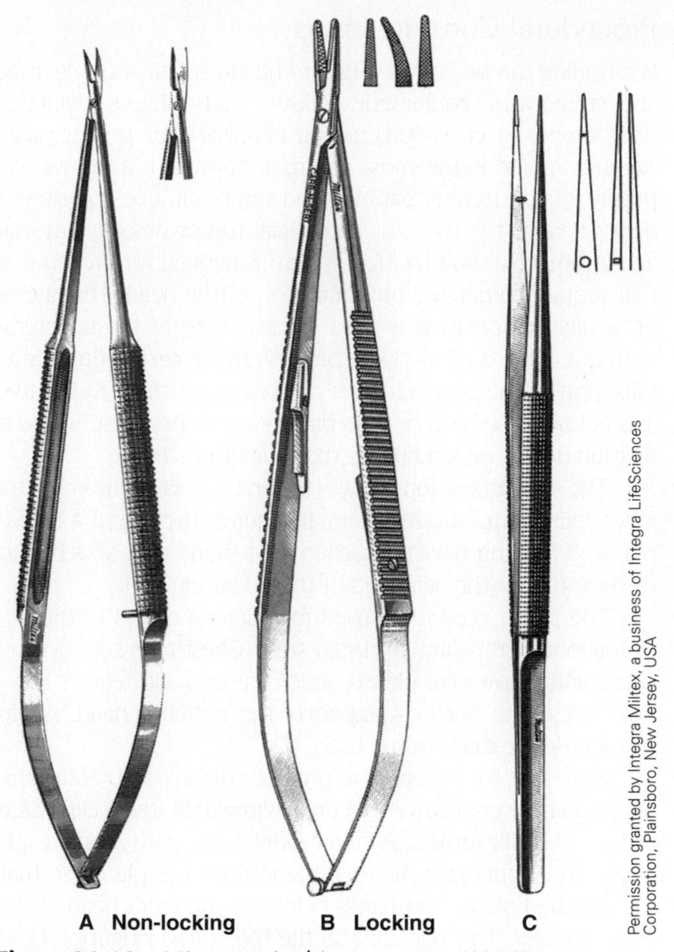

Figure 24-10 Microsurgical instruments: (A) Microsurgery scissors, (B) Jacobson microvascular needle holder, (C) Rhoton micro forceps

  - Operating microscope with increased illumination
  - Variable magnification of the operative field
- Nd:YAG or CO_2 laser. The CO_2 laser is able to deliver variable amounts of precise energy for removal of small amounts of tissue in tight places. The Nd:YAG laser delivers diffuse energy for better coagulation of bleeding vessels around the target tissue.
- Operative ultrasound machine. This instrument emits sound waves that penetrate the brain and bounce back to the machine to generate an image. It is used to locate lesions that lie deep beneath the surface of the **cerebrum** and evaluate the completeness of tumor resection.
- Frame-based or frameless stereotaxis systems. These systems can precisely deliver an instrument to a target at any point within a defined space. The target space is defined by CT or MRI scanning with reference points attached to the head. Various monitoring devices and amplifiers are used in conjunction with these systems.
- Cavitron Ultrasonic Aspirator (CUSA). This device emits a variable ultrasonic energy field that emulsifies abnormal tissue while preserving normal neural tissue. Saline ejected from the tip of the handheld unit liquefies the tissue, which is then aspirated back to the unit. This instrument is used when a moderate to large amount of tissue is to be removed.

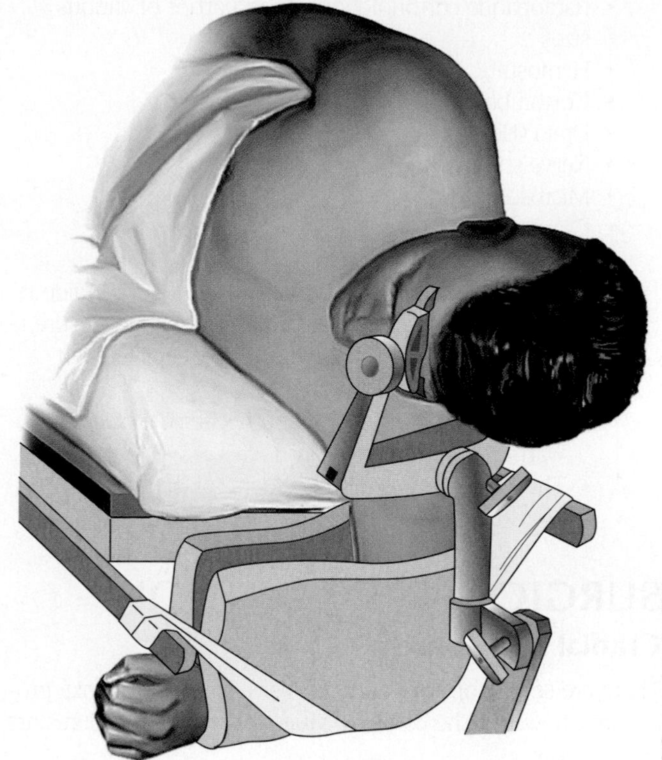

Figure 24-11 Pin fixation device

- Heating and cooling unit and temperature monitoring devices
- Bipolar and monopolar electrosurgical units
- Neuroendoscope, light source, recorder, and monitor
- Nitrogen source for power equipment (piped in or portable tank)
- Mayfield overhead table
- Headlight and fiberoptic light source
- C-arm and monitor
- Fluid warming units and Cell Saver autotransfusion machine

Routine Supplies

- Basic pack
- Ray-Tec and laparotomy sponges
- Hemostatic agents (Gelfoam, Avitene, Surgicel, bone wax)
  - Disposable bipolar cord (for attachment to nondisposable bipolar forceps)
  - Monopolar electrosurgical pencil

- Radiopaque cottonoid strips and patties of various sizes
- Hemostatic clips (MRI compatible)
- Cotton balls
- Drain (HemoVac)
- Nerve stimulator
- Microscope drape
- C-arm drape
- Ultrasound wand drape
- Suture material (surgeon's preference). Silk or braided nylon for the dura; polyglactin 910 for wound closure; monofilament nylon or stainless steel clips for skin
- Medications and solutions
  - Antibiotic solution of surgeon's choice mixed with warm saline for irrigation
  - Thrombin for use with Gelfoam for hemostasis

SURGICAL INTERVENTION

Cranial Procedures

There are several options available for a variety of cranial procedures; however, the commonalities for these procedures are listed below.

Practical Considerations

- Make sure CT or MRI scans, arteriograms, or plain film studies are in the room before the procedure begins.
- Always test drills and saws before procedure.
- Cut Surgicel and Gelfoam into same sizes of cottonoids. Gelfoam is usually soaked in thrombin.
- A 10-mL syringe filled with saline should be available to flush the Frazier suction tip as it becomes clogged with debris.
- Keep close track of all small countables such as dura needles and cottonoids.

Procedural Considerations

Positioning can be complex due to headrests, fixation devices, and stereotactic equipment. Pillows, pads, sheets, blankets, wide tape, and chest rolls are all necessary for proper positioning. Supine is the most common approach; it allows exposure of the frontal, parietal, and temporal lobes. A simple donut headrest is used for superficial tumor or clot removal, and a three-pin skull fixation system is needed for procedures that require complete immobilization of the head. The lateral or semilateral position is used for exposure of the unilateral temporal lobe, occipital lobe, brain stem, or **cerebellum.** Stabilization of the body requires a beanbag or chest rolls, tape, and pillows. The head may be placed onto a headrest or into a fixation device, depending on the type of procedure.

The sitting position allows bilateral access to the occipital lobe, brain stem, or cerebellum. It requires the use of a three-pin skull fixation device attached to a frame that attaches to the side rails of the head end of the operating table.

The prone position is used for bilateral access to the occipital lobe, cerebellum, or brain stem. Chest rolls support the chest, and pillows are placed under the legs and feet. A Mayfield horseshoe headrest supports the patient's head. A pin fixation device may also be used.

Eyes and ears should be protected from prep solutions. Draping consists of towels secured with small towel clips, skin clips, or 3-0 silk sutures. A craniotomy drape with a plastic adhesive sheet built into the round fenestration is placed so that the attached plastic bag hangs below the patient's head at the surgeon's feet. This bag collects the blood and irrigation fluid that runs down from the operative site and funnels it through suction tubing into a suction canister.

If the Mayfield table is used, it is placed over the patient with its edge just below the patient's chin before draping begins. The craniotomy sheet is placed over the table, and instrumentation is then brought up and placed onto the draped Mayfield table.

The physician marks the incision site with a marking pen and injects it with 1% lidocaine with epinephrine for hemostasis.

Procedure 24-1 Craniotomy

Surgical Anatomy and Pathology	• Craniotomy involves incising the cranium for access to the brain. • The cranium encloses and protects the brain and is covered with skin, subcutaneous tissue, galea aponeurotica, and periosteum.	• The cranium consists of eight bones: 1. One frontal bone, forming the forehead, nasal cavity, and orbital roofs 2. Two parietal bones on each side of the skull, just posterior to the frontal bone, forming a large portion of the sides and roof of the cranium 3. One occipital bone, forming the back and a large portion of the floor of the cranium

PROCEDURE 24-1 (continued)

4. Two temporal bones, forming a small portion of the sides and floor of the cranium
5. The sphenoid bone, forming portions of the base of the cranium, sides of the skull, and base and sides for the orbits
6. One ethmoid bone that forms portions of the roof and walls of the nasal cavity, the floor of the cranium, and the walls of the orbits (Figure 24-12)

- Three layers of protective tissue called the cranial **meninges** cover the brain and

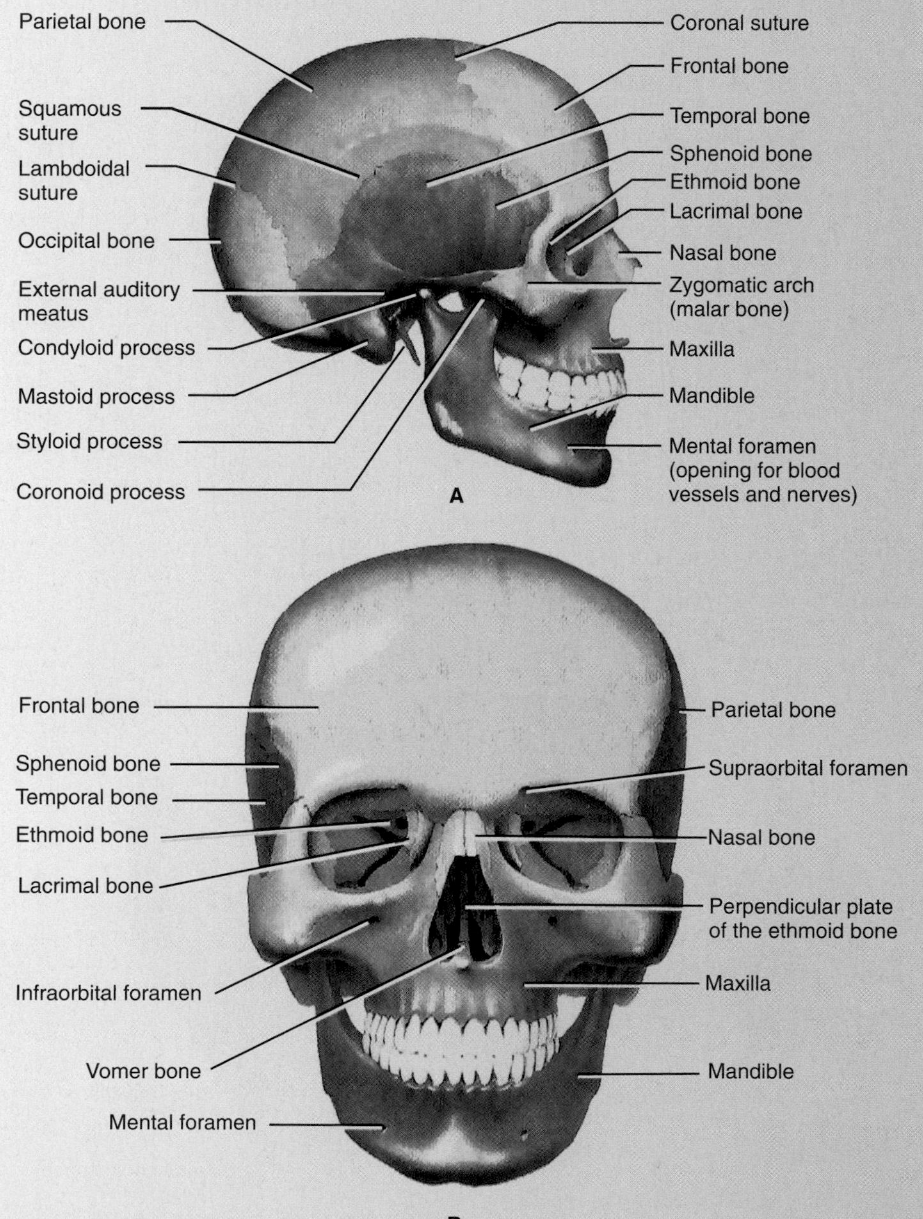

Figure 24-12 Cranial bones: (A) Lateral view, (B) anterior view

(continues)

PROCEDURE 24-1 (continued)

spinal cord. The outermost layer, referred to as dura mater, is composed of tough fibrous connective tissue. The middle layer is the arachnoid, which is a serous membrane. The layer closest to the brain is the pia mater; it contains blood vessels and nerves to provide nourishment to the neural tissue underneath. The space created between the arachnoid mater and the pia mater is referred to as the subarachnoid space, an area that contains cerebral spinal fluid (Figure 24-13).

- The cerebrum represents the largest portion of the human brain. Its surface is covered with convolutions (gyri) that are separated by shallow depressions (sulci) and deep grooves (fissures) into specific lobes, each with complex functions and named for the cranial bone that covers it (Figure 24-14).
- The cerebellum is the second largest structure of the brain and is located posterior to the medulla oblongata and inferior to the cerebrum's occipital lobe. The structure of the cerebellum is similar to that of the cerebrum.
- The brain stem connects the brain to the spinal cord and consists of the midbrain, pons, and medulla oblongata (Figure 24-15).
- The **circle of Willis** (Figure 24-16) is a ring of arteries that give rise to the various branches supplying blood to the brain.
- The cranial nerves are 12 pair of nerves that, with the exception of the first and second, originate in the brain stem (Figure 24-17).

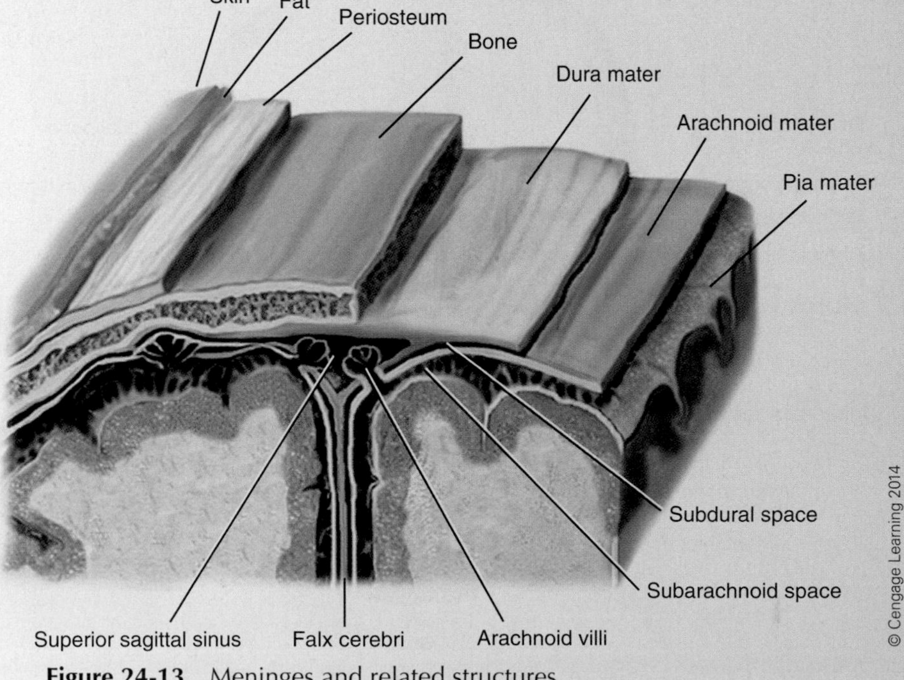

Figure 24-13 Meninges and related structures

PROCEDURE 24-1 (continued)

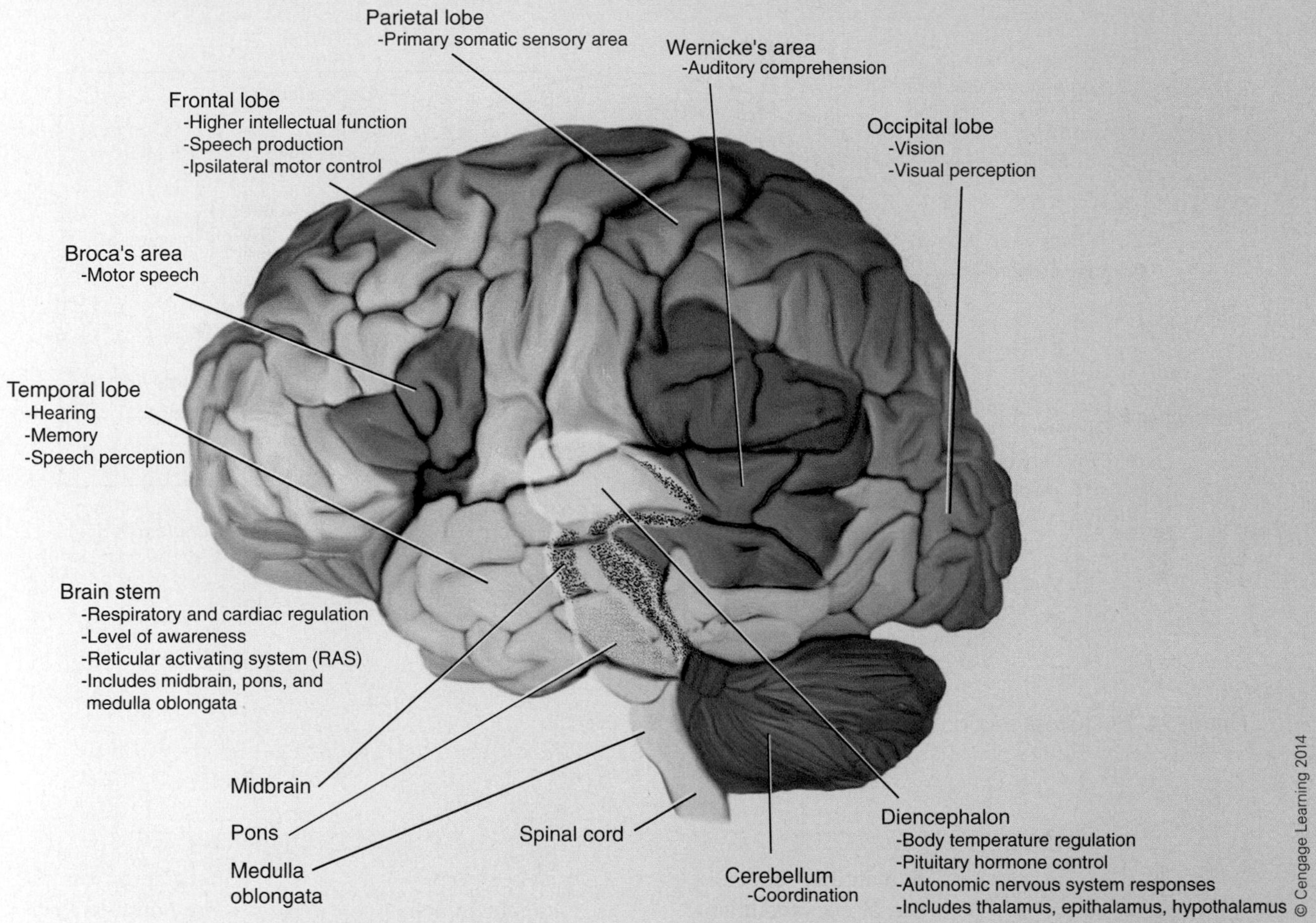

Figure 24-14 Functions of the cerebrum, brain stem, and cerebellum

They are responsible for sensory and motor functions of the body (Table 24-1).

- Primary and secondary neoplasms can affect the nervous system. Primary neoplasms arise from neural tissues or the meninges. Secondary neoplasms are metastatic lesions from other parts of the body.
- Symptoms for patients with intracranial neoplasms include compression of cranial nerves, destruction of brain tissue, irritation of cerebral cortex resulting in seizures, and increased **intracranial pressure**.
  - Benign tumors can usually be excised totally through craniotomy. These tumors include craniopharyngiomas, epidermoids, dermoids, hemangiomas, meningiomas, acoustic neuromas, and pituitary microadenomas. Malignant tumors, such as the astrocytomas or **gliomas**, usually cannot be totally excised, but as much tumor as possible is removed. A brief overview of the types of tumors is shown in Table 24-2.
- Head injuries that require craniotomy include **epidural**

(continues)

PROCEDURE 24-1 (continued)

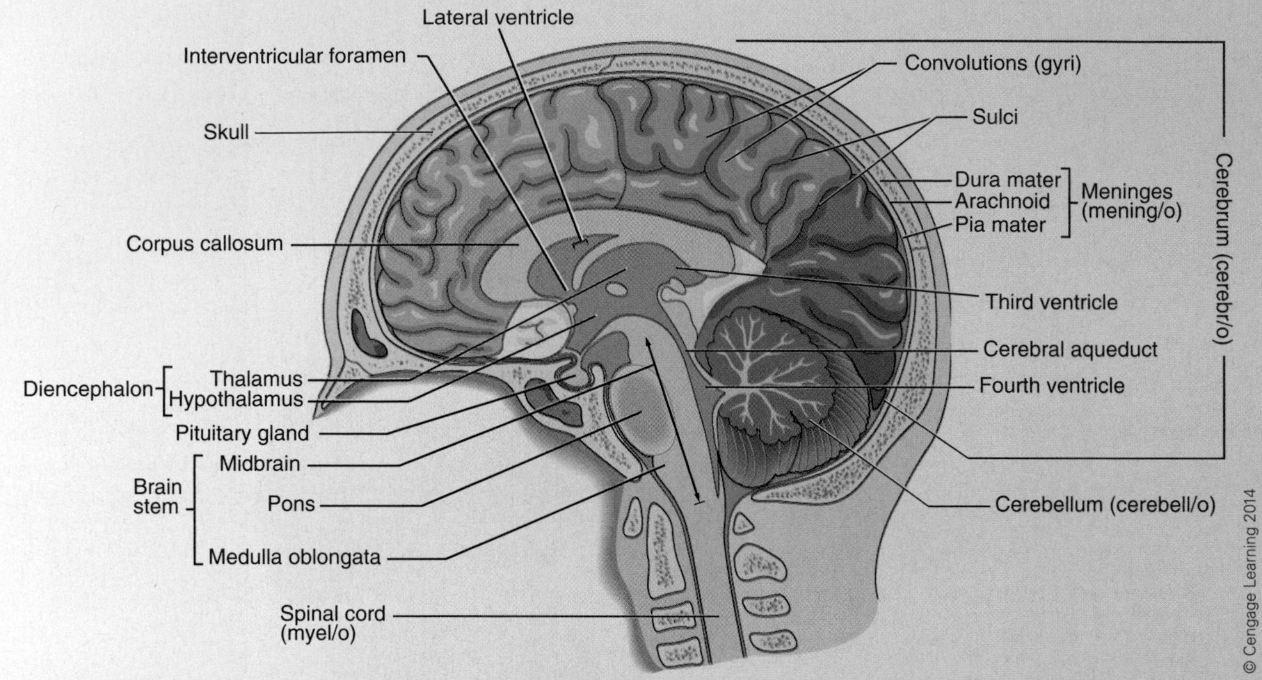

Figure 24-15 Cross-section of the brain

hematoma, subdural hematoma, and brain injury, including hemorrhage.

- A brain **abscess** requires surgical drainage to relieve pressure if the abscess is not treated in its early stages. A brain abscess arises from any of several causative factors, among them secondary infection from a primary infection such as bacterial endocarditis, direct contamination of the brain from a penetrating wound, and bone fragments or debris from traumatic injury.
- An epidural hematoma may result from a fractured skull or blow to the head. The pressure of blood from this arterial bleeding strips the dura away from the skull, causing more bleeding as the tiny veins from the dura to the skull are torn. There may be a symptomless period as the hematoma enlarges to a size sufficient to compress the cerebrum, resulting in a gradual loss of consciousness that can progress to coma and death without surgical intervention. Craniotomy is performed to relieve the resultant pressure of the hematoma, as well as to debride the area and control bleeding.
- A subdural hematoma occurs in relation to severe head injuries (Figure 24-18). When veins bridging the cerebral cortex to the venous sinuses are torn or the cortex is lacerated, hemorrhage occurs.

PROCEDURE 24-1 (continued)

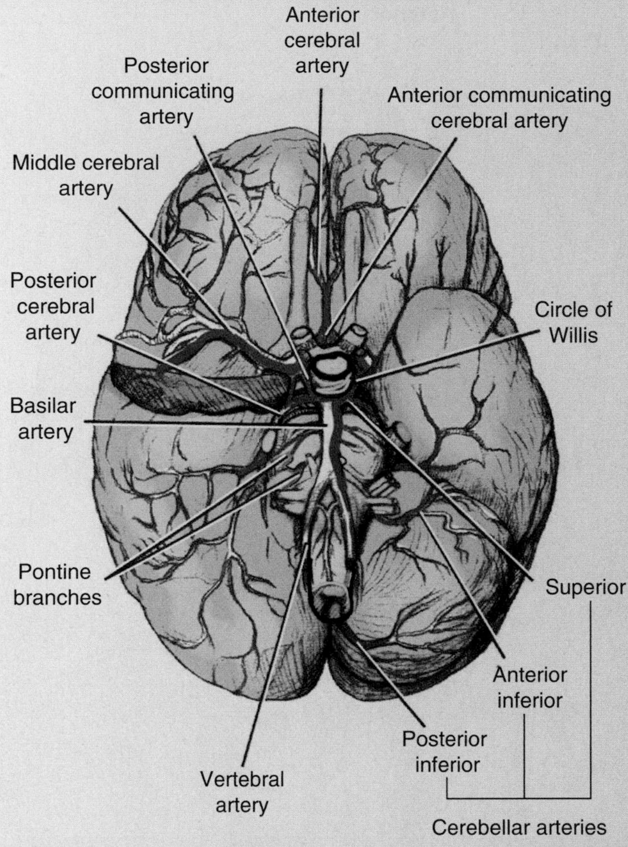

Figure 24-16 Circle of Willis

- Arteriovenous malformations (AVMs) are congenital defects causing abnormal communication between arteries and veins that divert blood from surrounding brain tissue. The surgery involves microsurgical resection of the malformation. Many AVMs have associated aneurysms, increasing the danger of hemorrhage. High-resolution MRI confirms the existence of an AVM, but selective cerebral angiography is usually necessary to identify details of the lesion.

Preoperative Diagnostic Tests and Procedures	• Tumors are diagnosed with CT (Figure 24-19) and high-resolution MRI. • Cerebral angiography is used to show the vascularity of tumors and aids in determining the type of tumor. It is also used for detection of AVMs.
Equipment, Instruments, and Supplies Unique to Procedure	• #10, #15, and #11 knife blades • Marking pen • Rubber bands for Dandy clamps • Glidel wafers for placement into tumor bed • Telfa for specimen • Dressings: inner contact gauze (e.g., petroleum gauze), 4 × 4 sponges, Kerlix

(*continues*)

PROCEDURE 24-1 (continued)

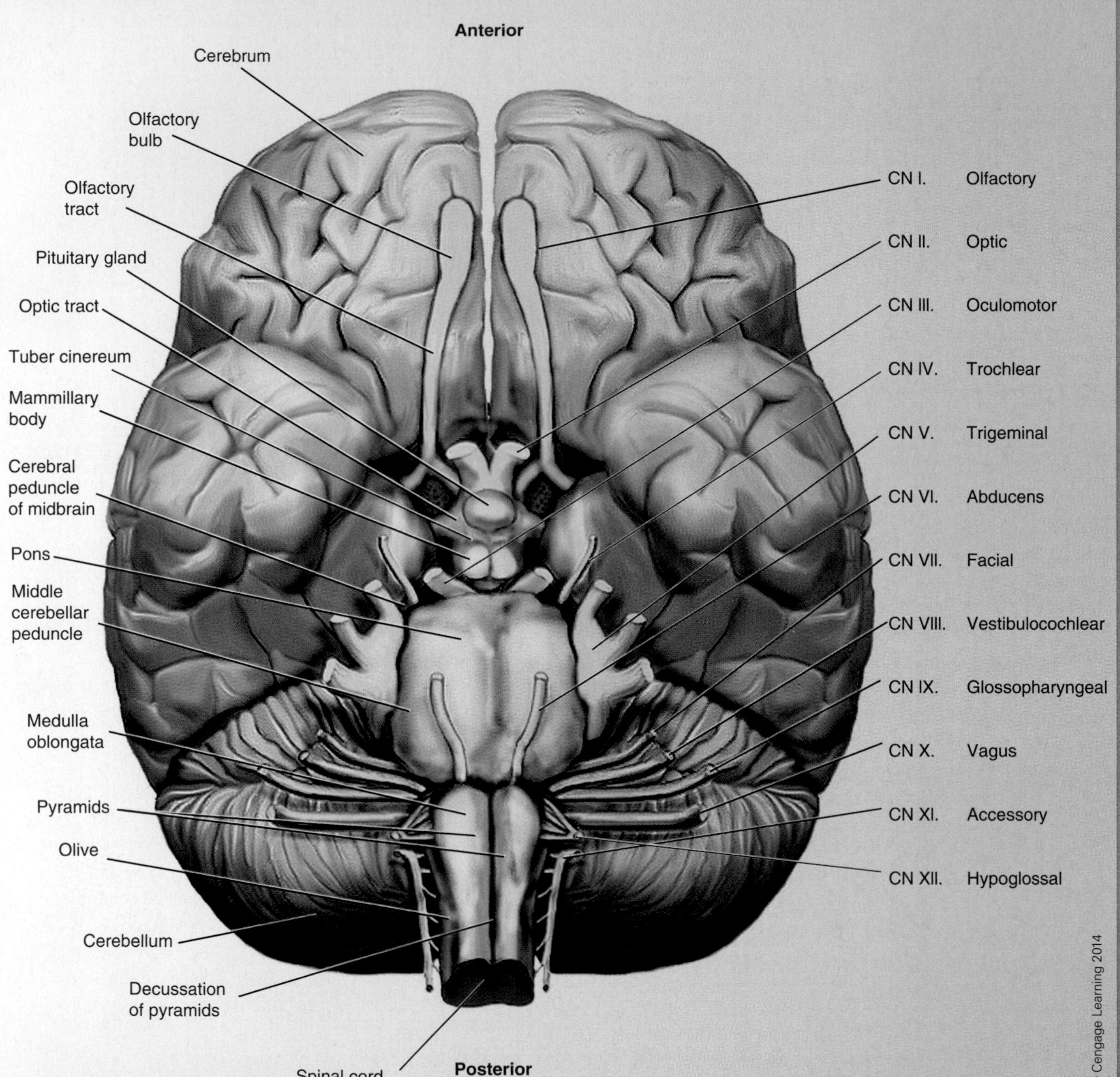

Figure 24-17 Cranial nerves and related structures

Preoperative Preparation

Position

- Depends on approach; see page 1142 "Procedural Considerations"

Anesthesia

- General

Skin prep

- Area around incision site is shaved and hair is saved for patient.
- After the initial prep with iodophor scrub, the surgeon may paint with alcohol and/or iodophor paint.

Draping

- See page 1142 "Procedural Considerations"

Procedure 24-1 (continued)

Table 24-1 Cranial Nerves and their Functions

Nerve (Type)	*Function*	*Target*
Olfactory (sensory)	Smell	Olfactory epithelium
Optic (sensory)	Vision	Retina
Oculomotor (mixed)	Motor: movement of eyeball and eyelid, pupil constriction	Levator palpebra superioris
	Sensory: proprioception	Superior rectus Medial rectus Inferior rectus Inferior oblique
Trochlear (mixed)	Motor: movement of eyeball	Superior oblique
	Sensory: proprioception	
Trigeminal ophthalmic (sensory)	Sensation from skin in region above orbit	Upper eyelid, eyeball, lacrimal glands, nasal cavity, side of nose, forehead
Trigeminal maxillary (sensory)	Sensation from skin in region from orbit to mouth	Mucosa of nose, portion of pharynx, upper lip, upper teeth, palate
Trigeminal mandibular (mixed)	Sensory: sensation	Anterior two-thirds of tongue, lower teeth, mandibular muscles, cheek
	Motor: chewing	
Abducens (mixed)	Sensory: proprioception	Lateral rectus muscle
	Motor: movement of eyeball	
Facial (mixed)	Sensory: proprioception and taste	Anterior two-thirds of tongue, facial, scalp, and neck muscles; lacrimal, sublingual, submandibular, nasal, and palatine glands
	Motor: facial expression, tear and saliva secretion	
Vestibulocochlear (sensory)	Hearing and balance	Organ of Corti, semicircular canals, saccule, utricle
Glossopharyngeal (mixed)	Sensory: blood pressure regulation, taste, proprioception	Posterior third of tongue, pharynx, palate, carotid sinus, carotid body
	Motor: saliva secretion	
Vagus (mixed)	Sensory: sensation from visceral organs, proprioception	Pharynx, larynx, auricle, external auditory meatus, muscles of thoracic and abdominal organs
	Motor: smooth muscle contraction and relaxation, secretion of digestive fluids	
Accessory (mixed)	Sensory: proprioception Motor: swallowing, head movements	Voluntary muscles of pharynx, larynx, palate; sternocleidomastoid, trapezius muscles
Hypoglossal (mixed)	Sensory: proprioception Motor: tongue movement during speech, swallowing	Tongue muscles

(continues)

Procedure 24-1 (continued)

Table 24-2 Intracranial Neoplasms

Disorder	Incidence	Symptoms	Tests	Treatment	Mortality
All intracranial neoplasms		Headache, nausea and vomiting, personality changes, increased intracranial pressure	CT scan, MRI		
Glioma	40% of primary brain tumors—majority are malignant		CT scan, MRI		
Astrocytoma, grades I and II	30% of gliomas; most common ages 30–40	Symptoms present for long period of time	CT scan, MRI	Excision and radiation	
Astrocytoma, grades III and IV	55% of gliomas; most common ages 50–60	Above symptoms present for up to 6 months	CT scan, MRI	Excision and radiation; chemotherapy	Glioblastoma survival is usually less than 12 months
Oligodendroma	5% of gliomas; most common ages 30–50	Spontaneous hemorrhage in 40%; calcification present in 50%; occurs along with astrocytomas in 50%	CT scan, MRI	Excision and radiation; chemotherapy	
Ependymoma	7% of gliomas; most common in children and young adults			Excision and radiation	
Medulloblastoma	Most common in children			Excision; chemotherapy	
Meningioma			Marked enhancement on CT scan or MRI; angiography shows characteristic "blush"	Excision	Benign; these tumors recur if not completely excised
Acoustic neuroma	Increased incidence with familial history of neurofibromatosis	Loss of hearing, headache, vertigo, facial pain	MRI, CT, audiometry	Surgery	
Craniopharyngioma	Most common in the young	Headache, behavioral changes	MRI	Treated conservatively with surgery	Usually benign; location determines postoperative complications
Hemangioblastoma	Involves the cerebellum; occurs primarily in the young		MRI	Surgical excision; postoperative radiation when complete removal is not possible	

PROCEDURE 24-1 (continued)

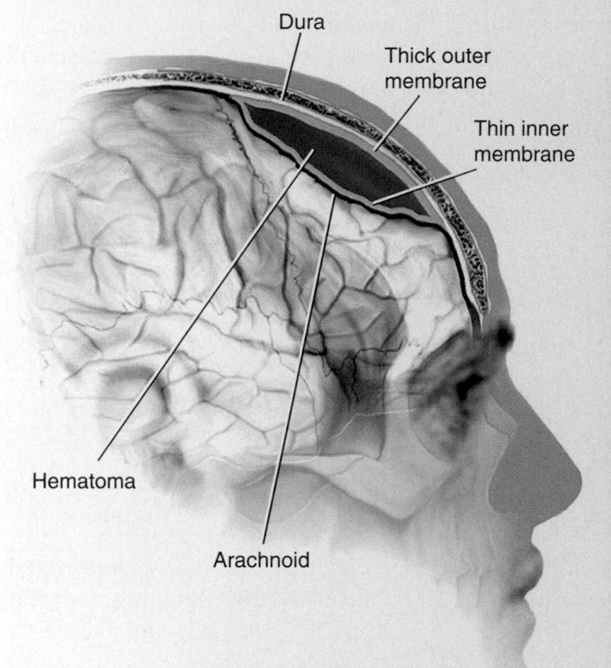

Figure 24-18 Subdural hematoma

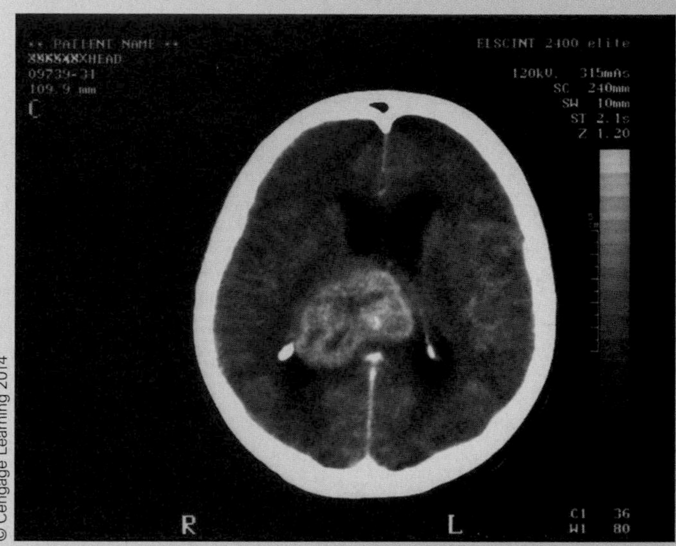

Figure 24-19 CT scan depicting a brain tumor

Practical Considerations	• See page 1142 "Practical Considerations"
Surgical Procedure	1. Digital pressure is applied to each side of the marked incision line for hemostasis, a U-shaped incision is performed, and Raney scalp clips are applied over the upper skin edges. **Procedural Consideration:** Quickly load Raney scalp clips as appliers are received from the surgeon. Bleeding from the scalp can be profuse.
	2. Dandy hemostatic clamps may be placed onto the lower skin edges and secured with rubber bands around the handles. **Procedural Consideration:** Dandy clamps should be passed to surgeon with tips pointing downward.
	3. The galea and periosteum are incised by electrosurgery, and the cranium is exposed. **Procedural Consideration:** Smoke should be evacuated with suction.
	4. After hemostasis has been achieved, the scalp flap is dissected away from the cranium, folded backward over a laparotomy sponge, and secured to the drape for retraction.
	5. Muscle and periosteum are stripped away from the cranium with a periosteal elevator and retracted.

(continues)

PROCEDURE 24-1 (continued)

6. Two or more burr holes are made into the cranium with an air-powered burr, such as the Midas Rex, or an electric-, battery-, or air-powered cranial perforator. Occasionally, burr holes are drilled manually with a Hudson brace and D'Errico bit (Figure 24-20).

   Procedural Consideration: Irrigate drill bit with saline to counteract heat generated by friction and to remove bone dust.

7. After the holes are drilled, they may be enlarged with a double-action rongeur or Kerrison rongeur. Any bleeding from the edges of the burr holes is controlled by bone wax and neurosurgical sponge.

   Procedural Consideration: Bone wax balls may be pressed against the tip of a #4 Penfield dissector and passed to the surgeon.

8. A small, straight bone curette is used to carve away the inner table and expose the dura.

9. The dura around the burr hole is separated from the cranium by a #3 Penfield dissector to prevent tearing of the dura mater when the flap is turned (Figure 24-21).

10. The cranium between the burr holes is cut with an electric-, battery-, or air-powered craniotome saw with dural guard attachment. Occasionally, the cranium is manually cut with a Gigli saw.

    Procedural Consideration: Irrigate the craniotome with saline.

11. After each burr hole has been connected, the bone flap is carefully lifted away from the dura with a periosteal elevator (Figure 24-22).

12. If muscle has been left attached, the bone flap is covered with a moistened laparotomy pad and retracted in a manner similar to the scalp flap; otherwise, it is removed.

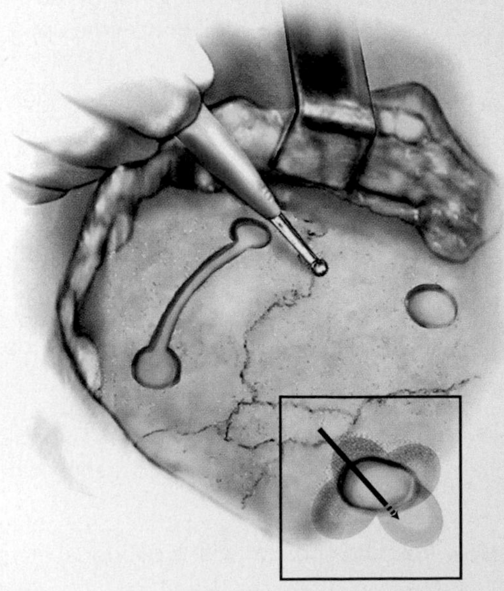

Figure 24-20 Bur holes

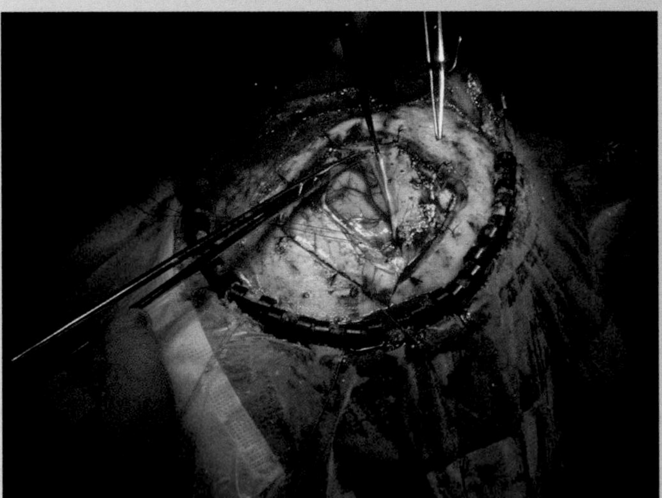

Figure 24-21 Opening dura

PROCEDURE 24-1 (continued)

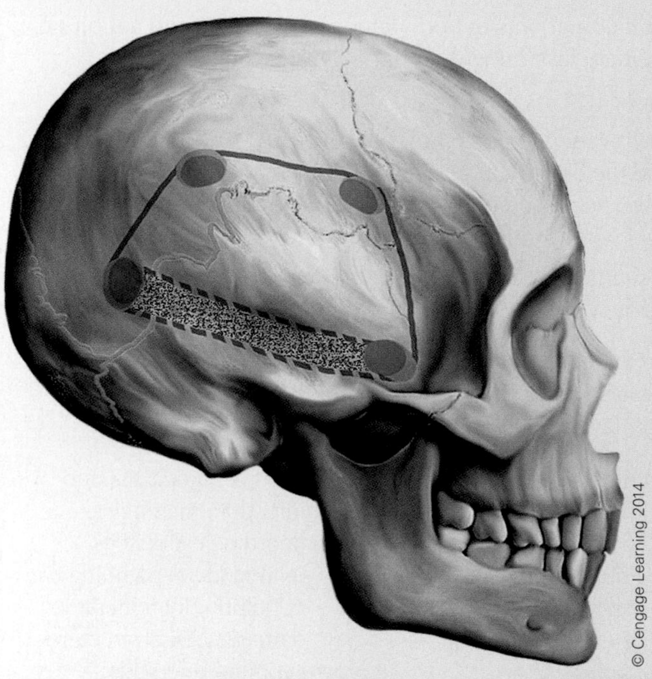

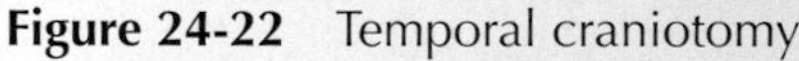

Figure 24-22 Temporal craniotomy

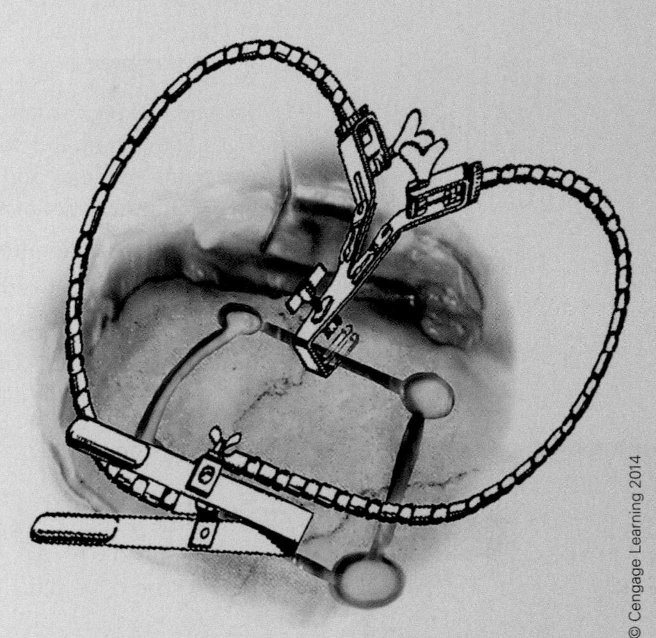

Figure 24-23 Self-retaining brain retractor

Procedural Consideration: Place bone flap in basin on back table to soak in betadine solution or normal saline and antibiotic.

13. Bleeding around the bone edges is controlled with bone wax; bleeding from the dura is controlled with the bipolar forceps and thrombin-soaked Gelfoam.
14. Holes may be drilled along the edges of the cranial defect with an air drill for epidural tacking to prevent postoperative epidural dead space.
15. Dural traction may be necessary to pull the dura away from the brain surface before incising. This is achieved with 4-0 braided nylon or dural hook.
16. A small incision is made into the dura with #11 or #15 blade and extended with Metzenbaum or dura scissors.
17. Cottonoid patties are placed under the dura with bayonet forceps as the dura is incised to protect the delicate brain tissue underneath, and 4-0 dural traction sutures are placed along the dural edges and tagged with mosquito hemostats for retraction.
18. Brain spoons are placed and held manually or attached to the Leyla-Yasargil self-retaining retractor (Figure 24-23).

    Procedural Consideration: Brain spoons should be moistened with saline before handing to the surgeon.
19. The pathological condition is treated, and hemostasis is achieved with warm saline irrigation, Surgicel, thrombin-impregnated Gelfoam, and bipolar cautery.

    Procedural Consideration: The microscope may be needed at this time.

(*continues*)

Procedure 24-1 (continued)

20. The brain is irrigated with copious amounts of body-temperature saline and antibiotic, and the dura is closed in an airtight fashion with a running 4-0 braided nylon or silk suture.

21. The Midas Rex or small air drill is used to place holes at strategic locations along the edges of the cranial defect and the bone flap, and the flap is secured to the cranium with titanium plates and screws. Some surgeons may prefer to wire the bone flap to the cranium with stainless steel wire.

    Procedural Consideration: A stainless steel brain spoon or periosteal elevator placed between the cranium and the dura prevents the drill from penetrating brain tissue.

22. A Hemovac drain is placed in the epicranium and brought up through the scalp through a small stab wound and secured with a 0 or 2-0 silk suture on a cutting needle. The wound is closed in layers.

Postoperative Considerations

Immediate Postoperative Care

- Care must be taken not to drop the head when removing it from the pin fixation device.
- Operative personnel should take precautions when moving the patient to the transport stretcher or ICU bed. The patient will have monitoring lines, urinary catheter and drainage bag, wound drains, or other important lines that can be easily pulled.

Prognosis

- Depends on the pathological situation and the condition the patient was in preoperatively
- Complications: Wound infection, meningitis, neurological deficits related to the pathological condition, intraoperative damage to vital structures, subdural or epidural hematoma, or intracerebral hemorrhage

Wound Classification

- Class I: Clean

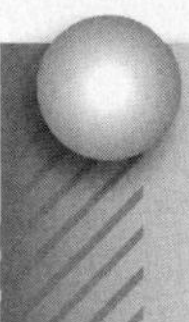

Pearl of Wisdom

Make sure saline irrigation is always body temperature. Always test the temperature of the saline before handing it to the surgeon. Keep close track of the amount of irrigation used.

Procedure 24-2 Craniotomy for Aneurysm Repair

Surgical Anatomy and Pathology

- Aneurysms are weak spots in the walls of arteries that over time will balloon out from the arterial wall, causing them to thin sufficiently. They can rupture, causing severe bleeding in and around the brain.
- Cerebral aneurysms are typically found at points of bifurcation in the arteries of the circle of Willis.
- Patients with cerebral aneurysm are generally asymptomatic until rupture unless the defect is large enough to press on surrounding structures, such as the optic chiasma or optic nerves. If the aneurysm ruptures, the patient will typically present with signs of meningeal irritation, focal signs of cerebral damage, and

PROCEDURE 24-2 (continued)

	uniformly bloody spinal fluid. • Cerebral aneurysms are typically found at points of bifurcation in the arteries of the circle of Willis. More than 85% of aneurysms occur in the carotid circulation, 30% of these arising from the internal carotid near the origin of the posterior communicating artery. Others arise from the anterior communicating artery, and some are positioned at the first major branch point of the middle cerebral artery. They often	occur in multiples, and vary in size from a small pea to a plum. • Patients with cerebral aneurysm are generally asymptomatic until rupture unless the defect is large enough to press on surrounding structures, such as the optic chiasma or optic nerves. If the aneurysm ruptures, the patient will typically present with signs of meningeal irritation, focal signs of cerebral damage, and uniformly bloody spinal fluid. Angiography will reveal the exact size	and location of the aneurysm. • The goal of surgical treatment for cerebral aneurysm is to isolate the aneurysm from the parent vessel by placing a specially designed clip across the neck of the aneurysm. If the aneurysm cannot be clipped in such a manner, the sac of the defect may be reinforced with synthetic materials such as polymethyl methacrylate or mesh gauze, or one of the feeding vessels may be ligated.
Preoperative Diagnostic Tests and Procedures	• Angiography will reveal the exact size and location of an aneurysm.		
Equipment, Instrumentation, and Supplies Unique to Procedure	• Aneurysm repair requires the use of microsurgical instruments with aneurysm clips and applicators, such as	those designed by Yasargil. • Carotid set for carotid artery exposure should be available for hemorrhage control.	• Papaverine • Aneurysm clips (temporary and permanent) • Refer to supplies for craniotomy
Preoperative Preparation	• Same as for craniotomy		
Practical Considerations	• Same as for craniotomy		
Surgical Procedure	1. The scalp and bone flaps are turned, and the dura is opened and retracted with dural sutures. **Procedural Consideration:** Follow the steps listed for craniotomy for entry into the cranium.		
	2. The Sylvian fissure is split by bipolar cautery dissection for separation of the frontal and temporal lobes.		

(continues)

Procedure 24-2 (continued)

3. Brain spoons are placed and secured to the Leyla-Yasargil or Greenberg self-retaining retractor. The optic nerves and optic chiasma are visualized.

4. The operating microscope is brought in and positioned, and the feeding vessels and the neck of the aneurysm are exposed with microsurgical dissection of surrounding structures.

   Procedural Consideration: Aneurysm clip appliers should be ready for loading and temporary clips should be available for use. Aneurysm clips will be selected at this time.

5. A temporary aneurysm clip may be utilized to test eventual placement of a permanent clip or to occlude the parent vessel if rupture occurs and the neck of the aneurysm cannot be visualized for clip placement (Figure 24-24).

   Procedural Consideration: Papaverine may be necessary to prevent vasospasm.

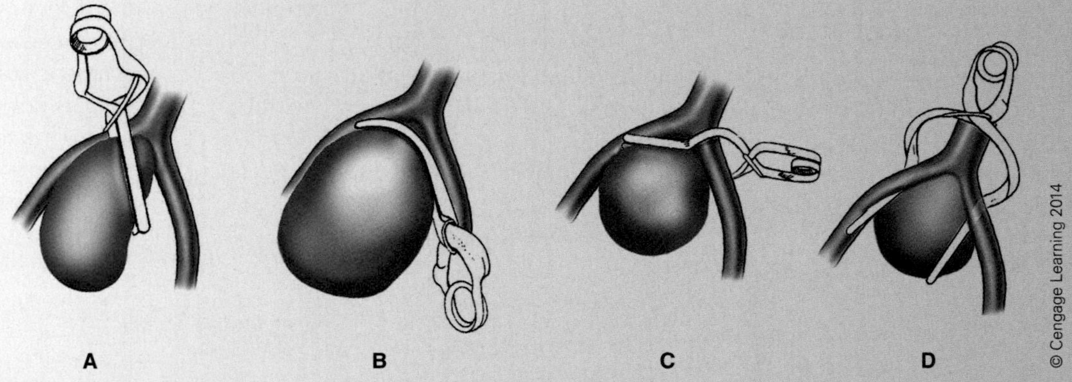

Figure 24-24 Cerebral aneurysm with clip (showing different configurations and types of clips)

6. After the patient's blood pressure has been lowered by the anesthesiologist, an angled, curved, or straight aneurysm clip is applied across the neck of the defect.

   Procedural Consideration: Once an aneurysm clip has been opened, it cannot be closed and used again.

7. The blood pressure is slowly raised, and the clip is checked for proper positioning and leakage. If necessary, an intraoperative angiogram can be performed with a C-arm.

8. The dura is closed, a drain is placed, and the bone flap and scalp flaps are secured in the usual manner.

   Procedural Consideration: Follow closure steps for craniotomy.

Postoperative Considerations

Immediate Postoperative Care

- Postoperative bleeding and intracranial pressure are monitored closely by ICU or recovery room personnel.
- See care for craniotomy.

Prognosis

- No complications: 24–48 hours monitoring in ICU; discharged after a few days. Overall prognosis is good to excellent.
- Complications: See those for craniotomy.

Wound Classification

- Class I: Clean

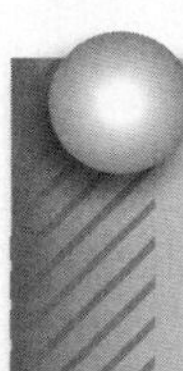

Pearl of Wisdom

Cerebral aneurysm procedures illustrate a common problem for the surgical technologist. The opening and closing portions of the craniotomy procedure are mostly concerned with bone, while the middle portion is concerned with soft neural tissue. In this case, the concern is microscopic. The surgical technologist must organize for wide variations in instrumentation, equipment, and passing technique.

Procedure 24-3 Cranioplasty

Surgical Anatomy and Pathology	• See information for craniotomy. • Cranioplasty is performed to repair defects in the skull resulting from a previous cranial procedure, trauma, or congenital anomaly. • Cranioplasty is also performed to relieve headache, prevent secondary injury to the brain, and for cosmetic effect.
Preoperative Diagnostic Tests and Procedures	• CT scans produce a computer-generated duplication of the defect.
Equipment, Instruments, and Supplies Unique to Procedure	• Methyl methacrylate • Closed mixing system • Antibiotic irrigation
Preoperative Preparation	**Position** • Depends on location of defect **Anesthesia** • General **Skin prep** • See that for craniotomy. **Draping** • See that for craniotomy.
Practical Considerations	• Repair of the defect can be performed immediately in clean cases. In contaminated cases, 6 months should pass before repair. • If cerebral edema or infection is a concern after craniotomy, the bone flap may not be replaced in the cranium immediately. Also, a flap can be removed to relieve intracranial pressure. The flap can be sterilized and stored in a bone bank within the facility or stored under the subcutaneous layer in the patient's abdomen for future placement. Refer to the craniotomy section for the procedure to reattach the bone flap using microplates and screws. • Titanium mesh and/or methyl methacrylate are the most common materials used for cranioplasty.
Surgical Procedure	1. The scalp flap is incised over the defect as for a craniotomy.
	2. If additional bone fragments exist due to injury, they are removed with a rongeur. **Procedural Consideration:** The surgical technologist should have a laparotomy sponge ready to clean the rougeur. Bone fragments should be kept for specimen.

(continues)

PROCEDURE 24-3 (continued)

3. The edges of the defect are trimmed to form a saucer-like ledge using rongeurs.

   Procedural Consideration: See Step 2.

4. Wound is irrigated with warm saline solution.

   Procedural Consideration: The surgeon may also use antibiotic irrigation.

5. The methyl methacrylate is prepared and dropped into a sterile bag. The wet cement is molded over the cranial defect.

6. The cement is removed from the defect to allow for it to harden.

   Procedural Consideration: Cool saline should be used on the plate while exothermic reaction takes place.

7. Once cool, excess material is trimmed away from the plate with bone rongeurs or cut with a saw.

8. A craniotome is sued to smooth the edges and allow the plate to blend gradually with the skull.

9. Holes are drilled in the plate and periphery of the skull defect. Sutures or small stainless steel wires are used to secure the plate.

10. The wound is irrigated and closed in routine fashion.

Postoperative Considerations

Immediate Postoperative Care

- Patient is transported to the ICU, where cardiac and neurological functions are monitored every hour for 24 hours.

Prognosis

- No complications: Moved to floor after 24 hours in the ICU. Discharged 3–4 days after procedure.
- Complications: Infection, wound breakdown, intracranial hemorrhage, sunken cranioplasty

Wound Classification

- Class I: Clean

PROCEDURE 24-4 Craniosynostosis Repair

Surgical Anatomy and Pathology

- **Craniosynostosis** is a premature closure of the cranial sutures of an infant. These sutures should remain open up to the age of 2 to allow for brain expansion. If the sutures fuse too early, the brain may be damaged because of insufficient space for growth.
- The sagittal suture is the most commonly affected suture, creating a long and narrow skull. Bilateral coronal suture craniosynostosis creates a short, high head. Unilateral coronal suture involvement flattens the frontal bone and orbit.
- Surgical intervention involves a linear strip craniectomy.

Preoperative Diagnostic Tests and Procedures

- Clinical diagnosis is made from the misshapen appearance of the head and is confirmed with radiographic studies.

PROCEDURE 24-4 (continued)

Equipment, Instruments, and Supplies Unique to Procedure	• Overbed warmer during induction and IV line placement		
Preoperative Preparation	**Position** • Supine using headrest **Anesthesia** • General	**Skin prep** • See that for craniotomy.	**Draping** • See that for craniotomy.
Practical Considerations	• Surgery is generally performed on the infant between 6 weeks and 6 months of age.	• Room temperature should be elevated to maintain infant's normal body temperature.	• Refer to Special Populations for considerations pertaining to pediatric patients.
Surgical Procedure	1. An incision is made midway between the anterior and posterior fontanelles from ear to ear posterior to the pinna.		
	2. The scalp is elevated off the skull with the periosteal elevator. **Procedural Consideration:** Care is used to leave the pericranium attached to the skull to minimize bleeding.		
	3. A burr hole is made using the Midas Rex. **Procedural Consideration:** The surgical technologist should irrigate the bone dust.		
	4. A craniotome is used to cut anteriorly to the anterior fontanelle on each side of the sagittal suture.		
	5. A Leksell rongeur is used to cut across the sagittal suture and connect the burr holes. **Procedural Consideration:** A sponge should be available to collect bone fragments from rongeur.		
	6. A Cobb periosteal elevator is used to dissect the sagittal suture off the underlying dura.		
	7. A burr hole is placed at the asterion on each side. The craniotome is used to make a cut just posterior to the coronal suture.		
	8. The parietal bone is fractured, leaving the periosteum intact.		
	9. The skin is closed with 3-0 and 4-0 absorbable sutures.		
Postoperative Considerations	**Immediate Postoperative Care** • Patient is transported to the ICU; stays for 1–2 days. • Possible blood transfusion for blood replacement	**Prognosis** • No complications: 3–7 days in hospital. Some require a molded helmet to guide skull development.	• Complications: Infection of brain, brain swelling, damage to brain tissue **Wound Classification** • Class I: Clean

Procedure 24-5 Craniectomy for Steriotactic Procedures

Surgical Anatomy and Pathology	• See information for craniotomy. • Craniectomy is the permanent removal of a section of the cranium using a burr hole to gain access to underlying structures. • Allows for the precise localization of subcortical targets without creating large scalp and bone flaps. • Intracranial masses (tumor, hematoma, abscess) and vascular malformations (arteriovenous malformations) can be successfully treated using stereotactic techniques. • Biopsy of intracranial tumors for treatment planning has been the primary focus of this technique, but stereotactic techniques are currently being utilized for the surgical treatment of movement disorders such as Parkinson's disease.
Preoperative Diagnostic Tests and Procedures	• MRI and CT scan • Scan is used to map intracranial lesions with pinpoint precision.
Equipment, Instruments, and Supplies Unique to Procedure	• Stereotactic system (Figure 24-25) • Computer equipment with monitor • Anspach or Midas Rex power instruments with attachments, or cranial perforator and craniotome
Preoperative Preparation	**Position** • See that for craniotomy. **Anesthesia** • Monitored anesthesia care **Skin prep** • See that for craniotomy. **Draping** • See that for craniotomy. • Sterile sleeve for navigation arm

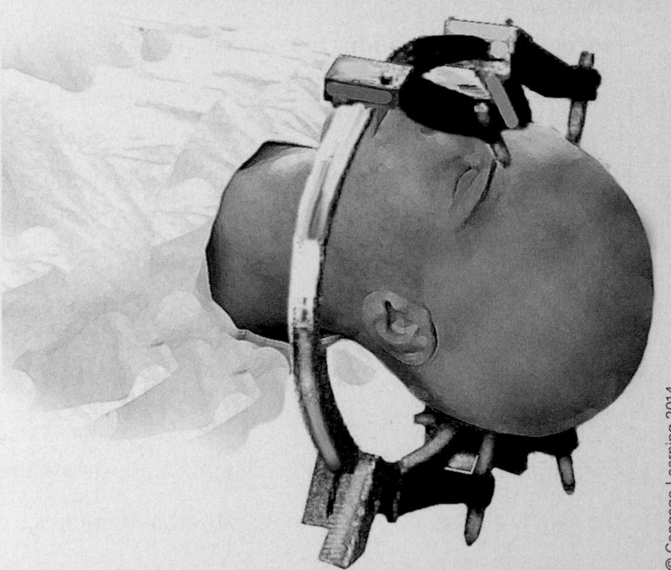

Figure 24-25 Stereotactic frame

Procedure 24-5 (continued)

Practical Considerations	• Stereotactic cranial surgery, in conjunction with CT, allows a probe to be guided to a specific location within the brain with minimal damage to normal neural tissue. • Fiducials are placed on bony landmarks or points around the skull before a preoperative MRI or CT scan. They are left in place for the operating room.
Surgical Procedure	1. Skull clamp is placed and an image-guided navigation arm is attached to the skull clamp. **Procedural Consideration:** This provides a fixed reference point. The arm should be out of the way for the surgical team to ensure it will not be bumped from its fixed point, disrupting the navigation system.
	2. The location of the fiducials is registered onto the computer, allowing the computer to align the preoperative images. The monitor shows the location of the navigation probe.
	3. After the registration process is complete, the fiducials are removed and the area is prepped and draped for surgery.
	4. An incision is made in the scalp with a #15 blade down to the skull (Figure 24-26A).
	5. The scalp is retracted with a small self-retaining retractor or scalp clips (Figure 24-26B).
	6. The periosteum is retracted with a periosteal elevator.

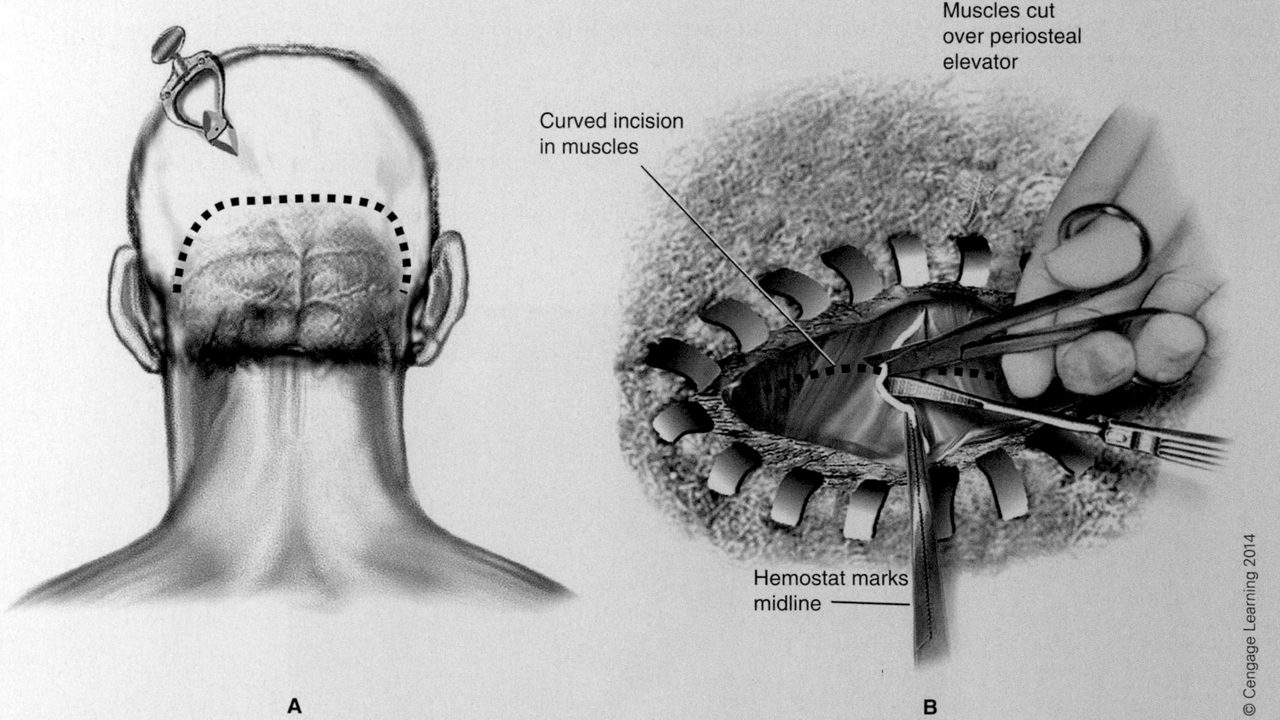

Figure 24-26 Posterior fossa craniectomy: (A) Transverse horseshoe incision is made over the occipital bone, (B) scale clips are placed and the muscle is cut

(continues)

PROCEDURE 24-5 (continued)

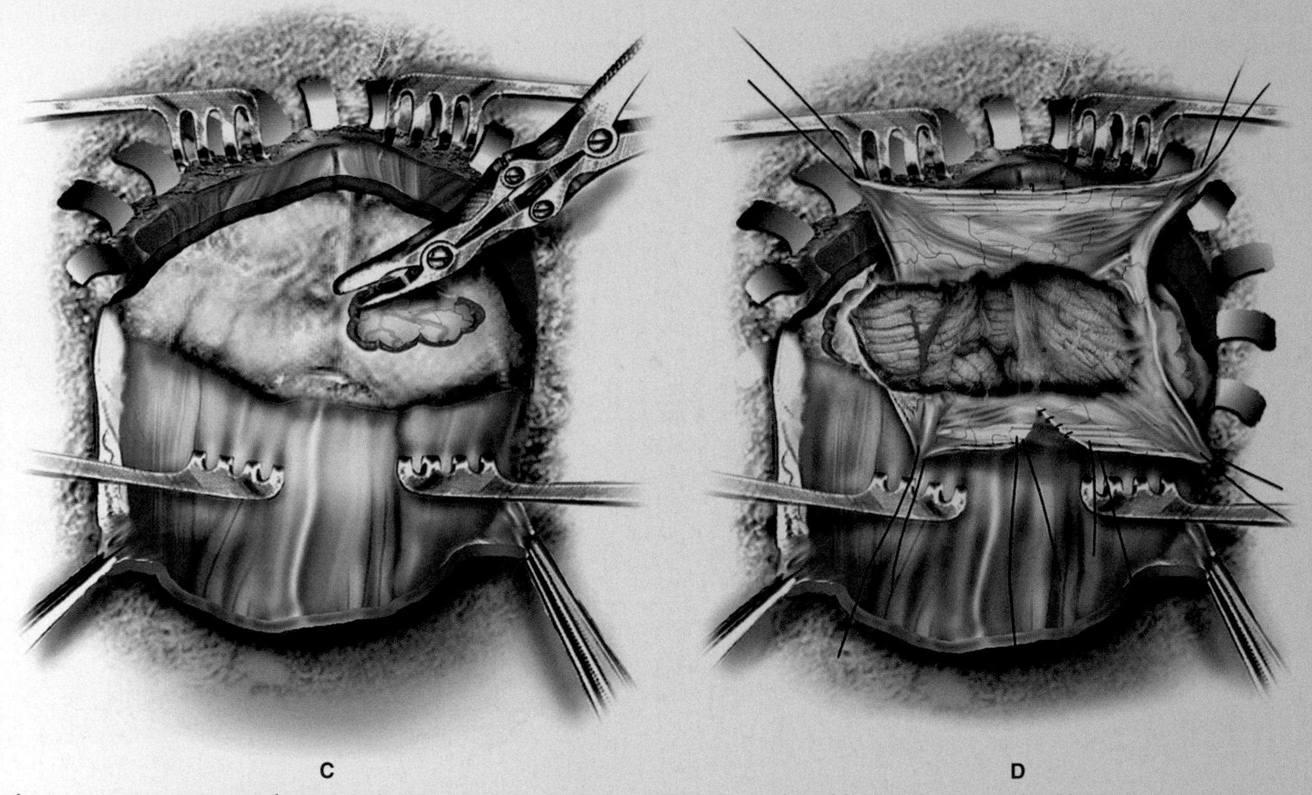

Figure 24-26 Posterior fossa craniectomy: (C) Retractors are positioned and bone is removed with a rongeur, (D) dura is opened and retracted, exposing the cerebellar hemisphere

7. A drill is used to create burr hole.
8. The burr hole is enlarged with a Kerrison rongeur (Figure 24-26C).
9. The dura is elevated with dural hook and incised with a #11 blade (Figures 24-26D and 24-27).

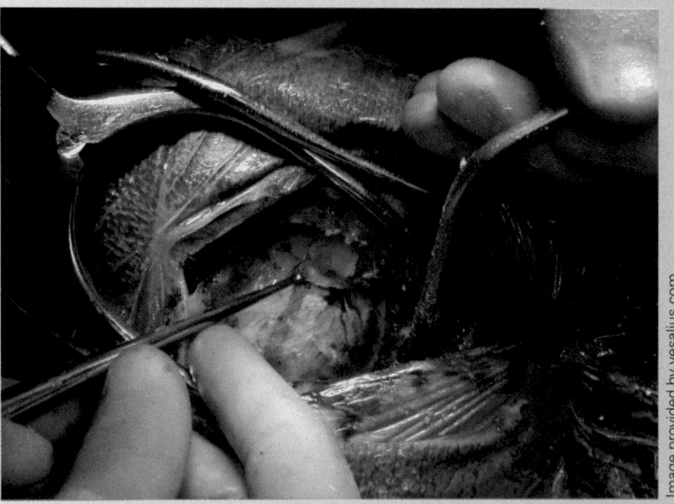

Figure 24-27 Dural exposure

Procedure 24-5 (continued)

10. Hollow cannulas, coagulating electrodes, cryosurgical probes, wire loops, and other biopsy instruments may be introduced to repair or excise a pathological condition.
11. Wound is closed in layers.

    Procedural Consideration: The bone is not replaced after a craniectomy.

Postoperative Considerations

Immediate Postoperative Care

- Patient is transported to the PACU.

Prognosis

- No complications: Patient will remain in the hospital for 2–3 days.
- Prognosis depends on outcome of procedure.
- Complications: See those for craniotomy.

Wound Classification

- Class I: Clean

Procedure 24-6 Ventriculoperitoneal Shunt Placement

Surgical Anatomy and Pathology

- Within the brain are a series of interconnected canals and cavities called ventricles. The first two ventricles are referred to as the lateral ventricles (right and left). The two large ventricles that are located in each cerebral hemisphere connect to the smaller third ventricles, by way of the interventricular foramen (foramen of Monro). The third ventricle connects to the even smaller fourth ventricle, located in the brain stem anterior to the cerebellum, by way of the cerebral aqueduct (aqueduct of Sylvius). The fourth ventricle is continuous with the central canal of the spinal cord (Figure 24-28).

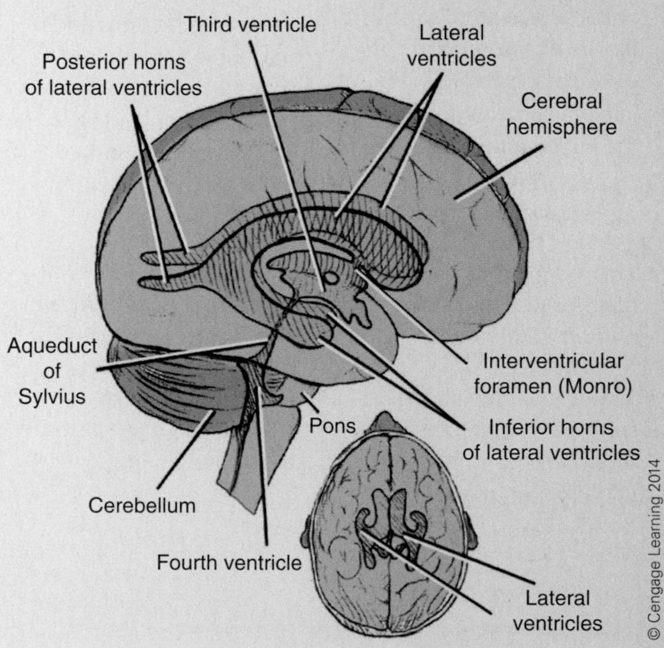

Figure 24-28 Ventricular system

(continues)

PROCEDURE 24-6 (continued)

	• The ventricles are filled with a clear, colorless fluid containing small amounts of protein, glucose, lactic acid, urea, and potassium, as well as a relatively large amount of sodium chloride. The fluid, known as cerebral spinal fluid (CSF), helps to support and cushion the brain and spinal cord and stabilizes the ionic concentration of the central nervous system. It also acts to filter the waste products of metabolism and other substances that diffuse into the brain from blood. • CSF is produced by specialized capillaries called choroid plexuses. The choroid plexuses are located in the lateral ventricles and the third and fourth ventricles. However, the choroid plexuses located in the lateral ventricles produce the largest amount of CSF. • CSF flows through the interventricular canal into the third ventricle. From the third ventricle, CSF flows through the aqueduct of Sylvius into the fourth ventricle, where a small portion enters the subarachnoid space through the fourth ventricular wall. CSF flows from the fourth ventricle into the central canal of the spinal cord and around the cord's surface, eventually surrounding the brain and spinal cord. • The CSF is reabsorbed by fingerlike projections of the arachnoid that project into the dural sinuses called arachnoid villi. This reabsorption occurs at approximately the same rate that CSF is formed, allowing for a constant CSF pressure. • The obstruction of the flow of CSF through the ventricular system and into the subarachnoid space (noncommunicating hydrocephalus), an increase in the amount of CSF normally produced (communicating hydrocephalus), or the improper absorption of CSF by the arachnoid villi causes CSF pressure to rise within the cranial cavity. Obstructive hydrocephalus in the infant may result from a congenital tumor or hemorrhage at the foramen of Monro, aqueduct of Sylvius, or the canal of exit from the fourth ventricle. • Childhood hydrocephalus may be a result of meningitis, tumors, hemorrhage, or aqueductal stenosis. Hydrocephalus in adults may be caused by obstructive tumors, meningitis, or hemorrhage. • Infants with hydrocephalus have an enlarged head circumference and present with enlarged and distended scalp veins. Increased intracranial pressure may cause optic atrophy.
Preoperative Diagnostic Tests and Procedures	• Hydrocephalus is diagnosed with history and physical examination and confirmed with CT scan. Ventriculography and ventriculoscopy may be employed if results are inconclusive.
Equipment, Instruments, and Supplies Unique to Procedure	• Scales to weigh soiled sponges to measure blood loss • Heating blankets • Midas Rex or Anspach systems to create a small burr hole • Tunneling device • Minor procedures set to place catheter into peritoneum • Shunt system of surgeon's choice • Manometer

Procedure 24-6 (continued)

Preoperative Preparation	**Position** • Supine with head turned slightly **Anesthesia** • General **Skin prep** • Area for cranial incision site is shaved. • Prep should extend from cranial incision site to the abdomen.	• After initial prep with iodophor scrub, the surgeon may paint with alcohol and/or iodophor paint. **Draping** • Towels for square draping from head to abdomen are secured with plastic adhesive drape.	• Nonfenestrated drape may be placed and holes cut in locations for incisions, split sheets may be placed with tails up and down, or fenestrated drape may be extended with scissors.
Practical Considerations	• Eyes and ears should be protected from prep solutions.	• Pediatric patients can quickly become hypothermic.	• Make sure diagnostic films are in the OR.

Surgical Procedure

1. A small linear incision is made, and a burr hole is drilled in the occipital or parietal bone with Hudson brace and D'Errico bit, cranial perforator, or Midas Rex or Anspach burr.

   Procedural Consideration: Shunt may be soaked in a saline and antibiotic mixture before use.

2. The dura is nicked and coagulated, and a ventricular catheter with stylet is placed into the posterior lateral ventricle. The stylet is removed, and a small bit of CSF is taken as specimen.

   Procedural Consideration: The surgical technologist should be loading the stylet into the catheter as the dura is nicked. A rubber shod may be necessary to clamp the end of the catheter closed after it is placed to prevent CSF loss. Intracranial pressure may be monitored with manometer.

3. The proximal portion of the ventricular catheter is connected to the reservoir. A tunneling device is used to make a tunnel from the burr hole to the abdomen, and the distal end of the shunt system is threaded under the skin and soft tissues to an incision in the abdomen.

   Procedural Consideration: Tunneling devices may be hollow CV tunnelers, Sarot clamps, or uterine dressing forceps. Long, heavy silk sutures will be used to draw the shunt system under the skin to the abdomen. For ventriculoatrial shunts, an incision is made in the neck and the internal or external jugular vein is exposed. A tunnel is made from the burr hole to the neck incision and the distal end of the shunt is threaded through the tunnel into the opened jugular vein and into the right atrium (Figure 24-29).

4. The peritoneum is exposed and opened, and the abdominal catheter is placed into the peritoneal cavity and secured with a purse-string suture. The wounds are irrigated with antibiotic solution and closed after patency of the system is verified.

5. The wounds are irrigated and the incisions are closed.

(*continues*)

PROCEDURE 24-6 (continued)

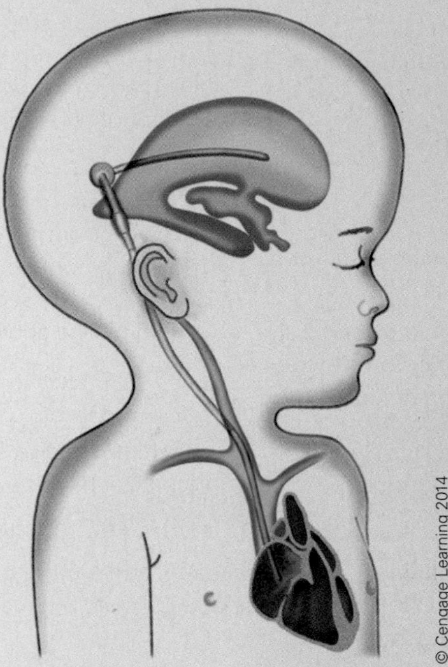

Figure 24-29 Ventriculoatrial shunt

Postoperative Considerations

Immediate Postoperative Care

- Incisions areressed with 4 × 4 dressing sponges.
- Check patency of shunt before patient leaves OR.

Prognosis

- No complications: Good if hydrocephalus has not been prolonged and severe
- Complications: Infection; children can outgrow shunt, requiring revision.

Wound Classification

- Class II: Clean-contaminated

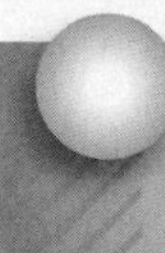

PEARL OF WISDOM

There are many different kinds of shunts. They vary in their pumping technique and the amount of pressure required to open the valve. The surgical technologist should know the technical details of all the shunts used in his or her facility.

Postoperative Considerations

PROCEDURE 24-7 Ventriculoscopy

Surgical Anatomy and Pathology

- See VP shunt.
- Patients considered for ventriculoscopy have enlarged lateral and third ventricles and normal-sized fourth ventricle.

Procedure 24-7 (continued)

Preoperative Diagnostic Tests and Procedures	• MRI
Equipment, Instruments, and Supplies Unique to Procedure	• Endoscopic equipment generally includes the following (specifics will vary according to surgeon's preference): • A 4.2-mm single-use disposable neuroendoscope with a 13-cm rigid shaft, or flexible neuroendoscope • Irrigation pump: Ringer's solution kept at body temperature is often used. The surgeon may want continuous irrigation at a very low flow rate (15 mL/min) or intermittent flow. • A #14 French peel-away sheath to cannulate the ventricle; the endoscope is then inserted through the sheath. • A #3 French Fogarty balloon catheter to enlarge the fenestration in the floor of the third ventricle
Preoperative Preparation	**Position** • Supine position with the head in pin traction, slightly elevated to minimize the loss of CSF and entry of air **Anesthesia** • General anesthesia **Skin prep** • See that for craniotomy. **Draping** • See that for craniotomy.
Practical Considerations	• Contraindications for the procedure include age (younger than 6 months; however, studies are being conducted on the effectiveness of ventriculoscopy on infants younger than 6 months) • Cause of hydrocephalus • Previous shunt placement, which can cause small ventricles • Meningitis
Surgical Procedure	1. The scalp incision is made and a 6–10-mm burr hole is created.
	2. The dura mater is opened.
	3. A #14 French peel-away catheter is used to cannulate the lateral ventricle. The stylet is removed, and the two peel-away tabs of the catheter are peeled downward and secured to the drapes, usually with staples to stabilize the catheter and prevent it from penetrating deeper into the ventricle. Another alternative is the use of an endosopic sheath with trocar; after insertion, the sheath is held in place with two Leyla retractor arms.
	4. The endoscope is passed through the sheath into the lateral ventricle.
	5. The scope is maneuvered into the third ventricle and the basilar artery is identified.
	6. At this point the surgeon may perform a ventriculostomy to reestablish the free flow of cerebral spinal fluid between the ventricles and subarachnoid space.
	7. A wire is inserted through the 2-mm working channel of the scope and used to create the initial opening in the floor of the third ventricle.
	8. The wire is removed and the #3 Fogarty balloon catheter is inserted through the opening in the floor. The balloon is slightly inflated to widen the opening/stoma to approximately 5 mm.
	9. The endoscope and sheath are removed.
	10. Gelfoam is packed into the burr hole and the scalp is sutured.

(*continues*)

Procedure 24-7 (continued)

Postoperative Considerations

Immediate Postoperative Care

- Patient is transported to the PACU.

Prognosis

- No complications: Patient remains in the hospital for 2 days. A CT scan is performed prior to patient discharge. A follow-up MRI is performed within 2 months of surgery.
- Complications: Fever, bleeding, and short-term memory loss

Wound Classification

- Class I: Clean

Procedure 24-8 Transphenoidal Hypophysectomy

Surgical Anatomy and Pathology

- The pituitary gland is about the size of a grape and is located at the base of the brain within the sella turcica, a small bony depression in the sphenoid bone.
- The pituitary gland is connected to the hypothalamus by a stalk called the infundibulum. The hypothalamus releases neurosecretory substances that stimulate the anterior pituitary gland to release hormones.
- The pituitary gland is considered the master gland.
- Tumors of the pituitary gland are usually benign, and are often responsible for the overproduction of specific pituitary hormones.
- There are two basic approaches in the surgical treatment of pituitary tumors.
  - Craniotomy is indicated if the tumor is large and pressing against the optic nerves and is similar to the technique previously described.
  - **Transphenoidal** resection is indicated for smaller tumors (Figure 24-30).

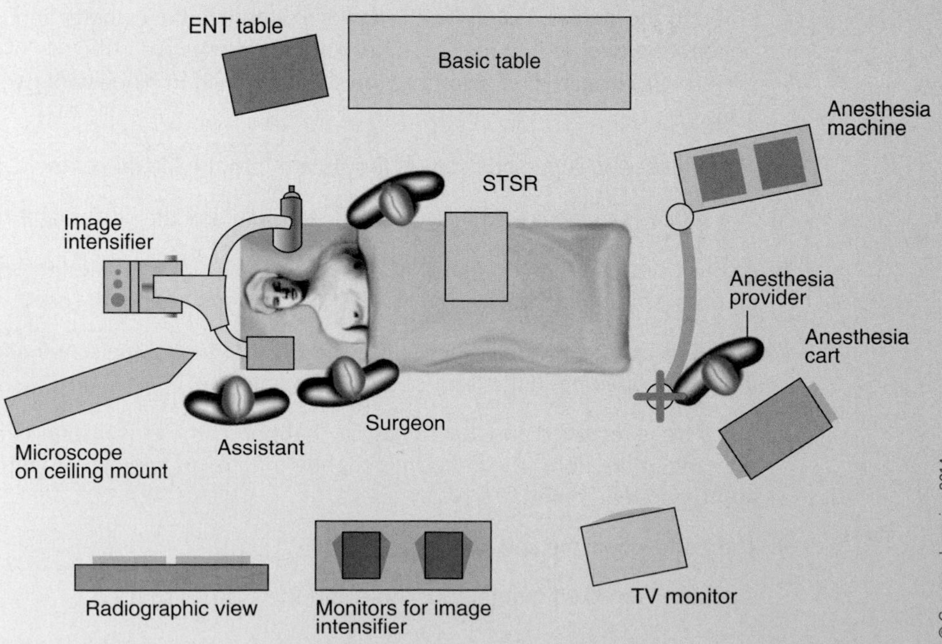

Figure 24-30 OR setup for transphenoidal hypophysectomy

PROCEDURE 24-8 (continued)

	• The sella turcica is easily approached through the sphenoid sinus, and complete tumor removal is possible for most tumors. • The transphenoidal approach to pituitary tumor removal offers several advantages. The cranium is not opened, so recovery time is much shorter. Pain may be considerably less for the patient, as well. Complications associated with manipulating the brain and vital structures are avoided.
Preoperative Diagnostic Tests and Procedures	• Endocrine function test • MRI
Equipment, Instruments, and Supplies Unique to Procedure	• Operating microscope and drape • C-arm and image intensifier with monitor and drape • Craniotomy set • Transphenoidal set • Nasal set (available) • Minor set for graft procurement • Drapes: towels, split sheet, medium sheet • Dressings: contact layer and 4 × 4 gauze for leg incision; nasal packing • Cocaine solution
Preoperative Preparation	**Position** • Semi-Fowler's **Anesthesia** • General **Skin prep** • The face and thigh are prepped with an antiseptic solution. The mouth and nose are usually not prepped. **Draping** • The thigh is square draped with towels and adhesive drape. • The face is draped with a split sheet to the mouth with tails up, and a flat sheet across the brow.
Practical Considerations	• The nasal mucosa is typically injected with lidocaine with epinephrine for hemostasis. Cocaine may be applied to the nasal mucosa. • An image intensifier that has been covered with a sterile drape is positioned in the lateral tilt with the beam aimed directly into the sella turcica.
Surgical Procedure	1. The surgeon injects the nasal mucosa and gingiva with lidocaine and epinephrine for hemostasis.
	2. The surgeon may approach the sella turcica with an incision in the upper gum margin just under the upper lip, or through the nasal cavity. **Procedural Consideration:** The surgical technologist should know which approach the surgeon will take in order to have the proper instrumentation available.
	3. An assistant may take the fascial graft from the thigh while the pituitary is being exposed. **Procedural Consideration:** The graft should be kept on the back table in saline to prevent it from drying out.
	4. After elevation of soft tissues by the periosteal elevator, the nasal septum is exposed and the mucosa is separated from septal cartilage. **Procedural Consideration:** The C-arm and microscope should be properly draped for visualization of the sella turcica.

(*continues*)

Procedure 24-8 (continued)

5. A special bivalved speculum designed for this procedure is inserted. After cartilage is resected and the floor of the sphenoid sinus is removed, the floor of the sella turcica is viewed. (Figure 24-31A)

   Procedural Consideration: All nasal instruments are kept isolated in a seperate Mayo stand.

6. The microscope is brought in, and the sella turcica is punched with the Kerrison rongeur and osteotome (Figure 24-31B).

   Procedural Consideration: The surgical technologist may be asked to gently tap on a small osteotome at the base of the sella turcica.

7. The dura is incised and the tumor is removed with pituitary curette, dissector, enucleator, and suction.

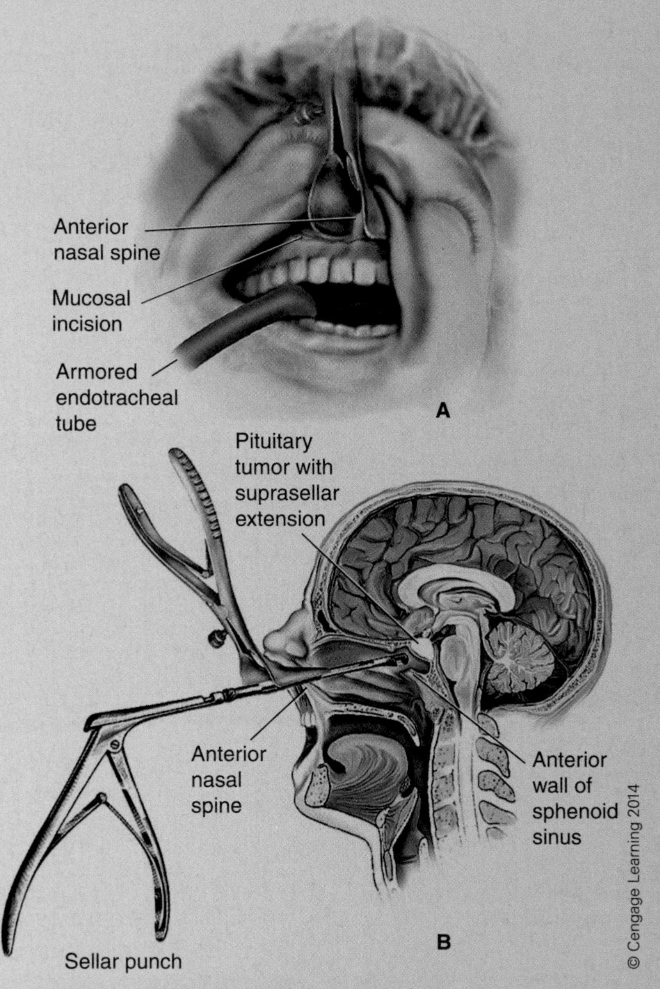

Figure 24-31 Transphenoidal approach to hypophysectomy: (A) Bivalved speculum is inserted, (B) floor of the sphenoid is removed with a sellar pouch

Postoperative Considerations

Immediate Postoperative Care

- Nasal packing with petroleum gauze will be the only dressing for the head. Petroleum gauze and 4 × 4 pads are typically used to dress the thigh incision.
- Patient is transported to the PACU.

Prognosis

- No complications: Discharged from hospital once packing is removed with no bleeding, usually 3–4 days.
- Complications: Wound infection; CSF leakage; meningitis

Wound Classification

- Class II: Clean-contaminated

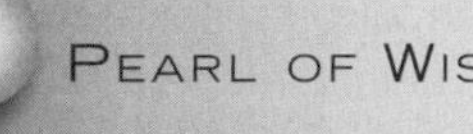

Pearl of Wisdom

Prepare separate Mayo stands for the nasal/oral phase and the surgical phase. Be sure that nasal speculums are not placed on the wrong Mayo stand, thereby contaminating the sterile field.

SPINAL PROCEDURES

Spinal procedures can be performed by either a neurosurgeon or an orthopedic surgeon. Neurosurgeons are almost always involved in cervical procedures, but both intervene in lumbar procedures. There are some differences in specialties; however, the commonalities for spinal procedures are discussed below.

Practical Considerations

- Make sure CT or MRI scans, or plain film studies are in the room before the procedure begins.
- Always test drills and saws before the procedure.
- Cut Surgicel and Gelfoam into same sizes of cottonoids. Gelfoam is usually soaked in thrombin.
- A 10-mL syringe filled with saline should be available to flush the Frazier suction tip as it becomes clogged with debris.
- Keep close track of all small countables.

Procedural Considerations

- Spinal procedures can be performed using a variety of positions depending on the approach. Positioning can be complex to accomplish proper alignment of the spine.
    - For spinal procedures performed in the prone position, the patient is anesthetized on the transport stretcher and rolled onto either the Wilson or Andrews frame or chest rolls. The Mayfield horseshoe headrest may replace the OR table's head section for cervical procedures.
    - Cervical procedures are still occasionally performed in the sitting position, with the head secured by pin fixation and arms extended onto padded armboards.
    - Anterior approaches to the spine are performed in the supine position, and the patient may be turned to the prone position to complete the procedure.
    - The anterior thoracic spine may be approached via thoracotomy in the lateral position.
- Certain spinal procedures may require electrophysiological monitoring.
- The operative area is prepped with iodophor scrub to the proper perimeters and blotted with a sterile towel. The circulator or the surgeon then applies iodophor paint.
- Draping begins with four folded towels placed by the surgeon. An adhesive drape often follows, and then the laparotomy or thyroid sheet is positioned.
- Two Mayo stands are often used, one for bone and one for soft tissue instruments.

PROCEDURE 24-9 Lumbar Laminectomy for Diskectomy with Spinal Fixation

Surgical Anatomy and Pathology

- The vertebral column of a normal adult is comprised of 33 vertebrae and is part of the axial skeleton. These 33 individual bones are separated into five regions. They are, from superior to inferior, cervical, thoracic, lumbar, sacral, and coccygeal (Figure 24-32).
- There are seven bones in the cervical region. The uppermost, or first, cervical vertebra (C1) is the atlas, which supports the skull. The second cervical vertebra (C2) is the axis, which is fused with the body of the atlas; it is responsible for allowing rotation, flexion, and extension of the head. The remaining five vertebrae (C3–C7), which are similar to each other in their structure, function in a supportive role of the skeleton.
- There are 12 bones in the thoracic region (T1–T12). They are larger and stronger than the cervical vertebrae and are the main support for the thorax, as each of the 12 ribs forming the thoracic cage articulates with each of the thoracic vertebrae.
- There are five lumbar vertebrae (L1–L5). The lumbar vertebrae have two main responsibilities. They provide support for a major portion of the weight of the body and allow for much of the flexibility of the trunk. Thus, the lumbar vertebrae are very large and have heavy bodies.
- The sacrum is formed by five individual bones that fuse to form one bone in adulthood. The sacrum is considered part of the pelvic girdle.
- The coccyx consists of four fused vertebrae. The coccyx serves as an important attachment for

(continues)

PROCEDURE 24-9 (continued)

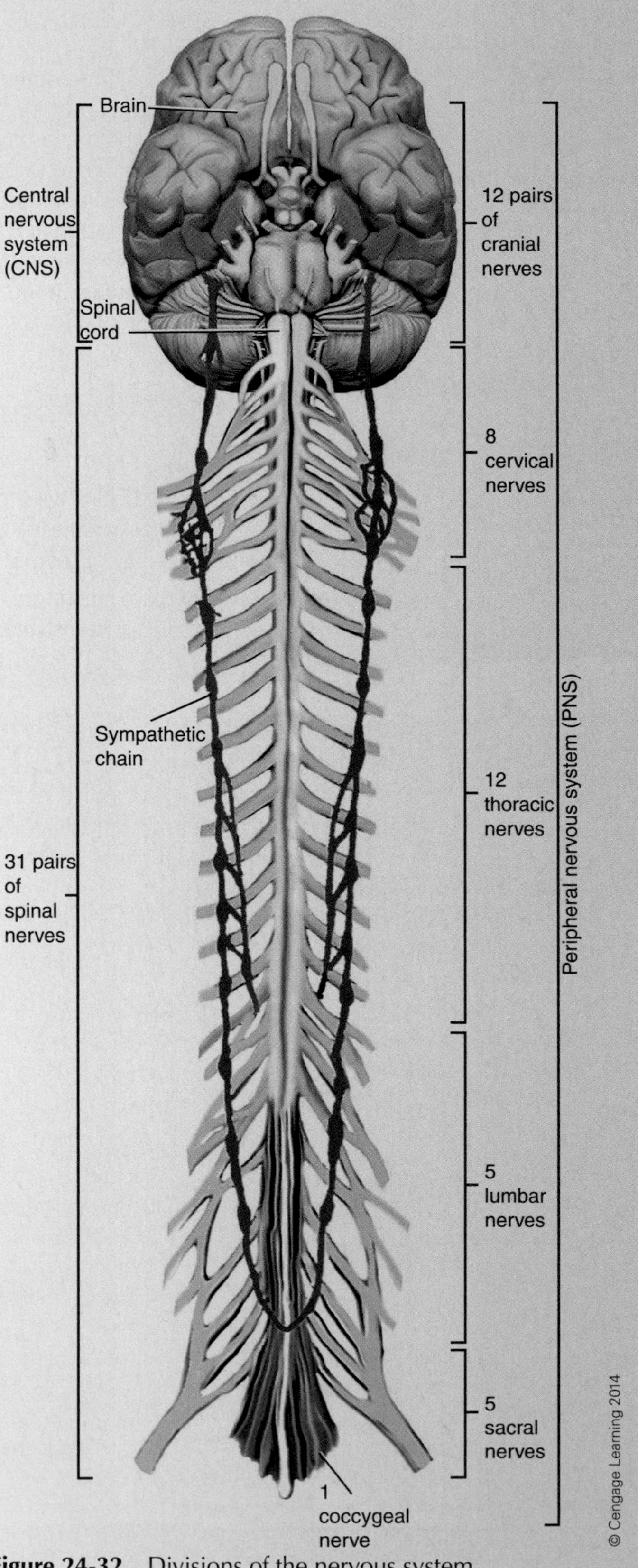

Figure 24-32 Divisions of the nervous system

PROCEDURE 24-9 (continued)

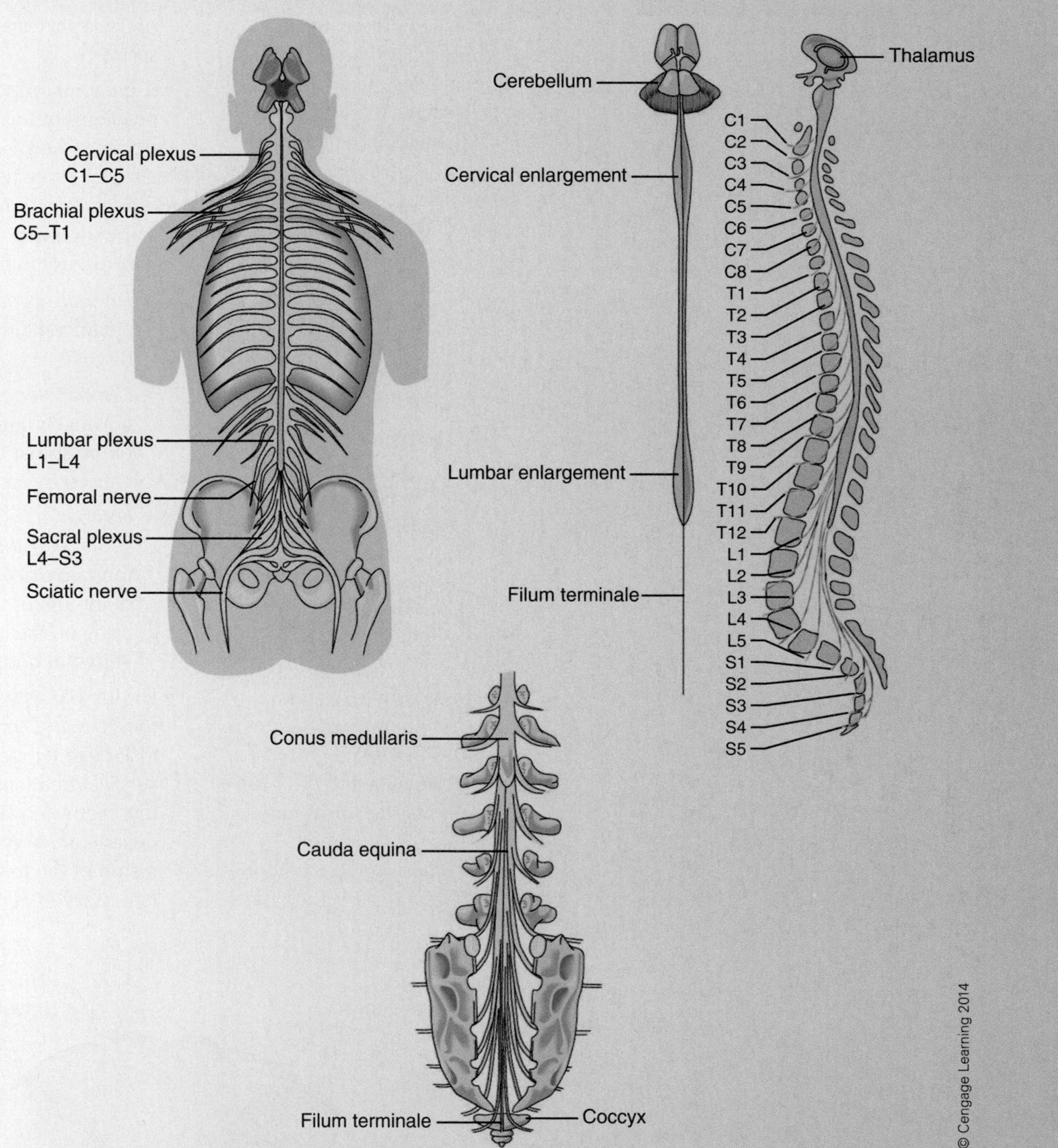

Figure 24-33 Spinal cord and spinal nerves

several hip and pelvic muscles (Figure 24-33).

- Each vertebra has a body or centrum anteriorly. Posteriorly, a neural arch encircles the opening for the spinal cord called the vertebral foramen. As the neural arch extends from the body on each side of the vertebra, it is referred to as the pedicle. The lateral extensions of the pedicles are called the transverse processes, which support the facets. The facets provide the articulating surfaces between the vertebrae. The bony surface extending posteriorly

(continues)

Procedure 24-9 (continued)

from the facet is the lamina. Laminae that extend from each side of the vertebra connect to form the spinous process of each vertebra.

- The spinal nerves pass through openings between adjacent vertebrae. These openings are referred to as the intervertebral foramina.
- Intervertebral disks are located between the vertebrae. The disk itself is comprised of fibrous connective tissue. Its tough outer layer is termed the annulus fibrosis, and the soft core is called the nucleus pulposus. The intervertebral disks bear most of the stress, in the form of pressure from gravity (body weight and lifting objects), that is transmitted to the vertebral column (Figure 24-34).
- When disk material extrudes through the annulus due to degeneration or trauma in the lumbar region, nerve roots may be compressed (Figure 24-35). This compression can, in severe cases, result in paraplegia or quadriplegia. In less severe cases, it may cause sensory loss in the upper extremities.
- In some cases, the disk does not extrude, but simply degenerates. This causes narrowing of the joint space, causing the cartilage at the end plates of the adjacent vertebrae to wear more quickly. Sometimes an **osteophyte**, or bony spur, may develop due to this increased mobility. When osteophytes form within the spinal canal, the cord may be compressed by the bony structure. This formation of osteophytes is called spondylosis.
- A great majority of the problems in this region occur in the L4–L5 and L5–S1 intervertebral spaces. Problems associated with lumbar disk disease include:
    - *Lumbar spondylosis:* advanced lumbar disk disease
    - *Lumbar stenosis:* advanced constriction of the spinal canal caused by spondylosis
    - *Lumbar spondylolisthesis:* forward displacement of the upper vertebral body on the lower vertebral body
- For lumbar as well as thoracic and cervical disk degeneration, surgical treatment involves removal of the degenerated disk and fusion of the joint when necessary. This is usually

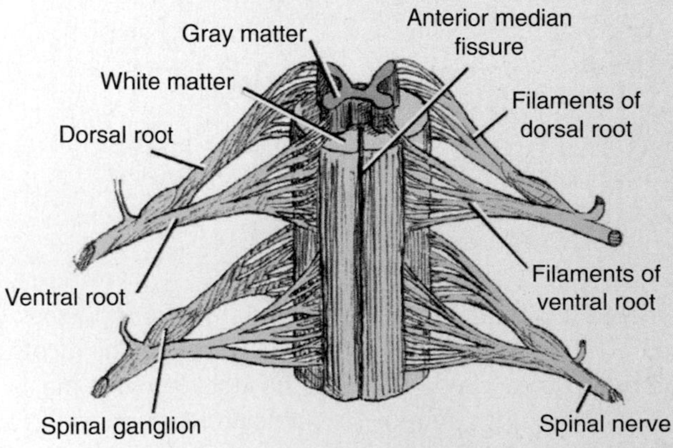

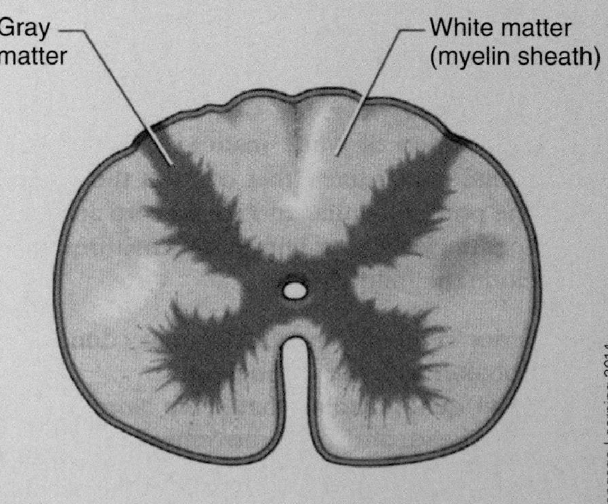

Figure 24-34 Spinal cord: (A) Anterior view, (B) cross-section view—white and gray matter

PROCEDURE 24-9 (continued)

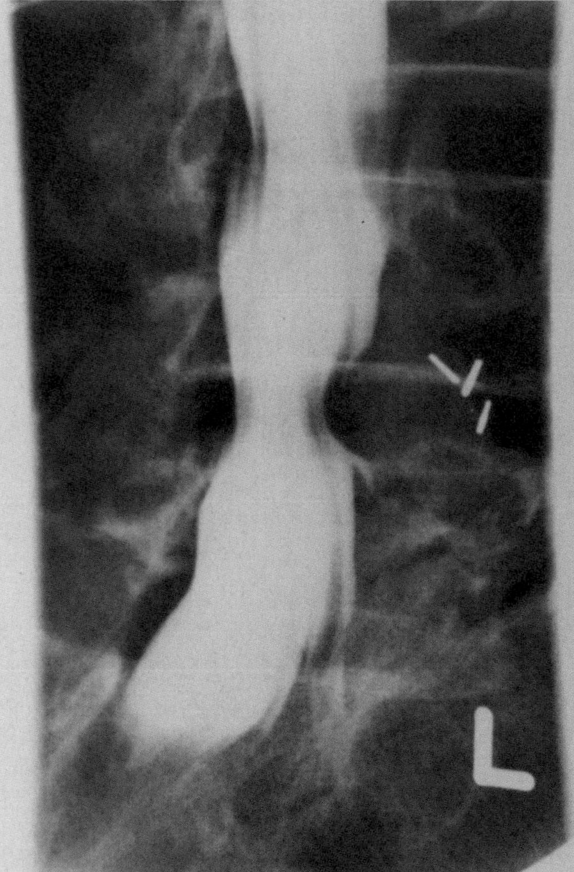

Figure 24-35 Lumbar myelogram depicting herniated disk

	achieved with a posterior approach and laminectomy. • Laminectomy for diskectomy is a common surgical procedure for the decompression of a nerve root that has been impinged by an extruded fragment of disk material	in the cervical, thoracic, or lumbar region of the spine. Due to its weight-bearing configuration, the lower lumbar region is affected the most often. Surgical treatment is often necessary to remove the extruded fragment and	**decompress** the nerve root. • Laminectomy or hemilaminotomy is also the surgical approach for spinal cord tumor and to provide exposure for insertion of pain control infusion pumps, cordotomy, and rhizotomy.
Preoperative Diagnostic Tests and Procedures	• For diagnosis, plain radiographic films of the spine are used to identify	bony changes in the lumbar region. CT or MRI scanning and	myelogram are useful in identifying lumbar disk herniations.
Equipment, Instruments, and Supplies Unique to Procedure	• Laminectomy set • Minor procedures set for soft tissue	• Fusion instruments listed previously • Hemovac drain	• Dresssings: Inner contact layer, 4 × 4 pads, ABD • Kerlix for Taylor retractor

(continues)

Procedure 24-9 (continued)

Preoperative Preparation	**Position** • Prone for bilateral laminectomy • Lateral can be utilized for unilateral laminectomy. • Fusion: Hip slightly elevated if needed for graft procurement	**Anesthesia** • General **Skin prep** • Depends on the level of the spine to be operated on; however, as an example of the L4-L5 region is operative site skin prep	is lower border of scapula to lower border of buttocks and bilaterally **Draping** • Square draped with towels and laparotomy drape
Practical Considerations	• When positioning on Wilson frame, make sure bony prominences are well padded and	breasts or penis and testicles are not impinged.	• The Wilson frame should be lowered completely before positioning.

Surgical Procedure

1. The interspace of the affected levels of the spine is approached posteriorly via a midline or paramedian incision with a #10 blade on a #3 knife handle.
2. The paraspinous muscles are separated from the spinous processes and laminae in the area with a periosteal elevator or osteotome. As the muscles are separated, sponges (Ray-tec opened and folded lengthwise) are packed around the margins to assist with hemostasis and to aid in blunt dissection.
3. After the muscles have been reflected, a retractor is placed to provide exposure.

   Procedural Consideration: Martin-Meyerding, Taylor, Adson-Beckman, or Angled Gelpi are examples of retractors used for exposure.
4. The spinous process is removed and rongeurs are used to remove the margin of the lamina above the interspace, the ligamentum flavum, and the medial margin of the adjacent facet. Care is taken not to damage the epidural veins when incising the ligamentum flavum (Figure 24-36).

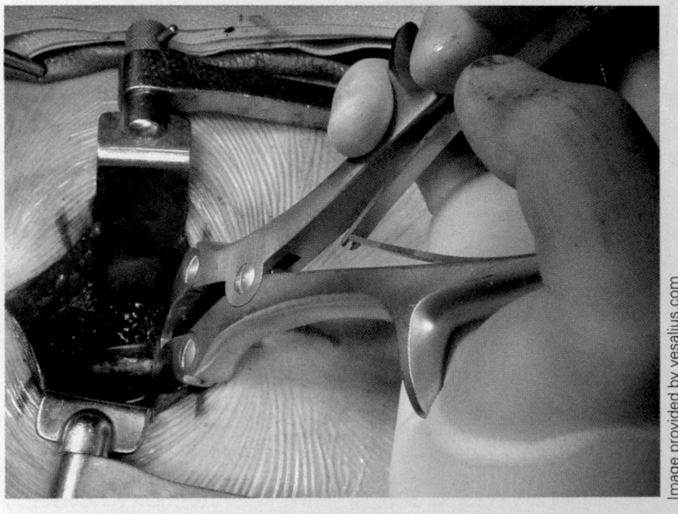

Image provided by vesalius.com

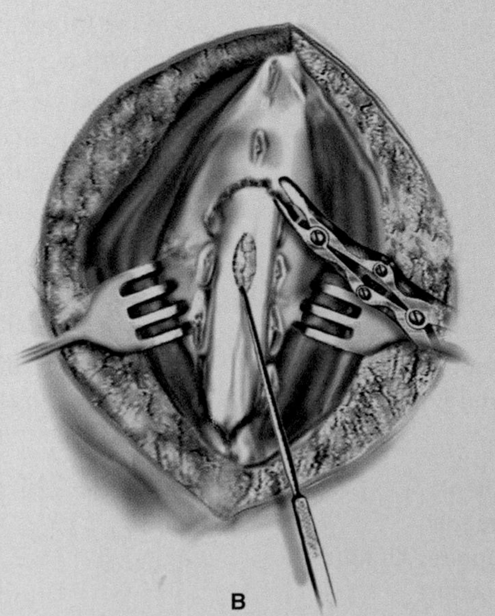

Figure 24-36a Laminectomy: (A) Spinous process excised, (B) completed bilateral multilevel laminectomy

PROCEDURE 24-9 (continued)

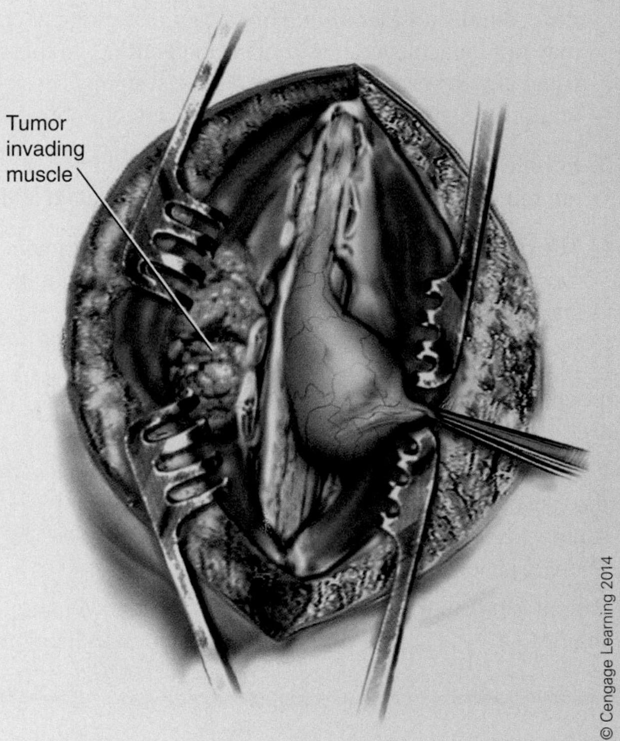

Figure 24-37 Spinal cord tumor

5. After the necessary amount of the lamina has been removed with a Kerrison rongeur, the dura and nerve root are carefully retracted medially with a nerve root retractor.

   Procedural Consideration: The surgical technologist should remove bone fragments from the rongeur with a sponge. The bone fragments can be saved to use to promote osteogenesis in fusion.

6. Pituitary rongeurs are then used to remove extruded fragments of disk material. If removing a spinal tumor, blunt and sharp dissection with scissors and a periosteal elevator will be performed (Figure 24-37).

   Procedural Consideration: The surgical technologist will need to remove disk fragments from the rongeur with a sponge and place into sterile specimen container. The disk material will be sent to pathologist.

7. Once the extruded disk material has been removed, the inner portion of the disk may be removed using rongeurs. Curettes are used in the intervertebral disk space to remove all remaining fragments of disk material. Care must be taken not to injure the aorta or vena cava that lie anterior to the vertebral column.

8. If the spine has been destabilized following laminectomy, fusion of the vertebrae may be performed. Fusion is achieved by placing struts of bone in and along the intervertebral spaces after curettage.

9. Curettage of the vertebral bodies assists in the formation of bony material after bone graft material is placed into the vertebral interspace. This bone is either taken from the iliac crest of the patient or homogenous banked bone is used.

(*continues*)

Procedure 24-9 (continued)

Procedural Consideration: For certain pathological conditions or fractures, stability may not be achieved by simple bone grafting. In these cases, stability is achieved by using any of several implanted device systems. These involve rods, cages, and plates and screws attached to nondamaged vertebra above and below.

10. Prior to wound closure, the wound is irrigated free of debris. All cottonoids and sponges are removed. Hemovac drains are typically placed in the wound before closure.
11. The paraspinous muscles are approximated with heavy-gauge polyglactin suture. The wound is closed in layers, and the skin is closed with monofilament nylon or stainless steel staples.

Postoperative Considerations

Immediate Postoperative Care

- Care is taken when turning the Patient back to the supine position to prevent injury to patient or staff.
- Patient is transported to the PACU.

Prognosis

- No complications: Generally if decompression is accomplished early enough, the results are favorable.
- Complications: Wound infection, destabilization of the spine, nerve root damage, and hemorrhage

Wound Classification

- Class I: Clean if no drain
- Class II: Clean-contaminated if drain is inserted

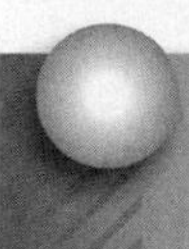

Pearl of Wisdom

For a laminectomy you will receive specimens that are bone and ligament. With the diskectomy, you will receive disk material. Disk material looks and feels somewhat like crabmeat. Always check the specimen materials as you take them from the rongeur. Report any suspicious looking specimen (e.g., lumen) to the surgeon immediately.

Procedure 24-10 Microdecompression Endoscopic Spinal Diskectomy

Background Information

- Performed for the same reason as an open lumbar laminectomy: decompression of an injured spinal disc.
- With the help of standard X-rays, fluoroscopy, and endoscopic instruments, the disk is removed and/or shrunk with the use of a laser.
- The procedure can also be performed for the removal of bony spurs.
- Advantages of the procedure include:
  - Small incision
  - No traumatic muscle dissection
  - No bone removal
  - No bone fusion
  - No manipulation of the nerves in the area
  - Minimal X-ray exposure
  - No hospitalization required
  - No postoperative scarring in or around the nerves
  - Patient can begin exercise program on the day of the procedure.

Procedure 24-10 (continued)

	• Cost of procedure is approximately 40% less than an open lumbar laminectomy.	• High success rate; approximately 90% of patients experience permanent pain relief.	
Preoperative Diagnostic Tests and Procedures	• CT scan, MRI, and/or myelogram reveals disk herniation		
Equipment, Instruments, and Supplies Unique to Procedure	• Small-diameter tube for introduction of instruments	• Endoscopic imaging equipment • Discotome	• Laser of surgeon's choice
Preoperative Preparation	**Position** • Most frequently lateral **Anesthesia** • Most often local/MAC	**Skin prep** • See previous	**Draping** • See previous
Practical Considerations	• Same as for spinal procedures		
Surgical Procedure	1. Local anesthetic is injected.		
	2. Skin incision is created with #15 blade.		
	3. Using X-rays, fluoroscopy, and endoscopic imaging for guidance, a small-diameter tube is inserted through the skin incision.		
	4. A variety of surgical instruments can be inserted through the tube, including the endoscope, micro-forceps, curettes, and discotome.		
	5. Using the discotome, the surgeon removes disk material to decompress and relieve the pressure on the nerve root.		
	6. The laser probe is used to shrink, tighten, and burn away other portions of the disk.		
	7. A probe is used to suction out small pieces of disk material.		
	8. The hollow tube is removed and a small bandage is applied over the incision.		
Postoperative Considerations	**Immediate Postoperative Care** • Patient is transported to the PACU. • Postoperative pain is minimal to none, thus requiring no medication.	**Prognosis** • No complications: Normal activity is resumed within 10 days to 3 weeks. • Complications: A few patients may have mild	muscle spasms; these can be relieved with the use of muscle relaxants and analgesics. **Wound Classification** • Class I: Clean

Procedure 24-11 Anterior Cervical Diskectomy and Fusion (ACDF): Cloward Technique

Surgical Anatomy and Pathology

- Certain spondylitic lesions, some fractures, and procedures for correction of spinal stenosis may require an anterior approach to the spine. Extreme cases require an anterior approach followed by a posterior approach. The anterior approach is especially useful for treatment of spinal stenosis at the cervical and thoracic levels.
- With cervical disk extrusion, symptoms may be chronic or **acute** (due to some injury). The patient may experience neck stiffness, soreness, and limited mobility, along with radicular symptoms. Some tenderness may occur over the brachial plexus. The normal curvature of the neck tends to be straightened somewhat in these patients (Figure 24-38).
- When osteophytes have formed in the foramen, cervical discomfort may occur in episodes over a period of months or years before radicular symptoms become evident.
- In some instances, radiographs will show narrowing in the disk space, indicating **extruded** disk, or disk degeneration (Figure 24-12). Radiographs will also show osteophytes that have formed.

There are two primary surgical treatments for cervical disk disease:

- Decompression of the nerve roots and/or spinal cord with a

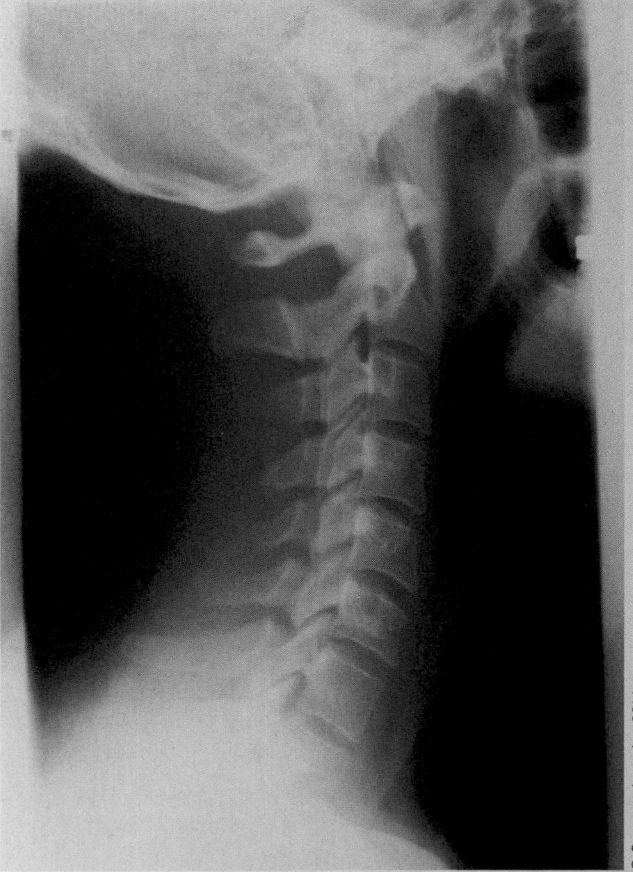

Figure 24-38 Lateral cervical x-ray

Procedure 24-11 (continued)

	posterior cervical laminectomy and diskectomy. • Anterior cervical diskectomy and fusion.	The anterior approach offers the advantage of a direct approach to the disk space without the removal of the lamina. After the	disk is removed, the disk space is filled with cancellous and cortical bone (fusion), usually from the iliac crest.
Preoperative Diagnostic Tests and Procedures	• See information for laminectomy.		
Equipment, Instruments, and Supplies Unique to Procedure	• Cloward Instruments (handheld and self-retaining retractors with detachable blades, vertebral spreader,	cervical drill with guards, bone dowel cutter, bone graft holder and impactor, bone curettes and rongeurs	• Minor set for soft tissue • Spinal needle • Cervical collar
Preoperative Preparation	**Position** • Supine with shoulder roll and head turned slightly away from the affected side • Hip elevated for graft procurement	**Anesthesia** • General **Skin prep** • Neck and iliac crest	**Draping** • Square draped with towels and covered with thyroid sheet
Practical Considerations	• The surgical technologist should be prepared for lateral X-ray for disk level identification.		
Surgical Procedure	1. An incision is made over the cervical disk space at the medial border of the sternocleidomastoid muscle with a #10 blade on #3 knife handle, and hemostasis is obtained with electrocautery.		
	2. The esophagus, carotid artery, and trachea are retracted medially. The periosteum of the anterior cervical vertebral bodies is stripped with a periosteal elevator, and a spinal needle is inserted into the vertebral space.		
	3. A lateral C-spine X-ray is taken to identify the proper level.		
	4. An incision is made over the iliac crest, and a bone graft is procured with a Hudson brace and dowel cutter or osteotome and mallet.		
	5. Blades are chosen for the Cloward self-retaining retractor, and the retractor is placed.		
	6. An incision is made into the disk space with a #15 blade loaded on a #7 knife handle, and disk material is removed with the pituitary rongeur and sent for specimen.		
	7. The vertebral spreader is placed into the disk space and opened to the desired width. Additional disk material is removed with small curettes, angled and straight. **Procedural Consideration:** A caliper may be used to ensure the vertebrae are distracted to the proper distance.		
	8. The depth of the intervertebral space is measured, and the cervical drill guard is inserted into the space. A hole is drilled into the guide with the Cloward drill on Hudson brace, and the drill and guide are removed.		

(continues)

Procedure 24-11 (continued)

9. The bone dowel is trimmed for size with the air drill and rongeur and placed into the disk space. The vertebral spreader is removed, and the bone graft is inspected for proper positioning.

   Procedural Consideration: An impactor and mallet are typically necessary to properly place the bone graft within the disk space.

10. The retractors are removed, and the wound is irrigated and closed in layers.

    Procedural Consideration: A lateral cervical X-ray may be obtained before closure to ensure proper bone graft placement.

11. The incisions are dressed with inner contact layers, 4 × 4 pads, and an ABD for the iliac crest.

Postoperative Considerations

Immediate Postoperative Care

- The surgical technologist should remain sterile and should not break down the back table or Mayo tray until the patient has left the OR.
- A cervical collar is placed.

Prognosis

- No complications: Hospital stay of 3–5 days; gradually return to normal activities; good prognosis
- Complications: Wound infection and nerve root damage

Wound Classification

- Class I: Clean

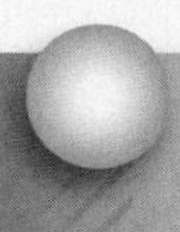

Pearl of Wisdom

In the classic Cloward procedure, the graft taken is 1 mm greater in diameter than the drill bit that matches it. This allows the normal muscle tension of the neck to hold the graft in place. Always check to see that the drill bit will fit just inside the graft taker.

Procedure 24-12 Posterior Cervical Decompression

Surgical Anatomy and Pathology

- The posterior cervical approach is used for laminectomy for decompression, intradural tumor removal, cordotomy, diskectomy, and fusion.
- See information for laminectomy and ACDF.

Preoperative Diagnostic Tests and Procedures

- See information for laminectomy.

Equipment, Instruments, and Supplies Unique to Procedure

- Mayfield skull clamp
- Cervical collar

Procedure 24-12 (continued)

Preoperative Preparation	**Position** • Prone with three-pin skull clamp **Anesthesia** • General	**Skin prep** • See that for ACDF.	**Draping** • See that for ACDF.
Practical Considerations	• OR bed is positioned in mild reverse Trendelenburg to encourage venous drainage.		
Surgical Procedure	1. A midline incision is made over the cervical spinous process. 2. Soft tissue dissection is completed. 3. Correct level placement is verified with X-ray. 4. A laminectomy is performed using a drill, Leksell rongeurs, curettes, and Kerrison rongeurs. 5. Disk is removed with pituitary rongeurs and curettes. 6. If fusion is required, follow steps above. 7. The wound is irrigated and closed in layers. 8. Dressings same as for Procedure 24-11 Cloward Technique		
Postoperative Considerations	**Immediate Postoperative Care** • See that for ACDF.	**Prognosis** • See that for ACDF.	**Wound Classification** • Class I: Clean

Procedure 24-13 Anterior Thoracic Decompression

Surgical Anatomy and Pathology	• A thoracotomy approach is popular for diskectomies in the thoracic region because of the small diameter of the thoracic spinal canal. An alternative approach is the removal of the medial segment of a rib and transverse process to expose the intervertebral disk. For these procedures, the rib is often used as autograft bone material and is packed into the disk space after the disk and cartilage plates have been removed and the vertebral bodies have been curetted. • An anterior/posterior thoracic approach may be utilized for the placement of rods and pedicle screws. The patient is first placed in a lateral thoracic position for the anterior approach, and a thoracic surgeon exposes the vertebral bodies through a thoracotomy. Screws and rods or fusion material is placed and secured, and the wound is closed in layers in the usual manner. The patient is then turned onto the Wilson frame to a prone position, prepped, and redraped. The posterior thoracic spine is exposed in the usual manner.
Preoperative Diagnostic Tests and Procedures	• Same as for laminectomy

(continues)

Procedure 24-13 (continued)

Equipment, Instruments, and Supplies Unique to Procedure

- See Procedure 22-7 Upper Lobectomy on page 1027
- Long rongeurs, curettes, and instruments are used for this approach due to the depth of the operative field.
- Jackson table if intraoperative fluoroscopy is needed, as beanbag will interfere.

Preoperative Preparation

Position
- Lateral with beanbag
- T1–T4—Right-side approach
- T5–T12—Leftside approach

Anesthesia
- General

Skin prep
- See that for thoracotomy.

Draping
- See that for thoracotomy.

Practical Considerations

- A double-lumen endotracheal tube may be used to allow for deflation of the lung.

Surgical Procedure

1. A thoracotomy incision is made and the latissimus dorsi and other muscles are transected.

   Procedural Consideration: A rib may be resected with a rib cutter to gain exposure.
2. The parietal pleura is opened and a thoracotomy retractor is placed.
3. A localization X-ray is taken to verify correct level.
4. The parietal pleura is cleared with blunt dissection.
5. Segmental vessels are ligated as necessary with hemoclips and transected to mobilize the aorta.
6. Diskectomy, decompression, or fusion is performed.
7. The wound is irrigated and a chest tube is placed. The ribs are reapproximated with a Bailey and sutured with heavy absorbable suture.
8. The fascia and subcuticular layers are closed in routine fashion.

Postoperative Considerations

Immediate Postoperative Care
- See that for thoracotomy.

Prognosis
- No complications: 3–4 days in hospital. Physical therapy started immediately with walking.
- Complications: See information for thoracotomy and ACDF.

Wound Classification
- Class II: Clean-contaminated

Procedure 24-14 Rhizotomy

Surgical Anatomy and Pathology

- Rhizotomy is a surgical procedure to sever nerve roots in the spinal cord.
- The procedure effectively relieves chronic back pain. For spinal joint pain, a facet rhizotomy may provide lasting low back pain relief by disabling the sensory nerve at the facet joint.
- Rhizotomy is also performed on patients with spasticity that is

PROCEDURE 24-14 (continued)

	insufficiently responsive to oral medications or injectable therapies. It is most commonly	performed for those patients with lower extremity spasticity that interferes with walking. It	is most commonly performed on children with cerebral palsy.
Preoperative Diagnostic Tests and Procedures	• Battery of tests to document the functional effects of spasticity		
Equipment, Instruments, and Supplies Unique to Procedure	• See information for laminectomy. • Intraoperative ultrasound	• Rubber pad to isolate nerve roots	• Electromyography equipment • Fentanyl for pain relief
Preoperative Preparation	**Position** • Prone **Anesthesia** • General	**Skin prep** • Same as for laminectomy	**Draping** • See previous.
Practical Considerations	• Surgeon may use laser or electrosurgical probe to sever nerves.		
Surgical Procedure	1. A 1- to 2-in. incision is made over L1.		
	2. A laminectomy is performed to gain access to the spinal cord and spinal nerve.		
	3. Ultrasound and x-ray technology is used to locate the tip of the spinal cord to find the natural separation of the sensory and motor nerves.		
	4. A special rubber pad is then placed to provide a division between these two nerve sets. The sensory nerve roots are tested and selectively eliminated; they are placed on top of the pad while the motor nerves will remain beneath the pad for their protection.		
	5. Once the sensory nerves have been exposed they are divided into three to five rootlets. These rootlets are then tested with electromyography recording the electrical patterns in the muscles. The severity of the damage is rated from 1 to 4, with the later being the most severe. Rootlets that are severely abnormal are severed, and the procedure is repeated between spinal nerves L2 and S2.		
	6. When testing and severing of the damaged nerves is complete, the dura mater is closed. A direct application of fentanyl is administered.		
	7. The wound is closed in layers.		
Postoperative Considerations	**Immediate Postoperative Care** • Patient is transported to the PACU; stays for 1–2 hours. **Prognosis** • No complications: Patient is transferred to	the ICU for an overnight stay and then to a room, where he or she will be monitored for 3 days. • Complications: Permanent paralysis of the legs and bladder, impotence, sensory loss and/or numbness,	wound infection, meningitis, and leakage of spinal fluid through the wound. **Wound Classification** • Class I: Clean

PERIPHERAL NERVE PROCEDURES

The nervous system of the human body is divided into two systems: the central nervous system (**CNS**), comprising the brain and spinal cord; and the peripheral nervous system (**PNS**), comprising the nerves that link the various parts of the body to the CNS. The PNS includes the cranial nerves that originate from the brain, and the spinal nerves that originate from the spinal cord. Trauma and various compression syndromes that affect the PNS often lead to surgery.

Practical Considerations

- The arm table will be used for hand and arm procedures.
- The surgeon will often sit. Sitting stools should be available.
- A pneumatic tourniquet is used frequently.
- Peripheral nerve procedures may be performed by a number of specialists, including the neurosurgeon, plastic surgeon, hand surgeon, and orthopedic surgeon.

Procedural Considerations

- Local, regional, or general anesthesia can be used.

PROCEDURE 24-15 Carpal Tunnel Release

Surgical Anatomy and Pathology	• Carpal tunnel syndrome is a condition of the hand in which the median nerve is compressed by the transverse carpal ligament. • Decompression of the nerve is achieved by incising part of the fibrous sheath of the ligament.		
Preoperative Diagnostic Tests and Procedures	• Symptoms noted on history and physical examination	• Electromyography	
Equipment, Instruments, and Supplies Unique to Procedure	• Drapes: three-quarters sheet, stockinette, extremity sheet	• Esmarch bandage	
Preoperative Preparation	**Position** • Supine with affected arm extended on arm table **Anesthesia** • Local, regional, or general	**Skin prep** • The arm is prepped circumferentially with iodophor **Draping** • Three-quarters sheet is placed on top of hand table.	• Stockinette is placed over hand (optional). • Arm is extended through extremity sheet. • Medium sheet may be needed to cover the legs.
Practical Considerations	• Procedure can also be accomplished endoscopically.		
Surgical Procedure	1. A small incision is made on the palmar surface of the hand with a #15 blade on #7 knife handle.		
	2. Hemostasis is achieved and the transverse carpal ligament is either stretched or cut to release the pressure being exerted on the median nerve.		

Procedure 24-15 (continued)

	3. The wound is irrigated and a simple closure is performed.
	4. The wound is dressed with initial contact layer and bulky dressing.
Postoperative Considerations	**Immediate Postoperative Care** • Ace bandage binds the bulky dressing to create a splint. • Patient is transported to the PACU. **Prognosis** • No complications: Overall results are good and patient can return to normal activities in a few weeks. • Complications: Median nerve damage and wound infection **Wound Classification** • Class I: Clean

Procedure 24-16 Ulnar Nerve Transposition

Surgical Anatomy and Pathology	• At the elbow, the ulnar nerve travels through a tunnel of tissue (the cubital tunnel) that runs under the medial epicondyle of the elbow. This is commonly referred to as the "funny bone." • Beyond the elbow, the ulnar nerve travels under muscles in relation to the ulna. As the nerve enters the hand, it travels through another tunnel (Guyon's canal). • The ulnar nerve gives feeling to the little finger and half of the ring finger. It also controls most of the little muscles in the hand that help with fine movements, and some of the bigger muscles in the forearm that create a strong grip.
Preoperative Diagnostic Tests and Procedures	• See information for carpal tunnel.
Equipment, Instruments, and Supplies Unique to Procedure	• Moist umbilical tape, vessel loops, or Penrose for retraction • See information for carpal tunnel.
Preoperative Preparation	**Position** • Supine with arm suspended or extended • See information for draping an extremity in Ch. 12.
Practical Considerations	• Ulnar nerve pain can be relieved with surgical intervention from two different surgical procedures. Ulnar nerve decompression is accomplished by cutting the ligament of Osborne where the nerve passes through the medial aspect of the elbow. Ulnar nerve transposition is an actual relocation of the ulnar nerve to a slightly more anterior location in the elbow. • The surgical technologist should be prepared to assist with bone reshaping if necessary.
Surgical Procedure	1. A long incision is made over the ulnar nerve.
	2. The nerve is dissected free from the surrounding soft tissues with Metzenbaum scissors and hemostatic forceps.

(continues)

PROCEDURE 24-16 (continued)

3. Moist umbilical tapes, vessel loops, or penrose tubing is passed around the freed segment of the nerve to aid in handling it for further dissection until the satisfactory length of nerve has been freed.
4. The muscle and fascia entered by the nerve at each end may be slit with scissors to prevent kinking of the nerve at these points.
5. A fascial flap overlying the medial epicondyle of the humerus is cut and elevated. The nerve is transposed beneath it.
6. The fascia is loosely reapproximated to the fascial edge remaining on the epicondyle.
7. The wound is closed in layers.

Postoperative Considerations

Immediate Postoperative Care

- Application of splint or cast material
- Transport to PACU

Prognosis

- No complications: Most patients enjoy complete pain relief following ulnar nerve decompression/ transposition.
- Complications: Nerve damage, new constriction points, infection and blood clots

Wound Classification

- Class I: Clean

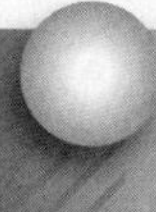

PEARL OF WISDOM

The surgical technologist will often be sitting opposite the surgeon, with the affected arm between them. Be sure all instruments and supplies are positioned where you can reach them before sitting. Once seated, do not stand up until the procedure is complete.

CASE STUDY Jamal is a 33-year-old truck driver. He went to his family physician because his right leg and buttock were hurting. The family physician examined him and referred him to a neurosurgeon. Jamal was examined again. He did not know of an incident that started the pain. Moving his legs with the knees bent did not bother him but lifting the leg with the knee straight caused sharp pain. Jamal had an MRI and was diagnosed with an L4–L5 herniated disk. He was scheduled for a lumbar discectomy.

1. Are a laminectomy and a diskectomy the same thing? Discuss your answer.
2. What instruments will be used for a diskectomy? Will a microscope be used?
3. What are the complications associated with lumbar surgery?

Questions for Further Study

1. What is the difference between a subdural and an epidural hematoma?
2. Which is the most dangerous type of intracranial hematoma, and why?
3. What is the difference between a craniotomy and a craniectomy?
4. Which approach is used for exploration of the posterior fossa, and why?
5. Why is a multilevel, bilateral laminectomy usually necessary for removal of an intradural spinal tumor?

BIBLIOGRAPHY

Association of Surgical Technologists. (2011). *Core curriculum for surgical technology* (6th ed.). Littleton, CO: Association of Surgical Technologists.

Black, P. M. (2002). Advances in neurosurgery. Retrieved from http://virtualtrials.com/black.cfm

Department of Neurobiology and Developmental Sciences, University of Arkansas. (2005). Gross anatomy of spinal cord and spinal nerves: A web-based tutorial. Retrieved from http://anatomy.uams.edu/

Goldman, M. A. (2007). *Pocket guide to the operating room* (3rd ed.). Philadelphia: F. A. Davis.

Lindsay, K., and Bone, I. (2004). *Neurology and neurosurgery illustrated* (4th ed.). St. Louis: Churchill Livingstone.

Oglivy, C. S. (n.d.). Combined modality treatment in the management of brain arteriovenous malformations [Online]. Retrieved from http://neurosurgery.mgh.harvard.edu/

Ropper, A. H., and Brown, R. H. (2009). *Adams and Victor's principles of neurology* (9th ed.). New York: McGraw-Hill.

Sabatini, R. M. E. (n.d.). The history of the electroencephalogram [Online]. Retrieved from http://www.cerebromente.org.br/

Shepherd, G. M. (1994). *Neurobiology.* New York: Oxford University Press.

Shier, D. N., Butler, J. L., and Lewis, R. (2009). *Hole's human anatomy and physiology* (12th ed.). New York: McGraw-Hill.

Spine Universe. (n.d.). Microdecompression endoscopic (arthroscopic) spinal discectomy [Online]. Retrieved from http://www.spineuniverse.com/

Thibodeau, G. A., and Patton, K. T. (2009). *Anthony's textbook of anatomy and physiology* (19th ed.). St. Louis: C. V. Mosby.

Tortora, G. J., and Derrickson, B. H. (2008). *Principles of anatomy and physiology* (12th ed.). Hoboken, NJ: John Wiley and Sons.

Appendix A

ANATOMY PLATES

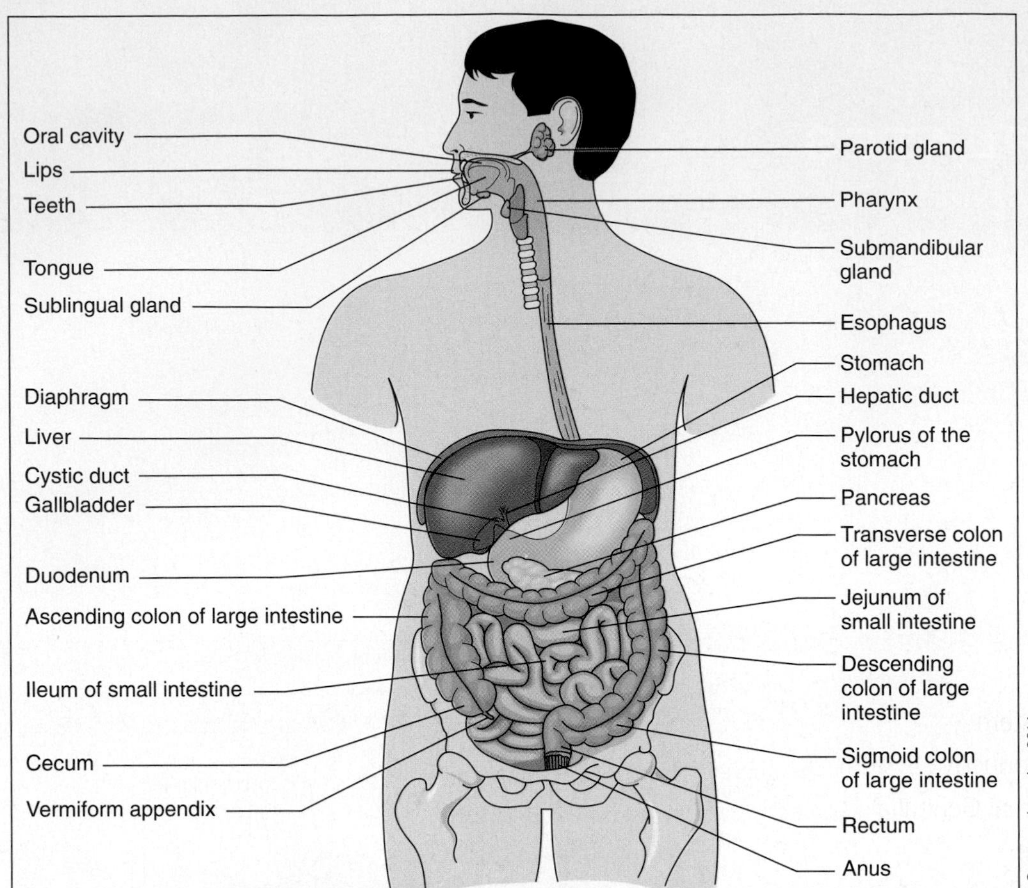

Plate 1 Digestive System

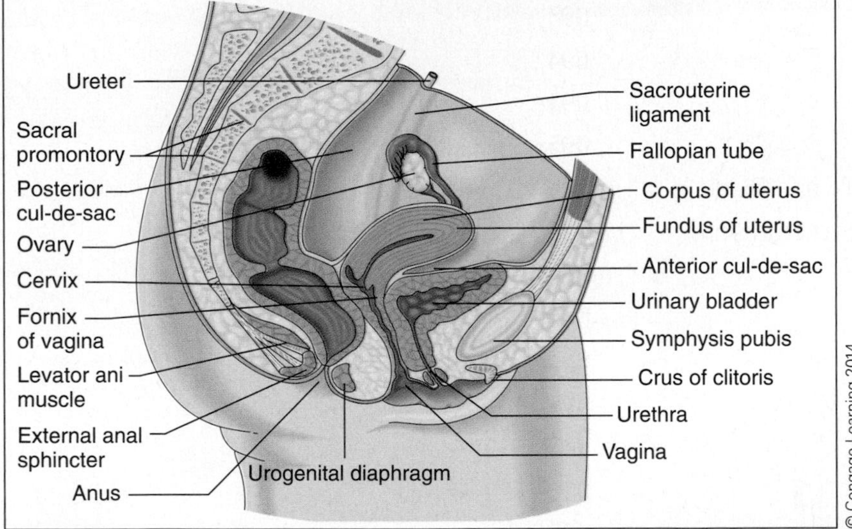

Plate 2A Female Reproductive System

Plate 2B Female External Genitalia

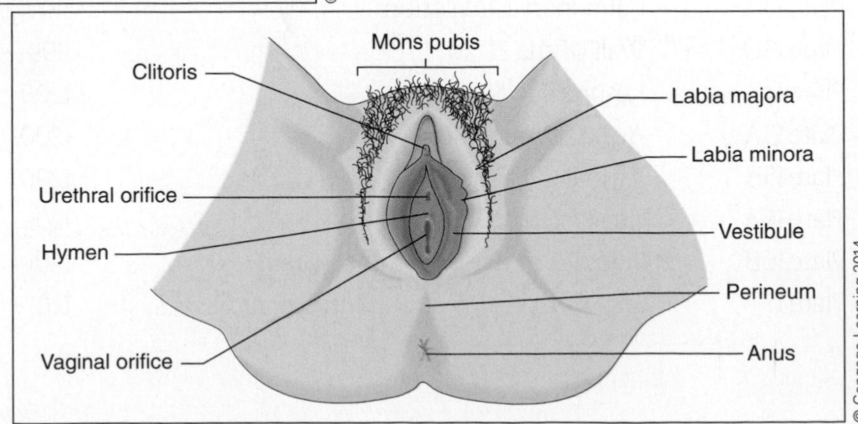

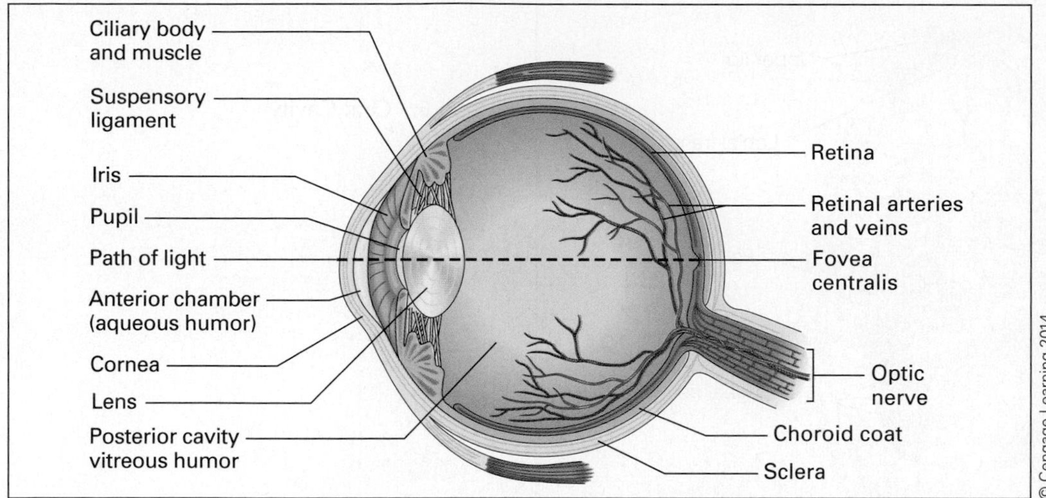

Plate 3 Eye Structure

Plate 4 Ear Structure

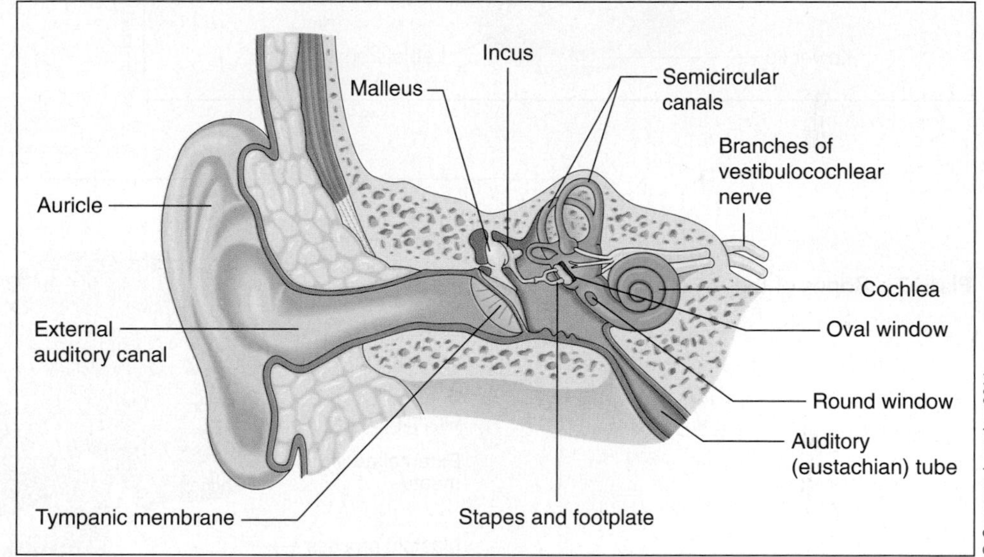

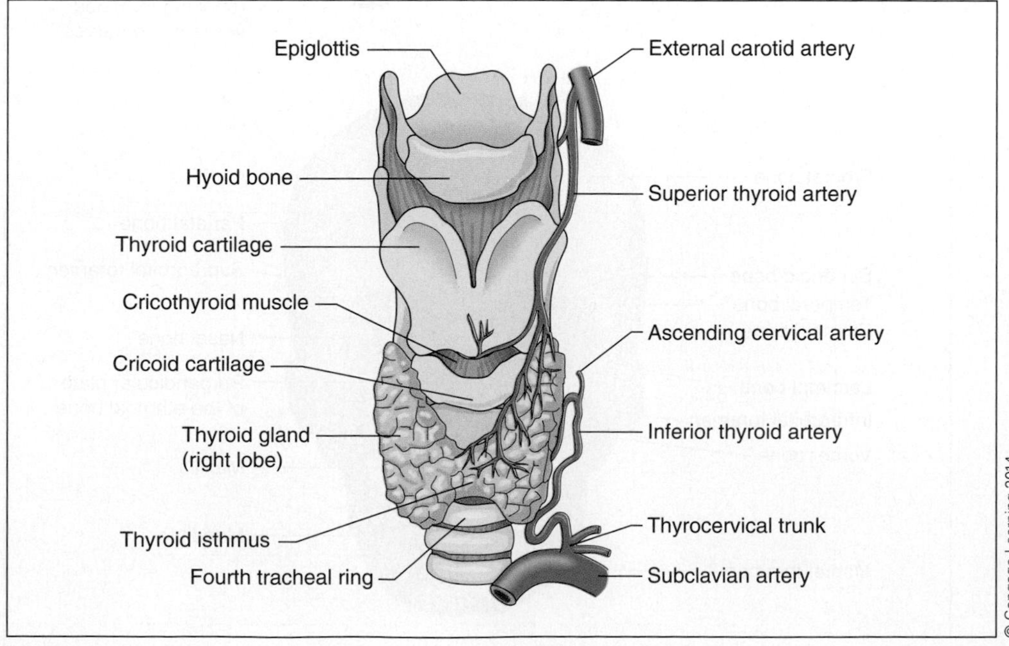

Plate 5 Thyroid

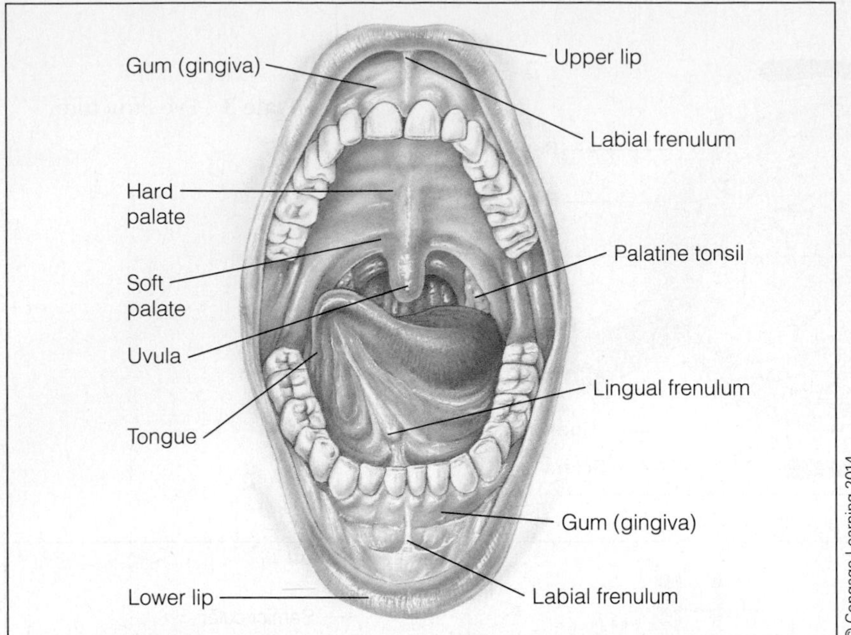

Plate 6 Oral Cavity

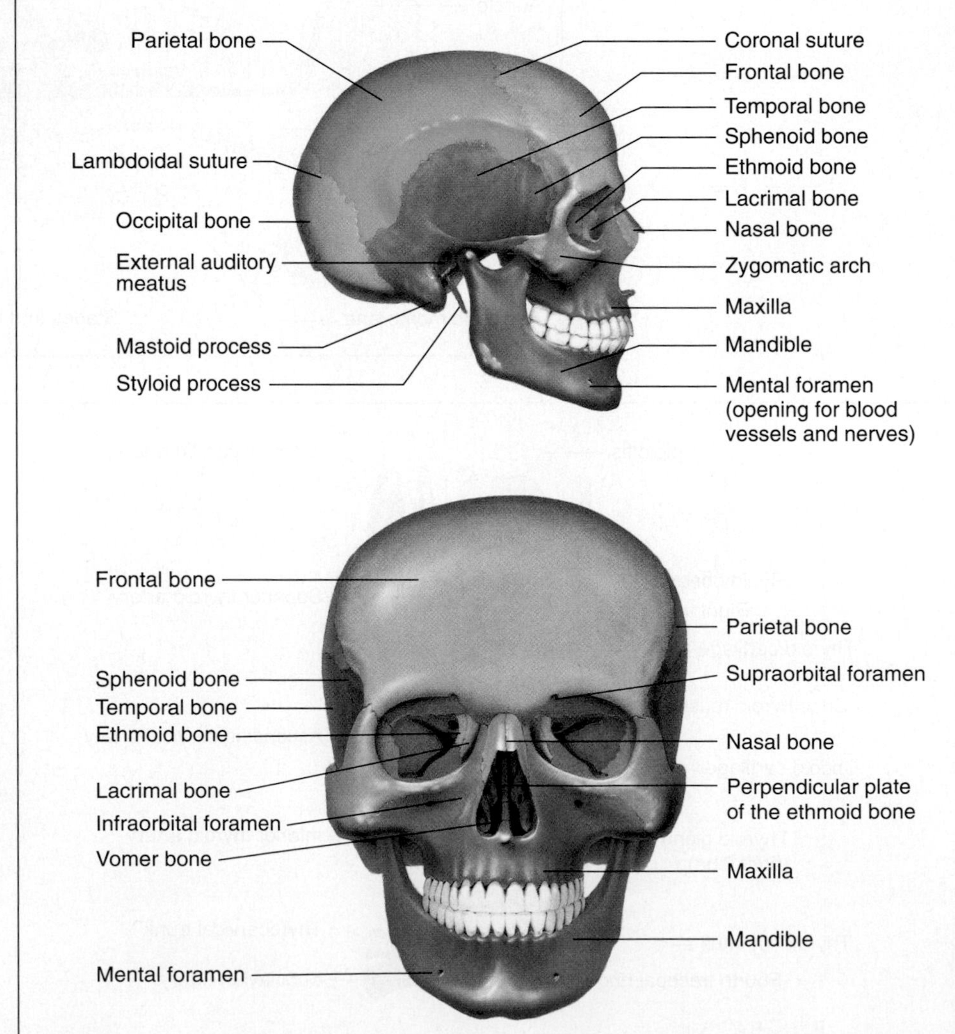

Plate 7 Bones of the Skull

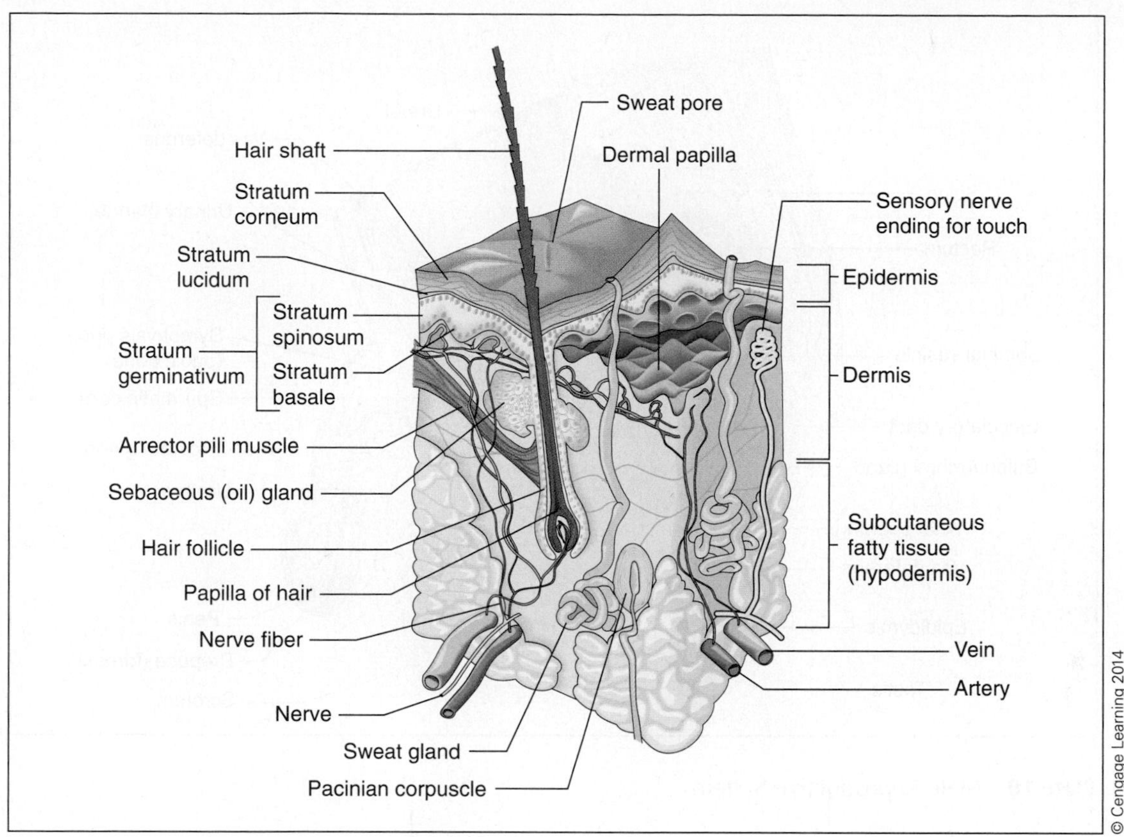

Plate 8 Skin Cross-section

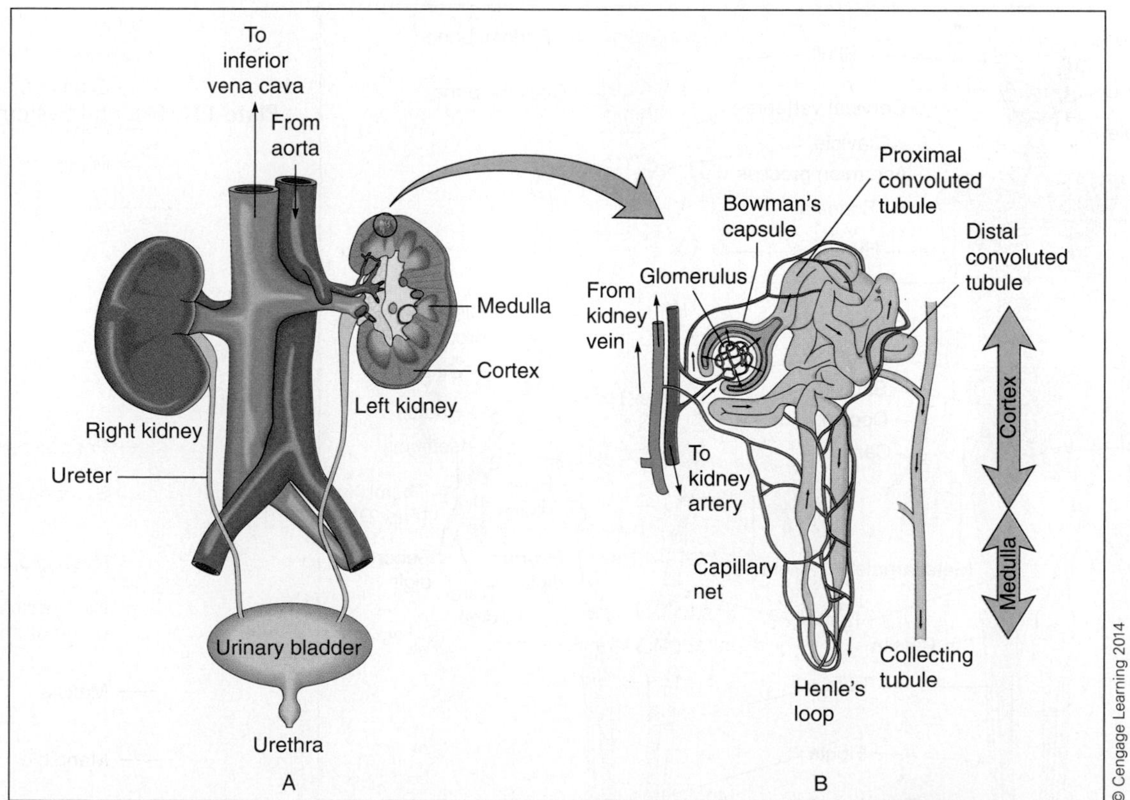

Plate 9A View of the Kidneys, Ureters, and Bladder

Plate 9B Nephron Unit and Related Structures (Arrows indicate the flow of blood through the nephron.)

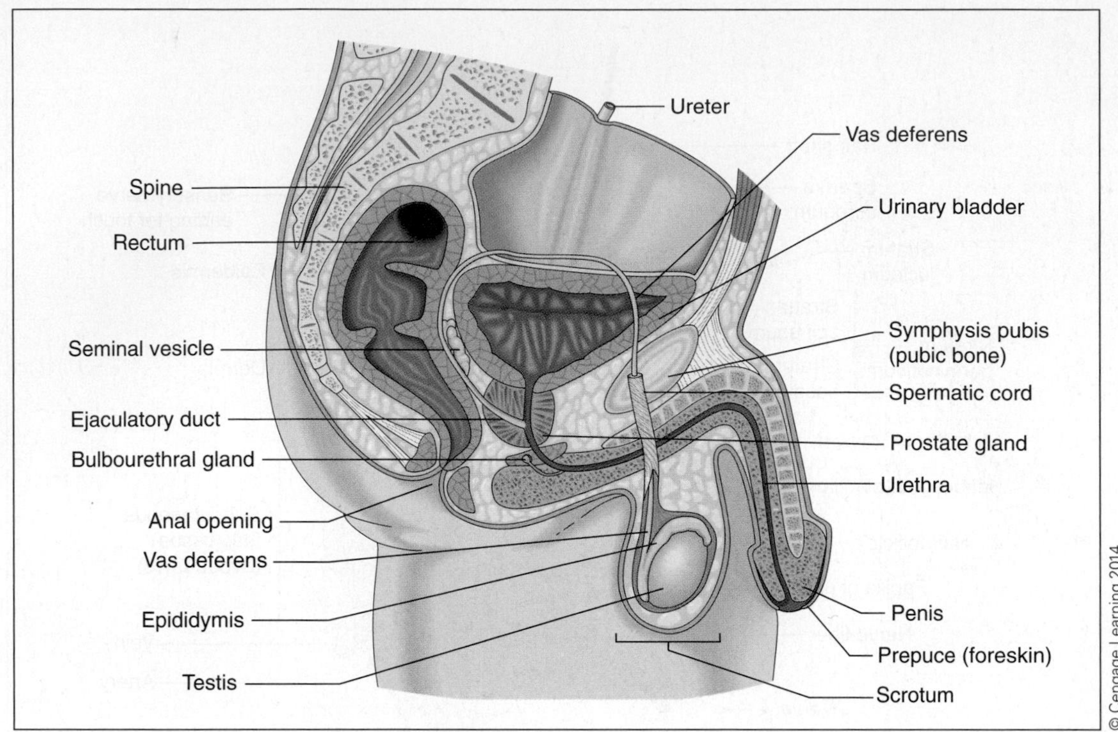

Plate 10 Male Reproductive System

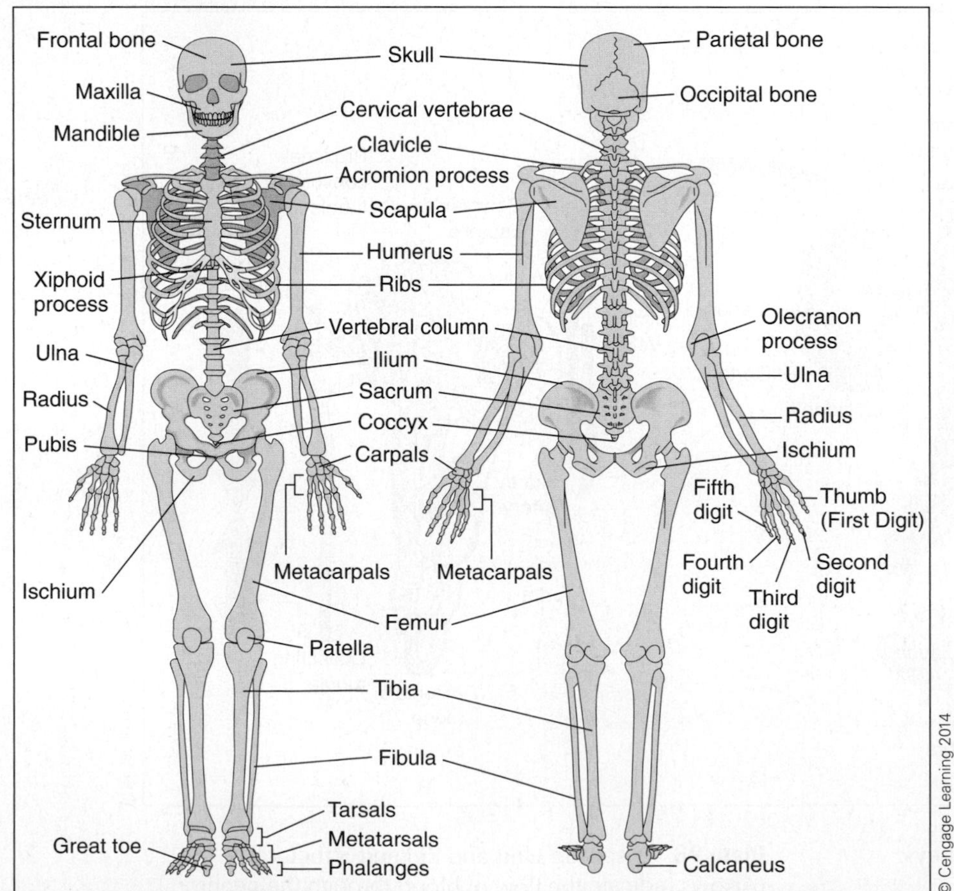

Plate 11 Skeletal System

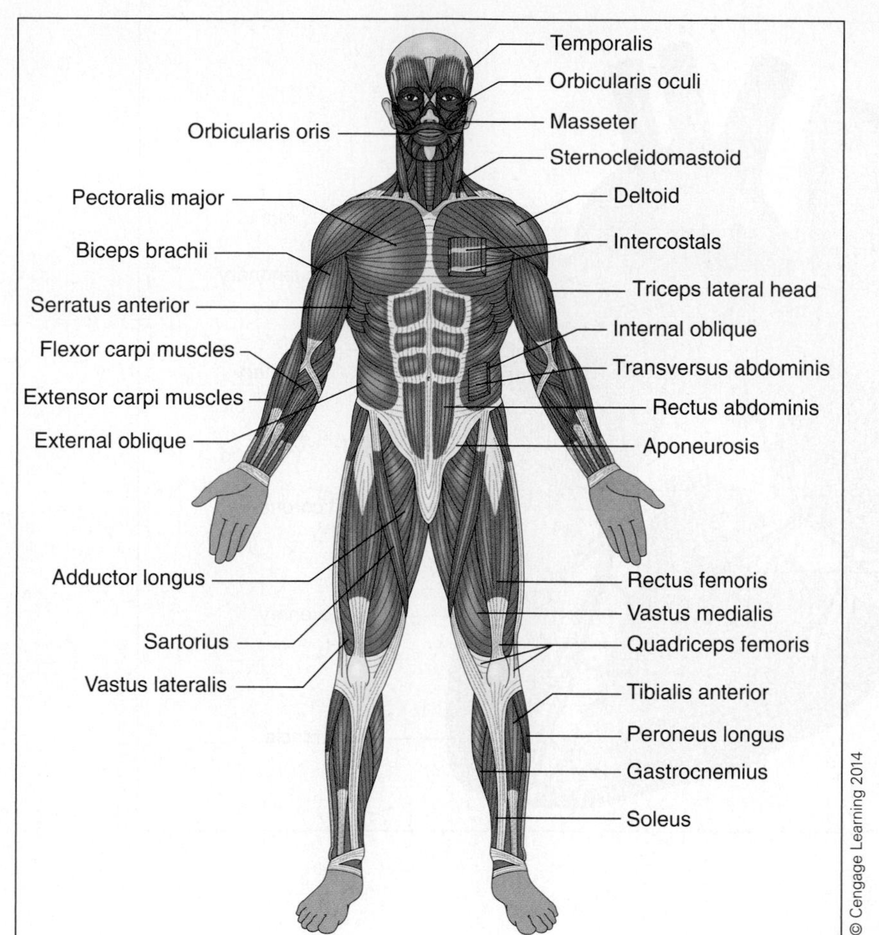

Plate 12A Skeletal Muscles—Anterior View

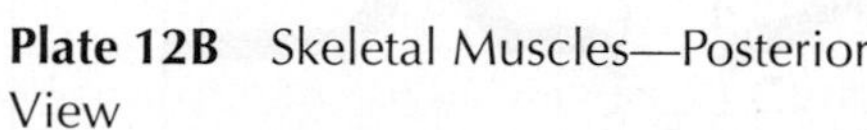

Plate 12B Skeletal Muscles—Posterior View

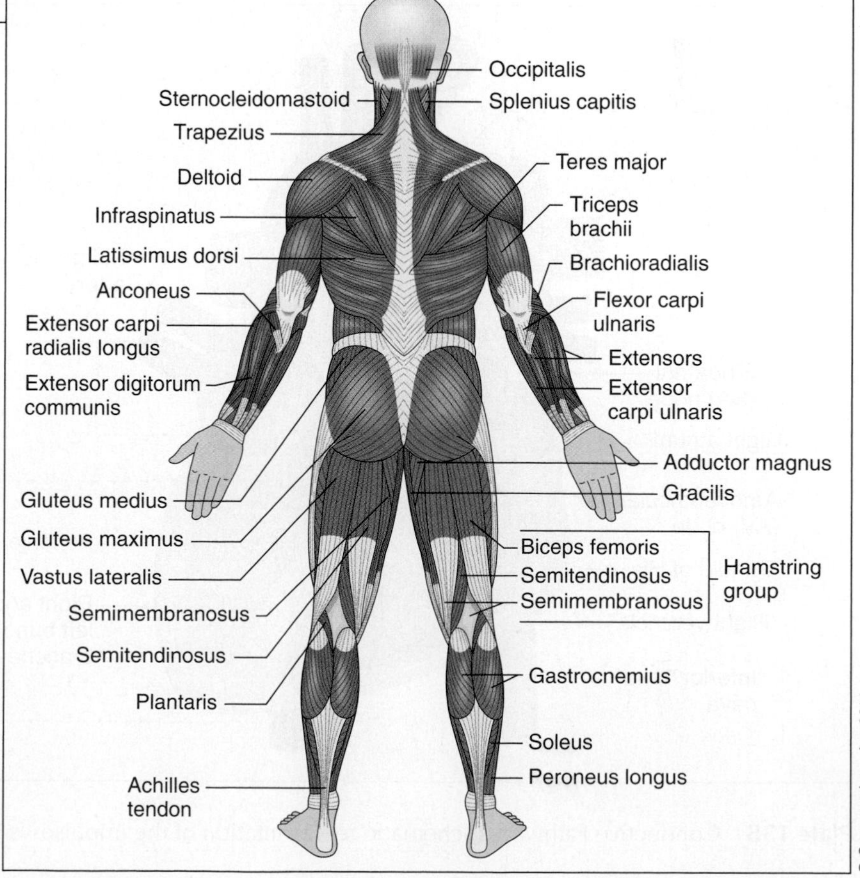

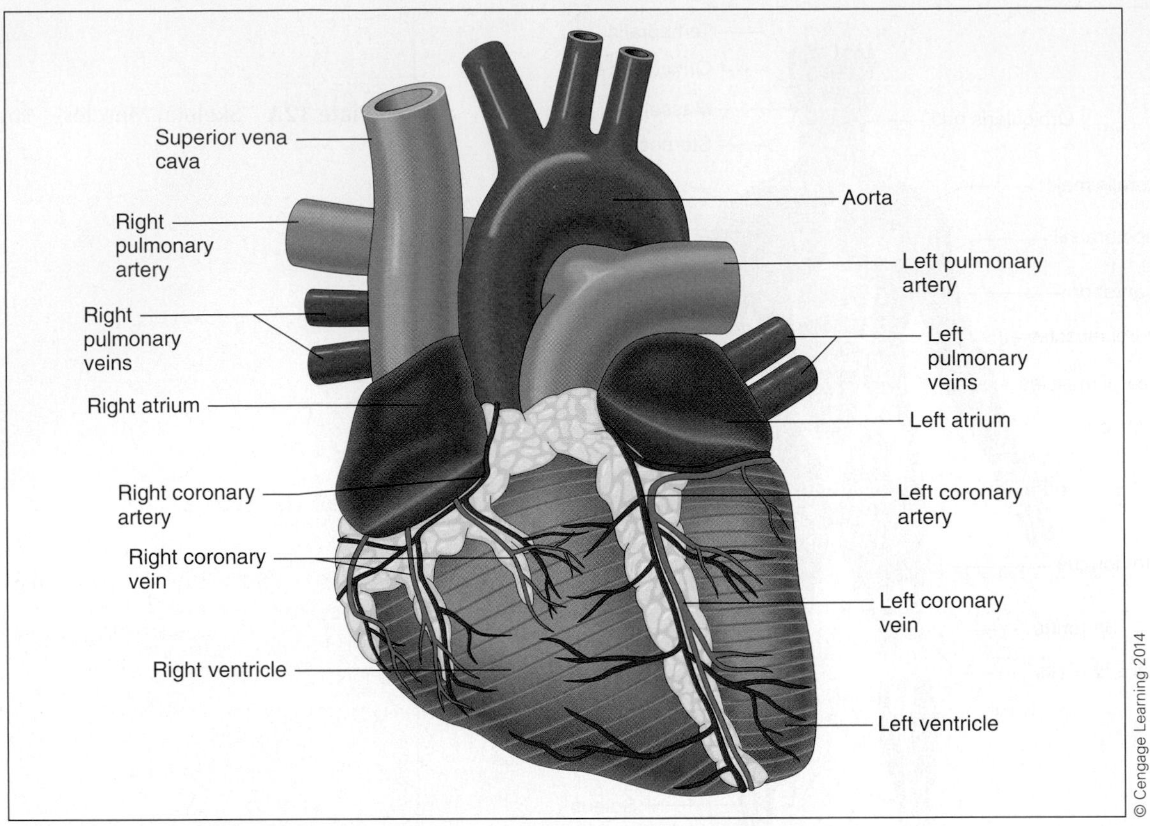

Plate 13A Heart—Anterior View

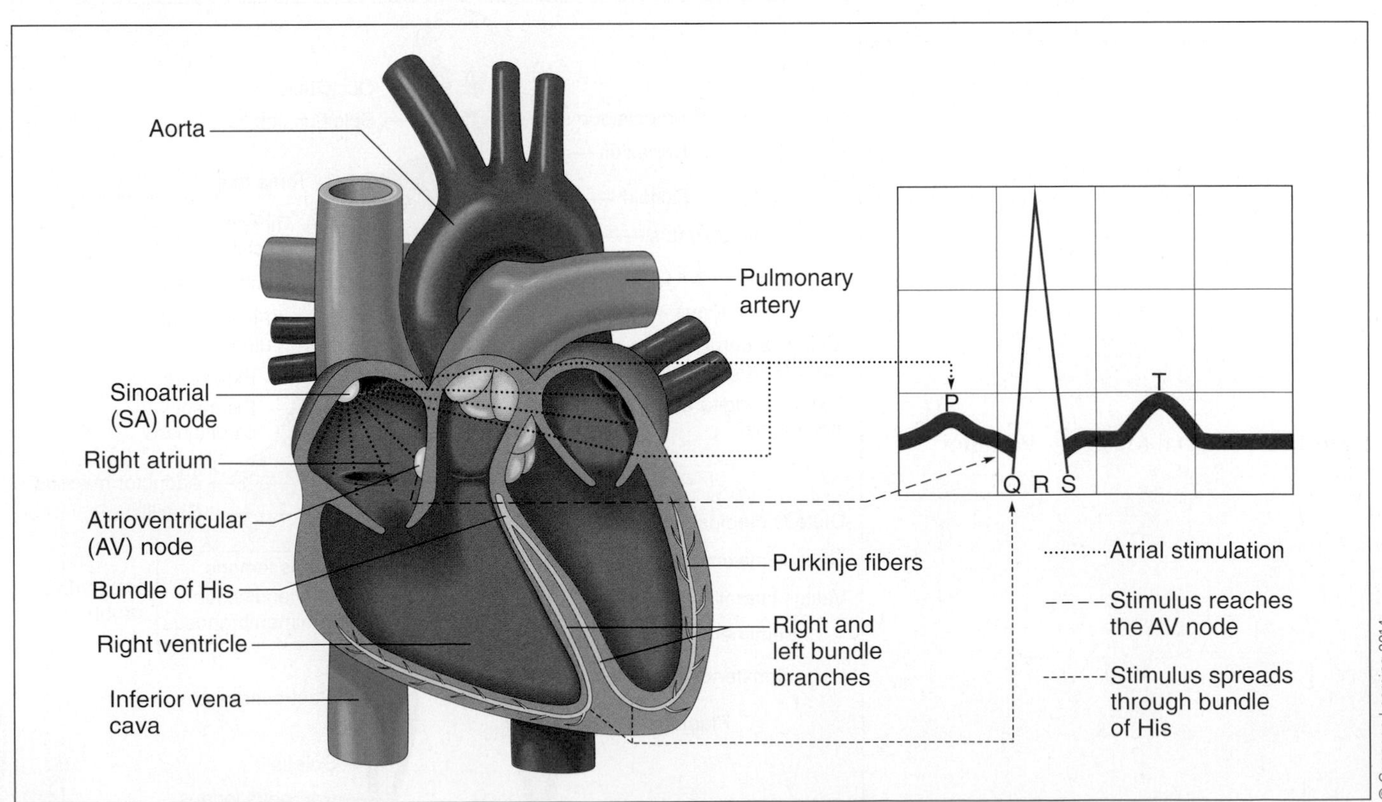

Plate 13B Conductive Pathways (Schematic representation of the impulses is shown on the right.)

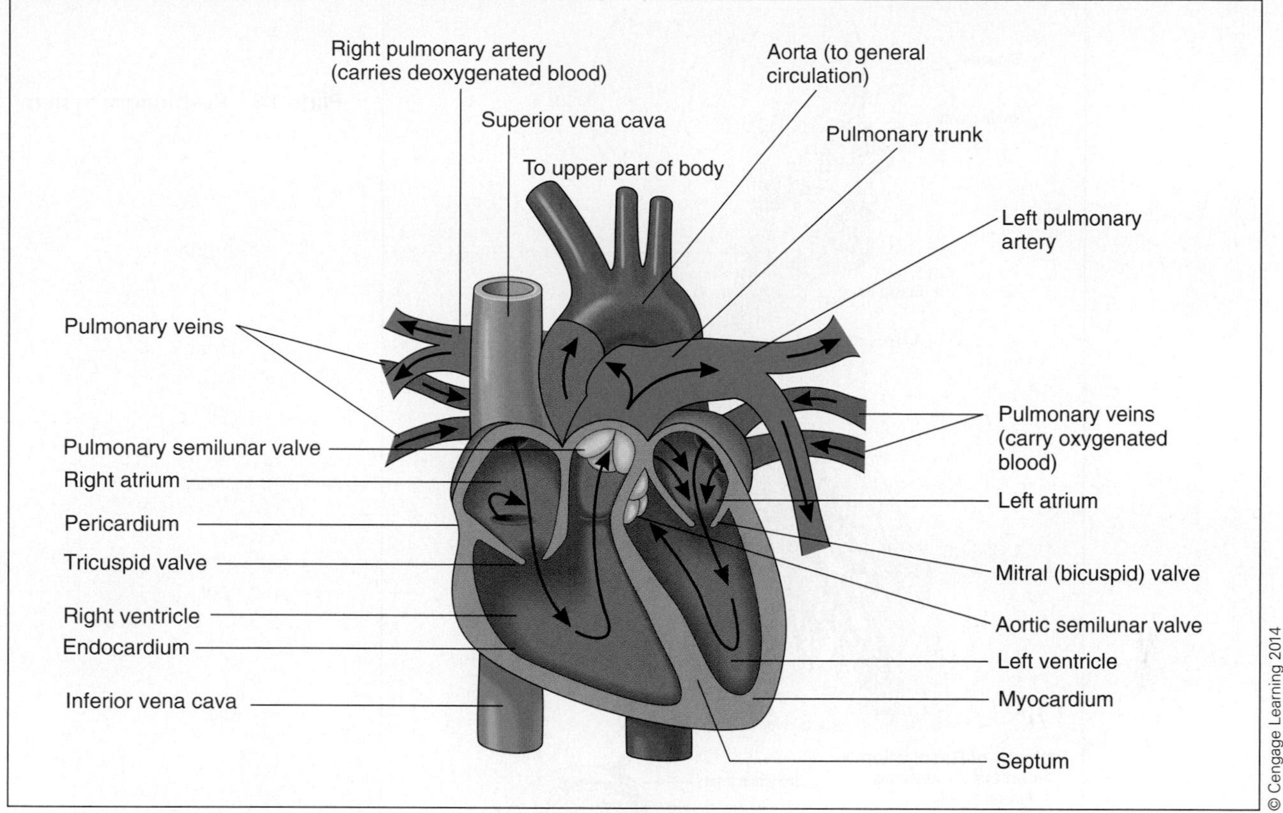

Plate 13C Pulmonary Circulation

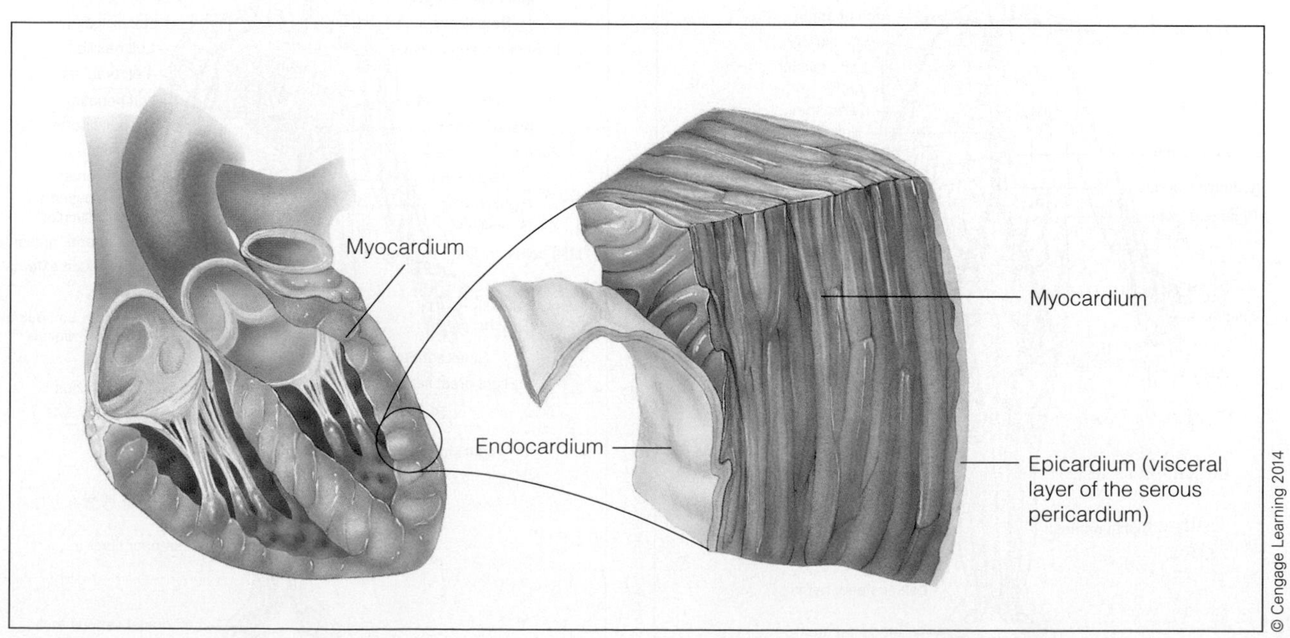

Plate 13D Wall of the Heart

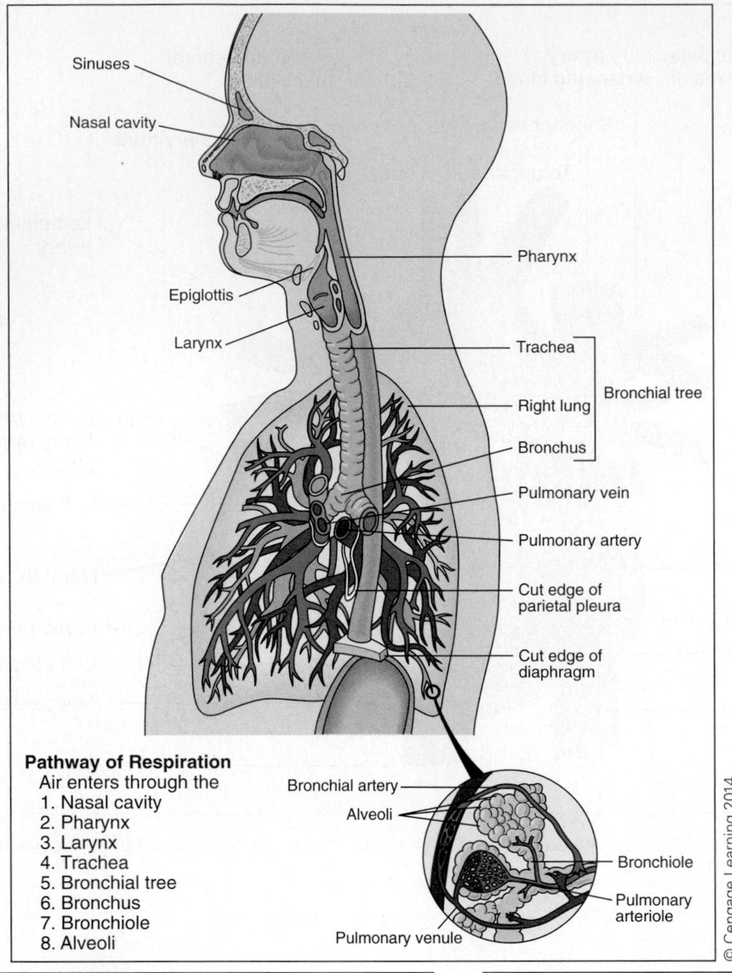

Plate 14 Respiratory System

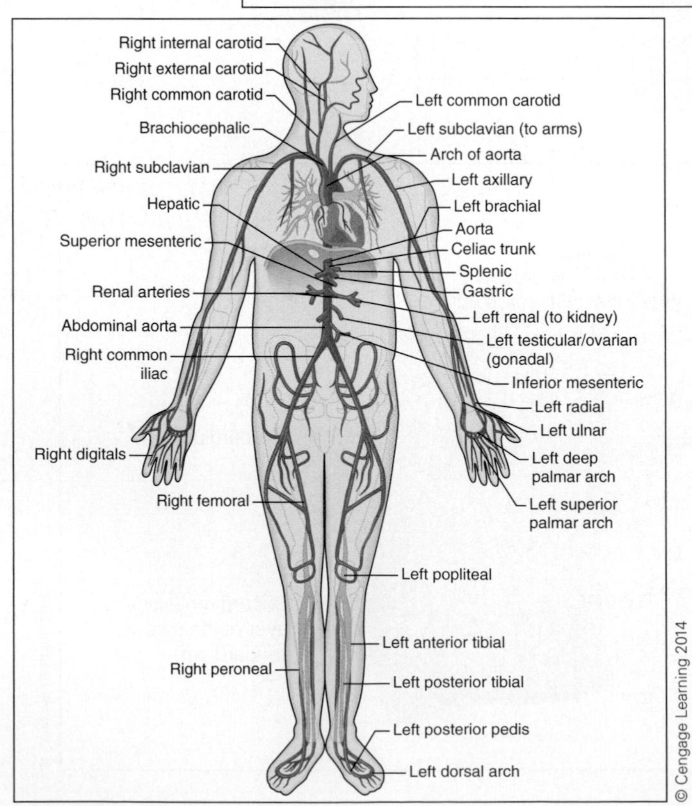

Plate 15A Arterial Circulation

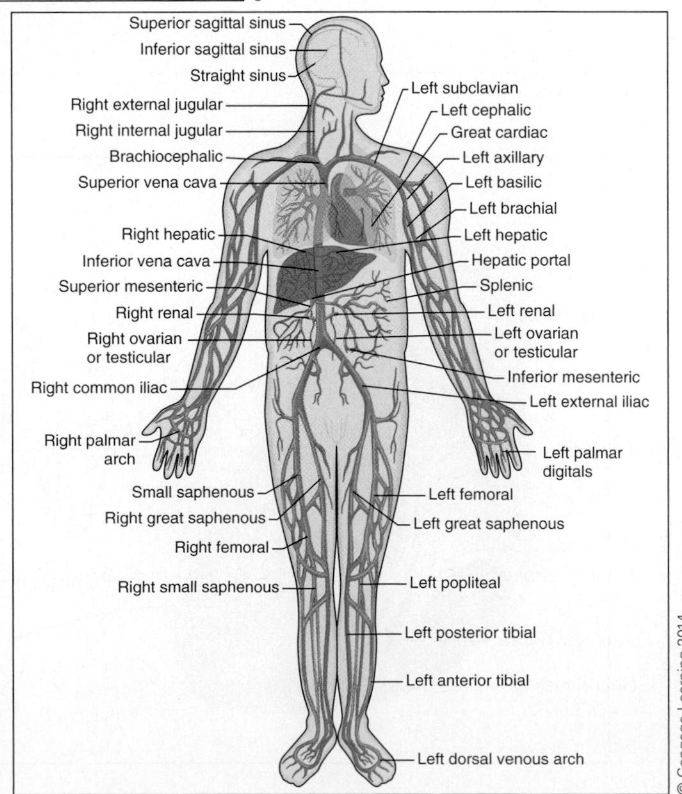

Plate 15B Venous Circulation

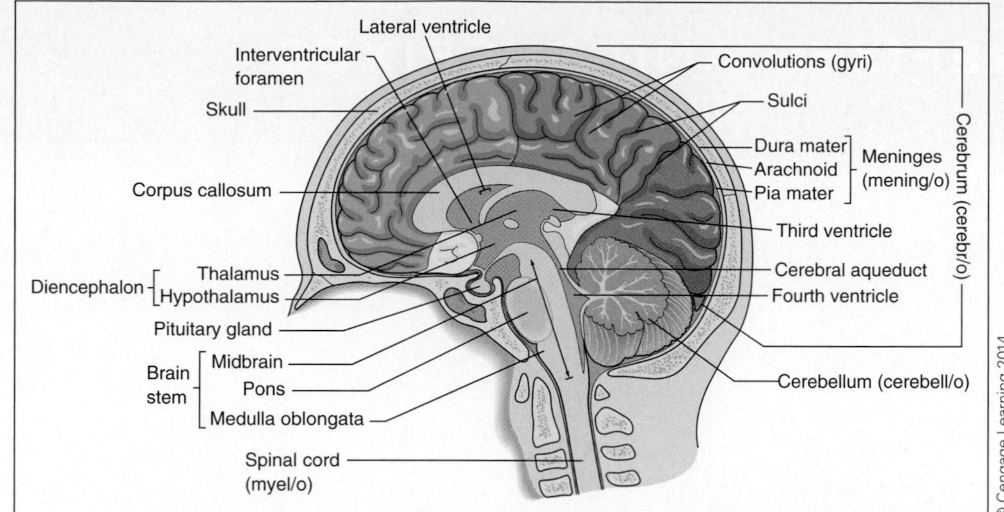

Plate 16A Cross-section of the Brain

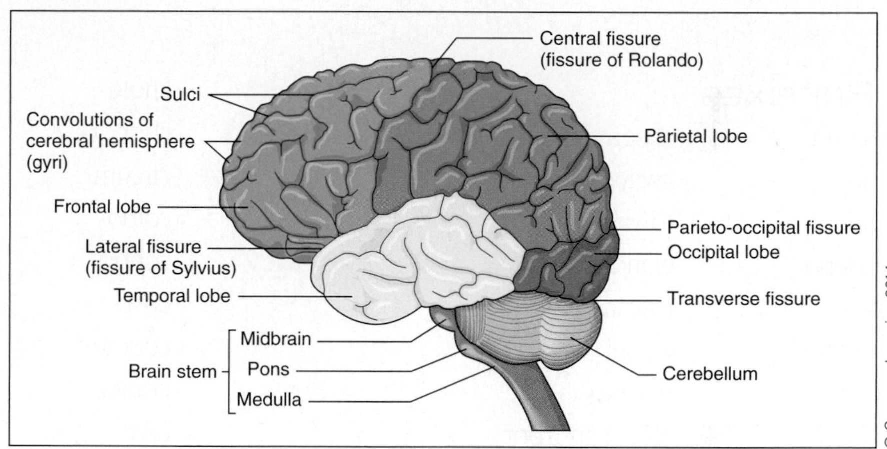

Plate 16B Lateral View of the Human Brain

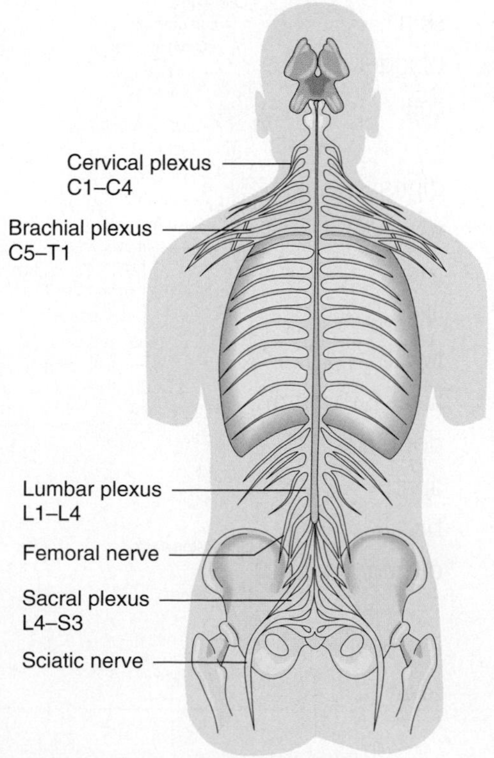

Cervical plexus C1–C4

Brachial plexus C5–T1

Lumbar plexus L1–L4

Femoral nerve

Sacral plexus L4–S3

Sciatic nerve

Cervical plexus
Nerve supply to muscles of neck and shoulder
Includes phrenic nerve that stimulates the diaphragm

Brachial Plexus
Includes Axillary, Radial, Median, Musculocutaneous, Ulnar

Lumbar Plexus
Includes Femoral, Obturator

Sacral Plexus
Includes Sciatic (largest nerve in the body), Peroneal, Tibial

Plate 17 Spinal Nerve Plexus and Important Nerves

APPENDIX B
COMMON PREFIXES AND SUFFIXES

PREFIXES

a-, an-	absent or deficient
ab-	away
ad-	toward
adeno-	gland
af-	toward
angio-	vessel
ante-	before
antero-	ahead, in front
anti-	against
arthro-	joint
aur-	ear
auto-	self
bi-	two
brachi-	arm
brachy-	short
brady-	slow
bucc-	cheek
carcin-	cancer
cardi-	heart
cephalo-	head
cerebro-	brain
cervi-	neck
cheilo-	lips
chole-	bile, gall
chondr-	cartilage
circum-	around
colpo-	vagina
contra-	opposed
cost-	ribs
counter-	against
cranio-	skull
cryo-	cold
crypt-	hidden
cut-	skin
cysto-	bladder, sac
cyto-	cell
dactyl-	digits
de-	remove
dento-	tooth
derm-	skin
di-	twice
dia-	across, through
diplo-	double
dis-	apart
dorsi-	back
dys-	difficult, painful
ecto-	external
ef-	away

endo-	within
entero-	intestine
epi-	upon
erythro-	red
eu-	good, well
ex-	away from, outside
extra-	beyond, in addition to
fasci-	fibrous tissue
fibro-	fibers, thread-like
gastro-	stomach
genito-	reproductive organs
glio-	connective tissue of the CNS
gloss-	tongue
glyco-	sugar
gnatho-	jaw
gon-	knee, seed
gyn-	female
hem-	blood
hemi-	half
hepato-	liver
hetero-	different
histo-	tissue
homeo-	unchanging
homo-	same
hydro-	water
hyper-	excessive
hypo-	beneath, deficient
hyster-	uterus
idio-	self
im-	into
in-	lacking
infra-	below
inter-	between
intra-	within
ipsi-	same
iso-	equal, same
juxta-	next to
kerat-	cornea, keratin
lacri-	tear
lacto-	milk
later-	side
leuko-	white
litho-	calculi
macro-	large
mal-	abnormal
malacia-	softening
mast-	breast
mega-	unusually large
meningo-	membranes covering the CNS
meno-	menstrual function
meso-	middle
meta-	beyond, change
micro-	small
mono-	one
muco-	mucous
multi-	many
myco-	fungi
myelo-	marrow, spinal canal (cord)
myo-	muscle
necro-	death
neo-	new
nephro-	kidney
neuro-	nerve
nocti-	night
noso-	disease
ocul-	eye
oligo-	few, deficient
onycho-	nails
oo-, ovi-, ovo-	ovum
oophoro-	ovary
ophthalm-	eye

ortho-	normal, straight
oseo-	bone
oto-	ear
ox-	pertaining to oxygen
pan-	all
para-	near
path-	disease
ped-	child, foot
per-	excessive, through
peri-	around
phag-	ingest
phleb-	vein
photo-	light
pleuro-	membranous lining of thoracic cavity
pneumo-	air, lung
pod-	foot
poly-	many
post-	following
pre-	before
presby-	old
pro-	in front of
procto-	rectum
pseudo-	false
psych-	mind
pulmo-	lung
pyelo-	pelvis of kidney
pyo-	pus
radio-	emission of radiation
re-	again
ren-	kidney
retro-	backward, behind
rhino-	nose
salpingo-	tube
sclero-	hard
scolio-	twisted
semi-	partial
sep-	poison
somato-	body
sono-	sound
sta-	stand still
sten-	narrow
sub-	under
super-	excessive
supra-	above
sym-	together
syn-	together
tachy-	rapid
thermo-	heat
tox-	poison
trach-	windpipe
trans-	through
tri-	three
ultra-	excessive
uni-	one
vas-	duct, vessel
viscero-	internal organs
xero-	dry

Suffixes

-algia	pain
-ase	enzyme
-cele	enlarged cavity, swelling
-centesis	removal of fluid via a surgical puncture
-cide	cut, kill, destroy
-clast	break
-dynia	pain
-ectasis	enlargement or stretching
-ectomy	surgical removal
-emia	relating to blood or a blood condition
-esthesia	sensation

-ferent	to carry
-gen	produces, originates
-glia	connective tissue of the CNS
-gram	written or recorded
-graph	writing or recording instrument
-graphy	the process of recording
-ia	state of
-ism	state of
-itis	inflammation
-lysis	breaking down, destruction, separation
-malacia	abnormal softening
-megaly	large
-meter	measure
-oid	like
-ology	study of
-oma	mass or tumor
-osis	abnormal condition, disease state
-ostomy	surgically creating a mouth or opening
-otomy	incision
-oxia	pertaining to oxygen
-penia	lack of
-pexy	fixation
-plasty	surgical repair
-pnea	related to breathing
-ptosis	drooping or prolapsed
-rrhagia	excessive flow
-rrhaphy	surgical repair of a defect
-rrhea	flow or discharge
-rrhexis	rupture
-sclerosis	abnormal hardening
-scopy	visual examination
-stenosis	abnormal narrowing
-taxia	order
-tripsy	to crush
-trophic	nutrition
-tropic	influencing change
-uria	related to urination or urine

APPENDIX C
MEASUREMENTS

Weights, Measures, and Equivalents

Apothecary System

Weight	
1 dram (ʒ) =	60 grains (gr)
1 ounce (℥) =	480 grains
1 pound (lb) =	16 ounces
Volume	
1 fluid dram =	60 minims (µ)
1 fluid ounce =	8 drams
1 pint (pt) =	16 ounces
1 quart (qt) =	2 pints

Metric System

Weight	
1 gram (gm) =	1,000 milligrams (mg)
1 kilogram (kg) =	1,000 grams
Volume	
1 liter =	1,000 cubic centimeters (cc)

Approximate Equivalents

Household, Metric, and Apothecary

1 teaspoon (tsp)	= 4 cc	= 1 fluid dram
1 tablespoon (tbsp)	= 15 cc	= ½ ounce
1 teacup	= 120 cc	= 4 fluid ounces
1 tumbler	= 240 cc	= 8 fluid ounces

Weights

Metric	*Apothecary*	*Metric*	*Apothecary*
0.4 mg =	1/150 grain	30 mg =	½ grain
0.6 mg =	1/100 grain	60 mg =	1 grain
1.0 mg =	1/60 grain	1 gm =	15 grains
10.0 mg =	⅙ grain	15 gm =	4 drams
15.0 mg =	¼ grain	30 gm =	1 ounce

Pounds to Kilograms Conversion

1 lb = 0.4536 kg	*1 kg = 2.2 lb*
lb	kg
5	2.3
10	4.5
20	9.1
30	13.6
40	18.1
50	22.7
60	27.2
70	31.7
80	36.3
90	40.8
100	45.5
110	49.9
120	54.4
130	58.9
140	63.5
150	68.0
160	72.6
170	77.1
180	81.6
190	86.2
200	90.7
210	95.3
220	99.5
230	104.3

- To convert kilograms to pounds: Multiply weight in kilograms by 2.2
- To convert pounds to kilograms: Divide weight in pounds by 2.2
- To convert centimeters to inches: Divide length in centimeters by 2.54

Linear Measures

1 millimeter (mm) =	0.04 inch (in.)
1 centimeter (cm) =	0.4 inch
1 decimeter (dm) =	4.0 inches
1 meter (m) =	39.37 inches
1 inch =	2.54 centimeters
1 foot =	30.48 centimeters

Celsius (centigrade) Fahrenheit Equivalents

Celsius	*Fahrenheit*	*Celsius*	*Fahrenheit*
36.0	96.8	39.0	102.2
36.5	97.7	39.5	103.1
37.0	98.6	40.0	104.0
37.5	99.5	40.5	104.9
38.0	100.4	41.0	105.8
38.5	101.3	41.5	106.7

- To convert inches to centimeters: Multiply length in inches by 2.54
- To convert degrees Fahrenheit to degrees Celsius: Subtract 32, then multiply by 5/9
- To convert degrees Celsius to degrees Fahrenheit: Multiply by 9/5 then add 32

Glossary

abandonment To leave a patient alone who is still in need of care or observation

Abbreviated Burn Severity Index (ABSI) A scale used to assess the severity of a burned patient's condition based on the patient's age and gender, presence of inhalation injury, depth of burn according to degree, and the percentage of the total body surface that has been burned

abduction Move away from the midline or turn outward

abscess Area of broken-down tissue containing pus and liquefied tissue

absorption To take in or soak up

AC joint *See* acromioclavicular joint

accreditation Process whereby businesses, educational institutions and programs, and health care organizations are determined to meet standards and performance criteria as established by an accrediting agency

Accreditation Review Council on Education in Surgical Technology and Surgical Assisting (ARC/STSA) A committee on accreditation that is under the large umbrella of the Commission on Accreditation of Allied Health Education Programs (CAAHEP), which oversees the accreditation processes of surgical technology education programs

acromioclavicular joint (AC joint) A part of the pectoral girdle located at the top of the shoulder that is an articulation between the lateral end of the clavicle and the flattened, small process located on the border of the acromion

acronym A word formed by the initial letters of the principal components of a compound term

ACTH *See* adrenocorticotropic hormone

active electrode Transfers concentrated electrical current into another medium (e.g., electrical current transformed into thermal energy)

acute Severe but of short duration

adduction Moving toward the midline or turning inward

adenocarcinoma Carcinoma derived from glandular tissue or in which the tumor cells form recognizable glandular structures

adhesion Abnormal attachment of two surfaces or structures that are normally separate

adhesive Type of surgical drape that is typically made of a thin, clear plastic material that has an adhesive backing and is applied to the skin; the drape may be impregnated with an antimicrobial iodine agent

adnexa Appendages or accessory structures of an organ

adrenocorticotropic hormone (ACTH) A hormone secreted by the anterior pituitary gland that stimulates the growth of the adrenal gland cortex and the secretion of corticosteroids. An increase in secretion occurs in response to a low level of circulating cortisol and to stress, fever, surgery, or hypoglycemia

advance directive Written instructions expressing the patient's wishes concerning the types and amount of medical treatment to be rendered in the event the patient can no longer make those types of decisions

adventitia The outermost layer of an artery composed of elastic connective tissue

aerodigestive tract Medical term for the throat

aesthetic Visually pleasing

affidavit Voluntary statement of facts sworn before an authority to be true

agonist Refers to an agent that stimulates or prolongs the response of a drug or a physiologic action

airborne bacteria Transported or spread by air; the surgical technologist is primarily concerned with airborne bacteria

alveolar process The part of the mandible or maxilla that forms the dental arch, which contains the sockets for the teeth

alveoli The terminal end of the bronchioles, grape-like clusters within the lung where the exchange of carbon dioxide and oxygen takes place

ambulatory surgical center Facility where patients are treated and released the same day; also known as outpatient surgery or same-day surgery center

amnesia Lack of recall

amphiarthrosis A joint that is slightly movable

anaphylaxis An immediate hypersensitivity reaction to a foreign protein or other specific substance

anastomosis Pathological, surgical, or traumatic formation of an opening between two normally separate organs or spaces

anesthesia Absence of sensation

aneurysm A sac formed by localized dilatation of the walls of an artery due to structural weakening

angina Intermittent or continuous cardiac pain caused by anoxia of the myocardium

antagonist Refers to an agent used to block the action of another drug or physiological action without producing any effect of its own

anterior chamber The cavity of the eye located anterior to the iris and containing the aqueous humor

anticipate To foresee or prepare for a situation before it occurs, such as the surgical technologist anticipating the surgeon's needs

antimicrobial Refers to an agent capable of killing some microorganisms and suppressing the growth of other types of microbes

antimuscarinic/anticholinergic Refers to an agent used to block parasympathetic effects such as salivation and bradycardia

aperture An opening

apical pulse The pulse taken at the apex of the heart

apnea Cessation of breathing

approximated Returned to proximity; brought together sides or edges

ARC/STSA *See* Accreditation Review Council on Education in Surgical Technology and Surgical Assisting

arrhythmia Absence of cardiac rhythm

arterial blood gases (ABGs) A method of monitoring blood oxygenation levels

arthrodesis Surgical fixation of a joint to relieve pain and provide support

ascites Abnormal collection of fluid in the abdominal cavity

asepsis Absence of microorganisms

aspiration Drawing in or out by suction

Association of Surgical Technologists (AST) The non-profit national professional membership organization for surgical technologists and surgical assistants

atria (pl.); atrium (sing.) Upper chambers of the heart that receive blood from the superior vena cava and inferior vena cava veins and the coronary sinus

augmentation Process of increasing; refers to size, quantity, degree, or severity

auscultation Use of the unaided ear or a stethoscope to listen to sounds within the body

autoclave Device to accomplish steam or gas sterilization

autoimmune diseases A disease such as rheumatoid arthritis that attacks the body's own tissues

autologous From oneself

avascular necrosis The consequence of temporary or permanent cessation of blood flow to the bones. The absence of blood causes the bone tissue to die, resulting in fracture or collapse of the entire bone.

back table Large movable table that is covered with a sterile drape for placement of sterile instruments, supplies, and equipment for surgical procedures

balanced salt solution (BSS) An irrigant used for the eye during eye procedures

bifurcation Division into two branches; "Y" shaped

bile A secretion of the liver that emulsifies fats, preparing them for further digestion and absorption in the small intestine

bioburden Amount of gross organic debris or the number of microorganisms on an object at any given time

biohazard Biologic material, which may be infective, that threatens humans or the environment

biological indicator A method for testing the sterilization capability of a sterilizer; contains microorganisms that are killed when exposed to a sterilization process; only method of guaranteeing the sterility of an item(s)

biopsy Removal of tissue or fluid from the body for pathological examination to determine a diagnosis

biotechnology The making of drugs in the laboratory using genetic engineering; also referred to as recombinant DNA technology

bipolar electrosurgery For this type of electrosurgery, both the active electrode and return electrode functions are performed at the site of surgery. The two tines of the forceps perform the active and return electrode functions. Only the tissue grasped is included in the electrical circuit. Because the return function is performed by one tine of the forceps, no patient return electrode is needed

Bowie-Dick test Specifically designed for use with a prevacuum steam sterilizer to test for air entrapment

breakpoints Points in the operating table that indicate where a section can be moved up or down

breech Intrauterine position of a fetus in which the buttocks or feet present first

BSS *See* balanced salt solution

buccal Pertaining to the cheek or mouth

calculi (pl.); calculus (sing.) Abnormal hard mass composed of minerals and salts; commonly referred to as a stone

calvarial Pertaining to the superior portion of the cranium where the fontanels of the infant are situated

cancellous bone A type of bone tissue found at the ends of bone and lining the medullary marrow cavity; composed of columns of trabeculae with large spaces in between; also referred to as spongy bone due to its appearance

capillaries The smallest blood vessels; composed of a single layer of endothelial cells where oxygen and carbon dioxide exchange occurs

capillary action Action by which liquid travels along an established path; often used in reference to suture in which infectious fluid travels along the length of the suture strand placed in a wound; also referred to as wicking

capnography Used in the anesthetic setting to provide a breath-by-breath analysis of expired carbon dioxide (end-tidal CO_2)

cardiac cycle Everything that occurs within the heart during a single heartbeat

cardiac dysrhythmias Refers to any type of abnormal heart rhythm

cardiopulmonary resuscitation (CPR) The act of manually providing chest compressions and ventilations to patients in cardiac arrest in an effort to provide oxygenated blood to the brain and vital organs, and reverse the processes that lead to death

carina The inferior tracheal cartilage that projects from the tracheal cartilage and bifurcates into the two primary bronchi

C-arm Type of portable fluoroscope, so named for its configuration

Cartesian coordinate geometry Refers to the 16th-century philosopher René Descartes, who invented coordinate geometry; also called *rectangular coordinate geometry*

cartilage A nonvascular fibrous connective tissue that is located in the joints, larynx, trachea, thorax, nose, and ear

cataract A pathological condition in which the crystalline lens has become opaque due to age or trauma

catheter A hollow, cylindrical tube that allows for the removal of fluids or air from the body, injection of fluids, removal of obstruction from ducts, or intravascular monitoring; may be plain tipped or may contain a retention balloon

catheterization The use or act of placing a catheter

cavitation Mechanical process used by ultrasonic cleaners during which air pockets implode to dislodge debris and soil from the crevices and serrations of surgical instruments and equipment

central nervous system (CNS) The system, composed of the brain and spinal cord, responsible for processing information to and from the peripheral nervous system. It is the main component that coordinates and controls the body's activities

central processing unit (CPU) Silicon chip located within the computer case that is responsible for coordinating the operations of the computer, managing the computer systems, and facilitating the exchange of data with the computer memory

central venous catheter A catheter passed through a peripheral vein and ending in the thoracic vena cava; it is used to measure venous pressure or to infuse concentrated solutions

cerebellum The portion of the brain located in the posterior cranial fossa posterior to the brainstem; consists of two lobes; functions include coordinating voluntary muscular activity

cerebrospinal fluid (CSF) The fluid that flows through the ventricles of the brain, subarachnoid space, and spinal canal; serves to protect these structures

cerebrum The largest section of the brain, divided by a fissure into the right and left cerebral hemispheres; at the bottom of the fissure the hemispheres are connected by the corpus callosum, and the surface of the hemispheres is convoluted and lobed; functions include motor functions, sensory functions, and functions associated with the many mental activities of the individual

cesarean section (C-section) A surgical procedure in which the abdomen and uterus are incised to deliver a baby

chalazion A small, red, inflamed lump that can be located on the inner or outer surface of the eyelid; caused by an inflammatory reaction to material trapped inside the meibomian gland in the eyelid

cheilo- Combining form that means lip

chelation A method of cleaning instruments in which the chosen cleaning solution uses the process of binding ions, such as iron and magnesium, in the solution to prevent their deposit on the surface of surgical instruments

chemical indicator Internal or external monitor that changes color when exposed to the sterilization process; only indicates that the sterilization process has occurred; it does not guarantee the sterility of the item

cholangiography A preoperative and intraoperative diagnostic tool in which a catheter is inserted into the common bile duct and contrast medium is injected to outline potential calculi under fluoroscopy

chole- Combining form that means bile

cholesteatoma A mass composed of cholesterol and epithelial cells that is either congenital or occurs as a complication of chronic otitis media; located in the middle ear

chondroradionecrosis One of the most serious complications of radiation therapy. It may progress or become fatal despite aggressive treatment measures.

chromic A suture material manufactured from the submucosa of sheep intestine or serosa of beef intestine treated with chromium salts to delay the rate of absorption

chromic gut *See* chromic

chronic wound Wound that persists for an extended period of time

cicatrix Scar

circle of Willis A complex vascular network located at the base of the brain and formed by the following interconnected arteries: internal carotid, anterior cerebral, posterior cerebral, basilar, anterior communicating, and posterior communicating

circuit The path that electricity travels between an energy source and its usage device(s)

circulator Nonsterile surgical team member who moves about the periphery of the sterile field

circumcision Surgical removal of the foreskin

circumferentially Circularly, or moving completely around an item, as in the circumferential prep of an extremity

claudication Severe pains in the muscle of the lower leg caused by poor circulation of blood to the muscle; usually caused by atherosclerosis

cleft Cleave, crack, or fissure

CNS *See* central nervous system

Code of Ethics Guidelines, usually expressed in a series of statements, that provide ethical standards of conduct for a profession

colonization The growth and collection of microbes into a group that lives in a particular area, such as the colonization of *S. aureus* in the nares of humans

comminuted fracture A type of bone fracture consisting of three or more fragments

compartmental syndrome Elevation of tissue pressure within a closed fascial compartment, causing a decreased arteriovenous pressure and decreased muscular perfusion.

competency (1) Skill; (2) ability; (3) statements that establish the level of skill or quality needed to be able to perform the job duties of a profession

compound fracture A fracture in which a bone fragment punctures the skin and exposes the bone; also referred to as an *open fracture*

compress To apply pressure

conduit Channel or pipe for conveying fluids

condyle Rounded projection/process at the epiphysis of a bone that articulates with another bone; serves as the point of attachment for ligaments

congenital Present at birth

contaminated Soiled with gross debris or by the presence of microbes

contraindication A reason why a specific procedure or drug may be undesirable or improper in a particular situation

contralateral The opposite side

contrast medium Solution injected into arteries, veins, or ducts during a radiographic exam that is radiopaque and therefore stands out in contrast to the surrounding tissues

Core Curriculum for Surgical Technology The recommended appropriate curriculum template for an educational program that provides the expected entry-level knowledge for the surgical technologist.

cortex Outermost part of a structure

cortical bone Type of bone tissue that is hard and dense, and that surrounds the marrow cavity; also referred to as *compact bone*

cottonoid Another name for neurosurgical sponge; used to protect delicate neural tissue and to assist with hemostasis

count Term used to describe the act of counting items used intraoperatively that could potentially be left in a surgical wound

CPR *See* cardiopulmonary resuscitation

craniosynostosis Premature closure of the cranial sutures of an infant

craniotomy Incision into the cranium

credentialing Process by which an agency or organization establishes a minimum knowledge base for a given health care profession and awards a credential to individuals who meet the minimum knowledge level

cryo- Prefix or combining form meaning cold

CSF *See* cerebrospinal fluid

curettage Removal of tissue with a blunt or sharp curette by scraping the surface; performed to remove abnormal tissue, to obtain tissue for examination and diagnostic purposes, or to remove tissue from infected areas

cylindrical Object with a tubular shape

cystoscopy The insertion of an endoscope through the urethra and into the bladder for the purpose of viewing for treatment and diagnosis
dacryo- Combining form referring to the lacrimal apparatus of the eye
dead space A space that remains in the tissues as a result of failure of proper closure of a surgical wound
debridement Removal of devitalized tissue and contaminants
decompress To remove pressure
decontamination room Room that typically contains sinks for gross decontamination, an ultrasonic washer, and a washer-sterilizer to decontaminate instruments and equipment
degrees of freedom The number of ways in which a robotic manipulator moves
dehiscence Partial or total separation of a layer or layers of tissue after closure of the wound
delayed union A delay in the healing of the ends of a fracture
dermatome Powered or manually operated surgical instrument used to cut thin slices of skin for grafting purposes
diabetes mellitus A disorder of the endocrine system that affects the production of insulin in the pancreas; either type I (in which the pancreas produces little or no insulin) or type II (in which the pancreas produces different amounts of insulin)
diarthrosis Freely movable joint
diathermy The use of high-frequency electromagnetic currents to cauterize blood vessels and destroy neoplasms
distraction Separation of joint surfaces by extension without injury or dislocation of the parts
DO *See* Doctor of Osteopathy
docho- Combining form meaning intestine
Doctor of Osteopathy (DO) A physician who treats patients in a holistic manner and emphasizes the use of manipulative techniques for correcting abnormalities thought to cause disease and inhibit recovery
donning To put on or dress in
Doppler Ultrasonic device used to identify and assess vascular status of peripheral arteries and veins by magnifying the sound of the blood moving through the vessel
drain Hollow, cylindrical device that is used to evacuate air and/or fluids from a surgical wound; may be passive or active
drug Agent used as a medicine for the diagnosis, treatment, cure, mitigation, or prophylaxis of a disease or condition
DUB *See* dysfunctional uterine bleeding
ductus arteriosus A fetal blood vessel that joins the aorta and pulmonary artery
dynamic equilibrium The individual's ability to adjust to displacements of the body's center of gravity
dysfunctional uterine bleeding (DUB) Abnormal uterine bleeding that is not due to a tumor, pregnancy, or infection; occurs when menstruation is not taking place
dyspnea Difficult or labored breathing
dystocia Difficult labor due to various reasons, such as cephalopelvic distortion, fetus size, or condition or position of fetus
ECG *See* electrocardiograph
-ectomy Suffix meaning removal of
EEG *See* electroencephalography
elective surgery Pertaining to a surgical intervention that does not require immediate intervention; the patient "elects" to have the surgery at a specific time
electrocardiogram (ECG) A record of the heart's electrical activity
electrocardiograph (ECG or EKG) A device used for recording the heart's electrical activity to detect transmissions of the electrical cardiac impulse through the tissues of the myocardium
electroencephalography (EEG) Display and recording of the brain's electrical activity by measurement of changes in electric potentials
electrons The negatively charged particles circling the nucleus of an atom
electrosurgical unit (ESU) Mechanical device that produces an electric current that is converted into thermal energy (heat) for the purpose of cutting or coagulating tissue
elliptical Curved or crescent shaped
embolus A piece of tissue, thrombus, air, or gas that circulates in the circulatory system until it becomes lodged in a vessel
emergent Surgical pathology that is life threatening
endoscope A general term used to describe the various types of flexible or rigid scopes used to view the body's internal structures
enterocolitis Inflammation of the small intestine and colon
enucleation En bloc removal of a structure; usually refers to the removal of the eye
epidural Above or outside the dura mater
epiglottis The small cartilaginous structure that acts like a lid and closes the passageway to the larynx to prevent food from entering the larynx and trachea during the act of swallowing
epiphysis The proximal portion of a long bone
episiotomy The surgical incision of perineum to enlarge the vaginal opening and prevent tearing of the perineum and muscles during delivery
epistaxis Nosebleed
ESU *See* electrosurgical unit

ethics Branch of philosophy dealing with good conduct and moral values

event-related sterility Sterility determined by how a sterile package is handled rather than time elapsed; the package is considered sterile until opened, or until the integrity of the packaging material is compromised

evisceration Interruption of a closed wound or traumatic injury that exposes the viscera

excision Surgical removal

exenteration Refers to total removal of; usually used in reference to the surgical procedure of total pelvic exenteration, which involves the removal of the vagina, uterus and cervix, fallopian tubes, ovaries, bladder, and rectum for surgical treatment of cancer

extracapsular cataract extraction A method for surgically removing a cataract through an incision in the side of the cornea and replacing the diseased lens with an intraocular implant

extrinsic muscles The six muscles of the eye that come from the bones of the orbit and function to move the eye in various directions

extruded Forced out of position

fenestration Opening

fimbria Finger-like structures that form on an edge, such as the fimbria of the fallopian tubes

first intention Type of healing that occurs with primary union that is typical of an incision opened under ideal conditions; healing occurs from side to side, dead space has been eliminated, and the wound edges are accurately approximated

fistulas Abnormal communication between two normally separate internal structures, or an abnormal communication between an internal structure and the body surface

flexion Bending of a joint

Fogarty embolectomy catheter A type of catheter that is small in diameter and is balloon-tipped; used to facilitate the removal of an embolus

free electrons The outermost electrons in the atom's orbit that can most easily be attracted away from the nucleus

French-eyed needle A type of needle in which the suture must be threaded by pulling the strand into a V-shaped area just above the eye

friable Easily torn or crumbled

frozen section A pathological method of diagnosis that involves freezing a tissue sample, slicing it into thin sections, staining it, and then viewing it under a microscope

Gelfoam Type of absorbable gelatin hemostatic agent that is made from purified pork skin gelatin; available in either pad or powder form, it is placed over an area of bleeding to control hemorrhage

generator Devices that convert mechanical energy to electric energy

generic Nonproprietary name for a drug that is often a shortened version of the chemical name and may include a reference to the intended use

Gerota's fascia A fibrous capsule that encircles the kidney to aid in keeping the kidney in the correct anatomical position and to cushion it from injury

Gibson incision A surgical incision that begins medial to the anterosuperior iliac spine and curves downward and medially, to slightly above the symphysis pubis; specifically designed for access to the lower portion of the ureter

glenoid fossa The socket in which the head of the humerus articulates to form the shoulder joint; a ball-and-socket joint

glioma Group of malignant tumors composed of glial cells

globe The eyeball in its entirety

glottis The small opening between the true vocal cords

golden hour Concept that medical treatment of a trauma victim within the first hour following injury improves patient outcomes

-gram Suffix meaning written record

Gram stain Laboratory method of identifying bacteria; bacteria that stain purple are referred to as *gram-positive*, and bacteria that do not retain the stain and appear red in color are referred to as *gram-negative*

-graph Suffix meaning producing a drawing or writing

gravida Refers to the pregnant female; the first pregnancy is referred to as gravida I; additional pregnancies are numbered sequentially

grounding pad A pad that is placed on a patient to complete the pathway for the electrical current back to the electrosurgical unit; also called the *dispersive electrode*

hand wash The mechanical and chemical washing of the hands to aid in removing transient microorganisms, dirt, and debris

health maintenance organization (HMO) Health care organization that serves as both the insurer and provider of medical services; typically, a group of physicians provides services to a population of clients who voluntarily enroll in the program

hematoma Localized collection of extravasated blood that is often clotted

hemolysis The destruction of erythrocytes

hemostasis The arrest of the escape of blood through natural or artificial means

hemostat A device or agent used as a coagulant

HEPA filter *See* high-efficiency particulate air (HEPA) filter

herniation Abnormal protrusion of an organ or other body structure through an opening in a covering membrane or muscle

high-efficiency particulate air (HEPA) filter Filter that is capable of removing bacteria as small as 0.5–5 mm; utilized in the operating room to aid in preventing the patient from acquiring a postoperative wound infection

hilum The medial border of the kidney that is convex and receives the renal blood vessels

HIV *See* human immunodeficiency virus

HMO *See* health maintenance organization

homeostasis The reactions in the body that act and counteract to maintain the body in a normal physiological state

homologous From the same species

human immunodeficiency virus (HIV) The virus that causes acquired immune deficiency syndrome (AIDS)

hyaline cartilage An elastic connective tissue that covers the ends of bones, supports the trachea and larynx, and connects the ribs to the sternum. It is covered by the perichondrium and calcifies as the individual ages

hyperthermia Abnormally high body temperature

hypertrophy Enlargement or overgrowth of a structure due to an increase in the size of its cells

hypnosis Altered state of consciousness that may be achieved by suggestion of another, an individual's own concentration, or with the use of a substance

hypospadias A congenital abnormality characterized by the urethral opening located on the underside of the penis or on the perineum of the male, or in the vagina of the female

hypothermia Abnormally low body temperature, typically defined as a core body temperature that is below 35°C

ICP *See* intracranial pressure

immediate-use steam sterilization A process of quickly sterilizing unwrapped items (such as a surgical instrument that has been dropped on the floor and is needed right away) using prevacuum or gravity steam sterilizers

immersion Placing an item in a container so it is completely covered by a liquid, such as immersing a surgical instrument in glutaraldehyde

immunocompetence Degree of function of an immune system that is designed to keep a patient from infection by pathogens

immunosuppressed patient Patient whose immune system has decreased due to disease, or intentionally decreased with immunosuppressive drugs for organ transplant patients to prevent organ rejection

in situ At the site of origin, or in its normal place

incident report Mechanism for reporting an incident, usually by completing a document describing what happened, related to any adverse patient occurrence

incision Cut made with a sharp instrument

incontinence Inability to control excretory functions

indication A reason to perform a specific procedure or prescribe a certain drug

indicator Tape, paper, vial, or other item used to confirm that a specific reaction has taken place (such as the chemical indicators for steam sterilization)

induction The second phase of general anesthesia, in which the patient is given induction drugs and intubated

indwelling A substance or item that remains in place either permanently or for a period of time

infarction An area of dead tissue caused by an inadequate supply of oxygenated blood

infiltrate Accumulation or diffusion of a foreign substance into tissue

inflammation The body's protective response to injury or tissue destruction

informed consent A situation in which a patient gives voluntary permission to another party (i.e., surgeon or anesthesia provider) to perform the procedures that have been explained; includes the risks, benefits, possible complications, and alternative treatment options

innominate An unnamed structure; for example, the innominate artery that branches from the arch of the aorta and divides into the right common carotid and right subclavian artery

insufflation Forcing powder, gas, or vapor into a body cavity

insulator Material that inhibits the flow of free electrons; typically prevents electron leakage and directs the flow to a destination

integrity Complete, with no breaks or tears

integumentary Pertaining to or composed of skin

intermediate-level disinfection Level of disinfection in which most microorganisms are killed except spores

intima Inner layer of the arterial vessel wall

intra-arterial measurement A method of ECG monitoring in which the intra-arterial catheter is inserted directly into the artery

intra-articular Within a joint

intracapsular cataract extraction A method for surgically removing a cataract by injecting alpha chymotrypsin into the posterior chamber to digest the suspensory ligament so that the diseased lens can be removed in its entirety

intracranial pressure (ICP) Pressure produced within the cranium; when elevated, represents a space-occupying lesion or brain edema

intraoperative Occurs during the surgical intervention

intravenous urogram (IVU) Diagnostic study that involves the injection of a contrast medium into a vein; the radiopaque material is filtered through the kidney and excreted, providing an outline of the entire urologic system; formerly called *intravenous pyelogram* (IVP)

ionizing radiation Process by which energy either directly or indirectly induces ionization of radiation-absorbing material or tissues; X-rays

iridotomy Incision of the iris for the creation of a new aperture in the iris when the pupil is closed

irrigation Washing with a stream of fluid

ischemia Lack of oxygenated blood supply to an area or organ of the body

isotope scanning Involves the intravenous injection of a radioactive isotope into the patient prior to an imaging study; also referred to as *nuclear medicine study* or *radionuclide imaging*

IVU *See* intravenous urogram

Joint Commission, The An independent, nonprofit national organization that develops standards and performance criteria for health care organizations

Julian date Calendar days that are sequentially numbered through the year; often used when maintaining sterilization records (i.e., February 1 would be the 32nd day of the Julian calendar)

Kaposi's sarcoma A cancer that produces painful external and internal lesions; internally, the lesions can cause complications, such as difficulty in swallowing (if present in the esophagus) or bowel obstruction (when present in the intestine)

kerato- Combining form or prefix indicating a relation to horny substances or to the cornea

kernicterus A potentially lethal disease of newborns caused by excessive accumulation of the bile pigment bilirubin

kinematics An attempt to understand the mechanism of injury and the action and effect of a particular type of force on the human body

labia (pl.); labium (sing.) Lips; a fleshy border

labial Side of tooth that is closest to the lips

laceration Cut or tear

lacrimal A facial bone that, along with the zygomatic bone and palate, helps to form the orbit of the eye

laminar airflow The unidirectional positive-pressure flow of air that captures microbes to be filtered

lap sponge A type of surgical sponge that is the largest and most absorbent of the sponges

laryngo- Combining form meaning larynx

laryngospasm Sudden involuntary contraction of the larynx capable of causing partial or total occlusion of the larynx

LEEP *See* loop electrosurgical excision

liability (1) An obligation to do or not do something; (2) An obligation potentially or actually incurred as a result of a negligent act

ligament A band of fibrous tissue composed of collagen that connects bone to bone

ligated The placement of a suture tie around a vessel or other anatomical structure for the purpose of constriction (i.e., to control hemorrhage from a blood vessel)

linen hamper Four-wheeled stand that can be lined with a biohazardous-marked bag for the collection of nondisposable linen during a surgical procedure

load The weight supported or force imposed

loop electrosurgical excision (LEEP) Surgical procedure that uses the electrosurgical unit coupled to a loop electrode on the cautery pencil; used to excise a cone of tissue to remove an area of neoplasia

lumen The opening in a tube or vessel

lysis Dissolution, loosening, or destruction of something

magnification Process of enlarging the size of an object with the use of a device such as a microscope

malar bone Cheek bone

malocclusion Abnormal alignment of the teeth of the upper jaw with those of the lower jaw

malpractice Professional misconduct that results in harm to another; negligence of a health care professional

malunion The joining of the fragments of a fractured bone in a faulty position, forming an imperfect alignment, shortening, deformity, or rotation

marrow Semisolid tissue found in the spaces of cancellous bone; there are two types: red bone marrow and yellow bone marrow

marsupialization Incision of a closed cavity with the suturing of the opened edges to the wall of the wound to form an open wound that will heal by second intention

mask A cover worn over the mouth and nose by surgical personnel to prevent blood and body fluids from splashing into those areas; also protects the patient from the surgical personnel's secretions

Maslow's hierarchy of needs A model developed by Maslow that expresses human development and progression using developmental stages that prioritize needs

mass The property of a body that causes it to have weight in a gravitational field

maxillofacial Pertaining to the face and maxilla

Mayo stand Small portable stand with a tray on top that is covered with a sterile drape and on which the instruments, equipment, and supplies that are most frequently used for the surgical procedure are placed; it is most often positioned over the patient's legs

mediastinum The area in the thoracic cavity in the middle of the thorax between the lungs

medulla Innermost part of a structure

meninges Three tissue membranes (called *dura mater, arachnoid, pia mater*) that enclose the brain and spinal cord
metacarpophalangeal joint (MPJ) A synovial hinge-type joint consisting of a metacarpal that articulates with a phalange; commonly referred to as a knuckle
modem A communications hardware device that enables the sending and receiving of data over a telephone line or cable; typically used to send e-mail or to access the Internet
monitor A visual interface for computers
monofilament suture Suture that is manufactured from one strand of natural or synthetic material
monopolar cautery Monopolar electrocautery in which the electrical circuit completes a path from the generator, to the patient, and then back again to the generator
moral principles Guides for ethical decision making that include the concern individuals have for the well-being of others, respect for individual autonomy, basic justice, prevention of harm to others, and refusal to take unfair advantage
morbidity Pertaining to disease
mortality Pertaining to death
mouse A hand device used to move a cursor on a computer monitor and select a file or function
mouth prop A self-retaining retractor used to keep the mouth open during oral or dental procedures
MPJ *See* metacarpophalangeal joint
myocardium The muscle of the heart that is composed of specially constructed cardiac muscle cells that contract and force blood from the heart's chambers
myoma A benign fibroid tumor of the uterus
myringo- Combining form referring to the tympanic membrane
National Board of Surgical Technology and Surgical Assisting (NBSTSA) Organization that is solely responsible for all decisions regarding certification, from determining eligibility to maintaining, denying, granting, and renewing the designation.
NBSTSA *See* National Board of Surgical Technology and Surgical Assisting
necrosis Tissue death
negligence Omission or commission of an act that a reasonable or prudent person would not do under the same conditions
neutral zone An area designated within the sterile field in which sharps may be safely placed by one person and retrieved by another
neutrons Subatomic particles equal in mass to protons but without an electrical charge
nonunion Failure to unite, as in a fractured bone that fails to heal completely
NPO Nothing by mouth; Latin acronym for *nil per os*
obstruction Hindrance or blockage of a passage
occiput anterior The most common relationship between the presenting fetal part and the maternal body pelvis
occlusion An obstruction
Occupational Safety and Health Administration (OSHA) Federal organization that is dedicated to protecting the health of workers by establishing standards that address issues related to safety in the workplace
ocutome A cutting system for posterior vitrectomy
olfaction Sense of smell
-oma Suffix meaning tumor
optional Surgical intervention that does not have to be performed in order to preserve life or limb
oropharynx Pertaining to the oral cavity and pharynx
OSHA *See* Occupational Safety and Health Administration
osteogenesis Development of bone tissue
osteophyte An abnormal bony growth
-ostomy Suffix meaning to create a new opening
oto- Combining form meaning ear
-otomy Suffix meaning to make an incision into
oxygenated Saturated with oxygen
packing Sterile fine-mesh gauze that is loosely placed in a chronic wound or one that has been left open to heal by second intention
PACU *See* postanesthesia care unit
palpation Examining by touch
pan- Combining form meaning *all*
parasympathetic nervous system (PNS) A division of the autonomic nervous system that slows the heart rate, relaxes sphincters of the body, and increases peristalsis in the GI tract
parenteral Taken into the body or administered in a manner other than through the digestive tract, as by intravenous or intramuscular injection.
parietal (1) Refers to the outer portion of a cavity or organ; (2) pertaining to the parietal bone of the cranium; (3) pertaining to the parietal lobe of the cerebrum
parity The classification used to indicate the number of live and stillborn births that a female has delivered at more than 20 weeks of gestation
patency The condition of being wide open
pathogen Microorganism that is capable of causing disease
pathology The study of the characteristics, causes, and effects of disease on the human body
pathology department The department responsible for testing and processing specimens, tissues, and body fluids to obtain a diagnosis
patient The person receiving medical treatment

Patient Care Partnership Replacing the AHA's Patients' Bill of Rights, this plain-language brochure informs patients about what they should expect during their hospital stay with regard to their rights and responsibilities

patient return electrode New term that replaces *dispersive (inactive) electrode;* also called a grounding pad

penetrating trauma Injury caused by a foreign object, such as a bullet or knife, that passes through tissue

perfusionist The individual responsible for running and maintaining the cardiopulmonary bypass machine during open heart procedures

pericardium A thin serous sac that surrounds the heart; it consists of the serous pericardium and fibrous pericardium

perineum The area between the posterior portion of the vagina or scrotum and the opening to the anus

peripheral nervous system (PNS) The part of the nervous system that is outside the central nervous system and comprises the cranial nerves excepting the optic nerve, the spinal nerves, and the autonomic nervous system

peritoneum A thin serous membrane that lines the abdominal cavity

permeability The condition of being permeable; capable of allowing the passage of fluids or substances

personal protective equipment (PPE) Attire worn to protect against exposure to physical and biological hazards

Pfannenstiel Surgical transverse incision made in the lower abdomen, usually employed when performing a cesarean section

pharmacodynamics The interaction of drug molecules with target cells, resulting in biochemical and physiological actions

pharmacokinetics The study of the movement of drugs through the body, involving absorption, distribution, biotransformation, and excretion

pharmacology The study of drugs and their actions

phrenic Pertaining to the diaphragm

physical need Any need or activity related to genetics, physiology, or anatomy

plasma (1) Liquid portion of body fluid; (2) an ionized gas made primarily of free electrons and having a neutral charge

pledget Small square of Teflon sutured over a hole in a vessel; it exerts external pressure over any small needle holes to prevent bleeding and to promote clotting; often used in peripheral vascular surgery

plethysmography An instrument for determining and registering variations in the volume of an extremity and in the amount of blood present in the extremity or passing through it; useful in patients with diffuse, small-vessel arterial disease

pleura A thin serous membrane that encloses the lung, composed of a single layer of mesothelial cells on top of a thin layer of connective tissue; it is divided into the visceral and parietal pleural layers

plume Smoke produced by laser or electrocautery that has been shown to contain biological material

pneumatic Pertaining to air

pneumothorax Abnormal accumulation of air in the pleural cavity

PNS *See* parasympathetic nervous system

PNS *See* peripheral nervous system

poly- Prefix meaning many or much

polymethyl methacrylate (PMMA) A chemical compound composed of a mixture of liquid and powder used for cementing prostheses during total joint arthroplasties; also referred to as bone cement

polyp Growth that protrudes from a mucous membrane; often precancerous growths

polysomnography Diagnostic test during which physiological variables are measured and recorded during sleep; often administered to individuals who suffer from some type of sleep disorder

polytetrafluoroethylene (PTFE) A synthetic coating used on certain types of nylon suture material to reduce the drag through tissue

portal venous system Venous system that carries blood to a second capillary bed prior to returning the blood to general circulation

postanesthesia care unit (PACU) Area where immediate postoperative care of the patient takes place before transfer to the hospital room or ICU

posterior chamber The area behind the iris, but in front of and behind the lens

postoperative Period of time after surgery when the patient is recovering

power The ability or capacity to perform or act effectively

PPE *See* personal protective equipment

preceptor Instructor or tutor who demonstrates the general rules of conduct and procedures and guides the students while they are practicing or performing

preoperative Period of time before the surgical procedure begins

prep Preparation, such as the skin prep of the patient

prepuce A fold of skin that forms a cover that can be pulled back, such as the foreskin of the penis and the fold around the clitoris

pressure The force per unit of area; applied evenly over a surface

primary suture line Main suture that approximates the wound edges for first intention healing to occur

professional An individual who has special education and experience in a given field and who meets certain competency-based and ethical criteria

prolapse To fall or slip out of normal anatomical position

prone A position in which the patient lies face downward

prophylaxis Prevention of a disease or condition

proprietary Organization or company that is owned and operated by an individual or corporation with the intent of making a profit that is returned to the investors; the profit is taxable

prostate-specific antigen (PSA) A protein produced and secreted by the prostate; elevated levels in the bloodstream may indicate cancer or another disease of the prostate

prosthesis Artificial device used to replace a body structure, aid bodily function, or give a cosmetic appearance; may be permanent or removable

protons An elemental particle with a positive charge equal to the negative charge of the electron

proximal Nearer to the origin of a structure

PSA *See* prostate-specific antigen

psychological need A mental requirement or necessity for fulfillment as a person

PTFE *See* polytetrafluoroethylene

radial hypoplasia A congenital condition caused by the failure of the radius and adjacent soft tissue to develop, causing the hand to be medially deranged; typically associated with deformities of the thumb; also referred to as radial dysplasia

ramus Smaller branch of a structure that extends from a larger branch that divides into two parts, such as the rami of the pubis

reduction Correction or placement of a body structure back into normal anatomical position

regurgitation Backward flow of fluid, in the opposite of a normal direction

replantation The replacement of an organ or other structure to the site from which it was previously lost or removed; also known as reimplantation

resident organisms Microorganisms that live on and within the body and that are beneficial for health; typically refers to bacteria that live below the skin surface in hair follicles and glandular openings; also referred to as *normal* or *resident flora*

resistance (1) Opposing or counteracting force; (2) a force that delays or impedes action

restricted area The areas of an operating department (including the sterile storage areas of the surgery department) that require proper OR attire, including the wearing of a mask

retract To draw back; to expose

retrobulbar Behind the eyeball or pons

retroperitoneal Referring to the space between the peritoneum and the posterior abdominal wall

Revised Trauma Score (RTS) A scoring system used to assess the severity of a traumatic wound and to determine the condition of a patient

Rh (Rhesus) factor Genetically determined blood group antigen that is present on the surface of erythrocytes of some individuals; if the antigen is present the individual is Rh+ (positive) and if absent Rh− (negative)

rhino- Combining form that means nose

rhinoplasty Surgical reshaping of the nose

ring stand A stand that is designed with one or two circular bands at the top to hold sterile basins

risk management The efforts of a health care provider organization to collect and utilize data to decrease the chance of harm to patients or staff or damage to property

roentgenography Radiography; X-rays

Safe Medical Device Act Established in 1990, this act requires medical device users to report to the manufacturer and/or FDA incidents that reasonably suggest that there is a probability that a medical device has caused or contributed to the death, serious injury, or illness of a patient

scalpel Another name for the surgical knife handle on which knife blades are attached

-schisis Root word pertaining to split or cleft

-sclerosis Suffix relating to hardening of a structure or tissue due to a pathological occurrence

scope of practice Professional duty limits based on state and federal law and on an individual's education and experience

sebum Oily substance produced by the sebaceous glands that reaches the skin through ducts that enter the hair follicle; aids with fluid regulation and acts to keep the skin and hair soft and pliable

second intention Healing that occurs when a wound fails to heal by primary union, or the wound is left open and allowed to heal from the inside to the outside by filling with granulation tissue

secondary suture line Sutures placed to support and ease the tension on the primary suture line, thus reinforcing the wound closure and obliterating any dead spaces

sedation State of being calm, usually effected by means of a sedative drug

sedative Agent that produces a soothing or quieting effect but does not cause the person to sleep

septic shock A state of shock produced by septicemia, when the body is overwhelmed by the pathogenic microorganisms and cannot adequately fight the infection

serrations Grooves located on the jaws of surgical instruments that are either longitudinal, cross-hatched, or horizontal

shoulder joint The ball-and-socket joint composed of the head of the humerus that rests in the glenoid fossa

sign Indication of a disease or condition perceived by the examiner

sinuses Dilated channels for venous blood

SMR *See* submucous resection

social need A need to fit into society and to be accepted by one's peers

spiritual need A need for a connection with a higher order

splenectomy Removal of the spleen

splenomegaly Abnormal enlargement of the spleen

splint A rigid device that is placed on one side of an extremity to immobilize and support while healing takes place; available in many forms (plastic, wood, metal, plaster)

split-thickness skin graft (STSG) A graft that involves the epidermis and approximately half the dermis; used when a large surface area needs to be covered

SSI *See* surgical site infection

stainless steel A type of metal that is a combination of carbon, chromium, iron, and other metals; most often used in the manufacture of surgical instruments

Standard Precautions Guidelines established by the Occupational Safety and Health Administration and the Centers for Disease Control and Prevention to reduce the risk of disease transmission from blood and body fluids

-stasis Suffix meaning stoppage or reduction of the flow of bodily fluids

stenosis Narrowing or constriction

stent (1) Device inserted to support luminous structures while still allowing passage of fluid; (2) external device applied to secure a skin graft or dressing in place

sterile attire Sterile garment and gloves donned during a surgical procedure

sterile field Area of sterility maintained by the surgical team during a procedure

sterile team member Member of the surgical team who has performed a surgical scrub, donned the sterile gown and gloves, and works within the sterile field

sterile technique Methods used to prevent contamination of the sterile field and prevent the patient from acquiring a postoperative wound infection

sterilization (1) Procedure to render an individual incapable of reproduction; (2) process by which all microorganisms, including spores, are destroyed

stoma An incised opening that is kept open for drainage or other purposes

strabismus A pathological condition involving a misalignment or deviation of the eyes that prevents them from working simultaneously to track visual objects

STSG *See* split-thickness skin graft

submucous resection (SMR) A surgical procedure to restore normal breathing; involves incising the mucous membrane lining of the nasal cavity, lifting the underlying perichondrium, removing underlying mucous membrane structures, and placing the mucous membrane back into position; also called a *septoplasty*

suction The act of sucking up air or fluids through a device, such as a tonsil suction tip

suction outlet A wall or ceiling connection for a suction device

supine A position in which the patient lies on his or her back, face upward, with arms usually placed on arm boards with the palms facing up

suprarenal glands Endocrine glands that rest on the superior portion of the kidneys; consist of a cortex and medulla; the cortex secretes steroid-type hormones essential to the control of fluid and electrolyte balance, and the medulla secretes epinephrine and norepinephrine

surgeon's preference card A list of the equipment, supplies, and surgical instrument set(s) that a surgeon prefers for each surgical procedure performed; used as a guide in collecting the items to be used for the surgical procedure; most surgery departments now have the cards stored on a computer, eliminating the need for handwritten cards

surgical conscience The basis for the practice of strict adherence to sterile technique by all surgical team members; involves a level of honesty and moral integrity that must be upheld

surgical scrub A hand and arm wash that is performed prior to donning the sterile gown and gloves; used for the purpose of removing as many microorganisms as possible and for arresting the growth of others; accomplished with the use of chemicals and mechanical action

surgical site infection (SSI) An infection of the surgical wound that was acquired during the course of the surgical procedure

swaged Strand of suture material with an eyeless needle attached by the manufacturer; the needle is continuous with the suture strand

switch A device used to open or close a circuit, thereby controlling the flow of electricity

symphysis A joint in which the two bony surfaces are joined by fibrocartilage (meniscus)

symptom Indication of a disease or condition perceived by the patient

syndactyly Webbed digits; congenital abnormality that occurs when the digits of the hands or feet fail to separate

synthesis The formation of a new entity out of previously existing ones

systole Represents the contraction phase of the cardiac cycle

T&A *See* tonsillectomy and adenoidectomy

tachycardia Fast heart rate that is greater than 100 beats per minute

tamponade Pathological compression of an anatomical part

teeth Small projections from the tip(s) of the jaw of certain surgical instruments; used to aid in grasping tissue or vessels

temporomandibular joint (TMJ) The joint formed by the mandible that articulates with the glenoid fossa in each temporal bone

tensile strength Amount of pull or tension that a suture strand will withstand before breaking; expressed in pounds

third intention Healing that occurs when two granulated surfaces are approximated; also referred to as *delayed primary closure*

thrombus Stationary blood clot within a blood vessel

TMJ *See* temporomandibular joint

tonsillectomy and adenoidectomy (T&A) Surgical removal of the tonsils and adenoids

topical As pertaining to anesthesia, an agent that is applied to the surface of the skin or anatomical structure (such as the eye) to produce a loss of feeling or sensation in the area of application; blocks the nerve conduction of superficial nerves

torsion A condition of being twisted

tort law Describes any civil wrong independent of a contract; allows for a remedy in the form of an action for damages

torticollis An abnormal contracted state of a muscle(s)

transient organisms Organisms that reside on the surface of the skin and are easily removed by hand washing

transsphenoidal Across or through the sphenoid bone

transurethral resection of the prostate (TURP) The partial or full removal of the prostate gland with a resectoscope that is placed through the urethra

trephine A cylindrical saw for cutting a circular piece of bone

tunic An investing membrane

TURP *See* transurethral resection of the prostate

ulcer A crater-like lesion that is usually circular in shape and penetrates the skin; may be very deep, resulting from infections or malignant disease processes

ultrasonic cleaner A machine used to remove minute organic particles and soil from the areas of instrumentation hardest to reach by manual or other mechanical methods of cleaning; the washer utilizes the process of cavitation for cleaning instruments

ultrasonography The use of high-frequency waves that are directed into the body and are reflected from the tissues to record an image for diagnostic purposes

UPPP *See* uvulopalatopharyngoplasty

ureteral Pertaining to the ureters that exit the kidney and transport urine from the kidney to the bladder

urethral Pertaining to the urethra, which travels from the bladder to the exterior of the body

urgent Surgical pathology requiring treatment within a relatively short period of time

urinalysis (UA) Laboratory examination of a urine specimen for diagnostic purposes

urinary tract infection (UTI) Inflammation or infection of one or more organs or structures of the urinary system

urine output Amount of urine collected and measured from a patient over a given amount of time; indicator of kidney function

UTI *See* urinary tract infection

uvulopalatopharyngoplasty (UPPP) Surgical procedure to treat intractable snoring and obstructive sleep apnea; involves removal of the redundant tissue of the fauces, tonsils, and a portion of the soft palate, including the uvula

valgus Bent or twisted away from the midline

valve A membranous fold in a passage that prevents backflow of material passing through it

venous compression device A device used for patients who are prone to the development of thrombophlebitis; a patient is fitted with intermittent venous compression boots that inflate and deflate every few seconds to promote the movement of venous blood in the leg(s)

ventricles The lower chambers of the heart that receive blood from the atria

Vesalius Father of modern anatomy who openly challenged and corrected the scientific anatomical writings of Galen by dissecting cadavers to illustrate anatomy

vesical trigone An important anatomical landmark of the bladder formed by the two ureteral openings at the posterolateral angles, and the urethral opening at the inferior angle

vessel loop Thin strips made of silicone that can be placed around a vessel, nerve, or duct for the purposes of retracting or isolating; the loops are colored for easy identification of the retracted structures

vestibule An opening that serves as the entrance to a passageway, such as the vestibule of the vagina

viscera Any organ of a body cavity; usually refers to the abdominal organs

vital signs Measurements of bodily functions essential to life, including temperature, pulse, respiration (TPR), and blood pressure

volatile agents A group of liquids that easily evaporate and, when inhaled, produce general anesthesia through interaction with the CNS

wraparound-style gown Sterile surgical gown that "wraps" around the individual to enclose the body from the neck to the middle of the lower leg, and is kept in place by ties and Velcro strips

xenograft Graft obtained from a dissimilar species

Index

Note: "b" indicates boxed material; "i" indicates an illustration; "t" indicates a table. Drugs appear under their generic names, with trade names in parentheses.

A

C

D

F

G

H

J

K

P

Q

R

S

T